Sampson's Textbook of Radiopharmacy

Sampson's Textbook of Radiopharmacy

FOURTH EDITION

Edited by
Tony Theobald
Formerly at the Department of Pharmacy,
King's College, London

On behalf of the UK Radiopharmacy Group

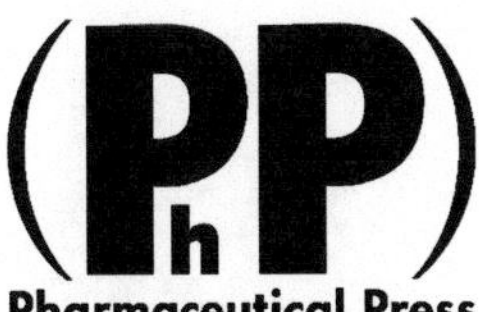

Published by the Pharmaceutical Press
66-68 East Smithfield, London E1W 1AW, UK

(PhP) is a trade mark of Pharmaceutical Press

Pharmaceutical Press is the publishing division of the
Royal Pharmaceutical Society of Great Britain

First, second and third editions published by
Gordon & Breach Science Publishers Ltd 1990, 1994, 1999
Fourth edition published by Pharmaceutical Press 2011
Made ASR in 2021

Typeset by Thomson Digital, Noida, India
Printed in Great Britain by TJ Books Ltd, Padstow, Cornwall

ISBN 978 0 85369 789 3

A catalogue record for this book is available from the British Library.

Contents

Preface

Some ten years have passed since the last edition of 'Sampson' was published and the science and art of radiopharmacy have changed considerably over the decade. The need for a new edition of this textbook was long felt by radiopharmacists and the current editor was invited to oversee the compilation of this edition by the United Kingdom Radiopharmacy Group. Many changes have occurred in practice since the last edition. The emergence of positron emission tomography (PET) and short-lived radiopharmaceuticals, new imaging modalities, new types of radiopharmaceuticals, changes in practice and regulation, and mergers of commercial suppliers have all influenced the way in which radiopharmacy is practised throughout Europe and other parts of the world, coupled with the recent global shortage of molybdenum-99 which has affected the supply of that most popular and versatile radionuclide, technetium-99m, for imaging studies.

This edition has been completely revised and rewritten with many new chapters covering topics gaining importance since the last edition. The contributors have been drawn from many parts of Europe and the Americas, thus giving a wide view of the state of radiopharmacy. The book is intended for advanced students and radiopharmacy practitioners and covers the various aspects of radiopharmacy, from physical principles through radiopharmaceutical chemistry, radiopharmacology, radiopharmaceutics and radiopharmacy practice, to new material on techniques in radiopharmaceutical research and development.

Thanks are due to many people who have made this book possible, including members of the United Kingdom Radiopharmacy Group. My thanks go particularly to a small group comprising Dr J Ballinger, Professor P Blower. Mr Guinness and Professor S Mather who were instrumental in advising on the content and choice of authors. My thanks go to the publishers for their understanding and support during the prolonged gestation of this volume. Lastly, thanks to my wife Patricia whose immeasurable patience and understanding enabled this work to reach the press.

Tony Theobald
Bishop's Castle, Shropshire, UK

About the editor

Tony Theobald is a Fellow of the Royal Pharmaceutical Society, whose career was in academic pharmacy at Chelsea and King's Colleges, University of London.

After completing his PhD on medicinal chemistry in the 1960s, his main teaching and research interests were the study of the quality and purity of medicines, and the design and formulation of radiopharmaceuticals. He was instrumental in devising and running numerous courses in radiopharmacy for practising radiopharmacists over a thirty-year period. He retired as Dean of the School of Health and Life Sciences at King's College in 2005, only to be asked to come back part-time to design and run a new Masters programme in Radiopharmaceutics and PET Radiochemistry in the School of Medicine.

Now fully retired, he took on the editorship of this volume at the request of the United Kingdom Radiopharmacists Group. His other interest is pharmacy history; he is a member of the British Society for the History of Pharmacy and has been studying the history of pharmacy in Shropshire for a number of years.

Contributors

Sue Ackrill BSc, MSc, MRPharmS, Radiopharmacist, Queen Elizabeth Hospital, Birmingham, UK

Erik Årstad BSc, MSc, MRSC, PhD, Senior Lecturer in Radiochemistry, Institute of Nuclear Medicine, University College London, London, UK

James R Ballinger PhD, Chief Radiopharmaceutical Scientist, Guy's and St Thomas' NHS Foundation Trust, London, UK

Stan Batchelor BSc, MSc, CPhys, CRadP, MInstP, MIPEM, MSRP, Head of Radiation Safety, Medical Physics Department, Guy's and St Thomas' NHS Foundation Trust, London, UK

Alison M Beaney DProf, MSc, MRPharmS, Regional Quality Assurance Specialist, North-East Region NHS, Newcastle, UK

Philip J Blower BA, DPhil, CChem, MRSC, Professor of Imaging Chemistry, King's College London, Division of Imaging Sciences, Rayne Institute, St Thomas' Hospital, London, UK

Pei-San Chan BSc, MSc, MRPharmS, Principal Radiopharmacist, Nuclear Medicine Department, Royal Free Hampstead NHS Trust, London, UK

Maggie Cooper PhD, Department of Nuclear Medicine, St Bartholomew's Hospital, London, UK

Jilly Croasdale BPharm, MRPharmS, Head of Radiopharmacy for Sandwell and West Birmingham NHS Trust, West Midlands, UK

Clemens Decristoforo MSc, PhD, Radiopharmacist, Clinical Department of Nuclear Medicine, Medical University Innsbruck, Innsbruck, Austria

Adriano Duatti PhD, Professor, Laboratory of Nuclear Medicine, Department of Radiological Sciences, University of Ferrara, Italy

Beverley Ellis BPharm, PhD, MRPharmS, CSci, CChem, MRSC, Consultant Radiopharmacist, Nuclear Medicine Centre, Central Manchester University Hospitals, Manchester, UK

Richard Fernandez BSc, Clinical Scientist, Guy's and St Thomas' NHS Trust, London, UK

Glenn Flux PhD, Physics Department, Royal Marsden Hospital, Sutton, Surrey, UK

Tony Gee PhD, Director PET and Radiotracer Development, GlaxoSmithKline plc, UK

David Graham BPharm MRPharmS, Chief Radiopharmacist, Aberdeen Royal Infirmary, Aberdeen, Scotland, UK

Adrian D Hall BSc, PhD, Physics Department, Royal Marsden Hospital, Sutton, Surrey, UK

Dr Neil G Hartman BPharm, MSc, PhD, Head of Radiopharmacy, Barts and The London NHS Trust, London, UK

Joseph C Hung PhD, BCNP, FASHP, FAPhA, Professor of Pharmacy, Professor of Radiology, Mayo Clinic College of Medicine; Director of Nuclear Pharmacy Laboratories, Director of PET Radiochemistry Facility, Mayo Clinic, Rochester, Minnesota, USA

Brian F Hutton BSc, MSc, PhD FACPSEM, Professor of Medical Physics in Nuclear Medicine, and Molecular Imaging Science, Institute of Nuclear Medicine, UCL and UCLH NHS Foundation Trust, London, UK

Russ Knapp Jr PhD, Manager, Nuclear Medicine Program, Nuclear Science and Technology Division, Corporate Fellow, ORNL, Oak Ridge National Laboratory (ORNL), Oak Ridge, Tennessee, USA

John E Lees BSc (Hons), PhD, CPhys, MInstP, Reader in Space Physics, Department of Physics and Astronomy, University of Leicester, Leicester, UK

Daniel R Lloyd PhD, Senior Lecturer, School of Biosciences, University of Kent, Canterbury, UK

Paul Maltby CSci MIPEM MRPharmS, Chief Radiopharmacist, Radiopharmacy Department, Royal Liverpool University Hospital, Liverpool, UK

Stephen J Mather PhD, FRPharmS, Professor, Centre for Molecular Oncology and Imaging, Institute of Cancer, Barts and The London School of Medicine and Dentistry, London, UK

Steve McQuarrie PhD, Professor, Faculty of Medicine and Dentistry, University of Alberta, Edmonton, Alberta, Canada

Alistair M Millar PhD, FRPharmS, Principal Radiopharmacist, The Royal Infirmary of Edinburgh, Edinburgh, Scotland, UK

Tom Murray MSc, PhD, MRPharmS, West of Scotland Regional Radiopharmacist, Radionuclide Dispensary, Western Infirmary, Glasgow, Scotland, UK

Joao Osso PhD, Head of Research and Development, Radiopharmacy Center, IPEN-CNEN-SP, São Paulo, SP, Brazil

Alan C Perkins BSc, MSc, PhD, CSci, FIPEM, ARCP, FRCR, Professor of Medical Physics and Honorary Consultant Clinical Scientist, University of Nottingham and Nottingham University Hospitals NHS Trust, Medical School, Queen's Medical Centre, Nottingham, UK

Roger D Pickett BPharm, PhD, MRPharmS, Specialist Scientist, GE Healthcare, Medical Diagnostics, Hemel Hempstead, UK

Jane Sosabowski, Department of Nuclear Medicine, St Bartholomew's Hospital London, London, UK

Richard Southworth BSc, PhD, Lecturer, Division of Imaging Sciences, King's College London, London, UK

James M Stone MBBS, MRCPsych, PhD, Clinical Senior Lecturer in Biological Psychiatry, Imperial College London, London, UK

Julie L Sutcliffe BSc, MSc, PhD, Associate Professor, Department of Biomedical Engineering, Division of Hematology-Oncology Director, Cyclotron and Radiochemistry Facility, Center for Molecular and Genomic Imaging, University of California, Davis, California, USA

Tony Theobald BPharm, PhD, FRPharmS, Bishop's Castle, Shropshire, UK

James Thom DipRadSci, BPharm, MRPharmS, Principal Radiopharmacist, Nuclear Medicine, Southampton University Hospitals NHS Trust, Southampton, UK

Henry F VanBrocklin PhD, Director of Radiopharmaceutical Research, Professor, Department of Radiology and Biomedical Imaging, University of California San Francisco, San Francisco, USA

Helen Whiteside BPharm, MRPharmS, Specialist Clinical Pharmacist – Radiopharmacy, Leeds Teaching Hospitals NHS Trust, Leeds, UK

Peter Williamson PhD, Division of Imaging Sciences, The Rayne Institute, St Thomas' Hospital, London, UK

Abbreviations

2D-DIGE	two-dimensional difference gel electrophoresis
2D-PAGE	two-dimensional polyacrylamide gel electrophoresis
2-FDG	2-fluorodeoxyglucose
2-FDM	2-fluorodeoxymannose
α-MSH	alpha-melanocyte-stimulating hormone
ACE	angiotensin-converting enzyme
ACPH	appropriate number of air changes per hour
ACTH	adrenocorticotrophic hormone
ADD	automated dose dispenser
ADME	absorption, distribution, metabolism and excretion
ALARA	as low as reasonably practical
ALI	annual limit of intake
AMS	accelerator mass spectrometry
ANP	authorised nuclear pharmacist
AO	atomic orbital
APCI	atmospheric pressure chemical ionisation
APF	4-azidophenacyl-fluoride
APIs	active pharmaceutical ingredients
ARSAC	Administration of Radioactive Substances Advisory Committee
ATP	adenosine triphosphate
ATSM	diacetyl-bis(N^4-methylthiosemicarbazone)
AUC	area under the curve
BBB	blood–brain barrier
BED	biologically equivalent dose
BER	base excision repair
bmim	1-butyl-3-methylimidazolium
BNMS	British Nuclear Medicine Society
Boc	*t*-butoxycarbonyl
BrudR	bromodeoxyuridine
BSC	biological safety cabinet
BUD	beyond-use date
CCD	charge coupled device
CCK	cholecystokinin
CCK2	cholecystokinin
CDR	complementarity determining region
cfu	colony-forming units
CGE	capillary gel electrophoresis
cGRPP	Current Good Radiopharmaceutical Practice
CHM	Commission on Human Medicines
CHMP	Committee for Medicinal Products for Human Use
CHO cells	Chinese hamster ovary
CIEF	capillary isoelectric focusing
CIT	β-carbomethoxy-3β-(4-iodophenyltropane)
CLDR	continuous low dose-rate
COPD	chronic obstructive pulmonary disease
COREC	Central Office for Research Ethics Committees
CPR	cardiopulmonary resuscitation
cps	counts per second
CSF	colony-stimulating factor
CSP	compounded sterile preparation
CTC	Clinical Trial Certificate
CTD	Common Technical Document
CTX	Clinical Trials Exemption
CZE/FSCE	capillary zone electrophoresis/free-solution CE
CZT	cadmium zinc telluride
Da	Dalton
DEDC	*N,N*-diethyldithiocarbamate
DG	Directorate General
DIPEA	*N,N*-diisopropylethylamine

DMARD disease-modifying antirheumatic drug
DMRC Defective Medicines Report Centre
DMSO dimethyl sulfoxide
dopa 3,4-dihyroxyphenylalanine
DOTA 1,4,7,10-tetraazacyclododecane-1,4,7,10-tetraacetic acid
DOTMP 1,4,7,10-tetraazacyclododecane-1,4,7,10-tetramethylene-phosphonic acid
dps disintegrations per second
DSB double-strand break
DTPA diethylenetriamine pentaacetic acid
EA Environment Agency
EANM European Association of Nuclear Medicine
EBRT external beam radiotherapy
EC electron capture
EDE effective dose equivalent
EDQM European Directorate of Quality of Medicines
EDTA ethylenediaminetetraacetic acid
EDTMP ethylenediaminetetramethylene phosphonic acid
EGF epidermal growth factor
EHT electrical high tension
ELISA enzyme-linked immunosorbent assay
EM Electromagnetic
EPC European Pharmacopoeia Commission
EPR enhanced permeability and retention
ESI electrospray ionisation
EU endotoxin unit
EU European Union
EUD equivalent uniform dose
eV electronvolt
EXAFS extended X-ray absorption fine structure
F-5′-FDA 5′-fluoro-5′-deoxyadenosine
FB *N*-succinimidyl 4-fluorobenzoate
FBA 4-fluorobenzaldehyde
FBA 4-fluorobenzoic acid
FBAU 5-bromo-2′-fluoro-2′-deoxyuridine
FBEM *N*-[2-(4-fluorobenzamido)ethyl] maleimide
FBP filtered back projection
FDAMA FDA Modernization Act
FDG-MHO FDGmaleiimidehexyloxime
FETNIM fluoroerythronitroimidazole
FHMA hydroxide macroaggregates
FHPG 9-[(1-fluoro-3-hydroxy-2-propoxy) methyl]guanine
FLT 3′-deoxy-3′-fluorothymidine
FMISO fluoromisonidazole
Fmoc fluorenylmethoxycarbonyl
FPA 2-fluoropropionic acid
FP-CIT *N*-3-fluoropropyl-2β-carboxymethoxy-3β-(4-iodophenyl) nortropane
FPyME 1-[3-(2-fluoropyridin-3-yloxy) propyl]pyrrole-2,5-dione
FSD full *scale* deflection
FWHM full width at half maximum height
GCP Good Clinical Practice
GDP Good Distribution Practice
GE gel electrophoresis
GEP gastroenterohepatic
GFR glomerular filtration rate
GIST gastrointestinal stromal tumour
GLP Good Laboratory Practice
GLP glucagon-like peptide
GM Geiger–Müller
GMP Good Manufacturing Practice
GPvP Good Pharmacovigilance Practice
GRP bombesin/gastrin releasing peptide
HAMA human anti-mouse-antibodies
HAS human serum albumin
HASS High Activity Sealed Radioactive Source
HATU *O*-(7-azabenzotriazol-l-yl)-1,1,3,3-tetramethyluronium hexafluorophosphate
HBsAg hepatitis B surface antigen
HCC hepatocellular carcinoma
HED *meta*-hydroxyephedrine
HEHA 1,4,7,10,13,16-hexaazacyclohexadecane-*N*,*N*′,*N*′,*N*″,N‴,*N*-hexaacetic acid
HEPA high-efficiency particulate air
HIDA scan hepatobiliary iminodiacetic acid scan
HIPDM *N*,*N*,*N*′-trimethyl-[2-hydroxy-3-methyl-5-iodobenzyl]-1,3-propanediamine
HMPAO hexamethylpropyleneamine oxime
HOMO highest occupied molecular orbital
HPGe high-purity germanium

HPLC high performance liquid chromatrography
HR homologous recombination
HSAB classification hard/soft acid base
HSE Health and Safety Executive
HVCZE high-voltage capillary zone electrophoresis
HYNIC hydrazinonicotinic acid; 6-hydrazinopyridine-3-carboxylic acid
HYNIC hydrazinonicotinic acid
IAEA International Atomic Energy Agency
IBZM (*S*)-3-iodo-*N*-[(1-ethyl-2-pyrrolidinyl)]methyl-2-hydroxy-6-methoxybenzamide
ICH International Conference on Harmonisation
ICRP International Commission on Radiological Protection
IDA iminodiacetic acid
IEF isoelectric focusing
IMBA *N*-(2-diethylaminoethyl)-3-iodo-4-methoxybenzamide
IMP Investigational Medicinal Product
IMPD Investigational Medicinal Product Dossier
IRMER Ionising Radiation (Medical Exposure) Regulations
IPD interstitial pulmonary disease
ISFET ion-selective field-effect transistor
IudR iododeoxyuridine
LA Licensing Authority
LAL *Limulus* amoebocyte lysate
LAN lanreotide
LC Liquid chromatography
LCM laser capture microdissection
LET linear energy transfer
LQ [model] Linear-quadratic
LRPRP leukocyte-rich platelet-rich plasma
LUMO lowest unoccupied molecular orbital
LUV large unilamellar vesicle
MAA macroaggregated albumin
MABG 1-(*m*-astatobenzyl)guanidine
MAG3 mercaptoacetyltriglycine
MALDI matrix assisted laser desorption ionisation
MCA Medicines Control Agency
MDA Medical Devices Agency
MDR multidrug resistance/resistant
mIBG *meta*-iodobenzylguanidine
MIRD Medical Internal Radiation Dosimetry [Committee of the Society of Nuclear Medicine]
MMP matrix metalloproteinase
MO molecular orbital
MPE medical physics expert
MS mass spectrometry
MTC medullary thyroid cancer
MTT 1-(4,5-demethylthiazoyl-2-yl)-3,5-diphenylformazan
MUGA multigated radionuclide angiography
n.c.a. no-carrier-added
NACWO Named Animal Care and Welfare Officer
NaI(Tl) thallium-activated sodium iodide
NBS *N*-bromosuccinimide
NET neuroendocrine tumour
NF nitrogen-fluorinated
NHEJ non-homologous end joining
NIMP Non Investigational Medicinal Product
NIOSH National Institute for Occupational Safety and Health
NIS sodium iodide symporter
NOTA 1,4,7-triazacyclononane-N,N′,N″-triacetic acid
NPSA National Patient Safety Agency
NPY neuropeptide Y
NTCP normal tissue complication probability
OMCL Official Medicines Control Laboratories
PANDA PET and NMR dual acquisition
PBBS peripheral benzodiazepine binding sites
PCR polymerase chain reaction
PEC primary engineering control
PEG poly(ethylene glycol)
PEO poly(ethylene oxide)
PET positron emission tomography
PHA pulse-height analysis
PHYP particulate hydroxypatite
PIC/S Pharmaceutical Inspection Co-operation Scheme
PPARγ peroxisome proliferator activated-receptor gamma

PPP	platelet-poor plasma
PRP	platelet-rich plasma
PRRT	peptide receptor radiation therapy
QA	quality assurance
QC	quality control
QWBA	quantitative whole body autoradiography
RBE	relative biological effectiveness/ efficacy
rCBF	regional cerebral blood flow
RCY	radiochemical yield
rhTSH	recombinant human thyroid-stimulating hormone
RIT	radioimmunotherapy
RNAi	RNA interference
RPA	Radiation Protection Adviser
RT-PCR	reverse transcriptase polymerase chain reaction
SAB	*N*-succinimidyl [^{211}At]astatobenzoate
SAPS	*N*-succinimidyl *N*-(4-astatophenethyl) succinamate
SCA	segregated compounding area
ScFv	single-chain variable fragments
SCK	shell cross-linked knedel-like (nanoparticles)
SDS	sodium dodecyl sulfate
SGMAB	*N*-succinimidyl 3-astato-4-guanidinomethylbenzoate
SI	Statutory Instrument
siRNA	short interfering RNA
SLN	sentinel lymph node
SOP	standard operating procedure
SPC	Summary of Product Characteristics
SPE	solid-phase extraction
SPECT	single-photon emission computed tomography
SSB	single-strand break
SST	somatostatin
SSTR	somatostatin receptor
SUV	unilamellar vesicle
SV40	Simian virus-40
TATE	Tyr^3-Thr^3-octreotide
TCEP	tris(2-carboxyethyl) phosphine
TCP	Tumour control probability
TETA	1,4,8,11-tetraazacyclotetradecane-*N*,*N*′,*N*″,*N*‴-tetraacetic acid
TFA	trifluoroacetic acid
THF	Tetrahydrofuran
TI	Transport Index
TIA	ischaemia/ischaemic attack
TIC	total ion current
TLC	thin-layer chromatography
TLD	thermoluminescent dosemeter
TOC	Tyr^3-octreotide
Toc	α-tocopheryl/α-tocopherol
TOF	time-of-flight
TPN	total parenteral nutrition
TRT	targeted radionuclide therapy
TSTU	*O*-(*N*-succinimidyl-*N*,*N*,*N*′,*N*′-tetramethyluronium tetrafluoroborate
VEGF	vascular endothelial growth factor
VIP	vasoactive intestinal peptide
VLLW	very low-level waste

1

What is radiopharmacy?

Tony Theobold

Radiopharmacy, the subject of this book, is the science and art (for there is still much of the craft about it) of the design, preparation, quality assurance and clinical pharmacy of radioactive medicines, called radiopharmaceuticals. The British and European Pharmacopoeias define a radiopharmaceutical as 'any medicinal product which, when ready for use, contains one or more radionuclides (radioactive isotopes) included for a medicinal purpose.'

Radiopharmacy draws on all the physical and biological sciences and is a truly interdisciplinary subject, ranging from the production and properties of the radionuclide, through its incorporation into a carrier, formulation and quality control, to adverse effects and drug interactions. It is a recognised health science specialty, employing pharmacists, chemists, physicists and life scientists, with all practitioners required to demonstrate adequate knowledge and practical competence through a number of accreditation schemes.

Some, but not all, of the knowledge required for good radiopharmacy practice will be found within the covers of this volume; it is a rapidly evolving discipline, both scientific and regulatory, so radiopharmaceutical scientists must be aware of advances and changes as part of their continuing professional development.

Radiopharmacy is unusual in being governed by two distinct sets of legislation and regulation: as radioactive substances on one hand, and as medicines on the other. The two sets of legislation may be in conflict, and a reasoned and justified compromise is sometimes necessary in practice.

The physical basis for using radiopharmaceuticals is twofold. For diagnostic applications employing imaging techniques, the radiopharmaceutical must act as a 'signal generator' by emitting radiation that is easily detected outside the body and that causes minimum damage or harm to the patient, and this implies the use of tracer quantities of the agent. By contrast, in therapeutic applications the radiations emitted from the radiopharmaceutical must act like a 'magic bullet' and be absorbed locally, imparting maximum damage to its target organ or tissue, and minimum damage elsewhere in the body.

A radiopharmaceutical, then, is a radioactive medicine and has two essential components; a radionuclide that emits an appropriate ionising radiation when it disintegrates, and a pharmaceutical ligand that binds the radionuclide and transports it to the target organ or tissue. Both components are necessary: a simple radionuclide itself will rarely be concentrated in the desired target; and the ligand by itself will not provide diagnostic information, nor will it have a therapeutic effect since the 'signal generator' or 'magic bullet' is absent. Some radiopharmaceuticals combine both components in a single molecule, such as ^{11}C-labelled raclopride, a dopamine receptor-binding molecule where the 'signal generator' is a radioisotope replacing the naturally occurring carbon at a specific position in the molecule.

The radionuclide

As mentioned above, a fundamental component of the radiopharmaceutical is the radionuclide (radioactive isotope) and the choice is governed by a number of factors:

- Suitable half-life (the time taken for the radioactivity to decay to one-half its initial value)
- Appropriate radiation (gamma photons for diagnostic imaging, alpha or beta particles for therapy)
- Ease of production and availability (by extraction from nuclear waste, or by bombardment with neutrons or charged particles)
- Suitable chemistry for bonding to the pharmaceutical ligand.

Medicinal radionuclides are characterised by their short half-lives (measured in hours or days), ease of production and ready availability. There are numerous chemical techniques for attaching the radionuclide to the ligand, some simple and others ingenious but complex. The radiations emitted are generally low-energy gamma photons ($\sim$100 keV) for imaging, or higher-energy particles ($\sim$1 MeV) for therapy. Very short-lived cyclotron-produced positron-emitting radionuclides are used in the technique of positron emission tomography (PET), which is now developing rapidly and is likely to become the major imaging modality in the future, replacing conventional SPECT (single-photon emission computed tomography) from its current leading position. These very short-lived radionuclides (with half-lives ranging from about 2 hours down to 2 minutes) must be produced, formulated as radiopharmaceuticals and administered to the patient as rapidly as possible for imaging, otherwise the radioactivity will have decayed to a low and almost undetectable level.

Ionising radiations

Ionising radiations can be harmful to living organisms – indeed, large radiation doses are used to sterilise standard pharmaceuticals and medical devices. Strict control is necessary in the production of radionuclides and radiopharmaceuticals to minimise the exposure of operators and medical staff to these radiations. Likewise to ensure the patient receives the minimum radiation dose commensurate with the value of the investigation. Much of the content of later chapters in this volume will deal with the properties of these radiations together with practical, regulatory, and legislative measures taken to protect operators, patients, and the general public from exposure.

Radiotracer and imaging fundamentals

Diagnostic nuclear medicine employs radiopharmaceuticals as tracers of biochemical processes, both normal and abnormal. As described above, imaging enables the clinician to view the distribution of the radiotracer within the patient's body and, through multiple time-lapse images, to follow the kinetics of the distribution and target uptake process.

Radiotracers

A tracer is a labelled molecule used to trace the progress of a process, *in vitro* or *in vivo*. A simple analogy would be for a plumber to throw a small amount of dye down a drain and look at the possible outfalls to see which one has a coloured outflow – not an environmentally friendly action but perhaps the only possible technique when the drains disappear underground and which illustrates the basic principle: add an easily detectable substance to a system and search for it after administration to see where, when, and how much is detectable in a specified place.

Coloured tracers have long been used in biology and physiology and some of the earliest studies on the metabolism of fatty acids were made with phenyl-substituted fatty acids, these being easily detectable through their ultraviolet absorption in spectrophotometry. But many other natural substances contain aromatic rings and the detection of the phenyl-fatty acid among all the others may be difficult. Also, it is possible that the fatty acid is metabolised and the aromatic phenyl group is transferred to other molecules so that its final location is not the same as the unlabelled fatty acid. This example suffers from several deficiencies: the label is not unique, the labelled molecule is different from the natural one, and metabolic processes may remove the label. Hence the characteristics of an ideal tracer may be summarised as follows:

- A unique label
- The labelled molecule is identical in all physical and chemical properties to the natural one
- The label is firmly fixed and does not come adrift during the investigation or experiment.

Isotopic labels fulfil all these criteria: they are easily detected and only the labelled molecules are so detected; there are no differences in properties (except for some small molecules labelled with deuterium, ^{2}H); and the covalent bonds fix the isotope firmly in the molecule. There is now a choice between stable and radioactive isotopes. For preliminary metabolic studies of new drugs in humans, the stable isotopic label (^{2}H or ^{13}C) is preferred to avoid radiation dosage to the volunteer, although this is changing with the introduction of ^{11}C-labelled drugs that can be studied by PET.

Radioisotopic tracers, or radiochemicals, are widely used in biology and medicine because their radioactivity is easily detected by fairly simple equipment and is not affected by other properties of the sample. The ideal characteristics of a radiotracer are:

- Chemical or biological properties are not changed.
- The signal (radioactivity) is easily detected.
- Minute amounts are employed that do not upset the kinetics of the system.
- Easy and complete mixing with indigenous chemicals – the mixing must be faster than the process being studied.
- Signal strength (radioactivity) must be proportional to concentration.

A radiotracer having these properties can be used with confidence to determine both the location and quantity of the substance being traced.

Many radiochemicals can be used as tracers, as can radiopharmaceuticals, but radiochemicals are not radiopharmaceuticals; they are sold expressly for experimental purposes and cannot be administered to humans. Radiopharmaceuticals, on the other hand, are licensed for administration to humans and comply with stringent standards for purity and sterility, among other properties. Most diagnostic radiopharmaceuticals can be regarded as radiotracers for human disease, indicating either normal or abnormal distribution and kinetics. Therapeutic radiopharmaceuticals can be regarded as selectively toxic agents, designed to kill off unwanted or cancerous cells in the body.

Molecular imaging

This term has come into use to describe the process of imaging an organ or receptor with a radiolabelled molecule, often formulated as a radiopharmaceutical. Many radiopharmaceuticals are molecular imaging agents. In essence, the labelled molecule is localised on specific receptors in the organ imaged, and the radiolabelled molecule is designed to have a high binding affinity for the target. There are many examples of molecular imaging agents, ranging from technetium-99m (^{99m}Tc) complexes for studying the condition of the brain, to ^{11}C-labelled agonists having exquisite sensitivity for disease states. Examples of molecular imaging agents will be found throughout this book.

Design and synthesis of radiopharmaceuticals

The design and synthesis of radiopharmaceuticals is an important aspect of radiopharmaceutical chemistry and radiopharmacology. The pharmaceutical ligand, carrying the 'signal generator' radionuclide must possess a number of essential and desirable properties:

- Accumulation, when radiolabelled, in the target organ or tissue
- Little or no accumulation in surrounding tissues, thereby giving a high target-to-background ratio
- Easy and quick radiolabelling
- Physical stability before and after radiolabelling.

In the case of radiopharmaceutical kits (in which the radionuclide is added to a sterile vial containing the pharmaceutical ligands, reagents and other ancillary substances), a great deal of formulation chemistry and art is required to produce a reliable system that will always produce the desired radiopharmaceutical, and these aspects are described in the radiopharmaceutical chemistry section of this book. Quality control methods for determining identity, purity, etc., are another important application of radiopharmaceutical and radioanalytical chemistry.

Dispensing and supply

Dispensing and supply of radiopharmaceuticals is restricted to hospital and licensed commercial radiopharmacies; there is no call for these articles in community or retail pharmacy and they are used only in the hospital setting within nuclear medicine or radiotherapy departments under the supervision of licensed clinicians. All aspects of procurement, dispensing and supply are strictly controlled in all countries, with regulation in the UK and USA being probably the most prescriptive and stringent, although all European Community nations are bound by the relevant Community legislation. Inspection of premises and facilities is undertaken, but curiously, there are at present no national or internationally recognised qualifications in the UK and most practitioners are self-taught or have learnt their craft under the supervision of a senior colleague. In the USA, radiopharmacy is recognised as a special discipline and practitioners can undertake examination for certification by the Board of Pharmaceutical Specialities, an independent organisation. There are numerous other unofficial qualifications: the European Postgraduate Specialisation Certificate in Radiopharmacy, and many national short courses and other specialist courses sponsored by International Atomic Energy Agency (IAEA). The VirRad website (www.virrad.eu.org) is an invaluable source of information and interactive learning about radiopharmacy and is recommended to all readers of this book; registration is free and gives access to a large number of discussion forums and learning aids.

The radiopharmacy

Another distinct characteristic of the radiopharmacy is its location, generally within or close to a nuclear medicine department and often not associated with the conventional hospital pharmacy. The staff, too, is often independent of the pharmacy organisation and is not restricted in the UK to registered pharmacists or pharmacy technicians.

Operations

The operations in a radiopharmacy fall in two distinct categories: procurement and production of radiopharmaceuticals, and maintenance of quality (materials, environment, facilities and people).

Nearly all radiopharmaceuticals are administered by injection, usually intravenously, as this route offers the most immediate access to the target organs or tissues, avoiding reflux and vomiting and incomplete absorption from the gastrointestinal tract (also, the radioactive material is then safely contained within the body).

Parenteral administration requires a sterile injectable formulation, and all pharmacopoeial injections are required to be sterile. Most radiopharmaceuticals must be treated differently from conventional parenteral preparations for a number of reasons. Firstly, the limited half-life of the radionuclide effectively precludes manufacture and quarantine until a satisfactory sterility test result is obtained, a process that can take from 7 to 14 days. Secondly, many of the ingredients are not stable to heating and the preparation cannot be sterilised by heating in an autoclave. These limitations mean that a rapid aseptic assembly or dispensing procedure must be used and the finished product released without the 'seal' of a sterility test. In these circumstances the quality of the manufacturing or dispensing unit environment is paramount: the design and operation of the facility must conform to strict standards specified by regulation and good manufacturing practice. All operators must be fully trained and demonstrate their competence at working in an aseptic environment through competency tests at regular intervals.

But this is only half of the picture: these materials are radioactive and constitute a health hazard. Precautions must be taken and procedures developed to reduce the radiation exposure to operators, to prevent ingestion of radioactive material, and to prevent contamination of the working area and the general environment enjoyed by the public at large. It turns out that conditions normally employed to keep microbial organisms out of the aseptic dispensing area will effectively aid the spread of radioactive contamination and increase the likelihood of ingestion of radioactive material. A compromise is often necessary here, usually by design of special cabinets or enclosures which provide containment of adventitious radioactive material (through spills, formation of aerosols, etc.). Thus the two objectives of patient safety and operator and public protection must be satisfied and demonstrated through numerous environmental monitoring (microbiological and radiation) schemes and records – a system of parametric release for the final radiopharmaceutical. A full account of current rules, practice, and recommended procedures appears in the section on the Practice of Pharmacy.

The daily routine

The daily routine will be similar in most medium to large radiopharmacies. Since the radiopharmaceuticals will be required in the clinics in the first part of the morning, production and dispensing will commence much earlier. In some commercial radiopharmacies and cyclotron units production may start in the middle of the night to ensure that materials are despatched and transported to their site of use in time for administration.

Radiation hygiene

The principles and practice of radiation hygiene are described in several chapters of this book as this is a topic that affects all operations and the business of the radiopharmacy, The central body here is the International Commission on Radiological Protection (ICRP), now based in Canada, an independent organisation that offers advice to regulatory bodies. The over-riding principle is public (and operator) protection through keeping radiation exposure *as low as reasonably achievable* – the ALARA principle.

Standards for radiopharmaceuticals

Like all medicinal substances, there are standards for the quality of radiopharmaceuticals. These may be published in the pharmacopoeias, and comprise part of a marketing authorisation specification in the case of licensed products. In the case of 'specials' and research materials, standards are set in the scientific journals, research papers or monographs. The radiopharmacy has a duty to ensure that all its products comply with the recognised standards, and must have appropriate testing equipment and procedures to ensure compliance.

Technetium radiopharmaceuticals

The majority of diagnostic radiopharmaceuticals contain technetium-99m as the radionuclide, and this is obtained daily by 'milking' of a generator system (see Chapter 21 for details). (At the time of writing there is a world shortage of the parent radionuclide molybdenum-99, and supplies of the daughter technetium-99m (^{99m}Tc) are somewhat limited.) This radionuclide is bound to the pharmaceutical ligand by injection of a sterile solution of the radionuclide into a sterile 'kit' vial containing all the ligands, reagents and other ingredients necessary to produce the final radiopharmaceutical. These manipulations constitute a 'closed' procedure in which none of the ingredients or components is exposed to microbial contamination, but the process is still carried out in an aseptic environment (an isolator, or laminar flow cabinet). Once reconstituted, according to the daily dispensing schedule, the radioactivity is measured and the vial and its protective lead shielding 'pot' are labelled; a small sample may be taken for some simple quality control tests and the completed radiopharmaceuticals are delivered to (or collected by) the receiving department. Strict controls are operated on the type of packaging and mode of transport, especially if the radioactive material is to be delivered to a remote site along a public highway.

Other radiopharmaceuticals

Non-technetium radiopharmaceuticals may be prepared at the same time, or shortly after. These range from simple dispensing of aliquots from a sterile stock solution into sterile vials, essentially under the same conditions as for technetium agents, to complex chemical manipulation and radiolabelling of biological molecules such as peptides and proteins or polysaccharides and oligosaccharides. These agents require special equipment, operator expertise, and a strict aseptic manipulation regime because many stages of their preparation cannot be regarded as 'closed' procedures; for example, the purification of radiolabelled peptide by high performance liquid chromatography (HPLC). Sometimes the quality control tests are very time consuming, and the manufacture must start early in the day to ensure that the product is passed fit for use in the afternoon clinic.

Blood labelling

Another complex and time-consuming operation is the labelling of a patient's (autologous) blood and other cells, ready to be re-injected later that day. Such cell labellings are carried out in a separate aseptic enclosure and extra precautions are necessary to prevent infection of operators – and other patients – by bacteria and viruses that may be present in the blood samples of the previous patient.

Procurement, storage and disposal

Materials, both radioactive and 'cold', are received in the radiopharmacy each day and each one has to be checked for identity, leakage and radioactive contamination. A record or log is maintained of all goods received, which are then stored under appropriate conditions: lead-shielded enclosure, cupboard or refrigerator for radioactive materials; ambient or cold storage for reagents and kit vials. Waste radioactive materials (used syringes, vials, tissues, etc.) must be stored separately and disposed of by an authorised route as specified in the licence to hold and use radioactive materials.

Cyclotron units

The processes and procedures just described will be very similar in a cyclotron unit dedicated to the production of very short-lived positron-emitting radionuclides (^{18}F, ^{11}C, ^{13}N, ^{15}O) incorporated into radiopharmaceuticals for PET studies. The main difference lies in the higher degree of automation in production and quality control necessary to reduce the radiation exposure of staff from the highly energetic 0.51 MeV annihilation photons from these radionuclides and the very large quantities of radionuclide that have to be produced to compensate for the rapid decay of radioactivity. The production process must obviously be a rapid one in view of the short half-lives of these radionuclides (e.g. that of ^{11}C is 20 minutes). The same pattern of work is undertaken as in a conventional radiopharmacy with the same attention to aseptic manipulations, the environment and quality assurance. Automation of synthesis and formulation is very common in these units.

Radiopharmaceuticals in the clinic

Radiopharmacy involvement does not stop at the point of delivery of the product to the clinic; radioactive residues are returned for disposal and any abnormal biodistributions or adverse reactions are reported in case the radiopharmaceutical itself is at fault. These reports are collated at national centres and anonymised summaries are circulated to all contributors for information and checking. Annual summaries are often published in the *European Journal of Nuclear Medicine.*

The majority of radiopharmaceuticals are used as diagnostic agents in nuclear medicine. After injection and a period of waiting until the biodistribution is complete, an image is taken of the distribution of radioactivity in the appropriate region of the body. Some clinical procedures require the administration of a drug to modify the normal response and others may be affected by the medicines currently taken by the patient; many examples of these are described in Chapter 31. The radiopharmaceutical is acting as a radioactive tracer of a normal or abnormal biochemical process and its location is measured or detected externally by some form of camera system. There are two main types of imaging system used: SPECT and PET.

SPECT

SPECT stands for single-photon emission computed tomography and is a technique whereby an image of the distribution of radioactivity (more properly, the emitted radiation) is made with a gamma camera. This consists of a collimator (a thick sheet of lead having many parallel holes) placed in front of a large scintillation crystal of sodium iodide that is backed by an array of photomultipliers to convert the scintillations into electrical pulses for further processing. The collimator allows gamma photons to reach the detector only if they travel normally to the scintillation crystal; otherwise they are absorbed by the lead. This is the only practical way of 'focusing' high-energy photons – mirrors and lenses are not effective as the photons just pass through. Electronic processing of the pulses from the photomultipliers produces a two-dimensional image of the distribution of radioactivity throughout the depth of the field of view. Images are taken at a number of angles to give an approximate representation of the three-dimensional distribution. By use of more complex collimators and software processing of the information, a more complete three-dimensional image may be obtained, and this can be viewed as a series of 'slices' or as a rotating object, thus enabling better visualisation of the radioactivity distribution.

PET

By contrast, the PET camera produces three-dimensional images routinely. PET stands for positron emission tomography and employs short-lived positron-emitting radionuclides – ^{11}C, ^{13}N, ^{15}O, ^{18}F being the most usual. They emit positrons (positively charged anti-particles of the electron) which are annihilated by combining with an ordinary electron and converted to two gamma photons of energy 0.511 MeV emitted in opposite directions. The camera is a circular array of detectors which register both gamma photons, and electronic processing results in a complete distribution of radioactivity within the subject.

Conclusion

This short introduction has attempted to describe the main features of radiopharmacy science and practice and the basic principles underlying the use of radiopharmaceuticals as tracers. Much more detail will be found in the following chapters. The book also contains a glossary of technical terms which, it is hoped, will aid the reader in understanding the sometimes jargon-laden world of radiopharmacy.

The Literature of radiopharmacy

As befits a multidisciplinary subject, there are few journals devoted exclusively to radiopharmacy, the material being published in a variety of clinical and scientific journals. The following list includes the journals most frequently consulted by radiopharmacists. Most are available on-line to recognised subscribers, either through professional bodies or universities.

- *American Journal of Hospital Pharmacy*
- *Applied Radiation and Isotopes*
- *Bioconjugate Chemistry*
- *Bioorganic & Medicinal Chemistry Letters*
- *Bioorganic Chemistry*
- *Clinical Nuclear Medicine*
- *European Journal of Nuclear Medicine and Molecular Imaging*
- *European Journal of Pharmaceutical Sciences*
- *Journal of Labelled Compounds and Radiopharmaceuticals*
- *Journal of Nuclear Cardiology*
- *Journal of Nuclear Medicine*
- *Journal of Nuclear Medicine Technology*
- *Journal of Organic Chemistry*
- *Journal of Organometallic Chemistry*
- *Journal of Pharmaceutical Sciences*
- *Journal of Radioanalytical and Nuclear Chemistry*
- *Nuclear Medicine and Biology*
- *Nuclear Medicine Communications*
- *Nuklearmedizin*
- *Quarterly Journal of Nuclear Medicine and Molecular Imaging*
- *Radiochimica Acta*
- *Seminars in Nuclear Medicine*

SECTION A

Physics applied to radiopharmacy

2

Nuclear structure and radioactivity

Richard Fernandez

Nuclear structure

Elementary particles and atoms

All matter, whether living or inert, is composed of molecules. Molecules are themselves formed from combinations of elements. The smallest constituent of an element exhibiting identical chemical properties is the atom, and for this reason atoms are often termed the 'building blocks' of matter.

The atom consists of three types of elementary particles: protons, neutrons and electrons. Classically, the atom of any given element consists of a positively charged nucleus, comprising positively charged protons and electrically neutral neutrons (collectively termed nucleons) surrounded by negatively charged electrons. Properties of the elementary particles are detailed in Table 2.1.

The physical size of the atom is of the order of tenths of a nanometre (10^{-10} m) and that of the nucleus is of the order of a femtometre (10^{-15} m). The electron configuration of the atom determines the chemical properties of the element, whereas the nuclear composition determines the stability of the nucleus and the radioactive decay process.

Electronic structure of the atom

In the simplest model of the atom, first proposed by Bohr in 1913, electrons orbit the nucleus, analogous to the planets orbiting the sun, but occupying discrete energy states or 'shells' around the nucleus.

Each shell is referred to as the *K* shell, the *L* shell, the *M* shell and so on, with the electrons in the *K* shell closest to the nucleus. According to quantum theory each individual shell is designated by a unique quantum number. This is an integer value and is referred to as the *principal quantum number*, *n*. For the innermost shell, the *K* shell, $n=1$, for the *L* shell $n=2$, and for the *M* shell $n=3$. From quantum theory the maximum number of electrons permitted in each shell is $2n^2$. Therefore the *K*, *L* and *M* shells contain a maximum of 2, 8 and 18 electrons, respectively.

Within each shell, electrons can exist in various subshells depending on their spin states (each subshell has its own set of subsidiary quantum numbers related to spin) – quantum theory necessitates that no two electrons in a given subshell can occupy the same spin state, i.e. no two electrons can have all quantum numbers identical.

Table 2.1 Properties of elementary particles

Particle	Symbol	Charge (*e*)[a]	Mass (u)[b]
Proton	P	+1	1.00726
Neutron	n	0	1.00867
Electron	e	−1	0.00055

[a] $1e = 1.6 \times 10^{-19}$ coulombs.
[b] $1u = 1$ universal mass unit $= 1.66 \times 10^{-27}$ kg.

Figure 2.1 is a schematic representation of a neutral atom with 6 protons in the nucleus and 6 orbiting electrons occupying the *K* and *L* shells.

When the atom is in its most stable, i.e. lowest, energy state (also termed the ground state) electrons occupy the lowest possible shells, closest to the nucleus.

The attractive electrostatic force binds the electrons to the nucleus. Energy is therefore required to excite electrons from lower to higher, unoccupied energy levels. This energy may be supplied, for example, by incident radiation interacting with the atom. If sufficient energy is transferred to the electrons, they can be removed completely from the atom – termed *ionisation*. The energy required to ionise electrons is referred to as the binding energy and is measured in electronvolts (eV). An electronvolt is equivalent to 1.6×10^{-19} J.

Electrons in different shells have different binding energies. Electrons closest to the nucleus have the greatest binding energy (in the keV range) and electrons in higher shells, farther from the nucleus have lower binding energy (in the eV range). This is analogous to

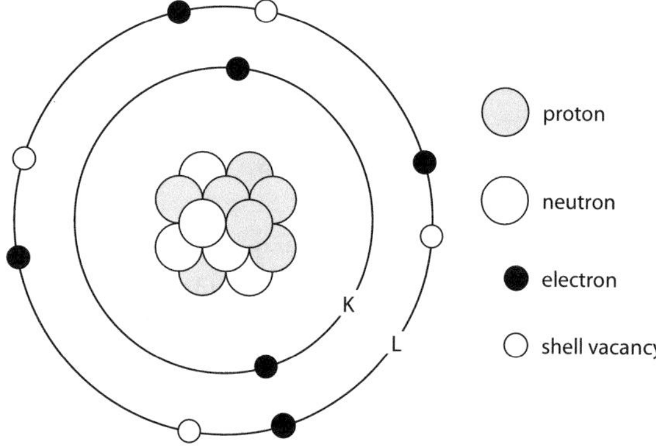

Figure 2.1 Structure of a neutral atom.

when two opposing magnetic poles are placed close together – the closer they are brought to each other, the greater the amount of energy required to pull them apart.

Electrons may be transferred or shared between atoms to form molecules. Examples of these chemical bonds are ionic (or electrovalent) bonds when electrons are transferred and covalent bonds when electrons are shared; the typical energy is of the order of a few electronvolts.

Nuclear structure

Neutral atoms have no overall charge as the number of electrons is equal to the number of protons. The number of protons in the nucleus is termed the *atomic number*, *Z*. The number of neutrons in the nucleus is denoted by *N*. The summation of *Z* and *N* gives the total number of nucleons in the nucleus and is referred to as the *mass number*, *A*. A particular element with chemical symbol X is typically represented by the notation $^{A}_{Z}X$. In this notation *N* is usually omitted since it can be simply calculated from $A - Z$. In the literature, the atomic number is often also omitted, since for a particular element *Z* is the same for all atoms of that element and the simple notation ^{A}X is used.

Nucleons are bound together by the *strong nuclear force*, which acts to overcome the repulsive electrostatic force between the protons in the nucleus. The nuclear force is a short-range force, the extent of its influence being limited to the nucleus itself, resulting in the very small size and very high density of the nucleus.

Nucleons can be thought of as existing in discrete energy shells, similar to electrons in the Bohr atomic model. In the same way that electrons orbiting the nucleus have an associated binding energy, nucleons in the nucleus also have a binding energy. However, unlike electrons, which have binding energy of up to a few keV, the energy required to separate an individual nucleon from a stable nucleus is much higher, of the order of a few MeV.

Nuclear stability and radioactivity

The stability of a nucleus is determined by its composition of neutrons and protons. The term *nuclide* is used to describe a particular nuclear composition. For stable, low-atomic-number nuclides, the ratio of neutrons to protons (*N*/*Z*) is approximately 1. Examples include $^{4}_{2}He$, $^{12}_{6}C$ and $^{16}_{8}O$. With increasing atomic number, *N*/*Z* increases to approximately 1.5, i.e. more neutrons than protons are required to ensure nuclear stability. In heavy nuclei an excess of neutrons is required as they provide only (attractive) nuclear force, unlike protons which provide both nuclear force and (repulsive) electrostatic force. Examples of stable, high-atomic-number nuclides include $^{197}_{79}Au$ and $^{208}_{82}Pb$.

Figure 2.2 is a diagram showing the relationship between proton and neutron number and nuclear stability for known nuclides.

Nuclides with an excess or deficiency of protons/neutrons relative to the stable element are energetically unstable. This is because there is insufficient binding energy to hold the constituent nucleons together. These unstable nuclides lie above or below the line of stability. They are termed *radioactive* as they transform to a more stable nuclide (and approach the line of stability) through the emission of radiation. The various modes of radioactive decay and types of emitted radiation are discussed subsequently.

Most elements have a mixture of stable and unstable *isotopes*. Isotopes are nuclides which have the same atomic number, and therefore identical chemical properties, but which have different numbers of neutrons. For example ^{11}C, ^{12}C and ^{14}C are all isotopes of carbon. In this example, ^{11}C and ^{14}C (among others) are termed *radioisotopes* as these nuclei are radioactive and convert to more stable states through the emission of radiation. Radioactive nuclides, also termed *radionuclides*, can occur naturally (e.g. ^{14}C) or they can be produced artificially in a nuclear reactor or cyclotron.

Kinetics

Radioactive decay

Radioactive decay is the spontaneous transformation of an unstable nucleus into a nucleus in a more stable state. The process of radioactive decay is governed by the laws of probability and the number of unstable nuclei decaying within a fixed time interval follows a *Poisson* distribution. The unstable, radioactive nuclide is termed the *parent* nuclide and, following the decay process, the resulting nuclide is termed the *daughter* nuclide. The daughter nuclide itself may be radioactive and therefore may subsequently undergo further nuclear transformation until a more stable state is eventually reached. An example of this is the molybdenum–technetium decay process. Parent nuclide molybdenum-99 (^{99}Mo) decays to daughter nucleus technetium-99m (^{99m}Tc) with the emission of beta radiation. Technetium-99m exists in a metastable state, denoted by the 'm', and subsequently decays to ^{99}Tc with the emission of gamma radiation.

The unit of radioactivity is the *becquerel* (Bq), named after Henri Becquerel who first discovered radioactivity in 1896. The becquerel is defined as one nuclear disintegration per second and therefore has units of s^{-1}.

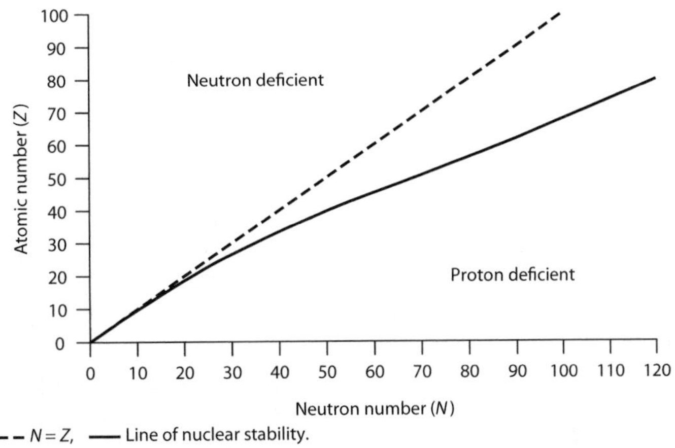

Figure 2.2 Diagram of *Z* versus *N* and nuclear stability.

Decay rate and half-life

Radioactive decay is a random process and consequently for a particular radioactive sample containing identical radioactive nuclei, at any instant of time we are unable to specify exactly which nuclei will undergo transformation. Rather, there is a *probability* associated with the number of nuclei decaying at any time. For N identical radioactive nuclei, the probability of a particular nucleus decaying in unit time is given by λ. The activity A of the sample, i.e. the number of nuclei decaying per unit time, is given by $N\lambda$. This is a fundamental property of radioactive decay – the number of nuclei decaying per unit time is proportional to the number of nuclei present at that instant in time. This can be written as

$$A = \frac{dN}{dt} = -N\lambda \tag{2.1}$$

The negative sign is inserted to indicate that N decreases with time. λ is termed the *decay constant* or *decay rate*; it is specific to the radionuclide and has units of s^{-1}. Equation (2.1) may be rearranged to give

$$\frac{dN}{N} = -\lambda\,dt$$

Since it is assumed that the probability of a nucleus decaying is independent of its age, i.e. that λ is independent of time and is therefore a constant, we can write

$$\int \frac{dN}{N} = -\lambda \int dt$$

At time $t=0$ the number of radioactive nuclei is N_0 and at some subsequent time t the number is N. Solving the above equation yields

$$\ln_e\left[\frac{N}{N_0}\right] = -\lambda t$$

or

$$N = N_0 \exp^{(-\lambda t)} \tag{2.2}$$

Equation (2.2) eloquently shows the exponential nature of the radioactive decay process.

The activity of a radioactive sample (measured in becquerels) is a more useful quantity than the number of radioactive nuclei. Using equation (2.1) to substitute for N and N_0 in equation (2.2) gives

$$A = A_0 \exp^{(-\lambda t)}$$

where A_0 is the initial activity of the sample at time $t=0$.

The radioactive *half-life* ($T_{1/2}$) is defined as the time taken for half the number of radioactive nuclei to decay. This can be obtained by substituting $N=N_0/2$ into equation (2.2) above and rearranging to give

$$T_{1/2} = \frac{\ln_e(2)}{\lambda} \tag{2.3}$$

For a particular radionuclide, half-life is constant and characteristic of that radionuclide. Half-life varies greatly between different radionuclides – some have extremely short half-lives measured in fractions of a second, while others have half-lives of millions of years. Half-lives for radionuclides commonly used in clinical practice are listed in Table 2.2.

Specific activity is defined as the radioactivity per unit mass of the element or compound and typically has units of Bq/gram or MBq/mole (or multiples of these). The maximum possible specific activity, termed the 'carrier-free' specific activity, is when all the atoms present in sample are radioactive, i.e. there are no stable atoms present. For a given mass of radioactive sample the carrier-free specific activity can be calculated for a particular radionuclide by obtaining

Table 2.2 Half-life of radionuclides used in clinical practice (Pearce 2008)

Radionuclide	Half-life	Radionuclide	Half-life
Carbon-11	20 min	Oxygen-15	122 seconds
Chromium-51	27.7 days	Phosphorus-32	14.3 days
Fluorine-18	110 min	Rhenium-186	3.7 days
Gallium-67	78.3 hours	Rhenium-188	17 hours
Iodine-123	13.2 hours	Samarium-153	1.9 days
Iodine-125	59.4 days	Strontium-89	50.6 days
Iodine-131	8.02 days	Technetium-99m	6.01 hours
Indium-111	67.3 hours	Thallium-201	3.04 days
Krypton-81m	13 seconds	Yttrium-90	64 hours

the tabulated half-life and substituting for λ using equations (2.1) and (2.3). It is important that specific activity is not confused with radioactive *concentration* which is simply the radioactivity per unit volume.

Radiation

The term *radiation* refers to the process of emission of energy and includes both particulate and electromagnetic forms. Particulate radiation carries energy in the form of kinetic energy and examples include, among others, alpha particles and beta particles. Electromagnetic radiation on the other hand carries energy by oscillating electrical/magnetic fields. X-rays and gamma rays are examples of electromagnetic (EM) radiation and are emitted with discrete energy, specific to the atom or radionuclide.

Alpha particles

An alpha (α-) particle is essentially a helium-4 (^{4}He) nucleus as it consists of two protons and two neutrons tightly bound together. The binding energy of these nucleons is high enough to ensure that the α-particle behaves as if it were a fundamental particle. The α-particle has a charge of $+2e$, mass number of 4 and atomic number of 2. Due to its charge and mass the α-particle has a high linear energy transfer (LET) compared with other forms of radiation. LET is defined as the amount of energy deposited per unit length of the path traversed by the radiation; it is expressed in units of keV/μm and relates to the biological damage caused. Owing to the high LET of α-particles, ingestion of an alpha emitter, polonium-210 being a relevant example, can have lethal consequences.

Beta particles

Beta particles (β^-) are high-energy electrons and are emitted from an unstable nucleus when a neutron converts to a proton. Since β-particles have only a single charge and are much lighter than α-particles, they have a much lower LET and can therefore penetrate further before absorption. Beta particles can be emitted with a range of energies up to a finite maximum.

X-rays and gamma rays

Both X-rays and gamma (γ-) radiation are part of the electromagnetic spectrum and therefore have an associated energy and wavelength. However the origin of their production differs as X-rays arise from *electronic* transitions whereas γ-rays result from *nuclear* transitions.

Incident radiation can cause ionisation or excitation of electrons in the atom and this creates vacancies in the inner shells. Electrons in outer, higher-energy shells promptly fill the vacancy, with the difference in binding energy between the two shells released as X-radiation. These X-rays are termed *characteristic* X-rays as they are specific to each element as different nuclides have different electron binding energies. As an alternative to characteristic X-ray emission, the energy released when an outer-shell electron fills a vacancy in a lower shell can be transferred to another outer electron. This ionised electron (or Auger electron) results in a *second* vacancy in the outer shell. Figure 2.3 shows schematically the processes of

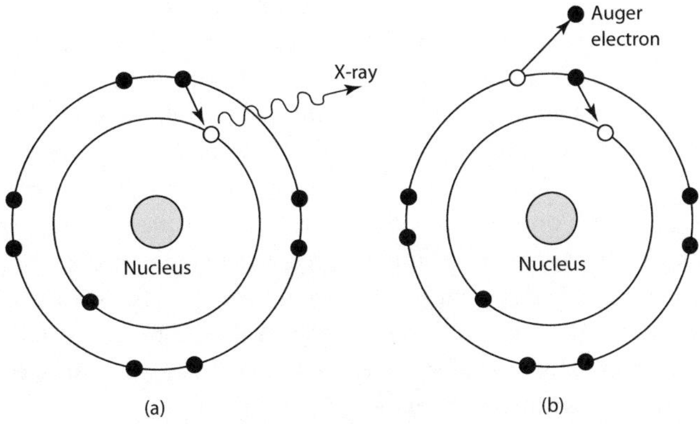

Figure 2.3 Characteristic X-ray emission (a) and Auger electron emission (b) for a K-shell vacancy.

characteristic X-ray and Auger electron emission for an inner-shell vacancy.

When the *nucleus* converts from an energetically unstable state to a more stable, lower-energy state, the difference in energy is released as a γ-ray. The excited energy states of the nucleus are referred to as isomeric states and are unique to the particular radionuclide. Consequently the energy of the γ-radiation emitted from the de-excitation process (termed *isomeric transition*) is specific to the radionuclide. For example, the γ-ray emitted when ^{99m}Tc reverts to its ground state has energy 140 keV, whereas for ^{81m}Kr the associated γ-ray has energy 191 keV.

Decay processes

There are a number of different modes of radioactive decay, some of which have been alluded to above. These modes include alpha and beta decay, electron capture, isomeric transition and internal conversion and spontaneous fission. All of these various decay processes are bound by the fundamental physical laws of conservation of charge, mass and energy.

Alpha decay

Emission of an α-particle occurs in unstable nuclei with a high atomic number ($Z > 80$). The α-particle ejected from the nucleus carries away energy released in the process as kinetic energy. The decay process can be written as:

$$^{A}_{Z}X \rightarrow {}^{A-4}_{Z-2}Y + {}^{4}_{2}\alpha$$

Note that total mass number and total atomic number on the right-hand side of the expression are equal to the corresponding mass and atomic number on the left side of the expression, satisfying the requirement for conservation of both mass and charge. The daughter product is a different element from the parent (transmutation) as atomic number has decreased by 2. Following α-particle emission, the daughter nucleus (often termed the *recoil* nucleus) may still be energetically unstable and undergo subsequent transitions with further emission of radiation.

An example of this decay process is the decay of uranium-238 (^{238}U) by α-particle emission to thorium-234 (^{234}U):

$$^{238}_{92}U \rightarrow {}^{234}_{90}Th + {}^{4}_{2}\alpha$$

Other examples of radionuclides that emit α-particles are ^{235}U and ^{210}Po.

An alternative to alpha decay for heavy nuclides is *fission*, whereby the unstable nucleus breaks down into two roughly equal fragments. Fission can occur spontaneously, but is more usually induced by bombardment of the target nucleus by charged particles in a nuclear reactor.

Beta decay

β⁻ emission

This mode of radioactive decay occurs when a nucleus has an excess of neutrons relative to more stable neighbouring nuclides. A more stable state is achieved by a neutron in the unstable nucleus converting to a proton. This is accompanied by the emission of a β-particle, necessary for the conservation of charge. The process of β^- decay may be represented as:

$$^{A}_{Z}X \rightarrow {}_{Z+1}^{A}Y + {}_{-1}^{0}\beta + \overline{\nu}$$

The anti-neutrino ($\overline{\nu}$) also emitted in the process is the 'anti-particle' to a neutrino. Both neutrino and anti-neutrino have neither mass nor charge and are not discussed further as they have no relevance in nuclear medicine. The excess energy resulting from the nuclear transition is characteristic of the radionuclide, and is shared between the β-particle and the antineutrino. Beta particles can therefore be emitted with a range of energies from zero up to a finite maximum depending on the particular nuclide.

Following β-particle emission, as for alpha decay, the daughter nucleus may be in an excited energy state and may convert to a more stable state by the immediate emission of one or more γ-rays. An example of beta decay is the molybdenum-technetium decay process where molybdenum-99 (^{99}Mo) decays to technetium-99m (^{99m}Tc) with a 66 hour half-life and the emission of a β-particle followed immediately by an additional γ-ray of typical energy 740 keV:

$$^{99}_{42}Mo \rightarrow {}^{99m}_{43}Tc + \beta^- + \gamma$$

β^+ *or positron emission*

The converse of β^- decay occurs in positron emission. An unstable nucleus with a higher proton-to-neutron ratio than more stable neighbouring nuclides converts to a more stable energy state through the conversion of a proton to a neutron with the emission of a positron (and neutrino). This process may be written as:

$$^{A}_{Z}X \rightarrow {}_{Z-1}^{A}Y + {}_{+1}^{0}\beta + \upsilon$$

The positron β^+ is the *anti-particle* of the electron, having identical mass but opposite charge of $+e$. As for β-particles, the excess energy arising from the nuclear transition is shared between the positron and the neutrino and consequently positrons are emitted with a range of energies up to a finite maximum.

The positron loses its kinetic energy through interactions in a medium and subsequently annihilates with a free electron, yielding two γ-ray photons. These two photons are emitted at 180° to each other, each with initial energy 511 keV (equivalent to the rest mass of an electron from Einstein's famous equation $E = mc^2$). The coincident detection of these two 511 keV γ-rays is the objective of positron emission tomography (PET) imaging.

The most widely utilised positron emission process in PET is the decay of fluorine-18 (^{18}F) to oxygen-18 (^{18}O) with the release of a positron:

$$^{18}_{9}F \rightarrow {}^{18}_{8}O + \beta^+$$

Electron capture

When a neutron-deficient nuclide has insufficient energy for positron emission, the excess of protons may be reduced by the 'capture' of an orbital electron. A proton in the nucleus combines with an electron, typically from an inner shell due to its proximity to the nucleus, and converts to a neutron with the emission of a neutrino. Since the latter is without charge and mass and therefore virtually undetectable, the process of electron capture would be undetectable externally. However the vacancy created by the captured electron results in rearrangement of atomic electrons and subsequent characteristic X-ray or Auger electron emission from the daughter nucleus. In some cases γ-ray emission can also accompany characteristic X-ray/Auger emission if the daughter nucleus is left in an excited energy state. This consequence is useful for nuclear medicine applications and accordingly many radionuclides that decay by electron capture are utilised in nuclear medicine including ^{51}Cr, ^{67}Ga, ^{111}In and ^{123}I.

Isomeric transition

This decay process occurs where a daughter nuclide (arising from previous radioactive decay) in an excited energy state decays to a more stable state through the emission of a γ-ray. Unlike all the aforementioned decay processes, there is no change in mass number or atomic number during isomeric transition. The reversion to a lower-energy state by isomeric transition is not necessarily instantaneous and the nucleus can exist in the excited state for a measurable length of time. This prolonged state is referred to as a *metastable* state and is usually denoted by the letter m following the mass number in the notation ^{Am}X. This is an extremely useful process for nuclear medicine imaging as the metastable daughter nucleus decaying by isomeric transition emits only gamma radiation, thus reducing the radiation dose to the patient. The most widely utilised radionuclide in nuclear medicine imaging is technetium-99m (^{99m}Tc) which has a half-life of 6.01 hours and decays by emission of a γ-ray with energy 140 keV. This decay process is represented as:

$$^{99m}_{43}Tc \rightarrow {}^{99}_{43}Tc + \gamma$$

Technetium-99 decays via β^- emission with a half-life of 2.1×10^5 years and so can essentially be treated as stable.

An alternative to the emission of a γ-ray by the isomer is the process of *internal conversion* in which the excited nucleus transfers its excess energy directly to an orbital electron. The electron is ejected if the excitation energy is greater than the binding energy of that particular shell. Although β-particles and conversion electrons are essentially the same fundamental particle, both their origin and their emitted energy differ. Beta particles originate from the nucleus and are emitted with a continuous distribution of energies up to a finite maximum, whereas conversion electrons are orbital, atomic electrons emitted with discrete energy characteristic of the binding energy levels of the particular nuclide.

As for the electron capture process, subsequent rearrangement of atomic electrons, to fill the vacancy created by the ejected conversion electron, results in characteristic X-ray or Auger electron emission.

The ratio of the number of conversion electrons to observed γ-rays is termed the conversion coefficient. Internal conversion is undesirable in imaging applications as the electron emission adds to the effective dose of the patient without imparting any diagnostic information. For this reason, a low conversion coefficient is desirable for radionuclides intended for use in diagnostic imaging.

Decay schemes

A decay scheme diagram is a useful way of illustrating the decay process for radionuclides. The following conventions are followed for representing decay scheme diagrams:

- Parent and daughter nuclei are identified by bold, adjacent horizontal lines. Increasing Z values are represented from left to right. The vertical distance between the lines is proportional to the energy released in the process.
- β^- decay is identified by a left-to-right diagonal arrow, i.e. $Z \searrow Z+1$.
- β^+, electron capture (EC) and alpha decay are identified by right-to-left diagonal arrows, i.e. $Z \swarrow Z-1$ or $Z \swarrow Z-2$, respectively.
- Excited energy states are represented by horizontal lines directly above the daughter ground state.
- Vertical arrows between energy levels indicate γ-ray emissions.

Figure 2.4 shows simplified decay scheme diagrams for a number of clinically used radionuclides.

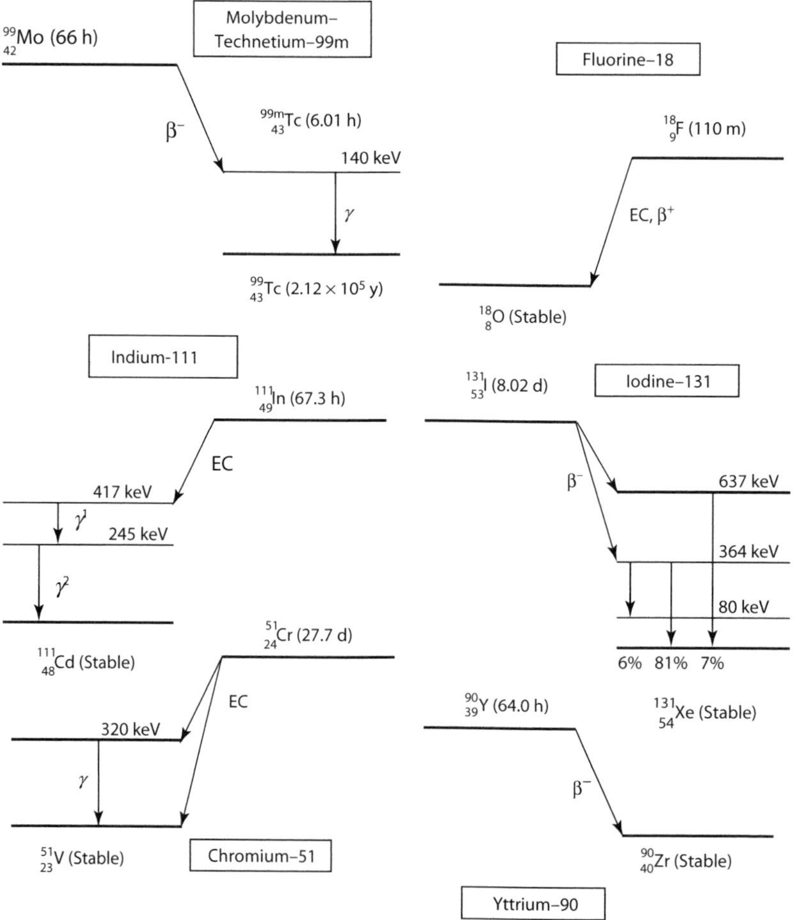

Figure 2.4 Simplified decay schemes for some clinically useful radionuclides.

Interaction of radiation with matter

The interaction of radiation with matter is important as it has implications both for radiation protection, since it determines how energy is deposited in the medium (whether shielding material or tissue), and instrumentation design, since it determines how the radiation is detected and measured. Particulate and EM radiation interact with matter via different mechanisms and are therefore considered separately.

Particulate radiation

Particulate radiation loses kinetic energy through electrostatic interactions with atoms in the absorbing material. The primary mechanisms for this are through *ionisation* and excitation of atomic electrons and the production of *bremsstrahlung* radiation.

Ionisation

Ionisation is the process of stripping of electrons from the atom. This occurs where particulate radiation transfers sufficient energy to orbital electrons to completely remove them from the atom, resulting in the formation of ion pairs. The number of ion pairs formed per millimetre is termed the *specific ionisation*. Owing to their higher mass and charge, α-particles have a specific ionisation of the order of 100 times greater than that of β-particles. Ionisation is the most prevalent mechanism of interaction for α-particles.

The high specific ionisation of α-particles means that they have an extremely short range in an absorbing material – a sheet of paper is sufficient to absorb α-particles. Beta radiation, being more penetrating due to its lighter mass and single charge, requires a few millimetres of aluminium for complete absorption.

Positrons cause ionisation in a similar way to beta radiation as they have almost identical physical properties. However, when the positron has expended all of its kinetic energy through ionisation, combination with a free electron results in two 511 keV annihilation photons. Shielding of the high-energy gamma radiation associated with positron annihilation requires a few centimetres of lead.

Excitation is the less prevalent mechanism for particulate radiation and occurs when incident radiation has insufficient energy for ionisation. Instead of being ejected, orbital electrons are excited to higher energy states.

Electrons liberated through particulate ionisation may themselves have sufficient energy to cause *further* excitation and ionisation of other atomic electrons – termed *secondary* ionisation.

Bremsstrahlung

Charged particles whose path is in close proximity to the nucleus can interact directly with the nucleus. Due to the strong electrostatic force exerted by the nucleus, the incident charged particle is deflected. This interaction causes rapid deceleration of the particle and as a consequence it loses kinetic energy. This energy is released as EM radiation, termed bremsstrahlung or 'braking' radiation, and is emitted as a continuous spectrum of X-rays. The energy of the bremsstrahlung radiation ranges from almost zero (where the charged particle is only slightly deflected) up to a maximum equal to the initial energy of the incident particle (where the charged particle is virtually stopped).

The intensity of bremsstrahlung radiation emitted in a particular medium with atomic number Z is proportional to Z^2. For this reason in X-ray tubes, in which electrons are accelerated across high voltages to bombard a target, the target material is chosen to have a high Z. Conversely, in clinical applications where shielding of beta radiation is required, materials with low Z (such as glass and Perspex) are typically chosen to minimise the secondary bremsstrahlung radiation produced.

Figure 2.5 is a schematic diagram showing the processes of ionisation and bremsstrahlung radiation.

Electromagnetic radiation

Particulate and electromagnetic radiation differ not only in their form but also in the way in which they interact with matter. The former causes primary ionisation whereas the latter causes secondary or indirect ionisation. It is the resulting secondary electrons that are responsible for the radiobiological effects caused by γ-ray, X-ray and bremsstrahlung radiation.

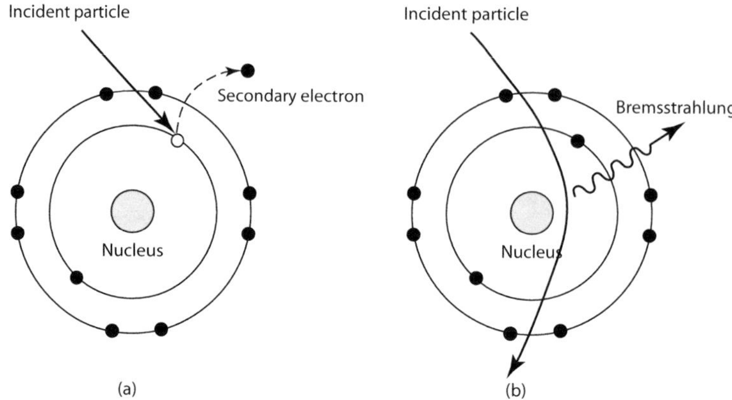

Figure 2.5 Ionisation (a) and production of bremsstrahlung radiation (b) when particulate radiation interacts with matter.

Gamma radiation interacts with matter via three mechanisms: the photoelectric effect, Compton scattering and pair production. The prevalence of each of these interactions is dependent on the energy of the incident gamma radiation.

Photoelectric effect

In this interaction all of the energy of the incident γ-ray is completely absorbed by the atom and transferred to an inner-shell electron, which is subsequently ejected. The energy imparted to the electron, called a photoelectron, is the difference between the γ-ray energy, E_γ, and the binding energy of the particular electron shell. The number of photoelectrons produced is proportional to Z^3 and inversely proportional to $E_\gamma{}^3$. This latter property means that radionuclides emitting low energy γ-rays are not suitable for diagnostic imaging as the γ-rays will be stopped in tissue by the photoelectric effect, causing unnecessary patient dose and providing no diagnostic benefit.

The ejected photoelectron subsequently causes ionisation, excitation and bremsstrahlung radiation as described in the previous section. Rearrangement of atomic electrons to fill the vacancy created by the photoelectron can additionally result in subsequent characteristic X-ray or Auger electron emission.

Compton scattering

For a particular absorbing material, Compton scattering dominates at higher γ-ray energies. Compton scattering occurs where a γ-ray imparts only a fraction of its energy to an outer-shell electron, termed the recoil electron, and continues onwards but scattered at a particular angle to its incident direction. The energy transferred is independent of Z or the density of the absorbing material – that is, Compton scattering is strictly a photon–electron interaction.

The maximum recoil electron energy occurs when the γ-ray is scattered at 180° to its incident direction (i.e. back-scattered). As the γ-ray loses only a small fraction of its initial energy when undergoing Compton scattering, it may subsequently undergo multiple Compton scattering events as it traverses the absorbing medium until its energy is sufficiently reduced for it to be completely absorbed via the photoelectric effect.

Pair production

An incident γ-ray photon with sufficiently high energy passing close to the electrostatic field of the nucleus can create an electron–positron pair. The incident γ-ray photon, which disappears in this process, must have energy greater than 1.022 MeV (twice the rest mass energy of the electron/positron) in order for electron–positron pair creation to be possible.

Any energy that the incident γ-ray has in excess of 1.022 MeV is shared between the electron and positron as kinetic energy. The electron and positron subsequently lose their kinetic energy through ionisation and excitation of atoms. The positron finally combines with a free electron, resulting in the creation of two 511 keV annihilation γ-ray photons.

Attenuation of electromagnetic radiation

When a beam of X-ray or gamma radiation traverses an absorbing medium, photon energy is transferred to matter via the various mechanisms detailed above. For each individual X-ray or γ-ray photon a series of interactions occurs involving secondary electrons and resulting secondary photons (e.g. characteristic X-rays, scattered or annihilation photons) of progressively less energy.

The probability of a particular interaction depends on the energy of the incident radiation and on the composition and thickness of the absorbing medium. For the latter, as would be expected, the thicker the absorber the greater the probability that an interaction will occur. The actual *type* of interaction that occurs depends on the energy of the radiation and absorber composition (density, atomic number) in a more complex way, as alluded to above.

At photon energies typically found in nuclear medicine, the prevalent interactions in tissue are photoelectric absorption and Compton scattering. In the former, the photons are absorbed and completely eliminated; in the latter, the photons are deflected from the direction of the incident radiation. Both interactions have the same effect of reducing the intensity of the beam traversing the absorbing medium.

For an incident narrow beam of mono-energetic radiation with initial intensity I_0, the residual intensity I after travelling through material of thickness d is given by

$$I = I_0 \exp^{(-\mu d)}$$

where μ is termed the *linear attenuation coefficient* and has units of cm^{-1}. Note that this equation showing that EM radiation is attenuated exponentially is similar in form to that for radioactive decay, given in equation (2.2). The linear attenuation coefficient includes the effect of all the interactions detailed previously (photoelectric, Compton scattering and pair production) and is characteristic of the photon energy and the composition of the absorber.

The *half-value thickness* $D_{1/2}$, analogous to half-life, is defined as the thickness of absorbing material that reduces the intensity of a beam of radiation to half its initial value and can be written as

$$D_{1/2} = \frac{\ln_e(2)}{\mu}$$

It follows that the half-value thickness also depends on both the absorbing material and the energy of the radiation. Table 2.3 gives the half-value thickness for water (equivalent to soft-tissue density) and lead for a number of radionuclides used commonly in nuclear medicine.

A reduction in the incident radiation intensity by 99% is effected by approximately seven half-value thicknesses ($[1/2]^7 = 0.008$). Table 2.3 shows that for ^{99m}Tc, 0.2 cm of lead is required for 99% reduction in radiation intensity. For ^{131}I, which has a higher energy γ-ray (364 keV compared with 140 keV), 1.8 cm of lead is required for the same reduction in radiation intensity. The 511 keV annihilation photons resulting from the positron emission by ^{18}F require 2.8 cm of lead for an equivalent absorption of the gamma radiation.

Table 2.3 Half-value thickness for radionuclides used in nuclear medicine (Short 1999; Cherry *et al.* 2003)

Radionuclide	Half-value thickness (cm)	
	Water	Lead
Gallium-67	4.7	0.07
Krypton-81m	5.0	0.06
Technetium-99m	4.5	0.03
Indium-111	5.1	0.07
Iodine-123	4.6	0.04
Iodine-131	6.3	0.25
Thallium-201	4.3	0.03
Fluorine-18 (511 keV γ-rays)	7.1	0.41

References

Cherry SR *et al.* (2003). *Physics in Nuclear Medicine*, 3rd edn. Philadelphia: Elsevier Science, Philadelphia.

Pearce A (2008). *Recommended Nuclear Decay Data*. NPL Report IR6. Teddington: National Physical Laboratory. ISSN 1754-2952

Short MD (1999). Basic Principles of Radionuclide Physics. In: Samson C, ed. *Textbook of Radiopharmacy*, 3rd edn. New York: Gordon and Breach Science Publishers, 1–17.

Further reading

Martin A, Harbinson S (2006). *An Introduction to Radiation Protection*, 5th edn. London: Hodder Arnold.

Saha GB (2004). *Fundamentals of Nuclear Pharmacy*, 5th edn. New York: Springer-Verlag.

Walker B, Jarritt P (1995). Basic Physics of Nuclear Medicine. In: Murray IPC, Ell PJ, eds. *Nuclear Medicine in Clinical Diagnosis and Treatment*. Edinburgh: Churchill Livingstone, 1279–1289.

3

Radiation protection

Stanley Batchelor

Introduction

This chapter gives an overview of the basic radiation protection measures needed to work safely with radioactive materials with a description of what the International Commission on Radiological Protection (ICRP) recommends in different grades of radionuclide laboratories. It also explains the requirements of United Kingdom law that exists to protect the patient, worker, members of the public and the environment from risks of radiation exposure. Finally, subjects such as personnel monitoring, decontamination and radioactive waste disposal are covered.

Most legislation stems from world governments taking due notice of the ICRP recommendations and so, although there will be some variation to that described in this chapter, the differences in developed countries should not be too marked. Certainly in the European Community the legislation of member states will be very similar as they will be in accordance with European Directives. An underlying principle of ICRP is that of keeping radiation exposure to as low as reasonably achievable (ALARA) or as low as reasonably practical (ALARP), and this is a common theme through all European legislation.

General methods of reducing radiation dose

Radiation dose is received by direct irradiation from a source external to the body or from radioactive material absorbed into the body. The former is reduced by correct optimisation of the three well-known dose saving factors:

- Time
- Distance
- Shielding.

The first factor, *time*, is pretty obvious: the shorter the exposure to a radiation source the less dose is received. This means that all radioactive sources should be returned to their shielded containers as soon as possible; bins full of hot waste should be removed and placed away from workers whenever possible; workers should proceed with their work as quickly as they are able *but without adding an undue risk of error or spill*. 'Cold runs' can also be carried out where a procedure using high activities is being performed for the first time.

The second factor, *distance*, is often not appreciated fully. The intensity of, and hence the absorbed dose from, a radioactive source varies inversely as the square of the distance from the source (the inverse square law). So on doubling the distance, the dose rate drops to one-quarter. However the effect is even more dramatic at short distances. If the fingers, for example, are touching the external surface of a glass vial containing a gamma emitter, the dose may be one hundred times higher than that experienced by using tongs of reasonable length. Making a 10-fold increase in distance between source and finger means a 100-fold reduction in absorbed dose. (It must also be remembered that the inverse square law is quite approximate once distances become comparable to the dimensions of the source.) Some people criticise the use of tongs, saying that they are able to handle items more quickly without them, thereby gaining in the time factor what they lose in the distance factor. There are two flaws in this argument: the first is that the gain does not compensate, and the second that if they persevere with tongs (and other dose-saving devices) they will find they quickly get used to them and perform the operations no slower than before.

The third factor, *shielding*, may appear obvious to many but there are many small points that make this subject quite complex at times. The electrons from beta emitters can be completely absorbed with a centimetre or so of Perspex (beta energy does not go up and up but has a finite maximum for any radionuclide). Gamma emitters show an exponential absorption with any absorber but this absorption depends on the energy of the gamma radiation and the atomic number and density of absorber. For low gamma energies the absorption varies as the cube of the atomic number, whereas for higher energies it is independent of atomic number. This means that for low-energy gamma/X-ray emitters such as ^{125}I only a very small thickness of lead will reduce the intensity of radiation by a factor of 10, whereas for the higher-energy emitters such those as in positron emission tomography (511 keV annihilation photons) or $^{22/24}$Na may need several if not tens of millimetres just to reduce the dose by a factor of 2. Refer to Table 3.1 on the radiation and shielding properties for commonly encountered radionuclides.

ICRP guidance on radiation protection and general radiation protection measures required

No new facilities or significant modification of existing facilities should be designed and brought into use without expert advice from the employer's Radiation Protection Adviser (RPA). This is one of the roles of the RPA detailed in the Ionising Radiation Regulations 1999 (HMSO 2000b). The facilities required will depend on the nature of the hazard involved.

The ICRP (ICRP 1989) classifies laboratories in which radioactive materials are used as being of low, medium or high hazard. This designation takes account of the risks of contamination for the various procedures. In order to determine which hazard category a given procedure comes into, a 'weighted activity' is calculated. This is the activity actually encountered multiplied by two modification factors – one for the radionuclide (Table 3.2) and one for the type of operation to be carried out (Table 3.3). The 'weighted activity' is then compared with the values given in Table 3.4, from which the hazard category of the laboratory is determined.

Requirements for the different laboratories

The standards required in low-, medium- and high-hazard laboratories are summarised below.

A low-hazard laboratory requires: no structural shielding, cleanable floor and bench surfaces, no fume cupboard for radiation work activities, standard ventilation and plumbing, and simple hand wash facilities.

Upgrading this to a medium-hazard laboratory requires in addition: continuous, cleanable flooring, good room ventilation, fume cupboard and some decontamination facilities. This room is likely to be a supervised or may possibly be a controlled area.

Table 3.1 Radiological data for radionuclides encountered in nuclear medicine and positron emission tomography centres

Radionuclide	Decay mode	Principal emission energy (MeV) (beta energies are maximum energies)	Half-life[a]	First tenth value layer (mm Pb)[b]	Annual limit of intake[c] (MBq)
Radionuclides encountered in nuclear medicine					
^{57}Co	EC	E_γ 0.122, 0.136	271 d	0.7	21
^{58}Co	β^+	E_β 0.475; E_γ 0.811	70.8 d	28	10
^{67}Ga	EC	E_γ 0.093, 0.185, 0.300	78.3 h	5.3	71
^{89}Sr	β	E_β 1.463	50.5 d	5000 (estimate)	3.6
^{99}Mo	β	E_β 1.232; E_γ 0.740, 0.141	66.0 h	20	17
^{99m}Tc	IT	E_γ 0.141	6.02 h	0.9	690
^{111}In	EC	E_γ 0.171, 0.245	2.83 d	2.5	65
^{123}I	EC	E_γ 0.027, 0.159	13.2 h	1.2	95
^{131}I	β	E_β 0.606; E_γ 0.364	8.04 d	11	1.8
^{127}Xe	EC	E_γ 0.172, 0.203, 0.375	36.4 d	—	—
^{133}Xe	β	E_β 0.346; E_γ 0.081,0.033	5.25 d	0.7	—
^{201}Tl	EC	$E_{X/\gamma}$ 0.075 ave.; E_γ 0.167	73.1 h	<0.9	211
^{32}P	β	E_β 1.71	14.3 d	range 6000 air	6
^{51}Cr	EC	E_γ 0.320; E_X 0.005	27.7 d	7	526
^{125}I	EC	E_γ 0.035; $E_{X/\gamma}$ 0.030 ave.	60.1 d	0.06	1.3
Radionuclides encountered in positron emission tomography					
^{11}C	β^+, EC	$E_{\beta+}$ 0.960; E_γ 0.511	20.4 min	13.5	880
^{13}N	β^+, EC	$E_{\beta+}$ 1.198 E_γ 0.511	10 min	13.5	not listed
^{15}O	β^+, EC	$E_{\beta+}$ 1.732 E_γ, 0.511	2.03 min	13.5	not listed
^{18}F	β^+, EC	$E_{\beta+}$ 0.633 E_γ 0.511	110 min	13.5	215

[a] min, minutes; h, hours; d, days; y, years.

[b] These data are taken from tables published from multiple sources; they may not take account of low-energy (20 keV) X- or gamma emissions. Where a radionuclide is a pure beta emitter the range in air is given.

[c] Mostly taken from ICRP Publication 68 (ICRP 1994) Dose Coefficients for Intakes of Radionuclides by Workers and ICRP Publication 72 (ICRP 1996) Age dependent Doses to members of the Public from Intake of Radionuclides: Part 5 Compilation of Ingestion and Inhalation Dose Coefficients. These values are minimum values giving the most pessimistic case. Radionuclides in certain forms, or taken in through a different route, may have a higher ALI than that shown.

Table 3.2 Weighting factors for different radionuclides

Radionuclide	Weighting factor
^{89}Sr, ^{125}I, ^{131}I	100
^{11}C, ^{13}N, ^{15}O, ^{18}F, ^{32}P, ^{51}Cr, ^{57}Co, ^{58}Co, ^{59}Fe, ^{67}Ga, ^{99}Mo, ^{99m}Tc, ^{123}I, ^{111}In, ^{201}Tl	1.0
^{3}H, ^{14}C, ^{81m}Kr, ^{127}Xe, ^{133}Xe	0.01

Table 3.3 Weighting factors for different activities

Operation performed	Weighting factor
Simple storage area	0.01
Radioactive waste: decay storage or storage prior to consignment	0.01–0.1
Diagnostic procedures (scans, sample counting), radioactive patients (diagnosis) in a waiting room or on wards	0.1
Dispensing and administering radionuclides, ward therapy patients, normal chemical operations	1
Complex operations, radiopharmaceutical preparation	10

A high-hazard laboratory may require structural shielding, floor surface as before but welded to walls, special plumbing, forced ventilation, and enhanced fume cupboard facility – depending on the nature of the hazard. This room is likely to be a 'Controlled Radiation' area. A controlled radiation area is defined within UK legislation (HMSO 2000a) as an area where special protection procedures must be followed in order to restrict exposure such that 3/10 of any relevant dose limit is not exceeded (refer to Regulation 16 (1) in the Ionising Radiations Regulations 1999 if more detail of this definition is required).

Table 3.4 Hazard category depending on weighted activity

Weighted activity (MBq)	Category
Less than 50	Low hazard
50–50 000	Medium hazard
Greater than 50 000	High hazard

A radiopharmacy hot room with a $^{99}Mo/^{99m}Tc$ generator will be a high-hazard area laboratory. A low-level assay room preparing, for example, glomerular filtration rate (GFR) samples would be a low-hazard laboratory. A cell labelling room could be either a medium-hazard or possibly a high-hazard area (although some of the higher specification features of the high-hazard laboratory may still be present due to the need for higher standards of cleanliness, etc., required).

General design requirements of rooms for using unsealed radioactive sources

Security

It is a legal requirement that radioactive sources are kept locked away. This means fridges and other stores that contain radioactive materials must be lockable. See later in this chapter for more about security.

Ventilation

Ventilation systems should function so that they do not extract radioactive material from one room and expel it into another room. This can occur either by design (i.e. using part of the extracted air to mix with external air) or by the location of the exhaust duct outlet position. This should be checked at commissioning. In some cases, such as dispensing for iodine therapy, a fume hood operating at a negative pressure is needed for protection of the worker. In other cases, such as sterile production, it is appropriate to have a fully exhausted laminar vertical flow system under positive pressure.

Space

It is essential that there is adequate space in work areas in rooms where radionuclides are handled. Workers must be able to safely perform their tasks without risk of collision and subsequent spills. Low-activity assay work areas must be separated from areas involving higher-activity work. Sensitive beta or gamma counting or imaging equipment (or whole body counters) should not be sited physically close to high-energy sources such as molybdenum/technetium generators or stock amounts of positron-emitting radionuclides. The interference between such high- and low-activity work can invalidate results or significantly restrict the use of the facility for either purpose.

Washing facilities

It is important that workers have convenient access to hand-washing facilities; these may usefully be sited close to the exit of the room. Taps should be able to be operated without using the hands (e.g. elbow or foot controls). Disposable towels for drying are preferred and a mains-operated monitor should be located reasonably close to the sink. The monitor should be left turned on so that staff are able and encouraged to use it without touching the controls and also the monitor will not have flat batteries – a common finding in audits. In addition, a personnel monitoring logbook should be kept with the monitor, preferably mounted on a dedicated, small inclined shelf under the monitor with a pen attached so that record keeping is made as easy as possible.

Designated sinks

In situations where large amounts of radioactivity are used, the designated sink for aqueous waste disposal should be connected as directly as possible to a main sewer. Although this is not always possible, one should still trace back the route of such drainpipes to determine whether there are any problems that can be foreseen as a consequence of the disposal. Examples that have been encountered (not infrequently) include:

- Lengths of pipe that do not empty due to insufficient downward gradient on the pipe
- Hand wash basins situated further down the pipe run which are lower than the designated sink, so that if a blockage did occur waste would come into the hand wash basin before appearing in the bottom of the designated sink
- Large-volume ‘traps’ on the waste outlet that are designed for holding materials to encourage dilution. These result in a delay in complete discharge of radioactive materials and therefore cause unnecessary irradiation to staff in the laboratory. Such traps on sinks designated for aqueous radioactive waste disposal are not generally acceptable to the regulator.

Solid waste

Some form of solid radioactive waste store is necessary. This may be a dedicated room where the volume and/or the amounts of radioactivity so dictate, or it may be a cupboard within a room used for another purpose. This waste will be stored for a given length of time prior to being despatched off site either as radioactive waste or possibly (for short-half-life material such as technetium-99m) as non-active waste (clinical or black bag, etc.) The store may need shielding unless the waste is very low level. Even if radiation levels are only moderately low, the exposure of staff or public is not acceptable nor is it within the ‘ALARP’ principle, so it is necessary to reduce this with shielding and/or by removal as soon as possible after production.

Benching

Medium- and high-hazard category laboratories should have a bench design with a raised lip at the front and coved at the back onto the wall to contain spills. There should be no gaps in joining of parts of the bench top as these would allow absorption of radioactive contamination into the joins. It is important that these features are still employed even if the worker employs a spill tray covered with disposable liner. The benching should be resistant to corrosion by chemicals and also be easily decontaminated. The bench must also be able to support the loading of lead shields.

Area designation

Controlled areas are required in the technetium generator suite of the radiopharmacy. Other rooms such as the blood labelling room, aseptic dispensing room and quality control laboratory may or may not be controlled areas depending on the nature of work undertaken, the activities handled and the local decisions made between the RPA and staff involved. These rooms will almost certainly be supervised areas if they are not controlled areas. The radionuclide store is likely to be a controlled area unless the amounts of radioactive material stored are low and well shielded. Sometimes it is more practical to control the entire suite or the entire suite past an entry/collection point where local deliveries may be made. The status of such rooms must be clearly signed and they should be fully described in local rules. It is customary to control an entire room rather than declare only part of it to be controlled, although this latter option is always available. An example of this would be the area behind a shield or in a fume cupboard, where only the hands can enter. In this case that area alone *may* be controlled on the basis of the dose limit for an extremity being likely to be exceeded. Rooms that are controlled radiation areas because of their potential for contamination, as well as direct radiation exposure, such as the radiopharmacy, will require the entrance to be via a 'step over' barrier. This not only serves to act as a convenient point at which to put on disposable overshoes and use monitoring facilities, but also draws attention to the special nature of the area being entered. It also demonstrates to a regulator that control of potential contamination is being appropriately managed.

Liquid waste disposal – delay tanks and storage

'Delay' tanks may be used in some hospitals for the reduction of environmental impact of the discharged iodine from cancer patients treated with radioiodine. This is unlikely to be required purely as a result of radiopharmacy activities. There currently appears to be further controversy between regulators as to whether delay tanks are justified in many situations in healthcare.

It is important to be aware of the local licensing conditions under which the site has to operate (see the later part of this chapter). If the hospital does not have the ability to store aqueous radioactive waste then it is important that the way such unwanted liquid waste is handled be agreed with the RPA and local Environment Agency inspector at the outset. In cases like this the waste must be disposed of at the moment it is declared as aqueous liquid waste.

Wall shielding

On safety grounds, it is rarely justified to shield rooms containing the radionuclides used in nuclear medicine imaging. However, it is possible for imaging to suffer if there are high radioactivities in rooms adjoining the imaging room. Such interference can result from patients being imaged in adjoining imaging areas, from an injected patient waiting in an adjoining room or from a radiopharmacy situated too close to imaging facilities. Hence wall shielding is sometimes found to be required. The amount of shielding needed is generally up to 2 mm thickness of lead, which should reduce any such effects by more than 100-fold. The use of leaded doors in nuclear medicine is not usually appropriate (except in SPECT, where they would be needed for X-ray attenuation).

Local shielding

By 'local shielding' is meant a shield placed over a radiation-emitting area so that control of dose rate at its source is effected, thereby making the rest of the room safer for work (as opposed to shielding a large area such as an entire wall). Local shielding should be applied wherever a significant reduction in dose may be possible. Obvious examples of sources for which local shielding is appropriate are ^{99}Mo/^{99m}Tc generators (both primary shields in which they are shipped and additional secondary shields in which the assembly is placed on delivery to the suite), multidose vials for patient administrations, individual diagnostic and therapeutic patient doses and flood sources for gamma camera quality control. Multidose vials containing ^{99m}Tc-labelled products are easily shielded using 2–4 mm thickness of lead pot. Iodine-131 therapy doses need much more protection (the tenth value thickness is 11 mm) and additional shielding to the pot used for transit may be deemed necessary when the sources are locked away in a shielded/isolated store. This is because what can be deemed acceptable for a short exposure duration may not be so acceptable during a longer-term exposure situation (see 'Shielding of the generator' below). Distance can also be usefully employed to reduce the dose rate, as well as time by storing the source in a room that has close to zero occupancy (see later).

Other shielding solutions are employed for operational procedures. Manipulation of radioactive materials must take place behind a body and eye shield, often termed an 'L shield' (Figure 3.1) Note that there is a bottom to the shield to protect the workers' lower body and to make the shield more stable. It is essential that the benching is able to safely accommodate the weight of the shielding. Commercial benching can be specified to take various loads. The shield acts both to attenuate radiation and as a guard to stop the operator becoming contaminated. Radioactive waste (whether solid or liquid) will also require local shielding. Distance may be used for bulky items such as sacks of clinical radioactive waste. When this is considered appropriate, it can be accomplished through the use of an entire dedicated room or by

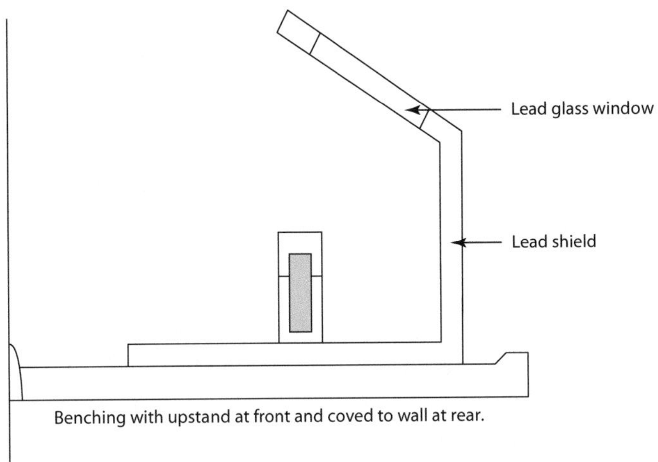

Figure 3.1 Typical shield for operational shielding of sources.

promptly depositing the waste in the institution's central radioactive waste store. Sometimes both shielding and distance (using a locked room) are required – e.g. for the waste from an iodine therapy in-patient. Ventilation of such areas must not be overlooked.

Radionuclide manipulation and administration

It is important that protective devices are used when vials and syringes containing radioactive materials are handled. For gamma emitters, tungsten is generally used in commercial protective products as it has a higher atomic number and density than lead, thereby providing more attenuation for the same thickness. Some lead-glass shields can provide better visibility. Perspex syringe shields are generally used for shielding beta emitters as they not only absorb the β-particles but also minimise the Bremsstrahlung X-radiation produced, which occurs when a shielding material of high atomic number is used. However, with sufficient thickness of lead the attenuation can be great enough to absorb all the beta radiation and most of the Bremsstrahlung. It is important that the operator does not become too complacent when using syringe shields. The radiation emitted from the ends of the shield results in a far lower overall protection than might be expected from the thickness of lead in the shield.

Shielding of the generator

Radiation protection has to follow the 'as low as reasonably practical' principle ('ALARP') The application of this principle to the shielding requirements for the transport of a new generator does not necessarily equate to its application during storage and use. For example, upon delivery the generator needs to be moved without lifting equipment and hence the weight of the primary shield has to take this into account. The primary shield may be depleted uranium as this offers more attenuation than lead (thickness for thickness) due to its higher atomic number and density. However, once placed within its secondary shield, the assembly (i.e. both the primary shielded generator and the secondary shield around it) is not required to be moved until the generator is removed. So what satisfies ALARP during transit (hours of personnel exposure at a significant distance) is different from what is needed during use (days of exposure at potentially closer personnel distance). Dose rates around the secondary shield should be measured for dosimetry validation. Adjoining rooms should not be overlooked if the generator is placed in proximity to a dividing wall and further shielding has to be added if required and environmental dosemeters used to integrate the dose at wall surfaces over a long period of use. Typically, total shielding of the order of 80–100 mm lead may be needed. All shielding within the radiopharmacy must be easily cleanable – this generally means that exposed lead surfaces are coated with paint or some other material.

Robotic systems

There has been some development of robotic systems so that automated formulation may be achieved, thereby reducing the hand doses of radiopharmaceutical staff. These systems need to overcome the

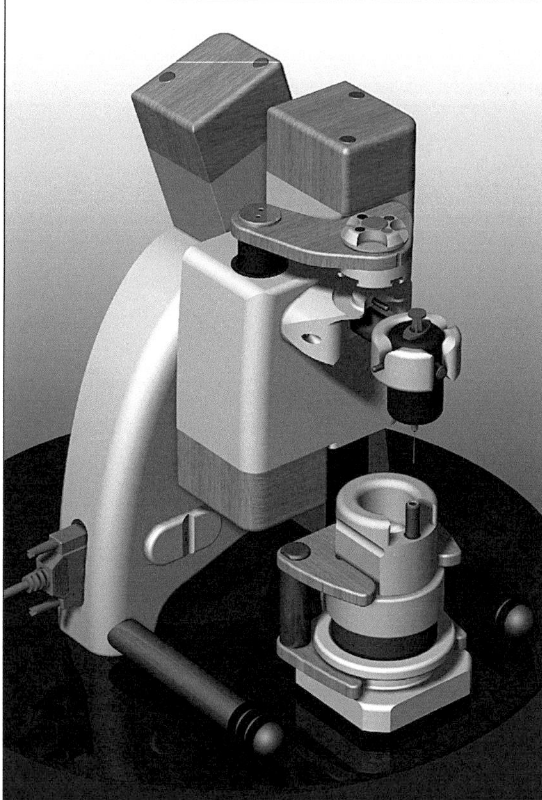

Figure 3.2 Remote fill station for use in PET. (Photograph courtesy of Amercare Ltd.)

potential contamination problems that seem to occur in the early generations of this equipment. Simplified, automated syringe filling stations are being developed to aid in manual manipulations. An example of such a device, an automated dispenser for PET, is shown in Figure 3.2. This, at least, may reduce the significant radiation dose that is received from the unshielded end of syringe shields, etc.

General procedures

The access allowed to the radiopharmacy for cleaning staff and other service personnel must take into account the hazards to which such staff may be exposed. If the area remains controlled or supervised when they need access, such workers must follow local rules. There must be clear marking, with an appropriate radiation trefoil warning symbol, of bins that are used for the accumulation of solid radioactive waste. It is also required that there be a clear written sign stating the nature of the bin's contents and that it must not be inadvertently removed by cleaning staff. Unintended radioactive waste leaving the premises as ordinary or clinical waste can result in legal action being taken against the employer by the Environment Agency due to the failure to keep waste secure and dispose of it via an appropriate waste stream.

Concise overview of legislation for protection of worker

In the UK the main items of legislation that will be relevant to workers using radioactive materials in a radiopharmacy are:

1. The Ionising Radiation Regulations 1999
2. The Ionising Radiation (Medical Exposure) Regulations 2000 (IRMER)
3. The Radioactive Substances Act 1993
4. The Environmental Permitting Regulations 2010
5. The High Activity Sealed Radioactive Source and Orphan Sources Regulations 2005 (HASS)
6. Carriage of Dangerous Goods and Use of Transportable Pressure Equipment Regulations 2007 (HMSO 2007)
7. The Medicines (Administration of Radioactive Substances) Act 1978 (and amendments in 1995 and 2006)

The Ionising Radiation Regulations 1999 (HMSO 2000b)

These regulations come under the umbrella of the Health and Safety at Work Act 1973. They are principally there to protect the worker from exposure to ionising radiation in the workplace. They are enforced by the Health and Safety Executive (HSE), which may issue Improvement and/or Prohibition Notices if it feels that working practices are a significant threat to workers or the public.

The main features of these regulations are:

1. Employers must notify the HSE 28 days prior to working with radiation of their intention to *start* such work. They must also do this if they are significantly changing the way they are working with radiation (e.g.

starting work with radioactive substances after working with X-ray generators, such as going to PET from CT).

2. The employer must have access to the services of a suitably qualified and trained Radiation Protection Adviser (RPA) unless the work falls under the category of this not being necessary. For radiopharmacy situations an RPA would be required. The RPA must be accredited by a body that has been accepted by the HSE as fit to perform this accreditation (e.g. RPA 2000; this is currently the only body accepted by the HSE).
3. The employer must have performed a suitable and sufficient written radiation risk assessment for all work they are undertaking. This risk assessment is pivotal in determining whether the area needs to be given special status (see controlled areas below) and also whether environmental or personal monitoring needs to be undertaken.
4. All doses must be 'as low as reasonably practical' – the ALARP principle. This means that where it is reasonable and practical to reduce a significant dose and it is cost-effective to do so, then this must happen. Employees' and public doses must, in any event, be within the specified dose limits. Prosecution can occur for employers not keeping radiation doses ALARP – even if they are within dose limits. These limits are absolute – exceeding them is illegal and prosecution is then a high probability. Limits are: 20 mSv for whole body* (*effective dose*); 500 mSv for extremities, skin,* etc.; 1 mSv for the fetus and public; 13 mSv for the abdomen of a woman of reproductive capacity during a 3-month interval; 5 mSv per 5 years for a person who may be exposed to ionising radiation as a result of the exposure of someone else. (The limits marked * apply only to what are termed 'classified radiation workers', who are persons who have been formally assessed as being fit to work with radiation and are *likely* to exceed 3/10 of the limits above.)

Other staff, the majority (>95%) of healthcare workers, are just ordinary radiation workers and have limits of 3/10 of these (i.e. 6 mSv for body, 150 mSv for extremities, etc.). Also, medical exposures are not subject to these dose limits although they need to be optimised and justified under the IRMER.

5. The employer must ensure that they have suitable contingency plans to cover cases where a reasonably foreseeable accident with radiation occurs.
6. The employer must also ensure that all the employees working with radiation are suitably trained. The degree of training will vary with the nature of the work performed. For workers formulating and dispensing in the radiopharmacy this may be a one-day radiation protection course, whereas for supervisory staff this may last several days.
7. Areas where work with radiation takes place have to be assessed as to whether they should be controlled or supervised. A supervised area is any area where a public dose limit may be exceeded and a controlled area is any area where 3/10 of the dose limits may be exceeded. These areas are required to have clear demarcation and work in them must follow local rules and/or systems of work (depending whether they have a controlled area within them). If local rules exist then a suitably trained Radiation Protection Supervisor needs to ensure radiation workers understand and follow the local rules.
8. The employer has a duty to monitor the workplace and workers for radiation exposure, unless prior assessment has shown that the workers' radiation dose does not justify this. For workers in a radiopharmacy this monitoring will be necessary (see later in this chapter) and this may be both whole body and extremity. Records of such monitoring must be kept for statutory periods, which vary depending on the nature of the record. The time for which contamination records should be kept is not specified in the Radioactive Substances Act but there is detailed guidance for the retention of other records in the Medical and Dental Guidance Notes, Appendix 9 (IPEM 2002).
9. There are many other requirements such as leak testing of sealed sources (e.g. those that are used to test the isotope calibrator); the need to account for the radioactive materials held and

to keep them secure; the need to notify HSE if there are uncontrolled dispersals or losses of material; and the need to move materials around premises in a secure and safe manner. There is also a duty on the installer of equipment that exposes patients to radiation to ensure that a critical examination is performed (to verify that safety devices and warning devices are functioning) and for employers to ensure that quality assurance is performed. Overexposures due to equipment failure must be reported to the HSE if they exceed specified levels.

Failure to conform to these regulations can result in the issue of an Improvement Notice by the HSE. If improvement fails to be implemented then a prohibition notice may be issued that requires the activity to cease immediately (these may be issued straight away if the non-compliance is deemed serious enough). If the issue escalates to prosecution (or such a major breach dictates this to occur after an incident has occurred) then substantial fines and custodial sentences are also likely. The associated Approved Code of Practice is also useful (HSC 2000).

The Ionising Radiation (Medical Exposure) Regulations 2000 (and Amendment Regulations 2006) (HMSO 2000a, 2006)

In England these regulations are now enforced through the Care Standards Commission and they require the employer to have in place measures to ensure that patients' radiation exposures are controlled through sound procedures, referred with adequate clinical information, performed by adequately trained, approved and identified practitioners and operators using equipment that is sound and fit for use.

Employers must have written procedures that cover:

- Identifying the patient
- Ascertaining the status of pregnancy
- A framework for naming who is a practitioner (justifies the procedure) and
  - who is an operator (performs the practical aspect of the exposure)
- Quality assurance and audit procedures
- Procedures for recording target doses (diagnostic reference levels)
- Procedures for overexposure of patients
- Other considerations such as the need for clinical audit, medical legal procedures, etc.

There must also be protocols that describe how the procedures are to be performed.

The training requirements for the operator and practitioner are set out in a schedule attached to the regulations.

Radiology, nuclear medicine and radiotherapy activities are required to have an appropriately experienced medical physics expert (MPE) whose role is to advise on the patient radiation dosimetry and radiation physics aspects of the procedures – these are separate from the role of the Radiation Protection Adviser (RPA).

These regulations chiefly apply to routine diagnostic procedures, therapy procedures (both unsealed source therapy, e.g. iodine-131 for Ca thyroid and hyperthyroidism and for external beam radiotherapy/brachytherapy) and also research procedures.

An inventory for equipment that controls radiation exposure must be kept – this must include all of the following:

- Make and type of equipment
- The year of manufacturer *and* of installation
- Serial number and name/model of equipment.

For a radiopharmacy this would include the isotope calibrator as this directly affects the activity and hence radiation dose delivered to the patient. It could also include any other hardware or software that could affect the dispensed radiopharmaceutical dose delivery procedure.

The Radioactive Substances Act 1993 (HMSO 1993) and the Environmental Permitting Regulations 2010 (HMSO 2010)

There is a legal obligation for UK users of radioactive materials to comply with the Radioactive Substances Act 1993 (RSA93) unless working under an exemption order (but this is very unlikely to apply to a hospital with a radiopharmacy). The purpose of this act is to ensure control over radioactive material and resulting radioactive waste. Because this waste is potentially harmful, it is important that it is stored, used and disposed of safely, and that it is not produced in unnecessary quantities. Control is therefore necessary over the use and storage of radioactive materials as well as over the waste produced.

Environmental Permitting requirements under RSA93 and EPR 2010

The Environment Agency (EA) provides a regulatory system of registration and authorisation for the use, accumulation and disposal of radioactive materials. The act is policed by the EA whose inspectors have the right of access to premises to determine whether a user is complying with the act. For a user such as a hospital to obtain permits they must submit an application to the EA, which assesses it, and if satisfied, issues the appropriate permits. Applying for, keeping or changing these site/employer specific documents generally involves the payment of a significant fee unless the variation requested is very minor in nature.

Applications must include:

- Details of organisation and premises and radioactive materials to be held.
- Justification case – why do you need to use radioactive material and what steps will you take to minimise the production of radioactive waste?
- Form of waste you are requesting to store or dispose of, i.e. solid, liquid, gas, organic scintillant.
- Maximum amounts, storage times and volumes of each waste requested.
- Accumulation of waste – use of decay storage to reduce the waste discharged into the environment by taking advantage of natural radioactive decay.
- Assessment – calculation of the maximum radiation dose to a critical group from the requested disposal.
- Demonstration that the organisation will be working to Best Practical Means and Best Available Technology. The EA will want to see that a review has been done that shows the work cannot be done in an equivalent way using either no radioactivity, less activity or a less damaging radionuclide.
- Evidence that there is management control of the use of radionuclides and that there are adequate written procedures in place that relate to the licence conditions of use.

This application process is usually undertaken by the Radiation Protection Adviser or his support team although the act does not specifically mention the term 'RPA'.

Disposal of radioactive waste

Record keeping

Record keeping is an important part of complying with permits, and requires very explicit records of stock and waste (e.g. activity levels, volumes and the time waste has been stored).

Solid waste

Radioactive waste from the radiopharmacy is characterised according to activity and is treated as follows:

- Solid waste less than 0.4 Bq/g is exempt under the act, so this can go out as non-radioactive waste. It may still be toxic waste and be bound by other requirements.
- Low level: 400 kBq in 0.1 m^3 and 40 kBq per article (or for ^{14}C and tritium, 4000 kBq in 0.1 m^3 and 400 kBq per article) may be disposed of as normal refuse. (A volume of 0.1 m^3 is specified as it is considered equivalent to 'one dustbin'; this is commonly termed *dustbin level waste*.) Again, if the waste is toxic for other reasons (such as clinical waste) then it may not be possible for it to be disposed of as dustbin type waste.
- Incineration: transfer to external contractor under certain conditions. The activity here must be within that allowed on the permit.
- Transfer to an authorised company/body may occur. This route is generally used by hospitals for the disposal of sealed sources (including spent gamma camera flood sources and sample counter checking standards). The waste may then be processed or sent to secure storage for decay.

Liquid waste

Drains may be used, but the disposal route must be known and designated and records must be kept of all disposals; monthly totals again must comply with site limits.

Organic solvents

Transfer off-site may occur, but the amounts transferred have to be within the limits of the permit.

Inspection process

Inspectors can visit whenever they wish, although prior notice is normally given. If an inspector feels that the conditions of the authorisation or registration are not being met, he or she is empowered to issue an Enforcement Notice which details how the employer is not fulfilling the conditions of the site licence. The employer is given a date by which improvements must be made; if it is not met, prosecution is likely. Penalties can range from sizeable fines to imprisonment of relevant corporate person.

The High Activity Sealed Radioactive Source and Orphan Sources Regulations 2005 (HASS) (HMSO 2005)

These regulations place duties on the owners of radioactive sealed sources so that they are kept and used in a secure manner. These regulations require an increasing raft of security measures to be in place depending on the activity of the radioactive sealed source. Different activity values apply to different radionuclides due to their differing radiotoxicity. The measures in place include physical measures (e.g. door locks and door frames to a specified standard), security checks on staff who have access to the sources, information and site security plans about the sources, evidence of adequate financial arrangements in place for eventual disposal of the source at the end of its working life or if the organisation ceases to exist for any reason, and so on. Although these regulations do not apply to unsealed sources, the Environment Agency expects the advice of the police to be followed where the hazard is similar.

Carriage of Dangerous Goods and Use of Transportable Pressure Equipment Regulations 2009

These regulations are enforced through the Department for Transport and define the requirements for the transport of radioactive materials in the UK. They define many roles (carrier, driver, consigner, packer, etc.) and detail the responsibilities that these roles carry. They also define radionuclide specific activity levels for exemption and excepted packages (i.e. excepted gives partial exemption from some of the regulations) and further classify packages into Type A, Type B, etc. The need for the correct documentation to accompany such packages is also strictly defined. Quality assurance programmes that show that the whole transport process is being controlled have to be in place and emergency procedures have to be rehearsed so that, should an accident happen whereby the integrity of the containment or shielding is threatened or breached, the staff involved are well versed in the emergency procedure. Placarding of vehicles and signage on packages is also defined. In recent years the regulations have changed several times in the UK with promises that further changes will occur every few years. The Department for Transport is also inspecting hospitals performing such activities with increasing frequency.

The transport of radioactive materials may also require a Dangerous Goods Safety Adviser (see Chapter 30 on packaging and transport of radiopharmaceuticals).

Medicines (Administration of Radioactive Substances) Regulations 1978 (HMSO 1978)

Clinicians (doctors and dentists) require a licence from the Department of Health if they intend to administer a radioactive material to a patient for the purposes of diagnosis, therapy or research. The licences are specific for a purpose, for a site and for a doctor, and run for a finite period of time (5 years). Hence, if a doctor wishes to practise on a new site they must apply for a new licence. If they wish to perform a specific research project they must apply for a specific licence and this has to be renewed if the time expires or if the number of patients originally asked for has been reached.

The application for the licence has to have the signature of the applicant as well as the supporting scientist, the radiopharmacist and the RPA who are testifying that they feel able to support the applicant in their application.

These regulations are enforced though the Department of Health.

Specific hazards

Hazards from contamination and specific hazards from iodine ingestion

The very low annual limit of intake (ALI) for ^{131}I (see Table 3.1) reflects the danger of ingestion of this radionuclide. Part of the reason for this very low ALI is that the thyroid gland is avid for iodine – ingestion of a small amount results in a very high percentage being taken up by the gland. Iodine is also found in the salivary and pituitary glands, ovaries, muscle and bile (Underwood 1977). Approximately, the committed dose equivalent from thyroidal ingestion of either ^{125}I or ^{131}I is 1 mSv/kBq. Uptake of iodine in the thyroid gland before or after contamination can be blocked using stable iodine. There are a number of possible methods for achieving this, but one must beware of potential side-effects and it is recommended that a medical adviser be consulted. Administration of potassium iodate is often thought to be the simplest method and the suggested daily dose has been reported to range from '>5 mg per day' (Prime 1985) to 100 mg (Bolton 1985). The delay in administration after ingestion affects the effectiveness of this treatment. A 100 mg dose given within 3–4 hours after ingestion is reported to reduce uptake by more than 50% (NCRP 1977). This ionic blocking works by the mechanism of the 'Wolff–Chaikoff block'. This involves the blocking of the organic binding of iodine and its incorporation into hormones caused by large doses of iodine; it is usually a transient effect, but in large doses and in susceptible individuals it can be prolonged and cause iodine myxoedema. Note that workers should not routinely take excess stable iodine prior to performing iodination procedures.

It is strongly recommended that iodine be manipulated inside fume cupboards when there is even a slight possibility of volatility. Such a state can accidentally be created by deviations from recommended procedures, such as unintended pH changes. An exception to this could be the manipulation of the very small amounts of radioiodine in, for example, radioimmunoassay procedures. It is suggested that the wearing of two pairs of gloves, possibly of different materials, when working with radioiodine is good practice as there is evidence that some iodine-labelled materials do penetrate some gloves (Connor, McLintock 1997). It is also suggested that if liquid radioactive iodine waste is being stored, this should be done by preparing a solution of 25 g sodium thiosulfate and 2 g sodium iodide in 1 litre of 1 mol/l sodium hydroxide and then adding the waste to this solution as it arises. Spills of radioiodine can be made safer by adding a solution of 5% sodium thiosulfate before carrying out the decontamination.

The thyroid glands of workers handling megabecquerel quantities of radioiodine materials should regularly be checked; good practice would be at least weekly or preferably a few hours after a procedure. Although this can be done very accurately using a dedicated thyroid uptake probe system, a contamination monitor with a sodium iodine scintillation crystal a few millimetres thick with a ratemeter display will suffice. Data on the fraction of ^{125}I remaining for up to 60 days after ingestion with normal thyroid function are given in Appendix 3 of *Health Physics Aspects of the Use of Radioiodines*. (Prime 1985).

Hazards from contamination and specific hazards from phosphorus-32 ingestion

As Table 3.1 shows, ^{32}P has the third lowest annual limit of intake (ALI) in the listing. In the form of sodium phosphate it can irradiate important cells related to the blood – indeed it is used in this form to treat polycythaemia vera (a potential side-effect of this radionuclide therapy is the induction of leukaemia; therapeutic amounts are in the region of only 200 MBq, so the ingestion of any amount is of significant concern).

For dosimetry purposes phosphorus is assumed to be deposited in the endo-osteal cells of the skeleton and retained on the bone surfaces; hence there is also a risk of bone cancer after irradiation. Jackson,

Dolphin (1966) give details of a model used to describe the whole body retention of phosphorus. Airborne ingestion via droplets is a hazard in processes such as centrifuging, blending or transfer of liquids using syringes. It is wise to perform a simple wipe test when a shipping container is opened. This enables contamination to be detected at source from a previous, perhaps undetected, incident. Such an incident could leave a dried residue on the surface of the vial, creating an invisible, insidious hazard.

Staff should also be aware that Eppendorf tubes have an attenuation for the α-particles from ^{32}P of only 30–50 % that for average glass vials. Indeed, the surface dose rate from such tubes containing tens of megabecquerels of ^{32}P can be several millisieverts per minute. An operator handling a few tens of these tubes a day, each for less than a minute, could receive more than the dose limit to the skin of the fingers (500 mSv per year). Additional shielding should be used by placing the Eppendorf tubes behind a 10 mm thick Perspex shield or in Perspex sample blocks, which are obtainable commercially. A 1 MBq spot of ^{32}P contamination, spread over 1 cm^2, can give a skin dose 1.82 Sv per hour (Ballance *et al.* 1992). Curran (1986) also provides a similar consistent estimate for skin contamination with ^{32}P.

Radiation protection in radioiodine therapy

Up to 0.1% of ^{131}I activity administered to patients has been found to be released into the air from a therapy ward (Lassmann *et al.* 1994). This reinforces the need for all such areas to be well ventilated. It has also been calculated that patients returning home, after being hospitalised for two days following radioiodine therapy, may give up to 0.2 kBq to the thyroids of family members, resulting in an equivalent dose to the thyroid of up to 4.7 mSv for adults and 20 mSv for children (Wellner *et al.* 1998). However, other workers have performed practical measurements on families of radioiodine therapy patients in their own homes at various times post treatment that have indicated that ingested doses are nowhere near this high level and generally give rise to acceptable doses, even to children in the family (Barrington *et al.* 2008).

Security of radioactive sources

These regulations are to some extent described in the section concerning the HASS (High Activity Sealed Radioactive Source) regulations above. It is worth emphasising, however, that it is not only the HASS regulations that make it mandatory to use and keep radioactive material securely. The Ionising Radiation Regulations 1999 and the Radioactive Substances Act 1993 (and Exemption Orders under the Act) as well as the Carriage of Dangerous Goods and Use of Transportable Pressure Equipment Regulations 2009 all require radioactive sources (sealed or unsealed) to be kept, used and transported in a secure manner.

These regulations require:

- Locking sources away in a suitable store (it is seldom acceptable to justify to Regulators for a source not being in a locked store by saying that the door to the room is locked).
- Having records readily available so that any suspected loss is readily ascertained.
- Reporting any loss, theft or uncontrolled release (thresholds are defined at which notification is mandatory).
- Not storing sources with certain other materials that may increase the likelihood of dispersal (e.g. inflammables, explosives, etc.).
- Leak testing, etc., as described above.

Personnel monitoring

Staff working in radiopharmacies or PET radiochemistry laboratories may be designated as classified radiation workers, Whether they are so designated will probably depend on the volume of work they are individually required to do. Staff in an average-sized radiopharmacy will probably not be designated as classified workers as they will be unlikely to exceed 3/10 of any relevant dose limit, whereas those in a very large radiopharmacy may very well be classified workers. If staff are classified it is more likely to be due to the extremity dose (hand) than a whole body dose.

Both classified and non-classified staff working with radioactive patients or radiopharmaceuticals should wear a personal dosemeter to give an estimate

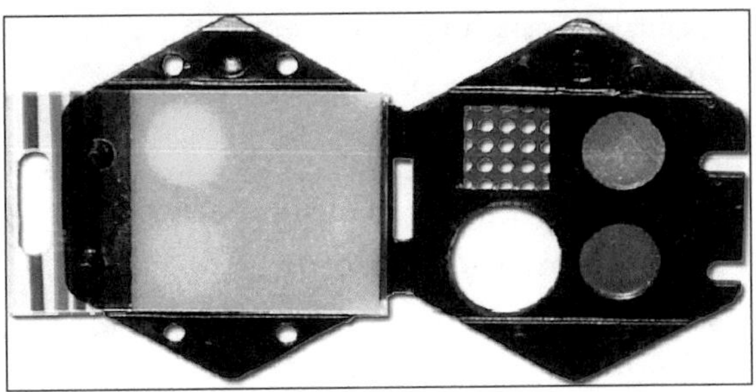

Figure 3.3 Opened-up personal dosemeter showing filters and detecting material (on left). (Photograph courtesy of Landauer, Inc.)

of effective dose and many will wear a dosemeter on an extremity to monitor their skin/extremity dose.

Personal dosemeters are usually in the form of a badge that is clipped or pinned to the clothing or in a form that can be worn on extremities, being mounted in a finger stool or ring. They generally work using either a crystalline material (which is able to absorb the radiation energy and either give it up later when heated or exposed to laser light) or a small film (using the latent exposure effect on a photographic emulsion). They contain filters so that the differential exposure of the sensitive material can be used to assess radiation type/energy and exposure situations. A typical whole body dosemeter is shown in Figure 3.3.

The importance of where to wear the extremity dosemeter

Whereas it may not be crucial exactly where on a hand these dosemeters are worn if the dose received is significantly less than 10% of a dose limit, it does become important as the dose approaches the dose limit (or 3/10 of the limit if staff are not classified). This is because the dose received in most situations is not uniform across the hand. Under legislation that is consistent with the recommendations of ICRP103, the dose to the skin can only be averaged over 1 cm^2, whereas before 1999 it could be averaged over 100 cm^2. There have been several articles dealing with the determination of regional factors that relate the hand dose to the exposure of the hand from different work activities (Williams *et al.* 1987; Batchelor *et al.* 1991a,b; Batchelor *et al.* 1994; Allen *et al.* 1997). If the work activity is similar to this published work, the dose to the finger tip may be estimated from the dose measured on a ring dosemeter. Sometimes a finger stool may be used and this may be on the finger receiving the highest dose, in which case no further consideration is necessary. If this is not the case, again a factor may be employed to ensure that dose limits are not being exceeded and that a person who is not classified is not receiving more than 3/10 of a dose limit.

Williams *et al.* (1987) showed that when the TLD was worn on the proximal phalanx of the middle finger or on one of the adjacent fingers, the dose so recorded was about 30% less than that received from the mean dose to the whole hand.

Batchelor *et al.* (1991a,b, 1994) carried out a more detailed study of the distribution of dose to the hands in dispensing, injecting and formulating in nuclear medicine and also for radiochemistry formulation, dispensing and injecting in clinical PET. The results showed that choice of location of the dosemeter can give a result between 33% and 200% of the mean hand dose

The work of Batchelor *et al.* (1991a) also showed that pre-placing a short (95 mm) butterfly cannula in a vein before handling the radioactive syringe can reduce doses to 47% and 72% of the doses received without using these devices for the left and right hands, respectively. Employing an unnecessarily long catheter will actually increase the dose received due to the activity in the tubing exposing the operator.

It is important that the hands are regularly checked for contamination. There are two reasons for this:

- Firstly, the dose to the skin and possible subsequent ingestion are a particular hazard that can be reduced if decontamination measures are taken as soon as contamination is detected.
- Secondly, a contaminated dosemeter will show a very high dose if the contamination is left on the surface of the dosemeter. This is generally not the skin dose received as the TLD shields the skin and also the dosemeter would be removed after work with radiation has ceased, although the irradiation of the dosemeter continues. This can lead to a dose limit *apparently* being exceeded and an incorrect report to a regulatory body.

Extremity dosemeters are also of value in assessing new techniques and in checking that 'ALARP' is being followed when a member of staff starts performing a new work activity. Wearing the dosemeter for a transient period only is useful. There are now also available electronic extremity dosemeters that can log dose/time events and hence show at what stage of a procedure these doses were received. Some workers (Guy *et al.* 2005) have incorporated a cine file from a simple small camera connected to a laptop alongside this electronic real-time dosemeter so that a visual record is available of what operations were being performed when a high dose was received.

Electronic personal dosemeters usually employ detecting elements that are either Geiger or solid-state and the whole instrument is pocket sized. Some have even been produced the size of a credit card and include bar codes to provide area access information.

It is important with all dosemeters that due consideration for energy response is made so that the instrument is suitable for its use or allowance is made for poor energy response for the radiation being measured.

Dosemeters must not be kept in an area of increased (above background) radiation level while not being used. This may sound obvious advice but it is not rare for dosemeters to be found inside investigation rooms, etc. Similarly, it is important that the hands of the person distributing or collecting these devices are not contaminated with radioactivity.

Communication of results to individuals wearing dosemeters

It is imperative that individuals are informed of their results as soon as possible after their dosemeters are returned for processing. In the case of an external service this may be one to two months after the end of the monitoring period. It is found that if people are aware of their doses and can compare them with those received by others then there is a general tendency for their dose to decrease over time. If the system is such that viewing their dose is not made easy then the reverse is true. Similarly a policy of telling workers their dose only when there is a problem also tends to encourage complacency in the workers' attitude to the ALARP principle. A radiation protection supervisor who undertakes his or her duties conscientiously is invaluable in ensuring that doses to staff are kept as low as possible.

Special considerations in positron emission tomography (PET) radiochemistry laboratories

PET procedures generally have the potential to result in a higher dose to the operator.

The reasons for this are simple:

- Each disintegration is accompanied by the emission of positrons which, if unshielded, result in a high skin dose.
- Each emission eventually results in *two* γ-ray photons (photons from the annihilation of the positrons).
- These photons, having energies of 511 keV, are harder to shield than those from ^{99m}Tc.

Unsurprisingly, this has implications for the design and operation of PET facilities.

The specific γ-ray constant for PET nuclides (i.e. ^{18}F, ^{15}O, ^{13}N, ^{11}C) is an order of magnitude higher than that for ^{99m}Tc and it should be remembered that this does not allow for the skin dose that would be received from the positrons (specific γ-ray constants relate only to gamma emission).

The tenth value thickness in lead is *15 times* greater for the PET 511 keV γ-ray photons compared to those from ^{99m}Tc. It is therefore not surprising that distance is used in design wherever possible, as the amount of lead needed to reduce dose rates considerably is much greater (and sometimes less practical) than when using most other conventional nuclear medicine radionuclides.

Concrete density equivalent bricks are available and a two-course wall (approximately 200 mm) gives an attenuation of just under a factor of 10; a single course gives only a factor of 2.

PET facilities frequently include a cyclotron on-site, unless there is one nearby with spare capacity to supply the PET tracers. A dedicated PET tracer-producing cyclotron operates generally in the region of 10–11 MeV and often has its own primary shield, which may be operated on hydraulic rams. These machines, though often located in a vault, are actually designed to be able to function alongside other rooms. Allowance must be made for service work as there is a considerable level of activity remaining in the target area after bombardment (not just the intended PET tracer; there may be high activities from induced radionuclides in the cyclotron for several hours after the end of bombardment). Indeed, this induced activity has to be declared on the operator's 'site licence' issued by the Environment Agency or the Scottish Environment Protection Agency in the UK.

The automated chemistry to facilitate the production of the more routine PET tracers (e.g. ^{18}F-labelled FDG [fluorodeoxyglucose]) may result in release of volatile by-products during synthesis and this also has to be allowed for in the arrangements agreed with the regulatory bodies. It is essential to fit a monitoring system on the extractor from the cyclotron room, the chemistry unit and any shielded fume cupboards ('hot cells') so that data can be continuously logged and emissions automatically recorded. Additionally an abatement system can be deployed whereby such emissions are reduced through storage and decay.

Hand doses of the PET radiochemist/radiopharmacist have the potential to be high and so it is advisable to monitor hand doses and to employ devices to reduce doses received as much as possible.

Possible dose-saving measures are:

- Use of large Perspex syringe shields that protect the skin from positrons and also employ distance to reduce dose. These can be more effective than a lead or tungsten shield.
- An arrangement for assaying each patient dose with the $H_2{}^{15}O$ tracer remaining in the lead transit pot to avoid direct unshielded manipulation (Marsden *et al.* 1994). Due to the short half-life of ^{15}O (2 minutes) it is necessary for high activities to be administered to patients and even higher activities to be dispensed in the radiochemistry laboratory. This can potentially lead to high operator doses if the syringe of $H_2{}^{15}O$ is removed from its shield and assayed in a radionuclide calibrator in the normal way. To avoid this, the tracer, inside its shielded pot, is placed at a defined point alongside the exterior shield of a radionuclide calibrator ionisation chamber and an appropriate modified activity calibration factor is employed.
- Possible modifications to delivery systems for the automated chemistry, so that tracers are delivered straight into the collection vial within a radionuclide calibrator (Batchelor *et al.* 1994).

All of these measures generally require some local skill and expertise together with on site workshop facilities.

Pregnancy and working with radiation

The dose to the fetus should be as low as reasonably practicable. The ICRP (ICRP 2007) recommends that a fetus should receive no more radiation than a member of the public and so should not receive more than 1 mSv during the declared term of pregnancy. This gives a risk of 3.0×10^{-5} or about 1 in 33 000 of developing a fatal malignancy up until the age of 15 years, which compares with the natural risk of 1 in 1300. A fetal dose of 1 mSv can be interpreted as broadly equivalent to a dose at the surface of the abdomen of a pregnant woman of about 2 mSv for X-rays, but a lower level, possibly 1.3 mSv for higher-energy radiation from radionuclides such as ^{99m}Tc and ^{131}I, and here advice from the RPA will be required.

Most of the routine activities performed by technologists in nuclear medicine would not result in an external radiation dose of this magnitude. However, where a radiopharmacist or technologist is dealing with potential or actual contamination (including volatility/aerosol droplets), and is in the presence of a high radiation field, this dose could be exceeded. Hence it is advised that it best for staff known to be pregnant who are working in nuclear medicine to avoid the following tasks (Harding, Mountford 1993):

- Dealing with radioactive spills
- Using aerosols or unshielded krypton generators
- Imaging very ill patients
- Preparing radionuclide therapy doses.

Because of the potential for an incident, it would seem prudent that a radiopharmacist, working single-handed, should not continue working with radioactivity while pregnant. The radiopharmacist may still be involved in supervising the work of a colleague, as being several metres away from the formulation process should reduce risks to an acceptable level. The anxiety factor that an expectant mother may have in this situation, even after being given reassurance, should be remembered. It is often possible for the person to change duties with a colleague and work in a non-radiation area, where the source of the anxiety can be removed entirely.

In assessing potential fetal doses it may be helpful to consult the 'Notes for Guidance on the Clinical Administration of Radiopharmaceuticals and the Use of Sealed Radioactive Sources' (HPA 2006) Other useful publications are ICRP (2001) and ICRP (2003). There are also many leaflets that give advice to the worker and manager (HSE 2001; HPA 1988)

Monitoring for contamination

In this section, practical advice is given on monitoring for radioactive contamination.

For both controlled and supervised areas, there should be routine systematic contamination monitoring of surfaces at regular intervals as well as at the end of individual work procedures involving radionuclides. In any situation where monitoring is carried out – i.e. routine or in contamination incidents, the following points are important:

- Select the appropriate monitor for the radionuclide used. (Note that tritium [^{3}H] is generally not detectable except by wipe test – see below). Switch the monitor on and check battery status.
- Measure the background count rate in an area not used for handling radionuclides. Record the result.
- Remove gloves used during the work procedure, wash hands and monitor them. Record the measured count rate.
- Monitor all work surfaces (including the interior of fume cupboards if appropriate), tools and laboratory equipment used in the work procedure, items removed from the work area during the procedure, and floors. Systematically move the monitor probe over each surface/article, without touching, and record the maximum count rates encountered.
- For both hands and work surfaces, etc., convert any reading significantly above background to an equivalent contamination level (in Bq/cm^2). If contamination persists, carry out decontamination procedures as described in the appropriate section below. Monitoring should be carried out before and after each stage of the decontamination procedure.
- Tritium should be monitored using wipe tests; surfaces should be swabbed using filter papers; these are then transferred to a vial containing organic scintillant and the activity is measured on a scintillation counter. It should be assumed that 10% of the contamination is transferred to the swab. Results of wipe tests should be recorded.

Decontamination procedures

Decontamination can be described as any process that will reduce the level of any radionuclides from a contaminated surface. It is important to realise that it will usually be impossible to remove all the contamination.

It is difficult to be prescriptive since the decontamination procedures employed will depend largely on the individual circumstances prevalent at the incident. This protocol, therefore, gives a general and adaptable set of procedures for dealing with surface and personal contamination. Further information can be obtained from Mountford (1991).

Personal contamination

In incidents involving suspected personal contamination, the RPA or other radiation safety staff should be informed first. It is advisable to undertake personal decontamination as a first priority before other decontamination procedures are carried out.

Contaminated persons must not leave the designated area or laboratory where the incident is assumed to have occurred to avoid the risk of spreading contamination to other areas.

Persons assisting in personal decontamination should wear protective clothing.

Eye contamination

Suspected contamination in the eyes should be treated immediately by irrigating outwards with copious amounts of sterile eye wash solution. Ensure that the fluid does not spread to other parts of the body – in particular the orifices. The Appointed Doctor should be consulted.

Ear contamination

Trained hospital staff should be asked to syringe out contaminated ears with water at body temperature (37°C).

Nasal contamination

The contaminated person should blow their nose into paper tissues and expectorate into a disposable cup. The products should be monitored.

If nasal contamination is still high, irrigation should be considered under medical supervision. The subject should be seated in front of a designated sink or hand basin with a waterproof cover over the trunk and lap. A receptacle should be placed in the sink to collect the irrigation fluid (saline or sterile water). The subject should tilt their head forward over the sink so that the nasal bone is approximately vertical – the irrigation fluid should flow back out of the nostrils rather than into the frontal sinuses or nasopharynx. An irrigation tube should be placed just inside the nostril and the flow of the irrigation fluid controlled by pinching the tube.

Contamination of nails

As much as possible of the contaminated nail should be cut away with scissors and retained for monitoring. The area immediately around and under the nail should be decontaminated following the procedure for skin below. Alternatively, calamine lotion can be applied, allowed to dry, then brushed off with the hand inside a plastic bag to collect the contaminated dust powder.

Skin/hair contamination

If the contamination is localised to an area of the body, then decontamination should be restricted to that localised area only. This should avoid the spread of contamination to other parts of the body, particularly the eyes and orifices. Showers should not be used – they are more likely to dilute but spread contamination to other areas of the body, risking ingestion via the orifices.

The first stage for more major contamination is the careful removal of outer clothing followed by normal washing of hands, face and, if necessary, hair using water and mild soap in the hand washing basin (*not* the waste disposal sink). It will not be feasible to collect the water as liquid radioactive waste.

Where local areas of personal contamination persist, detergent and soft nail brushes should be used. Care should be taken not to be too abrasive to the point of injury to the skin since this will increase the risk of allowing the contamination into the body. If necessary, affected areas of hair should be trimmed and the clippings retained for monitoring.

For serious contamination of the hands only, a saturated solution of potassium permanganate followed by decolorisation by 5% sodium bisulfite solution may be considered. No other chemical treatments should be used on the skin.

Clothes and shoes removed should be checked for contamination. Contaminated articles should be sealed in a plastic bag and retained for decontamination before being returned to the owner.

Contaminated wounds

Any foreign objects should be removed from the wound. The surrounding skin should be decontaminated following the procedure described above. Bleeding from the wound should be encouraged by applying pressure above the wound to occlude the venous system – this will aid dispersal of the contaminant. The wound should then be irrigated using saline or sterile water, taking care not to spread contamination, and dried by wiping away from the edges. Monitor before and after bleeding and irrigation. Small skin tags should be cut away. The wound should be surgically excised if gross beta-contamination is left.

Mouth/Internal contamination

If contamination of the mouth is suspected, any dentures should be removed for separate cleaning. The person should be warned not to swallow. The mouth should be rinsed immediately with water at the hand basin and the teeth should be brushed away from the gums. If ingestion is suspected, the RPA and the Appointed Doctor should be consulted immediately.

Surface contamination

The following principles should be followed:

- Stop any operations that might add to the contamination.
- Take obvious containment measures.
- Warn others not to enter the area in which material has been spilled.
- Mark the area using chalk or marker pen.
- Inform the Radiation Protection Supervisor.
- Using the laboratory spills kit, carry out decontamination of personnel following the procedures set out above.
- Put on (fresh) protective gloves, protective clothes and overshoes.

Table 3.5 shows the contents of a typical spill kit. Table 3.6 shows useful methods for decontaminating equipment.

Table 3.5 Decontamination spill kit

Object	Comments
Protective clothing	
Overalls/lab coat	Overalls are more appropriate if the spill presents a very serious hazard to clean up staff
Gloves	Different pairs may be indicated for different situations
Face masks	
Wellington-type boots	
Disposable overshoes	These may be heavy duty or lightweight These should not be absorbent the whole way through from outside to inside onto shoe/sock
Decontamination agents	
Soap	As a liquid to quickly make into solution and as a bar
Cetrimide solution	Concentration should be written on container
'Swarfega'	
Potassium permanganate	
Sodium bisulfite	
Saline	Several sealed containers each of 500 mL
Sterile water	As above
Calamine lotion	
Potassium iodate/iodide	Tablets or solution (monitor expiry date)
Other proprietary agents (Decon, Lipsol, Camtox, Countoff, RBSA 350)	
Miscellaneous equipment	
Large warning sign capable of standing up on ground	Trefoil plus worded warning – 'Do not Enter, Radioactive Contamination'
Contamination monitor	Keep one monitor with kit for speed of access in emergency (remember to keep within calibration)
Radiation hazard adhesive tape	
Coloured rope to control access	To be used with adhesive tape to keep in place
Impermeable material to cover floor.	
Absorbent tissue, large/small rolls	
Polythene waste bags with radiation warning symbol	Minimum size 2 L
Plastic bucket	
Tweezers and tongs (various sizes)	1 pair, medium size (e.g. blades about 125 mm long)
Notebook, pen	
Scissors	
Soft brush	
Marker pen	

Table 3.6 Decontamination procedures for polythene, plastics, glassware, trays, sinks and metal tools

Object	Procedure
Paintwork, polished linoleum, epoxy resin floor coverings	Clean with detergent and water, in severe cases with a long half-life contaminant, remove paint with paint stripper or consider physical removal of surface. If the half-life is short, covering with impermeably coated paper or strong polythene sheeting may be appropriate. For all removals of radioactive waste, consider disposal before creation of the waste
Glassware	Clean immediately with detergent. Ammonium citrate or chelating agents such as EDTA may be useful
Plastics	Dilute nitric acid may be useful since it usually does not attack plastics. Care is needed if using ketonic solvents and certain chlorinated hydrocarbons that dissolve plastics. Note that no organic solvents have any effect on polythene
Metal tools, trays, workbenches and sinks	Use a heavy-duty detergent followed if necessary by specific chelating agents. If lipids are involved, 1,1,1-trichloroethane or EDTA mixed with Swarfega may be used. An abrasive cleaner can be used as a last resort

General order of decontamination

1. Decontamination will start with contaminated floors, bench surfaces and articles nearest to the entry route into the area.
2. Particular attention should be paid to areas known to be highly contaminated. Areas should be decontaminated as the operator reaches them following the specific procedures set out below.
3. At each stage in the treatments, monitoring should be carried out to assess the success of the operation.
4. Portable articles may, if necessary, be wrapped up and removed from the area for more efficient procedures to be used later.
5. Suitable thickness lead pots (see Table 3.1) may be used to secure any solid radioactive materials found in the contaminated area.
6. Having decontaminated the floor and bench surfaces the operator may then start on the walls.
7. In cases where there are several operators or the area to be decontaminated is large, this may be started before the other surfaces have been finished.
8. If it becomes necessary during these procedures to remove or replace any protective clothing worn by the operator, this should be done in such a way as to prevent personal contamination. The items replaced should be deposited in a receptacle.
9. When all decontamination procedures have been completed, all materials used including floor coverings should be carefully collected into separate receptacles as solid and liquid radioactive waste.
10. The entire area including all personnel involved should be re-monitored at the end with any residual readings recorded.

Specific decontamination procedure

Absorb spilt liquid using absorbent, disposable paper tissues or cloths. Place used ones in the waste disposal sink if convenient, otherwise in a strong plastic bag. Continue until the area is dry. Dry spills should be removed by wet methods, using wet absorbent paper to prevent dispersion.

The first treatment is with the mildest cleaning agent, e.g. water or solvents to remove grease. Copious amounts of cleaning agent and absorbent materials should be used without risking the spread of the contamination. If the first treatment is not sufficient then the use of detergent for a second treatment in the same manner is advised.

Monitor the contaminated area, taking care that the monitor itself does not become contaminated. If the reading exceeds, further decontamination is needed.

Ascertain the correct decontaminating agent for the surface/radionuclide. Using the appropriate solution, wash the area thoroughly using disposable tissues, working inwards towards the centre, and avoiding use of large volumes of liquid. Take care to avoid the spread of contamination. Dry the area, and re-monitor. If contamination persists, a Radiation Safety Physicist should be informed.

For more serious spills it may be appropriate for the contingency plan to direct staff to summon the Radiation Protection Adviser at the outset (or that person's team), who may be more appropriate to deal with a more hazardous situation.

Radioactive waste arising from decontamination procedures

All disposals arising from decontamination procedures should be fully recorded (i.e. date, radionuclide, and an estimate of the activity disposed).

Spillage in transit

Movement of radionuclides within an establishment must be by trained members of staff and in carrying boxes specifically designed for the purpose. However, if a spill does occur in transit it is important to stop people entering the contaminated area. Staff should stay with the spill and they should ask someone to contact their RPS or department manager (or RPA). The hospital switchboard may also have emergency contact details of the radiation safety team.

Management of radioactive waste

Any producer of radioactive waste in the UK has, by law, to ensure that they are minimising the volume and activity of waste that they create. Also, to ensure that radioactive waste is minimised at the point of transfer to a waste company, it is generally necessary for it to be separated at creation into bins according to half-life. If the half-life is too long for decay storage to make a significant difference (tritium, carbon-14) disposal should take place as soon as possible. In nuclear medicine it is useful to allow radioactivity to decay to lower levels. Technetium-99m, for example, can be left to decay until it is below the definition of being radioactive under the Radioactive Substances Act 1993 (i.e. 0.4 Bq/g). Use of non-radioactive methods should be promoted where possible, and care should be taken that waste that may be clearly identified as non-active (e.g. packaging after checking for contamination) is not be put in the active waste bin.

The waste should also be 'streamed' according to its activity level. Very low-level waste (VLLW) is waste that may go out with normal refuse to landfill provided special conditions are met. Above this level, waste may be low-level waste and this may be incinerated by a licensed company that is named on the user's authorisation. Other solid sources (particularly sealed sources) may go to an external organisation for special disposal. This may require a special authorisation from the Regulator if it is not built into the user's authorisation and falls outside of the relevant exemption orders.

It is important to be able to demonstrate that at any time one can show the amount of waste in storage. The easiest way of doing this is in some form of spreadsheet so that automatic correction for decay occurs each time the file is accessed. Hard-copy records of disposals should also be available together with copies of waste consignment notes.

Features of a radioactive waste store

The store should have adequate space, be secure, be easily decontaminated and be adequately ventilated and shielded, unless it is isolated and a radiation risk assessment has demonstrated this is not necessary. When bags are despatched to the waste contractor, the correct streaming should prevent all but the minimum amount of re-handling.

Radioactive waste from nuclear medicine departments may often also be clinical waste. The biological hazards need to be taken into account as well as the radiological ones. Further reference is made to the HHSC publication *The Management of Radioactive Waste in Laboratories, Handbook No 19* (McLintoch 1996), which gives clinical waste a further five categories of subdivision. These subdivisions then determine, from a clinical waste perspective alone, how the material may be disposed of (no choice but incineration or possible landfill routes, and so on).

Transport of radioactive waste

Radioactive waste will need to be transported within the organisation or from the central store to the contractor's disposal point.

It is important that the waste is moved between rooms and to the central store in a manner that does not cause spillage or contamination of adjacent areas. Hence when the waste is ready to be moved on to the next stage of the disposal cycle a further precaution of 'double containment' should be taken. This means that it should be double-bagged (clear heavy-gauge polythene with trefoil is good as a copy of the transport documents can be added between the clear bags to facilitate auditing at a later stage). While it is in the store waiting to be picked up by a contracted waste company, a rigid outer container should be used so that any spillage is contained should a bag become torn. If this container is lined with absorbent material, it will help prevent contamination spreading from the container.

The containers should have appropriate labels describing their contents, and their security is also important. They should not be left unattended in a courtyard for any length of time. The entire procedure needs to be governed by local rules, as it is in itself a work activity involving radiation.

The transport of waste off site by a contractor does not remove the responsibility from the waste producer to ensure that certain legal criteria are being met ('duty of care'). Generally, radioactive waste from laboratories and hospitals will come within the category of excepted packages under the transport regulations. This means that they still come under the regulations but are exempt from certain requirements of the regulations provided certain conditions are met. An obvious exception to this could be the disposal of certain closed sources.

It must also be remembered that certain waste (e.g. used liquid scintillation solvent) must conform to the special waste regulations.

'Excepted package' conditions

Even for radioactive waste that comes under excepted packages, it is required that:

- Consignment notes must be correctly filled out that identify each container of the shipment. It is likely that each bin containing several bags will be an excepted package and so it will be a minimum requirement that the total activity of each of the nuclides present is documented.
- The dose rates at the surface of the container must be less than 5 μSv/h.
- There must not be a level of non-fixed contamination on the external surface that exceeds 0.4 Bq/cm^2.
- The warning label declaring that the package contains radioactive material must only be on the inside part of the package.
- The package should remain intact during the conditions it is likely to meet during routine transportation. This means that if another package rolls over on it or if it moves suddenly during heavy braking of the vehicle, it should retain the contents without contamination.

Further information on transport of radioactive materials should be obtained from the employer's Radiation Protection Adviser.

References

Allen S *et al.* (1997). Comparison of radiation safety aspects between robotic and manual systems for the preparation of radiopharmaceuticals [Abstract]. *Nucl Med Commun* 18: 295.

Ballance PE *et al.* (1992). *Phosphorous 32: Practical Radiation Protection*. HHSC Handbook No. 9. Leeds: H and H Scientific Consultants Ltd.

Barrington SF *et al.* (2008). Measurement of the internal dose to families of outpatients treated with 131I for hyperthyroidism. *Eur J Nucl Med Mol Imaging* 35: 2097–2104.

Batchelor S *et al.* (1991a). Radiation dose to the hands in nuclear medicine. *Nucl Med Commun* 12: 439–444.

Batchelor S *et al.* (1991b). Radiation dose distribution to the hands of a radiopharmacist. *Pharm J Hosp Pharm Suppl* 247: 38–39.

Batchelor S *et al.* (1994). Staff and patient dosimetry issues in clinical positron emission tomography. Abstracts of the World Congress on Medical Physics and Biomedical Engineering, Physics in Medicine and Biology, 39a (part2) (abstract OS32-3.4), 820.

Bolton, AE (1985). *Radioiodination Techniques: Review 18*. Amersham: Amersham International plc.

Connor, KJ, McLintock, IS (1997). *Practical Radiation Protection. Radiation Protection: Handbook for Laboratory Workers No 14*, 2nd edn. Leeds: H and H Scientific Consultants Ltd, 17–22.

Curran AR (1986). Calculation of the dose to the basal layer of the skin from beta/gamma contamination. *J Soc Radiol Protect* 1: 23–32.

Guy MJ *et al.* (2005). Development of a combined audio-visual and extremity dose monitoring software tool for use in nuclear medicine. *Nucl Med Commun* 26(12): 1147–1153.

Harding LK, Mountford PJ (1993). Editorial: Pregnant employees in a nuclear medicine department. *Nucl Med Commun* 14: 345–346.

Health & Safety Commission (2000). *Approved Code of Practice and Guidance to IRR99, 'Work with Ionising Radiation' L121*. London: Health & Safety Commission. ISBN 0-7176-1746-7.

HMSO (1978). The Medicine (Administration of Radioactive Substances) Regulations 1978. ISBN 0-11-084006-2.

HMSO (1993). Radioactive Substances Act 1993 Chapter 12.

HMSO (2000a). The Ionising Radiation (Medical Exposure) Regulations 2000.

HMSO (2000b). The Ionising Radiation Regulations 1999 Statutory Instrument 1999 number 3232. ISBN 0-11-085614-7.

HMSO (2005). The High Activity Sealed Radioactive Source and Orphan Sources Regulations 2005.

HMSO (2006). The Ionising Radiation (Medical Exposure) (Amendment) Regulations 2006.

HMSO (2007). The Carriage of Dangerous Goods and Use of Transportable Pressure Equipment Regulations 2007.

HMSO (2010). The Environmental Permitting Regulations 2010 (SI 2010 No 675).

HPA (1988). *Diagnostic Medical Exposures: Advice on Exposure to Ionising Radiation during Pregnancy*. London: Health Protection Agency. ISBN 0-85951-420-X.

HPA (2006). *Notes for Guidance on the Clinical Administration of Radiopharmaceuticals and the Use of Sealed Radioactive Sources*. London: Health Protection Agency.

HSE (1999). *Work with Ionising Radiation. Ionising Radiation Regulations 1999. Approved Code of Practice and Guidance*. London: HSE Books. ISBN 0 7176 1746 7.

HSE (2001) Working Safely with Ionising Radiation: Guidelines for Expectant or Breastfeeding Mothers. http://www.hse.gov.uk/pubns/indg334.pdf (accessed 28 June 2010).

ICRP (1989). *Radiological Protection of the Worker in Medicine and Dentistry*. ICRP publication 57. Oxford: Pergamon Press. [*Annals of the ICRP* 20(3): 1–83].

ICRP (2001). *Doses to the Embryo and Fetus from Intakes of Radionuclides by the Mother*. ICRP Publication 88. Oxford: Pergamon Press. [*Annals of the ICRP* 31(1–3): 19–515].

ICRP (2003). *Biological Effects after Prenatal Irradiation (Embryo and Fetus)*. ICRP Publication 90. Oxford: Pergamon Press. [*Annals of the ICRP* 33(1–2): 5–206].

ICRP (2007). *The 2007 Recommendations of the International Commission on Radiological Protection*. ICRP Publication 103. Oxford: Pergamon Press. [*Annals of the ICRP* 37(2–4): 1–332].

IPEM (2002). *Medical and Dental Guidance Notes: A good practice guide on all aspects of ionising radiation protection in the clinical environment*. York: Institute of Physics and Engineering in Medicine. ISBN 903613 09 4.

Jackson S, Dolphin GW (1966). The estimation of internal radiation dose from metabolic and urinary excretion data for a number of important radionuclides. *Health Phys* 12: 481–500.

Lassmann M. *et al.* (1994). Measurement of 131I-activity to air emitted from a radioiodine therapy ward. In: Koelzer, W, Maushart, R, eds. *Strahlenshultz: Physik und Messtechnik*. Koln: TUV Rheinland, 719–722.

Marsden PK *et al.* (1994). A system for measuring and injecting PET radiopharmaceuticals [abstract]. *Nucl Med Commun* 15: 259.

McLintoch IS. (1996). *The Management of Radioactive Waste in Laboratories, Handbook No. 19*. Leeds: H and H Scientific Consultants Ltd.

Mountford PJ (1991). Techniques for radioactive decontamination in nuclear medicine. *Semin Nucl Med* 21(11): 82–89.

NCRP (1977). *Protection of the Thyroid Gland in the Event of Release of Radioiodine*. Report No. 55. Washington, DC: National Council on Radiation Protection and Measurement. ISBN 0-913392-37-5.

Prime D. (1985). *Health Physics Aspects of the Use of Radioiodines*. Science Reviews Occupational Hygiene Monograph No. 13. Leeds: H and H Scientific Consultants.

Underwood E. J. (1977). *Trace Elements in Human and Animal Metabolism*, 4th edn. New York: Academic Press.

Wellner U *et al.* (1998). The exposure of relatives to patients of a nuclear medical ward after radioiodine therapy by inhalation of ^{131}I in their home. *Nuklearmedizin* 37: 113–119.

Williams ED *et al.* (1987). Monitoring radiation dose to the hands in nuclear medicine: the location of dosemeters. *Nucl Med Commun* 8: 499–503.

4

Detection of radiation

Alan C Perkins and John E Lees

Introduction

Radioactive substances produce ionising radiation as a result of nuclear transformation. In nuclear medicine the radiation emitted from the radionuclide, for example a γ-ray, is used as the 'reporter signal' for imaging, or a β-particle can be used to deliver a therapeutic dose to tumour cells. Radioactivity is defined in the British Pharmacopeia (BP) as 'the number of nuclear transformations per unit time in a given amount of the [radioactive] preparation'. The SI unit of radioactivity is the becquerel (Bq). This is equivalent to an average transformation rate of one atom per second. When undertaking any practices involving the human administration of radiopharmaceuticals it is essential to use sensitive instrumentation for the detection and measurement of radioactive emissions. This allows a practical measure for dispensing the low amounts required for diagnostic uses and an accurate measure of therapeutic levels of radioactivity. This is also especially important for experimental work contributing to scientific knowledge relating radiation doses to biological effects.

For applications with low levels of radioactivity, measurement of the amount is nearly always as a count rate in counts per second (cps) or counts per minute (cpm). The becquerel is a relatively small unit for radiopharmaceutical work, so that the multiples kBq (10^3 Bq), MBq (10^6 Bq) and GBq (10^9 Bq) are used in practice. It is worth noting that the former unit of the curie (Ci; equivalent to 37 GBq) and its submultiples mCi (37 MBq) and μCi (37 kBq) are still used in the USA and in many other countries. It is also important to note that some instruments are calibrated to produce a reading in units of exposure or dose in sieverts, for example dosemeters that normally read in μSv or mSv.

The absolute measurement of radioactivity is difficult and time consuming and requires equipment that is only available in specialist laboratories such as the National Physical Laboratory (NPL) in the UK. The BP sets limits of ±10% (or 15% in some cases) for the radioactivity of most licensed radiopharmaceuticals. In practice in the radiopharmacy it is generally necessary to measure the radioactivity of dispensed radiopharmaceuticals to a precision within about 2–5%.

Detector principles and properties

Ionising radiations have the property of producing ions when they interact with matter. These radiations can be subdivided into directly ionising and indirectly ionising radiation. Directly ionising radiation includes alpha- and beta-radiation. These consist of highly energetic ionised particles that interact directly with atoms to produce charged ion pairs. Indirectly ionising radiation includes X- and gamma-radiation. These consist of photons that interact primarily with orbiting electrons that can be ejected and then interact with other atoms to produce charged ions.

Radiation detectors generally function in two ways:

1 The radiation causes ionisation within a medium it is passing through and the ions produced are detected and measured.
2 The radiation causes electronic excitation in atoms or molecules, which then dissipate this excess energy by some mechanism that can be detected and measured.

Three main types of counting systems are used for the quantitative determination of radioactivity: gas ionisation chambers (e.g. Geiger–Mueller or GM detector), scintillation detectors (e.g. sodium iodide crystals or liquid scintillants) and semiconductors (e.g. lithium-drifted germanium). Each detector is suitable for a certain situation. The most common types of measuring instruments include GM counters, ionisation chambers, scintillation detectors and thermoluminescent detectors. No one instrument is suitable for measuring every type and energy of radiation. Ionisation detectors include GM detectors and gas-filled ionisation chambers and are based on the collection of the charged ions produced by the radiation passing through a gas-filled chamber. Scintillation detectors use visible photon energy that is emitted from a scintillant when an excited electron returns to its normal state. Photographic detectors use the excited electron energy to produce a latent image in the emulsion grains. Most personal radiation monitors depend on electron excitation, e.g. film badges and thermoluminescent dosemeters (TLDs) described subsequently.

The instruments that are available to measure ionising radiation vary in their sensitivity to radiation, the type and energy of radiation to which they respond, and the time required to obtain the reading. The performance of an instrument generally varies with the nature and volume of the detector. Most instruments require calibration with a 'standard' source of known activity to ensure that it is performing within accepted limits and that it is working in a reproducible manner. The factors governing the choice of a detector are described below.

Sensitivity

Instruments of various sensitivities are required for different purposes. It is necessary to measure high amounts of radioactivity for the assay of therapeutic amounts of radioactivity, e.g. iodine-131, while very low amounts have to be measured in surveys of surface contamination and levels of natural background radiation.

Response to different radiation types

The types of radiation to be measured in a clinical environment include X-rays, γ-rays, α- and β-particles and possibly neutrons. No instrument is capable of measuring all of these radiations. In the radiopharmacy the most commonly used radiopharmaceuticals emit γ-rays and β-particles. Some instruments are designed so that they can measure X-rays and γ-rays plus β-particles; then, by placement of a simple filter in front of the detector, only the X-rays and γ-rays are detected, the contribution from the β-particles being given by subtraction of the second reading from the first.

Energy of the radiation

The energy of the radiation being measured affects the response of an instrument. Instruments generally do not respond equally to equal doses at all energies of radiation, even if the radiation is all of one type. Some instruments have peaks in their response curves; that is, at some energies they are particularly sensitive to the radiation and therefore give a high reading that can make accurate measurement and interpretation of the results difficult.

Detector volume

The volume of the detector affects the sensitivity of the instrument. The larger the volume of the detector, the more sensitive the instrument, providing the cross-section of the radiation beam is big enough to irradiate the whole of the detector.

Source geometry

In addition to the volume of the detector itself, the efficiency of most radiation instruments varies with the detector–source geometry. Radiation intensity decreases with distance from the source according to the inverse square law and, whenever comparisons are to be made between activities of a number of sources, care must be taken to ensure that the source–detector distance and geometrical configuration remain the same. This is particularly important in the radiopharmacy when measuring different samples of radioactivity. The accuracy of the measurement may depend upon the tube or vial size, and for accurate measurements of different samples it is often necessary to adjust sample sizes to the same volume before measurement or assay.

Time to obtain the reading

The time taken to obtain the reading has to be considered when selecting an instrument. If the level of radiation is constant, or changes only slowly, an instrument with a fairly long time constant will be acceptable. However, such an instrument would give a dangerously false reading if used to measure a pulse of radiation, such as that from an X-ray computed tomography scanner ('CT' scanner), where the X-ray beam is on for periods of much less than a second. Such an instrument would not have time to respond fully, or at all, and would not, therefore, record the full dose of radiation received.

Another application in which the time for the readout can be very important is in personal dosimetry. It is common for a personal dosemeter to be worn for a week or a month before being processed and read, so there is a considerable delay before the result is known. This may be unacceptable if the radiation levels to which the worker is exposed vary greatly, or if there is the possibility of accidental irradiation that must be detected and corrected. In such cases it is usual for an additional instrument to be used, such as an electronic personal dosemeter. This will give an immediate readout of any radiation dose that has been encountered and may be set with an audible warning that will sound if levels exceed a pre-set level.

Calibration

A counting instrument must be used under the same conditions as those for which it was designed and calibrated. For example, large-volume detectors are usually calibrated with the radiation source normal to (i.e. at right angles to) the window of the detector, and with the whole volume of the detector exposed. If either of these two conditions is not met, the calibration of the instrument will not apply, and the reading obtained will be inaccurate. Each instrument used for making measurements needs to be calibrated prior to use, and then at regular intervals as part of an ongoing programme of quality control.

Dead time

Every instrument requires time for processing of the individual detected events. This occurs within both the detector volume and the electronic circuits. A characteristic of counting systems is that some radiation passing through the detector may be missed because the system is processing a previously detected event. This is known as the detector dead time or pulse resolving time. The dead time for a GM tube is of the order of 50–200 μs and for sodium iodide and semiconductor detectors is in the range 0.5–5 μs. Dead-time effects can result in a loss of counting efficiency at increasing levels of activity. For any given instrument it is very important to know the level of activity when significant dead time effects occur. The count rate response should be linear over the working range of the counting system.

The following sections describe the common types of detectors used in nuclear medicine and radiopharmacy.

Gas-filled ionisation detectors

The operating principle of all ionisation detectors is fairly simple. The detector consists of a gas-filled chamber containing two electrodes (one is usually the chamber wall) that are maintained at a suitable potential difference by a high-voltage supply (extra high tension or EHT) (see Figure 4.1). When ionising radiation (e.g. a γ-ray) enters the chamber it may interact with electrons in the gas molecules. The interaction energy is sufficient to strip an electron from the molecule, leaving a positive ion. The negatively charged electrons, being light and highly mobile, drift rapidly towards the positively charged anode, which then acquires a small negative charge. The magnitude of the charge depends on the number of electrons

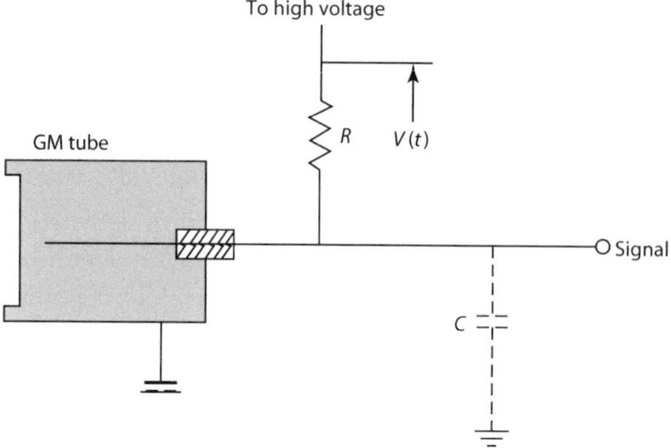

Figure 4.1 Schematic diagram of a gas-filled Geiger–Mueller ionisation chamber.

collected and is proportional to the number of ionising photons or particles that enter the chamber. The charges are small and require electronic amplification for their detection and display of their value. When small numbers of ionising particles are to be measured, ionisation detectors are designed to generate an electrical pulse for each ionising event. Electronic equipment is used to detect, amplify and count these pulses so that the count rate (e.g. counts per minute, cpm) is directly proportional to the amount of radiation entering the detector and to the radioactivity of the source emitting the radiation. The Geiger–Mueller (GM) detector is an example of this family of pulse detectors. The GM detector is often referred to as a 'GM counter', but it is simply a detector – the counting is always done by the associated electronics. The electronic counting circuit is called a scaler.

These devices form the basis of a number of commercial ionisation chambers used for the routine measurement of radioactivity and determination of radiation exposure doses. The effect of electrode potential is illustrated in Figure 4.2. As the voltage (EHT) is increased, all the primary ions formed by the initial ionising event are collected and a further increase in EHT does not affect the count rate (region I, saturation) or charge collected. If the EHT is

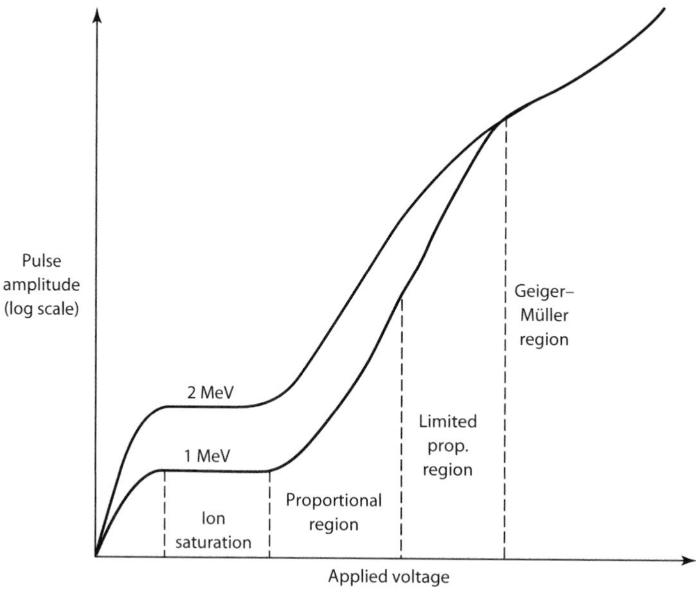

Figure 4.2 Voltage–response curve for ionisation chambers. This shows the effect of the voltage differences between electrodes on the electric current recorded by an ionising chamber per ionisation event detected.

increased beyond this plateau the primary ions are accelerated and generate secondary ions by collision with gas molecules. These secondary ions are collected and so the count rate or charge increases (region II, proportional region). Further increase in EHT generates more secondary ions until saturation is achieved (region III, Geiger–Mueller region). At these voltages a single ionising particle generates an avalanche of secondary ions, and the GM tube produces a single large pulse that is independent of the initial particle energy. Increasing the EHT beyond the Geiger plateau causes spontaneous electron emission and may cause damage to the detector.

Choice of instrument

The choice of an instrument for a particular application is dependent upon a number of factors. Some instruments vary in sensitivity with the direction of the incoming radiation and are calibrated for radiation from one direction only. Some are inaccurate if subjected to interference from electric or magnetic fields. Some give a rapid but not very accurate reading, while others have good accuracy but take longer to produce a reading. The larger instruments must be rested on a firm surface, or may only be read in certain orientations. Most instruments vary in sensitivity with radiation energy, and this is generally the most difficult problem to deal with.

X-rays and γ-rays below about 100 keV

In this region, energy dependence is often the dominating difficulty. GM tubes are always energy dependent, but this dependency may be reduced over part of the range by the use of appropriate filters. Ionisation chambers are preferred for their accuracy, but they must have thin walls if the energy of the radiation to be measured is less than about 20 keV.

X-rays and γ-rays above 100 keV

Measurements in the range from about 0.1 to 3 MeV pose the least problems of energy dependence. Within this range, it is possible to use most GM tubes, as well as ionisation chambers.

Detection efficiency

For beta-emitting nuclides, the gas ionisation detectors can provide quite acceptable counting efficiencies for all but the weakest emitters, with typical counting efficiencies for ^{32}P being 30% with a GM counter.

Low-energy gamma-emitting nuclides can be detected using gas ionisation detectors, particularly detectors filled with high-atomic-number counting gases, such as krypton and xenon. Indeed, for X-ray emitters (i.e. those nuclides decaying by electron capture), a gas ionisation detector may be more efficient than a crystal scintillation detector. For high-energy gamma photons (above 500 keV), gas-filled detectors are virtually useless, having detection efficiencies less than 0.1%. Crystal scintillation detectors are excellent in the energy range from 50 keV to 2 MeV, but at higher energies these also have lower detection efficiencies. To some extent, this decline in counting efficiency can be offset by increasing the size of the crystal, although this soon becomes a very expensive way of achieving relatively small increases in efficiency. Most semiconductor detectors have rather low counting efficiencies at best, and above 100 keV cannot be regarded as serious competitors for the crystal scintillation detectors.

Radionuclide activity calibrators

The radionuclide activity calibrator is an example of an ionisation chamber filled with gas, normally argon. This is a microprocessor-controlled device comprising the chamber with a central access space, into which the vial of active material can be inserted and an electrometer that can be set to give a direct readout of radioactivity in MBq or mCi units (Figure 4.3). This device is usually interfaced to an electronic printer that can print the label for the activity together with other essential information on the radiopharmaceutical preparation. The user can enter details of the radionuclide to be measured as a calibration factor and the individual preparation label can be printed with the nature of the radiopharmaceutical, the recorded activity, the time of measurement, the volume of solution and an expiry time. Some devices are auto-ranging, that is they select the optimum measuring range and measurement integration time for the amount of radioactivity being measured.

It is worth noting that this instrument is commonly referred to as the 'radionuclide dose calibrator' since in pharmacies it is common practice to dispense

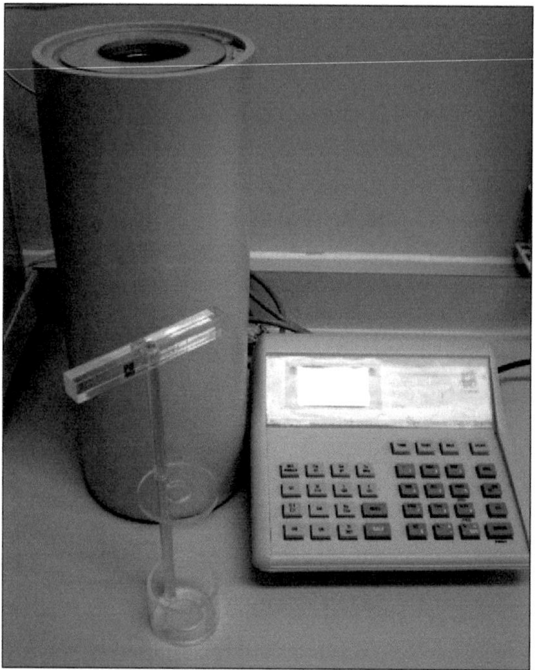

Figure 4.3 Photograph of a radionuclide activity calibrator.

individual doses of a drug. However, strictly speaking this term is incorrect because the instrument measures activity and not radiation dose! It is essential practice to check the nature and amount of radioactivity of all preparations leaving the radiopharmacy and for the radioactivity to be re-checked on receipt or prior to injection into the patient. Separate measuring instruments are used at clinic locations for this purpose. It is good practice to check that all instruments remain in calibration by measuring a standard sample, such as caesium-137, with a relatively long physical half-life. A decay correction can then be applied if necessary. It is also worth noting that operation of the radionuclide calibrator may change from day to day as a result of changes in atmospheric pressure. It may be necessary to perform a manual readjustment of the instrument to bring the calibrator back within the specified tolerance limits set by measuring with a standard source.

Scintillation detectors

Scintillation detectors are highly sensitive devices that are particularly suitable for the measurement of small amounts of radioactivity used in nuclear medicine procedures. They are found in a various devices in radiopharmacy and nuclear medicine ranging from contamination monitors to gamma cameras and have the following characteristics:

- Very short resolving time (less than 1 microsecond)
- High detection efficiency (up to 95% with some radiations)
- A response directly proportional to particle or photon energy.

Scintillation detectors can be constructed for the measurement and detection of alpha-, beta- and gamma-radiation, although the materials used are quite different for each type of radiation. The underlying physical mechanism is similar. For this reason the general principles of scintillation counting are discussed before describing the commonly used scintillation systems.

Scintillants and scintillation crystals

A scintillant or scintillator is a substance that emits a weak flash of light (scintillation) of very short duration whenever it is struck by an ionising radiation (e.g. an α-particle) or photon (e.g. a γ-ray). The intensity of the scintillation is proportional to the amount of energy dissipated to the molecules of the scintillator by the photons. The scintillations are detected by a light cell or photomultiplier that converts the light energy into electrical pulses that are then amplified and counted.

Different scintillators are used for the detection of various types of radiation. Alpha particles can be detected by zinc sulfide arranged as a thin layer on the photomultiplier window. Beta particles, especially low-energy particles from soft beta emitters such as ^{3}H and ^{14}C, are detected efficiently by dissolving the radioactive sample in a suitable liquid scintillant and placing the mixture in a glass tube near the photomultiplier. Gamma and X-ray photons are best detected with crystals of thallium-activated sodium iodide (NaI(Tl)), which is dense enough to absorb energetic photons.

The basic scintillation mechanism is the same in all these scintillation materials. The incoming particle or photon loses energy in the scintillator and this is then transferred to the scintillant ions or molecules, causing excitation of electrons to a higher energy; on return to the ground state, the excess energy is emitted as visible photons.

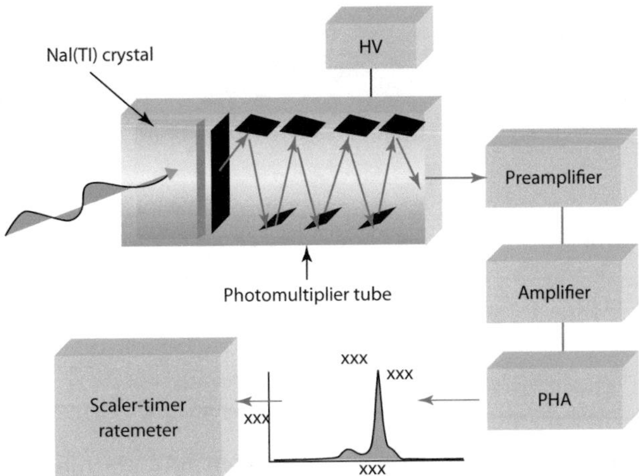

Figure 4.4 Schematic diagram of a single-crystal photomultiplier scintillation detector and associated electronics. HV = high voltage; PHA = pulse-height analyser.

Instrumentation

The basic components of a scintillation counting system are the scintillator, photomultiplier, high-voltage supply and counting electronics. A schematic diagram of a single-crystal photomultiplier device used for the detection of gamma radiation is shown in Figure 4.4. The photomultiplier (PM) must be supplied with a stable source of high voltage (HV). The scintillation flashes fall on the photocathode of the photomultiplier tube and cause the emission of photoelectrons. These electrons are accelerated by the HV applied between a series of electrodes of the photomultiplier tube, known as dynodes At each dynode secondary electron multiplication occurs, producing successive amplification of the electron current. The overall gain, or multiplication factor, depends on the number of dynode stages and the applied HV, so that the heights of the pulses produced by the tube depend on the applied voltage.

Pulses from the PM tube are passed to a preamplifier that is usually a transistorised follower circuit and brought to a suitable level for transmission to the main amplifier and analyser circuits. Amplified pulses are analysed in a number of ways before registration and counting on the scaler. Since the photomultiplier output pulse height is proportional to the energy of the particles or photons, the output from the linear amplifier is also directly proportional to these energies, and the spectrum of amplified pulse heights will be very similar to the energy spectrum of the radiation. With the choice of suitable analyser circuits, the pulse-height spectrum can be investigated by pulse-height analysis (PHA). Although the crystal and photomultiplier are protected from background radiation by lead shielding and from extraneous light by a thin (gamma-transparent) aluminium casing around the crystal, thermal election noise increases appreciably as the HV is increased. For high-activity gamma sources, the optimum HV can be determined by inspection of the source and background count–voltage curves.

Beta scintillation counting

For the assay of a sample containing beta emitters it is necessary to suspend or dissolve the activity in a liquid scintillant. The radioactivity-containing sample is mixed with an aromatic solvent (e.g. benzene or toluene) and fluors (fluorescent dye) known as a 'cocktail'. The samples are placed in small transparent or translucent (glass or plastic) vials that are loaded into an instrument known as a liquid scintillation counter. Beta particles emitted from the sample transfer energy to the solvent molecules, which in turn transfer their energy to the fluors that dissipate the energy by emitting light. In this way, each beta emission results in a pulse of light that may be detected using photomultiplier tubes. The scintillation cocktails often contain additives that shift the wavelength of the emitted light to make it more easily detected. High-energy beta emitters such as ^{32}P may also be counted in a scintillation counter without the cocktail. This technique is known as 'Cherenkov counting'.

Table 4.1 Physical properties of crystal scintillators used in nuclear medicine instrumentation

Scintillator	Atomic number, Z	Density, ρ (g/cm^3)	Decay time (ns)	Wavelength (nm)	Relative light output (% of NaI(Tl))
NaI (Tl)	50	3.67	200	415	100
CsI (Tl)	54	4.5	1000	550	45
CsI (Na)	54	4.51	630	420	85
$LaBr_3$:Ce	47	5.3	25	360	160

Gamma scintillation counting

For the majority of the common gamma-emitting radionuclides used in nuclear medicine (such as ^{99m}Tc, ^{123}I, ^{131}I, ^{111}In, ^{201}Tl), thallium-activated sodium iodide (NaI(Tl)) crystals are used for scintillation detection in combination with a photomultiplier tube (Figure 4.4). The efficiency of detection depends on a number of factors, of which the following are the most important.

- **Gamma photon energy:** highly energetic photons may pass completely through the crystal without energy dissipation. Low-energy photons may be absorbed in the outer layers of the crystal away from the photomultiplier tube.
- **Crystal size and geometry:** a large crystal will absorb high-energy photons more efficiently than a small crystal, but the size is limited by the optical transmission of scintillations. For this reason, larger crystals are commonly used for more energetic gamma emitters such as ^{131}I. The shape of the crystal will also influence detection efficiency. A gamma-emitting source placed near the surface of a cylindrical crystal will give a lower count rate than the same source placed inside a well drilled in the centre of a similar crystal.
- **Photomultiplier high voltage:** at low voltages, the potential between successive dynodes is not sufficient to produce an electrical pulse. Pulses are produced at higher voltages; at excessive voltage, spontaneous electron emission and thermal noise contribute greatly to the observed count rate.

For imaging purposes and in probe detectors, an increasing range of scintillation crystals are used. The demand for high-performance imaging in terms of increased sensitivity and spatial resolution has led to the introduction of a number of new scintillators. Some basic physical properties of the main scintillation crystals are given in Table 4.1.

Pulse-height analysis

One of the main advantages of the direct proportionality between the voltage and the initial gamma energy is that it is possible to plot the energy of the gamma events by pulse-height analysis. A spectrum is usually plotted to show the number of detected events on the y-axis and the energy (or analyser voltage) on the x axis (Figure 4.5). The low-energy region of a spectrum is generally known as the area of Compton scattering and the principal peak is known as the photopeak. By setting the level of upper and lower discriminators it is possible to set a window so that the activity within the peak may be determined. Since the energy spectrum of each radionuclide is unique, this allows production of a gamma

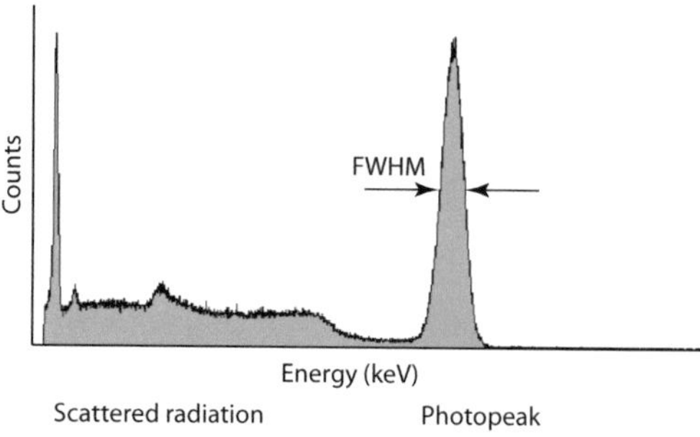

Figure 4.5 Gamma spectrum produced by a multichannel analyser unit. The energy resolution of the system can be expressed as the full width at half maximum (FWHM) of the photopeak.

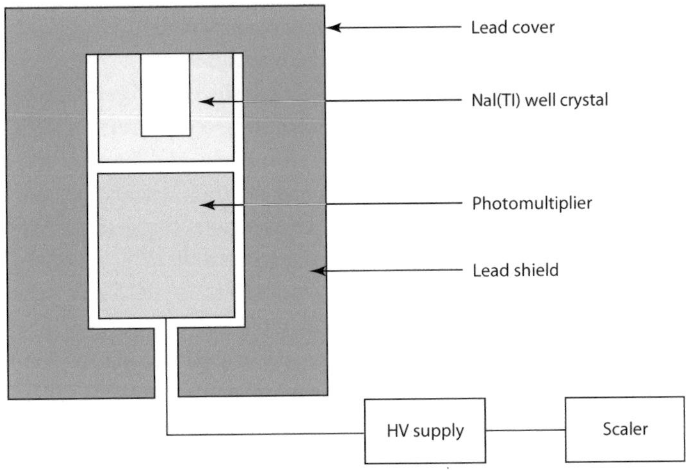

Figure 4.6 Schematic diagram of a well scintillation counter.

spectrum that may be used for analysis of radiochemical purity. Alternatively, spectrum analysis may be used for the identification of the composition of complex mixtures of different radionuclides. The energy resolution of the system is the ability to differentiate between the peaks of different gamma energies. This is usually determined by measuring the full width of the gamma peak at half the maximum height (FWHM) and expressed as a percentage of the maximum value.

For simple detection and counting of gamma activity (as in radiochemical analysis, chromatogram scanning, and radioimmunoassay with ^{125}I-labelled materials) a thin-walled NaI(Tl) well crystal can be used with a scaler-timer equipped with a HV supply, photomultiplier detector inputs, and a lower discriminator, or threshold. The well detector is used since the crystal almost completely surrounds the sample and therefore provides high detection efficiency. A schematic diagram of a well counter and photograph of an automatic well counter are shown in Figures 4.6 and 4.7, respectively. Typical hand-held survey monitors are shown in Figure 4.8.

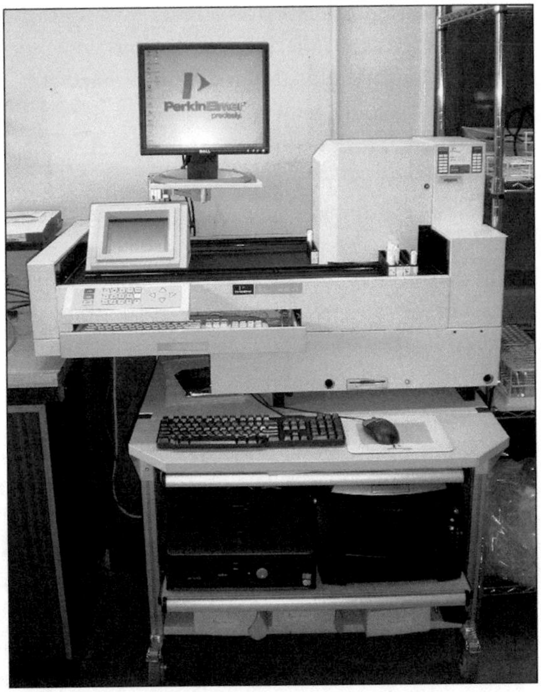

Figure 4.7 Photograph of an automatic sample counter.

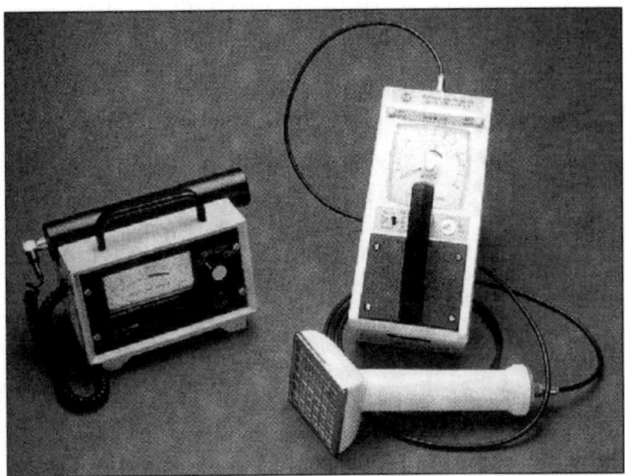

Figure 4.8 Hand-held survey monitors for determination of the levels of laboratory radioactivity and surface contamination. Left: scintillation detector. Right: GM detector.

Solid-state detectors

Solid-state detectors offer many advantages for measurement of high-energy gamma rays over either gas detectors or scintillation counters, one major advantage being their higher energy resolution. The dimensions of solid-state detectors can be much smaller than the gas detector of equivalent performance as they normally have densities approximately 1000 times greater than commonly used gases. Solid-state detectors come in a variety of materials, but they are predominantly based on silicon or germanium. Other materials in use or under development include diamond and semiconductor compounds such as CdTe, CdZnTe, GaAs, SiC and AlGaAs.

Radiation impinging on a solid-state detector results in the direct creation of a number of electron–hole pairs, unlike in a scintillator which has the intermediate optical photon generation process. The number of electron–hole pairs generated in the detector is related to the energy of the incident photon (particle) and the material's properties. Electrons and holes are swept away under the influence of the electric field controlled by a bias voltage applied across the device. The resulting charge is collected to give a measure of the incident energy and, in the case of imaging detectors, the position of interaction. Detectors based on silicon and germanium are typically operated at low temperatures to improve the signal to noise and energy resolution.

The energy resolution of semiconductor detectors can be described by the sum of the three independent terms under the square root sign in equation (4.1). The first term relates the variance of the number of primary electron–hole pairs, where F is the Fano factor, E is the incident energy (eV) and ω is the energy required to generate an electron–hole pair.

$$\Delta E = 2.36\omega\sqrt{\frac{FE}{\omega} + R^2 + A^2} \qquad (4.1)$$

The second term, R^2, relates to the readout noise and arises from the loss of charge during collection, drift or transfer. The last term, A^2, is associated with the amplifier noise (pre-amplifier, main amplifier and signal processing electronics) with A in units of electronvolts. To achieve Fano limited energy resolution the partial quadratic sum of R and A must obviously be minimised.

For silicon and germanium, the Fano factors (at an operating temperature of 77 K) are 0.143 and 0.129, respectively, and the accepted values for electron–hole pair creation energy, ω, are 3.76 eV and 2.96 eV. Therefore, if the detector were Fano limited (R and A equal to zero in equation (4.1)) then the energy resolution, at 59.5 keV would be 0.422 keV for Si and 0.355 keV for Ge.

Silicon diodes are available as compact, real-time personnel dosemeters. These devices continuously monitor the radiation environment, unlike film or thermoluminescent dosemeters, and can give higher levels of protection for the user. However, the response of this type of device is dependent on the energy of the incident photon, with the sensitivity decreasing for higher-energy radiation. This effect can be taken into account by using metallic absorbers around the detector to provide 'energy compensation'.

For efficient detection of high-energy gamma rays (>200 keV) with excellent energy resolution, germanium detectors are the only viable choice. Unlike silicon detectors, which cannot be thicker than a few millimetres, germanium can have sensitive thicknesses of several centimetres, and therefore can be used as a total absorption detector for gamma rays up to few MeV. Widely available types are lithium-doped germanium, Ge(Li) and high-purity germanium (HPGe) detectors. A major disadvantage of germanium detectors, however, is the requirement to operate them at liquid-nitrogen temperatures (77 K).

Diamond has many interesting properties for use in radiation detectors; the detectors can be operated at room temperature, have low noise and intrinsic high radiation tolerance, and have near 'tissue equivalent' absorption. High-quality diamond for detectors is slowly becoming available as manufacture and costs issues are being resolved.

Compound semiconductor devices offer alternatives to silicon and germanium detectors and have the potential to overcome some of the limitations of these widely used materials. The most widely investigated compound semiconductors, CdTe, CdZnTe and HgI_2, can all operate at room temperature with respectable energy resolution and good detection efficiency. The higher effective atomic number of the compound materials translates into significantly

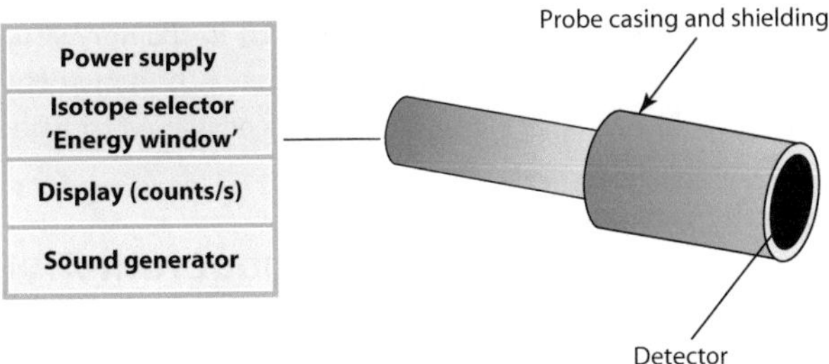

Figure 4.9 Schematic diagram of the main components of a gamma probe system suitable for use during surgery.

better photoelectric absorption and hence higher detector efficiency per unit thickness. Widespread adoption of these materials for radiation detectors for medical application will require improvements in manufacture and processing to reduce the costs to levels competitive with silicon and germanium.

Solid-state detectors have mostly been used in electronic autoradiography units, and probe systems for intraoperative detection. However, this type of detector is now becoming more frequently used for imaging such as in small gamma cameras, scintimammography units and digital X-ray systems. The most widely known imaging devices based on silicon are charge coupled devices (CCDs), found in many high-end consumer cameras and CMOS devices typically used in web cameras. These imaging devices offer very good spatial resolution and digital output. CCD-based cameras for dental imaging utilise a scintillator (Gadox or CsI) to covert the X-rays and gamma rays to optical photons that the device can image efficiently. Simpler direct imaging and use of lower levels of activity are some of the main benefits of these devices.

Probe systems

Since the very beginning of clinical nuclear medicine practice, probe systems have been used for monitoring radiopharmaceutical uptake in vivo. The very first clinical investigations were based on the use of Geiger counters to monitor the uptake of radioiodine in the thyroid gland (thyroid uptake). Subsequently, probe systems have used single NaI(Tl) scintillation crystals with a photomultiplier since these are recognised as being the most sensitive form of radiation detector. The first imaging systems were the rectilinear scanners. These were based on the mechanical scanning of collimated probes across the length of the patient.

Probe systems have been used for a range of applications in intensive care and surgical exploration. Intraoperative probe systems consist basically of two component parts, the hand-held detector and the electronic processing and display unit; these two are usually coupled together by an electrical cable (Figure 4.9). At the tip of the probe is a collimated detector element that provides the directional properties of the system. This is mounted on a shaft that widens to form the handle and often contains some electronics such as the pre-amplifier unit. The majority of commercial probe systems are manufactured from high-grade metal such as stainless steel or anodised aluminium that may be cleaned and sterilised often using ethylene oxide gas (Figure 4.10). At least one prototype

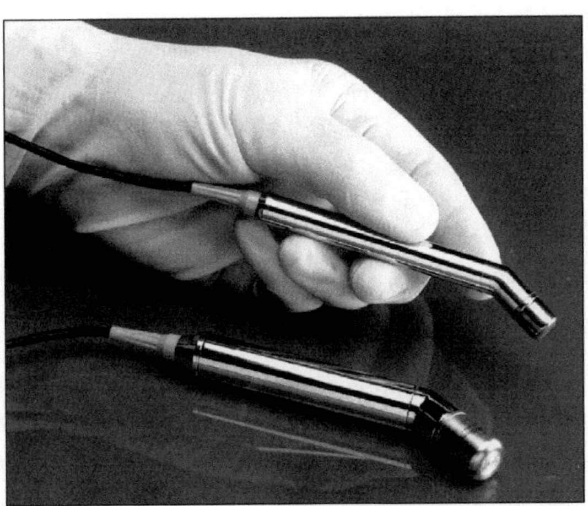

Figure 4.10 Photograph of hand-held surgical probes. These can be sterilised or placed in a sterile sheath for intraoperative use.

commercial system has a 'single-use' disposable handle and cable.

The probe is designed to be as slim as possible to facilitate access through small surgical incisions. The active detector element is generally a scintillation crystal, NaI(Tl) or CsI(Na), coupled to a photodiode or photomultiplier tube, or a solid-state detector, usually CdTe with adjacent signal pre-amplification, built into the handle. In the case of scintillation detectors the design should facilitate good optical coupling of the detector crystal to the electronics, since the use of long fibreoptic cables has been found to be unreliable.

With both scintillation and solid-state devices, increasing the diameter of the detector increases sensitivity but reduces spatial resolution. Scintillation detectors tend to be physically larger but have much higher sensitivity. The higher sensitivity of scintillation devices arises from a combination of increased intrinsic detection efficiency and the efficiency of collection of the electrical signal from the detector. CdTe detectors collect charge less efficiently as detector size increases. A 1 mm thick CdTe crystal has an intrinsic stopping power of about 50%, and typical probes that use 2–3 mm thick CdTe wafers do not show exponential increases in overall efficiency due to falling charge collection efficiency.

Accurate spatial localisation of the sites of tracer uptake depends upon the directional properties of the probe. This is primarily affected by the degree of collimation, which usually comprises 5–10 mm thickness of tungsten. Although it is desirable for the probe to be physically small, significant errors may result if there is insufficient shielding around the detector.

The electronic unit will provide the electrical power source, usually in the form of rechargeable batteries, signal processing circuitry, a pulse-height analyser and some form of display. Different probe systems have different means of output (digital count-rate meters, scalers and audible outputs). Audible outputs generally produce a series of clicks or tone bursts with the frequency proportional to count rate, and this is the main means of relaying the count rate to the surgeon while his vision is focused on the operating field. A threshold or 'squelch' control is usually available, which can be set to a level below which there is no audible output. However, a digital display is recommended since this facilitates a numerical reading that may be recorded in the surgical notes. Since the electronics are not connected to the mains supply during operation, leakage currents to the patient are well below 10 mA and are not considered to be hazardous.

Personal radiation dosemeters

All personnel working with radioactive materials and ionising radiations are required to wear personal radiation dosemeters as part of health and safety regulations. These are basically one of three types, electronic, thermoluminescent, and film as shown in Figure 4.11. These monitors are usually calibrated by a dose-monitoring service and results are provided in microsieverts (μSv). The more traditional type is the film badge dosemeter. This uses a small piece of X-ray film sandwiched between two plastic covers containing a combination of filters (Figure 4.12). The badge is worn for a period of time and with appropriate calibration the density of the film exposure can be related to the absorbed dose.

One of the simplest and most reliable radiation monitors is the thermoluminescent personal dose monitor. The dosemeters are usually supplied in the form of a whole-body monitor or a finger badge. The active component is lithium fluoride powder placed in a specially designed holder that incorporates screening materials to differentiate between the different radiations received. When ionising radiation interacts with the crystals it causes electrons in the atoms to jump to higher energy states, where they remain trapped due to the influence of impurities such as

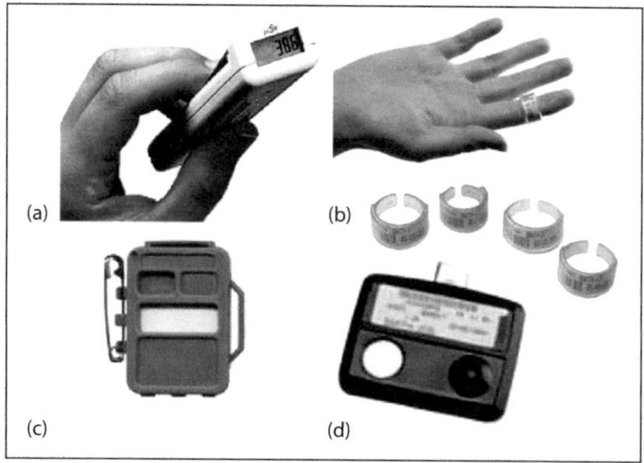

Figure 4.11 Personal dosemeters: (a) electronic dosemeter, (b) TLD finger monitors, (c) film badge, (d) TLD body monitor.

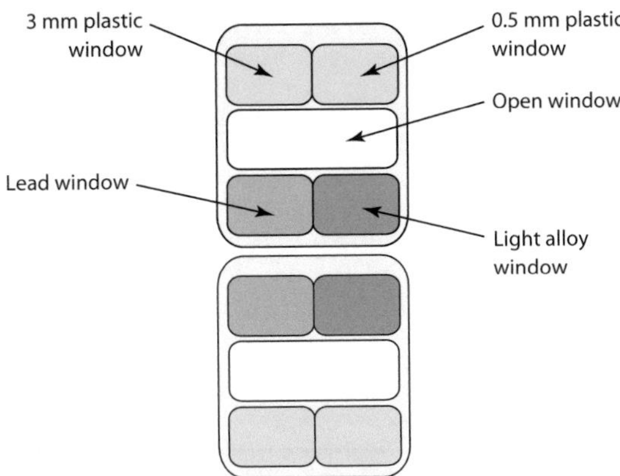

Figure 4.12 A schematic diagram of the casing of the film badge dosemeter. The filters are used to discriminate the different types and energy of radiation.

manganese or magnesium in the crystal, until heated. After the designated period of wearing, the badge is returned and the exposure reading is taken. Heating the crystals causes the electrons to drop back to their ground state, releasing energy in the form of light photons equal to the energy difference between the trapped state and the ground state. The light output is converted into an absorbed dose level.

Electronic dosemeters are usually solid-state devices that are used for general monitoring of personal radiation doses. These have the advantage of providing an immediate reading on a digital display. They can also be set with an audible output and an alarm that can be triggered at pre-set level. These are particularly useful when undertaking a risk assessment of individual procedures that may result in significant radiation doses to personnel.

All staff monitoring and record keeping of personal radiation doses should be undertaken by an approved monitoring service with the support of the hospital radiation protection officers, normally the radiation protection supervisor (RPS) and radiation protection adviser (RPA).

Further reading

Brown BH *et al.* (1999). *Medical Physics and Biomedical Engineering*. Bristol: IOP Publishing. ISBN 0-7216-8341X.

Cherry SR *et al.* (2003). *Physics in Nuclear Medicine*. Philadelphia: Saunders.

Knoll GF (2000). *Radiation Detection and Measurement*, 3rd edn. New York: Wiley. ISBN 0-471-07338-5.

Sharp PF *et al. Practical Nuclear Medicine* 3rd edn. London: Springer 2005. ISBN 185233-875-X.

5

Physics applied to radiopharmacy: imaging instruments for nuclear medicine

Brian F Hutton

Introduction

Central to the role of nuclear medicine is the ability to obtain an image that accurately reflects the spatial distribution of an administered radioactive tracer and its variation in time. Traditionally the Anger gamma camera has been the standard instrument used for planar imaging, permitting static, dynamic or gated acquisition. Of more interest now is the ability to obtain images of the three-dimensional distribution of activity by means of emission tomography. This involves either single-photon emission computed tomography (SPECT) based on detection of the gamma emissions from a single photon-emitting radionuclide (e.g. ^{99m}Tc) or positron emission tomography (PET) which relies on the detection of dual photons that arise from positron annihilation. Both PET and SPECT are now available combined with X-ray computed tomography (CT), which aids in localisation and can also be used for attenuation correction. In this chapter a basic overview of these imaging systems will be presented, primarily for systems designed for human use. There is also increasing interest in imaging systems used for preclinical imaging in small animals; these systems are based on similar principles and will be covered briefly. The chapter concludes with a brief overview of current developments in nuclear medicine instrumentation. References have been limited to key papers, reviews and book chapters. For a general coverage see Cherry *et al.* (2003).

The gamma camera

The instrument most commonly used for imaging in nuclear medicine is the Anger gamma camera (Anger 1958), whose performance has improved since its inception but whose design is largely unchanged. Emitted photons are detected in a scintillation detector (usually NaI with thallium impurities), in which visible light is emitted as a result of the photon interaction and is detected by a photomultiplier. In practice the detector is usually a single large crystal of dimension typically around 500 mm × 400 mm × 9.5 mm. The emitted light travels in all directions and is detected by an array of photomultiplier tubes, optically coupled to the scintillator, in which the light is further converted to a small electrical signal and amplified. The distribution of light across the photomultiplier array provides an estimate of the spatial location of the photon interaction; the summed light signal is proportional to the energy deposited in the crystal during interaction. The availability of an energy signal permits discrimination of photons that have undergone Compton scattering prior to detection, because these photons will have lower energy; since these photons are deflected, their origin is uncertain. The remaining essential component is a collimator, without which the origin of the emitted gamma photon would be unknown. The collimator consists of a lead or tungsten 'honeycomb' with long narrow holes that ideally permit only photons travelling normal to the scintillator to be detected (Figure 5.1). A range of collimators is available, each designed to provide optimum image quality for specific emission energy.

The acquired data are normally digitised so that each detected photon whose energy falls within a selected range, so as to minimise scatter, is simply added to a picture element (pixel) that corresponds to the physical location on the detector. Each pixel accumulates counts proportional to the activity exposed to that pixel. A visible image is constructed by converting the summed counts in the array of pixels to a corresponding array of display elements, where shades of grey or colours are used to represent the range of acquired counts. The result is a planar image of the activity distribution being viewed.

The image quality that is obtained with a gamma camera is a consequence of the instrument design. The most important parameters are the spatial resolution and sensitivity of the system. Spatial resolution describes the ability to discriminate points of activity that are closely spaced (i.e. the ability to image fine detail in the activity distribution). Sensitivity refers to the fraction of emitted photons that are acquired; typically the acquired counts are relatively low, resulting in an observed mottle or noise that is a direct result of the limited statistics. In most cases the sensitivity can only be improved to the detriment of spatial resolution and vice versa. The spatial resolution is limited by two factors: (1) the intrinsic ability of the detector to correctly estimate the location of a photon interaction in the crystal, usually 3–4 mm FWHM (FWHM is the full width at half maximum value for an image of a point source, the normal measure of spatial resolution); (2) the limited angle of acceptance defined by the collimator geometry (by far the primary effect as resolution at 10 cm is typically ~8 mm; this geometric resolution worsens linearly with distance from the collimator). The resolution could be improved by narrowing the collimator holes, but this would reduce the number of detected photons, i.e. worsen sensitivity. The number of acquired counts could be increased by acquiring for a longer time; this is clearly limited for practical reasons. Alternatively, administering a larger activity of radionuclide would increase the photon flux, but this is limited by the acceptable radiation dose delivered to the patient. Even when optimised, nuclear medicine images are typically blurred (i.e. of limited resolution) and somewhat noisy (i.e. of limited sensitivity) compared with other modalities such as X-ray CT.

A further parameter of interest is the energy resolution or ability to discriminate energies of the detected photons. In the case of NaI(Tl) this is 9–10%; i.e. for the single-energy emission of ^{99m}Tc an energy window width of 20% is required to capture 95% of the detected primary photons (with approximately 35% of the total detected counts being scattered photons).

Emission tomography (general)

As outlined above the standard Anger camera is a planar imaging instrument which does not permit identification of the origin of emission at depth in tissue (like planar radiography). However, by acquiring information at multiple angles around the patient a three-dimensional distribution of the activity distribution can be mathematically reconstructed; this is referred to as tomography (similar to CT). The method of acquiring data is different for single-photon

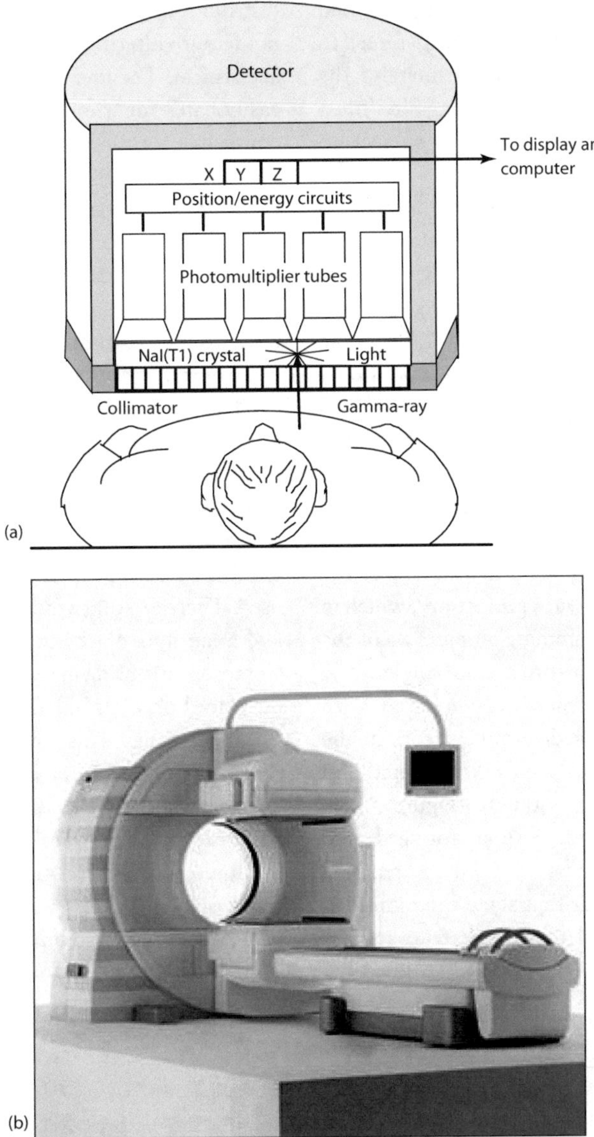

Figure 5.1 (a) Schematic of gamma camera operation showing collimator, crystal and photomultiplier assembly. (b) Commercial dual-head gamma camera (Siemens Healthcare). Most systems are mounted on a stable gantry to facilitate SPECT and some also incorporate a CT system.

emitters (SPECT) or positron emitters (PET), but the principles of tomographic reconstruction are similar for both (and for CT); it is therefore logical to consider this separately.

There are essentially two methods available for reconstruction from projections: filtered back projection (FBP) and iterative methods, both being routinely used (see Hutton *et al.* 2006; Tsui, Frey 2006). Both methods are based on the assumption that the origin of emission can be 'modelled' given knowledge of the acquired projection counts. The simplest model assumes that all photons must originate along lines perpendicular to the point where measured; given no knowledge of the depth of origin, the best that can be done is to simply back project the measured counts, distributing these along the perpendiculars (Figure 5.2a). This results in a build-up of counts due to consistent measurement at different angles, but data remain blurred. This blurring can be exactly rectified by use of an appropriate filter (the ramp filter) to produce an analytical solution. Unfortunately, the process amplifies noise and so a smoothing filter must also be applied. The technique is also subject to streaking and sensitive to missing data.

The alternative is to use an iterative approach, most commonly maximum likelihood–expectation maximum (ML-EM) reconstruction (Lange, Carson 1984) or an accelerated version of this, e.g. ordered subsets EM (OS-EM) (Hudson, Larkin 1994). The principles of the iterative methods can be considered as an extension to the back projection described above. If instead of simply back projecting measured projections, an initial guess is made regarding the distribution of activity (usually assuming this to be uniform), one can estimate what would be acquired for this activity distribution using the inverse of the back projection process (forward projection), which in its simplest form involves summing along rows of the image orthogonal to each projection angle. The estimated projections can then be compared with the actual measurements to determine errors in the estimate; the resultant errors are back projected and used to correct the original estimate (Figure 5.2b). The process continues with further forward and back projection until the estimated and measured projections are in agreement; at that stage the estimated activity distribution should match the true activity distribution. The appeal of this method is that it does not require filtering (and has usually better noise characteristics). The method is also very flexible and can easily cater for a much more complex model of the emission process including attenuation, scatter and variation in resolution at distance from the detector (Tsui *et al.*, 1994; Hutton *et al.*, 1997; King *et al.* 2004). The accelerated OS-EM algorithm is in widespread clinical use particularly in PET where the improved noise characterisation in low-count background regions facilitates lesion detection (see Hutton *et al.* 1997).

The image quality obtained in emission tomography, as in planar imaging, depends on a number of factors. There is the usual trade-off between noise and resolution (or contrast); for FBP this is largely controlled by choice of filter, but for ML-EM or OS-EM the result depends on the number of iterations used. There are other factors that affect image quality and quantitative accuracy. Emitted photons undergo Compton scattering in tissue, which results not only in misplaced photons but also loss of counts (referred to as attenuation). This loss is significant, resulting in typically only 10% of emitted photons leaving the body (<5% for PET). Correction for attenuation is therefore an important consideration. In addition, the limited resolution results in loss of contrast for small objects (and at times inability to detect small objects); motion also limits contrast but also can give

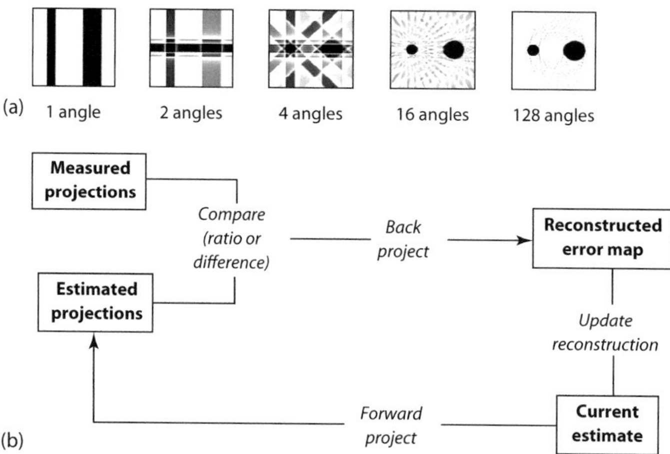

Figure 5.2 (a) Simple illustration of reconstruction by filtered back projection. The cancellation of back projection errors as the number of projection angles increases can be seen. (b) Schematic of iterative reconstruction: the reconstructed image is obtained by ensuring that estimated projections match the measured projections.

rise to additional serious artefacts. Some of these factors will be discussed in more detail in relation to SPECT or PET.

Single-photon emission computed tomography (SPECT)

In the case of SPECT the most commonly used system involves the rotation of one or more gamma cameras around the patient, acquiring planar images at multiple angles (see Figure 5.5). For the set of acquired angles, each row of the acquired planar images can be selected to reconstruct a single cross-sectional slice. As outlined above, reconstruction can be performed using either FBP or iterative methods. The attraction of the rotating gamma camera is that the same instrumentation can be used for both planar and tomographic acquisition, providing great flexibility. The use of an Anger camera for SPECT places extra demands on the system. The camera must have a good uniformity as errors are amplified in SPECT; a small uniformity defect at the centre of the detector can give rise to a serious defect on reconstruction. In addition, the rotational stability of the system must be ensured (both electronic and mechanical stability caused problems in early systems). Both uniformity of detector response and the alignment of the electronic and mechanical centre of rotation should be checked regularly as part of routine quality control procedures.

Correction for attenuation in SPECT is not trivial, especially when there is non-uniform attenuation as in the chest. Approximate correction (Chang 1978) can be implemented post reconstruction in the case of uniform attenuation, sufficient for visual interpretation. However, in the case of non-uniform attenuation there is need to acquire a measured transmission map; correction then can be achieved by incorporating this known attenuation directly into the model used for iterative reconstruction. There have been various approaches for transmission measurement using gamma-emitting sources (see review by Bailey 1998), although the commercial application of these systems has proved to be unreliable (O'Connor, Kemp 2002). Recently, combined SPECT/CT systems have become available wherein the CT provides an improved transmission map as well as a means of anatomical localisation. The CT values must be converted to attenuation coefficients appropriate for the gamma emission energy of the specific radionuclide, normally using a bilinear function. Care should be taken that the CT does not contain artefacts (e.g. streaking) or metallic implants as these can result in errors in the attenuation correction. Misalignment between emission and transmission data can also be problematic (e.g. due to acquisition at different respiratory phases).

Correction for other factors affecting SPECT quantification continues to be a research topic. There have been numerous suggestions for methods to correct for scatter (see, for example, reviews by Buvat *et al.* (1994) and by Zaidi and Koral (2006)), but many are difficult to implement in a clinical setting. Probably the most popular method involves the acquisition of additional energy windows above and below the photopeak, which are used to estimate the scatter within the photopeak window (Ogawa *et al.* 1994). Unfortunately, subtraction of scatter enhances noise although image quality can be improved by simply adding the measured scatter in the forward projection during iterative reconstruction. Partial volume effects are particularly problematic for SPECT given the limited spatial resolution (at best the resolution is equivalent to the planar resolution at the centre of rotation; typically 12–16 mm using parallel-hole collimators; at best 8 mm for brain SPECT using a fanbeam collimator). Corrections for partial volume effects have been devised for brain SPECT using aligned high-resolution anatomical images, but, in general, correction is difficult and rarely exact. Only recently has more careful attention been given to motion effects, particularly those due to involuntary motion as a result of respiration. Owing to the slow acquisition involving detector rotation, effects of motion can be somewhat unpredictable.

Positron emission tomography (PET)

Imaging using positron emitters is always tomographic and the principles of acquisition are unique to this modality. When a positron is emitted, it travels a short distance in tissue, loses energy, and eventually interacts with an electron, the two particles annihilating with emission of two 511 keV gamma photons that travel in opposite directions. PET is designed using a ring of

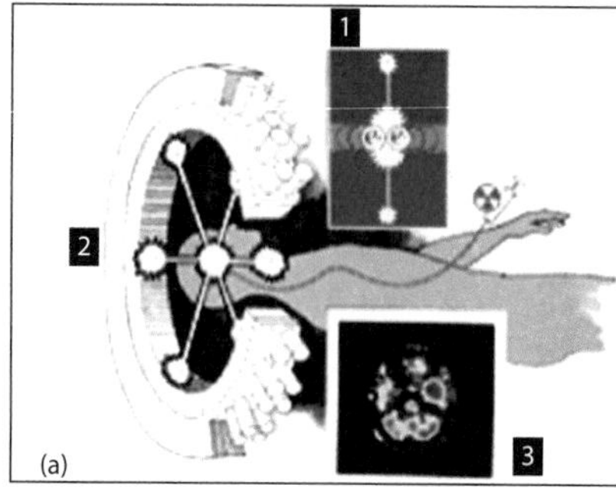

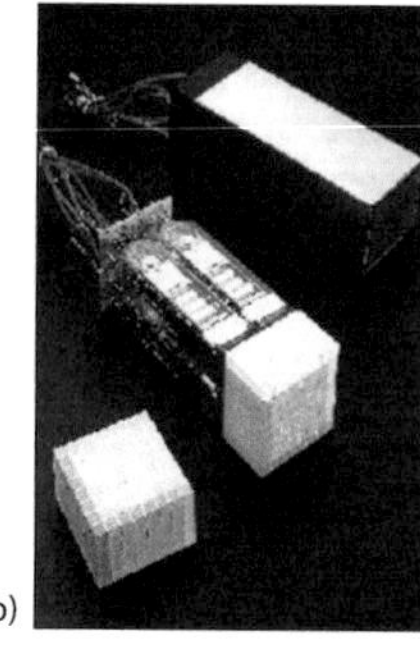

Figure 5.3 (a) PET detects the two collinear gamma photons that are emitted when a positron annihilates with an electron (1). The two photons are detected in coincidence, permitting localisation of a line-of-response (2). The activity distribution (3) is determined normally via iterative reconstruction. (b) Most PET detectors utilise a block design with multiple crystals connected to a small number of photomultiplier tubes.

small detectors around the patient, specifically designed to detect events only when pairs of gamma photons arrive within a short time of each other (i.e. in coincidence; in practice typically within 8–12 ns). When an event is detected (assumed due to a single positron emission) the line joining the two detectors defines the origin of the annihilation without the need for physical collimation (Figure 5.3a). The lack of a physical collimator results in approximately 100 times higher sensitivity than in a typical SPECT system.

The scintillators used for PET are not NaI (although PET systems have previously been designed using this material) but are selected to have high stopping power and fast light output. Table 5.1 lists properties of detector materials in commercial use at the time of writing compared with NaI(Tl); lanthanum bromide ($LaBr_3$) is included as a promising new detector material (Moses, Shah 2005). A variety of detector designs have been suggested, although the most commonly used system is currently based on block detectors where a small array of detectors is coupled to a small number of photomultiplier tubes which, like the Anger camera, decode the interaction location based on the detected light distribution (Figure 5.3b). The set of acquired projection lines (or lines of response) at first appears quite different from the data acquired in SPECT, but in fact these can easily be reordered so as to represent a set of parallel projections. Consequently reconstruction is very similar to that used for SPECT. Many PET studies are performed by acquiring the whole body (or at least neck to thigh); this is achieved by acquiring for a set time (2–4 minutes) in each of several bed positions. These bed positions are spaced so as to achieve constant sensitivity along the patient's length (typically requiring 6–7 bed positions).

A specific property of PET is that owing to the coincidence detection of dual photons the probability

Table 5.1 Comparison of scintillation materials used for PET

	Density (g/cm^3)	Relative light output (%)	Decay time[a] (ns)
NaI(Tl)	3.67	100	230
BGO	7.13	30	300 (60)
LSO	7.35	80	40
GSO	6.31	40	60 (600)
$LaBr_3$	5.06	165	16

[a] Secondary component in brackets.

BGO, bismuth germanate; LSO, lutetium oxyorthosilicate; GSO, gadolinium oxyorthosilicate.

of event detection is affected only by the total attenuation along a line of response and is independent of the location along that path; consequently, attenuation measured externally for that specific line of response provides an exact correction for the attenuation along that path. The ease of correcting for attenuation resulted in PET being considered 'quantitative', although the modality is subject to problems similar to those affecting SPECT (scatter, resolution, motion). A limitation to the original approach to the attenuation correction was noise from the transmission measurement that propagated into the reconstructed emission images; consequently transmission measurements traditionally occupied almost the same time as the emission measurement. Nowadays PET is supplied with CT, permitting high-quality transmission measurement of the whole body in less than a minute (Beyer *et al.* 2000). As in the case of SPECT, the CT data must be converted to appropriate attenuation coefficients; also artefacts and areas of abnormally high attenuation can give rise to artefactual PET activity distribution. Mismatch of emission and transmission can still occur as the measurements are sequential and respiration and heart motion remain involuntary. The availability of dual modality PET/CT has revolutionised the clinical use of PET. ^{18}F-fluorodeoxyglucose (FDG), though somewhat non-specific, has very high sensitivity for lesion detection, but localisation can be difficult. The addition of high-resolution CT not only enables accurate localisation but also the combined information can further clarify diagnosis. As a result virtually all PET systems are now supplied as PET/CT configurations.

Early PET systems included lead septa that separated the axial planes, permitting a set of two-dimensional (2D) acquisitions and 2D reconstruction. However, it is now more common for these septa to be removed so that data acquisition and reconstruction are both performed in three dimensions. A consequence is that there is increased scatter, potentially similar to the fraction encountered in SPECT. As with SPECT, there are several approaches to scatter correction, typically now implemented as standard processing by the suppliers. Note that scatter in PET can give rise to events outside the patient boundary, unlike SPECT in which scatter is limited to the area within the body boundary. One type of event unique to PET is random coincidence, a result of detecting two photons in coincidence that derive from independent positron sources. These events are a further source of error, but they are corrected either on the basis of calculating the random coincidence rate with knowledge of the recorded single event rate (photons detected without a second photon being necessarily detected in the coincidence timing window) or by direct measurement using a delayed coincidence window (see, for example, Wernick and Aarsvold listed in Further Reading for detail). The main consequence is that random events correction and scatter correction both contribute to the noise in the final reconstruction. Partial volume effects are less serious than experienced in SPECT owing to the better resolution (typically around 4–6 mm FWHM). Motion has a more noticeable effect, however. Research continues on methods to detect and correct for motion.

A significant contributor to the high quality of PET images is the reconstruction algorithm. Iterative algorithms are now implemented to permit full 3D reconstruction that can incorporate a model of emission that includes attenuation, scatter and resolution as well as detector normalisation and correction for random events. A feature of iterative reconstruction is that noise is proportional to signal and reduction of noise in low-count areas greatly enhances the ability to detect low-contrast lesions, a common requirement of ^{18}F-FDG studies. See Bailey *et al.* (2005) for a useful coverage of PET.

Preclinical imaging

In recent years there has been growing interest in the development of instrumentation specifically for imaging of small animals. This is proving important in streamlining the preclinical development of suitable tracers by permitting ultra-high-resolution imaging of tracer kinetics and distribution without the need for dissection of multiple animals. These systems have further appeal in being able to evaluate pharmaceutical distribution as well as monitoring response to drug administration. The use of these systems is likely to expand further in response to an increasing need for efficient evaluation of new potential therapies tailored for specific diseases or tumour types. Both PET and SPECT systems are commercially available as well as CT and MRI. Performing dual or multiple modality studies is therefore quite feasible.

Micro-PET

Several systems have been designed for preclinical PET, most notably deriving from work of Simon Cherry. Recent systems have been based on scaled-down versions of clinical systems based on block detectors. A particular concern in systems with small detector ring radius is the uncertainty in line-of-response as a result of interaction at depth in one of several crystals, with degraded resolution as a consequence. Some recent designs attempt to correct for this effect using some form of depth encoding, usually using multiple crystal layers.

The highest resolution achievable to date has been of the order of 1 mm; in fact the theoretical limit of resolution for PET is due to physical limitations of positron emission. On emission, a positron travels a finite distance prior to annihilation, this distance being dependent on the positron emission energy. For ^{18}F the range is relatively small (mean 0.6 mm), for more energetic positron emitters such as ^{82}Rb this can be more significant. What is measured is the point of annihilation rather than the point of positron emission. The main limitation in resolution, however, is due to the fact that there can be some loss of momentum during annihilation, which results in a small angular deviation from the expected collinear emission of dual photons ($\sim$0.2°). Though small, this angular deviation is sufficient to introduce a spatial uncertainty in localisation that limits the achievable resolution to around 1 mm. As with clinical systems micro-PET is combined with micro-CT and more recently MRI (see Rowland, Cherry 2008).

Micro-SPECT

Surprisingly, preclinical SPECT systems can significantly out-perform PET as there are no physical limitations to the achievable resolution similar to those influencing micro-PET. At the time of writing, resolution of 0.35 mm had been demonstrated (Beekman, van der Have 2007). The main contributor to this excellent spatial resolution has been the pinhole collimator, whose properties are very well suited to imaging of small animals. Unlike parallel-hole collimators, the pinhole can be utilised to provide both high resolution and high sensitivity provided it is used close to a small object. The pinhole collimator operates on the same principle as the optical pinhole camera. An inverted and magnified image of the object is obtained on the detector when the pinhole aperture is placed close to the object and the aperture–detector distance exceeds this distance. As a result of the magnification, the resolution achieved can be significantly less than the intrinsic resolution of the detector (the effective intrinsic resolution component is reduced by the magnification factor). By using a large number of small-diameter apertures, the sensitivity can be maintained. The example illustrated in Figure 5.4 is of the U-SPECT system (MILabs), in which 75 pinholes with gold inserts view a small volume of a mouse, the final whole-body image being obtained by translating the animal's position relative to the collimator. Alternative systems image the whole animal with lower magnification, sometimes permitting overlap of acquired images (multiplexing) which is decoded during reconstruction (Wirrwar *et al.* 2001). The principles of reconstruction are identical to those used in human systems, mainly based on the same iterative reconstruction algorithms.

Recent developments

There continue to be developments in instrumentation for nuclear medicine. This section describes a few recent developments at the time of writing that are likely to influence the range of instrumentation available for clinical and preclinical use.

Detector components

There is a continuing search for better detector materials that permit improved performance. There is currently strong interest in the scintillator lanthanum bromide (see Table 5.1 for properties). This material has very good stopping power and fast, high light output. There is also increasing interest in using solid-state detectors such as cadmium zinc telluride (CZT) (see Wagenaar 2004); their stability and cost have improved to a stage where these detectors are becoming economically viable. These developments are complemented with development of readout systems as an alternative to photomultiplier tubes. Examples are avalanche photodiodes, silicon PM tubes, electron-multiplying CCDs and silicon drift

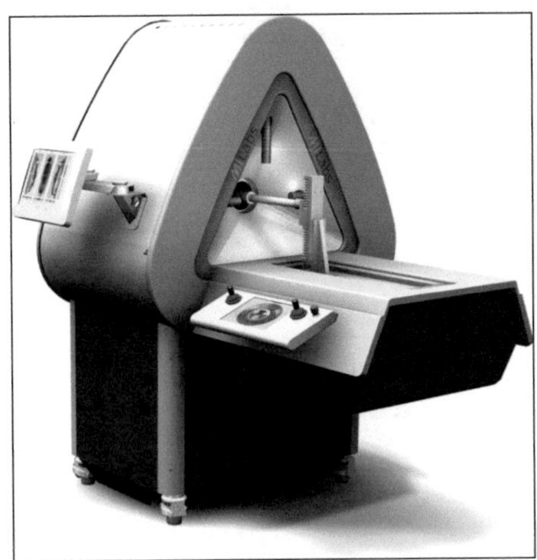

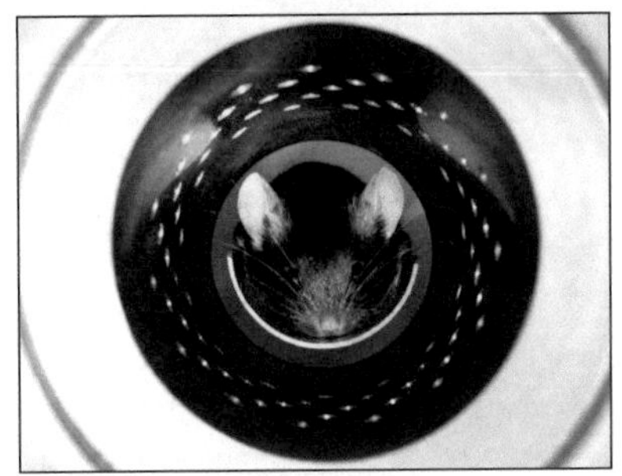

U-SPECT: 75 pinholes
Resolution: 0.35 mm

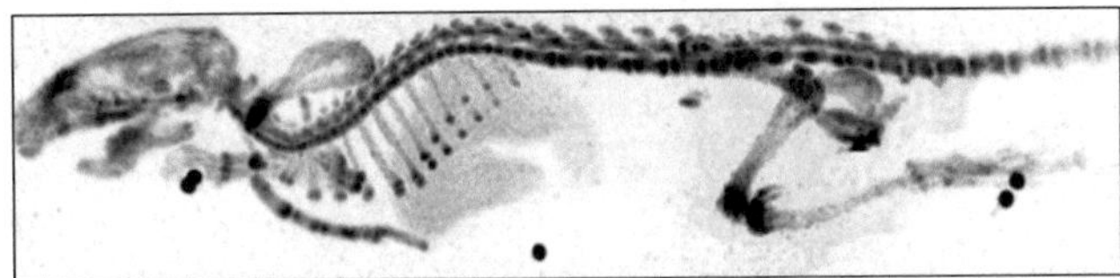

Figure 5.4 Preclinical SPECT using 75 pinholes with three detectors (MILabs, the Netherlands). The system images a very small volume and performs a 'rectilinear' scan of the animal to provide a whole-body SPECT study. Reproduced with permission from F. Beekman, MILabs, The Netherlands.

diodes (see Pichler, Ziegler 2004 for review). Though detailed description is beyond the scope of this chapter, all of these systems offer promise for future detectors; some are already in use in laboratory settings. An intrinsic resolution of 1 mm is readily achievable. The challenge remains to design systems that take best advantage of this improvement in intrinsic resolution as conventional parallel-hole collimators dominate performance. There is now interest in utilising alternative collimators including multiple-pinhole, crossed-slit and slit-slat collimators.

Organ-specific SPECT systems

There is a current trend to design systems optimised for specific purposes (Patton *et al.* 2007). Clearly better performance can be achieved than for the more general-purpose but flexible conventional systems. Of particular interest has been recent development of systems dedicated for cardiac studies, mainly driven by the need for high throughput of myocardial perfusion studies to meet clinical demand. Examples of these systems are the CardiArc and MarC systems, both of which utilise rotating slit-slat collimators (parallel holes in the axial direction but pinhole in the transaxial direction) with resultant improvement in sensitivity (about threefold).

A further novel system is D-SPECT (Figure 5.5), which utilises nine CZT detectors that each rotate around their axes so as to acquire data within programmable arcs; the combination of wide-beam collimation and region-centric acquisition permits a sensitivity gain of up to 8 and hence either a significant reduction in acquisition time, or reduced radiation dose. Other suggested approaches involve use of multiple pinholes or multiple-segment slant-hole collimators. Again central to the success of these systems are the iterative reconstruction algorithms that are tailored to the specific geometry of acquisition. In particular the inclusion of resolution models in these algorithms is proving to be useful in providing not only enhanced reconstructed resolution but also improved noise properties; the commercial interest in improving noise has been to permit reduction in imaging time and more efficient system utility. Other dedicated systems for breast scanning are also under development. Systems for brain imaging were developed in the past and may resurface to meet the growing demand for

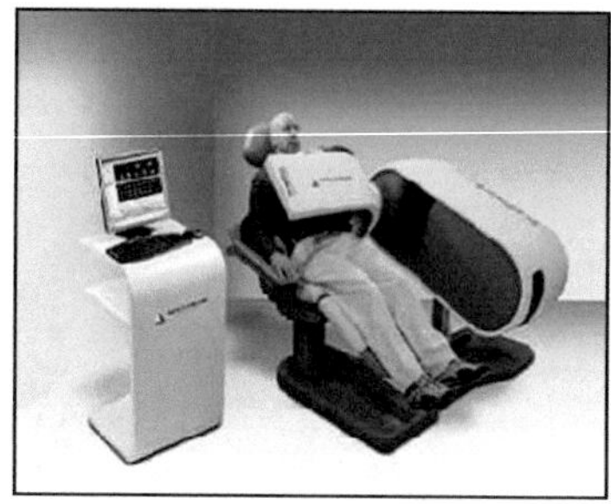

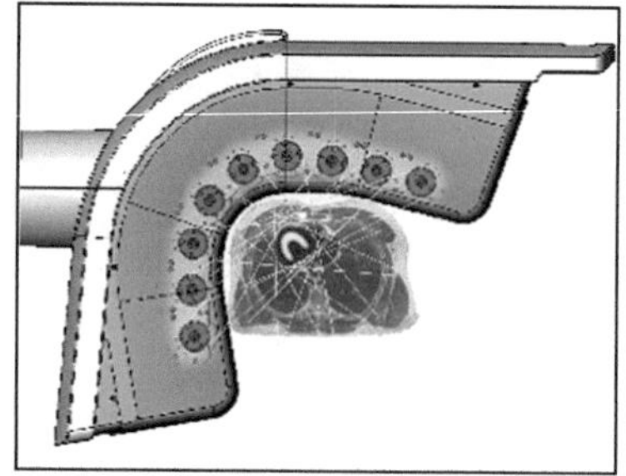

Figure 5.5 Example of system designed specifically for cardiac SPECT (D-SPECT, Spectrum Dynamics, Israel). Nine CZT detectors acquire counts during programmed rotation so as to maximise counts from the cardiac region. To optimise sensitivity, the rotation of each detector is programmed in a scan pattern that centres on the heart. Reproduced with permission from D-SPECT, Spectrum Dynamics, Israel.

brain studies on the basis of the recent resurgence of specific tracers for neurological applications (e.g. various studies of receptor systems and amyloid deposits).

Recent PET developments

Of particular interest in PET has been the reintroduction of systems that utilise time-of-flight information. When the two annihilation photons are emitted, they both travel at the speed of light but, depending on the location of the annihilation, there will be a time difference in their detection. If this time difference could be measured accurately, the exact location of the annihilation could be determined without reconstruction. However with current technology the measurement of this small time difference is limited (500–600 picoseconds) so the location can only be estimated to within around 8 cm. Nevertheless this additional information can be incorporated in the reconstruction model with a resultant improvement in signal-to-noise ratio, which is particularly beneficial in large patients (where statistical quality can be a concern). Time-of-flight PET systems were built in the 1980s based on barium fluoride detectors, but these tended to be unstable; more recently the main suppliers have released systems based on newer detector materials (e.g. LYSO) (Karp *et al.* 2008).

A further development of interest is the recent introduction of PET/MRI, at this time specifically for application in the brain. Several preclinical systems have been designed before (Shao *et al.* 1997) that exploit the use of readout technologies that, unlike conventional PM tubes, can operate near or within strong magnetic fields employed by MRI systems. Optical fibres are also used to transfer the scintillation light from detectors outside the main magnetic field prior to decoding. The first commercial human system was released in 2007. Work is also in progress to develop SPECT/MRI systems.

References

Anger HO (1958). Scintillation camera. *Rev Sci Instrum* 29: 27–33.

Bailey DL (1998). Transmission scanning in emission tomography. *Eur J Nucl Med* 25: 774–787.

Bailey DL *et al.*, eds. (2005). *Positron Emission Tomography: Basic Sciences*. London: Springer.

Beekman F, van der Have F (2007). The pinhole: gateway to ultra-high-resolution three-dimensional radionuclide imaging. *Eur J Nucl Med Mol Imaging* 34: 151–161.

Beyer T *et al.* (2000). A combined PET/CT scanner for clinical oncology. *J Nucl Med* 41: 1369–1379.

Buvat I *et al.* (1994). Scatter correction in scintigraphy; the state-of-the-art. *Eur J Nucl Med* 21: 675–694.

Chang LT (1978). A method for attenuation correction in radionuclide computed tomography. *IEEE Trans Nucl Sci* 25: 638–643.

Cherry SR *et al.* (2003). *Physics in Nuclear Medicine*. New York: Elsevier Health Sciences.

Fulton R *et al.* (1994). Use of 3D reconstruction to correct for patient motion in SPECT. *Phys Med Biol* 39: 563–574.

Hudson HM, Larkin RS (1994). Accelerated image reconstruction using ordered subsets of projection data. *IEEE Trans Med Imaging* 13: 601–609.

Hutton BF *et al.* (1997). A clinical perspective of accelerated statistical reconstruction. *Eur J Nucl Med* 24: 797–808.

Hutton BF *et al.* (2006) Iterative reconstruction methods. In: Zaidi H, ed. *Quantitative Analysis in Nuclear Medicine Imaging*. New York: Springer, 107–140.

Karp JS *et al.* (2008). Benefit of time-of-flight in PET: experimental and clinical results. *J Nucl Med* 49: 462–470.

King MA *et al.* (2004). Attenuation, scatter and spatial resolution compensation in SPECT. In: Wernick MN, Aarsvold JN, eds. *Emission Tomography: The Fundamentals of SPECT and PET*. San Diego, CA: Elsevier.

Lange K, Carson R (1984). EM Reconstruction algorithms for emission and transmission tomography. *J Comput Assist Tomogr* 8: 306–316.

Moses WW, Shah KS (2005). Potential for $RbGd_2Br_7$:Ce, $LaBr_3$:Ce, $LaBr_3$:Ce, and LuI_3:Ce in nuclear medical imaging. *Nucl Instrum Methods Phys Res A* 537: 317–320.

O'Connor MK, Kemp B (2002). A multicenter evaluation of commercial attenuation compensation techniques in cardiac SPECT using phantom models. *J Nucl Cardiol* 9: 361–376.

Ogawa K *et al.* (1994). Accurate scatter correction in single photon emission CT. *Ann Nucl Med Sci* 7: 145–150.

Patton JA *et al.* (2007). Recent technologic advances in nuclear cardiology. *J Nucl Cardiol* 14: 501–513.

Pichler BJ, Ziegler SI (2004). Photodetectors. In: Wernick MN, Aarsvold JN, eds. *Emission Tomography: The Fundamentals of SPECT and PET*. San Diego, CA: Elsevier.

Rowland DJ, Cherry SR (2008). Small-animal preclinical nuclear medicine instrumentation and methodology. *Semin Nucl Med* 38: 209–222.

Shao Y *et al.* (1997). Simultaneous PET and MR imaging. *Phys Med Biol* 42: 1965–1970.

Tsui BMW, Frey E (2006). Analytic image reconstruction methods. In: Zaidi H, ed. *Quantitative Analysis in Nuclear Medicine Imaging*. New York: Springer, 82–106.

Tsui BMW *et al.* (1994). The importance and implementation of accurate 3D compensation methods for quantitative SPECT. *Phys Med Biol* 39: 509–530.

Wagenaar DJ (2004). CdTe and CdZnTe semiconductor detectors for nuclear medicine imaging. In: Wernick MN, Aarsvold JN, eds. *Emission Tomography: The Fundamentals of SPECT and PET*. San Diego, CA: Elsevier.

Wirrwar A *et al.* (2001). High resolution SPECT in small animal research. *Rev Neurosci* 12: 187–193.

Zaidi H, Koral K (2006). Scatter correction strategies in emission tomography. In: Zaidi H, ed. *Quantitative Analysis in Nuclear Medicine Imaging*. New York: Springer, 205–235.

Further reading

Wernick MN, Aarsvold JN, eds. (2004). *Emission Tomography: The Fundamentals of SPECT and PET*. San Diego, CA: Elsevier.

Zaidi H, ed. (2006). *Quantitative Analysis in Nuclear Medicine Imaging*. New York: Springer.

6

Production of radionuclides

Steve McQuarrie

Introduction

No textbook on radiopharmacy would be complete without a chapter on alchemy. This chapter is where the reader will find information on the conversion of one element into another and where the 'radio' part of radiopharmacy comes from. Although one of alchemy's best known goals was the transmutation of lead into gold, it was the discovery of radioactivity by Becquerel in 1896 and the Curies in 1898 and Ernest Rutherford's series of experiments on radioactivity in 1911 that led to the realisation that elements could be transmuted. In 1919 Rutherford managed to bombard a nitrogen nucleus with an alpha (α-)particle (from radon), transforming it into a nucleus of oxygen followed by the emission of a proton (Rutherford 1919). The dream of medieval alchemists, the transmutation of the chemical elements, had finally been achieved.

The key to producing radioactive elements, or radionuclides, is to find a mechanism for altering the nucleus of an atom to make it unstable. Through the process of radioactive decay, the radionuclide returns to a stable form, and it is this process of decay that allows the radiopharmaceutical scientist to visualise the location of the radionuclide (and hopefully, the molecule to which it is attached). Two methods for producing radionuclides will be discussed in this chapter; a nuclear reactor in which a neutron is used to initiate the required nuclear reaction, and a cyclotron in which a charged particle such as a proton is added into a nucleus, transforming it into the desired radioactive product.

The material in this chapter should provide sufficient information for the radiopharmaceutical scientist to:

- understand the principles of nuclear transformation
- understand and work with equations that can be used to determine how much of a radionuclide can be produced
- understand the principles of cyclotron operation as they apply to radionuclide production
- evaluate the specifications of a cyclotron in order to select the most appropriate one for their anticipated needs
- understand the principles of radionuclide production in a nuclear reactor and
- understand and evaluate some of the confounding issues related to radionuclide production in both a nuclear reactor and a cyclotron.

Nuclear reactions

The production of fluorine-18 (^{18}F) by a cyclotron will be used as an example, in which a proton is introduced into the nucleus of the non-radioactive element oxygen-18 (^{18}O). This nuclear reaction is typically written in short hand as $^{18}O(p, n)^{18}F$ which may be translated as:

target atom(incoming particle,
outgoing particle)product atom

Several factors dictate how much ^{18}F can be produced from ^{18}O and these include the number of target atoms, the number of protons, the energy of the proton, and the probability of occurrence of the desired nuclear reaction.

Based on the relationship between the proton energy and the production cross-section described below, it is important to select a proton energy that will maximise the production of the desired product while avoiding the production of unwanted contaminants. However, other factors must be considered when selecting the energy of the bombarding particle. The first is based on the fact that both the bombarding particle (proton) and the target nucleus (^{18}O) are positively charged, so that the incoming particle must have sufficient energy to overcome this electrostatic repulsion or Coulomb barrier. The Coulomb barrier is related to the charge of the two particles and is given by the equation:

$$B = \frac{Zze;^2}{4\pi\varepsilon_0 R} \tag{6.1}$$

where B = the Coulomb barrier for the reaction, Z = the atomic number of the target, z = the atomic number of the bombarding particle, e = the elementary charge (1.6×10^{-19} C), ε_0 = the permittivity of free space ($8.854 \times 10^{-12}\,C^2\,N^{-1}\,m^{-2}$), and R = the distance between the charges (m).

The distance between the charges (R) can be estimated from the experimentally determined nuclear radius $\langle R_0\ (a^{1/3})\rangle$, where $R_0 = 1.2 \times 10^{-15}$ m, so that $R = R_0(A^{1/3} + a^{1/3})$ where A = the mass number of the target and a = mass number of the bombarding particle. The conversion from joules to MeV is $1\,J = 6.24 \times 10^{12}$ MeV. Equation (6.1) can then be simplified as:

$$B = \frac{1.2\,Zz}{(A^{1/3} + a^{1/3})}\ \text{MeV} \tag{6.2}$$

Example 1

In the case $^{18}O(p, n)^{18}F$, the Coulomb barrier is

$$\begin{aligned} B &= \frac{1.2 \times 8 \times 1}{(18^{1/3} + 1^{1/3})}\ \text{MeV} \\ B &= 2.65\ \text{MeV} \end{aligned} \tag{6.3}$$

However, nuclear reactions can take place for proton energies below this value due to an effect known as quantum mechanical tunnelling (Heyde 2004).

A second effect that relates proton energy to the likelihood of a particular nuclear reaction occurring is the conservation of energy. In any nuclear reaction, the total energy must be conserved, which means that the total energy, including the rest mass of the starting products (^{18}O and p) must equal the total energy, including the rest mass of the final products (^{18}F and n). The observed change in energy is called the Q-value and its value may be positive or negative. If the sum of the rest masses of the starting products exceeds that of the rest masses of the final products, the Q-value of the reaction is positive, with the decrease in rest mass being converted into a gain in kinetic energy. The mass deficit energy equivalent Q is given by:

$$Q\ (\text{MeV}) = 931.494\ 043\ \Delta M \tag{6.4}$$

where

$$\Delta M = (m_b + M_T) - (m_e + M_p)\ \text{amu} \tag{6.5}$$

and m_b is the bombarding particle mass, M_T is the target mass, M_P is the product mass, m_e is the emitted particle mass.

If $Q < 0$ the reaction is endoergic; conversely, if $Q > 0$ the reaction is exoergic. If the reaction is endoergic, then sufficient energy must be added to the nuclear reaction in an amount greater than the Q-value. The threshold for an endoergic nuclear reaction will then be the Coulomb barrier energy plus the Q-value. If the reaction is exoergic, energy is released as a result of the nuclear reaction and the threshold energy will be just that of the Coulomb barrier.

Example 2

Calculation of the Q-value for the $^{18}O(p, n)^{18}F$ reaction (data from NNDC 2003a and NIST 2010) using

$$\begin{aligned} m_b &= 1.007\,825\,032\ \text{amu} \\ M_T &= 17.999\,160\,4\ \text{amu} \\ M_P &= 18.000\,937\,7\ \text{amu} \\ m_e &= 1.008\,664\,915\,60\ \text{amu} \end{aligned}$$

Using the expanded form of equation (6.4):

$$\begin{aligned} Q\,(\mathrm{MeV}) &= 931.494\,043\,[(m_b + M_T) - (m_e + M_p)] \\ &= 931.494\,043\,(19.006\,985\,43 - 19.009\,602\,62) \\ &= -2.44\,\mathrm{MeV} \end{aligned} \tag{6.6}$$

A service offered by the National Nuclear Data Center at Brookhaven National Laboratory provides an interactive online estimate of Q-values (NNDC 2003b).

The threshold energy for the ^{18}O(p, n)^{18}F nuclear reaction is made up of both the Coulomb barrier (2.65 MeV) and, because this reaction is endoergic, the Q-value (2.44 MeV), which must also be taken into account. The bombarding proton should then be at least 5.1 MeV in order for this reaction to be energetically possible. However, due to quantum mechanical tunnelling through the Coulomb barrier, this energy requirement is lower and the accepted value for the threshold energy is 2.574 MeV (NNDC 2003b). For a more comprehensive description of the nuclear reaction threshold, including a discussion on the conservation of momentum, the reader is referred to the introductory book by Heyde (2004).

Yield of a nuclear reaction

This section illustrates the methodology used to determine the amount of a radionuclide that can be produced. An equation will be developed that will permit the user to estimate the yield of a nuclear reaction; the production of ^{18}F via the ^{18}O(p, n)^{18}F reaction will again be used to illustrate the application of this equation.

The nuclear cross-section may be described as the probability that the desired nuclear reaction will occur. If one visualises a proton as a sphere and the ^{18}O nucleus as another sphere, then it is possible to imagine that a nuclear reaction can only occur if these two spheres overlap. Once this happens, an intermediate nucleus comes into existence that has the mass of the target nucleus plus the mass of the bombarding particle. This intermediate nucleus or compound nucleus exists as an excited nucleus that can decay in a variety of ways; in this example, through the emission of a neutron. This whole process occurs over a very short time and appears instantaneous to the observer. This probability is expressed in units of barns, where 1 barn $= 1 \times 10^{-24}\,\mathrm{cm}^2$. This expression arose from the fact that the probability for the proton to interact with the ^{18}O atom is proportional to the cross-sectional area of its nucleus, which when compared to the size of the proton, appeared 'as big as a barn'. In the case of the ^{18}O(p, n)^{18}F reaction, the maximum cross-section is about 500 mb or $0.5 \times 10^{-24}\,\mathrm{cm}^2$ (Figure 6.1). The peaks in this figure represent an increased likelihood of ^{18}F formation at a particular energy but the overall production yield is related to the area under this curve when integrated from the maximum energy of the proton entering the ^{18}O target to the reaction threshold (2.574 MeV). In order to estimate the amount of ^{18}F that can be made, the following series of equations are introduced to illustrate the important considerations when designing a particular production scheme. These will then be simplified in order to make them more accessible for radiopharmaceutical applications.

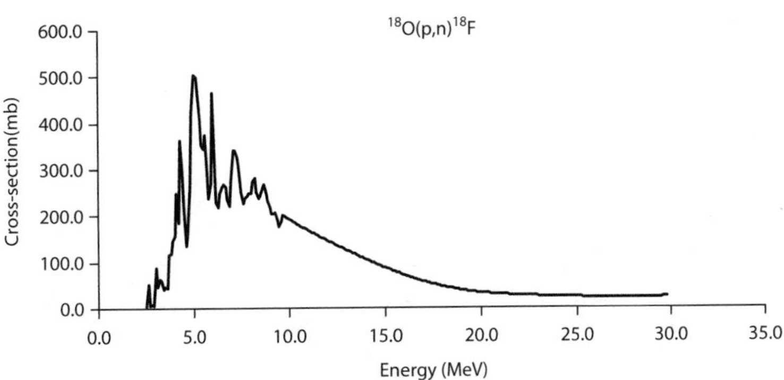

Figure 6.1 Cross-section for the ^{18}O(p,n)^{18}F reaction. (Data from IAEA-1.)

The rate of production for a radionuclide depends on several factors including the nuclear reaction cross-section (a function of bombarding particle energy), the energy of the bombarding particle, the number of bombarding particles and the thickness of the target (number of target atoms). The rate of production (R) is expressed by:

$$R = n_t I \int_{E_f}^{E_0} \frac{\sigma(E)}{\mathrm{d}E/\mathrm{d}x} \mathrm{d}E \qquad (6.7)$$

where R = the number of nuclei (^{18}F) formed per second; n_t = the number of target atoms (^{18}O) in nuclei per cm^2; I = the bombarding particle flux (p) per second and is related to beam current; $\sigma(E)$ = the reaction cross-section, or probability of interaction, expressed in cm^2, and is a function of energy (see Figure 6.1); E = the energy of the bombarding particles; x = the distance travelled by the bombarding particle; the integration is carried out from the initial energy (E_0) to the final energy (E_f) of the bombarding particle along its path through the target atoms; and dE = the differential loss in energy and dx = the differential distance travelled by the particle.

However, when radionuclides are made, they are also decaying. This leads to a modification of equation (6.7) to include a decay term ($-\lambda N$) so that the overall rate of production is given by:

$$A(t) = n_t I \int_{E_f}^{E_0} \frac{\sigma(E)}{\mathrm{d}E/\mathrm{d}x} \mathrm{d}E - \lambda N \qquad (6.8)$$

where $A(t)$ = the activity at time t; t = the time since the start of bombardment or irradiation time; λ = the decay constant of the product; and N = the number of radioactive nuclei produced in the target.

To simply this relation and make it more generally usable, equation (6.8) will be modified to:

$$Y_{\mathrm{EOB}} = A_{\mathrm{SAT}} I (1 - e^{-\lambda t}) \qquad (6.9)$$

The term I in equation (6.9) represents the number of bombarding particles (protons) in the production equation and, for the purposes of this equation is measured as beam current in microamperes (μA). A_{SAT} represents the maximum amount of activity that could be produced if you irradiated the target forever; in practice irradiating a target for 3 half-lives will produce 87.5% of this maximum. A_{SAT} is obtained by the integration of equation (6.7) over the energy range experienced by the proton as it loses energy during its pass through the target. Rather than performing this integration, its value can be read off a graph (or table) that has been previously calculated. (For ^{18}O(p,n)^{18}F see http://www-nds.iaea.or.at/medical/o8p18f0.html.) The relevant data for the ^{18}O(p, n)^{18}F reaction are shown Figure 6.2. The final term ($1 - e^{-\lambda t}$) is often referred to as the saturation factor and accounts for the fact that while the radionuclide is being produced, it is also decaying away.

Going back to our example for the production of ^{18}F, a sample calculation will be performed to calculate the amount of ^{18}F that can be made from irradiating 95% enriched ^{18}O-water using 50 μA of 16 MeV protons. Assumptions are that all of the protons are stopped within the water target and the irradiation time is 1 hour. Use equation (6.9) to

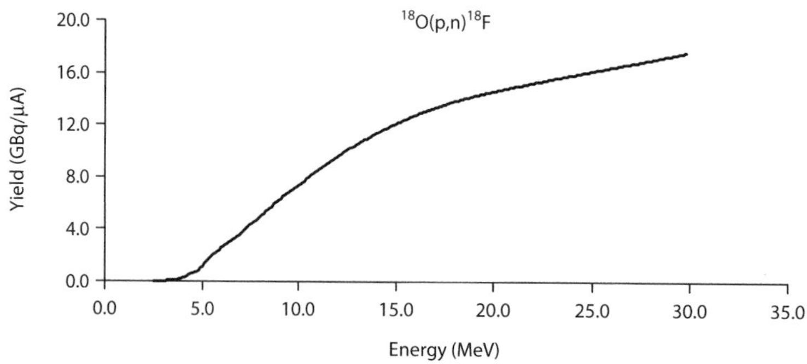

Figure 6.2 Yield (in GBq/μA) calculated from the recommended cross-sections for the ^{18}O(p,n)^{18}F reaction. (Data from IAEA-2.)

calculate the yield, where $A_{SAT} = 12.8$ GBq/μA (from IAEA-2), $I = 50$ μA, $\lambda = \ln 2/(\text{half-life } ^{18}\text{F}) = 0.693/110$ minutes $= 0.0063\ \text{min}^{-1}$.

$$Y_{EOB} = 12.8\ \text{GBq}/\mu\text{A} \times 50\ \mu\text{A}\ (1 - e^{-0.0063\times 60}) \\ = 201\ \text{GBq}$$

(Note: the exponent must be dimensionless – use the same time units for both λ and t.)

To take into account that the target is only 95% enriched in ^{18}O, the answer must be multiplied by 0.95, yielding 191 GBq. The 5% ^{16}O in the target material will lead to a radioactive contaminant ^{13}N via the ^{16}O(p,α)^{13}N reaction. This radionuclidic impurity is generally not an issue because (1) it decays away with a shorter half-life (10 minutes) and (2) subsequent radiochemical trapping and syntheses are designed for fluorine chemistry so that ^{13}N will not be incorporated into the final radiopharmaceutical.

Some of the commonly used radionuclides are listed in Table 6.1, including their half-lives and the usual nuclear reactions used in their production. Note that when ^{123}I is produced from ^{124}Xe, this is a multistage reaction in which first ^{123}Xe is made and collected followed by its decay into ^{123}I, the desired product. Ease of recovery and separation from other unwanted radioisotopes of iodine are the main advantages of this production route.

A discussion of the source of bombarding protons and a short review of the physical aspects of the target environment appear in the next section.

Cyclotrons

In the previous section we saw the necessity for a source of high-energy charged particles that are required to initiate the nuclear reaction leading to the desired radionuclide. These particles are raised to the appropriate energy by causing them to travel at very high speeds and they are then smashed into a target nucleus with enough energy to transform it, typically into the desired radioactive nucleus. The machines that perform this feat are collectively known as particle accelerators and all particle accelerators operate on the principle of the interaction between electrical charges. Like charges repel each other and unlike charges attract. As most radionuclides produced for medical applications use cyclotrons to provide the high-energy bombarding particles, the following discussion will focus on their design and operation.

A cyclotron operates on the principle of the attraction and repulsion of charged particles. A simplified depiction of a cyclotron will be used to illustrate the basic principles behind its operation using a proton as the accelerated bombarding particle. The acceleration of the proton takes place inside the cyclotron where the accelerating force is generated by the cyclotron 'dees' (Ds) (Figure 6.3). Imagine a proton that has been introduced into the middle of the cyclotron and that one of the dees is positively charged and the other negatively charged. The positively (or negatively) charged proton will be attracted to the oppositely charged dee and repelled from the like-charged dee,

Table 6.1 Common radionuclides produced by charged-particle accelerators

Radionuclide	Half-life	Production reaction	Radionuclide	Half-life	Production reaction
^{11}C	20.3 min	^{14}N(p,α)	^{64}Cu	12.7 h	^{64}Ni(p,n) ^{64}Zn(α,2n)
^{13}N	9.97 min	^{16}O(p,α)	^{86}Y	14.7 h	^{86}Sr(p,n)
^{15}O	2.03 min	^{15}N(p,n) ^{14}N(d,2n)	^{123}I	13.2 h	^{123}Te(p,n) ^{124}Xe(p,pn) → ^{123}Xe → ^{123}I
^{18}F	110 min	^{18}O(p,n) ^{nat}Ne(d,α)	^{124}I	4.2 d	^{124}Te(p,n)

d, day; h, hour; min, minute.

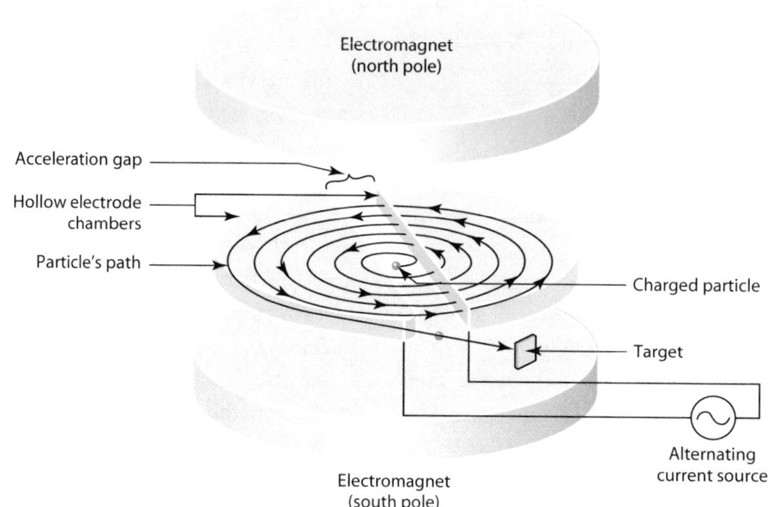

Figure 6.3 Schematic diagram of a cyclotron illustrating a simplified dee structure (shown as hollow electrode chambers). The magnetic field is in the vertical plane to the circulating particles.

during which the proton will gain energy. If this process is repeated many times, the proton will gain the necessary energy to cause the nuclear reaction. The energy gained from each push/pull is related to the magnitude of the electric charge on each of the dees and the charge of the accelerated particle. However, the accelerated proton will travel in a straight line and would exit the cyclotron after only one push/pull cycle, in this case not having gained enough energy to cause a nuclear reaction.

Ernest Lawrence came to the rescue to solve this dilemma when, in 1929 after reading about the work of a Norwegian engineer, Rolf Wideröe (Waloschek 2002), Lawrence was inspired to think about how one could use the same accelerating potential multiple times instead of just once. He solved this problem when he realised that in order for this acceleration process to continue, the proton must be bent within the cyclotron in order to experience another round of acceleration. Lawrence thought to use a magnetic field to force the proton into a circular path, leading it through the dees many times until it had reached the appropriate energy to cause a nuclear reaction.

Lawrence started construction on his cyclotron in early 1930, and in January 1931 Lawrence and his graduate student, M. Stanley Livingston met with their first success (Lawrence, Livingston 1932). The first cyclotron was about 4.5 inches (~11.5 cm) in diameter and used a potential of 1800 volts to accelerate hydrogen ions up to energies of 80 000 electronvolts (eV). In summer 1931 they built an 11-inch (~28 cm) cyclotron that achieved particle energy of a million electronvolts. Ernest Lawrence was awarded the 1939 Nobel Prize in Physics 'for the invention and development of the cyclotron and for results obtained with it, especially with regard to artificial radioactive elements'. The modern cyclotrons used for the production of medically useful radionuclides are based on these same design principles and today produce proton beams with energies that typically range from 10 to 19 million electronvolts (MeV).

How does it all work? A brief description of the acceleration process is given next in order to provide an understanding of another critical aspect of a cyclotron: the radiofrequency field used to push/pull the protons around the inside of the cyclotron. Lawrence realised that if a constant accelerating voltage were used on the dees then the acceleration process would stop after one period when the positively charged proton approached the positively charged dee (and was repelled instead of experiencing further acceleration). He realised that the push/pull force exerted by the dees must be timed such that as the protons cross the space between the dees, the accelerating potential will change in a manner to keep the acceleration process going. A radiofrequency field is used to provide this ever-changing push/pull on the proton and is timed to provide the appropriate acceleration across the dee gap where the acceleration takes place. A typical value of the dee voltage is 50 kV so that the proton would receive $2 \times 50\,\text{kV} = 100\,\text{kV}$ of acceleration push/pull per orbit. For the proton to reach an energy of 16 MeV under these conditions, the proton would stay in the cyclotron for 160 orbits.

This acceleration process takes place in high vacuum so that the protons being accelerated will not collide with gas molecules inside the cyclotron, which would prevent their further acceleration and ultimately remove their potential to produce radionuclides. Cyclotrons typically operate under vacuum conditions in the range of 1×10^{-6} torr, where 1 torr = 1 mmHg = 133.322 Pa.

Once the proton has reached the appropriate energy it is usually steered out of the cyclotron towards the target where the radionuclide is to be produced, such as an ^{18}O target for the production of ^{18}F. As negative-ion cyclotrons are commonly used for the production of medical radionuclides, the extraction process for this type of cyclotron will be briefly discussed. The negatively charged ions (H atoms with 2 electrons) are constrained by the magnetic field to move in a circular path within the cyclotron; however, if the negatively charged ions were to become positively charged, the magnet field would have the reverse effect and cause the ions to bend in the opposite direction and be steered out of the cyclotron. These electrons are removed by passing the ion beam through a very thin carbon foil, leaving only the positively charged protons. After the protons leave the cyclotron, they are directed to the target where the appropriate nuclear reactions are initiated to produce the required radioactive products (such as ^{18}F).

How one gets the protons into the cyclotron in such a manner that leads to their efficient acceleration is a problem whose solution is a closely guarded secret of the major cyclotron manufacturers. In many cases this is a two-step process, the first being the production of protons from hydrogen gas, followed by an extraction process in which the protons are directed into the cyclotron. In general terms the source of protons is provided by hydrogen gas that is 'leaked' into the high vacuum environment of the cyclotron. This hydrogen must first be given a charge so that it can be steered and focused by electric and magnetic fields (remember that it is possible to control the path of particles if they are electrically charged). In the case of negative-ion cyclotrons (the most common type used for radionuclide production), the hydrogen molecule is converted into atomic hydrogen and the atoms are given a second electron by streaming the gas through an electron beam, perpendicular to the flow of gas. The two common types of ion sources used to produce protons for a cyclotron are the hot filament Penning ion gauge (PIG) type (Rickey, Smythe 1962) and the cusp type (Leung *et al.* 1983).

The second step involves removing the protons from the ion source and directing them into the cyclotron so that they can be accelerated to the appropriate energy. In the case of an external ion source, the protons enter in at right angles to the accelerating region of the cyclotron, and must be bent into the plane of acceleration and then given a push to get them moving in the right direction. Conceptually this is similar to a child sliding down a circular slide; their vertical potential energy at the top of the slide is converted into horizontal velocity at the bottom of the slide (Figure 6.4). Once the proton enters the gap between the dees, it is accelerated as described above. A high capacity vacuum pump in the ion source removes the uncharged gas, and helps maintain the high vacuum in the cyclotron.

Inside the cyclotron target is where all the action takes place. It is here that the transmutation process manifests itself, where the target atoms are transformed into the desired radionuclides. If we

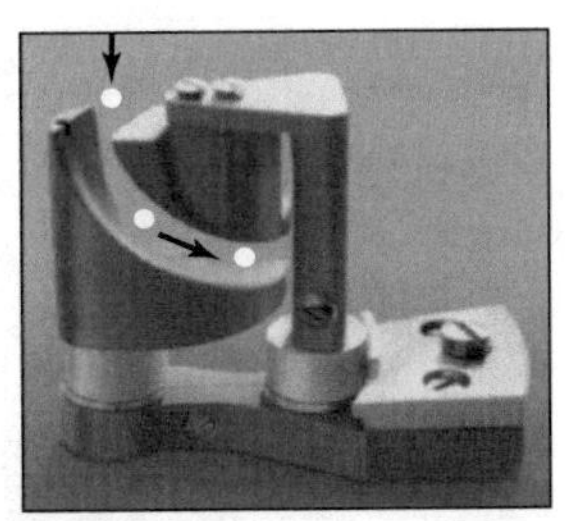

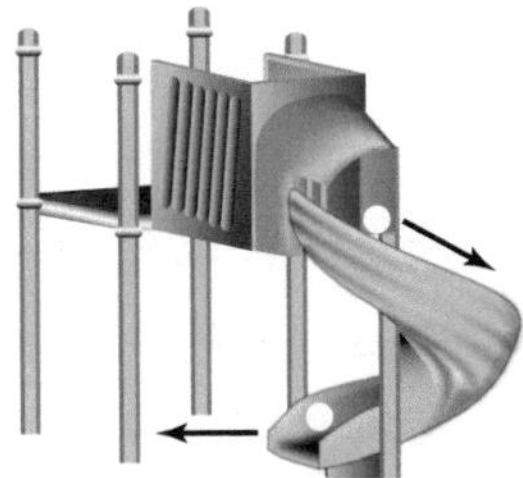

Figure 6.4 The drawing on the left illustrates a proton (·) entering from the top and being electromagnetically steered into horizontal plane where it can be accelerated by the dees. The schematic diagram of a slide on the right shows a proton sliding down to illustrate this change in direction process.

understand that the purpose of a cyclotron target is to ensure that the conditions for the required nuclear reaction are optimal, then the following conditions must be met. The target body housing the target atoms should be designed to keep the target atoms in the proton beam during irradiation and facilitate the removal of the radioactive products at the end of bombardment. The target body should be constructed from a material that will not react with either the target atoms or the resulting radionuclide(s) that are produced. The target body should be capable of withstanding the expected increase in temperature and pressure experienced during irradiation. For example, if a 15 MeV proton beam at 100 μA was absorbed in the target, this would impart heat energy at a rate of about 1.5 kW. Thus, efficient cooling of the target is mandatory to prevent molecular dispersion in gas targets, liquid targets from boiling away, or solid targets from melting; all these processes tend to remove the target atoms from the proton beam and hence negatively impact production yield.

A schematic diagram of a cyclotron target used to produce ^{18}F is shown in Figure 6.5. Several components illustrated in this figure are common to most external targets:

- The vacuum foil (A) is used to separate the high vacuum in the cyclotron from the pressure inside the target. Design considerations usually demand that this foil be made as thin as possible to reduce the energy loss to the proton passing through it; these foils are usually cooled with helium gas. Because of its high tensile strength, a metal alloy known as Havar is usually used to make these thin foils. Some targets may also have a target foil (B) to separate the target material from the helium foil cooling subsystem.
- The target body holds the target atoms in such a way as to maximise the production and recovery of both the target material and the radionuclide. The target body must also be electrically isolated to permit assessment of the number of protons entering the target (the beam current). This parameter is used to optimise radionuclide production and to estimate to amount of the radionuclide being made.
- The recovery system is designed to remotely load and unload the targets for radiation safety considerations and to efficiently recover the sometimes expensive enriched target material. The recovery system is frequently connected directly to automated chemistry modules that are used to manufacture radiopharmaceuticals and at the same time recover the enriched target atoms.

When making ^{18}F from an ^{18}O-water target, each of the above considerations must be taken into account. Target bodies have been made from materials such as aluminium, silver, niobium and tantalum, each

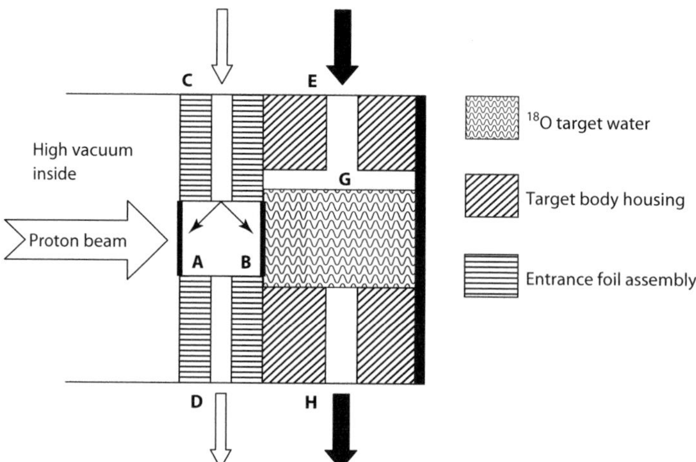

Figure 6.5 Schematic of an ^{18}O-water target used to produce ^{18}F; where A and B are the vacuum and target entrance foils, C and D are the helium cooling ports for the foils, E and H are the enriched water loading and unloading ports, respectively. G is the reflux headspace on top of the water target.

with its own advantages and disadvantages. Silver is a good choice for heat removal, but the target body requires more maintenance to remove chemical contaminants that can affect downstream chemistry. Niobium and tantalum are more inert and require much less maintenance but do not remove the heat produced during irradiation as efficiently. Most modern water targets for ^{18}F now use niobium targets as adequate heat removal can be achieved with high-flow water cooling. Note that all water targets use the in-target boiling/reflux method to optimise heat removal from the target (Berridge, Kjellstrom 1988) (G in Figure 6.5).

Another consideration that may impact on subsequent radiopharmaceutical labelling of bioactive compounds is that of chemical contaminants produced in the cyclotron target. For example, during the production of ^{18}F in an ^{18}O-water target, the formation of water-soluble contaminants has been observed, which affected the reactivity of ^{18}F and resulted in a decrease in labelling yield of radiopharmaceuticals (Kilbourn *et al.* 1985; Solin *et al.* 1988). In the last few years, refractory metals such as niobium and tantalum have been the materials of choice for chamber targets for the irradiation of aqueous targets. The use of these metals has lengthened the maintenance interval of targets without sacrificing the reactivity of fluoride (Zeisler *et al.* 2000; Berridge *et al.* 2002; Satyamurthy *et al.* 2002). Although entrance foils of these materials would be also favourable for the production of fluoride, the materials' weak mechanical properties limit their use as foils, making them unsuitable for the routine production of ^{18}F under pressurised conditions. One solution is the use of niobium-coated Havar foils for the production of reactive fluoride under high-power irradiation conditions (Wilson *et al.* 2008). These foils combine the robust mechanical properties of Havar with the excellent chemical inertness of niobium.

Nuclear reactors

Another method routinely used to produce radionuclides for the radiopharmaceutical sciences uses neutrons from a nuclear reactor to initiate the appropriate nuclear reaction. In this section a review of the production nuclear reactions, equations used to estimate their yield and some considerations on sample preparation are presented.

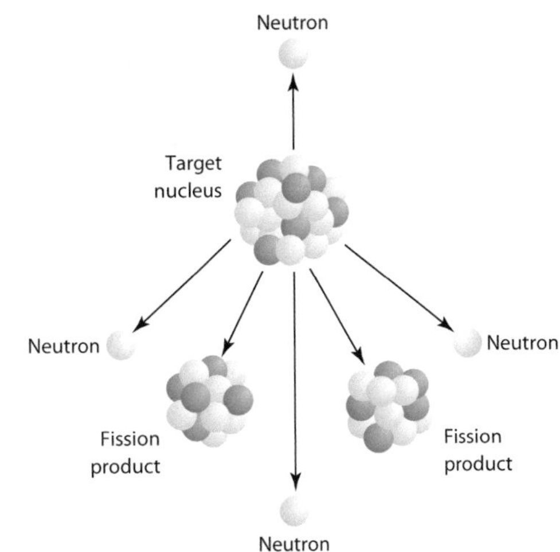

Figure 6.6 Schematic diagram of nuclear fission.

Nuclear reactors operate on the principle of nuclear fission (see Atomic Archive 2008), a process in which a fissionable nucleus such as ^{235}U is split into two smaller fragments resulting in the release of energy and 2 or 3 additional neutrons. This process is illustrated schematically in Figure 6.6. The resulting neutrons from this process can be used to initiate another nuclear reaction leading to the desired product, generally by the (n, γ) reaction. The other route used to obtain radionuclides from a nuclear reactor is based on the creation of radioactive fission products during the fission process (Figure 6.6). Both production methods, with selected examples will be reviewed in the following sections.

(n,γ) Production

The neutrons produced from the fission process yield on average about 2.3 neutrons per event. These neutrons are emitted over a large energy range; however, it is the very low-energy neutrons, known as thermal neutrons, which are most commonly used for this type of radionuclide production.

In addition to keeping the chain reaction going in the nuclear reactor, some of these thermal neutrons are used to produce radionuclides. In a manner analogous to that of charged particle production, a neutron (instead of a proton) is inserted into the target nucleus to create a radioisotope; this process most often results in the emission of a gamma (γ-) ray. This (n,γ) reaction is also commonly referred to as radiative capture. For example, a common radionuclide produced by the (n,γ) reaction is:

$$^{59}\text{Co}(\text{n},\gamma)^{60}\text{Co} \quad (\sigma = 36 \text{ barns})$$

Note that the product radionuclide is an isotope of the target element itself and hence cannot be chemically separated. Therefore, the specific activity is limited by the neutron flux available in the reactor.

A special case of the (n,γ) reaction can be used in which a short-lived intermediate radionuclide is produced which then decays into the desired product. An example of this is the production of ^{131}I through the irradiation of ^{130}Te. The simplified reaction equation is:

$$^{130}\text{Te}(\text{n},\gamma)^{131}\text{Te}; \quad \text{and then} \quad ^{131}\text{Te} \rightarrow {}^{131}\text{I}+\beta^-$$

In this case, the product can be chemically separated from the target as it is a different element from the starting material (Te). This two-stage method has the potential of producing carrier-free ^{131}I, leading to the added benefit of high-specific-activity radiopharmaceuticals. Table 6.2 lists some commonly used radionuclides in the radiopharmaceutical sciences that are produced in a nuclear reactor.

Yield calculations

As developed above, the probability of the desired radionuclide being formed is governed by the cross-section, the number of target nuclei and the number of bombarding particles, in this case neutrons. Similarly to the argument developed for protons, the neutron cross-section varies with the energy of the neutrons. In general, a slower-moving neutron has a greater probability of causing the desired nuclear reaction. These slow-moving neutrons are called thermal neutrons. The other difference when using neutrons to initiate the nuclear transformation is that there is no coulomb barrier to overcome.

Owing to the many confounding factors involved in the production of radionuclides using a nuclear reactor, only an estimate of the desired radionuclide yield (Y) will be presented (equation 6.10).

$$Y = N\phi\sigma(1 - e^{-\lambda t}) \tag{6.10}$$

where N = the total number of atoms present in the target; φ = the neutron flux in neutrons cm^{-2} s^{-1}; σ = the cross-section in cm^{-2}; t = time in seconds from the start of irradiation; and $(1 - e^{-\lambda t})$ is the decay term.

Equation (6.10) illustrates that, for a constant target size, the main factor affecting the yield of a radionuclide is the neutron flux, where typical neutron fluxes are around 10^{14} neutrons cm^{-2} s^{-1}.

In practice, the activity induced in the target under irradiation will be less than the activity calculated using equation (6.10). Some of the main confounding factors are summarised below.

- The self-shielding effect in the target.
  Self-shielding will reduce the product yield when the target has a high activation cross-section (σ) and the geometry of the target material is such that target nuclei in the centre of the sample experience a reduced neutron flux due to neutron absorption by the outer layer of target material.

Table 6.2 Common radionuclides produced in a nuclear reactor

Radionuclide	Half-life	Production reaction	Radionuclide	Half-life	Production reaction
^{3}H	12.3 y	^{6}Li(n,α)	^{131}I	8.0 d	^{130}Te(n,γ)^{131}Te → ^{131}I or ^{235}U(n,f)
^{14}C	5730 y	^{14}N(n,p)	^{133}Xe	5.3 d	^{35}U(n,f)
^{99}Mo	66 h	^{98}Mo(n,γ) or ^{235}U(n,f)	^{137}Cs	30.0 y	^{35}U(n,f)

α = alpha particle, n = neutron, p = proton, γ = gamma ray, f = fission.
y, year; d, day; h, hour.

- There is generally a variation in the neutron flux (φ) in the reactor, either due to core design or the effect of neighbouring samples.
- Transformation of the product due to subsequent neutron capture, particularly if this subsequent transformation has a high thermal neutron cross-section. This burn-up (or conversion to the product radionuclide) of the target nuclei may be a problem for the longer irradiation times of targets with high activation cross-sections, such as in the production of ^{60}Co. Irradiation times may be as long as 3 years.

The amount of activity actually produced in the target compared with the activity calculated using equation (6.10) depends on the cumulative effects of the confounding factors referred to above. The experimental yield should be empirically determined by a test irradiation.

Fission production

The other source of radionuclides arises from processing the fission products of ^{235}U. These fission products fall into two groups, one light group with mass number around 95 and a heavy group with mass number around 140. Analogously to the production of ^{131}I presented above, some fission products undergo successive decays, leading to production of the desired product via a fission-initiated decay chain. Some important fission products that have found widespread use in radiopharmacy are ^{90}Sr, ^{99}Mo and ^{131}I. Both ^{90}Sr and ^{99}Mo are used in the generator systems to produce ^{90}Y and ^{99m}Tc, respectively. These generator systems and their principles of operation are described elsewhere in this book.

Sample preparation

The target material should be selected to maximise the production of the desired radionuclide and may include enriched isotopes to reduce unwanted radionuclidic impurities. Selection of the physical form of the target should be based on optimising sample cooling and reducing neutron self-absorption effects while facilitating post-irradiation handling. Under irradiation conditions, the target material should be stable and not explosive, pyrophoric, or volatile in nature.

Encapsulation of the target material must take into account the physical parameters that exist in the high neutron flux in the special sample ports in the reactor core. The target material is encapsulated inside a container that will maintain an appropriate environment for the sample during irradiation; not only must it provide for physical containment of the sample during irradiation using a leak-tight seal but the capsule should also be chemically inert and easily cooled. Post-irradiation considerations include use of a container that does not become radioactive and is designed to facilitate handling of intensely radioactive targets.

Common containers are made from aluminium, Zircaloy and stainless steel. Aluminium is a popular choice because it has a low absorption cross-section for neutrons, and the radionuclides produced in aluminium are very short lived and contribute little to the radiation field from the irradiated target material. Aluminium also has good thermal conductivity, so that heat produced within the target is easily transferred to the coolant system.

One of the advantages of radionuclide production using a nuclear reactor is the ability to irradiate large volumes of target material in multiple irradiation sites. This leads to the production of large amounts of the radionuclide and, as the production of other radionuclides is possible in the other sites within the reactor, the simultaneous production of many different radionuclides is routinely achieved. This unique aspect of reactor production has led to the economic production of this class of radionuclides and their subsequent adoption as medical and industrial tracers.

Conclusion

This chapter has presented information that should be sufficient to allow the radiopharmacist to understand the basic concepts of how artificial radionuclides are produced. This information, coupled with the resource material from other chapters, should assist the radiopharmacist in the design of radiopharmaceutical synthesis methods and their ultimate use as tracers for better understanding of human physiology at the molecular level, in both healthy and disease states.

References

Atomic Archive (2008). *Nuclear Fission: Basics*. http://www.atomicarchive.com/Fission/Fission1.shtml (accessed 11 May 2010).

Berridge MS, Kjellstrom R (1988). Fluorine-18 production: new designs for [^{18}O] water targets. *J Labelled Comp Radiopharm* 26: 188.

Berridge MS, Voelker KW *et al.* (2002). High-yield, low pressure [^{18}O]water targets of titanium and niobium for [^{18}F] production on MC-17 cyclotrons. *Appl Radiat Isot* 57: 303–308.

Heyde K (2004). *Basic Ideas and Concepts in Nuclear Physics: An Introductory Approach*. Baton Rouge: CRC Press.

IAEA-1 (2003). *Recommended Cross Sections for $^{18}O(p,n)^{18}F$ reaction*. http://www-nds.iaea.or.at/medical/o8p18f0.html (accessed 11 May 2010).

IAEA-2 (1999). *Charged-particle Cross Section Database for Medical Radioisotope Production*. http://www-nds.iaea.or.at/medical/ (accessed 11 May 2010).

Kilbourn MR *et al.* (1985). An improved [^{18}O]water target for [^{18}F]fluoride production. *Int J Appl Radiat Isot* 36: 327–328.

Lawrence EO, Livingston MS (1932). The production of high speed light ions without the use of high voltages. *Phys Rev* 40: 19–35.

Leung KN *et al.* (1983). Extraction of volume produced H^- ions from a multicusp source. *Rev Sci Instrum* 54: 56–62.

NIST (2010). *Atomic Weights and Isotopic Compositions for All Elements*. Gaithersburg, MD: National Institute of Standards and Technology. http://physics.nist.gov/cgi-bin/Compositions/stand_alone.pl?ele=&all=all&ascii=ascii&isotype=all (accessed 11 May 2010).

NNDC (2003a). *Atomic Mass Adjustment*. Upton, NY: National Nuclear Data Center, Brookhaven National Laboratory. http://www.nndc.bnl.gov/amdc/masstables/Ame2003/mass.mas03 (accessed 11 May 2010).

NNDC (2003b). *Q-value Calculator*. Upton, NY: National Nuclear Data Center, Brookhaven National Laboratory. http://www.nndc.bnl.gov/qcalc/ (accessed 28 June 2010).

Rickey M E, R Smythe R (1962). The acceleration and extraction of negative ions in the C.U. cyclotron. *Nucl Instrum Methods* 18–19: 66–69. doi:10.1016/S0029-554X(62)80010-X.

Rutherford E (1919). Collision of alpha particles with light atoms; an anomalous effect in nitrogen. *The Philosophical Magazine* 37(222): 537–587.

Satyamurthy N *et al.* (2002). Tantalum [^{18}O]water target for the production of [^{18}F]fluoride with high reactivity for the preparation of 2-deoxy-2-[18F]fluoro-D-glucose. *Mol Imaging Biol* 4: 65–70.

Solin O *et al.* (1988). Production of [^{18}F] from water targets. Specific radioactivity and anionic contaminants. *Appl Radiat Isot* 39: 1065–1071.

Waloschek P, ed. (2002). *The Infancy of Particle Accelerators: Life and Work of Rolf Wideröe*. Braunschweig: Vieweg & Sohn/DESY-Report 94-039. http://www.waloschek.de/pedro/pedro-texte/wid-e-2002.pdf (accessed 11 May 2010).

Wilson JS *et al.* (2008). Niobium sputtered havar foils for the high power production of reactive [^{18}F]fluoride by proton irradiation of [^{18}O]H_2O targets. *Appl Radiat Isot* 66(5): 565–570.

Zeisler SK *et al.* (2000). A water-cooled spherical niobium target for the production of [^{18}F]fluoride. *Appl Radiat Isot* 53: 449–453.

SECTION B

Radiopharmaceutical chemistry

7

Radiopharmaceutical chemistry: basic concepts

Philip J Blower

Introduction

A radiopharmaceutical is essentially a partnership between two components – a radionuclide providing the signal or cytotoxic effect, and a vehicle to deliver it selectively to a specific tissue in response to specific physiological conditions or gene expression patterns. The useful radionuclides come from all parts of the periodic table (see Figure 7.1), including the 'organic' elements characterised by covalent bonding (carbon, nitrogen, oxygen, phosphorus, sulfur, and the halogens) and all the metallic groups and periods including both transition and non-transition elements (Blower 2006). The types of molecules or targeting entities are also very wide-ranging and non-exclusive: we may be dealing with a small organic molecule, a metal coordination complex, a polymer, a particulate or nanoparticulate material, a biomolecule such as a protein, a peptide, a carbohydrate, a lipid, etc., or a combination of any of these. Multiplying these two sources of diversity generates a field of enormous breadth that cannot be covered fully in a specialist volume such as this. The purpose of this chapter is to provide an overview of the general concepts and principles that underpin radiopharmaceutical chemistry, with reference to other texts and reviews to provide background in specific areas as necessary. It is followed by a more detailed exposition of the chemistry of the key radionuclides.

The challenge for the radiopharmaceutical chemist is not only to make imaginative use of these diverse chemical resources to incorporate a suitable radionuclide into a suitable targeting vehicle (Blower 2006), but also to devise a methodology to make the synthesis of the radiopharmaceutical feasible under the rather restrictive conditions imposed by the radioactivity itself and the regulatory environment associated with the use of the materials in humans (Blower 2006).

In the radiopharmaceutical 'partnership', the role of the radionuclide in achieving selective, targeted delivery varies from peripheral to central. At one extreme, it may be merely a passenger with little influence on the targeting, as for example in bioconjugates such as radiolabelled monoclonal antibodies (Dearling, Pedley 2007; Goldenberg, Sharkey 2007). For the purposes of this chapter, this type of radiopharmaceutical is referred to as 'radionuclide-tagged'. At the other extreme, the radionuclide may be part of a

1	2	3	4	5	6	7	8	9	10	11	12	13	14	15	16	17	18
1 H																	2 He
3 Li	4 Be											5 B	6 C β^+	7 N β^+	8 O β^+	9 F β^+	10 Ne
11 Na	12 Mg											13 Al	14 Si	15 P T	16 S	17 Cl	18 Ar
19 K	20 Ca	21 Sc	22 Ti	23 V	24 Cr	25 Mn	26 Fe β^+	27 Co	28 Ni	29 Cu β^+T	30 Zn	31 Ga $\gamma\beta^+$	32 Ge	33 As β^+	34 Se γ	35 Br β^+T	36 Kr γ
37 Rb β^+	38 Sr T	39 Y T	40 Zr β^+	41 Nb	42 Mo	43 Tc $\gamma\beta^+$	44 Ru	45 Rh	46 Pd	47 Ag	48 Cd	49 In γ	50 Sn T	51 Sb	52 Te	53 I $\gamma\beta^+$T	54 Xe
55 Cs	56 Ba	57 La *	72 Hf	73 Ta	74 W	75 Re T	76 Os	77 Ir	78 Pt	79 Au	80 Hg	81 Tl γ	82 Pb T	83 Bi T	84 Po	85 At T	86 Rn
87 Fr	88 Ra T	89 Ac †															

*Lanthanides	57 La	58 Ce	59 Pr	60 Nd	61 Pm	62 Sm T	63 Eu	64 Gd	65 Tb T	66 Dy	67 Ho T	68 Er	69 Tm	70 Yb	71 Lu T
†Actinides	89 Ac	90 Th	91 Pa	92 U	93 Np	94 Pu	95 Am T	96 Cm	97 Bk	98 Cf	99 Es	100 Fm	101 Md	102 No	103 Lr

Figure 7.1 Periodic table showing main applications of radioisotopes. Useful radionuclides (shaded) are drawn from all sections of the periodic table. Some elements have radionuclides useful for multiple applications: γ – single-photon imaging; β^+ – PET imaging; T – radionuclide therapy. Therapeutic nuclides may be beta, alpha or secondary electron emitters, and may also give imageable emissions not shown.

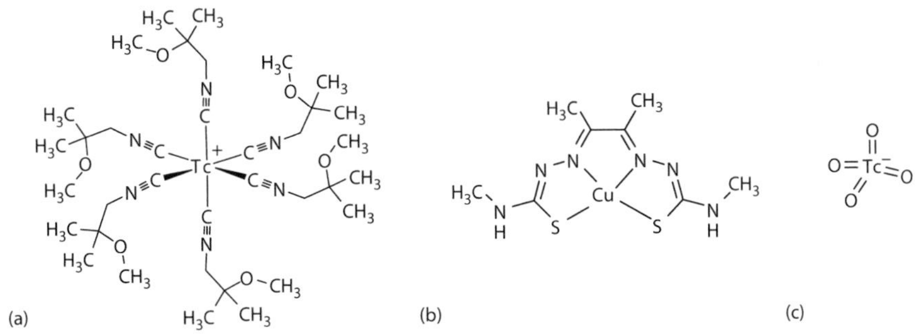

(a) (b) (c)

Figure 7.2 Examples of radionuclide-essential radiopharmaceuticals. (a) ^{99m}Tc-sestamibi: accumulation in mitochondria in the heart is associated with its positive charge (provided by the Tc^{+} ion) and its lipophilicity (provided by the alkyl groups of the ligands). (b) ^{64}Cu-ATSM: the redox properties, lipophilicity and planar shape (all provided by the copper^{2+} ion/ligand combination) are believed to govern its selective uptake in hypoxic cells (Vavere, Lewis 2007). (c) [^{99m}Tc]pertechnetate: accumulation in thyroid is due to the similarity with iodide, by virtue of the monoanionic charge and the size and close-to-spherical symmetry of the ion, making it a substrate of the thyroid sodium iodide symporter (Chung 2002; Lewis 2006).

construct whose targeting properties are intrinsic to, and dependent on, the chemistry of the inorganic radioactive element itself. Such radiopharmaceuticals are here referred to as 'radionuclide-essential'. This is the case, for example, in the copper bis(thiosemicarbazone) complexes for measuring blood flow and hypoxia (oxygen deficiency in tumours, heart disease, etc.) by PET, where the redox activity of the copper is the key to the targeting properties (Figure 7.2) (Vavere, Lewis 2007). Other radiopharmaceuticals lie in between or have features of both. For example, the radiolabel attached to a peptide radiopharmaceutical (Signore *et al.* 2001; Win *et al.* 2007; De León-Rodríguez, Kovacs 2008; Lucignani 2008) may not provide targeting but it may assist in other ways, e.g. by altering excretion pathways or enhancing stability against peptide degradation *in vivo*.

Organic versus metallic

To understand and contribute to radiopharmaceutical chemistry across its full breadth one requires an appreciation of basic organic and coordination chemistry as well as biological chemistry, and it is beyond the scope of this book to provide this background. The reader is referred to standard undergraduate-level organic, physical and inorganic chemistry text books for the necessary grounding. It is, however, worth drawing attention to the essential difference between the chemistry of the organic and metallic radionuclides as it affects their labelling chemistry. Those elements familiar in organic chemistry form single or multiple covalent bonds (four for carbon, three for nitrogen, two for oxygen, one for hydrogen and halogens) that are kinetically stable (e.g. to hydrolysis) and conform closely to well-established rules governing bond numbers, angles, etc. This allows us to visualise molecules as collections of atoms linked by well-defined covalent bonds represented by lines in the conventional structural representation (e.g. as in Figure 7.2). Labelling with carbon-11, by replacing a carbon-12 atom in an organic molecule with no alteration at all to the native structure, is the 'purest' form of radiolabelling. Labelling of carbon-based molecules with halogen radionuclides (group 17) usually involves slightly more structural modification: halogen radionuclides are typically incorporated into small organic molecules and biomolecules by the formation of a single covalent carbon–halogen bond, by replacement of a hydrogen atom or other organic element in the native structure. The change in structure is still relatively minor, although the modest change in size of the atoms and the dipoles of the bonds can have significant effects on the pharmacology (see Figure 7.3). By contrast, metallic radionuclides are not restricted to formation of simple single covalent bonds, and cannot simply replace another atom in an organic molecule or biomolecule. Often the metal bonding cannot readily be represented by lines representing covalent bonds. The metal typically has to be surrounded by, and bonded to, several atoms or groups (known as ligands).

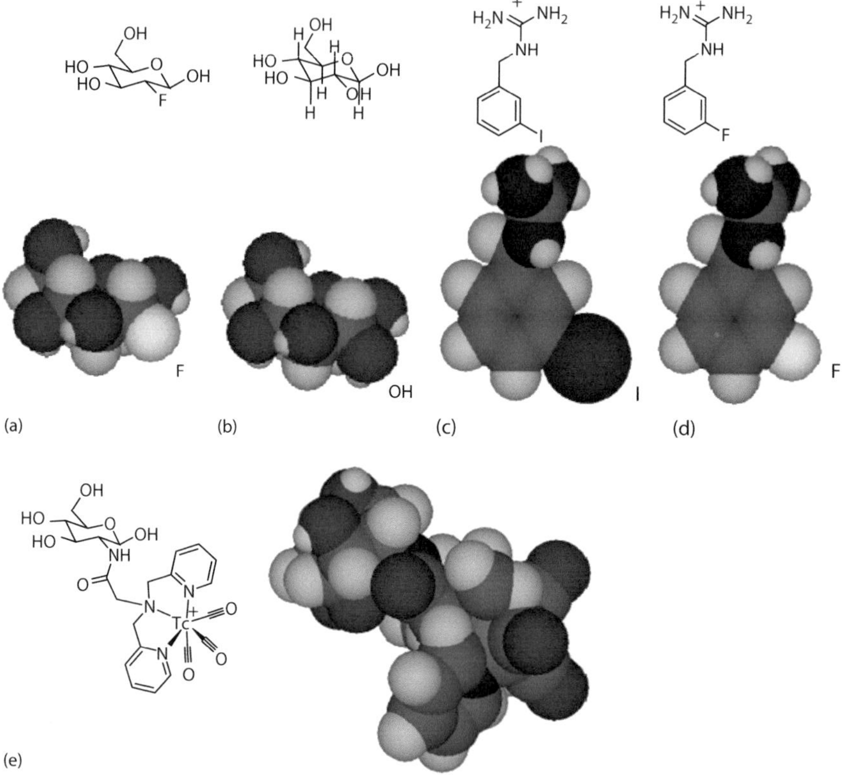

Figure 7.3 Examples of structures of small-molecule radiopharmaceuticals, using space-filling representations to illustrate the scale of modification to the molecules caused by introduction of the radiolabel. (a, b) 2-[^{18}F]Fluoro-2-deoxyglucose (FDG, a), in which an OH group in glucose (b) is replaced by fluoride, showing the comparable size of F and OH groups. (c, d) *meta*-[^{123}I] Iodobenzylguanidine (mIBG) and its ^{18}F-labelled analogue, showing the relative size of I and F atoms. (e) Glucose conjugate of a technetium tricarbonyl complex (Bowen, Orvig 2008), showing the overwhelming modification to glucose due to conjugation to the technetium complex compared to F-labelling in (a).

The metal is most often formally positively charged and the bonds are formed by donation of pairs of electrons by the ligands. Consequently, when a biological molecule is labelled with a metallic radionuclide, the metal brings with it a retinue of ligands, usually chelating ligands in the form of bifunctional chelators (see below; these are themselves usually organic molecules), leading to a much larger and more significant structural alteration on labelling (Figure 7.3). The kinetic stability with which these ligands are bound to the metal varies enormously between metals and types of ligands, and the oxidation state (a formality defining the number of electrons associated with the metal, and hence its charge) and coordination number (the number of ligands the metal prefers to bind) can vary, adding further to the complexity of design. Metallic radionuclides are thus often not suitable for labelling small molecules unless the metal is intrinsic to the design and function. The modification is less significant if the molecule to be labelled is a larger molecule such as a peptide or a protein, and this is typically the setting in which metallic radionuclides are used.

PET versus single-photon imaging

PET and SPECT rely on different nuclear decay phenomena leading to different detection and imaging physics, and consequently each has commonly discussed advantages and disadvantages in respect of resolution, sensitivity, quantification and so on (see other chapters). However, a more fundamental comparison arises from the *chemical* nature of the radionuclides concerned. The most important positron emitters are grouped in the top right-hand corner of the periodic table – C, N, O, F, covalently bonding elements that, as discussed above, are readily incorporated into small organic molecules like metabolites or drugs (Welch, Redvanly 2003; Schubiger *et al.* 2006). On the other hand, the most important gamma emitters are broadly speaking heavier elements, mostly metals, which are not. Rather, they are more suitable for use in labelling larger biomolecules (peptides and proteins) using bifunctional chelators. (Blower 2006; Dearling, Pedley 2007; Goldenberg, Sharkey 2007; Win *et al.* 2007; Bowen, Orvig 2008; De León-Rodríguez, Kovacs 2008; Lucignani 2008). On the whole, gamma-emitting radionuclides (with the exception of iodine-123) are chemically unsuitable for labelling small organic metabolites and drugs. To exploit the potential of molecular imaging with both small molecules and large biomolecules, both kinds of radioelements are needed. Therefore, both PET and SPECT imaging technologies are required, and they are mutually complementary.

Hydrophilic versus hydrophobic

The assembly of, and interactions between, biomolecules and other cellular structures (membranes, organelles, proteins, carbohydrates, DNA), and compartmentation of cell functions by lipid bilayer membranes, is rooted at some level in the contrast between hydrophilic and hydrophobic molecules or parts of molecules. In turn, hydrophilicity and hydrophobicity of molecules or parts of molecules originates in the dipolar nature, or lack of it, of the covalent bonds within them. Bonds between two atoms of very different electronegativity (e.g. C and O, H and O, H and N, H and F) are highly polarised because electron density is drawn towards the more electronegative atom. Thus these bonds are typically polarised with an accumulation of negative charge at the oxygen, nitrogen or fluorine. The dipole of one molecule is attracted to the dipole of another, creating a mechanism for non-covalent bonding between molecules (Figure 7.4). Hydrogen bonding is an extreme form of this.

These bonds are weaker and more kinetically labile than most intramolecular covalent bonds, but they are strong enough to have great significance. For example, hydrogen bonding accounts for phenomena such as the anomalously high boiling point of water and the interactions between peptide bonds that direct the secondary structure of proteins. Molecules (and ions) that interact strongly with the dipole of water are described as hydrophilic. By contrast, molecules or parts of molecules that contain predominantly bonds between atoms of comparable electronegativity (e.g. C–C and C–H bonds) are not dipolar. They do not interact strongly with water or other polar molecules, and consequently behave as if they have a repulsion for water. Water molecules interact much more strongly with other water molecules than with non-polar groups. Intimate mixing of water with non-polar molecules or groups requires the breaking of hydrogen bonds between water molecules and consequently adoption of a more ordered (lower entropy) arrangement of water molecules at the interface. This is both enthalpically and entropically unfavourable, and the new bonds formed between the non-polar groups and water molecules are too weak to overcome this. Consequently, systems

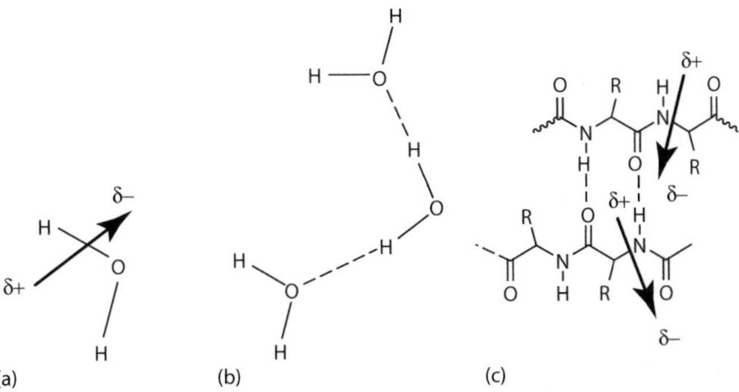

Figure 7.4 Dipoles and hydrogen bonding. (a) dipole (arrow) in the water molecule; (b) hydrogen bonding between water molecules due to the dipole; (c) hydrogen bonding between peptide chains due to the dipoles (arrows) in the peptide bonds.

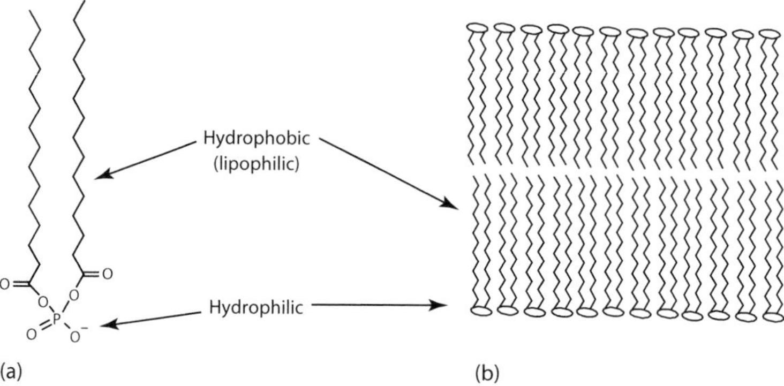

Figure 7.5 Hydrophobic and hydrophilic groups. (a) A phospholipid. (b) Assembly of phospholipid molecules to form a lipid bilayer (as in cell membranes, liposomes, etc.). Lipophilic molecules such as ^{99m}Tc-sestamibi and ^{64}Cu-ATSM (Figure 7.2) are able to penetrate the cell membrane by virtue of their lipid solubility, whereas hydrophilic polar and ionic species generally cannot.

containing both polar and non-polar groups tend to separate in the manner of 'like attracts like' – hydrophilic groups associate with each other and with water, and hydrophobic (non-polar) groups associate with each other and avoid water.

The phenomenon of association of hydrophobic groups with each other is often known as 'hydrophobic bonding', although of course it is not a type of bonding at all. Rather, it is due to the presence of stronger attractions between nearby water molecules, 'squeezing' the non-polar molecules out of this environment. These interactions manifest themselves in phenomena such as the insolubility of non-polar molecules in water, the folding of proteins by association between hydrophobic regions or patches, and of hydrophilic regions with water (secondary and quaternary structure), recognition of signalling molecules by receptors (see Chapters 15 and 16) and the formation of lipid bilayer membranes that give rise to cellular compartmentation (see Figure 7.5). They can be put to use in analytical methods such as solvent extraction and reversed-phase HPLC (see Chapter 35), and in the design of radiopharmaceuticals to influence their ability to penetrate cells (exploiting lipid solubility to traverse cell membranes) or control excretory pathways – as a rough rule of thumb, hydrophobic species tend to be excreted by the hepatobiliary system and hydrophilic ones via the kidney (see Chapter 15). Further discussion of intermolecular interactions is beyond the scope of this book and is given in the early chapters of many biochemistry texts.

Metal complexes

The chemistry of the metal ions is more flexible, and less bound by rigid 'rules', than that of the organic elements. It is usually most convenient to view metals as behaving as if positively charged (to an extent depending on their oxidation state) and seeking to gain electrons by complexing with ligands. Ligands comprise molecules or ions that have non-bonding 'lone pairs' of electrons that are available to form dative bonds with the metal. The ligand is viewed as donating a pair of electrons to form this bond. In principle, any atom, ion or molecule that has a non-bonding pair of electrons can function as a ligand in a metal complex (OH^-, H_2O, Cl^-, $N(CH_3)_3$, CH_3S^-, etc., but not, for example, alkane hydrocarbons, hydrogen, or positive metal ions). Each metal has its own preferences for oxidation state, which can to some extent be predicted from its position in the periodic table (e.g. +7 for technetium and rhenium, +3 for iron, +1 for silver). Some metals are stable in more than one oxidation state and consequently can readily give and take electrons to and from other molecules in reduction–oxidation ('redox') reactions. The process of removing an electron from a metal to raise its oxidation state is known as oxidation, and the reverse as reduction. Other metals have such a strong preference for a particular oxidation state (e.g. Na^+, K^+, Rb^+, Zn^{2+}, In^{3+}) that, at least under biological conditions, redox reactions are out of the question. Each metal in each different oxidation state has its own characteristics that govern its behaviour:

- Thermodynamic preferences for type of ligand ('hard' ligands such as most electronegative and least polarisable atoms – fluorine, oxygen, nitrogen, or 'soft' ligands such as the least electronegative and most polarisable atoms such as sulfur, phosphorus and carbon).
- Coordination number: the number of ligand atoms bound to the metal, from 2 – as in the heavy metals silver, gold, cadmium, mercury – to 9 or more (lanthanides and actinides); these preferences are governed partly by the electronic structure of the metal and partly by the size of the metal ion (larger radius leads to larger coordination number).
- Geometric arrangement of ligands (see Figure 7.6).
- Kinetic lability towards the making and breaking of metal–ligand bonds with timescales varying from picoseconds (as in the exchange of water molecules in the coordination sphere of sodium) to years in the most inert transition metal complexes with macrocyclic ligands.

For further discussion of these characteristics among the metals, reference to standard inorganic chemistry texts is suggested.

Metallic radionuclides must be securely attached to targeting molecules by means of their ligands, so the metal–ligand bonds must be resistant to breaking over the timescale of the application. Many individual metal–ligand bonds do not have the required kinetic stability and so additional measures must be taken in designing ligands to overcome this. The main design tool is to exploit the chelate effect (see below). Further discussion of this topic requires a little background discussion of concepts of stability and lability. The fundamental theory is presented in standard general and physical chemistry texts, and a brief discussion in context follows.

Thermodynamic and kinetic stability

The term 'stability' is used in many different contexts with different meanings. Any dynamic system, for example a simple solution containing hydrated metal ions M and ligands L, will have a preferred arrangement at which it will ultimately arrive, given enough time. Once it has reached that preferred arrangement, it is said to be at equilibrium and no further significant change will occur. For example, the system may reach a state in which nearly all the metal ions are associated with ligand molecules in solution to form a complex:

$$M + L \rightleftharpoons ML$$

In this process the double half-arrow indicates a dynamic equilibrium, with both forward and backward reactions occurring. The formation of complex ML may be strongly favoured, in which case most of the free (hydrated) metal will be converted to it, or it

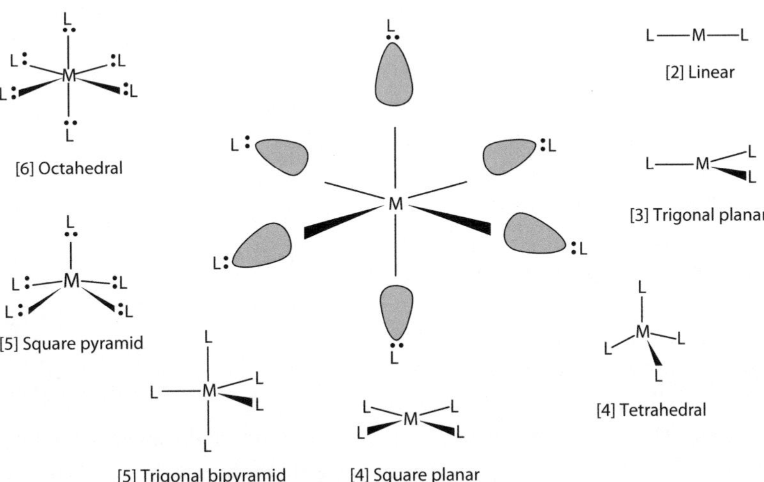

Figure 7.6 Interaction of ligands with metal centres via lone (non-bonding) pairs of electrons, and geometries associated with different coordination numbers. Coordination numbers are given in square brackets.

may not be favoured, in which case most of the metal will remain free (hydrated). If the complex formation is strongly favoured, the rate of formation (forward reaction) will be faster than the reverse reaction. Once the association and dissociation processes are in balance and the system has reached equilibrium, the extent of complex formation can be expressed by an equilibrium constant K. In this case, because the process is the *association* of metal and ligand, the equilibrium constant is known as an *association constant*, K_a, defined as:

$$K_a = \frac{[ML]}{[M][L]}$$

where the square brackets mean 'concentration of' the species within them. Thus if ML formation (association) is strongly favoured, K_a will be large ($\gg 1$), and if dissociation is favoured, K_a will be small ($\ll 1$). K_a is a measure of the thermodynamic stability of the complex ML. Often the same property is expressed instead in terms of a *dissociation constant* K_d, which is the inverse of K_a:

$$K_d = \frac{[M][L]}{[ML]}$$

A small K_d indicates a strong ('thermodynamically stable') complex. Since these constants are often very large or very small numbers, it is convenient to refer to their logarithms ($\log_{10} K$) instead of the numbers themselves. If the ligand is well matched to the preferences of the metal, the complex will have a large K_a (or a small K_d). For example, microorganisms have evolved to secrete iron-binding agents into their surroundings to extract traces of iron. These ligands are finely tuned for their purpose with $\log_{10} K_a$ of 30–40 or more. Clearly, to link a metal to a targeting molecule with sufficient stability to exist *in vivo*, it is advisable to design the ligand such that K_a is as large as possible.

Unfortunately, the biological milieu is much more complicated than the simple association reaction referred to above. Biological media such as blood plasma contain molecules that will act as ligands for the metal M, and hence will compete with L, displacing it from the metal. This would break the link between the radiolabel and its targeting vehicle, rendering the radiopharmaceutical useless. Often these competing ligands are present in much higher concentration than L or ML. For example, serum albumin binds very strongly to copper, and transferrin binds very strongly to iron-like metals. Moreover, biological fluids also contain other metals (e.g. zinc, calcium), and also protons, which may compete with the radiometal M for binding to L. Since radiopharmaceuticals are used at very low *in-vivo* concentration (e.g. 1 pmol/L), and the native competitors exist at relatively high concentration, under these conditions even complexes with very high association constants cannot hope to survive. If dissociation of ML occurs, the metal is much more likely to be bound by a native ligand such as albumin or transferrin than by L, and L is more likely to bind to a native metal or proton than to re-attach to M (this is simply entropy at work). Thus, under biological conditions, even complexes with the highest association constants will not be thermodynamically stable. If the system is allowed to reach equilibrium *in vivo* (which sooner or later it will be), extensive dissociation is inevitable.

Therefore, in order to succeed in making a complex that will survive *in vivo* for long enough to perform its task, we must do everything we can to *delay* the inevitable destruction of the complex. That is, we must minimise the *rate* of the dissociation process – i.e. make the complex *kinetically stable.* Mechanistic routes to the thermodynamic end point (dissociation) must be blocked or made as difficult as possible. The rate of a reaction is described using a rate constant k. The rate of reaction between a metal M and a ligand L depends on the frequency of encounters between M and L in solution, which is proportional to the concentration of each, and on the fraction of those encounters that result in association. For the association reaction

$$\text{Rate} = k_a[M][L]$$

and for the dissociation reaction

$$\text{Rate} = k_d[ML]$$

the rate constants are related to the equilibrium constants:

$$K_a = k_a/k_d \quad \text{and} \quad K_d = k_d/k_a$$

The optimal strategy for linking a radiometal to a targeting vehicle will then involve designing the ligand such that the ML complex has a small value of k_d, while at the same time keeping k_a large enough to make the radiolabelling step (association) feasible, at high yield, in a few minutes under mild conditions. This is not easy – those features of ligand design that promote slow dissociation also promote slow association, because the same barrier must be surmounted going in either direction.

Chelating ligands and the chelate effect

The most useful way to design a ligand so as to increase its K_a and decrease k_d is to exploit the *chelate effect*. By linking ligands together, usually by means of an organic carbon chain, in such a way that two or more donor atoms can coordinate to the metal at the same time without straining natural bond angles, the fractional concentration of free metal ion in the solution at equilibrium can be decreased by many orders of magnitude. Moreover, the dissociation rate constant k_d can be decreased, also by many orders of magnitude. Ligands containing two donor atoms or groups are described as *bidentate*, those with three are *tridentate*, and so on. Such ligands are termed chelators (derived from Greek *chelos*, a claw) or chelating agents, and their metal complexes are termed chelates or chelate complexes. The enhancement of thermodynamic and kinetic stability caused by chelation is known as the chelate effect. Broadly speaking the strength of the effect increases as the number of donor groups increases, provided they can all coordinate at the same time without strain (Figure 7.7). Some examples relevant to radiopharmacy are shown in Figure 7.8.

The origin of the chelate effect is easy to visualise qualitatively. Thermodynamically, the main driver is the relatively favourable entropy change associated with association – for example, a single hexadentate ligand with a metal, compared to six monodentate ligands. This can be simplistically illustrated by reference to a complex of an iron-like metal interacting with the iron binding protein transferrin:

Six monodentate ligands:

$$ML_6 + \text{transferrin} \rightleftharpoons M(\text{transferrin}) + 6L \text{ (two molecules become seven)}$$

One hexadentate ligand:

$$ML + \text{transferrin} \rightleftharpoons M\ (\text{transferrin}) + L \text{ (two molecules become two)}$$

The entropy change in the former case is more favourable than in the second: the increase in the number of particles allows the system to become more disordered and hence arrive at a more probable state.

Kinetically, one may visualise the increased association rate constant in terms of the likelihood that encounters between M and L will lead to complex formation. In an encounter between a metal and a monodentate ligand, the ligand may approach the metal in different orientations, some of which allow the donor atom to contact the metal while others shield the donor atom from the metal. If the ligand is bidentate, there is a greater probability that the encounter will allow contact between one of the donor atoms and the metal, so a higher fraction of encounters will lead to complexation. Moreover, once the first donor has coordinated with the metal, the second is held in close proximity (at a higher 'effective concentration'), leading to higher probability of its coordination. Conversely, dissociation of a chelate will be slowed: breaking the first metal–ligand bond leaves the second intact, so the dissociated donor group is not free to diffuse away and has a high

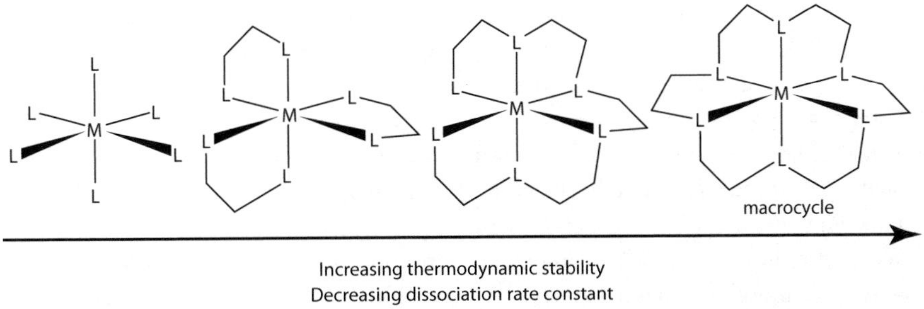

Figure 7.7 Qualitative schematic summary of the chelate and macrocyclic effects.

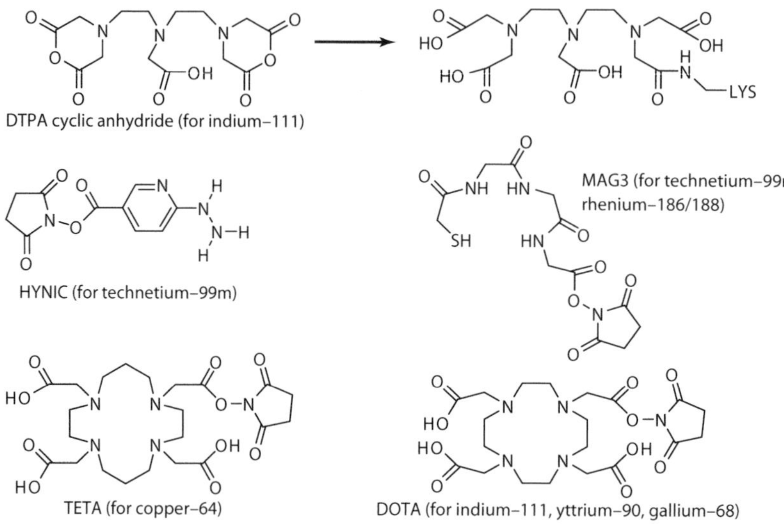

Figure 7.8 Some examples of bifunctional chelators and macrocycles (Blower *et al.* 1996; Prakash, Blower 1999; Fichna, Janecka 2003; Win *et al.* 2007; Bowen, Orvig 2008; De León-Rodríguez, Kovacs 2008; Lucignani 2008).

probability of re-association. The probability of dissociation is therefore much reduced.

The chelate effect is generally maximal when the rings formed by the coordination of two donor atoms to the metal are five-membered, as shown in Figure 7.7 – this is the arrangement that brings the donor groups into closest proximity with the metal with minimal additional strain in the ligand. Occasionally six-membered rings are required to provide the necessary flexibility to accommodate the geometric preferences of the metal.

A further enhancement of thermodynamic and kinetic stability of complexes is generally attainable by linking the ends of a chain of donor groups together (Figure 7.8) to make a *macrocyclic* chelator. This is known as the *macrocyclic effect*. Macrocyclic complexes are often extremely resistant to dissociation (see Chapter 13, copper radionuclides) because the structures are rather rigid and a great deal of strain in the ligand may need to be overcome in order to break the first metal–donor bond. This exceptional kinetic stability comes at a cost: the same barriers due to ligand strain are present during *formation* of the complex, often leading to slow complex formation and consequently a need for harsh labelling conditions. Labelling of DOTA conjugates with gallium-68 is a case in point: the Ga–DOTA conjugate complex is highly inert (more so than is necessary for a physical half-life of 68 minutes – its dissociation half-life is measured in years under physiological conditions) but heating is required to accomplish labelling efficiently in a short time (Win *et al.* 2007; De León-Rodríguez, Kovacs 2008)

Bifunctional chelators

Chelating ligands may be used to make either radionuclide-essential metal complex radiopharmaceuticals or radionuclide-tagged radiopharmaceuticals. In the latter case the chelating agent must have a second, reactive structural element to enable it to form a covalent link to the targeting vehicle (a protein, a peptide, etc.) to form a *bioconjugate*. Bifunctional chelators are chelating agents that have such a reactive group. The bifunctional chelator serves as a prosthetic group. The reactive groups present in biomolecules, through which they can be linked to a prosthetic group, are nearly always nucleophilic amino acid side-chains (the ω-amino group of lysine, or the N-terminal α-amino group, or the thiol group of cysteine). Therefore, the reactive group of a bifunctional chelator is usually an electrophilic group such as an active ester, isothiocyanate, maleimide, etc. A selection of examples are shown in Figure 7.8. Chelators designed to suit specific metals are discussed in succeeding chapters (Chapters 8, 9 and 13). The principles underlying design and synthesis of bioconjugates for radiolabelling are discussed in more detail in Chapter 14.

Radionuclide survey of the periodic table

The following is an overview of properties of radioelements in relation to their location in the periodic table and their uses in nuclear medicine.

Group 1

Group 1 of the periodic table consists of monovalent metals (lithium, sodium, potassium, rubidium, caesium, francium) whose chemistry is restricted to the formation of hydrated M^+ ions in aqueous solution. That is, each metal ion is surrounded by a shell of water molecules that constantly and rapidly exchange with water molecules in the bulk aqueous medium (exchange half-life is of the order of picoseconds). Their preference for existing in this state is so great that in aqueous solution they do not interact significantly with other ligands or functional groups, nor do they form covalent bonds. Thus, there is no chemistry by which they can be introduced into targeting molecules in a stable manner. Their applications are therefore restricted to those in which they mimic biological group 1 metals, i.e. sodium and potassium. The only clinically useful radionuclide in this group is rubidium-82 (^{82}Rb, a positron emitter, half-life 1.3 minutes), which forms hydrated Rb^+ that mimics the potassium ion K^+ in being transported by transmembrane potassium transporters, e.g. the Na^+/K^+-ATPase pump that maintains potassium concentration and electrical potential gradients across cell membranes (Machac 2005) In practice this use is restricted to myocardial perfusion imaging by PET, in which Rb^+ is accumulated quickly in cardiomyocytes of well-perfused myocardium via the Na^+/K^+-ATPase pump (Chapter 13).

Group 2

These metals form only M^{2+} ions and interact mainly with anionic oxygen ligands such as carboxylate, carbonate and phosphate. These interactions are kinetically labile compared with most organic chemical covalent bonds. Thus, like the group 1 metals, they cannot be incorporated into targeting molecules, and their use is restricted to mimicking the normal biological functions of calcium. This provides opportunities for targeted radionuclide therapy of bone metastases using the beta emitter strontium-89 (^{89}Sr), which, when administered as $SrCl_2$ (i.e. aqueous solution containing Sr^{2+} ions), is taken up in mineralising bone (Lin, Ray 2006). This mimicking of calcium is currently being evaluated for the alpha emitter radium-223 as a very potent radionuclide therapy for bone metastases (McDevitt *et al.* 1998).

Groups 3–12: the transition metals

The chemistry of the group 3 metals is governed by an extreme preference for the formation of M^{3+} ions (e.g. Y^{3+}). These do not exist as stable hydrated metal ions in aqueous solution except under strongly acidic conditions, because the polarising effect of the M^{3+} on coordinated water molecules results in release of protons to form hydroxides. However, they do interact strongly with polydentate chelating ligands containing anionic oxygen (carboxylates and phosphonates especially) and nitrogen donors. The tendency to form M^{3+} complexed by such ligands is not restricted to group 3, but is also exhibited by iron, chromium, cobalt, gallium, indium and the lanthanides (see below). Despite the similarity in coordination preferences shared by the M^{3+} ions, it is unrealistic to carry the analogy too far. While the complexes formed have high thermodynamic stability, their kinetic lability depends strongly on the particular metal and on the design of the chelator. Thus, for example, In^{3+} forms complexes with DTPA derivatives that have sufficient kinetic stability for imaging biomolecules labelled with ^{111}In, but the Y^{3+} analogue is too labile for analogous therapeutic applications (Virgolini *et al.* 2002). Moreover, the size of the ion affects the preferred coordination number, and hence the structure and biological properties. For example, Ga^{3+} and In^{3+} are both chelated strongly by DOTA (Virgolini *et al.* 2002; De León-Rodríguez, Kovacs 2008), but in the case of indium all of the carboxylate groups are bound to the metal, while in the case of gallium only two are coordinated leaving the other two free to interact with other biomolecules. The '3+ metals' are discussed in more detail elsewhere (Chapter 9).

The remaining transition metals (groups 4 to 12: titanium to zinc, zirconium to cadmium and hafnium to mercury) are characterised by a departure from the relatively hard and fast preferences for particular charge/valency states and ligand types exhibited by groups 1, 2 and 3. They can exist in a range of oxidation states (most notably from −1 to +7 in the case of rhenium and technetium), each with its own preference for ligand type, coordination number, and kinetic reactivity. Most important in this group in terms of clinical utility is technetium-99m (^{99m}Tc), which is discussed in detail later. Other transition metals gaining in importance include rhenium (^{186}Re, ^{188}Re) (Prakash, Blower 1999) and copper ($^{60,61,62,64,67}Cu$) (Blower *et al.* 1996). A wide range of ligands and chelators have been designed that form highly inert complexes of metals in certain oxidation states, which are stable for long enough *in vivo* for imaging and radionuclide therapy. Many bifunctional chelator systems have been developed from these to allow labelling of biomolecules with these elements. In addition, other characteristic properties of the transition metals, such as their participation in redox and electron transfer reactions, can be harnessed to achieve targeted delivery, for example to trap the radionuclide within cells by bioreductive mechanisms. This has been used in the design of copper radionuclide complexes for imaging of perfusion and hypoxia (Blower *et al.* 1996; Vavere, Lewis 2007).

Group 13

The group 13 elements all share clearly metallic characteristics, with a strong tendency to form hard 3+ cations (with similar coordination characteristics to the group 3 metals). This tendency diminishes down the group, to the extent that while ^{67}Ga, ^{68}Ga and ^{111}In resemble iron and can be chelated by polydentate nitrogen/oxygen ligands like the group 3 metals, the heaviest member, thallium, has a preference for the 1+ oxidation state (Tl^+) and its biological transport is reminiscent of the group 1 metals. Thallium-201 is used as a myocardial imaging agent by virtue of its uptake via the Na^+/K^+-ATPase pump (Bhatnagar, Narula 1999).

Group 14

The character of the group 14 elements varies from clearly covalent and tetravalent at the top of the group (carbon) to strongly metallic and with more ambivalent oxidation state at the bottom (lead, which behaves as a metal ion, Pb^{2+}, but also forms covalent molecules containing tetravalent lead analogous to carbon). Thus, carbon-11 (^{11}C) is able to replace ^{12}C in the native structure of the molecule and is particularly useful as a label for small organic molecules such as neuroreceptor ligands (Schubiger *et al.* 2006). In contrast, the heavier members tin and lead are treated by radiopharmaceutical chemists as metals, forming cations Sn^{2+} and Pb^{2+}. Tin and lead are used in the form of metal chelates, usually with polydentate oxygen/nitrogen ligands. Experimental examples are therapeutic use of ^{117m}Sn-DTPA complex for bone metastases (McEwan 1997; Li *et al.* 2001) and ^{212}Pb linked to biomolecules via polydentate bifunctional chelators (Su *et al.* 2005).

Group 15

Group 15 elements again exhibit a range of properties from covalent and predominantly trivalent nitrogen, to increasingly ready access to higher oxidation states and metallic behaviour lower down the group. Thus the positron emitter ^{13}N is used exclusively in its trivalent form as a component of covalent molecules (although the complexity of these is severely restricted by the short half-life of this radionuclide (10 minutes), and the only widely used form is ammonia, NH_3), while ^{32}P is used exclusively in its pentavalent state (which is favoured under aerobic biological conditions) in the form of phosphate and polyphosphates, as a beta-emitting radiotherapy nuclide targeted towards bone mineral and bone marrow (Silberstein 2005). Bismuth, although forming relatively stable pentavalent compounds such as bismuthates, also behaves as a 3+ metal and is treated as such in radiopharmaceutical chemistry, linked to biomolecules using polydentate nitrogen/oxygen chelators for use in targeted alpha emitter therapy (Yang, Sun 2007).

Group 16

Group 16 has few useful radioisotopes to offer to nuclear medicine. The most important is the positron emitter oxygen-15 (^{15}O), but its half-life is so short (2 minutes) that, with few exceptions (Miller *et al.*

2008), it is not useful in any form other than H_2O, for PET imaging studies of perfusion.

Group 17

Group 17 offers a rich source of highly versatile radionuclides, and the more important members of the group are discussed extensively elsewhere in this volume. Their chemical behaviour consists of either formation of stable monoanions (fluoride F^-, chloride Cl^-, bromide Br^-, iodide I^- and astatide At^-), or covalent incorporation into organic molecules and proteins, usually by formation of a single covalent bond with carbon (e.g. mIBG and FDG, see Figure 7.3). The natural biodistribution and function of the monoanions are exploited for imaging bone lesions with PET (^{18}F fluoride, which becomes incorporated into bone mineral) (Fogelman *et al.* 2005) or thyroid sodium/iodide symporter activity with SPECT (^{123}I- and ^{131}I-iodide) or PET (^{124}I-iodide) (Chung 2002; Lewis 2006). The covalent character is exploited in an extremely wide variety of labelled biologically active small molecules and proteins, for both imaging and therapy purposes (Adam, Wilbur 2005). The monovalency means that either fluorine or iodine can replace hydrogen or a hydroxyl group while maintaining the approximate shape of the molecule. While fluorine is small, the relatively large atomic radius of iodine, lower down the group, means that this substitution can have significant effects on steric properties (see Figure 7.3) and lipophilicity, and these effects need to be taken into account in the design of radiopharmaceuticals. While fluorine is restricted to the monocovalent and monoionic forms, iodine is relatively easily oxidised to higher oxidation states such (IO^-, IO_3^-, IO_4^-) but these have found no biomedical uses to date.

Bromine isotopes (^{76}Br, ^{77}Br) have potential applications in PET and radionuclide therapy, again in the form of covalent molecules with carbon–bromine bonds, often based on analogous fluorine- and iodine-labelled compounds (Adam, Wilbur 2005).

Astatine is the heaviest member of the group and has no stable isotopes. It is potentially useful for alpha emitter therapy (^{211}At) (Zalutsky, Pozzi 2004; Adam, Wilbur 2005), again usually in the form of organic molecules or proteins, labelled by means of carbon–astatine bond formation analogously to iodine. Astatine can reach higher oxidation states even more readily than iodine, reflecting increasingly metallic tendencies exhibited by the heavier of the p-block elements (groups 13–18), but again this property has not been exploited with any vigour to date. Indeed, the chemistry of astatine remains relatively mysterious because of the lack of stable isotopes and the highly toxic nature of its radioisotopes.

Group 18

Group 18 comprises the noble gases (helium, neon, argon, krypton, xenon, radon). Being 'noble' these cannot be incorporated into any targeting molecules and are useful only in the form of the elemental gas for lung ventilation studies. The gaseous state is exploited in the design of the krypton-81m (gamma emitter, half-life 13 seconds) generator, from which the gas is eluted from a solid support with air directly into the inhaled airstream (see Chapter 20) (Lambrecht *et al.* 1997).

Lanthanides

The nature of the lanthanides is similar to that of the group 3 and group 13 metals, in that they all form 3+ cations with a high affinity for oxygen/nitrogen chelators. Although they all conform to this pattern, and can be effectively chelated by the same chelator (most popular is DOTA, see Figure 7.8), there is a contraction in ionic radius towards the right of the period (the 'lanthanide contraction'), which affects the coordination number and can lead to significant differences in behaviour of bioconjugates in which the same chelator is used. Most important are samarium-153 (beta emitter), holmium-166 (beta emitter) and terbium-149 (alpha emitter) (Rosch, Forssell-Aronsson 2004).

Actinides

The actinides form very large (high-ionic-radius) ions with high coordination number and high charge. The only actinide to have been investigated with any serious intent for use in nuclear medicine is the alpha emitter actinium-225 (Miederer *et al.* 2008). Its ionic radius is larger than that of the other useful metals and it requires O/N chelating molecules containing a higher than usual number of chelating groupings.

References

Adam MJ, Wilbur DS (2005). Radiohalogens for imaging and therapy. *Chem Soc Rev* 34: 153–163.

Bhatnagar A, Narula J (1999). Radionuclide imaging of cardiac pathology: a mechanistic perspective. *Adv Drug Deliv Rev* 37: 213–223.

Blower P (2006). Towards molecular imaging and treatment of disease with radionuclides: the role of inorganic chemistry. *Dalton Trans*, 1705–1711.

Blower PJ *et al.* (1996). Copper radionuclides and radiopharmaceuticals in nuclear medicine. *Nucl Med Biol* 23: 957–980.

Bowen ML, Orvig C (2008). 99m-Technetium carbohydrate conjugates as potential agents in molecular imaging. *Chem Commun*, 5077–5091.

Chung J-K (2002). Sodium iodide symporter: its role in nuclear medicine. *J Nucl Med* 43: 1188–1200.

De León-Rodríguez LM, Kovacs Z (2008). The synthesis and chelation chemistry of DOTA-peptide conjugates. *Bioconjugate Chem* 19: 391–402.

Dearling JLJ, Pedley RB (2007). Technological advances in radioimmunotherapy. *Clin Oncol* 19: 457–469.

Fichna J, Janecka A (2003). Synthesis of target-specific radiolabeled peptides for diagnostic imaging. *Bioconjugate Chem* 14: 3–17.

Fogelman I *et al.* (2005). Positron emission tomography and bone metastases. *Semin Nucl Med* 35: 135–142.

Goldenberg DM, Sharkey RM (2007). Novel radiolabeled antibody conjugates. *Oncogene* 26: 3734–3744.

Lambrecht RM *et al.* (1997). Radionuclide generators. *Radiochim Acta* 77: 103–123.

Lewis MR (2006). A "new" reporter in the field of imaging reporter genes: correlating gene expression and function of the sodium/iodide symporter. *J Nucl Med* 47: 1–3.

Li Z *et al.* (2001). Synthesis and structural characterization of the promising therapeutic agent Sn-117m DTPA. *J Nucl Med* 42: 77.

Lin A, Ray ME (2006). Targeted and systemic radiotherapy in the treatment of bone metastasis. *Cancer Metastasis Rev* 25: 669–675.

Lucignani G (2008). Labeling peptides with PET radiometals: Vulcan's forge. *Eur J Nucl Med Mol Imaging* 35: 209–215.

Machac J (2005). Cardiac positron emission tomography imaging. *Semin Nucl Med* 35: 17–36.

McDevitt MR *et al.* (1998). Radioimmunotherapy with alpha-emitting nuclides. *Eur J Nucl Med* 25: 1341–1351.

McEwan AJB (1997). Unsealed source therapy of painful bone metastases: an update. *Semin Nucl Med* 27: 165–182.

Miederer M *et al.* (2008). Realizing the potential of the actinium-225 radionuclide generator in targeted alpha particle therapy applications. *Adv Drug Deliv Rev* 60: 1371–1382.

Miller PW *et al.* (2008). Synthesis of C-11, F-18, O-15, and N-13 radiolabels for positron emission tomography. *Angew Chem Int Ed* 47: 8998–9033.

Prakash SD, Blower PJ (1999). The chemistry of rhenium in nuclear medicine. In: Hay R *et al*, eds. *Perspectives on Bioinorganic Chemistry*. Stamford, CT:, JAI Press. 4: 91–143.

Rosch F, Forssell-Aronsson E (2004). Radiolanthanides in nuclear medicine. *Metal Ions in Biological Systems*, Vol 42: *Metal Complexes in Tumor Diagnosis and as Anticancer Agents*. New York: Marcel Dekker, 77–108.

Schubiger PA *et al.* (2006). *PET Chemistry: The Driving Force in Molecular Imaging*. New York: Springer.

Signore A *et al.* (2001). Peptide radiopharmaceuticals for diagnosis and therapy. *Eur J Nucl Med* 28: 1555–1565.

Silberstein EB (2005). Teletherapy and radiopharmaceutical therapy of painful bone metastases. *Semin Nucl Med* 35: 152–158.

Su FM *et al.* (2005). Pretargeted radioimmunotherapy in tumored mice using an in vivo Pb-212/Bi-212 generator. *Nucl Med Biol* 32: 741–747.

Vavere AL, Lewis JS (2007). Cu-ATSM: a radiopharmaceutical for the PET imaging of hypoxia. *Dalton Trans*, 4893–4902.

Virgolini I *et al.* (2002). Experience with indium-111 and yttrium-90-labeled somatostatin analogs. *Curr Pharm Design* 8: 1781–1807.

Welch MJ, Redvanly CS (2003). *Handbook of Radiopharmaceuticals: Radiochemistry and Applications*. Chichester: Wiley.

Win Z *et al.* (2007). Somatostatin receptor PET imaging with Ga-68-labeled peptides. *Q J Nucl Med Mol Imaging* 51: 244–250.

Yang N, Sun H (2007). Biocoordination chemistry of bismuth: recent advances. *Coord Chem Rev* 251: 2354–2366.

Zalutsky MR, Pozzi OR (2004). Radioimmunotherapy with alpha-particle emitting radionuclides. *Q J Nucl Med Mol Imag* 48: 289–296.

8

Fundamentals of technetium and rhenium chemistry

Adriano Duatti

Introduction

Technetium-99m (^{99m}Tc) has been the most important radionuclide for nuclear medicine. It is likely that, without ^{99m}Tc radiopharmaceuticals, nuclear medicine would not have experienced the tremendous growing during the last thirty years. Beside the ideal nuclear properties of the gamma-emitting nuclear isomer, a key factor in determining the success of ^{99m}Tc imaging agents was the development of sophisticated chemical methods for designing and preparing new radiopharmaceuticals having specific targeting properties. Fundamental studies on the chemistry of Tc complexes (Schwochau 2000; Liu 2004) led to a precise characterisation of the molecular structure of ^{99m}Tc radiopharmaceuticals that, in turn, constitutes the basic information for understanding the biological behaviour of a tracer at the molecular level. In this respect, the molecular studies on ^{99m}Tc agents can be viewed as a first example of the application of the new paradigm of diagnostic medicine that is currently dubbed 'molecular imaging'.

The chemistry of the element technetium is extremely rich and elegant and, therefore, can be described using a general theoretical framework. Recently, the surge in the use of radiolabelled compounds for therapeutic applications has attracted interest in radionuclides having useful nuclear characteristics for therapy. The β^--emitting radionuclide rhenium-188 (^{188}Re) is among the most promising candidates and an increasing number of studies are currently devoted to the development of therapeutic ^{188}Re radiopharmaceuticals. Since the element rhenium belongs to the same group as technetium, it shares with its congener some common chemical characteristics. In this chapter, an overview of the fundamental concepts of technetium and rhenium chemistry is presented. Emphasis is mostly given to those aspects relevant for understanding labelling methods and the properties of the corresponding radiopharmaceuticals. For this purpose, a general approach based on the use of molecular orbital theory has been employed. This picture offers significant advantages over more conventional descriptions, particularly for the illustration of the molecular structure and reactivity of the various metallic species.

General

In the past twenty years, the radionuclide technetium-99m has played a fundamental role in the development of nuclear medicine particularly because it possesses almost ideal nuclear properties for diagnostic applications. This metastable nuclear isomer decays through the emission of a nearly monochromatic γ-radiation of 140 keV that is particularly well suited for imaging with conventional gamma cameras based on doped sodium iodide crystals. Moreover, the 6.06-hours decay half-life of ^{99m}Tc allows the easy preparation of ^{99m}Tc radiopharmaceuticals, but at the same time avoids the delivery of an excessive radiation exposure to the patient. A similar situation is found with the radionuclide ^{188}Re that is currently attracting high interest because its nuclear properties appear suitable for therapeutic applications of ^{188}Re radiopharmaceuticals.

The two elements technetium and rhenium (Earnshaw, Greenwood 1997; Cotton *et al.* 1999) belong to the same group 7 of the transition metal series of the periodic table along with manganese. It is commonly observed in all groups of the transition series, the chemical properties of the first lighter member differ significantly from those of the other two heavier members. In contrast, the remaining two elements of the group show many chemical similarities though their characteristics cannot be always considered superimposable. It turns out, therefore, that the chemistry of manganese deviates radically from that of technetium and rhenium, while these latter elements exhibit similar chemical behaviour. The usual explanation of these observations is dubbed 'lanthanide contraction' and refers to a phenomenon through which the size of the external orbitals becomes dramatically contracted as a result of the high speed of the outer electrons approaching that of light (in essence, a relativistic effect). The most important consequence of this effect is that the ionic radii of the lower two elements of the groups are found to be almost equal when they are measured with the elements in the same oxidation state. This fact has important implications in the design of radiopharmaceuticals labelled with the two radionuclides ^{99m}Tc and ^{188}Re. In particular, it has been demonstrated that a pair of ^{99m}Tc and ^{188}Re complexes having exactly the same chemical composition, molecular geometry and stability, and differing only in the metallic centre, always display the same biological behaviour. Such a combination of biologically equivalent complexes in radiopharmaceutical chemistry is referred to as a 'matched pair' (Liu, Hnatowich 2007; Liu 2008).

However, it turns out that the chemical similarities between technetium and rhenium are much less pronounced than usually claimed. In fact, there are some fundamental differences that may have a dramatic impact on the preparation of the corresponding radiopharmaceuticals. All these can be traced back to the value of the standard reduction potentials ($E°$). It was found that, on the average, $E°$ for a redox process involving the reduction of a technetium compound is approximately 0.20 mV higher than that for the corresponding rhenium compound. This apparently tiny difference has a tremendous effect on the reaction yields because of the exponential form of the Nernst equation. It follows, therefore, that the preparation of a rhenium radiopharmaceutical occurring through the reduction of the metallic centre is usually less favoured than that for the corresponding technetium radiopharmaceutical. Moreover, since differences in $E°$ values can be qualitatively explained by the variation in both energy and spatial distribution of atomic orbitals, it is expected that this difference in the electronic density around the two metallic ions may also lead to changes in the molecular geometry between complexes belonging to the same class of analogous rhenium and technetium complexes.

The tetraoxo anions $[M(VII)O_4]^-$ (M = Tc, Re)

The common starting materials for the preparation of both ^{99m}Tc and $^{186/188}Re$ radiopharmaceuticals are the tetraoxo anions $[MO_4]^-$ (M = Tc, Re), which constitutes the most stable chemical form of these elements in aqueous solution. A general procedure is schematically illustrated in Figure 8.1.

In Figure 8.1, R stands for a suitable reducing agent or combination of reducing agents, and L for a coordinating ligand or a combination of ligands able to stabilise the reduced oxidation state in the final complex ML_n (n = integer number). In ^{99m}Tc and ^{188}Re radiopharmaceutical preparations, the most common reducing agent is $SnCl_2$ with only a few exceptions. Although usually 100 micrograms is sufficient to reduce the Tc(VII) metallic centre in $[^{99m}TcO_4]^-$ to lower oxidation states, far larger amounts of $SnCl_2$ and more drastic reaction conditions are generally required to obtain the same result with $[^{188}ReO_4]^-$, a requirement imposed by the lower $E°$ value of this latter species.

A number of different approaches have been proposed to overcome the problem of the reduction of $[^{188}ReO_4]^-$, and these are all based on the addition to the radiopharmaceutical preparation of some suitable reagent capable of favouring the electron transfer between the reducing agent and the metal centre. Despite differences in the reagents employed, these methods have a common chemical foundation that can be illustrated by simple thermodynamic considerations.

Essentially, the value of the standard reduction potential, $E°$, is related to the standard free energy of a reaction, $\Delta G°$, according to the equation:

$$-zFE° = \Delta G° = \Delta H° - T\Delta S \qquad (8.1)$$

$$[MO_4]^- + R + L \longrightarrow ML_n$$

Figure 8.1 The reduction of $[MO_4]^-$ (M = Tc, Re).

where zF is the amount of charge transferred per mole of substance, $\Delta H°$ is the standard heat of reaction (standard enthalpy), T is the absolute temperature (K) and $\Delta S°$ is the standard entropy. Negative values of $\Delta G°$ (corresponding to positive values of $E°$) indicate that the reaction is thermodynamically favoured. Thus, dropping the value of $\Delta G°$ (or equivalently, increasing the value of $E°$) may lead to a significant increase of the reaction yields. This can be obtained by acting on the various parameters in equation (8.1). The term $\Delta H°$ is related to the balance of bond energies involved in the formation of the final products, and it is usually difficult to modify. Similarly, only very high temperatures may have some effect on the standard free energy, and these are usually incompatible with the requirements of a radiopharmaceutical preparation. The term $\Delta S°$ is related to the changes in molecular geometry in passing from the starting compound to the final products. Specifically, in ^{188}Re preparations, geometry is always converted from the starting tetrahedral geometry of the perrhenate anion into the final geometry of the product, which usually ranges between a square pyramidal and an octahedral arrangement (see next section). It turns out that this unavoidable geometrical modification has a strong negative effect of the reduction process since it corresponds to a decrease in entropy and, consequently, to an increase of $\Delta G°$ (decrease of $E°$).

A reagent capable of improving the reduction yield of $[^{188}ReO_4]^-$ usually corresponds to a ligand that can weakly bind the Re^{+7} centre, thus forming some intermediate Re(VII) species having a molecular geometry identical, or closely similar, to that of the final product. In this situation, the reduction process no longer requires dramatic changes of the molecular geometry in going from the starting Re^{+7} to the final reduced metallic centre and, as a consequence, the entropy factor does not have the same negative effect. This phenomenon is well known in inorganic chemistry and is dubbed 'expansion of the coordination sphere'.

Many different reagents have been employed as reduction enhancers, mostly belonging to the class of polyoxo anions. Three of them are particularly worthy of mention. In the presence of Sn^{2+} ions, *diphosphonates* are able to form complexes with rhenium of unknown structure and in which the metal oxidation state remains undetermined. Despite this limitation, ^{188}Re-diphosphonate complexes can be utilised as intermediate complexes for the preparation of ^{188}Re-radiopharmaceuticals in satisfactorily high yield (Faintuch *et al.* 2003). Similarly, *ethylenediamine-tetraacetic acid* (EDTA) was found to react with $[^{188}ReO_4]^-$ in the presence of Sn^{2+} ions to give rise to an intermediate ^{188}Re(III)-EDTA complex. Although the structure and the metal oxidation state of the supposed $^{188}Re^{3+}$ complex have not yet been elucidated, the preliminary formation of this intermediate compound was found to strongly increase the radiochemical yield of the final ^{188}Re-radiopharmaceutical (Seifert, Pietzsch 2006). Probably the most striking example of a ligand capable of expanding the Re(VII) coordination sphere is given by the *oxalate* ion, $[C_2O_4]^{2-}$. This anion, derived from the simplest dicarboxylic acid, when added to a radiopharmaceutical preparation starting from $[^{188}ReO_4]^-$, sharply increase the radiochemical yield also under very mild reaction conditions (Bolzati *et al.* 2000).

Geometries of Tc and Re complexes

Although four-coordination is limited to the tetraoxo anions, which possess a tetrahedral geometry (*t*) (Figure 8.2a), common arrangements for Tc and Re complexes range from five- to six-coordination corresponding to square pyramidal (*sp*) and trigonal bipyramidal (*tbp*) geometries (Figure 8.2b and c), and to octahedral geometry (*oh*) (Figure 8.2d), respectively.

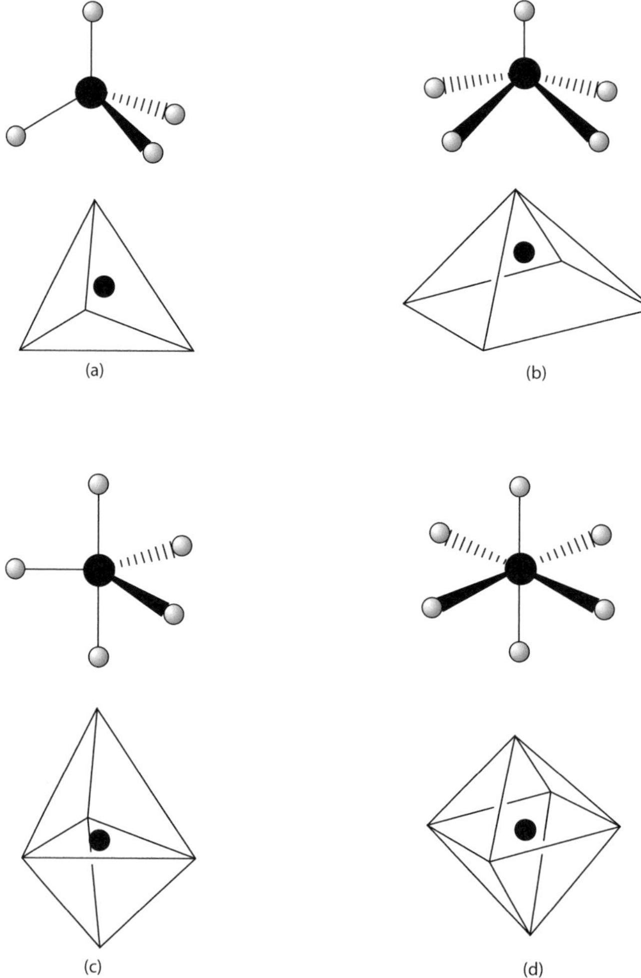

Figure 8.2 Common geometries for Tc and Re complexes: (a) tetrahedral (*t*), (b) square pyramidal (*sp*), (c) trigonal bipyramidal (*tbp*), (d) octahedral (*oh*).

Generally, in *sp* geometry, the metal ion occupies a position inside the square pyramid that lies above the basal square plane. This arrangement imparts a characteristic reversed umbrella-shaped form to the resulting complexes (Figure 8.2b). Conversely, in *tbp* and *oh* geometries, the metallic atom is usually placed in the equatorial plane, though some distortion is possible when the actual molecular structure deviates from the ideal symmetry.

Metallic functional groups for Tc and Re

The common approach to the description of the chemistry of metallic elements is to classify the various complexes based on the formal oxidation state of the metal centre. In radiopharmaceutical chemistry, this procedure does not appear particularly useful for explaining the most important characteristics of ^{99m}Tc and $^{188/186}$Re radiopharmaceuticals and, thus, an alternative approach is followed here, which stems from Hoffman's theory of orbital fragments (Albright *et al.* 1985). The key concept of this theory is that of *inorganic functional groups* (Tisato *et al.* 2006), which is fully analogous to the well-established concept of *organic functional groups* in organic chemistry. Essentially, the basic idea is to view a specific category of metal complex as composed of some characteristic metallic functional group coordinated to some suitable ligands. As with an organic functional group, its inorganic analogue represents a chemical motif characterising a particular class of complexes. Obviously, it should always include the metal tightly bound to some specific atom or groups of atoms, thus forming a characteristic moiety. Usually, this moiety exhibits a high stability and its electronic properties are responsible for the peculiar chemical behaviour of the resulting complexes. Accordingly, a simple knowledge of the energy levels of the inorganic functional group (*fragment orbitals*) is sufficient to describe the chemical properties of the whole complex. Metallic functional groups (also called metallic *cores*) relevant for ^{99m}Tc and $^{188/186}$Re radiopharmaceuticals are the $[M{\equiv}O]^{3+}$ (M-monoxo), $[M{\equiv}N]^{2+}$ (M-nitrido or M-nitride), $[M{=}N{-}R]^{3+}$ (M-imido), $[M{=}N{=}N{-}R]^{2+}$ (M-hydrazido, M-diazenido) and $[O{=}M{=}O]^{+}$ (M-dioxo) groups, where the metal formal oxidation state is +5, the $[M(YS_3)]$ (Y = N, P) group, where the metal formal oxidation state is +3, and the $[M(CO)_3]^+$ (M-carbonyl) group in which the metal oxidation state is +1 (M = Tc, Re). In the following sections, the electronic and chemical properties of these functional groups are discussed.

Electronic description of metallic functional groups

The chemical and geometrical properties of a coordination complex always originate from its inner electronic structure (Chang 2005; Atkins, de Paula 2006). A basic assumption of orbital fragment theory is that the electronic behaviour of a whole complex can be simply traced back to the electronic properties of its characteristic metallic functional group. Actually, the electronic distribution of the metallic motif dominates and controls the structure of the resulting complex. Thus, to achieve a deeper description of the chemical features of Tc and Re radiopharmaceuticals, and of the underlying labelling methods, it would be convenient to devise some suitable electronic picture of the most common metallic functional groups.

Fragment theory explains the formation of a single complex as resulting from the bonding interaction between a characteristic metallic functional group and some set of suitable ligands. Accordingly, the molecular orbitals (MOs) of the metallic fragment play a critical role in determining its chemical reactivity. In particular, the most important orbitals are the so-called *frontier orbitals*, which are defined as the set including the *highest occupied molecular orbital* (HOMO) and the *lowest unoccupied molecular orbital* (LUMO). Since metal–ligand interactions can usually be classified as Lewis acid–base interactions, where the metal behaves as a Lewis acid (electron acceptor) and the ligand behaves as a Lewis base (electron donor), the LUMO holds a fundamental role in determining the chemical reactivity of a metallic fragment.

There are a number of standard theoretical methods for obtaining HOMOs and LUMOs. The most common approaches employ a linear combination of atomic orbitals (AO) of the atoms composing the metallic fragment. These combinations afford the energy levels of the fragment and allow determination of the corresponding fragment orbitals. A simple rule enables us to calculate the number of MOs resulting from the combination of n atomic orbitals (n = integer number). This rule states that when n AOs are superimposed according to the symmetry of the molecule, this combination should afford exactly the same number of MOs. These new orbitals usually belong to the two categories of low-energy bonding and high-energy antibonding MOs, though the formation of localised MOs and non-bonding orbitals is also possible. A further classification of MOs is based on their symmetry properties with respect to the metal–ligand bond axis. Specifically, MOs lying on the bond axis and as a consequence not changing sign after a 180° rotation around it, are classified as σ orbitals. Conversely, MOs changing sign after the same rotation must be perpendicular to the bond axis and are classified as π orbitals. According to this, ligands generating σ- or π-type MOs when overlapping their orbitals with metallic AOs, are classified as σ- or π-donors (π-acceptors), respectively.

In the following sections, the chemical properties of the most relevant Tc and Re functional groups required for a deeper understanding of the various labelling methods and of the behaviour of the corresponding radiopharmaceuticals will be illustrated. The approach will always be an attempt to correlate the chemical and structural properties of a specific class of complexes with the electronic features of the characteristic metallic functional group.

The isoelectronic metal oxo, $[M{\equiv}O]^{3+}$, and metal nitrido, $[M{\equiv}N]^{2+}$, functional groups [M = Tc(V), Re(V)]

The $[M{\equiv}O]^{3+}$ (M-oxo, M = Tc, Re) and $[M{\equiv}N]^{2+}$ (M-nitrido or M-nitride, M = Tc, Re) functional groups are composed of the metal bound to a single heteroatom through a multiple bond (Bandoli *et al.* 2001; Boschi *et al.* 2005; Bandoli *et al.* 2006). In aqueous solution, the metal oxo group is usually produced when a residual oxo oxygen atom remains bound to the metal atom during the reduction process of the $[MO_4]^-$ anion. In contrast, formation of the metal nitrido group requires the reaction of the tetraoxo anion with some suitable donor of nitrido nitrogen atoms, $[N]^{3-}$, in the presence of a reducing agent. It was found that a large number of molecules containing the hydrazine-like moiety, >N—N<, behave as suitable sources of nitrido groups. Common donors of nitrido nitrogen atoms employed in chemical synthesis of nitrido complexes are sodium azide (NaN_3), diethyldithiocarbazate ($H_2N{-}N(CH_3){-}C({=}S)SCH_3$) and succinic dihydrazide ($H_2N{-}NH{-}C({=}O){-}(CH_2)_2{-}C({=}O){-}NH{-}NH_2$).

The formal oxidation state for the metal is +5, for the oxo oxygen atom −2, and for the nitrido −3. Accordingly, the outer valence electron configuration for the metal is d^2, that for the heteroatom is p^6, and the two resulting moieties are isoelectronic (in total, eight valence electrons). The symmetry-adapted combinations of metal d orbitals and heteroatom p orbitals, calculated for a square pyramidal geometry, generate the corresponding fragment orbitals and energy levels. These are pictorially illustrated in Figure 8.3.

Evidently, both $[M{\equiv}O]^{3+}$ and $[M{\equiv}N]^{2+}$ groups possess the same type of fragment orbitals. In particular, the eight valence electrons can be accommodated in the lowest energy σ and π bonding orbitals, thus giving a total bond order of three (triple bond). The HOMO is an n non-bonding orbital, and the LUMO is composed of a pair of π* antibonding orbitals. These LUMOs are the critical frontier orbitals controlling the reactivity of the metallic fragment. The forms of these orbitals are depicted in Figure 8.3. It is apparent that the regions of highest electronic density are sharply positioned along the internal axes of a *sp* geometry and this nicely accounts for the geometrical features of the resulting complexes. The only difference between the M-oxo and M-nitrido groups lies in the energy of the corresponding LUMOs. Since the N^{3-} group is the strongest π-donor ligand, the LUMOs of the $[M{\equiv}N]^{2+}$ fragment have higher energies than those of the $[M{\equiv}O]^{3+}$ fragment. The remaining high-energy σ* antibonding orbital plays a minor role in determining the chemical behaviour of these metallic fragments.

The forms and energies of LUMOs of the $[M{\equiv}O]^{3+}$ and $[M{\equiv}N]^{2+}$ groups nicely account for their chemical reactivity. Since these empty frontier orbitals are antibonding in character and lie at relatively high energies, the corresponding metallic fragments can be classified as soft Lewis acids exhibiting a marked electrophilic behaviour. Therefore, their preferred interaction is with soft Lewis bases containing

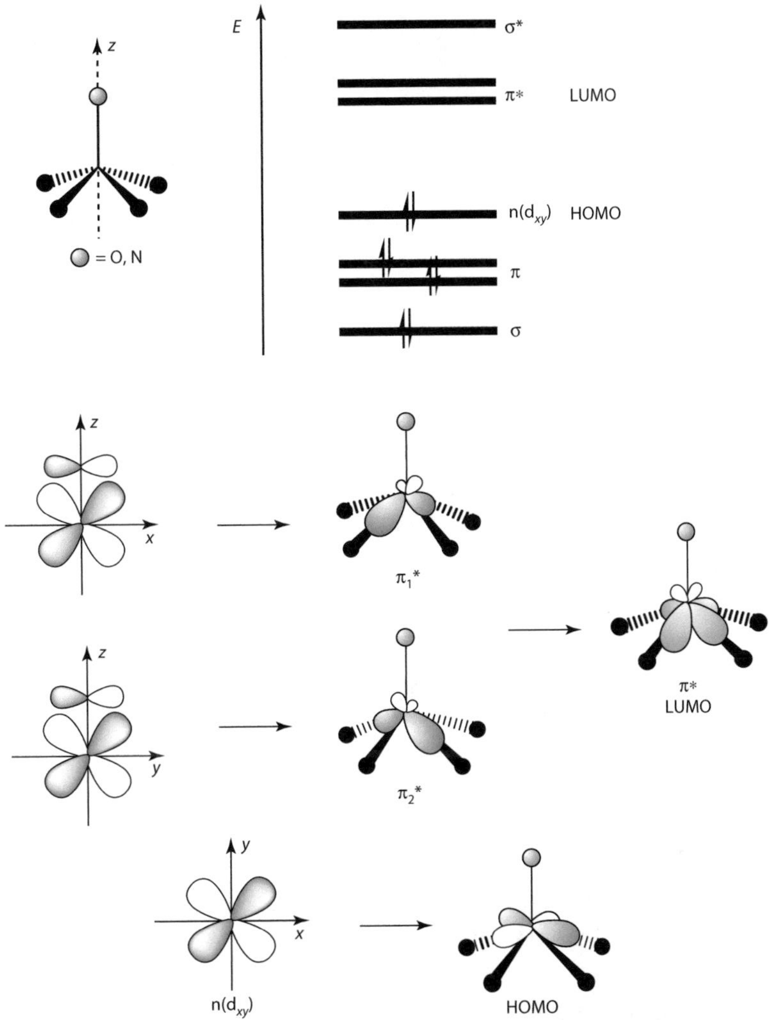

Figure 8.3 Fragment orbitals for the metallic functional groups $[M{\equiv}O]^{3+}$ and $[M{\equiv}N]^{2+}$ (M = Tc, Re).

electrons in high-energy orbitals. Accordingly, the most suitable coordinating ligands are those including negatively charged donor atoms like S^-, O^- and N^-. As a general rule, when four donor atoms are coordinated to these cores the resulting geometry is *sp* where the oxo or nitrido group occupies an apical position and the four donor atoms span the four positions on the basal plane of the square pyramid. The simplest example of this category of complexes is the tetrahalogeno derivatives $[M(Y)X_4]^-$ (M = Tc, Re; Y = O, N; X = Cl, Br) and the mixed halogeno-phosphino compounds $[ReOCl_3(P')_2]$ and $[M(N)Cl_2(P')_2$ (P′ = tertiary monophosphine). It should be noted that the nitrido complexes $[M(N)X_4]^-$ contain the metal in the +6 formal oxidation state. Of particular interest are multidentate ligands ranging from bidentate to tetradentate chelating systems. The general structures of these ligands are illustrated in Figure 8.4.

In dealing with multidentate ligands, significant differences between the oxo and nitrido cores always arise. For instance, tetradentate ligands form highly stable *sp* complexes with the oxo-metal fragment. In particular, stability follows the order $[N_2S_2] > [N_3S]$. Conversely, this category of ligands hardly bind to the nitrido-metal core, presumably because of the strong distortion of *sp* geometry imparted by the encumbering electronic density around the M≡N triple bond. As a consequence, *sp* nitrido complexes are easily formed with bidentate ligands yielding symmetrical nitrido complexes as illustrated in Figure 8.5a.

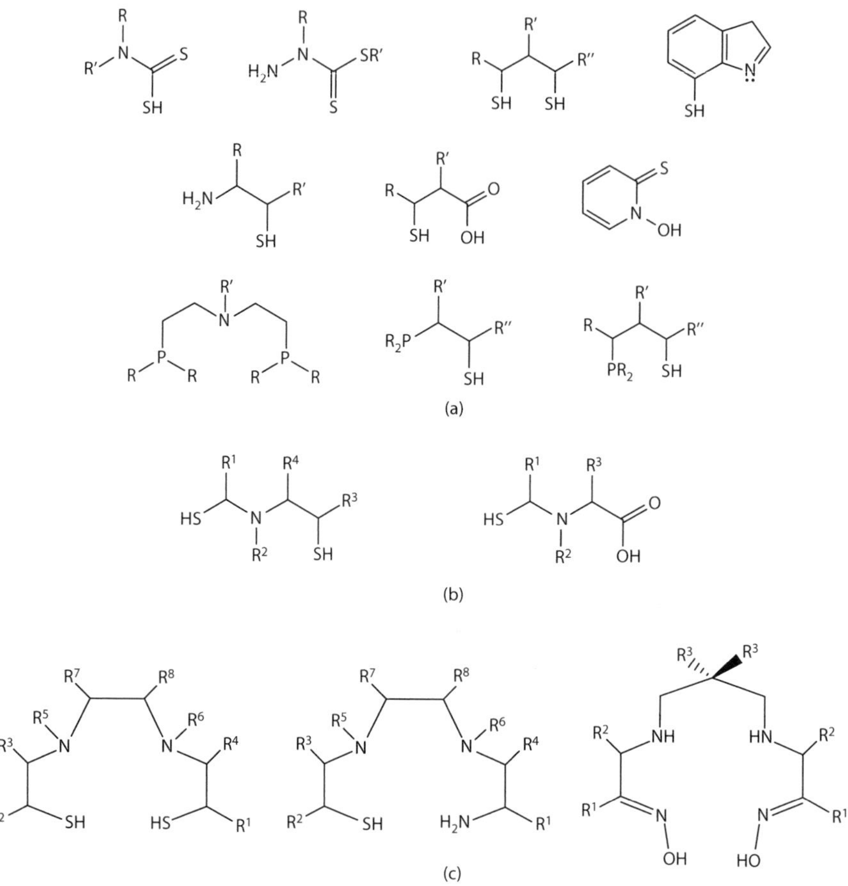

Figure 8.4 Types of multidentate chelating ligands for the $[M{\equiv}O]^{3+}$ and $[M{\equiv}N]^{2+}$ (M = Tc, Re) functional groups: (a) bidentate ligands, (b) tridentate ligands, (c) tetradentate ligands (R, R′, R″, R^{1-8} = H, organic functional group).

Tridentate ligands of the type [XNS] (X = O, S) bind to both the oxo and nitrido groups, but a remarkable difference between the composition of the resulting complexes is usually observed. Specifically, the tridentate ligand binds the oxo core as a dianionic $[^{-}XN(H)S^{-}]$ chelating system yielding *sp* complexes where the remaining fourth coordination position is occupied by a halogen atom (Cl^-, Br^-) (Figure 8.5b). The same coordination mode is adopted when these ligands bind to the nitrido core, but the crucial difference is that the donor halogen atom in the fourth coordination position is replaced by a π-acceptor ligand like a monophosphine (Figure 8.5c).

The combination of π-donor and π-acceptor coordinating atoms bound to the same metallic fragment has far richer consequences for the nitrido core than for the isoelectronic oxo analogue. Usually, the $[M{\equiv}O]^{3+}$ group exhibits a lower stability towards π-acceptor ligands because of the ability of these species to remove the oxo oxygen atom through the formation of the corresponding oxide with the concomitant reduction of the metallic centre. This is more likely to occur with the $[Tc{\equiv}O]^{3+}$ group due to the higher standard reduction potential of technetium with respect to rhenium. Conversely, removal of the nitrido group is rather difficult and, as a result, this core affords interesting examples of mixed complexes containing different combinations of π-donor and π-acceptor coordinating atoms. For instance, when the coordinating set is composed of two π-donor and two π-acceptor atoms the coordination arrangement switches from *sp* to trigonal bipyramidal (*tbp*). Interestingly, this conversion leads to a sharp separation between the positions spanned by the two types of ligands within the *tbp* geometry. In particular, π-acceptor atoms always reside at the two axial positions of the *tbp* structure, the three donor atoms including the nitrido group being on the equatorial

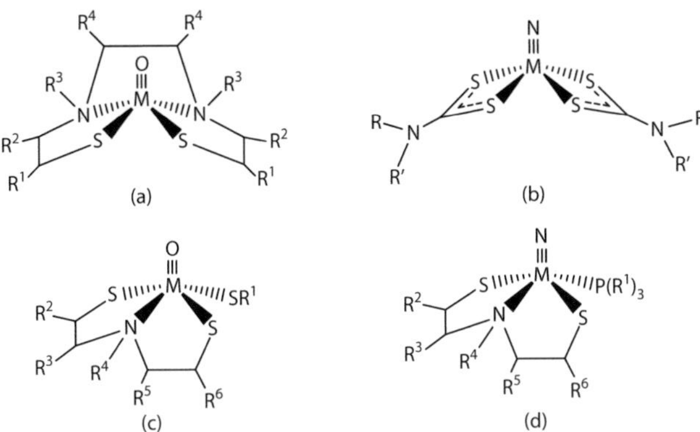

Figure 8.5 Types of square pyramidal metal oxo and metal nitrido complexes with different multidentate ligands (R, R′, R^{1-7} = H, organic functional group).

plane. Figure 8.6 shows an example of this class of *tbp* nitrido Tc(V) complexes with bidentate, mixed π-acceptor–π-donor phosphinothiol ligands. The coordination arrangement of the resulting bis-substituted complexes contains a $[Tc{\equiv}N]^{2+}$ group and the two negatively charged sulfur π-donor atoms placed in the equatorial plane of the trigonal bipyramid, and the two neutral phosphorus atoms occupying the two axial positions perpendicular to the same plane.

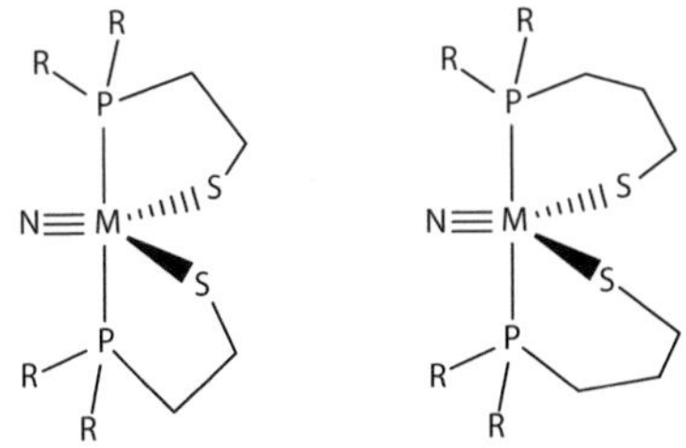

Figure 8.6 Trigonal bipyramidal (*tbp*) nitrido Tc(V) complexes with bidentate phosphinothiol ligands having a π-acceptor and a π-donor as coordinating atoms (R = organic functional group).

The high stability of the ligand environment composed by two π-acceptor and two π-donor atoms bound to a $[Tc{\equiv}N]^{2+}$ group can be conveniently exploited to afford bis-substituted complexes incorporating two different bidentate ligands coordinated to the same metal centre. This can be simply obtained by changing the connectivity between π-donor and π-acceptor atoms in bis-substituted *tbp* complexes as illustrated in Figure 8.7. The resulting complexes will possess the same arrangement of coordinating atoms, but the ligand system will be composed of a bidentate,

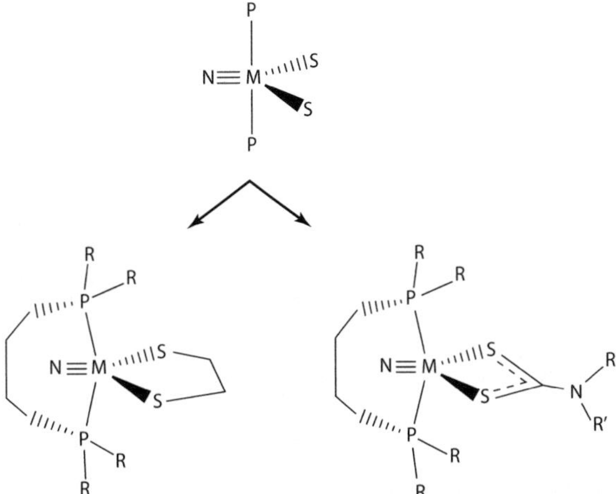

Figure 8.7 Examples of formation of asymmetrical nitrido Tc(V) heterocomplexes (R, R′ = organic functional group).

fully π-acceptor ligand and a bidentate, fully π-donor ligand, thus yielding bis-substituted asymmetrical complexes (*heterocomplexes*). Examples of asymmetrical nitrido Tc(V) heterocomplexes with various bidentate ligands are reported in Figure 8.7.

The metal dioxo functional group, *trans*-[O=M=O]$^+$ (M = Tc, Re)

The combination of two terminal oxygen atoms coordinated to the metal centre in a reciprocal *trans* position affords another functional group for Tc and Re in the +5 oxidation state (Tisato *et al.* 1994; Bandoli *et al.* 2001). The frontier orbitals for this group are particularly simple because the bonding of the two oxygen atoms captures almost all the metallic orbitals leaving empty only those placed in the plane perpendicular to the O=M=O axis as illustrated in Figure 8.8.

Since dioxo complexes always assume an octahedral geometry, hybridisation of metallic s, p_x, p_y, p_z, d_{z^2} and $d_{x^2-y^2}$ affords six d^2sp^3 hybrid orbitals lying along the internal axes of an octahedron. By placing the O=M=O moiety along the *z*-axis, two hybrid d^2sp^3 metal orbitals pointing towards the apical

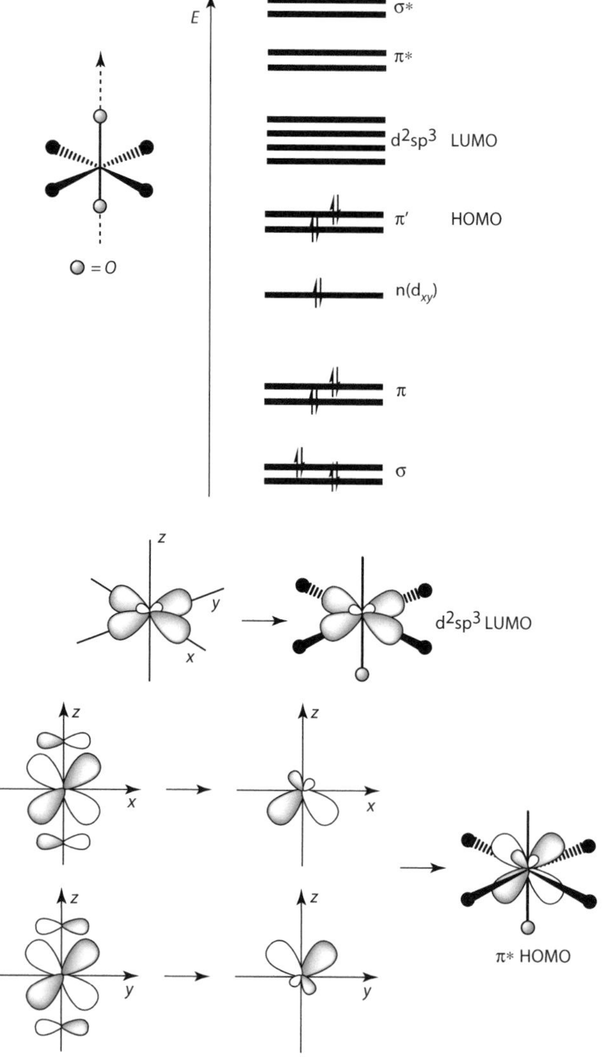

Figure 8.8 Fragment orbitals for the metallic functional group *trans*-[O=M=O]$^+$ (M = Tc, Re).

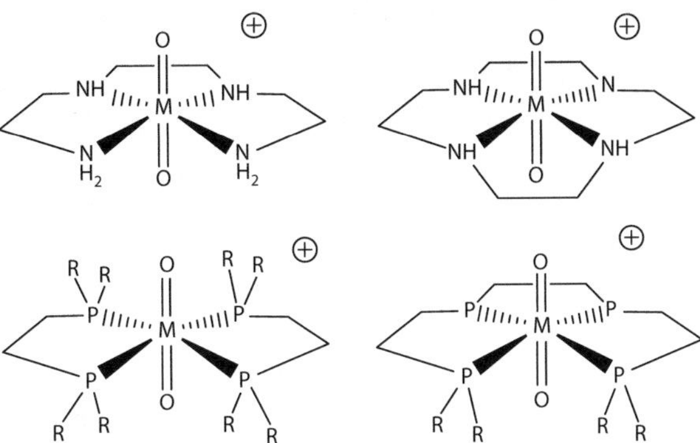

Figure 8.9 Examples of complexes with the *trans*-$[O{=}M^V{=}O]^+$ (M = Tc, Re) group (R = organic functional group).

positions on this axis can be used to form σ-bonds with the p_z orbitals of the two *trans* oxygen atoms (Figure 8.8). This interaction is completed by the superposition of the two metallic d_{xz} and d_{yz} orbitals with the four p_x and p_y orbitals on the two oxo groups, thus yielding a total of four σ and π bonding MOs, four σ* and π* antibonding MOs, and two πs′ MOs that are mostly localised on the two opposite metal–oxo bonds, respectively (Figure 8.8). The residual d_{xy} metal orbital is left as non-bonding orbital. Apart from the two high-energy σ* and π* antibonding orbitals and the remaining four d^2sp^3 hybrid orbitals, the other MOs and the non-bonding d_{xy} (in total, 7 MOs) can accommodate the 14 valence electrons (12 electrons from the two oxo groups plus 2 metal electrons) of the *trans*-$[O{=}M^V{=}O]^+$ (M = Tc, Re) group. According to this picture, the frontier orbitals of the metal *trans*-dioxo core are composed by the filled π′ HOMO orbitals and the four empty d^2sp^3 hybrid orbitals lying on the equatorial plane of the octahedron (Figure 8.8). This set of LUMOs largely determines the chemical behaviour of the *trans*-dioxo fragment.

It turns out that the formation of σ bonds with σ-donor atoms constitutes the preferred interaction of the dioxo functional group and that σ-donor ligands are the most suitable type of coordinating ligands. An important class of *trans*-dioxo complexes is obtained when four nitrogen donor atoms occupy the equatorial positions of the octahedron, thus yielding an N_4 coordinating system as illustrated in Figure 8.9. Linear and cyclic polyamines are suitable chelating ligands for the *trans*-$[O{=}M^V{=}O]^+$ core, though it is usually easier to bind to this group to an open N_4 chain than to introduce it into a cyclic N_4 ring. Similarly, a linear P_4 chelating system affords another class of stable *trans*-dioxo complexes through the σ donor interaction with four phosphorus atoms (Figure 8.9). For instance, bidentate and tetradentate tertiary phosphines form stable complexes with the *trans*-$[O{=}M^V{=}O]^+$ (M = Tc, Re) group. In these compounds, the strength of this metal-to-phosphorus bond is always enhanced by the additional π-acceptor interaction between the empty π orbitals of the π-acid phosphine ligands and the filled d_{xy} non-bonding orbitals of the metallic fragment. This back-donation of electron density from the metal group to the ligand is able to further stabilise the resulting complexes.

An interesting example of sterically controlled conversion between monoxo and dioxo cores is given by Tc(V) complexes with amino-oxime ligands (Figure 8.10). This N_4 chelating system can bind the $[Tc{\equiv}O]^{3+}$ group as a trianionic tetradentate ligand

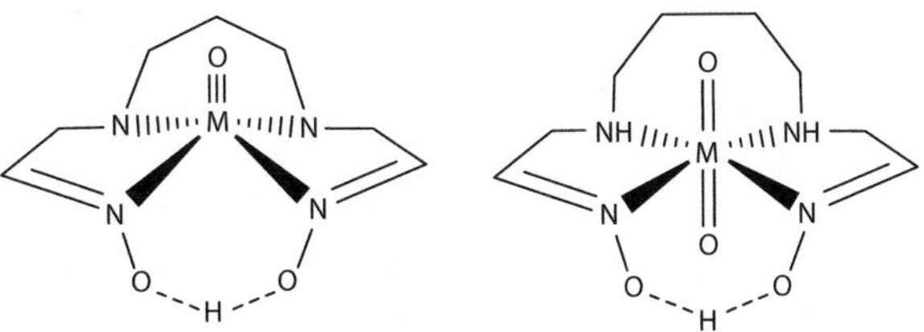

Figure 8.10 The N_4 amine-oxime ligand system for monoxo and dioxo groups.

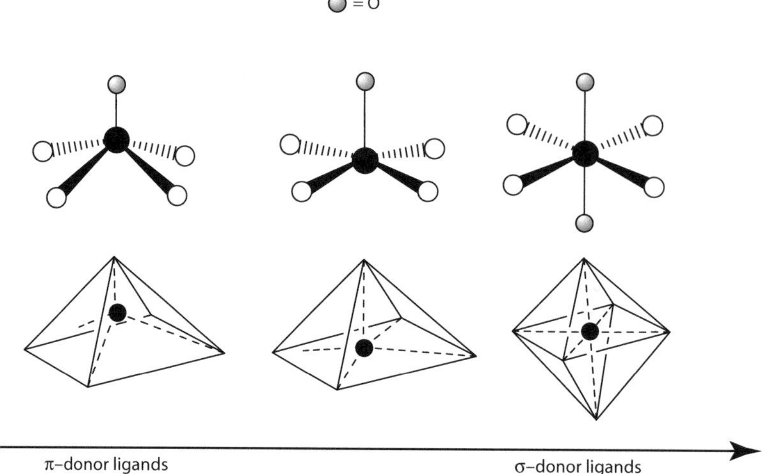

Figure 8.11 Reaction pathway of conversion of *sp* monoxo complexes into *oh trans*-dioxo complexes.

through two neutral and two negatively charged nitrogen atoms, the third negative charge being generated through deprotonation of one hydroxyl group. The concomitant formation of a hydrogen bond bridging the two hydroxyl oxygen atoms gives rise to a closed ring surrounding the metal centre. Depending on the dimension of this ring, the resulting complex can switch between *sp* and *oh* geometries, thus yielding either monoxo or dioxo complexes, respectively. Specifically, when the size of the ligand cycle is small and does not allow inclusion of the metal ion, the system assumes an *sp* arrangement with the metal lying above the plane of the square pyramid. Conversely, when the ring size is increased by adding a carbon atom to the ligand cycle as shown in Figure 8.10, the metal ion can be incorporated into the ring and the system assumes *oh* geometry. This geometrical conversion changes the electronic properties of the metal centre allowing the binding of another oxygen atom in *trans* position to the first oxo group.

It should be noted that the conversion between *sp* and *oh* geometries always involves lowering of the metal centre from the interior of the square pyramid towards the basal plane defined by the four atoms coordinated to the $[Tc{\equiv}O]^{3+}$ group. There exists a close relationship between the donor properties of these atoms and the value of the displacement of the metal centre from the basal plane (Δ). As a general rule, soft donor atoms favour an increase of Δ, thus causing a progressive distortion of the square pyramid towards the reversed umbrella-shaped form. Conversely, hard donor atoms cause a reversal of this process, achieving an almost ideal *sp* geometry with the metallic centre occupying the basal square plane. In the final stage of this process, the attack of a water molecule *trans* to the oxo group, followed by the loss of two protons, leads ultimately to the formation of the *trans*-$[O{=}M^{V}{=}O]^{+}$ core with the concomitant transformation of *sp* into *oh* geometry (Figure 8.11). It is interesting to note that the same behaviour is also observed with the $[M{\equiv}N]^{2+}$ fragment, though the stronger π-donor character of the nitrido nitrogen atom prevents the complete conversion of *sp* to *oh* geometry.

The metal imido, $[M{=}NR]^{3+}$, and metal hydrazido (diazenido), $[M{=}N{=}NR]^{2+}$, functional groups [M = Tc(V), Re(V), R = organic functional group]

Primary amines (H_2NR) and monosubstituted hydrazine derivatives (H_2N-NHR) can bind Tc and Re in the +5 oxidation state to form the $[M{=}NR]^{3+}$ (M-imido) and $[M{=}N{=}NR]^{2+}$ (M-hydrazido, M-diazenido) functional groups (M = Tc, Re; R = organic functional group), respectively (Tisato *et al.* 1994; Eikey, Mahdi 2003; Young-Seung *et al.* 2006). Though the $[M{=}NR]^{3+}$ group is formally considered isoelectronic with the metal oxo and nitrido groups, its electronic properties differ significantly from those of the two

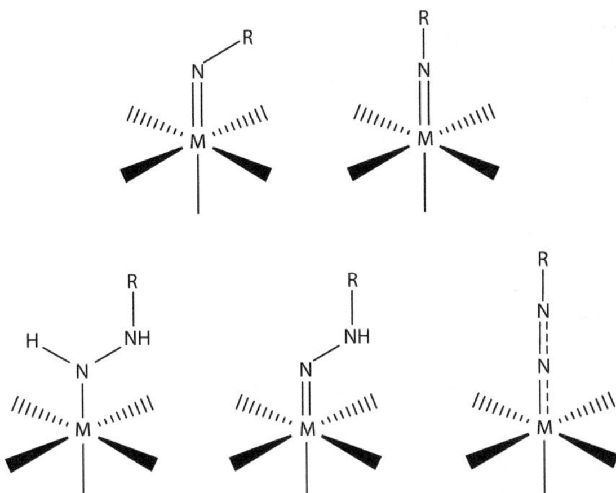

Figure 8.12 Possible arrangements for M-imido and M-hydrizido functional groups (R = organic functional group).

previously described cores, as clearly demonstrated by the fact that M-imido complexes usually exhibit an *oh* structure. Depending on the nature of the R group appended to the nitrogen atom, the M-N-R arrangement may assume either a linear or bent configuration. In particular, electron-withdrawing groups favour a bent structure where the N atom has sp^2 hybridisation and the M—N bond is double bond in character. Conversely, electron-donating groups force the system to achieve a linear configuration where the N atom has sp hybridisation and the M–N bond has a partial triple bond character (Figure 8.12). It should be noted that the preference between the linear or bent arrangements can also be influenced by the coordination environment around the metal centre.

Similarly, the M-hydrazido group may exist in different configurations though it is not always simple to establish those factors controlling the stability of the various arrangements schematically illustrated in Figure 8.12.

The metal M(III)(4+1) functional group (M = Tc, Re)

Stable Tc and Re complexes possessing a *tbp* geometry are obtained when tetradentate lantern-type YS_3 (Y = N, P) ligands (Figure 8.13) coordinate the metal centre, in the +3 oxidation state, through the neutral Y atom and the three negatively charged sulfur atoms

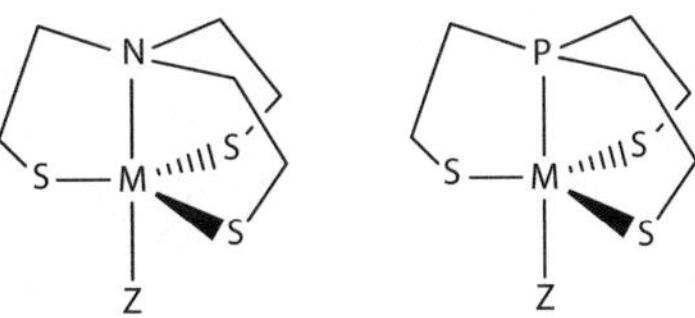

Figure 8.13 General structure of M(III)(4+1) (M = Tc, Re) complexes (Z = C≡N—R, PR_3; R = organic functional group).

(Pietzsch *et al.* 2001; Schiller *et al.* 2005; Mirtschink *et al.* 2008).

The resulting neutral metallic fragment [$M(YS_3)$] exhibits a selective chemical reactivity only towards π-acceptor ligands like tertiary monophosphines (PR_3) and isocyanides (R—N≡C). This leads to the formation of bis-substituted complexes composed of a tetradentate ligand and a monodentate π-acceptor ligand occupying the residual axial position of the *tbp* structure (hence, the name 4+1 complexes).

The electronic structure of the M(4+1) fragment reveals the essential features of the orbital distribution in a *tbp* geometry. In particular, a convenient picture of the energy levels posits that, in a *tbp* symmetry, there exists a separation between the orbitals involved in the bonding along the axial positions and those forming bonds on the trigonal plane. Thus, considering the *tbp* equatorial plane as lying on the *xy* plane, hybridisation of the metallic s, p_x and p_y, orbitals (sp^2) can be used to account for the three σ bonds on the same plane. Similarly, hybridisation of the metallic d_z^2 and p_z orbitals affords two hybrid dp orbitals describing the σ bonding along the two axial positions, though, in the M(4+1) fragment, only one of these dp orbitals is used to represent the M—Y bond. This leaves the π d_{xy}, $d_{x^2-y^2}$, and d_{xz}, d_{yz} orbitals and the remaining hybrid dp σ orbital to enter the set of fragment frontier orbitals (Figure 8.14). Since the total electron count for the M(4+1) fragment is 12 electrons (8 electrons from the YS_3 ligand plus 4 metal electrons), the HOMOs correspond to the filled d_{xz} and d_{yz} orbitals and the LUMO to the hybrid dp orbital (Figure 8.13).

The σ character of the frontier dp LUMO provides hints on the chemical reactivity of the M(4+1) metallic group. Evidently, monodentate σ donor ligands appear as obvious candidates for coordination to this group. However, the existence of a pair of filled d_{xz} and d_{yz} orbitals having a close energy also indicates

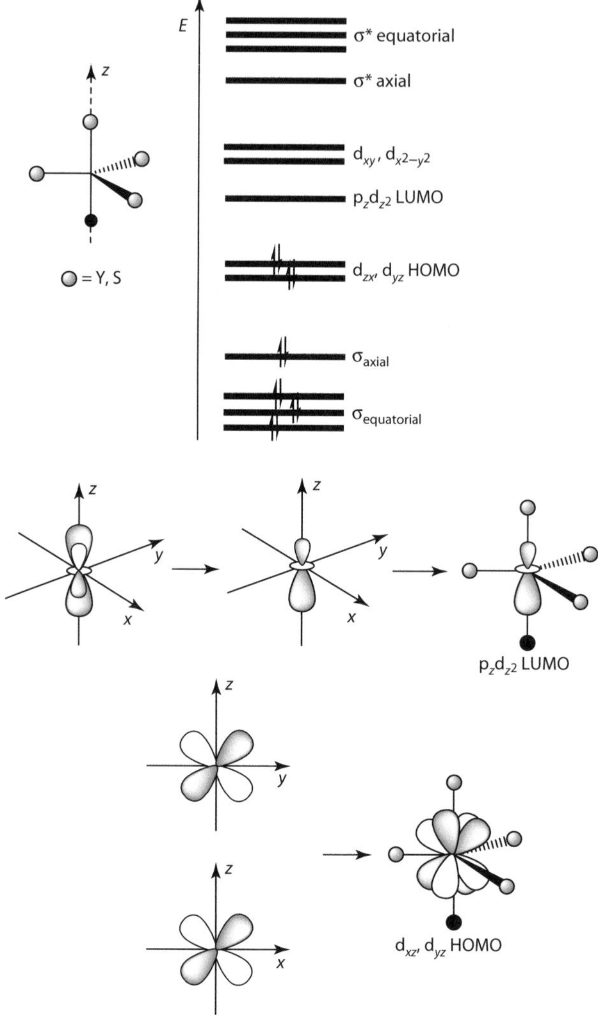

Figure 8.14 Fragment orbitals for the metallic functional group M(4+1) (M = Tc, Re).

that π interaction may play a critical role in determining the nature of the most suitable ligand. Actually, ligands possessing π orbitals that can overlap with the d_{xz} and d_{yz} orbitals usually give rise to a stronger coordination bond with the M(4+1) moiety. Specifically, π acceptor ligands constitute the most important class of coordinating agents for the M(4+1) fragment because of their ability to accept electronic density from the metal through back donation. It should be noted that the two metal π orbitals span both axial positions of the *tbp* structure (Figure 8.14) and, as a consequence, they may allow a kind of electronic communication when shared between the two axially positioned ligands. In particular, when both axial ligands are π acceptors the resulting complexes exhibit a higher stability. This suggests that PS_3 type ligands form more stable complexes than NS_3 type ligands.

It is worthy of note that *tbp* complexes for Tc and Re are relatively rare, and that *oh* complexes are more common. Usually, these latter species contain a combination of σ,π-donor and π-acceptor coordinating atoms that can be also incorporated in a single molecule to afford multidentate mixed donor–acceptor ligands. Figure 8.15 shows some illustrative examples of *oh* Tc(III) and Re(III) complexes.

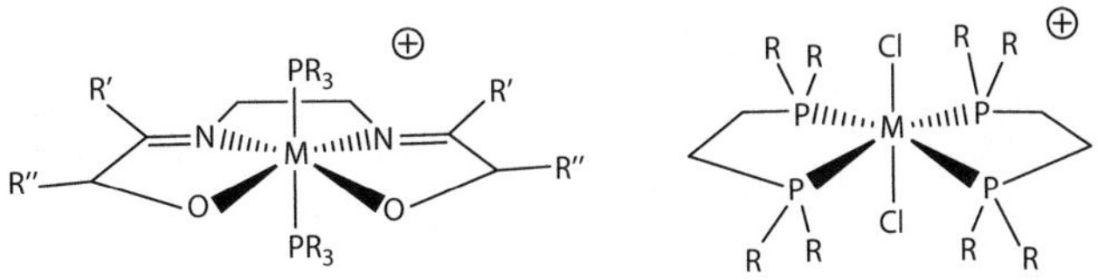

Figure 8.15 Representative examples of *oh* M(III) complexes (M = Tc, Re; R, R′, R″ = organic functional group).

The metal $[ML_6]^+$ functional group (M = Tc, Re)

A simple M^+ (M = Tc, Re) ion with a formal oxidation state +1, constitutes an important metallic fragment in Tc and Re chemistry. Obviously, this formal ion cannot exist as a free species and can be isolated only when embedded into the structure of a coordination complex. In particular, when six identical, monodentate, neutral σ ligands (L) are bound to the M(I) centre, the resulting $[ML_6]^+$ complex can be conveniently considered as a true inorganic functional group (Schwochau 2000; Bandoli *et al.* 2001). However, the electronic properties of the M^+ ion are fully sufficient to explain the chemical behaviour of this category of complexes. It turns out that the description of the electronic structure of the M^+ fragment is particularly simple. Since M(I) complexes usually possess an *oh* geometry, the frontier orbitals of the M^+ group can easily be obtained by considering the five d orbitals and the four s, p_x, p_y and p_z orbitals belonging to the next upper energy level. Mixing these latter metallic orbitals with d_z^2 and $d_{x^2-y^2}$ provides six hybrid d^2sp^3 σ orbitals pointing towards the vertexes of the octahedron. The remaining d_{xy}, d_{xz} and d_{yz} can be considered as non-bonding orbitals having a π-symmetry. If six σ-donor atoms are coordinated to the M(I) centre, the resulting orbital distribution is as shown in Figure 8.16. Considering a

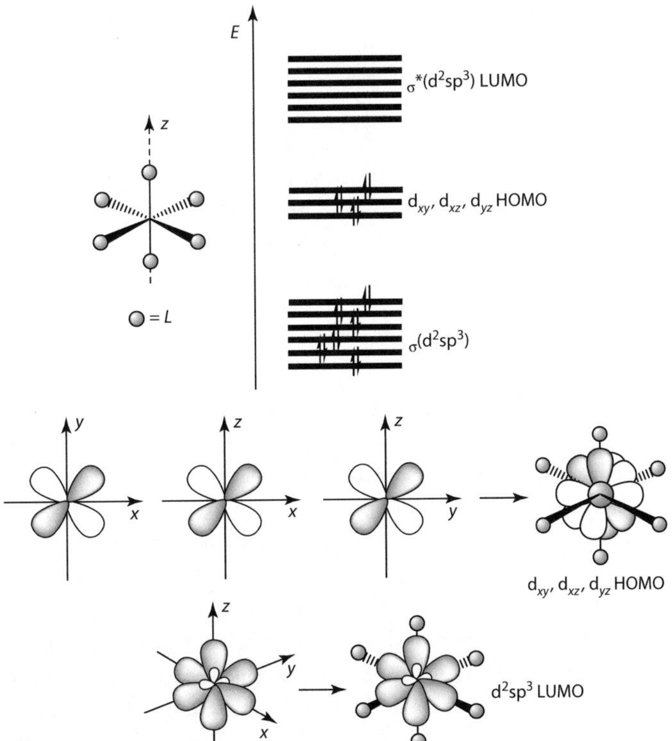

Figure 8.16 Fragment orbitals for the metallic functional group $[ML_6]^+$ (M = Tc, Re; L = monodentate σ-donor ligand).

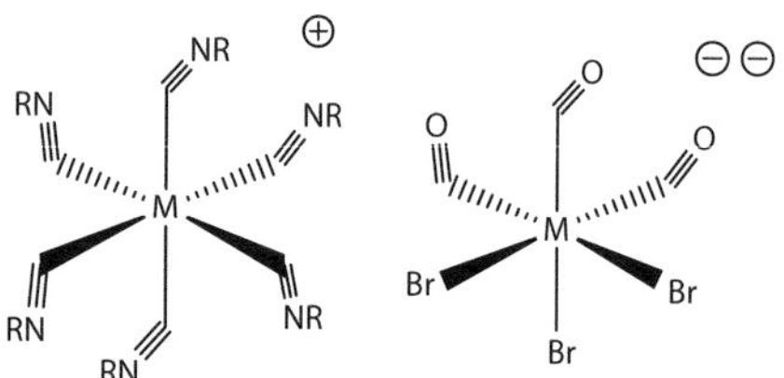

Figure 8.17 Representative examples of $[ML_6]^+$ complexes with π-acceptor ligands (R = organic functional group).

total electron count of 18 electrons (12 electrons from the six L ligands plus 6 metal electrons), the HOMOs correspond to the filled d_{xy}, d_{xz} and d_{yz} orbitals and the LUMOs to the high-energy d^2sp^3 σ* antibonding orbitals.

The orbital diagram illustrated in Figure 8.16 indicates that the chemical behaviour of the $[ML_6]^+$ fragment is largely dominated by the filled set of d_{xy}, d_{xz} and d_{yz} orbitals having a π symmetry. For instance, these orbitals can efficiently overlap with empty π orbitals on some suitable π-acceptor ligand. This interaction involves a redistribution of electronic density from the metal to the acceptor ligand with the concomitant strengthening of the metal–ligand bond. Therefore, π-acid ligands can afford the most stable coordination set for the M(I) centre. Representative examples of this class of complexes are the isocyanide and carbonyl derivatives shown in Figure 8.17.

The metal tris-carbonyl, [*mer*-M(CO)$_3$]$^+$ (M = Tc, Re), functional group

Another interesting example of a metallic fragment containing the metal atom in the +1 oxidation state is provided by the metal tris-carbonyl, [*mer*-M(CO)$_3$]$^+$ (M = Tc, Re), functional group (Alberto *et al.* 1999; Schibli, Schubiger 2002; Alberto 2007). This group can be easily produced in aqueous solution by reacting the tetraoxo anion $[MO_4]^-$ with carbon dioxide in the presence of the borohydride anion $[BH_4]^-$. Alternatively, this fragment is formed through the reaction of the potassium salt of the boranocarbonate anion, $[H_3BCO_2]^{2-}$, with $[MO_4]^-$, though when M = Re the further addition of the amino-borane Lewis adduct, $BH_3{\cdot}NH_3$, is used to improve the reaction yield (Park *et al.* 2006). When formed in aqueous solution, the M-carbonyl core is usually bound to three water molecules to yield the mixed aquo-carbonyl complex $[M(CO)_3(H_2O)_2]^+$. The three water molecules are only weakly bound to the metallic centre and can easily be replaced by some stronger coordinating ligand to afford substituted carbonyl complexes in which the tris-carbonyl moiety is always preserved.

Generally, complexes incorporating the metal tris-carbonyl moiety exhibit an *oh* geometry. Therefore, the electronic description of the $[M(CO)_3]^+$ core can be easily derived from that illustrated previously for *oh* $[ML_6]^+$ complexes. In binding to the M^+ ion, the three CO ligands assume a reciprocal *mer* configuration and can overlap a σ orbital with three adjacent metallic d^2sp^3 hybrid orbitals, thus forming three σ bonding and three σ* antibonding MOs. This leaves three d^2sp^3 hybrid orbitals pointing towards the opposite equilateral face of the octahedron. In addition, carbon monoxide is a strong π-acceptor ligand and possesses an empty π* antibonding orbital having the same symmetry of the metal d_{xy}, d_{xz} and d_{yz} orbitals. Overlapping of three CO π* orbitals with d_{xy}, d_{xz} and d_{yz} affords three π bonding and three π* antibonding MOs. Since there are 12 valence electrons for the $[M(CO)_3]^+$ core (6 electrons from the CO ligands plus 6 metal electrons), the filled π bonding MOs can be identified with the frontier HOMOs and the remaining σ d^2sp^3 with the LUMOs (Figure 8.18). This description is in close agreement with the π-acceptor properties of the CO ligands because the electron density on the HOMOs is ultimately redistributed to the ligands through the π interaction.

Evidently, the existence of three d^2sp^3 LUMOs sharply regulates the chemical behaviour of the $[M(CO)_3]^+$ fragment and suggests that ligands containing σ-donor atoms are the most preferred coordinating systems. Actually, a neutral nitrogen atom appears to strongly interact with the $[M(CO)_3]^+$ core as demonstrated by the large number of tris-carbonyl complexes with primary and secondary amines. In particular, multidentate nitrogen-containing ligands offer some convenient chelating sets, particularly when employed in conjunction with negatively charged oxygen atoms as in amino acids. For example, histidine has been found to be among the strongest coordinating ligands for the $[M(CO)_3]^+$ group as it acts as a tridentate

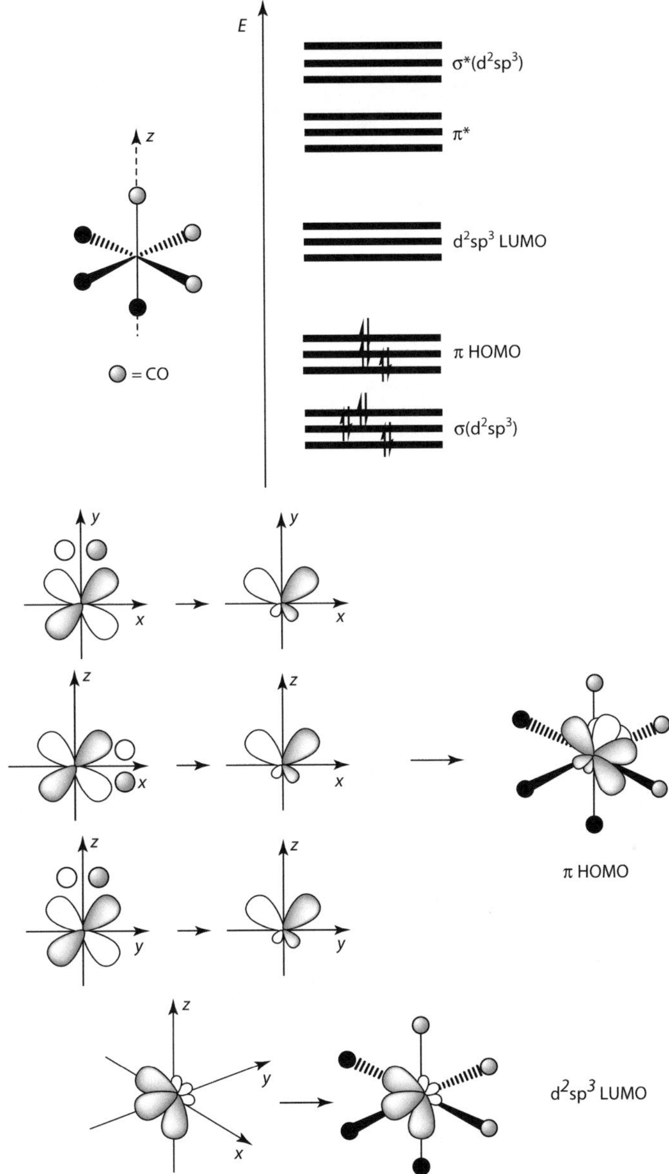

Figure 8.18 Fragment orbitals for the metallic functional group $[M(CO)_3]^+$ (M = Tc, Re).

chelating agent through the amino and heterocyclic nitrogen atoms and the deprotonated carboxylic oxygen atom (Figure 8.19). However, the number of possible ligands for this group is extremely high and some representative examples of them and of the resulting complexes are given in Figure 8.19. Usually, tridentate ligands yield the most stable complexes, but a combination of monodentate and bidentate ligands have been also employed. As outlined above, essentially these ligands interact with the $[M(CO)_3]^+$ fragment through the formation of σ bonds. But π-acceptor ligands can also be used, though it should be always taken into account that this π interaction has to be shared with the carbonyl groups and, consequently, may have some impact on the stability of the metallic fragment itself.

An interesting class of carbonyl derivatives is given by mixed carbonyl-cyclopentadienyl complexes as

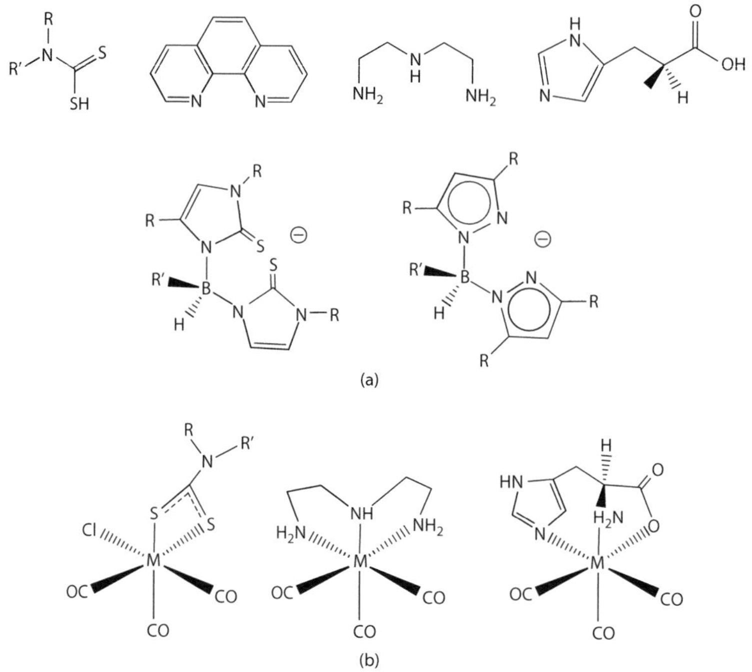

Figure 8.19 Examples of (a) ligands and (b) complexes of the $[M(CO)_3]^+$ functional group.

illustrated in Figure 8.20. In these complexes, cyclopentadiene (Cp) is coordinated to the $[M(CO)_3]^+$ fragment as a mononegative anion (Cp^-) after deprotonation of the aromatic ring. Usually, this deprotonation is strongly hampered in aqueous solution, a fact that drastically limits the development of the aqueous chemistry of cyclopentadienyl complexes. Recently, it was reported that appending a ketone group to the Cp ring, as shown in Figure 8.20, greatly improves the loss of a hydrogen from the ring. These findings may open new routes to the synthesis of a large class of cyclopentadienyl complexes in aqueous conditions. The carboxylic group appended to the cyclopentadienyl ring is just another example of a derivative prepared in aqueous solution and also could be used for further functionalisation.

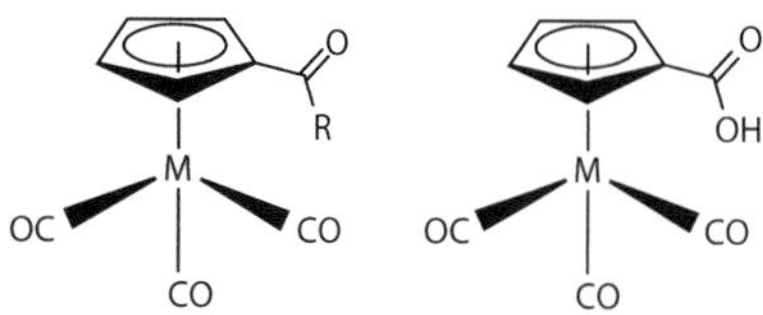

Figure 8.20 Structure of metal tris-carbonyl complexes containing a cyclopentadienyl ring.

Some relevant examples of ^{99m}Tc and ^{188}Re radiopharmaceuticals

During recent decades, the various functional groups described in the previous sections have been widely employed to develop a large number of ^{99m}Tc radiopharmaceuticals exhibiting different biodistribution properties and selective accumulation in some target tissues. Some of these compounds have received final marketing authorisation from regulatory authorities and are currently used as important diagnostic tools in hospital nuclear medicine departments. Conversely, a significant number of ^{99m}Tc radiopharmaceuticals have not been yet approved for commercial distribution despite the fact they have shown interesting diagnostic properties potentially useful for clinical application. In this section, the molecular structures of the most important examples of both commercial and experimental ^{99m}Tc radiopharmaceuticals, grouped on the basis of their characteristic metallic functional fragment, are briefly described (Zolle 2007).

In Figure 8.21, the chemical structures of ^{99m}Tc radiopharmaceuticals containing the $[Tc{\equiv}O]^{3+}$ group are reported. This class of imaging agents includes the

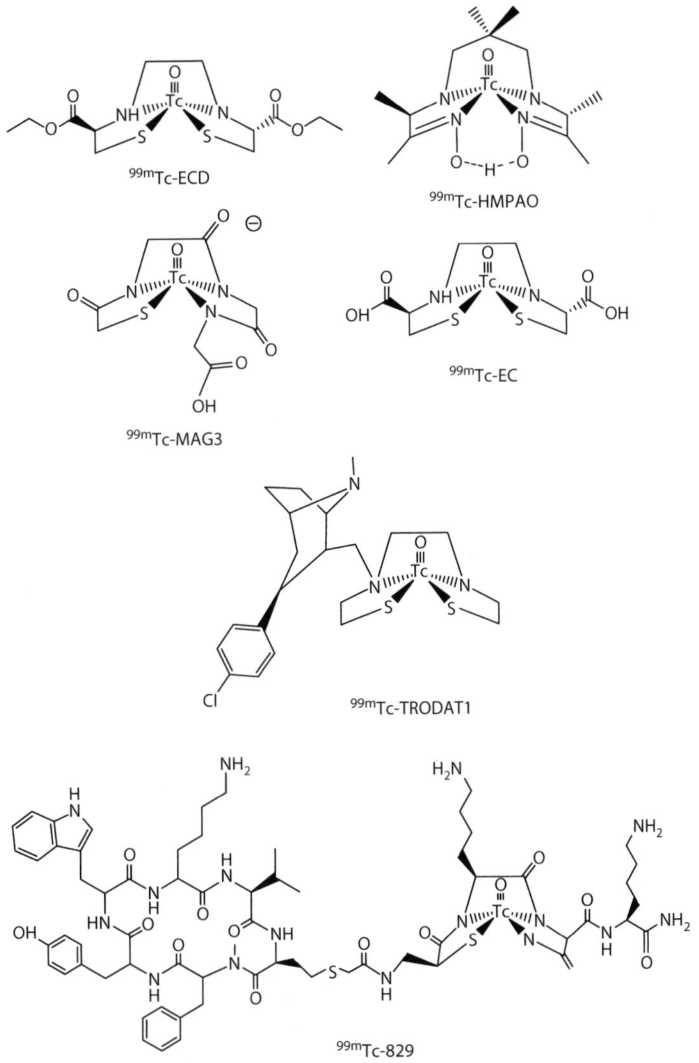

^{99m}Tc-ECD

^{99m}Tc-HMPAO

^{99m}Tc-MAG3

^{99m}Tc-EC

^{99m}Tc-TRODAT1

^{99m}Tc-829

Figure 8.21 Relevant examples of ^{99m}Tc radiopharmaceuticals containing the $[Tc{\equiv}O]^{3+}$ core.

highest number of ^{99m}Tc radiopharmaceuticals, ranging from the two brain perfusion imaging agents ^{99m}Tc-HMPAO (Ceretec) and ^{99m}Tc-ECD (Neurolite) (Koyama *et al.* 1997), the two kidney perfusion imaging agents ^{99m}Tc-MAG3 (Technescan) (Eshima, Taylor 1992) and ^{99m}Tc-EC (not approved) (Kabasakal 2000), the compound ^{99m}Tc-TRODAT1 (not approved) for imaging D2 receptors in the central nervous system (Kung *et al.* 2003), and the peptide-based conjugate complex ^{99m}Tc-829 (^{99m}Tc-NeoTect or NeoSpect) for imaging somatostatin receptor expressing tumours (Cyr *et al.* 2007).

Although there are no approved ^{99m}Tc radiopharmaceuticals containing the $[Tc{\equiv}N]^{2+}$ group, two classes of these complexes have demonstrated very interesting properties, particularly for cardiac imaging. The symmetric nitrido compound ^{99m}TcN-NOET (CisNOEt) was the first neutral heart perfusion imaging agent showing prolonged retention in the myocardial tissue (Vanzetto *et al.* 2004) (Figure 8.22). Recently, the monocationic asymmetric nitrido complex ^{99m}TcN-DBODC has been found to possess a remarkably high heart/liver ratio, thus allowing collection of high-quality perfusion images of myocardium (Cittanti *et al.* 2008).

The most important example of a ^{99m}Tc radiopharmaceutical containing the *trans*-$[O{=}Tc{=}O]^{+}$ core is given by the monocationic compound

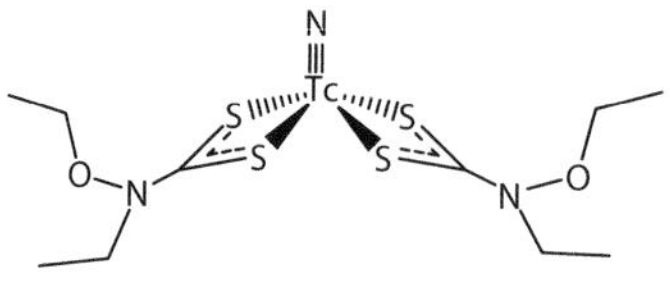

^{99m}TcN–NOET

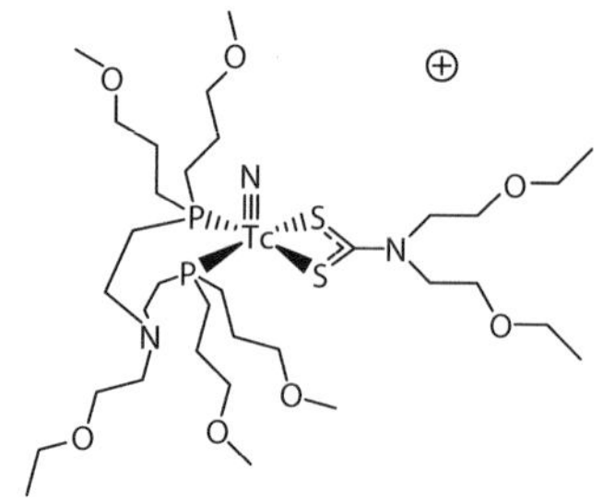

^{99m}TcN–DBODC

Figure 8.22 Relevant examples of ^{99m}Tc radiopharmaceuticals containing the $[Tc{\equiv}N]^{2+}$ core.

^{99m}Tc-tetrofosmin (Myoview) (Heo, Iskandrian 1994), widely employed for heart perfusion imaging (Figure 8.23). The peptide-based dioxo conjugate complex ^{99m}Tc-demotate has been recently reported and is currently under evaluation as imaging agent for detecting somatostatin receptor-expressing tumours (Maina *et al.* 2002).

Complexes containing ligands derived from hydrazinonicotinic acid (HYNIC) provide the most interesting examples of ^{99m}Tc radiopharmaceuticals containing the $[M{=}N{=}NR]^{2+}$ core (see Figure 8.24). This core appears particularly suitable for the efficient labelling of proteins and peptides, as is nicely demonstrated by the two agents ^{99m}Tc-HYNIC-Annexin V (not approved) and ^{99m}Tc-HYNIC-TOC (not approved). The tracer ^{99m}Tc-HYNIC-Annexin V is employed for *in-vivo* imaging of apoptosis as it incorporates the protein Annexin V covalently bound to the carboxylic group of HYNIC, which selectively binds phosphatidylserine residues expressed on the surface of apoptotic cells (Blankenberg *et al.* 2006). The peptide-based complex ^{99m}Tc-HYNIC-TOC is employed for imaging somatostatin receptor-expressing tumours (Guggenberg *et al.* 2004).

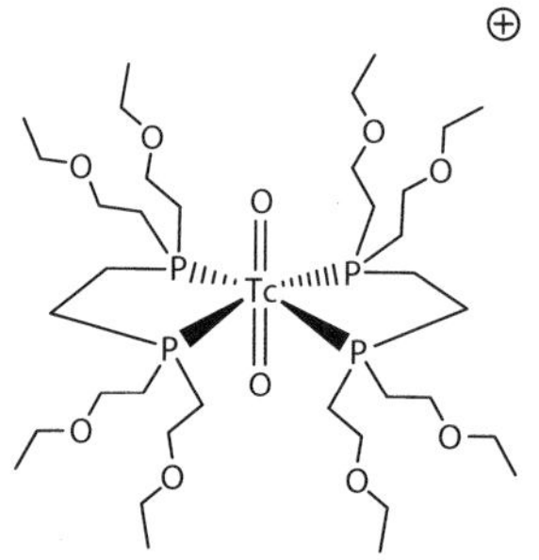

^{99m}Tc–Tetrofosmin

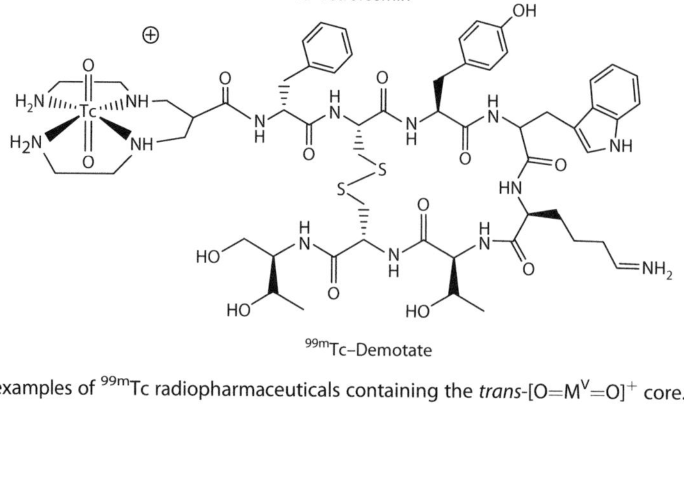

^{99m}Tc–Demotate

Figure 8.23 Relevant examples of ^{99m}Tc radiopharmaceuticals containing the *trans*-$[O{=}M^{V}{=}O]^{+}$ core.

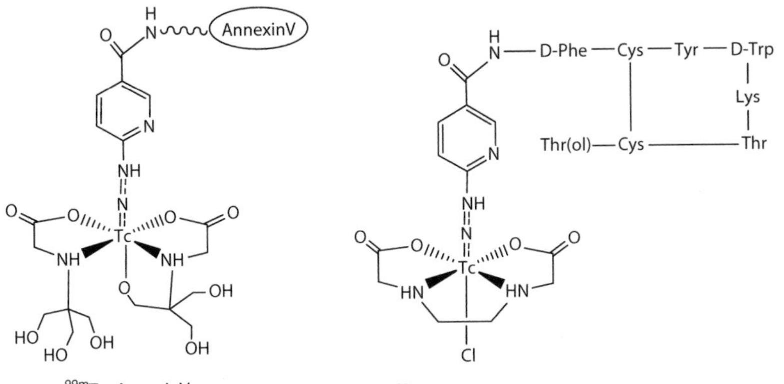

^{99m}Tc–AnnexinV

^{99m}Tc–HYNIC–TOC

Figure 8.24 Relevant examples of ^{99m}Tc radiopharmaceuticals containing the Tc(III) ion.

The neutral Tc(III) heptacoordinated complex ^{99m}Tc-teboroxime (CardioTec) was the first market approved cardiac perfusion imaging agent (Leppo *et al.* 1991) (Figure 8.25). It shows a high transient cardiac uptake followed by a fast washout. Another example of a ^{99m}Tc radiopharmaceutical containing the Tc(III) ion is represented by the monocationic heart perfusion tracer ^{99m}Tc-furifosmin or ^{99m}Tc-Q12 (TechneCard) (Gerson *et al.* 1994) (Figure 8.25).

The monocationic octahedral complex ^{99m}Tc-MIBI or ^{99m}Tc-sestamibi (Cardiolite) provides the most significant example of a ^{99m}Tc radiopharmaceutical containing the metal in the +1 oxidation state (Figure 8.26). This agent is routinely employed for imaging myocardial perfusion and can surely be considered as among the most successful radiopharmaceuticals (Heo, Iskandrian 1994).

In recent years, a huge number of ^{99m}Tc complexes containing the $[^{99m}Tc(CO)_3]^+$ core have been reported, a result that has been favoured by the introduction of a freeze-dried kit formulation for the preparation of the intermediate $[^{99m}Tc(CO)_3(H_2O_3]^+$ complex (Isolink). Though none of these compounds has yet revealed potentially useful properties for diagnostic applications, the search in this specific area is progressing and this group is mostly utilised

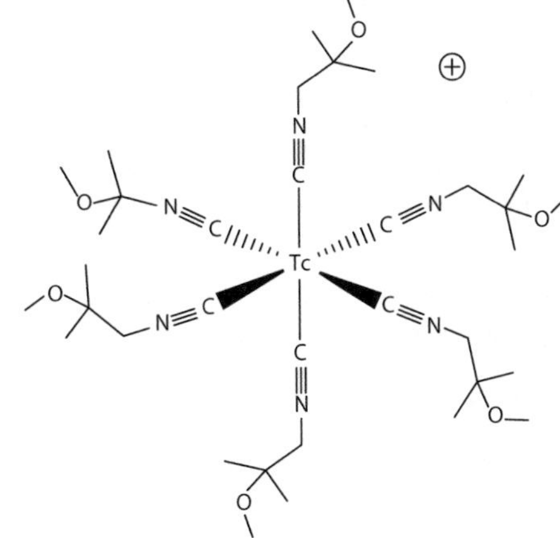

Figure 8.26 A ^{99m}Tc radiopharmaceutical containing the Tc(I) ion.

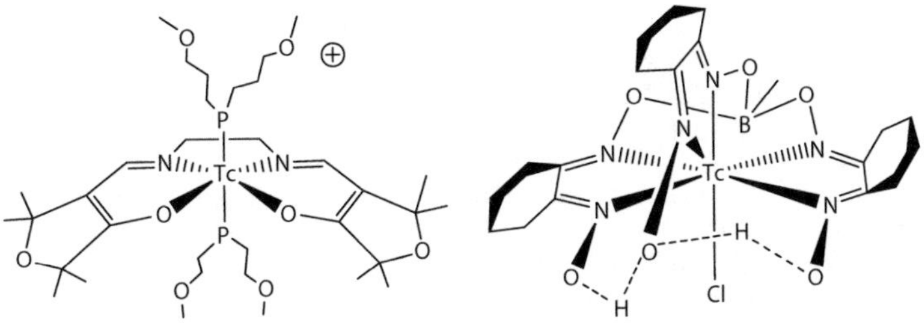

^{99m}Tc–Q12

^{99m}Tc–Teboroxime

Figure 8.25 Relevant examples of ^{99m}Tc radiopharmaceuticals containing the $[M{=}N{=}NR]^{2+}$ core.

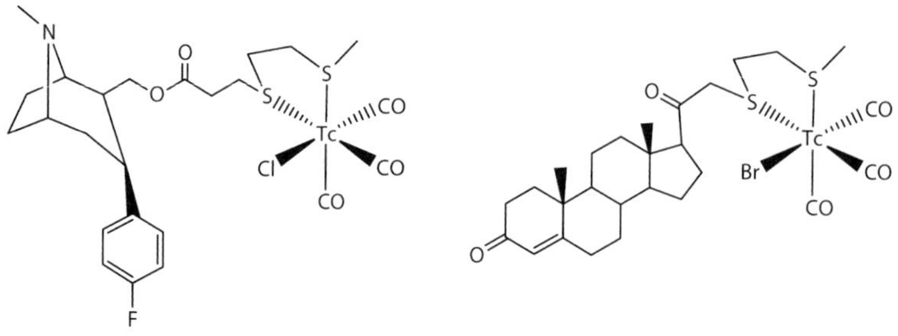

^{99m}Tc–TROTEC–1

Figure 8.27 Relevant examples of ^{99m}Tc radiopharmaceuticals containing the $[Tc(CO)_3]^+$ core.

for labelling biologically active molecules. A few examples of ^{99m}Tc-carbonyl radiopharmaceuticals are illustrated in Figure 8.27 (Hoepping *et al.* 1998; Schibli, Schubiger 2002).

References

Alberto R (2007). The particular role of radiopharmacy within bioorganometallic chemistry. *J Organometal Chem* 692: 1179–1186.

Alberto R *et al.* (1999). Basic aqueous chemistry of $[M(OH_2)_3(CO)_3]^+$ (M = Re, Tc) directed towards radiopharmaceutical application. *Coord Chem Rev* 190–192: 901–919.

Albright TA *et al.* (1985). *Orbital Interactions in Chemistry.* New York: Wiley-Interscience.

Atkins P, de Paula J (2006). *Physical Chemistry.* New York: Oxford University Press.

Bandoli G *et al.* (2001). Structural overview of technetium compounds (1993–1999). *Coord Chem Rev* 214: 43–90.

Bandoli G *et al.* (2006). Structural overview of technetium compounds (2000–2004). *Coord Chem Rev* 250: 561–573.

Blankenberg FG *et al.* (2006). Radiolabeling of HYNIC-annexin V with technetium-99m for in vivo imaging of apoptosis. *Nat Protoc* 1: 108–110.

Bolzati C *et al.* (2000). An alternative approach to the preparation of ^{188}Re radiopharmaceuticals from generator-produced $[^{188}ReO_4]^-$: efficient synthesis of ^{188}Re(V)-*meso*-2,3-dimercaptosuccinic acid. *Nucl. Med. Biol* 27: 309–314.

Boschi A *et al.* (2005). Development of technetium-99m and rhenium-188 radiopharmaceuticals containing a terminal metal–nitrido multiple bond for diagnosis and therapy. *Top Curr Chem* 252: 85–101.

Chang R (2005). *Physical Chemistry for the Biosciences.* Herndon, VA: University Science Books.

Cittanti C *et al.* (2008). Whole-body biodistribution and radiation dosimetry of the new cardiac tracer 99mTc-N-DBODC. *J Nucl Med* 49: 1299–1304.

Cotton FA *et al.* (1999). *Advanced Inorganic Chemistry*, 6th edn. New York: Wiley-Interscience.

Cyr JE *et al.* (2007). Isolation, characterization, and biological evaluation of *syn* and *anti* diastereomers of [^{99m}Tc]technetium depreotide: a somatostatin receptor binding tumor imaging agent. *J Med Chem* 50: 4295–4303.

Earnshaw A, Greenwood N (1997). *Chemistry of the Elements*, 2nd edn. Oxford: Butterworth-Heinemann.

Eikey RA, Mahdi MA-O (2003). Nitrido and imido transition metal complexes of groups 6–8. *Coord Chem Rev* 243: 83–124.

Eshima D, Taylor A Jr (1992). Technetium-99m (^{99m}Tc) mercaptoacetyltriglycine: update on the new ^{99m}Tc renal tubular function agent. *Semin Nucl Med* 22: 61–73.

Faintuch BL *et al.* (2003). Complexation of ^{188}Re-phosphonates: *in vitro* and *in vivo* studies. *Radiochim Acta* 91: 607–612.

Gerson MC *et al.* (1994). Kinetic properties of ^{99m}Tc-Q12 in canine myocardium. *Circulation* 89: 1291–1300.

Guggenberg EV *et al.* (2004). Radiopharmaceutical development of a freeze-dried kit formulation for the preparation of [^{99m}Tc-EDDA-HYNIC-D-Phe1, Tyr3]-octreotide, a somatostatin analog for tumor diagnosis. *J Pharm Sci* 93: 2497–2506.

Heo J, Iskandrian AS (1994). Technetium-labeled myocardial perfusion agents. *Cardiol Clin* 12: 187–198.

Hoepping A *et al.* (1998). TROTEC-1: a new high-affinity ligand for labeling of the dopamine transporter. *J Med Chem* 41: 4429–4432.

Kabasakal L (2000). Technetium-99m ethylene dicysteine: a new renal tubular function agent. *Eur J Nucl Med* 27: 351–357.

Koyama M *et al.* (1997). SPECT imaging of normal subjects with technetium-99m-HMPAO and technetium-99m-ECD. *J Nucl Med* 38: 587–592.

Kung HF *et al.* (2003). Radiopharmaceuticals for single-photon emission computed tomography brain imaging. *Semin Nucl Med* 33: 2–13.

Leppo JA *et al.* (1991). A review of cardiac imaging with sestamibi and teboroxime. *J Nucl Med* 32: 2012–2022.

Liu G, Hnatowich DJ (2007). Labeling biomolecules with radiorhenium: a review of the bifunctional chelators. *Anticancer Agents Med Chem* 7: 367–377.

Liu S (2004). The role of coordination chemistry in the development of target-specific radiopharmaceuticals. *Chem Soc Rev* 33: 445–461.

Liu S (2008). Bifunctional coupling agents for radiolabeling of biomolecules and target-specific delivery of metallic radionuclides. *Adv Drug Deliv Rev* 60: 1347–1370.

Maina T *et al.* (2002). [^{99m}Tc]Demotate, a new ^{99m}Tc-based [Tyr3]octreotate analogue for the detection of somatostatin receptor-positive tumours: synthesis and preclinical results. *Eur J Nucl Med Mol Imaging* 29: 742–753.

Mirtschink P *et al.* (2008). Modified "4 + 1" mixed ligand technetium-labeled fatty acids for myocardial imaging: evaluation of myocardial uptake and biodistribution. *Bioconjug Chem* 19: 97–108.

Park SH *et al.* (2006). Novel and efficient preparation of precursor [$^{188}Re(OH_2)_3(CO)_3]^+$ for the labeling of biomolecules. *Bioconj Chem* 17: 223–225.

Pietzsch HJ *et al.* (2001). Mixed-ligand technetium(III) complexes with tetradendate/monodendate NS(3)/isocyanide coordination: a new nonpolar technetium chelate system for the design of neutral and lipophilic complexes stable in vivo. *Bioconj Chem* 12: 538–544.

Schwochau K (2000). *Technetium: Chemistry and Radiopharmaceutical Applications.* Weinheim: Wiley-VCH.

Schibli R, Schubiger PA (2002). Current use and future potential of organometallic radiopharmaceuticals. *Eur J Nucl Med Mol Imaging* 29: 1529–1542.

Schiller E *et al.* (2005). Mixed-ligand rhenium-188 complexes with tetradentate/monodentate NS3/P ('4 + 1') coordination: relation of structure with antioxidation stability. *Bioconj Chem* 16: 634–643.

Seifert S, Pietzsch HJ (2006). The ^{188}Re(III)-EDTA complex: a multipurpose starting material for the preparation of relevant ^{188}Re complexes under mild conditions. *Appl Radiat Isot* 64: 223–227.

Tisato F *et al.* (2006). The preparation of substitution-inert ^{99}Tc metal-fragments: promising candidates for the design of new ^{99m}Tc radiopharmaceuticals. *Coord Chem Rev* 250: 2034–2045.

Tisato F *et al.* (1994). Structural survey of technetium complexes. *Coord Chem Rev* 135: 325–397.

Vanzetto G *et al.* (2004). Tc-99m N-NOET: Chronicle of a unique perfusion imaging agent and a missed opportunity? *J Nucl Cardiol* 11: 647–50.

Young-Seung K *et al.* (2006). A novel ternary ligand system useful for preparation of cationic ^{99m}Tc-diazenido complexes and ^{99m}Tc-labeling of small biomolecules. *Bioconj Chem* 17: 473–484.

Zolle I, ed. (2007). *Technetium-99m Pharmaceuticals: Preparation and Quality Control in Nuclear Medicine.* Berlin Heidelberg: Springer.

9

Trivalent metals and thallium

Adrian D Hall

Introduction

Groups 3 and 13 of the periodic table contains several transition elements of relevance to radiopharmacy. Group 13 comprises boron, aluminium, gallium, indium and thallium. However, there is no universally accepted convention for the layout of the periodic table, and there are a number of differences in the way the group 3 elements are categorised. Whilst scandium and yttrium are always classified as belonging to group 3, there are four common conventions that categorise members of the lanthanide and actinide series differently. Some versions of the periodic table include lanthanum and actinium (the first members of the lanthanide and actinide series respectively) as group 3 elements, some include lutetium and lawrencium (the last members of the lanthanide and actinide series), some include all 30 lanthanide and actinide elements and some include none. As far as this text is concerned, where the chemistry of those lanthanide and actinide elements finding application in radiopharmacy is similar to that of other group 3 metals, they will be considered here.

The chemical behaviour of many of the elements in these groups is predominantly controlled by the tendency to form ions with an overall charge of 3+ (tripositive cations). However, due to its small ionic radius, boron tends to lack cationic chemistry and thallium readily forms Tl^{+} rather than Tl^{3+} oxidation states, by virtue of the inert electron pair in its valence shell. This tendency of the elements in these groups to form tripositive cations results in much of their radiopharmaceutical chemistry being based upon coordination compounds. In coordination chemistry, a ligand binds to a cationic metal ion to form a coordination complex, in which electrons are donated from electron-rich donor atoms (Lewis base) to the electron-deficient metal ion (Lewis acid). As a result of their high charge densities, group 3 and group 13 metal ions behave as Lewis acids (electron acceptors), and form most stable bonds with ligands containing weakly polarisable donor atoms, such as oxygen. Some important atomic properties of the group 3 and group 13 cations are shown in Table 9.1. Iron is included for comparative purposes, as an example of a biologically relevant tripositive cation.

Table 9.1 Selected atomic properties of some trivalent cations

Cation	Electronic structure of M^{3+}	Ionic radius of M^{3+} (Å)	Coordination number of aquo M^{3+}
Fe^{3+}	[Ar]3d^{10}	0.65	6
Ga^{3+}	[Ar] 3d^5	0.62	6
In^{3+}	[Kr]4d^{10}	0.80	6
Y^{3+}	[Kr]	0.90	6–9
Sm^{3+}	[Xe] 4f^5	1.08	6–9
Ho^{3+}	[Xe] 4f^{10}	1.02	6–9
Lu^{3+}	[Xe] 4f^{14}	0.98	6–9

The majority of radionuclides with physical properties suitable for use in either diagnostic or therapeutic radiopharmaceuticals are metals (Jurisson *et al.* 1993). There is an inherent difference between radiopharmaceuticals labelled with metals and with non-metals, as most radiopharmaceuticals labelled with non-metals have the radionuclide covalently attached to the pharmaceutical, whereas metal-containing radiopharmaceuticals hold the metal in the form of a coordination complex (Liu 2004). In this latter case, the biodistribution properties of the radiopharmaceutical may be controlled either by the design of the coordination complex itself, or by attachment of the complex to a large biomolecule.

With the exception of radiopharmaceuticals consisting of simple salts, one of the most important factors in the design of a radiopharmaceutical is its stability. In the case of radiopharmaceuticals containing non-metallic radionuclides, the overall stability is likely to be controlled by the metabolism of the pharmaceutical component of the radiopharmaceutical, whereas with metal-containing radiopharmaceuticals, the overall stability is more likely to be affected by the properties of the coordination complex. The factors affecting stability of coordination complexes are discussed in more detail below.

Factors affecting stability of coordination complexes

The chemical properties of a metal that determine its interaction with donor atoms of ligands include size (either the ionic radius, or the radius of the hydrated metal ion), polarisability (see section on hard/soft donor atoms), redox properties, desolvation energy, stability of the metal complex (both thermodynamic and kinetic), the rate of reaction with the ligand and the geometry of the complex.

The molecular species that surround a metal ion and that are chemically bonded to the metal are termed ligands (Kauffman *et al.* 1983), while the atoms in the ligand that interact with the metal ion are termed donor atoms. This, plus the number of ligand molecules surrounding the metal ion, the polarisability of both metal and donor atoms, the stereochemistry of the resulting complexes and their thermodynamic and kinetic stabilities are the fundamental factors involved in studies of metal complexation.

Ligand denticity and the chelate effect

The denticity of a ligand is defined as the number of coordination sites on the metal that the ligand is able to fill. Thus, ligands that contain one (set of) donor atom(s) capable of binding to a metal ion are known as monodentate ligands, while ligands containing two are referred to as bidentate, those with three as tridentate, and so on. It is well established that multidentate ligands form more stable complexes with a given metal ion than do multiple monodentate ligands using the same donor atom, an effect known as the chelate effect (Hancock, Martell 1989). This is directly attributable to a decrease in the entropy of reaction resulting from the different stoichiometry involved in formation of the metal complex. This effect explains why, for a metal ion possessing six coordination sites, the stability constant for formation of the complex with different ligand types varies as:

$$\text{metal}-(\text{monodentate})_6 < \text{metal}-(\text{bidentate})_3 < \text{metal}-(\text{tridentate})_2 < \text{metal}-(\text{hexadentate})_1$$

It is thus easy to see that, providing the ligand geometry allows, the highest-stability complexes are produced from interaction of high-order multidentate ligands with metal ions.

Hard/soft donor atoms

Of the major determinants in the rational design of compounds designed for the specific complexation of particular metal ions, the selection of donor atoms is a well-established area (Pearson 1963; Schwarzenbach 1961), whereas the influence of ligand design is less well understood.

A preliminary indication of suitable donor atoms for selected ligands may be obtained using the Hard/Soft Acid Base (HSAB) classification of Pearson (1963). This divides metal ions and donor atoms into hard, soft, and intermediate groupings (see Table 9.2), and is based on the observation that hard metals are best chelated by hard donor atoms, while soft metals prefer soft donors. However, this simple classification is not infallible, and problems are often encountered with prediction of complex stabilities – for example, in ligands containing neutral oxygen donors. Such donor atoms occur not only in water, but also in ligands containing alcohol, amide, ether or ketone moieties. The relative coordinating abilities of oxygen in such groupings are quite different and, while there are indications as to selectivity effects based on metal ion size (Hancock 1986), it is clear that this area represents an important variable in ligand design that has received little attention to date.

Table 9.2 Classification of metal ions and donor atoms into hard, soft and intermediate groupings

	Soft	Intermediate	Hard
Acids	Cu^+, Ag^+, Au^+	Fe^{2+}, Cu^{2+}, Zn^{2+}, Sn^{2+}	H^+
	Br^+, I^+		Li^+, Na^+, K^+
	Br_2, I_2		Be^{2+}, Mg^{2+}, Ca^{2+} Fe^{3+}, Ga^{3+}, In^{3+}, Al^{3+}, La^{3+}
Bases	I^-, SCN^-, H^- R-SH, R-NC	Br^- SO_3^{2-}	HO^-, F^-, Cl^- PO_4^{3-}, CO_2^- SO_4^{2-}, CO_3^-

Thermodynamic stability

The thermodynamic stability of a metal complex is determined by the equilibrium constant (known as the stability or formation constant) for the reaction of a metal ion (M^{m+}) and a ligand (L^{n-}) to form the metal–ligand complex $ML^{(m-n)+}$, according to the reaction:

$$M^{m+} + L^{n-} \rightleftharpoons ML^{(m-n)+}$$

Since the metal ion exists as a hydrated aquo ion in aqueous solution, the equation should be more correctly written as:

$$M(H_2O)_x^{m+} + L^{n-} \rightleftharpoons M(H_2O)_{x-1}\,L^{(m-n)+} + H_2O$$

The coordination of a metal ion by a number of ligand molecules occurs in successive steps, for which individual stepwise stability constants may be determined, as indicated below:

$$\begin{aligned} M^{3+} + L^- &\rightleftharpoons ML^{2+}: & K_1 &= [ML^{2+}]/([M^{3+}][L^-]) \\ ML^{2+} + L^- &\rightleftharpoons ML_2^+: & K_2 &= [ML_2^+]/([ML^{2+}][L^-]) \\ ML_2^+ + L^- &\rightleftharpoons ML_3: & K_3 &= [ML_3]/([ML_2^+][L^-]) \end{aligned}$$

This gives the value of the overall stability constant, β_3, as $K_1 \cdot K_2 \cdot K_3$. Since this stability constant merely indicates the equilibrium distribution of metal and ligand between the various metal complexes, addition of a second ligand (possessing a higher stability constant for the metal ion than the first ligand) to this system would be expected to move the position of equilibrium in favour of the second ligand, i.e. causing dissociation of the original metal–ligand complexes. However, this simple explanation considers only the final position of equilibrium, rather than also considering the rate at which equilibrium is attained. This is controlled by the kinetic stability of the complex, as detailed below.

Kinetic stability

The kinetic stability of a metal complex is an indication of the rate at which ligands will associate with or dissociate from the metal ion. This rate is largely determined by the strength of the electrostatic interaction between metal and donor atom(s) of the ligand. The strength of such interactions is governed, at least partly, by the outer electron configuration of the metal, and is predicted to be highest for those metals having filled (or half-filled) outer orbitals, which therefore display spherical symmetry.

The kinetic stability of a metal ion may be assessed from the rate of exchange of water molecules within the primary hydration sphere of the metal. This reaction does not possess any thermodynamic driving force, and simply reflects the strength of electrostatic interactions between metal and solvent. The rate constants for such water exchange reactions have been shown to span a range of more than 15 orders of magnitude (Martell 1978). For metals possessing spherical symmetry, there is a direct correlation between rate of water exchange and charge density (Geier 1965). It is thus possible to estimate relative kinetic stabilities for a range of metal ions, which is of considerable importance when designing complexes for *in-vivo* use. In the nuclear medicine setting, high kinetic stability *per se* is not a prerequisite but, rather, adequate stability over the time course of the investigation (taking into account thermodynamic stability and any transchelation). Indeed, there are instances in which serum stabilities of metal complexes have been shown to follow an order different from that predicted from thermodynamic stability constants, an observation which is explained on the basis of differing kinetic stabilities and affinities for plasma proteins (Cole *et al.* 1986). Thus, the decision whether adequate stability will be achieved will depend, at least in part, on the half-life of the nuclide under consideration.

Transchelation

In addition to the problems of thermodynamic and kinetic stability, a further problem is posed in the *in-vivo* situation by the possibility of transchelation of the metal ion from the complex under investigation to a plasma component. This will inevitably lead to an altered biodistribution with concomitant problems regarding accurate estimation of uptake in various organs.

Problems associated with transchelation may be expected to arise from two major sources: plasma proteins having a role in the transport of one or more endogenous metal ions, or low-molecular-weight species capable of forming complexes with the metal ion.

Of the plasma proteins, the two classes that would be expected to present the greatest problems are the transferrins (Crichton 1990) and serum albumin. The transferrins are a group of metal binding glycoproteins that have evolved as specific iron-sequestering agents to maintain iron in a soluble form. Transferrin is a relatively small protein, with a molecular weight of approximately 80 kDa, that contains two binding sites for iron and other similar metal ions. The high affinity of transferrin for iron maintains the concentration of other forms of iron in the plasma at an extremely low level. Given that iron is an essential nutrient for growth, maintaining levels of available iron at a very low level produces a powerful antibacterial and antifungal effect. The closely related protein lactoferrin also has a molecular weight of approximately 89 kDa with two metal ion-binding sites and is found in a number of epithelial secretions including milk, seminal fluid, tears and nasal secretions; as a result of having an affinity for iron that is even higher than that of transferrin, it reduces levels of available iron in these secretions to the point at which opportunistic infections are unlikely to occur. However, the transferrins will also accommodate a range of different metal ions including Cu(II), Zn(II), Pt(II), Cr(III), Co(III), Ga(III), In(III), Mn(III), Sc(III) and a range of trivalent lanthanide elements including Ho, Er, Tb, Eu, Nd, Pr and Gd (Aisen 1980). The thermodynamic stability of transferrins for iron and similar metal ions is, by necessity, high, in order to prevent loss of metal to other plasma components, with subsequent toxicity associated with Fe^{2+}/Fe^{3+} redox cycling. Furthermore, over 60% of the metal-binding sites on transferrin are normally unoccupied, allowing transchelation to occur readily. Metal complexes intended for nuclear medicine applications should, therefore, have stabilities high enough to prevent exchange with transferrin over the time course of the study.

Serum albumin may pose a similar problem with some metal ions. One of the important functions of albumin is its ability to bind and transport a variety of low-molecular-weight species in the plasma. These include fatty acids, calcium, some steroid hormones, bilirubin and some plasma tryptophan. In addition, approximately, 10% of the plasma copper is bound to albumin. While the metal-binding sites on serum albumin appear not to be as specific nor of such high stability as those on transferrin, the relatively high concentration of albumin in plasma may enhance metal ion exchange from some complexes.

Another protein that plays a role in the observed biodistribution of the group 3 metal cations is ferritin. This is a large protein, responsible for iron storage, and capable of storing approximately 4500 Fe^{3+} ions in the form of a ferric oxide-hydroxide core. Ferritin is present in most cells, but is present at the highest concentrations in the Kupffer cells of the liver and in macrophages.

Gallium

Gallium possesses an electronic configuration ($3d^{10}\,4s^2\,4p^1$), which ensures that most of its chemistry is confined to the +3 oxidation state. Gallium is considered to be a 'hard' metal under the Pearson classification, with its coordination chemistry dominated by ligands carrying oxygen and nitrogen donors (Green, Welch 1989).

Much of the (radiopharmaceutical) chemistry of gallium has been developed from the close similarity between Ga^{3+} and Fe^{3+} (high-spin ferric iron). Both have similar ionic radii (Ga^{3+} 0.62 Å; Fe^{3+} 0.65 Å), both have coordination numbers of 6 and electronic configurations that give stable, spherical symmetrical tripositive cations. A direct consequence of this is that both cations have remarkably similar charge densities, which is one of the dominant influences controlling metal ion selectivity by ligands (Hancock, Martell 1989). The interaction with ligands is thus dominated by electrostatic forces, a behaviour which contrasts markedly with that of the transition metals, where incompletely filled outer orbitals in the cation result in the bonding with ligands being highly directional, and hence affecting the stereochemistry of the resultant metal complexes.

As with many hard metal ions, the free, hydrated (uncomplexed) gallium ion is stable in aqueous solution only under acid conditions, showing a strong tendency towards hydrolysis as the pH is raised. This results in the formation of a range of insoluble gallium hydroxy complexes which, unlike most other metal hydroxy complexes, are amphoteric and redissolve with the formation of gallate ions [$Ga(OH)_4^-$] as the pH is raised further. As a result of this hydrolysis, in order to keep gallium in solution between pH 3 and 8 at concentrations likely to be encountered in nuclear medicine applications, the addition of stabilising ligands is required.

Due to this predisposition towards extensive hydrolysis, complexes of gallium with multidentate ligands must normally be prepared via ligand exchange reactions, since the low rate of complexation by multidentate ligands is often too slow to prevent gallium hydrolysis, even at low pH (Moerlein, Welch 1981). For such ligands to be useful in the nuclear medicine setting, they must possess a high enough stability (thermodynamic and/or kinetic) to prevent both hydrolysis of the gallium ion *in vivo* and transchelation from the ligand to transferrin.

Three radionuclides of gallium have found clinical application, ^{66}Ga, ^{67}Ga and ^{68}Ga. Some of the nuclear characteristics of these nuclides are shown in Table 9.3. Both ^{66}Ga and ^{67}Ga are cyclotron-produced nuclides, while ^{68}Ga is generator-produced. Of these nuclides, ^{67}Ga has historically found the greatest application in nuclear medicine practice, although the use of ^{68}Ga is expected to increase significantly as a result of the increasing commercial

Table 9.3 Selected nuclear characteristics of commonly used gallium radionuclides

Nuclear characteristic	^{66}Ga	^{67}Ga	^{68}Ga
Typical production method	^{66}Zn (p, n) ^{66}Ga	^{68}Zn (p, 2n) ^{67}Ga	$^{68}Ge/^{68}Ga$ generator
Decay process	EC (43%)/β^+ (57%) $\rightarrow$ ^{66}Zn	EC (100%) $\rightarrow$ ^{67}Zn	EC (11%)/β^+ (89%) $\rightarrow$ ^{68}Zn
Physical half-life	9.5 hours	78.3 hours	68 minutes
Gamma emissions (abundance)	511 keV (114%)	93 keV (38%) 184 keV (24%) 300 keV (22%)	511 keV (178%)

availability of $^{68}Ge/^{68}Ga$ generators. This generator system has the advantage of having a very long working life owing to the long physical half-life (275 days) of the ^{68}Ge parent nuclide. Early generators had the disadvantage of eluting the gallium as an EDTA complex, which could only be used for a limited range of clinical applications without requiring time-consuming processing to remove the gallium from the complex. The $^{68}Ge/^{68}Ga$ generator systems now available produce gallium in an ionic form, which is much more amenable to direct incorporation into radiopharmaceuticals.

While ^{68}Ga is a high-efficiency positron emitter, the 68-minute physical half-life may be too short for some applications where uptake of the radiopharmaceutical into the target site is relatively slow. In an attempt to overcome this restriction, ^{66}Ga has been investigated as an alternative positron-emitting nuclide with a rather longer half-life. However, the decay characteristics of ^{66}Ga make it far from ideal for use as a diagnostic imaging agent (the long range of the high-energy positrons reduces spatial resolution in PET imaging, and the multiple gamma photons emitted can increase the detection of coincidence events by the PET scanner). Despite this, a number of radiopharmaceuticals have been labelled with ^{66}Ga, including monoclonal antibodies, albumin and blood cells. Furthermore, ^{67}Ga is itself not an ideal radionuclide for diagnostic imaging, despite its relatively widespread use. The abundance of gamma photons suitable for imaging is rather low (see Table 9.3), and necessitates the use of three times as much ^{67}Ga as ^{111}In to obtain equal count rates at a fixed detector geometry.

Gallium radiopharmaceuticals

Gallium-67 citrate (see Figure 9.1) is the most commonly used gallium-labelled radiopharmaceutical, and is used for the detection of infection, chronic inflammation in a number of autoimmune diseases, as well as detection, staging and identifying the response to treatment of a number of soft-tissue tumour types. The mechanism of localisation of uptake of gallium in tumours and areas of inflammation is intimately linked to the rapid transchelation of gallium from the citrate complex to plasma transferrin. Once gallium citrate is administered into the bloodstream of a patient, the citrate complex rapidly dissociates and the gallium is distributed between transferrin and gallate ions in plasma. At typical plasma concentrations of gallium achieved in a nuclear medicine study, over 99% of the gallium would be expected to be bound to transferrin within 40 minutes of administration, with less than 0.5% being present as gallate. Rapid infusions of large amounts of gallium may initially lead to high plasma concentrations of gallate before the gallium has time to bind to transferrin, and this may be related to the nephrotoxicity sometimes observed with gallium administration. However, if the transferrin binding of gallium is reduced for any reason (low plasma transferrin concentrations or increased concentrations of competing metal ions which would preferentially bind to transferrin), the gallate concentration increases significantly, and in some circumstances has been postulated to be responsible for the altered biodistribution of gallium on a nuclear medicine scan (Hattner, White 1990).

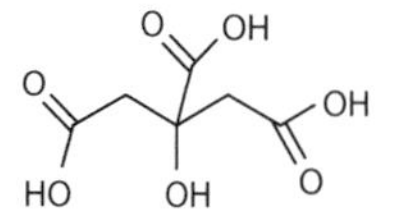

Figure 9.1 Structure of citric acid.

In those tissues containing lactoferrin (breast, nasopharynx, etc.), gallium will be selectively transchelated from transferrin to lactoferrin, owing to the binding constant of lactoferrin for gallium being about 90 times higher than that of transferrin. Lactoferrin is also present at increased levels in areas of infection and inflammation, and is thought to be secreted by activated neutrophils. This secreted lactoferrin is taken up by activated macrophages, and a subsequent ATP-mediated process causes bound metal ions to dissociate from the lactoferrin through induction of a conformational change in the lactoferrin molecule. Any dissociated gallium would then be rapidly converted into intracellular gallate, which would then be efficiently accumulated in ferritin. This combination of events provides a rational explanation for the localisation mechanism of gallium in inflammation and infection (Figure 9.2).

The mechanism of gallium uptake in tumours is less clear, and it is likely that there are several competing mechanisms operating in different tumour types. In some tumours, the gallium uptake has been shown

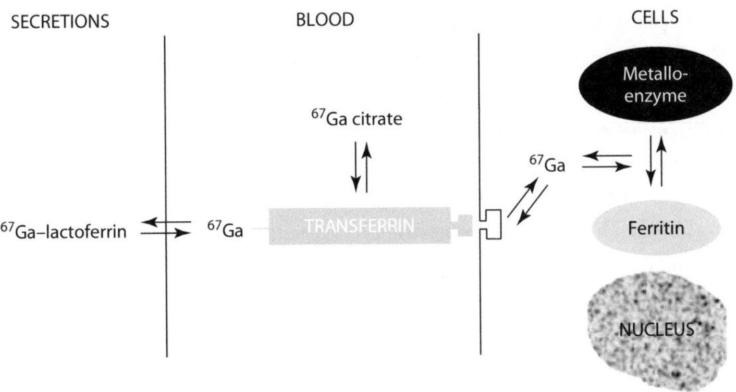

Figure 9.2 Diagrammatic representation of transferrin-mediated uptake mechanism for gallium.

to be linked to the presence of transferrin receptors on the surface of the tumour cells, with gallium uptake being directly proportional to the extent of expression of transferrin receptors. However, there are other tumour types where gallium uptake appears to be by a transferrin-independent mechanism. It is not entirely clear what this mechanism is, but is may involve direct cellular uptake of gallate ions.

To date, the use of ^{68}Ga radiopharmaceuticals has been somewhat limited by the scarcity of radiopharmaceuticals with appropriate physicochemical properties and biological behaviour. Given the short (68-minute) physical half-life of ^{68}Ga, any clinical application of this radionuclide requires a radiopharmaceutical that can be easily (quickly) radiolabelled, and which demonstrates both rapid localisation at the target site and residence times sufficiently long for performance of the imaging procedure. Although a number of molecules have been used in limited numbers of patients over the past 20 years, the current use of ^{68}Ga is based mainly on the use of radiolabelled peptide somatostatin analogues, derivatised with a macrocyclic chelating agent, 1,4,7,10-tetraazacyclododecane-N,N',N'',N'''-tetraacetic acid (DOTA) (see Figure 9.3), for detection and staging of neuroendocrine tumours.

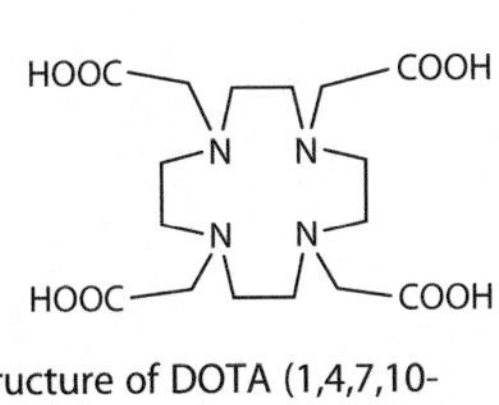

Figure 9.3 Structure of DOTA (1,4,7,10-tetraazacyclododecane-N,N',N'',N'''-tetraacetic acid).

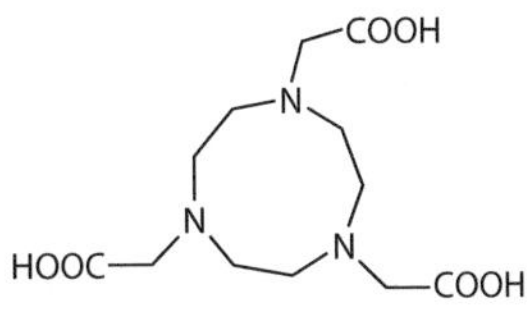

Figure 9.4 Structure of NOTA (1,4,7-triazacyclononane-N,N',N''-triacetic acid).

Although radiolabelling these molecules with ^{68}Ga is reasonably straightforward, they do require heating in order to achieve acceptable labelling efficiencies and radiochemical purities. This does have the disadvantage that it can significantly reduce the amount of radioactivity available at the end of labelling through radioactive decay. However, a novel radiopharmaceutical has recently been reported (Velikyan *et al.* 2008) that uses a radiolabelling procedure that is capable of achieving labelling efficiencies of over 95% in as little as 10 minutes, and that requires no additional pre-administration purification, using a chelating agent based on NOTA (see Figure 9.4). Although this agent has not yet been used in human subjects, it is perhaps an indicator of the approaches that may become more commonplace as the use of ^{68}Ga inevitably increases in the coming years.

Indium

Indium is positioned below gallium in the periodic table, and as a result of its outer electron configuration, shares many properties with gallium, including the tendency to form predominantly In^{3+} cations in aqueous solution. As with gallium, indium will undergo extensive hydrolysis as the pH is raised above about pH 3.5, to form a mixture of indium hydroxy complexes, of which the most prevalent at neutral pH is $In(OH)_3$. However, in contrast to gallium, indium is much less amphoteric in nature, and formation of soluble higher-order hydroxy complexes is much less pronounced as the pH is raised above pH 7.4. This can cause potential problems, as indium is a very toxic metal, with toxicity similar to that of mercury, and much of the toxicity is attributable to the insoluble hydroxy complexes (Luckey, Venugopal 1977).

Three radionuclides of indium have found clinical application, ^{111}In, ^{113m}In and ^{114m}In. Some of the nuclear characteristics of these nuclides are shown in Table 9.4.

Of the three nuclides of indium listed above, both ^{111}In and ^{114m}In are cyclotron-produced, while ^{113m}In is generator-produced. Of these, ^{111}In is the most widely used, primarily because of its good imaging characteristics, and this has led to the use of ^{113m}In declining markedly in the past 30 years. While the 115-day physical half-life of ^{113}Sn would give the ^{113}Sn/^{113m}In generator a useful working life of between 6 and 9 months, the relatively short physical half-life of the daughter ^{113m}In restricts the range of applications to those where the radiopharmaceutical accumulates rapidly at the target site. Furthermore, the energy of the ^{113m}In gamma photons is rather higher than is optimal for most commercial gamma camera systems. The potential attraction of ^{114m}In is that, following decay to the ground state (^{114}In) via isomeric transition, the subsequent decay of ^{114}In results in the emission of high-energy β-particles (2 MeV) in high abundance (97%). These β-particles could potentially be used for therapeutic applications, while the ^{114m}In gamma photon provides a mechanism for visualising the distribution of the therapeutic radiopharmaceutical. Indium-111 has also been used for therapeutic applications to a limited extent, as the decay process results in the emission of low energy (3 keV) Auger electrons in high abundance (100%). While these electrons have very short path lengths, typically less than 10 μm (or one cell diameter), there is the potential for them to cause cell death through mechanisms such as double-stranded DNA breaks if the radiopharmaceutical is internalised into the cell.

Indium radiopharmaceuticals

Indium-containing radiopharmaceuticals may be divided into two broad categories – those composed of bidentate ligands, which have inherently low stability, and those composed of hexadentate ligands, which have higher stability. Under many circumstances in nuclear medicine, complexes of high stability are desirable, in order to prevent or minimise the effects of transchelation. However, in the case of the bidentate indium ligands, a relatively low stability is desirable.

Bidentate ligands

Two of the most common indium complexes based on bidentate ligands are indium-oxine (8-hydroxyquinoline) (Figures 9.5 and 9.6) and indium tropolone (2-hydroxy-2,4,6-cycloheptatrien-1-one) (Figure 9.7). These have been used extensively to label blood cell components, such as leukocytes and platelets (see Chapter 24 on cell labelling for further details). Both of these complexes are neutral and lipophilic in nature, and are able to readily diffuse across the cell membrane of the isolated blood cells. Once inside the cell, the complex will dissociate and the indium will be transchelated by a cellular component with a higher

Table 9.4 Selected nuclear characteristics of commonly used indium radionuclides

Nuclear characteristic	^{111}In	^{113m}In	^{114m}In
Typical production method	^{112}Cd (p, 2n) ^{111}In	^{113}Sn/^{113m}In generator	^{114}Cd (p, n) ^{114m}In
Decay process	EC (100%) → ^{111}Cd	IT (100%) → ^{113}In	IT (95.7%) → ^{114}In EC (4.3%) → ^{114}Cd
Physical half-life	67.9 hours	99.5 minutes	49.5 days
Gamma emissions (abundance)	171 keV (91%) 245 keV (94%)	393 keV (64%)	190 keV (95.7%)

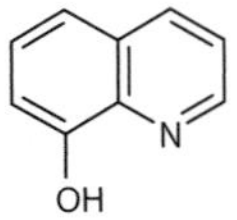

Figure 9.5 Structure of oxine (8-hydroxyquinoline).

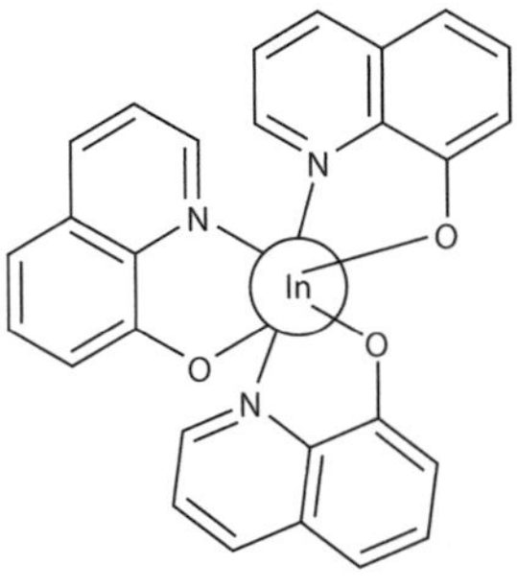

Figure 9.6 Structure of indium-oxine complex.

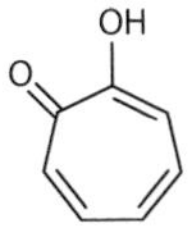

Figure 9.7 Structure of tropolone (2-hydroxy-2,4,6-cycloheptatrien-1-one).

affinity for the indium ion. The unbound oxine or tropolone molecules are then free to diffuse back out of the cell, leaving the indium trapped within the cell.

Hexadentate ligands

The most commonly used radiopharmaceuticals based on hexadentate indium ligands are proteins and peptides, derivatised with acyclic or macrocyclic aminopolycarboxylate ligands such as DTPA (diethylenetriamine pentaacetic acid) and DOTA. A typical example is pentetreotide, a DTPA-derivatised octapeptide analogue of the peptide hormone, somatostatin. The structure of the compound is shown in Figure 9.8.

In general, the approach to producing a radiopharmaceutical carrying a suitable hexadentate ligand is based on the concept of modifying the biological molecule with a bifunctional chelating agent, (Liu, Edwards 2001; Liu 2008). This is a chemical entity with two reactive functional groups, one of which is capable of covalently binding to the biological molecule while the other is capable of forming a strong complex with a cation. The bifunctional chelator, once covalently bound to the biomolecule, has to be capable of forming a metal complex of high thermodynamic and kinetic stability in order to minimise the loss of radiometal via transchelation. Although the interaction of a ligand with a particular metal ion may be well established, care has to be taken when considering the chelation properties of the ligand when part of the bifunctional chelating agent. Figure 9.9 illustrates a generic approach to conjugation of a bifunctional chelator with a protein or peptide, in which a carboxylic

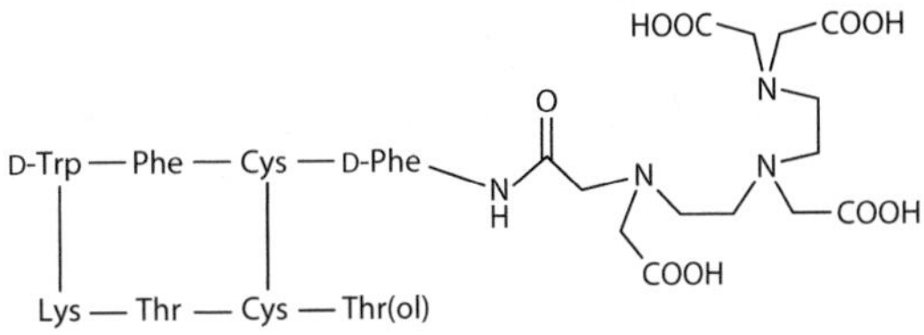

Figure 9.8 Structure of DTPA derivatised octreotide (pentetreotide).

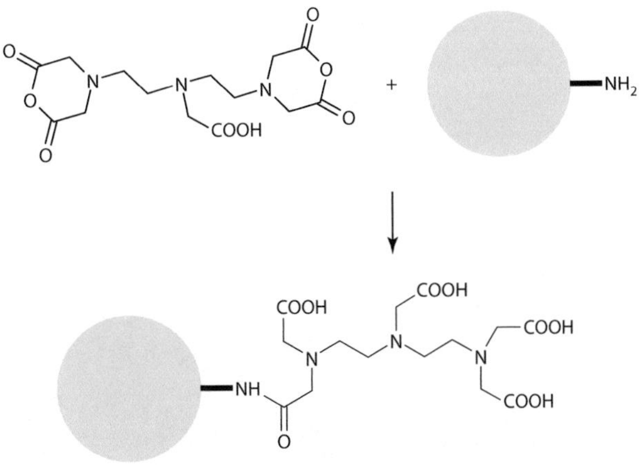

Figure 9.9 General approach to protein or peptide derivatisation with DTPA adducts.

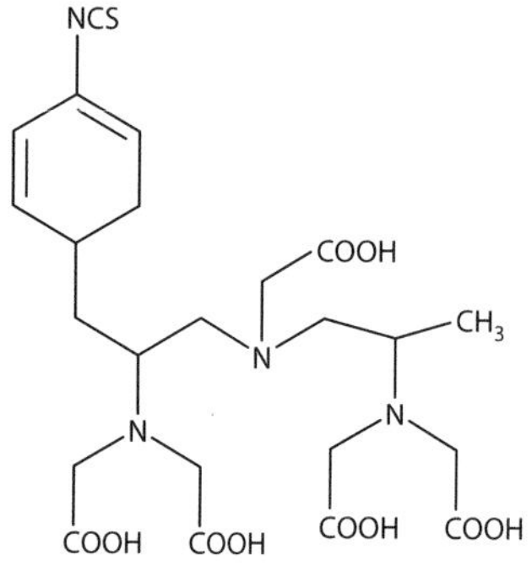

NCS COOH CH_3 N N N COOH COOH COOH COOH

Figure 9.10 Structure of *p*-SCN-Bz-DTPA.

acid group on the ligand interacts with an amine group on the protein or peptide to form an amide linkage.

Metal complexes formed between the resulting ligand and a metal ion may now exhibit altered kinetic and thermodynamic stabilities owing to the altered denticity of the ligand; that is, the fact that a carboxylic acid group is now unavailable for metal binding may adversely affect the stability of the resultant metal complex. In order to avoid this potential complication, an alternative approach is to synthesise a derivatised ligand, such as *p*-SCN-Bz-DTPA (see Figure 9.10), in which binding to the biomolecule is achieved via a reactive group introduced into the backbone of the ligand. This leaves all the donor groups on the ligand free for interaction with the metal ion, often resulting in a more stable complex, although the initial synthesis of the derivatised ligand may be rather more complex.

Yttrium

Yttrium is a group 3 element that possesses an inert gas outer electron configuration in the +3 oxidation state. However, the lanthanide contraction effect results in it having atomic and ionic radii lying closer to those of the lanthanides (dysprosium and terbium in particular) than the lighter group 3 metals, and this, together with its predisposition for forming compounds analogous to those of the lanthanide elements, results in it often being considered as a pseudo-lanthanide. Although yttrium favours a coordination number of 6, it can, due to its size, accommodate coordination numbers up to 9.

While the lanthanide elements form complexes with few ligands that do not exclusively carry oxygen donor atoms, yttrium – although still characterised as a 'hard' metal – also forms many complexes with ligands bearing nitrogen donor atoms. As with other 'hard' metal ions, uncomplexed yttrium undergoes hydrolysis in aqueous solution, although, in contrast to gallium, the hydrolytic reaction appears to stop following replacement of a single water molecule from the hydration sphere with a hydroxide ion, resulting in the predominant species in solution being $Y(OH)^{2+}(H_2O)_{5-8}$.

Problems with transchelation of yttrium *in vivo* are not as severe as for other tripositive cations. Despite initial studies that appeared to implicate transferrin in yttrium transport *in vivo* (Blank *et al.* 1980), subsequent studies could find no evidence of transchelation of yttrium from DTPA to transferrin (Hnatowich *et al.* 1985), the yttrium being either renally excreted or accumulated in the bone. Deposition of yttrium in the liver following intravenous administration of uncomplexed metal appears to be the result of direct uptake of a colloidal (hydroxy) form of the metal, which is cleared from the circulation by the reticuloendothelial system.

Three radionuclides of yttrium have found clinical application, ^{86}Y, ^{88}Y and ^{90}Y. Some of the nuclear characteristics of these nuclides are shown in Table 9.5.

Table 9.5 Selected nuclear characteristics of commonly used yttrium radionuclides

Nuclear characteristic	^{86}Y	^{88}Y	^{90}Y
Typical production method	^{86}Sr (p, n) ^{86}Y	^{88}Sr (p, n) ^{88}Y	$^{90}Sr/^{90}Y$ generator
Decay process	β^+ (33%) $\rightarrow$ ^{86}Sr EC (67%)	EC (100%) $\rightarrow$ ^{88}Sr	$\beta^- \rightarrow$ ^{90}Zr
Physical half-life	14.7 hours	106.6 days	2.67 days
Gamma emissions (abundance)	511 keV (66%) 628 keV (33%) 1076 keV (83%)	898 keV (94%) 1836 keV (99%)	Pure β^--emitter 2.28 MeV β^- (100%)

Of these nuclides, both ^{86}Y and ^{88}Y are cyclotron-produced, while ^{90}Y is generator-produced. Of these three, ^{90}Y is the most widely used and the only one currently available commercially. It is of particular interest as it is a pure beta emitter, and the high-energy (2.28 MeV) β-particle that is emitted during the decay process has a path length in tissue of 5.3 mm, making it useful in applications where radiation dose is to be delivered to a relatively large volume of tissue. However, the fact that ^{90}Y is a pure beta emitter also poses problems in terms of accurate assessment of the radiation dose being delivered to the patient. Although it is possible to obtain images using ^{90}Y, using bremmstrahlung imaging, such images are of rather low resolution and are not ideally suited to accurate quantification. In an attempt to overcome these problems, both ^{86}Y and ^{88}Y have been used as surrogates of ^{90}Y to image the distribution of a number of radiopharmaceuticals, but neither of these is ideal as a radionuclide for imaging. ^{86}Y is a positron-emitting nuclide, although positron emission only occurs with 33% abundance, and the simultaneous emission of high-energy gamma photons from the competing electron capture decay process makes it a less than ideal nuclide for PET imaging. ^{88}Y, in contrast, undergoes radioactive decay only by electron capture, although the high-energy photons emitted have too high an energy for efficient detection with standard gamma cameras, and the long physical half-life results in a comparatively high radiation dose being delivered to the patient. A feasibility study has looked at the use of ^{87}Y for determination of ^{90}Y biodistribution, although no clinical studies have been reported. ^{87}Y is also cyclotron-produced (using the $^{87}Sr(p, n)^{87}Y$ reaction) and has several advantages over ^{88}Y for single-photon imaging – its physical half-life of 3.3 days is more closely matched to ^{90}Y and it emits 485 keV gamma photons in 92% abundance. However, ^{87}Y decays to form ^{87m}Sr, which has a 2.8-hour physical half-life and emits 388 keV gamma photons in 82% abundance, and the concern is that the high affinity of strontium nuclides for metabolising bone tissue may lead to significant toxicity in some cases.

Yttrium radiopharmaceuticals

The major applications of ^{90}Y radiopharmaceuticals are as therapeutic agents for the treatment of a number of different types of cancer. The two most commonly used radiopharmaceuticals for these applications are Zevalin (ibritumomab tiuextan) and DOTATOC. Zevalin is an anti-CD-20 antibody, derivatised with the acyclic polyaminocarboxylate ligand DTPA (see Figure 9.11) and subsequently labelled with ^{90}Y, that has been shown to be effective for the treatment of refractory tumours in non-Hodgkin lymphoma. DOTATOC is an octapeptide derivative of the peptide hormone, somatostatin, derivatised with the macrocyclic aminopolycarboxylate ligand DOTA (see Figure 9.12). This has been shown to be highly effective in the treatment of a range of somatostatin receptor-positive neuroendocrine tumours (Breeman *et al.* 2001; Weiner, Thakur 2002). The use of these radiopharmaceuticals is considered in greater detail in Chapter 19.

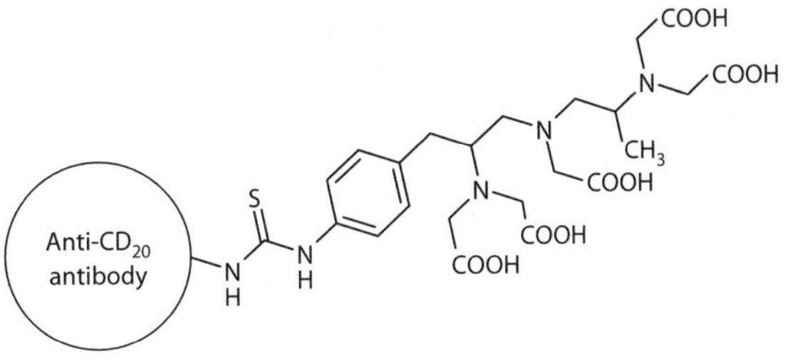

One major disadvantage of ^{90}Y radiopharmaceuticals is that the lack of any gamma emissions often means that a surrogate ^{111}In radiopharmaceutical has to be used to image biodistribution and to provide some estimates of delivered radiation dose from dosimetry measurements (Hindorf *et al.* 2007). However, there are concerns about the validity of such approaches. Although the coordination chemistry of In^{3+} and Y^{3+} is very similar, there have been a number of reports of radiopharmaceuticals labelled with the two metals exhibiting structural differences in solution (Deshmukh *et al.* 2005). This is mainly due to the size differences between In^{3+} and

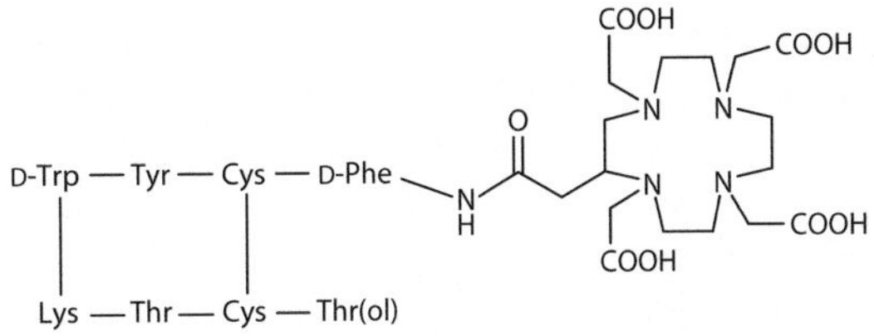

Figure 9.11 Structure of ibritumomab tiuxetan.

Figure 9.12 Structure of DOTA-derivatised octreotide.

Y^{3+}, which result in yttrium fitting the cavity in the macrocyclic DOTA ligand almost perfectly, forming an 8-coordinate complex in the process, while the smaller indium cation fits into the DOTA cavity less well and forms only a 6- or 7-coordinate complex. These differences in solution structure of the complexes can produce marked changes in the lipophilicity of the complexes, as well as in their kinetic or thermodynamic stability. However, given the fact that many radiopharmaceuticals derivatised with DOTA complexes are based on large biological molecules such as peptides and proteins, it is unclear how such structural differences in the metal complex will affect the overall behaviour of the radiopharmaceutical. It is, therefore, very important that the extent of any differences in biological behaviour of radiopharmaceuticals labelled with indium and yttrium is established before measurements on indium complexes are used to predict dosimetry for the corresponding yttrium radiopharmaceutical.

Lutetium

Lutetium is a lanthanide element, with a $[Xe]4f^{14}$ outer electron configuration. Since 4f electrons are not involved in bonding, the interactions between donor atoms and lanthanide metal ions are predominately ionic. Given the large ionic radius of the Lu^{3+} cation, in common with many of the lanthanide elements it exhibits a higher coordination number than many other group 3 cations. Few lanthanide elements form six coordinate complexes, with coordination numbers of 8 and 9 being more prevalent. The radionuclide of lutetium that is of most interest for radiopharmaceutical applications is ^{177}Lu. This is a reactor-produced radionuclide, which exhibits nuclear decay properties as shown in Table 9.6.

Table 9.6 Selected nuclear characteristics of lutetium-177

Nuclear characteristic	^{177}Lu
Typical production method	^{176}Lu (n, γ) ^{177}Lu
Decay process	$\beta^- \rightarrow {}^{177}Hf$
Physical half-life	6.65 days
Beta emissions (abundance)	176 keV (12%) 384 keV (9%) 497 keV (79%)
Gamma emissions (abundance)	113 keV (12%) 208 keV (11%)

The energy (and therefore, range) of the emitted β-particles has resulted in a significant interest in this radionuclide for therapeutic applications in cancer, particularly when used in combination with, or as an adjunct to, ^{90}Y-labelled radiopharmaceuticals. The use of ^{90}Y in the treatment of micrometastatic disease is suboptimal, as most of the energy will be deposited outside the tumour, increasing the radiation dose to surrounding normal tissue. With ^{177}Lu, however, most of the energy will be deposited within the micrometastases. Furthermore, the ability to directly image the biodistribution of the ^{177}Lu is a significant advantage in contrast to ^{90}Y.

Much of the clinical application of ^{177}Lu has been as one of a number of DOTA-derivatised peptides, the majority of which have been somatostatin analogues used for treatment of neuroendocrine tumours. Further details relating to these specific clinical applications may be found in a number of reviews, including those of Esser (2006) and Van Essen (2007). Although ^{177}Lu complexes of EDTMP (ethylenediamine tetramethylenephosphonic acid, Figure 9.13) have been used for palliation of pain from bone metastases, relatively little use has been made of radiopharmaceuticals based on acyclic ligands. Part of the reason for this is that exposure of such acyclic lutetium complexes to the low-pH environment of lysosomes following cellular uptake may result in liberation of lutetium from the complex, with the possibility of subsequent irreversible incorporation of the radiometal into bone. The use of macrocyclic ligands such as DOTA reduces the potential for toxicity from unwanted biodistribution, largely as a result of the macrocyclic complexes exhibiting significantly higher kinetic stability than acyclic complexes, despite their thermodynamic stabilities being relatively similar.

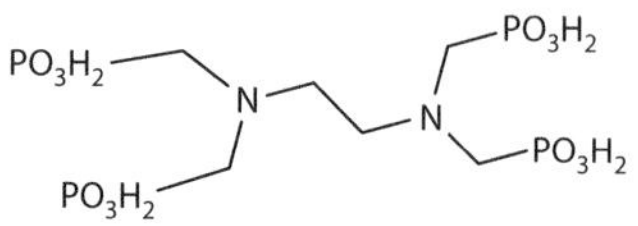

Figure 9.13 Structure of ethylenediamine tetramethylenephosphonic acid, EDTMP.

Samarium

Samarium is a lanthanide element, with a [Xe]4f^5 outer electron configuration. Samarium-153 is a reactor-produced radionuclide, with nuclear decay properties as shown in Table 9.7. As with ^{177}Lu and ^{166}Ho, the combination of emission of gamma photons suitable for imaging together with emission of β-particles makes ^{153}Sm attractive as a therapeutic radionuclide.

Although ^{153}Sm has been used for a variety of clinical applications, the most common application is as ^{153}Sm EDTMP for palliation of pain from bone metastases. The chemistry of a radionuclide is often an important factor controlling the accumulation and retention of radiopharmaceuticals within bone tissue. For example, those elements which form basic oxides/alkaline solutions when added to water and which typically adopt an oxidation state of +1 or +2, such as Sr^{2+}, tend to be mobile within biological systems. However, elements forming basic oxides and adopting oxidation states of +3 or +4 tend to form insoluble hydroxides, and are less mobile. This mechanism is important in the uptake of Sm^{3+} by bone, a process which involves interaction of the samarium cations with hydroxyapatite in bone to form insoluble hydroxide or phosphate complexes. These complexes are thermodynamically stable and exhibit essentially no subsequent mobilisation. Delivery of chelated forms of such metal ions to the hydroxyapatite surface of bone relies on the presence of multidentate carboxylate and phosphonate ligand systems, which can themselves bind to the hydroxyapatite, effectively forming a bridging complex. The metal ion then subsequently dissociates from the complex and binds directly to the hydroxyapatite as an insoluble hydroxide as described above. Both the rate and extent of transchelation of the metal ion from the radiopharmaceutical to the bone surface will depend on the comparative kinetic and thermodynamic stability of the soluble and bone-associated insoluble complexes (Volkert, Hoffman 1999).

In clinically used preparations of Sm-EDTMP, there is often a very large stoichiometric excess of EDTMP, typically of the order of 250 : 1 or greater. This large excess of ligand is required to prevent *in-vivo* formation of insoluble samarium hydroxyl complexes, which would localise in the liver. Although EDTMP forms thermodynamically stable complexes with samarium, such complexes are not kinetically inert, and will readily dissociate in the circulation unless there is a large excess of EDTMP ligand present.

Holmium

Holmium-166 may be produced from neutron irradiation of enriched ^{165}Ho, although if ^{166}Ho with a higher specific activity is required, the favoured production route is from a ^{166}Dy/^{166}Ho generator. Table 9.8 shows some selected nuclear decay characteristics of ^{166}Ho.

The decay properties of ^{166}Ho which result in emission of reasonably high-energy β-particles together with an imageable gamma photon, albeit in low abundance, make it suitable for use in

Table 9.7 Selected nuclear characteristics of samarium-153

Nuclear characteristic	^{153}Sm
Typical production method	^{152}Sm (n, γ) ^{153}Sm
Decay process	$\beta^- \rightarrow$ ^{153}Eu
Physical half-life	46.7 hours
Beta emissions (abundance)	640 keV (30%) 710 keV (50%) 810 keV (20%)
Gamma emissions (abundance)	103 keV (28%)

Table 9.8 Selected nuclear characteristics of holmium-166

Nuclear characteristic	^{166}Ho
Typical production methods	^{165}Ho (n, γ) ^{166}Ho ^{166}Dy/^{166}Ho generator
Decay process	$\beta^- \rightarrow$ ^{166}Er
Physical half-life	26.8 hours
Beta emissions (abundance)	1770 keV (48%) 1850 keV (51%)
Gamma emissions (abundance)	80 keV (6%)

therapeutic applications. Although ^{166}Ho is not as widely used as other radionuclides such as ^{90}Y and ^{177}Lu, ^{166}Ho has found application in a number of clinical settings (Rösch 2007). These include the use of ^{166}Ho-chitosan for treatment of liver tumours, ^{166}Ho-DTPA in liquid-filled balloons for brachytherapy in coronary artery restenosis, ^{166}Ho-ferric hydroxide macroaggregates for radiation synovectomy to treat chronic rheumatoid arthritis, and the use of ^{166}Ho-DOTMP for ablation of bone marrow in myeloma. Holmium-166 has also been used to radiolabel monoclonal antibodies using bifunctional chelating agents based on DTPA. As with other lanthanide elements, holmium tends to favour the formation of ionic complexes, principally with hard donor atoms.

The selection of DOTMP (1,4,7,10-tetraazacyclododecane-1,4,7,10-tetramethylene-phosphonic acid, Figure 9.14) for chelation of ^{166}Ho is based on the fact that DOTMP forms a kinetically inert complex with holmium with a stoichiometry of approximately 1 : 1, whereas many acyclic phosphonate ligands (such as EDTMP) with lower affinities for lanthanide metal ions require a stoichiometry of more than 250 : 1 for efficient chelation of the metal ion. Given the low specific activity of ^{166}Ho produced by neutron irradiation of ^{165}Ho, selection of a chelating agent with a lower affinity for the metal would require much larger quantities of ligand in order to produce a complex with the same overall stability. For a typical therapeutic dose of ^{166}Ho this may require several milligrams of holmium and, therefore, several hundred milligrams of an acyclic phosphonate ligand. However, the higher thermodynamic and kinetic stability of the DOTMP complex means that upon delivery to bone, there is no fixation of the holmium in the form of insoluble hydroxide as with samarium, and that the complex is more loosely bound to bone as a bridging complex

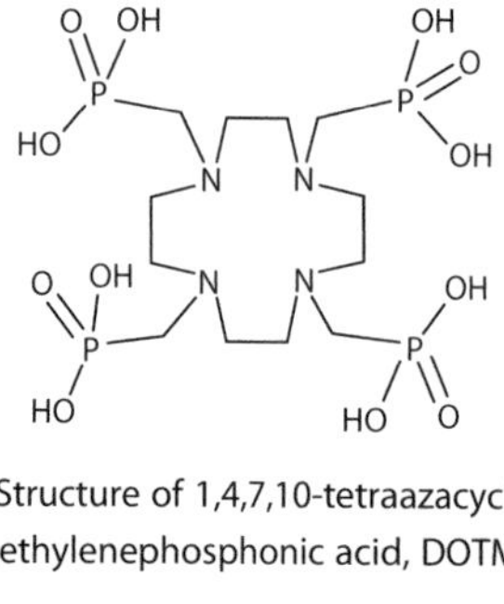

O OH
P
HO
OH
P
O
OH
N N
N N
O OH
P
HO
OH
P
HO O

Figure 9.14 Structure of 1,4,7,10-tetraazacyclododecane-1,4,7,10-tetramethylenephosphonic acid, DOTMP.

referred to previously. Despite the fact that ^{166}Ho-DOTMP binds effectively to bone, it is generally not used for treatment of skeletal metastases, as the higher-energy β-particles emitted tend to cause more suppression of bone marrow than would be seen with ^{153}Sm-EDTMP. However, this effect on the bone marrow is of fundamental importance in the treatment of myeloma, where ablation of myeloma cells within the bone marrow is required for treatment to be effective.

Practical considerations

Given the potential for a wide variety of divalent and trivalent cations to bind to many of the ligands on which the radiopharmaceuticals discussed in this chapter are based, it is vital that the levels of contaminating metal ions present during a radiolabelling procedure are kept to an absolute minimum. Failure to do so can lead to significantly reduced radiolabelling yields, as the quantities of contaminating metal ions can often exceed the amount of radiometal of interest. While it is inevitable that contaminating metal ions will be present in materials used for the labelling reaction, specifications for starting materials should be set so as to limit the amount of contaminating metal ions as far as possible. Furthermore, many radiometals are supplied in acid solution at low pH, so as to minimise the formation of hydrolysis products before the radiolabelling process has been completed. Special care should be taken if manipulating these acidic solutions with metallic components, such as syringe needles, as the low pH of the solutions is capable of stripping significant levels of metal ions from the needle. Such problems may be minimised by the use of needles constructed from acid-resistant grades of stainless steel or by using acid washed plastic components where possible.

One of the major differences between acyclic ligands, such as DTPA, and macrocyclic ligands, such as DOTA, lies in the lower kinetic stability of the acyclic complexes in comparison with the macrocyclic complexes, which has two effects in a radiopharmaceutical setting. Firstly, it results in the binding of metal ions to the acyclic ligands being rapid under mild conditions, which often enables high radiolabelling efficiencies to be achieved at room temperature. However, this low kinetic stability can lead to the radiometal dissociating from the chelate *in vivo*, resulting in accumulation at non-target sites via, for instance, transchelation to transferrin. This can lead to unacceptably high radiation doses being delivered to non-target tissues, particularly when using beta-emitting radionuclides such as ^{90}Y and ^{177}Lu. In contrast, macrocyclic ligands such as DOTA produce metal complexes which are much more kinetically inert, minimising the loss of radiometal *in vivo*. However, this inevitably means that the kinetics of formation of the complex are also slower, often requiring heating at temperatures close to 100°C in order to achieve radiolabelling yields that are sufficiently high to avoid the necessity of post-labelling purification of the radiopharmaceutical (Breeman *et al.* 2003). While this may be achievable for small molecules, including many peptides, exposure of larger proteins such as antibodies to such high temperatures can often lead to a complete loss of biological activity. This can lead to limitations in the use of some potential radiopharmaceuticals for therapeutic applications, depending on whether a suitable combination of high-stability ligand and acceptable radiolabelling conditions can be found.

References

Aisen P (1980). The transferrins. In: Jacobs A, Worwood M, eds. *Iron in Biochemistry and Medicine*, Vol. II. London: Academic Press, 87–129.

Blank ML *et al.* (1980). Liposomal encapsulated Zn-DTPA for removing intracellular ^{169}Yb. *Health Phys* 39: 913–920.

Breeman WAP *et al.* (2001). Somatostatin receptor-mediated imaging and therapy: basic science, current knowledge, limitations and future perspectives. *Eur J Nucl Med* 28: 1421–1429.

Breeman WAP *et al.* (2003). Optimising conditions for radiolabelling of DOTA-peptides with ^{90}Y, ^{111}In and ^{177}Lu at high specific activities. *Eur J Nucl Med Mol Imaging* 30: 917–920.

Cole WC *et al.* (1986). Serum stability of ^{67}Cu chelates: comparison with ^{111}In and ^{57}Co. *Int J Rad Appl Instrum B* 13: 363–368.

Crichton RR (1990). Proteins of iron storage and transport. *Adv Protein Chem* 40: 281–363.

Deshmukh MV *et al.* (2005). NMR studies reveal structural differences between the gallium and yttrium complexes of DOTA-D-Phe1-Tyr3-octreotide. *J Med Chem* 48: 1506–1514.

Esser JP *et al.* (2006). Comparison of [^{177}Lu-DOTA^0,Tyr3] octreotate and [^{177}Lu-DOTA^0,Tyr3]octreotide: which peptide is preferable for PRRT? *Eur J Nucl Med Mol Imaging* 33: 1346–1351.

Geier G (1965). Kinetische untersuchungen der komplexbildung von murexidmit Co^{2+}, Ni^{2+}, In^{3+}, Sc^{3+}, Y^{3+}. *Ber Bunsenges Phys Chem* 69: 617–627.

Green MA, Welch MJ (1989). Gallium radiopharmaceutical chemistry. *Int J Rad Appl Instrum B* 16: 435–448.

Hancock RD (1986). Macrocycles and their selectivity for metal ions on the basis of size. *Pure Appl Chem* 58: 1445–1452.

Hancock RD, Martell AE (1989). Ligand design for selective complexation of metal ions in aqueous solution. *Chem Rev* 89: 1875–1914.

Hattner RS, White DL (1990). Gallium-67/stable gadolinium antagonism: MRI contrast agent markedly alters the normal biodistribution of gallium-67. *J Nucl Med* 31: 1844–1846.

Hindorf C *et al.* (2007). Dosimetry for ^{90}Y-DOTATOC therapies in patients with neuroendocrine tumors. *Cancer Biother Radiopharm* 22: 130–135.

Hnatowich DJ *et al.* (1985). DTPA-coupled antibodies labelled with yttrium-90. *J Nucl Med* 26: 503–509.

Jurisson S *et al.* (1993). Coordination compounds in nuclear medicine. *Chem Rev* 93: 1137–1156.

Kauffman GB *et al.* (1983). Ligand. *J Chem Educ* 60: 509–510.

Liu S (2004). The role of coordination chemistry in the development of target specific radiopharmaceuticals. *Chem Soc Rev* 33: 445–461.

Liu S (2008). Bifunctional coupling agents for radiolabelling of biomolecules and target-specific delivery of metallic radionuclides. *Adv Drug Deliv Rev* 60: 1347–1370.

Liu S, Edwards DS (2001). Bifunctional chelators for therapeutic lanthanide radiopharmaceuticals. *Bioconjug Chem* 12: 7–34.

Luckey TD, Venugopal B (1977). Physiologic and chemical basis for toxicity. In: *Metal Toxicity in Mammals*, Vol. 1. New York, Plenum Press, 171–173.

Martell AE (1978). *Coordination Chemistry*. ACS Monograph 174, Volume 2. Washington DC: American Chemical Society.

Moerlein SM, Welch MJ (1981). The chemistry of gallium and indium as related to radiopharmaceutical production. *Int J Nucl Med Biol* 8: 277–287.

Pearson RG (1963). Hard and soft acids and bases. *J Am Chem Soc* 85: 3533–3539.

Rösch F (2007). Radiolanthanides in endoradiotherapy: an overview. *Radiochim Acta* 95: 303–311.

Schwarzenbach G (1961). The general, selective, and specific formation of complexes by metallic ions. *Adv Inorg Radiochem* 3: 257–285.

Van Essen M *et al.* (2007). Peptide receptor radionuclide therapy with radiolabelled somatostatin analogues in patients with somatostatin receptor positive tumours. *Acta Oncol* 46: 723–734.

Velikyan I *et al.* (2008). Convenient preparation of ^{68}Ga-based PET-radiopharmaceuticals at room temperature. *Bioconj Chem* 19: 569–573.

Volkert WA, Hoffman TJ (1999). Therapeutic radiopharmaceuticals. *Chem Rev* 99: 2269–2292.

Weiner RE, Thakur ML (2002). Radiolabeled peptides in the diagnosis and therapy of oncological diseases. *Appl Radiat Isot* 57: 749–763.

10

Radiohalogenation

Maggie Cooper

Introduction

Radiolabelled molecules are important for diagnosis and therapy of a variety of diseases. One of the most common ways of radiolabelling these molecules, particularly ones that are biologically interesting, is by radiohalogenation. However, it is rare to find a halogen present in a biological molecule, although a few contain chlorine. So, why the interest in radiohalogenation? Why not just replace one of the naturally occurring atoms such as carbon, oxygen or nitrogen with its radioactive isotope?

The halogen isotopes offer several advantages over the radioactive isotopes of these naturally occurring atoms. Although carbon-11, oxygen-15 and nitrogen-13 are all PET isotopes giving good images clinically, they have short half-lives (20, 2 and 10 minutes, respectively), which makes synthesis of biologically active molecules a challenge. In contrast, the halogen isotopes have a number of different emissions (positrons, β-particles, α-particles, γ-rays and Auger electrons), which can be used for both diagnosis and therapy. In addition, the longer half-lives of the radioactive halogens are appropriate both for synthesis and for clinical applications.

The wide variety of halogen isotopes means that they can be used for different purposes but, as a group, they are of particular importance because their chemistry is well understood, they form stable covalent bonds, their steric and electronic nature is unlikely to cause major changes to the biological activity of the compounds labelled with them, and lastly, high-specific-activity radiolabelling can be achieved (Wilbur 1992).

This chapter will look at the family of radiohalogens, their physical properties and methods of synthesis and then describe methods that can be used to radiolabel biologically relevant molecules with iodine, bromine and astatine using radiopharmaceutically relevant examples. Although fluorine is a vital member of the halogen family, it will be mentioned only briefly here as it is covered in more detail in Chapter 11.

Halogen radioisotopes

The halogens are a series of non-metallic elements from group 17 (formerly known as group 7) of the periodic table comprising fluorine, chlorine, bromine, iodine and astatine. Astatine is the only halogen that does not have a stable isotope. Radioisotopes of the other halogens have been produced and are of particular interest to the radiochemist due to their physical and chemical properties. The most commonly used of these radioactive halogens have been the iodine isotopes but, with the development of PET radiopharmacy, there is increasing interest in radiolabelling with the PET isotopes of bromine and fluorine. Astatine is interesting because it is an α-particle emitter so may have a role to play in therapy. The physical properties of each isotope are shown in Table 10.1 (Firestone *et al.* 1999).

Table 10.1 Table of pharmaceutically interesting halogen isotopes (Firestone *et al.* 1999)

Isotope	Half-life	Major route of decay
^{119}I	19.1 m	β^+
^{120}I	81.0 m	β^+
^{121}I	2.12 h	β^+
^{122}I	3.63 m	β^+
^{123}I	13.27 h	EC
^{124}I	4.18 d	EC (70%), β^+ (30%)
^{125}I	59.41 d	EC
^{126}I	13.11 d	EC (55%), β^- (44%), β^+ (1%)
^{127}I	Stable	
^{129}I	1.57×10^7 y	β^-
^{130}I	12.36 h	β^-
^{131}I	8.02 d	β^-
^{132}I	2.30 h	β^-
^{133}I	20.80 h	β^-
^{134}I	52.5 m	β^-
^{135}I	6.57 h	β^-
^{74m}Br	46 m	β^+
^{75}Br	96.7 m	β^+
^{76}Br	16.2 h	β^+
^{77}Br	57.04 h	β^+
^{79}Br	Stable	
^{18}F	109.8 m	β^+
^{19}F	Stable	
^{211}At	7.21 h	α (42%), EC (58%)

m, minute(s); h, hour(s); d, day(s); y, year(s).
EC, electron capture.

Radioisotopes of iodine

Iodine has several radioisotopes. The naturally occurring iodine-127 is not radioactive but can be useful for modelling radiolabelling reactions. Both iodine-123 and iodine-131 can be used for gamma scintigraphy. The short half-life ($t_{1/2} = 13.2$ hours) and medium energy gamma emission (159 keV) make iodine-123 the isotope of choice for gamma scintigraphy, amongst the iodine radioisotopes, but the cost can sometimes outweigh these benefits. Iodine-131 is more readily available and hence cheaper; it has three main medium-high energy gamma emissions (284 (6.1%), 364 (81.2%), 637 (7.3%) keV), which can be used for imaging studies. However, the high-energy gamma emissions can cause handling and radioprotection issues in the radiopharmacy and the long half-life ($t_{1/2} = 8$ days) and β^- particles (β^- maximum emission 606 keV (90%)) make its use in imaging limited to patients with malignancy. These disadvantages for imaging, however, become advantages for therapy, where the β^--particles can kill malignant cells and the location of the radiopharmaceutical in the body can be observed by gamma scintigraphy.

Iodine-125 is rarely used clinically due to the low energy gamma emission and long half-life (60 days, gamma emission 35 keV) but it is an extremely useful isotope for modelling radiolabelling reactions, for carrying out preclinical studies and for radioimmunoassay. It also has a role in Auger electron therapy and has been applied to radioimmuno-guided surgery (Mayer *et al.* 2000).

There are also five positron-emitting isotopes of iodine (^{119}I, ^{120}I, ^{121}I, ^{122}I and ^{124}I). Potentially the most useful of these is iodine-120 ($t_{1/2} = 1.4$ hours) due to the short half-life and availability via high- or medium-energy cyclotrons using proton beam energies (E_p) from 9 to 37 MeV ($^{122}Te(p,3n)^{120}I$, $E_p = 37 \rightarrow 32$ MeV) (Hohn *et al.* 1998a) and

(^{122}Te(p,n)^{120}I, $E_p = 15 \rightarrow 9$ MeV) (Hohn *et al.* 1998b). Although iodine-124 only has 24% positron emission, its longer half-life ($t_{1/2} = 4.18$ days) allows it to be used in dosimetric evaluation of iodine-131 therapeutic radiopharmaceuticals since its half-life matches the biological half-life of antibodies (Pentlow *et al.* 1991). Iodine-122 has only limited application due to its very short half-life ($t_{1/2} = 3.6$ minutes).

Other isotopes of iodine exist (^{126}I, ^{129}I, ^{130}I, ^{132}I, ^{133}I, ^{134}I and ^{135}I) but they have not been used clinically either because of their availability or because of their physical properties.

Radioisotopes of bromine

A number of isotopes of bromine exist but their clinical application has been limited to date. Although the energies of the gamma emissions of bromine-77 are quite high (239 keV (24%) and 521 keV (23%)) for imaging on conventional gamma camera, this isotope has been used for imaging in some studies (McElvany *et al.* 1982). More promising are the positron-emitting bromine isotopes, bromine-74m, bromine-75 and bromine-76. The 97-minute half-life of bromine-75 makes it attractive but it has fairly high-energy gamma emissions, which degrade image quality. In view of this, it offers little advantage over fluorine-18. Bromine-76 may be useful for labelling proteins due to its longer half-life (16 hours). Several potential applications have been reported in the literature (Höglund *et al.* 2000; Cho *et al.* 2005; Lee *et al.* 2006; Rowland *et al.* 2006), and it can be produced using a low-energy cyclotron and a copper(I) selenide pellet (^{76}Se(p,n)^{76}Br, $E_p = 16 \rightarrow 8$ MeV) (Tolmachev *et al.* 1998).

Radioisotopes of astatine

The only useful radioisotope of astatine is astatine-211; the others have unsuitable half-lives or decay characteristics. Astatine-211 is produced by bombardment of natural bismuth metal targets with α-particles in a ^{209}Bi(α, 2n)^{211}At reaction ($E_\alpha = 29 \rightarrow 28$ MeV, where E_α is the beam energy of the α-particles) using a high-energy cyclotron. It is an α-particle-emitting isotope (5.89 MeV) with a half-life of 7.2 hours (Vaidyanathan, Zalutsky 1996a); this makes ^{211}At an interesting candidate for therapeutic applications. The short tissue path length (50–80 μm, equivalent to only a few cell diameters) of α-particles means that, having a high linear energy transfer (LET), they give up their energy quickly to the targeted cells and so are more potent from a radiobiological perspective than β-particles. This also means that they are less toxic to adjacent normal tissue. In addition, α-particles are particularly cytotoxic to cancer cells since they tend to create DNA double-strand breaks, which are less easy for the body to repair (Kampf 1988). There is also evidence to suggest that cells, not directly targeted by the α-particle but adjacent to the targeted cell, are also killed owing to the so-called 'bystander effect' (Boyd *et al.* 2006). However, targeting still needs to be good to get effective tumour kill and, hence, many applications using α-particles have been focused on easily accessible tumour targets such as in haematological malignancies and intracavity delivery such as in ovarian carcinoma.

Radioisotopes of fluorine

Fluorine-18 is the most widely used PET radioisotope. It has the advantage of having a high positron abundance (97%), a half-life that is long enough for synthesis of simple radiopharmaceuticals (110 minutes) and low positron emission energy (635 keV), which gives good resolution when imaging. Fluorine-18 and its applications are covered in more detail elsewhere in this book (Chapter 11).

Radiolabelling with iodine

Several strategies have been employed to radiolabel compounds with iodine. The methods have developed over time to meet the needs of the radiochemist to optimise labelling efficiency and to reduce unwanted side-reactions. The ideal method for any given radiopharmaceutical will depend on many different factors and radiolabelling will need to be individually optimised.

Oxidative electrophilic radioiodination techniques are usually used for proteins, whereas nucleophilic substitution techniques are more often employed for small organic molecules.

Oxidative methods

Much of the early work carried out in the area of radioiodination was with proteins. Similar strategies to those used in conventional iodinations in organic synthetic chemistry can be applied to radioiodination, although account may need to be taken of factors such as the dilute conditions for radiolabelling and the presence of minor impurities from the production of the isotope itself. Optimisation of radiolabelling methods will need to be carried out to give rapid labelling in high radiochemical yields.

In general, direct iodination of proteins occurs on tyrosyl or to a lesser extent histidyl residues within a protein following electrophilic attack by a positive iodine species (Krohn *et al.* 1977). The point of attachment is at the most electron-dense part of the ring, i.e. at the *meta* position in the tyrosine ring.

It is worth noting that there are drawbacks to direct labelling even though it is by far the most commonly used method. There can be problems *in vivo*, particularly if the labelled molecule is taken up inside the cell. Rapid de-iodination can occur with efflux of iodine or an iodinated catabolite. This is a problem for three reasons: firstly, the iodine is not at the target site so is not in the right place for diagnosis or therapy; secondly, the radioactive iodine can cause radiation damage elsewhere in the body, particularly to the thyroid, which actively takes up iodine; and thirdly, free circulating iodine gives rise to high background counts that can obscure images in the target site. The same problem exists for the other halogens when they are used to directly label proteins.

Although the thyroid can be blocked using non-radioactive potassium iodide, there still remains the problem that the iodine is not at the target site. To overcome this problem, the protein can be indirectly labelled with a prosthetic group which is less prone to catabolism inside the cell.

Figure 10.1 shows a scheme of radioiodination of proteins on tyrosyl and histidyl residues.

O
CCHNH
CH_2
OH
$^*I^{\delta+}$
$^*I$

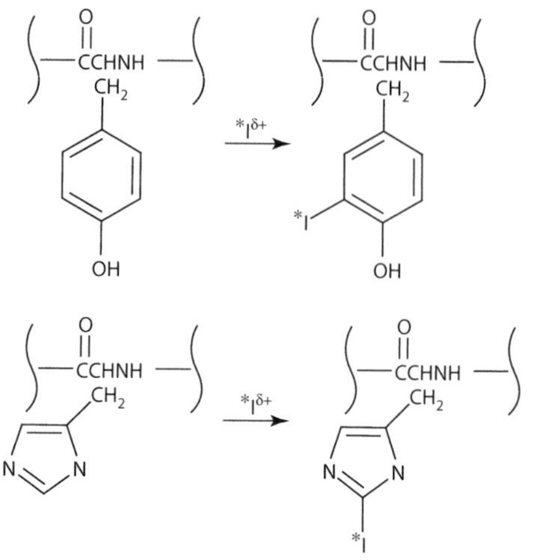

Figure 10.1 Radioiodination of protein on tyrosyl and histidyl residues (Seevers, Counsell 1982).

Molecular iodine

Some of the earliest methods for radioiodination involve the use of molecular iodine as this was commonly used for standard iodination reactions but, since radioactive iodine is usually available as sodium iodide, it was necessary to first carry out an oxidation reaction to obtain radioactive molecular iodine. A number of different oxidising agents have been proposed (Eisen, Keston 1949; Francis *et al.* 1951; Stadie *et al.* 1952; McFarlane 1956), but all these methods suffer from the disadvantage that the maximum possible radiochemical yield is 50% since half of the label ends up as ionic radioiodide. There are also radiation hazards to the operator, not least the fact that molecular iodine is highly volatile and will accumulate in the thyroid if inhaled.

Iodine monochloride (ICl)

In view of these difficulties, alternative labelling strategies were sought. The first method was to use iodine monochloride (McFarlane 1958), which is strongly polarised, having the iodine essentially in the form of I^+. When treated with radioactive sodium iodide it undergoes isotopic exchange with virtually all the radioiodine being converted to I^+. Hydrolysis of the radiolabelled iodine monochloride produces HOI, which will label proteins or other compounds. There is therefore the potential for 100% radiochemical yield. Iodine monochloride can also be used in electrophilic addition across a double bond, for example for radiolabelling of fatty acids (Robinson, Lee 1975).

Chloramine-T

Chloramine-T (*N*-chloro-*p*-toluenesulfonic acid) has been widely used as an oxidising agent for electrophilic

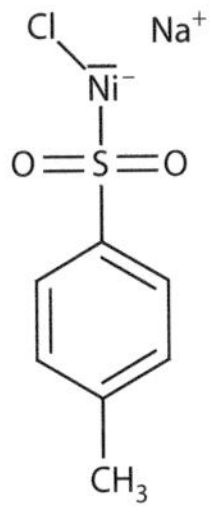

Figure 10.2 Structure of chloramine-T.

iodination reactions (Hunter, Greenwood 1962). In aqueous solution it forms HOCl, which in turn reacts with sodium iodide to give a positive iodine species, possibly H_2OI^+ (Hunter 1970). Figure 10.2 shows the chemical structure of chloramine-T.

In practical terms, the labelling is quite straightforward (Mather 2005). For labelling proteins, the protein can first be buffered using sodium phosphate buffer and radioactive sodium iodide then added. The reaction occurs rapidly (in less than 5 minutes) after the addition of a freshly prepared solution of chloramine-T and continues until the reaction is quenched, for example by addition of excess tyrosine or sodium metabisulfite. The radiolabelled product can be separated from unreacted iodine using thin-layer chromatography (TLC), solid-phase extraction (SPE) or liquid chromatography (LC) techniques. For small scale radiopharmaceutical production, carrying out the labelling in aseptic conditions can be a challenge since the solutions of chloramine-T and tyrosine/metabisulfite need to be freshly prepared; terminal sterilisation of the final product will normally be required.

A modified chloramine-T method was used to radiolabel the chimeric IgG1 anti-CD20 monoclonal antibody rituximab (Turner *et al.* 2003). The antibody has been used in a multicentre phase II clinical trial for relapsed or refractory indolent non-Hodgkin lymphoma.

One of the drawbacks of using chloramine-T is that the conditions for iodination are quite harsh and can cause damage to the compound being labelled, especially sensitive proteins. Undesirable side-reactions such as chlorination, oxidation of thiol and thioester groups and cleavage of tryptophanyl peptide bonds can occur. Carrying out the reaction on ice can help to avoid unwanted side-reactions.

To get round these problems, a proprietary polymer-bound *N*-chloro-*p*-toluenesulfonic acid called Iodobeads can be used (Hussain *et al.* 1995). Using this immobilised chloramine-T on polystyrene beads keeps the concentration of oxidising agent down, hence reducing unwanted side-reactions, although it does result in lower labelling yields. Another advantage is that the reaction is easily stopped by filtration of the reaction solution to remove the beads. These advantages overcome the problems of having to prepare small amounts of fresh solutions in an aseptic environment.

Iodogen

Iodogen (1,3,4,6-tetrachloro-3α,6α-diphenylglycoluril) is very useful for radioiodination of proteins and peptides since radioiodination occurs in milder conditions than those required for the chloramine-T reaction, giving rise to less oxidative damage, although sometimes at the expense of lower yields. The method was first developed by Fraker and Speck (1978) and is extremely simple and reliable.

Iodogen is almost insoluble in water, so it is necessary to first coat the inside of the reaction vessel with a solution of Iodogen in an organic solvent such as dichloromethane. Following evaporation of the solvent, the compound to be labelled can be added in a suitable buffer (e.g. 0.5 mol/L phosphate buffer, pH 7.4) to the reaction vessel. The reaction will begin following addition of sodium iodide and can be monitored by chromatographic techniques. The reaction will typically take 5–15 minutes and can be stopped by simply removing the solution from the reaction vessel. Figure 10.3 shows practical schematic of labelling using Iodogen.

The advantage of the Iodogen technique is that the radiolabelling can easily be carried out aseptically. The Iodogen tubes in which the reaction is to take place can be prepared in advance as a pharmaceutical batch and stored for up to a year in the dark at −20°C. The tubes can be checked in advance for sterility and apyrogenicity. The buffers required for the radiolabelling can also be prepared in advance and their quality tested.

Occasionally, problems can occur with uniformity of coating when tubes are prepared 'in house'; however, pre-coated Iodogen tubes are commercially available, so this problem can easily be avoided.

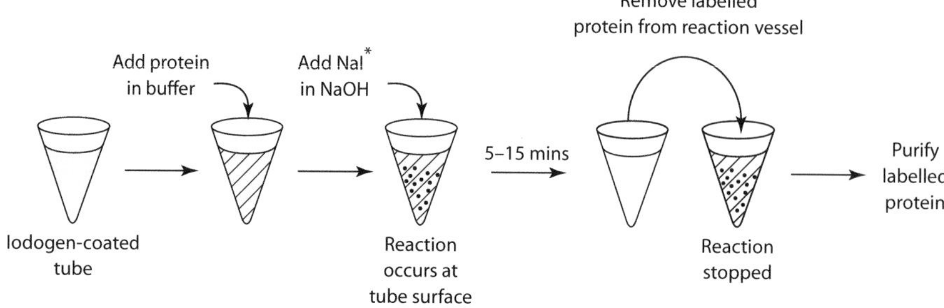

Figure 10.3 Radioiodination of proteins using the Iodogen method.

The anti-CD20 monoclonal antibody B1 (tositumomab) was labelled by the Iodogen method (Kaminski *et al.* 1993). This antibody is used for radioimmunotherapy of B-cell lymphoma and is commercially available as Bexxar.

N-Bromosuccinimide

Another technique for labelling monoclonal antibodies with large quantities of radioiodine is to use *N*-bromosuccinimide (NBS) as the oxidising agent (Mather, Ward 1987). In practice, it is similar to the method using chloramine-T; the antibody is first buffered using a suitable buffer (e.g. 0.1 mol/L phosphate buffer, pH 7.4) and then sodium iodide is added. After the addition of NBS, the reaction proceeds fairly rapidly (in less than 5 minutes) and can be stopped by addition of tyrosine or sodium metabisulfite. Yields tend to be fairly high (>90%), allowing simple purification and reduced radiation dose to the operator. This method has been used, for example, to radiolabel HMFG2, a monoclonal antibody that defines a tumour-associated glycoprotein antigen present in ovarian carcinomas (Ward *et al.* 1987). The radioiodinated antibody was used in both the detection and treatment of ovarian carcinomas.

From a pharmaceutical perspective, the method suffers the same drawbacks as the chloramine-T method in that solutions need to be freshly prepared, causing difficulties if it is necessary to perform the radiolabelling under aseptic conditions. Furthermore, the conditions for radiolabelling are still fairly harsh and damage to the protein can occur in some cases (Youfeng *et al.* 1982).

Other *N*-halosuccinimides can also be used for radioiodination, for example *N*-chlorotetrafluorosuccinimide and *N*-chlorosuccinimide. One approach has been to use *N*-chlorosuccinimide in trifluoromethanesulfonic acid (triflic acid) to iodinate non-activated and strongly deactivated arenes in a 'no carrier added' system with a radiochemical yield of 70% (Mennicke *et al.* 2000). This method relies on the compound being stable in triflic acid but has been used to radioiodinate benzamides and phenylpentadecanoic acid. One problem of this method of radioiodination is that an isomeric mixture of products can form. The substitution can be regioselective under some circumstances, depending on the secondary substituents.

Peracids

Peracids can be used as oxidants in radioiodination reactions. The advantages of using peracids are that no chlorinated by-products can be formed and it is less likely that over-oxidation of sensitive substrates will occur. The disadvantage is that radiochemical yields tend to be low (Moerlein *et al.* 1988).

The peracids can be added directly to the radioiodination reaction, although this is more likely to cause oxidative damage to the substrate. The preferred method is to use an organic acid (e.g. acetic acid) and to add a small quantity of hydrogen peroxide so that the peracid forms *in situ*.

For radiolabelling the dopamine D_2 receptor imaging agent, (*S*)-3-[^{123}I]iodo-*N*-[(1-ethyl-2-pyrrolidinyl)]methyl-2-hydroxy-6-methoxybenzamide ([^{123}I]IBZM), it was found that peracetic acid was a superior oxidant to chloramine-T. The [^{123}I]IBZM was prepared by adding peracetic acid to a mixture of BZM and sodium iodide (Kung, Kung 1989). The reaction took 2 minutes at room temperature and was terminated by the addition of sodium bisulfite. The yield was 90–95% and the radiochemical purity was 93–95%. This agent is useful for investigating patients with Parkinson disease and other psychiatric disorders. It is also been assessed for its role in monitoring addiction (Jongen *et al.* 2008).

Enzymatic methods

Enzymatic radioiodination is a milder method than the other oxidative techniques and so does not tend to damage protein (Kienhuis *et al.* 1991). It relies on the fact that peroxidases will iodinate tyrosine residues in the presence of small amounts of hydrogen peroxide. In view of this, lactoperoxidase has been employed for radioiodination of proteins since, in the presence of another enzyme system such as glucose oxidase, hydrogen peroxide will be produced *in situ* (Morrison, Bayse 1970). This method can also be used to radioiodinate histidine residues, but at a slower rate than tyrosine.

The lactoperoxidase/glucose oxidase enzyme method has been used to radiolabel recombinant human thyroid-stimulating hormone (rhTSH) with iodine-123 and iodine-125. This promising new radiopharmaceutical is being used to diagnose non-iodine-uptaking differentiated thyroid cancer metastases (Corsetti *et al.* 2004).

One drawback of using lactoperoxidase for radioiodination is that yields tend to be fairly low. This is due to the fact that during the reaction the lactoperoxidase itself is iodinated, which can lead to problems with purification of the labelled protein. This problem can be overcome by using lactoperoxidase–glucose oxidase-coupled beads (Enzymobeads). The insoluble beads can be easily removed from the reaction mixture at the end of the reaction (Tatum *et al.* 1979).

Prosthetic groups

In cases where the compound to be labelled does not have an activated aromatic group that can be easily labelled, or in cases where damage occurs to the protein when labelled under oxidative conditions, or in cases where de-iodination *in vivo* is a problem, an alternative is to radiolabel via a prosthetic group. Two approaches can be taken. The first is to radiolabel the prosthetic group and then attach it to the compound to be labelled. The second is to attach the prosthetic group to the compound and then radiolabel it. In either case, it is important that the incorporated prosthetic group does not affect the biological properties of the compound being labelled (Eckelman *et al.* 1976).

Bolton and Hunter (1973) developed an acylating agent for radioiodinating proteins. The prosthetic group, *N*-succinimidyl 3-(4-hydroxyphenyl)propanoate, is first radiolabelled using chloramine-T and then coupled, generally via the ε-amino group of lysine residues, to the protein. Figure 10.4 shows the scheme of iodination using the Bolton–Hunter agent.

To improve *in-vivo* stability, alternative prosthetic groups such as 3- and 4-radioiodinated benzoic acid and phenylalkyl carboxylic acid esters have been developed. When labelled in this way, proteins are less susceptible to loss of radioiodine *in vivo* than proteins directly labelled by electrophilic substitution (Vaidyanathan, Zalutsky 1990).

Another approach to improve *in-vivo* stability and to prevent rapid diffusion of iodotyrosine from the target cell (following internalisation and catabolism of radioiodinated monoclonal antibodies) has been to use radioiodinated diethylenetriamine pentaacetic acid-appended peptides containing D-amino acids (Govindan *et al.* 1999). These peptides can be synthesised using standard techniques, radiolabelled using chloramine-T, and then conjugated to disulfide

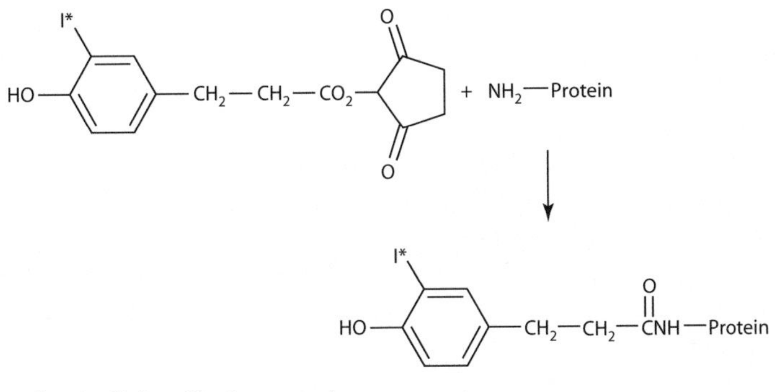

I*
HO—(benzene ring)—CH_2—CH_2—CO_2—(succinimide ring, O, O) + NH_2—Protein
↓
I*
HO—(benzene ring)—CH_2—CH_2—C(=O)NH—Protein

Figure 10.4 Iodination using the Bolton–Hunter reagent.

reduced monoclonal antibodies. Antibodies labelled in this way have shown good tumour uptake and retention in nude mice lung cancer models (Stein *et al.* 2003).

Exchange methods

For the radioiodination of small organic molecules, exchange methods are the most straightforward approach. Most often the exchange is of a metal atom (M) for a radioactive iodide atom (I*). These methods rely on the fact that the carbon–metal (C–M) bond is weaker than the carbon–hydrogen (C–H) bond, so that substitution of M by I* is easier than substitution of H by I*. The least complex of these exchange methods involves the substitution of stable iodine with radioactive iodide, but exchange with bromine, diazonium salts, boron, tin, silicon, thallium and germanium is possible.

Exchange for stable iodine

The exchange can be carried out in two ways, either by exchange in solvent or by exchange in melt.

Exchange in solvent

For exchange in solvent, it is important that both the organic material and the radioactive iodide dissolve in the solvent. One of the problems is that the final product will contain much stable iodine and it is not possible to separate the stable from the radioactive product at the end of the reaction; hence the specific activity of the final product will be low. In many cases, this does not present a problem and will depend to some extent on the biological activity and toxicity of the unlabelled compound *in vivo*. One reason for this is that the concentration of radioactive iodine used in the reaction is extremely low. This is particularly true when using iodine-123 and can make it extremely difficult to obtain non-carrier-added product as it is sometimes necessary to add stable iodine in order for the reaction to proceed. The reaction is normally carried out under reflux conditions. Under these conditions, some compounds will exchange very readily.

Iodine-123-labelled *N,N,N'*-trimethyl-[2-hydroxy-3-methyl-5-iodobenzyl]-1,3-propanediamine (HIPDM) has been used clinically as a regional cerebral perfusion imaging agent. [^{123}I]HIPDM can be prepared by a simple aqueous exchange reaction in a kit form from the unlabelled HIPDM in the presence of a reductant (sodium bisulfite) and oxidant (sodium iodate) (Lui *et al.* 1987).

Exchange in melt

For compounds that will not exchange under reflux conditions in solvent, exchange in melt can be carried out. The most basic of the melt methods is simply to heat the organic molecule up to its melting point and add the radioiodide. The compound must be stable at its melting point and be able to dissolve the radiodide.

In cases where radioiodide will not dissolve in the melted compound, a variation of the method can be used in which the exchange occurs in a melt of acetamide (Sinn *et al.* 1979). Acetamide melts at 82°C but is stable up to 200°C, so the reaction is typically carried out at 180°C.

A third type of exchange-in-melt method is to use ammonium sulfate. The compound is heated in ammonium sulfate to 120-160°C (this may actually be below the melting point of the substrate and is below the melting point of ammonium sulfate) for 1–4 hours.

Catalysts for exchange reactions

Radiochemical yields can be increased and reaction times decreased by the use of a catalyst. One of the most commonly used catalysts is copper metal or copper(I) salts (Klapars, Buchwald 2002).

Exchange for bromine

The advantage of using exchange for bromine is that very high specific activities can be achieved, as long as it is possible to separate the radioiodinated compound from the brominated precursor. As with the exchange for iodine, exchange for bromine can be carried out in solvent (for example acetone, aqueous acid, acetonitrile), in melt, or using an ammonium sulfate melt (Seevers, Counsell 1982).

One potential problem with exchange for bromine is that it is likely *in vivo* the bromo compound will bind as well, or better, to receptors than the corresponding iodo compound, so it is vitally important that the product is pure as even small amounts of the precursor will lower the effective specific activity at the receptor.

Exchange with diazonium salts

A standard method for preparation of iodinated compounds is to use iodine for diazonium salt exchange. Therefore, this approach lends itself to being used for radioiodination. The starting material is the corresponding aniline, which is converted to the diazonium salt by reaction with nitrous acid or alkyl nitrate. It may be necessary to protect other functional groups within the molecule to prevent their reaction under these harsh conditions. As above, a copper catalyst can be used to reduce reaction time.

A novel brain perfusion imaging agent, the α-methylated analogue of iodoamfetamine, *p*-[^{123}I and ^{131}I]iodo-α,α-dimethylphenethylamine (*p*-iodophentermine) was prepared by solid-phase isotopic exchange reaction of the diazonium salt with potassium iodide with a radiochemical yield of 40–60% (Kizuka *et al.* 1985).

Exchange with boron

Since organoboranes will react with molecular iodine under basic conditions, exchange with boron has often been used in standard organic synthesis to incorporate iodine into organic molecules. This method can be adapted for radioiodination, but care needs to be taken owing to the volatile nature of molecular iodine. Because of radiation safety concerns over the use of radioactive iodine in these reactions, methods have been developed using iodine monochloride or sodium iodide and chloramine-T. This method is useful both for alkyl compounds and for vinyl compounds.

Exchange with tin

Exchange with tin also occurs by direct substitution. It is the most commonly used exchange method for radioiodination. One of the advantages of using tin is that the carbon–tin bond is not very strong and so high radiochemical yields can be obtained. *In situ* oxidation of the sodium radioiodide can be achieved using chloramine-T or peracids (Moerlein *et al.* 1988).

One of the most important pharmaceutical examples using destannylation is in the synthesis of the [^{123}I]ioflupane (commercially available as DaTSCAN). DaTSCAN is used in the differential diagnosis of Parkinson disease from other disorders presenting with similar symptoms since ioflupane binds to dopamine transporters in the brains of humans. Figure 10.5 shows structure of ioflupane.

[^{123}I]Ioflupane is synthesised by the chloramine-T method by iodination of the trimethylstannyl precursor using sodium [^{123}I]iodide in a yield of 95% and with a radiochemical purity of 98% (Chaly *et al.* 1996).

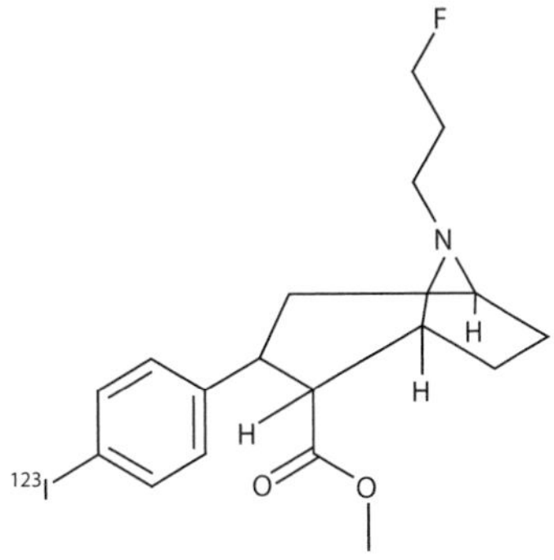

Figure 10.5 Structure of ioflupane, [^{123}I]FP-CIT.

Exchange with silicon or germanium

The carbon–silicon bond is similar to the carbon–tin bond, so organosilanes can be used in exchange reactions to give iodinated compounds. The reaction is usually carried out in protic solvents under acidic conditions at moderate temperatures (Vaidyanathan *et al.* 1996b).

Likewise, organogermanium compounds can be used. Again, chloramine-T is often used as the oxidising agent. Alkylgermanium precursors may be suited to specific applications since they have higher stability than organotin compounds and higher reactivity than organosilyl compounds.

Exchange with mercury and thallium

Organometallic precursors incorporating mercury or thallium can also be used in exchange reactions with radioiodine. The mercury precursors are more stable than their thallium counterparts. The exchange is usually carried out under carrier added conditions. However, Nicholl *et al.* (1997) prepared the melanoma imaging agent *N*-(2-diethylaminoethyl)-3-iodo-4-methoxybenzamide (IMBA) by reaction of halogen-free *N*-(2-diethylaminoethyl)-4-methoxybenzamide with thallium(III)-tris(trifluoroacetate) solution followed by exchange with previously evaporated [^{123}I]iodide. IMBA has shown good uptake in melanoma and metastases in mice. Images showed clear visualisation of the primary subcutaneous tumour and induced lung metastases (Edreira, Pozzi 2006).

The development of [^{131}I]mIBG

Radioactive *meta*-iodobenzylguanidine, [^{131}I]mIBG, is an important radiopharmaceutical in clinical use and is a good example of how the exchange methods

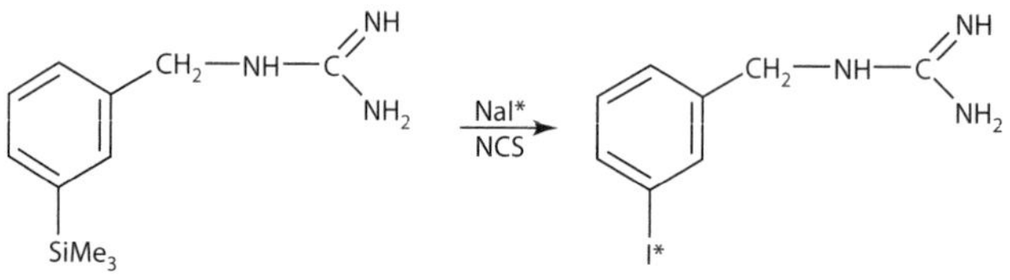

Figure 10.6 Synthesis of no-carrier-added [^{131}I]mIGB by iododesilylation of *m*-trimethylsilylbenzylguanidine using *N*-chlorosuccinimide (NCS) as the oxidant in trifluoroacetic acid (Vaidyanathan, Zalutsky 1993).

can be usefully employed and how variations in the methods used have improved yields and the specific activity of the product.

The agent [^{131}I]mIBG was first synthesised in 1980, in order to image the adrenal cortex and its neoplasms (Wieland *et al.* 1980). The radioactive material was prepared by radioiodide exchange of an aqueous solution of the non-radioactive *meta*-iodobenzylguanidine sulfate by the addition of carrier free Na[^{131}I]. The solution was refluxed for 72 hours, cooled and then passed through a glass column packed with Cellex D anion exchange cellulose to remove unreacted radioiodide and iodate.

However, this method was not very suitable for synthesis of [^{123}I]mIBG for imaging due to the long reflux time (72 hours) and the short half-life of ^{123}I. In addition, this initial method left a large quantity of non-radiolabelled mIBG, which reduced the specific activity (Mairs *et al.* 1994). Improvement to the radiolabelling method reduced the synthesis time to 1 hour (Mock, Weiner 1988), but use of a cuprous catalyst and radioiodine improved both the yield (99.9%) and the synthesis time (15 minutes) (Verbruggen 1987).

There still remained the problem, however, of the unreacted mIBG present in the final product, which reduced the difference in accumulation between target and non-target cells. Vaidyanathan and Zalutsky (1993, 1995), sought to prepare pure, no-carrier-added, radioactive mIBG in order to improve the target to non-target ratio (Figure 10.6). This was achieved for both [^{123}I]mIBG and [^{131}I]mIBG by iododesilylation of *meta*-trimethylsilylbenzylguanidine using *N*-chlorosuccinimide as the oxidant in trifluoroacetic acid.

No-carrier-added [^{123}I]mIBG has also been prepared by a copper sulfate-catalysed reaction of *meta*-bromobenzylguanidine (Samnick *et al.* 1999) by reaction for 10 minutes at 180°C similar to that of the improved synthesis of Verbruggen (1987).

Non-carrier-free [^{131}I]mIBG can also be prepared by radioiodide exchange of non-radioactive mIBG with [^{131}I]radioiodide using a copper catalyst and a temperature of 134°C. The crude mixture is purified by anion exchange chromatography in which the excess ^{131}I is retained on the column and pure [^{131}I]mIBG is eluted.

Similarly, [^{123}I]mIBG can be prepared in an exchange reaction catalysed by copper nitrate. Cold mIBG is mixed with the catalytic solution and ^{123}I in dilute sodium hydroxide. The reaction is carried out at 150°C for 45 minutes, after which time a phosphate buffer is added and the copper and iodide ions are removed by anion exchange.

Radiolabelling with bromine

Radiolabelling with bromine can essentially be carried out in the same way as radiolabelling with iodine. Proteins can be labelled directly by electrophilic substitution or indirectly using prosthetic groups. Similarly, exchange reactions can be used for nucleophilic substitution on organic molecules. The most commonly used method is substitution for tin, although in some circumstances it may be more convenient to carry out other exchange reactions.

It should be noted that bromine is more difficult to oxidise than either iodine or astatine. This being the case, labelling conditions for protein radiobromination often tend to be fairly harsh, using low pH and high levels of oxidant, and this can damage sensitive proteins. In view of this, indirect labelling methods may be preferred.

Other factors that may influence the choice of radiobromination method may be: radiolabelling yield, ease of purification of final labelled product (for example removing enzymes from enzymatic bromination of antibodies), ease of *in-vivo* catabolism of radiolabelled product (particularly directly labelled proteins), whether tyrosine or lysine residues are important in the recognition site of antibodies (this will influence whether a direct or indirect labelling method is chosen) and ease of synthesis of precursors for exchange reaction. Some examples of radiobromination reactions are given below. As discussed earlier, the main radioisotope of bromine used for radiolabelling is bromine-76 due to its 16-hour half-life and availability from low–medium energy cyclotrons. However, bromine-75 and bromine-77 have also been used in some studies.

Oxidative methods

Chloramine-T

Chloramine-T can be used for direct electrophilic substitution of proteins; bromination occurring at tyrosyl residues within the protein. Petzold and Coenen (1980) showed that the optimum labelling conditions were low pH (pH 1) and high concentrations of oxidant. This is appropriate for small organic molecules and peptides, but conditions may need to be modified at the expense of radiochemical yield in order to label proteins in this way without damaging them.

Enzymatic methods

Enzymes such as myelo-, chloro- and bromoperoxidases can, in the presence of small quantities of hydrogen peroxide, oxidise bromide to hypobromous acid and hence can be used for direct electrophilic substitution on tyrosyl residues of proteins (Senthilmohan, Kettle 2006). Although the conditions are fairly mild and unlikely to cause damage to the protein being labelled, it is worth noting that one problem with using enzymatic methods can be the difficulty of removing enzyme from the labelled product at the end of the radiolabelling (Höglund *et al.* 2000).

Lövqvist *et al.* (1995) labelled anti-CEA (carcinoembryonic antigen) antibodies using both the chloramine-T method and the bromoperoxidase method. They found that radiolabelling using chloramine-T resulted in low yields and poor immunoreactivity of the antibodies. However, using bromoperoxidase, yields of 70% ($\pm$10%) were obtained without significant loss of immunoreactivity.

Prosthetic groups

The most commonly used method for labelling monoclonal antibodies with bromine has been the use of prosthetic groups. There are several potential advantages of this approach. Firstly, harsh conditions can be confined to the radiolabelling step prior to conjugation of the prosthetic group onto the antibody. Secondly, attachment to the antibody can occur on lysine residues rather than labelling on tyrosine residues, which may be important for antigen recognition. Thirdly, the main catabolite of directly labelled antibodies is bromine, which is poorly excreted from the body. This gives rise to low tumour-to-background ratios on images due to high background activity caused by the bromine retained in the body. The use of prosthetic groups can overcome this problem since catabolism will occur via different routes (Höglund *et al.* 2000).

The simplest method involves using *N*-succinimidyl derivatives, which can be easily conjugated to the ε-amino group of lysine residues within antibodies using a method analogous to use of the Bolton–Hunter reagent discussed for radioiodination (Bolton, Hunter 1973).

Figure 10.7 shows a scheme of labelling of HPEM and then conjugation to the protein. For example, Mume *et al* (2005) radiolabelled the precursor, ((4-hydroxyphenyl)ethyl)-maleimide (HPEM), using the chloramine-T method before conjugation to an anti-HER2 antibody.

It is also possible to radiobrominate the precursor using exchange methods. The most commonly employed being exchange for tin using a trimethyltin precursor and chloramine-T as oxidant (Höglund *et al.* 2000).

An alternative to conjugation strategies involving *N*-succinimidyl derivatives is to use isothiocyanatobenzyl derivatives and conjugate to the ε-amino group of lysine residues via a thiourea bond. For example, Bruskin *et al.* (2004) used [^{76}Br](4-isothiocyanatobenzyl-amminio)-bromo-decahydro-*closo*-dodecaborate (bromo-DABI), labelled using chloramine-T as oxidant, as the prosthetic group for radiobromination of the anti-HER2/neu humanised antibody, trastuzumab.

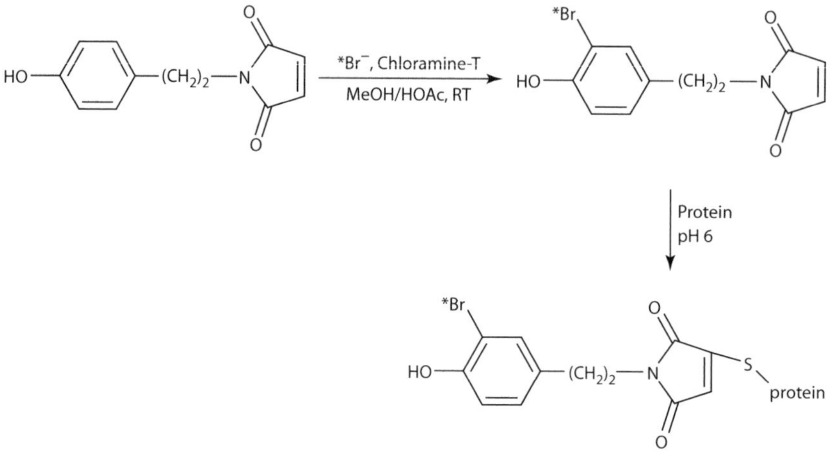

Figure 10.7 Radiobromination of HPEM and conjugation to protein (Mume et al. 2005).

Exchange methods

As for radiodination, exchange for tin is the most commonly used exchange reaction for radiobromination. Lundkvist *et al.* (1999) used this method for synthesis of a radioligand, 5-bromo-6-nitroquipazine, to study the serotonin transporter in the brain. Synthesis of the radioligand was via the *N*-t-BOC-protected 5-tributylstannyl-6-nitroquipazine precursor in a two-step synthesis which first involved exchange for tin using chloramine-T as oxidant.

A similar method was used by Rowland *et al.* (2006) to synthesise σ_2-receptor ligands. The σ_2-receptors often occur in high densities on tumour tissues and this receptor is thought to have a function in cell proliferation. Brominated σ_2-receptor ligands have been synthesised by de-stannylation of tributyltin precursors using peracetic acid as oxidant. These brominated ligands showed good uptake in breast tumours.

Although it is likely that brominated radiopharmaceuticals will predominantly be used for brain imaging studies they may also have a role in peripheral *in-vivo* molecular imaging. Several reported probes have been designed for use with *in-vivo* gene expression systems such as the type 1 thymidine kinase (HSV1-tk) gene system. Using ^{76}Br in such reporter probes may offer some advantage over other PET tracers due to the longer half-life allowing the opportunity for extended observation *in vivo*. The uracil analogue, 5-[^{76}Br] bromo-2′-fluoro-2′-deoxyuridine ([^{76}Br]FBAU) is one such reporter probe. The synthesis involves exchange for tin using peracetic acid as oxidant (Cho *et al.* 2005). [^{76}Br]FBAU was found to accumulate in glioma cells expressing HSV1-tk.

Exchange for halogen can also be used for radiobromination. Lee *et al.* (2006) synthesised several peroxisome proliferator activated-receptor gamma (PPARγ) antagonists using exchange for chlorine in melt using Cu^{2+} as catalyst. They chose this method due to difficulties in preparing the trimethyltin precursor. Similarly, de-iodination can be used as in the case of the epbatidine analogue norchlorobromoepibatidine, which was prepared by Cu^{+}-catalysed bromodeiodination exchange from the iodo analogue in reducing conditions at 190°C with 70% radiochemical yield and 98% radiochemical purity after purification (Kassiou *et al.* 2002).

Radiolabelling with astatine

Although many of the standard methods used for radioiodination can be applied to radiolabelling with ^{211}At, standard protein electrophilic methods cannot be used for labelling proteins due to the poor stability of astatotyrosine (Zalutsky, Pozzi 2004).

The most widely used procedure for labelling monoclonal antibodies and fragments is a two-step procedure that involves synthesis of *N*-succinimidyl 3- or 4-[^{211}At] astatobenzoate (SAB) from the corresponding *N*-succinimidyl trialkylstannylbenzoate precursor followed by coupling of SAB to ε-amino groups of monoclonal antibody lysine residues (Zalutsky *et al.* 1989). This method has been applied to the radiolabelling of several antibodies including rituximab (Aurlien *et al.* 2000), A33 (Orlova *et al.* 2002) and MX35 F(ab′)$_2$ (Elgqvist *et al.* 2006). Modifications of this approach have used other *N*-succinimidyl prosthetic groups such as *N*-succinimidyl *N*-(4-[^{211}At]astatophenethyl)succinamate (SAPS) or *N*-succinimidyl 3-[^{211}At]astato-4-guanidinomethyl-benzoate (SGMAB) but use of these groups does not seem to offer any particular advantage in terms of radiolabelling (Zalutsky *et al.* 2007). Radiolysis can be a serious problem when labelling monoclonal antibodies with ^{211}At, as can formation of by-products from reaction solvents such as chloroform, although the latter problem can largely be overcome by using methanol instead.

An interesting area in which ^{211}At may have an important role in the future is in sodium iodide symporter (NIS)-mediated radionuclide therapy. For example, Willhauck *et al.* (2008) have used a prostate specific antigen promoter to target NIS expression to prostate cancer cells. They then used ^{211}At-astatide, which is also transported by NIS to specifically target the prostate cancer cells. Similar gene therapy targeting strategies are likely to be explored in the future.

Radiolabelling with ^{211}At can be carried out using exchange reactions as with other radiohalogenation methodologies. Those using exchange for tin have already been mentioned with reference to radiolabelling monoclonal antibodies. In addition, exchange for silicon has been used for the synthesis of the mIBG analogue 1-(*m*-[^{211}At]astatobenzyl)guanidine (mABG) using *N*-chlorosuccinimide as oxidant. This method was an adaptation of the method used to synthesise mIBG and resulted in an 85% yield (Vaidyanathan, Zalutsky 1992).

Summary

While radioiodination has found a useful place in radiopharmaceutical synthesis and has been used to prepare many important radiopharmaceuticals such as [^{123}I]mIBG, [^{131}I]mIBG, [^{123}I]ioflupane (DaTSCAN) and [^{131}I]tositumomab (Bexxar), it is possible that in the future brominated and astatinated radiopharmaceuticals may also be commercially available. Particularly interesting is the potential role of the PET isotope ^{76}Br in brain imaging agents, where its 16-hour half-life may offer advantages over ^{18}F and the quality of the images may offer advantages over the use of ^{123}I. In addition, the use of ^{211}At in therapy, particularly in gene therapy using NIS, is an exciting possibility.

It has been shown that similar radiohalogenation techniques can be used for labelling with iodine, bromine and astatine. For proteins, electrophilic substitution is common using chloramine-T, Iodogen, *N*-halosuccucinimides or enzymes as oxidants, but prosthetic groups may be required to label proteins with bromine (owing to the harsh conditions required for electrophilic substitution with bromine) or astatine (due to the instability of astatotyrosine). For other molecules, exchange reactions such as exchange for halogen, boron, tin, germanium, thallium or mercury can be used, the most common method being exchange for tin. Catalysts such as copper salts can be used to improve synthesis.

Radiohalogenation techniques have been very useful in the development of radiopharmaceuticals and, with the progress of PET and gamma scintigraphy as well as new approaches to therapy, it is likely that they will continue to be important for some considerable time.

References

Aurlien E *et al.* (2000). Demonstration of highly specific toxicity of the alpha-emitting radioimmunoconjugate ^{211}At-rituximab against non-Hodgkin's lymphoma cells. *Br J Cancer* 83: 1375–1379.

Bolton AE, Hunter WM (1973). The labelling of proteins to high specific radioactivity by conjugation to a ^{125}I-containing acylating agent. *Biochem J* 133: 529–539.

Boyd M *et al.* (2006). Radiation-induced biologic bystander effect elicited in vitro by targeted radiophamaceuticals labelled with α-, and β-, and auger electron-emitting radionuclides. *J Nucl Med* 47: 1007–1015.

Bruskin A *et al.* (2004). Radiobromination of monoclonal antibody using potassium [^{76}Br] (4-isothiocyanatobenzyl-ammonio)-bromo-decahydro-closo-dodecaborate (Bromo-DABI). *Nucl Med Biol* 31: 205–211.

Chaly T *et al.* (1996). Radiosynthesis of [18F] N-3-fluoropropyl-2-β-carbomethoxy-3-β-(4-iodophenyl) nortropane and the first human study with positron emission tomography. *Nucl Med Biol* 23: 999–1004.

Cho SY *et al.* (2005). Evaluation of ^{76}Br-FBAU as a PET reporter probe for HSV1-tk gene expression imaging using mouse models of human glioma. *J Nucl Med* 46: 1923–1930.

Corsetti F *et al.* (2004). Radioiodinated recombinant human TSH: a novel radiopharmaceutical for thyroid cancer metastases detection. *Cancer Biother Radiopharm* 19: 57–63.

Eckelman WC (1976). Iodinated bleomycin: an unsatisfactory radiopharmaceutical for tumor localization. *J Nucl Med* 17: 385–388.

Edreira MM, Pozzi OR (2006). Iodide benzamides for the in-vivo detection of melanoma and metastases. *Melanoma Res* 16: 37–43.

Eisen HN, Keston AS (1949). The immunologic reactivity of bovine serum albumin labeled with trace-amounts of radioactive iodine (I131). *J Immunol* 63: 71–80.

Elgqvist J *et al.* (2006). Alpha-radioimmunotherapy of intraperitoneally growing OVCAR-3 tumors of variable dimensions: outcome related to measured tumor size and mean absorbed dose. *J Nucl Med* 47: 1342–1350.

Firestone RB *et al.* (1999). *Table of Isotopes*, 8th edn. New York: Wiley.

Fraker PJ, Speck JC (1978). Protein and cell membrane iodinations with a sparingly soluble chloramide 1,3,4,6-tetrachloro 3a,6a diphenylglycoluril. *Biochem Biophys Res Comm* 80: 849.

Francis GE *et al.* (1951). Labelling of proteins with iodine-131, sulfur-35 and phosphorus-32. *Nature* 167: 748–751.

Govindan SV *et al.* (1999). Labeling of monoclonal antibodies with diethylenetriaminepentaacetic acid-appended radioiodinated peptides containing D-amino acids. *Bioconj Chem* 10: 231–240.

Hohn A *et al.* (1998a). Nuclear data relevant to the production of ^{120g}I via the ^{120}Te(p,n)-process at a small-sized cyclotron. *Appl Radiat Isot* 49: 1493–1496.

Hohn A *et al.* (1998b). Excitation functions of (p,xn) reactions on highly enriched ^{122}Te: relevance to the production of ^{120g}I. *Appl Radiat Isot* 49: 93–98.

Höglund J *et al.* (2000). Optimized indirect ^{76}Br-brominiation of antibodies using N-succinimidylpara-[^{76}Br]bromobenzoate for radioimmuno PET. *Nucl Med Biol* 27: 837–843.

Hunter R (1970). Standardization of the chloramine-T method of protein iodination. *Proc Soc Exp Biol Med* 133: 989–992.

Hunter WM, Greenwood FC (1962). Preparation of iodine-131 labelled human growth hormone of high specific activity. *Nature* 194: 495–496.

Hussain AA *et al.* (1995). Chloramine-T in radiolabeling techniques. II. A nondestructive method for radiolabeling biomolecules by halogenation. *Anal Biochem* 224: 221–226.

Jongen C *et al.* (2008). SPECT imaging of D(2) dopamine receptors and endogenous dopamine release in mice. *Eur J Nucl Med Mol Imaging* 35: 1692–1698.

Kaminski MS *et al.* (1993). Radioimmunotherapy of B-cell lymphoma with [^{131}I]anti-B1 (anti-CD20) antibody. *N Engl J Med* 329: 459–465.

Kampf G (1988). Induction of DNA double-strand breaks by ionizing radiation of different quality and their relevance for cell inactivation. *Radiobiol Radiother* 29: 631–658.

Kassiou M *et al.* (2002). Preparation of a bromine-76 labelled analogue of epibatidine: a potent ligand for nicotinic acetylcholine receptor studies. *Appl Radiat Isot* 57: 713–717.

Kienhuis CB *et al.* (1991). Six methods for direct radioiodination of mouse epidermal growth factor compared: effect of non-equivalence in binding behavior between labelled and unlabelled ligand. *Clin Chem* 37: 1749–1755.

Kizuka H *et al.* (1985). Synthesis and evaluation of p-iodophentermine (IP) as a brain perfusion imaging agent. *Nucl Med Commun* 6: 49–56.

Klapars A, Buchwald SL (2002). Copper-catalyzed halogen exchange in aryl halides: an aromatic Finkelstein reaction. *J Am Chem Soc* 124: 14844–14845.

Krohn KD *et al.* (1977). Differences in the sites of iodination of proteins following four methods of radioiodination. *Biochim Biophys Acta* 490: 497–505.

Kung MP, Kung HF (1989). Peracetic acid as a superior oxidant for preparation of [^{123}I]IBZM: a potential dopamine D-2 receptor imagin agent. *J Labelled Comp Radiopharm* 27: 691–700.

Lee H *et al.* (2006). Synthesis and evaluation of a bromine-76-labeled PPARgamma antagonist 2-bromo-5-nitro-*N*-phenylbenzamide. *Nucl Med Biol* 33: 847–854.

Lövqvist A *et al.* (1995). ^{76}Br-labeled monoclonal anti-CEA antibodies for radioimmuno positron emission tomography. *Nucl Med Biol* 22: 125–131.

Lui B *et al.* (1987). Radioactive iodine exchange reaction of HIPDM: kinetics and mechanism. *J Nucl Med* 28: 360–365.

Lundkvist C *et al.* (1999). Characterization of bromine-76-labelled 5-bromo-6-nitroquipazine for PET studies of the serotonin transporter. *Nucl Med Biol* 26: 501–507.

Mairs RJ *et al.* (1994). Carrier-free ^{131}I-meta-iodobenzylguanidine: comparison of production from meta-diazobenzylguanidine and from meta-trimethylsilylbenzylguanidine. *Nucl Med Commun* 15: 268–274.

Mather SJ (2005). Radioiodination of antibodies. In: Celis JE, ed. *Cell Biology: A Laboratory Handbook*, 3rd edn. Burlington, MA: Academic Press, 539–544.

Mather SJ, Ward BG (1987). High efficiency iodination of monoclonal antibodies for radiotherapy. *J Nucl Med* 28: 1034–1036.

Mayer A *et al.* (2000). Radioimmunoguided surgery in colorectal cancer using a genetically engineered anti-CEA single-chain Fv antibody. *Clin Cancer Res* 6: 1711–1719.

McElvany KD *et al.* (1982). 16α-[^{77}Br]Bromoestradiol: dosimetry and preliminary clinical studies. *J Nucl Med* 23: 425–430.

McFarlane AS (1956). Labelling of plasma proteins with radioactive iodine. *Biochem J* 62: 135–143.

McFarlane AS (1958). Efficient trace-labelling of proteins with iodine. *Nature* 182: 53.

Mennicke E *et al.* (2000). Electrophilic radioiodination of deactivated arenes with N-chlorosuccinimide. *J Lab Comp Radiopharm* 43: 721–737.

Mock BH, Weiner RE (1988). Simplified solid state labelling of [^{123}I]m-iodobenzylguanidine. *Appl Radiat Isot (Int J Radiat Appl Instrum Part A)* 39: 939–942.

Moerlein SM *et al.* (1988). No-carrier-added radiobromination and radioiodination of aromatic rings using in situ generated peracetic acid. *J Chem Soc Perkin Trans I* 3: 779–786.

Morrison M, Bayse GS (1970). Catalysis of iodination by lactoperoxidase. *Biochemistry* 9: 2995–3000.

Mume E *et al.* (2005). Evaluation of ((4-hydroxylphenyl) ethyl)maleimide for site-specific radiobromination of anti-HER2 affibody. *Bioconjug Chem* 16: 1547–1555.

Nicholl C *et al.* (1997). Pharmacokinetics of iodine-123-IMBA for melanoma imaging. *J Nucl Med* 38: 127–133.

Orlova A *et al.* (2002). Comparative biodistribution of the radiohalogenated (Br, I and At) antibody A33. Implications for in vivo dosimetry. *Cancer Biother Radpharm* 17: 385–396.

Pentlow KS *et al.* (1991). Quantitative imaging of I-124 using positron emission tomography with applications to radioimmunodiagnosis and radioimmunotherapy. *Med Phys* 18: 357–366.

Petzold G, Coenen HH (1980). Choramine-T for no-carrier-added labelling of aromatic biomolecules with bromine-75, 77. *J Lab Comp Radiopharm* 18: 1319–1336.

Robinson GD, Lee AW (1975). Radioiodinated fatty acids for heart imaging: iodine monochloride addition compared with iodide replacement labeling. *J Nucl Med* 16: 17–21.

Rowland DJ *et al.* (2006). Synthesis and in vivo evaluation of 2 high-affinity ^{76}Br-labeled σ_2-receptor ligands. *J Nucl Med* 47: 1041–1048.

Samnick S *et al.* (1999). Improved labelling of no-carrier-added ^{123}I-MIBG and preliminary clinical evaluation in patients with ventricular arrhythmias. *Nucl Med Commun* 20: 537–545.

Seevers RH, Counsell RE (1982). Radioiodination techniques for small organic molecules. *Chem Rev* 82: 575–590.

Senthilmohan R, Kettle AJ (2006). Bromination and chlorination reactions of myeloperoxidase at physiological concentrations of bromide and chloride. *Arch Biochem Biophys* 445: 235–244.

Sinn H *et al.* (1979). A fast and efficient method for labelling radiographic contrast media with ^{121}I and ^{123}I. *Int J App Radiat Isot* 30: 511–512.

Stadie WC *et al.* (1952). Studies of insulin binding with isotopically labeled insulin. *J Biol Chem* 199: 729–739.

Stein R *et al.* (2003). Improved iodine radiolabels for monoclonal antibody therapy. *Cancer Res* 63: 111–118.

Tatum JL *et al.* (1979). Radioiodination of biologically active compounds: a simplified solid-state enzymatic procedure. *Invest Radiol* 14: 185–188.

Tolmachev V *et al.* (1998). Production of ^{76}Br by a low-energy cyclotron. *Appl Radiat Isot* 49: 1537–1540.

Turner JH *et al.* (2003). ^{131}I-Anti CD20 radioimmunotherapy of relapsed or refractory non-Hodgkins lymphoma: a phase II clinical trial of a nonmyeloablative dose regimen of chimeric rituximab radiolabeled in a hospital. *Cancer Biother Raiopharm* 18: 513–524.

Vaidyanathan G, Zalutsky MR (1990). Protein radiohalogenation: observations on the design of N-succinimidyl ester acylation agents. *Bioconjug Chem* 1: 269–273.

Vaidyanathan G, Zalutsky MR (1992). 1-(m-[^{211}At]astatobenzyl)guanidine: synthesis via astato demetalation and preliminary in vitro and in vivo evaluation. *Bioconjug Chem* 3: 499–503.

Vaidyanathan G, Zalutsky MR (1993). No-carrier-added synthesis of meta [^{131}I]iodobenzylguanidine. *Appl Radiat Isot* 44: 621–628.

Vaidyanathan G, Zalutsky MR (1995). No-carrier-added meta-[^{123}I]iodobenzylguanidine: synthesis and preliminary evaluation. *Nucl Med Biol* 22: 61–64.

Vaidyanathan G, Zalutsky MR (1996a). Targeted therapy using alpha emitters. *Phys Med Biol* 41: 1915–1931.

Vaidyanathan G *et al.* (1996b). No-carrier addd (4-fluoro-3-[131I]iodobenzyl)guanidine and (3-[^{211}At]astato-4-fluorobenzyl)guanidine. *Bioconjug Chem* 7: 102–107.

Verbruggen RF (1987). Fast, high-yield labelling and quality control of [^{123}I]- and [^{31}I]-mIBG. *Appl Radiat Isot (Int J Radiat Appl Instrum Part A)* 38: 303–304.

Ward BG *et al.* (1987). Localization of radioiodine conjugated to the monoclonal antibody HMFG2 in human ovarian carcinoma: assessment of intravenous and intraperitoneal routes of administration. *Cancer Res* 47: 4719–4723.

Wieland DM *et al.* (1980). Radiolabeled adrenergic neuron-blocking agents: adrenomedullary imaging with [^{131}I] iodoenzylguanidine. *J Nucl Med* 21: 349–353.

Wilbur DS (1992). Radiohalogenation of proteins: an overview of radionuclides, labeling methods, and reagents for conjugate labeling. *Bioconjug Chem* 3: 433–470.

Willhauck MJ *et al.* (2008). The potential of ^{211}Astatine for NIS-mediated radionuclide therapy in prostate cancer. *Eur J Nucl Med Mol Imaging* 35: 1272–1281.

Youfeng H *et al.* (1982). A comparative study of simple aromatic compounds via N-halosuccinimides and chloramines-T in TFAA. *J Lab Comp Radiopharm* 19: 807–819.

Zalutsky MR *et al.* (1989). Labeling monoclonal antibodies and F(ab$'$)$_2$ fragments with the α-particle-emitting nuclide astatine-211: Preservation of immunoreactivity and in vivo localizing capacity. *Proc Natl Acad Sci USA* 86: 7149–7153.

Zalutsky MR, Pozzi OR (2004). Radioimmunotherapy with α-particles emitting radionuclides. *Q J Nucl Med Mol Imaging* 48: 289–296.

Zalutsky MR *et al.* (2007). Targeted α-particle radiotherapy with ^{211}At-labeled monoclonal antibodies. *Nucl Med Biol* 34: 779–785.

Further reading

Coenen H *et al.* (2006). *Radioiodination Reactions for Pharmaceuticals: Compendium for Effective Synthesis Strategies*. Heidelberg: Springer.

Seevers RH, Counsell RE (1982). Radioiodination techniques for small organic molecules. *Chem Rev* 82: 575–590.

Wilbur DS (1992). Radiohalogenation of proteins: an overview of radionuclides, labeling methods, and reagents for conjugate labeling. *Bioconjug Chem* 3: 433–470.

11

Radiolabelling approaches with fluorine-18

Julie L Sutcliffe and Henry F VanBrocklin

Introduction

There has been a marked increase in the application of fluorine-containing molecules in a variety of life science fields, most notably the pharmaceutical industry (Ismail 2002; Maienfisch, Hall 2004). The substitution of fluorine for hydrogen or hydroxyl group in a bioactive molecule, a common strategy for the development of new drug candidates, has profound impact on the molecule's pharmacokinetic, pharmacodynamic and even toxicological properties. Fluorine, the most electronegative element and smallest halogen, has a van der Waals radius of 1.47 Å that is similar to that of oxygen (1.52 Å), accounting for its hydroxyl group-mimicking properties. The electronegativity also increases the carbon–fluorine bond strength relative to carbon–carbon, carbon–oxygen and carbon–hydrogen bonds. Additionally, fluorine substitution increases the lipophilicity, enhancing cellular absorption, and changes the molecular conformational structure, steric parameters that influence metabolic characteristics; yet fluorine is small enough to minimise loss of biological activity when interacting with binding or substrate pockets on receptors or enzymes (Smart 2001; Ismail 2002; Kirk 2008).

Long before the current interest in incorporating natural fluorine into bioactive molecules, fluorine-18 gained prominence in the development of positron-emitting radiotracers for positron emission tomography (PET) imaging. Fluorine-18 was discovered in 1936 at the Radiation Laboratory in Berkeley, California by proton irradiation of neon-20 (Snell 1937). Sodium [^{18}F]fluoride, the first fluorine-18 imaging agent, was applied to bone scintigraphy long before the development of PET imaging systems (Blau *et al.* 1962).

Fluorine-18 possesses favourable properties for both synthesis and imaging, and is now readily available in gigabecquerel (GBq) or curie (Ci) quantities from low-energy (10–20 MeV) cyclotrons throughout the world. With a half-life of 110 minutes, lengthy and/or multistep syntheses may be performed with sufficient quantities of labelled product available for delivery to PET imaging suites distant from the cyclotron and production facilities. The short half-life means that the theoretical specific activity of fluorine-18 is high, 63.7×10^9 GBq/mol (1.71×10^9 Ci/mol), leading to radiotracers with low mass (nanomoles or micrograms per mCi or MBq) per injected dose. The half-life is also sufficient for protracted PET imaging studies involving slow biochemical processes that may take several hours to observe. The combination of decay characteristics, positron emission of 97% and low positron energy (0.635 MeV), which allows the highest resolution imaging, together with the half-life make fluorine-18 the ideal isotope for PET imaging.

Production of fluorine-18

There are over 20 known nuclear reaction pathways for the production of fluorine-18 (Qaim *et al.* 1993), the most common being the $^{18}O(p,n)$ reaction on enriched oxygen-18 targets, water or gas, or the $^{20}Ne(d,\alpha)$ reaction on natural-abundance neon-20 gas (Helus *et al.* 1979; Ruth, Wolf 1979; Casella *et al.* 1980; Blessing *et al.* 1986; Ruth *et al.* 2001). Figure 11.1 shows the fluorine-18 products that are produced in the cyclotron along with the electrophilic and nucleophilic labelling agents needed for tracer preparation. Irradiation of oxygen-18 water with protons for 1–2 hours gives 185–370 GBq (5–10 Ci) of aqueous [^{18}F]fluoride ion. Gaseous targets may also be used to produce [^{18}F]fluoride ion. Proton irradiation of enriched [^{18}O]O_2 gas or deuteron irradiation of a neon-20 gas target produces fluorine-18 that sticks to the walls of the target. Recovery of the target gas after irradiation is followed by heating the target in the presence of a gas flush or water rinse of the target to release the [^{18}F]fluoride ion (Winchell *et al.* 1976; Nickles *et al.* 1982; Dahl *et al.* 1983; Blessing *et al.* 1986; Hamacher *et al.* 1986). As a result of the higher proton cross-section for oxygen-18 versus neon-20 (700 versus 115 millibarns), the yield of fluorine-18 from oxygen is more than twice that from neon.

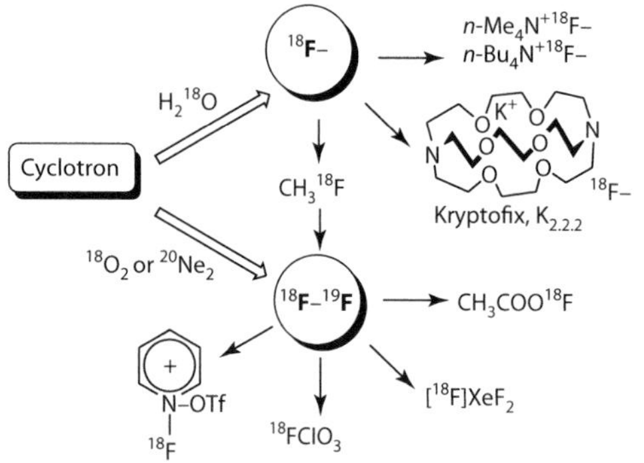

Figure 11.1 Fluorine-18 fluoride ion and fluorine-18 gas, key labelling precursors produced in the cyclotron target, shown in circles, with secondary nucleophilic and electrophilic labelling agents.

Oxygen-18 and neon-20 gas may also be used to prepare [^{18}F]fluorine gas (^{18}F-^{19}F). Deuteron irradiation of neon-20 gas doped with 0.1–2% [^{19}F]fluorine gas produces [^{18}F]fluorine gas directly in the target (Bida *et al.* 1980; Casella *et al.* 1980). The specific activity of the [^{18}F]fluorine gas will depend on the amount of [^{19}F]fluorine gas added into the target. A 'double-shoot' method was developed for the production of [^{18}F]fluorine gas from enriched oxygen-18 gas ($^{18}O_2$) (Nickles *et al.* 1984). The $^{18}O_2$ is loaded in the target and irradiated with protons. The fluorine-18 adheres to the target walls, allowing the recovery of $^{18}O_2$. Subsequent introduction of argon gas with up to 100 μmol of [^{19}F]fluorine gas into the target and irradiation with 20 μA protons for 10 minutes scrubs the [^{18}F]fluorine from the walls, forming [^{18}F]fluorine gas (^{18}F-^{19}F) by isotopic exchange.

An alternative method for the production of high-specific-activity [^{18}F]fluorine gas from [^{18}F]fluoride ion was developed by Bergman and Solin (Bergman, Solin 1997). The conversion, shown in Figure 11.1, involves the intermediate production of [^{18}F]fluoromethane ($CH_3{}^{18}F$) by nucleophilic [^{18}F]fluoro-for-iodo exchange on methyl iodide. Subsequent exchange of the fluorine-18 from the $CH_3{}^{18}F$ to fluorine gas is facilitated by electrolytic discharge. The resulting [^{18}F]fluorine gas has a specific activity 2–4 orders of magnitude greater than that of [^{18}F]fluorine gas produced *in situ* in the cyclotron target.

Direct fluorine-18 labelling strategies

There are two main approaches to labelling radiotracers with fluorine-18, direct fluorination and indirect fluorination. The direct approach involves incorporation of the fluorine-18 into the radiotracer or a protected intermediate in a single step. The indirect approach couples a 'directly' labelled intermediate, coined the 'labelled prosthetic group', to another molecule to form the desired labelled molecule. The indirect approach may be utilised to produce a library of labelled molecules from a common labelled prosthetic group or when direct labelling approaches are not possible owing to the chemical structure limitations or the stability of the molecule to the labelling conditions. Direct labelling of radiotracers or prosthetic groups may be accomplished by either nucleophilic or electrophilic fluorination conditions. Nucleophilic labelling reactions using [^{18}F]fluoride ion are more abundant, in large part owing to the greater availability of [^{18}F]fluoride ion and the high specific activity afforded to the final radiotracers.

Electrophilic fluorinating agents

The process whereby an electrophile, a positively charged species, interacts with an electron-rich molecule including an alkene, an aromatic ring or a carbanion, forming a covalent bond is an electrophilic reaction. In the case of electrophilic [^{18}F]fluorinations, $^{18}F^{+}$, in the form of [^{18}F]F_2 gas or other labelling reagents shown in Figure 11.1, is the electrophile that forms a carbon–fluorine bond introducing the label into the molecule. Several electrophilic fluorinating agents may be produced from [^{18}F]fluorine gas. Labelled xenon difluoride ($Xe^{18}F^{19}F$, [^{18}F]XeF_2, Figure 11.1) is formed by heating [^{18}F]fluorine gas in the presence of xenon gas (Chirakal *et al.* 1984). A series of nitrogen-fluorinated (NF) reagents may be prepared by the reaction of amines, quaternary salts, amides and sulfonamides with [^{18}F]fluorine gas. The NF agents include *N*-[^{18}F]-2-pyridone (Oberdorfer *et al.* 1988b), *N*-[^{18}F]fluoropyridinium triflate (Figure 11.1) (Oberdorfer *et al.* 1988a), *N*-[^{18}F]fluoro-*endo*-norbornyl-*p*-tolylsulfonamide (Satyamurthy *et al.* 1990), and most recently *N*-[^{18}F] fluorobenzenesulfonimide (Teare *et al.* 2007). These mild radiofluorinating agents react with metal-carbanions (R-Li, R-MgX) to provide alkyl or aryl fluorides (Satyamurthy *et al.* 1990). Perchlorofluoride ($^{18}FClO_3$, Figure 11.1), produced by passing [^{18}F]fluorine gas through a column of solid $KClO_3$, also reacts with aryl lithium compounds to give aryl fluorides (Ehrenkaufer, MacGregor 1983). The most widely used fluorinating reagent besides [^{18}F]fluorine gas is [^{18}F]acetyl hypofluorite ($CH_3COO^{18}F$, Figure 11.1) formed by passage of [^{18}F]fluorine gas through a column of acetic acid and potassium acetate (Fowler *et al.* 1982; Jewett *et al.* 1984; Chirakal *et al.* 1988). These reagents and [^{18}F]fluorine gas offer a limited yet useful range of reaction and reagent activities to make a variety of radio-tracers.

Electrophilic fluorination reactions

As seen in Figure 11.1, the [^{18}F]fluorine gas molecule is composed of one fluorine-18 atom and one fluorine-19 atom. Reaction of [^{18}F]fluorine gas with electron-rich substrates where only one fluorine is added into the molecule means that the maximum yield of radiolabelled product is only 50%, accounting for decay. The in-target production of [^{18}F]fluorine gas requires up to 100 µmol of fluorine-19 gas (Nickles *et al.* 1984), about 10^6 times the amount of fluorine-18 produced in the target. Therefore, several milligrams (equivalent to the amount of fluorine gas added to the target) of the precursor to be labelled will need to be used for each radiosynthesis. This may be costly, and a significant amount of carrier, fluorine-19, product will be produced. Thus, the specific activity of the fluorine-18-labelled compounds will be ~37 GBq/mmol (~1 Ci/mmol), 10^6-fold less than theoretical specific activity and 10^3–10^4-fold less than the nucleophilic [^{18}F]fluorination products. The resultant radiotracers may only be used to image processes that do not require high specific activity such as enzymatic activity. The Bergmann/Solin methodology for preparation of [^{18}F]fluorine gas from [^{18}F]fluoride ion does offer some improvement in the specific activity, but [^{19}F]fluorine gas must still be introduced into the discharge chamber for exchange with the [^{18}F] fluoride. Applying this methodology gives radiotracers with a specific activity of 0.37–3.7 TBq/mmol (10^2–10^3 Ci/mmol) at the low end of the range of specific activities typically seen for nucleophilic fluorination products (Bergman, Solin 1997).

Representative electrophilic fluorination reactions are shown in Figures 11.2 and 11.3. As seen in Figure 11.2, [^{18}F]acetyl hypofluorite adds across a double bond to give either of the two fluoroacetate intermediates. In many cases the acetate is hydrolysed, resulting in the addition of one fluorine to the molecule. With the production of FDG (Figure 11.2) the acetyl hypofluorite may react at either face of the alkene, giving either axial or equatorial fluorination (Adam 1982; Shiue *et al.* 1982; Diksic, Jolly 1983; Herschied *et al.* 1984). Subsequent acetate

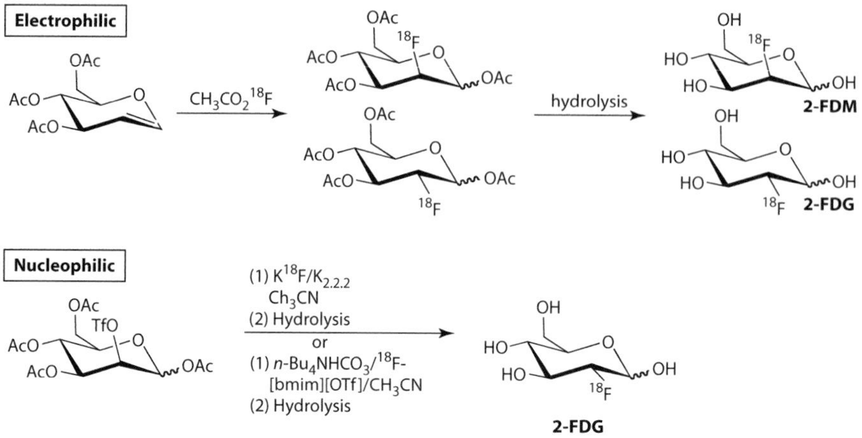

Figure 11.2 Synthesis of 2-[^{18}F]fluorodeoxyglucose (2-FDG). (2-FDM = 2-[^{18}F]fluorodeoxymannose).

hydrolysis yields two products, in this case 2-fluorodeoxyglucose (2-FDG) and 2-fluorodeoxymannose (2-FDM; a metabolically less reactive analogue). While altering the reaction conditions, especially the solvent, reduces the amount of 2-FDM by-product, the 2-FDG must still be chromatographically separated from 2-FDM. The FDG reaction proceeds similarly with [^{18}F] fluorine gas addition across the double bond giving a 3 : 1 mixture of the 1,2-difluoro intermediate (reaction not shown). Chromatographic separation followed by acid hydrolysis gives the desired 2-FDG (Ido *et al.* 1978).

Highly reactive [^{18}F]fluorine gas undergoes electrophilic aromatic substitution with hydrogen on phenyl rings. An example of this reaction is shown in Figure 11.3. The first reaction (A) demonstrates the non-selective reaction of [^{18}F]fluorine gas in hydrogen fluoride with dopa, 3,4-dihyroxyphenylalanine, a substrate for amino acid decarboxylase in dopaminergic neurons in the brain. The reaction gives 2-, 5- and 6-[^{18}F]fluorodopa analogues which are separable by HPLC. The product pattern is dictated by the steric environment and the activating groups that are situated around the ring. About 70% of the [^{18}F]fluorine was incorporated into this molecule (Firnau *et al.* 1986).

Alternatively, the regioselective introduction of electrophilic fluorine-18 may be facilitated by the [^{18}F]fluorodemetallation reaction with trialkyltin, trialkylgermanium or trialkylsilicon arenes (Adam *et al.* 1983, 1984; Coenen, Moerlein 1987). Electrophilic reaction B in Figure 11.3 illustrates the regioselective preparation of 6-[^{18}F]fluorodopa from the corresponding trimethylstannyl precursor. The acid, amine and hydroxy functional groups are protected for the [^{18}F]fluorination reaction and subsequently hydrolysed with concentrated hydrogen bromide to produce the 6-[^{18}F]fluorodopa in two steps. The overall decay-corrected yield is 26%, just greater than 50% of the maximum possible yield (Namavari *et al.* 1992).

The number of electrophilic reactions and compounds that have been radiolabelled with electrophilic fluorine-18 is limited, a direct consequence of the restricted availability and low specific activity of the [^{18}F]fluorine gas. Increased availability and specific activity will prompt the investigation of these and other, yet unexplored, electrophilic reactions.

Nucleophilic fluorinating agents

Nucleophilic reactions involve either the addition of an electron-rich nucleophile (anion) to a compound with an unsaturated double bond (alkene, carbonyl, imine, nitrile) or the substitution of a leaving group. Nucleophilic substitution reactions with [^{18}F]fluoride ion as the nucleophile are most common for introduction of fluorine-18 into radiotracers or their precursors. [^{18}F]Fluoride ion as it comes from the cyclotron in oxygen-18 water is a poor nucleophile as a result of water solvation owing to strong hydrogen bonding (Hefter, McLay 1988). With the exception of biomolecules (proteins, peptides, antibodies, DNA, RNA, etc.), most radiotracers are organic molecules

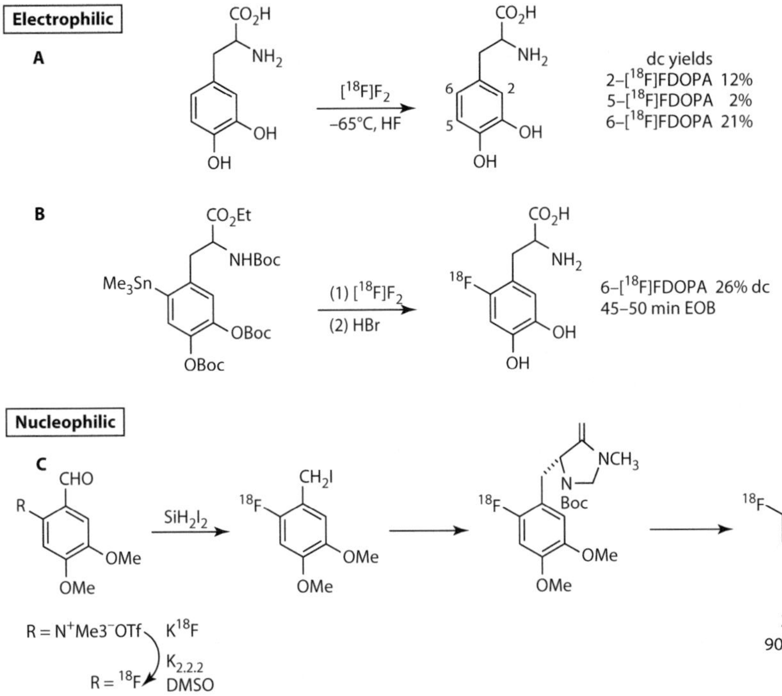

Figure 11.3 Preparation of $[^{18}F]$fluorodopa (*S*)-Boc-BMI = (*S*)-1-(*tert*-butyl)-3-methyl-4-imidazolidinone. (A: Firnau *et al.* 1984; Coenen *et al.* 1988. B: Dolle *et al.* 1998a; Fuchtner *et al.* 2002. C: Lemaire *et al.* 1991, 1994.)

that are only soluble in non-aqueous, dry organic solvents. Therefore, $[^{18}F]$fluoride ion must be dehydrated and coupled with a counter-ion that promotes solubility in organic solvents suitable for nucleophilic reactions.

The $[^{18}F]$fluoride ion must be exposed or 'naked' to be most reactive. Early labelling studies investigated evaporation of target water in the presence of an alkali earth metal (potassium, rubidium or caesium), forming the $[^{18}F]$fluoride salts. Low solubility of the $[^{18}F]$fluoride salts in organic solvents, especially the potassium $[^{18}F]$fluoride, limited this route for tracer synthesis (Tewson, Welch 1980; Attina *et al.* 1983a,b; Shiue *et al.* 1985, 1986). The use of crown ethers, e.g. 18-crown-6 (Irie *et al.* 1982, 1984) and subsequently, aminopolyethers, e.g. Kryptofix 2.2.2 ($K_{2.2.2}$; Figure 11.1), to complex the cation, especially potassium, has proved very successful for the phase transfer and nucleophilic $[^{18}F]$fluoride reactions (Block *et al.* 1986; Coenen *et al.* 1986; Hamacher *et al.* 1986). Tetraalkylammonium hydroxide and bicarbonate, (alkyl = methyl or butyl; Figure 11.1) have also been used as phase transfer agents for nucleophilic $[^{18}F]$fluorinations (Kiesewetter *et al.* 1986; Brodack *et al.* 1988; Culbert *et al.* 1995). While there has been little difference reported in the reactivity of these species when compared in identical nucleophilic substitution reactions (Korguth *et al.* 1988), most of the current $[^{18}F]$fluoride reactions are performed with $K_{2.2.2}/K^{18}F$. The evaporation of the target water in the presence of potassium carbonate and $K_{2.2.2}$ is more forgiving to excessive drying.

The sequence for processing aqueous $[^{18}F]$fluoride from the cyclotron follows. The aqueous $[^{18}F]$fluoride is either added directly to the potassium carbonate/ $K_{2.2.2}$ solution or trapped on an anion-exchange resin and eluted off with an aqueous acetonitrile–potassium carbonate/$K_{2.2.2}$ solution. The resulting aqueous acetonitrile potassium carbonate/$K_{2.2.2}$ $[^{18}F]$fluoride solution is azeotropically evaporated to dryness with heat, vacuum, a stream of nitrogen gas and addition of dry acetonitrile. Current $[^{18}F]$fluoride targets hold more than one millilitre of water, so resin trapping of $[^{18}F]$fluoride permits the recovery of the enriched oxygen-18 target water, reduces the evaporation time needed to remove several millilitres of water and allows the concentration of the $[^{18}F]$fluoride ion with the concomitant elimination of potential reaction-killing contaminants. The resin trapping has largely supplanted the direct addition of target water to the reaction prior to evaporation.

Once dry, the residue is dissolved in a variety of polar aprotic solvents such as acetonitrile, dimethyl sulfoxide, dimethylformamide, tetrahydrofuran, dichloromethane or *o*-dichlorobenzene and then added to the desired reactants. The choice of solvents provides a range of properties to facilitate reagent solubility and a variety of reaction temperatures. Reasonably dry reactions free of competing ions and protic solvents that will not solvate or hydrogen-bond the [^{18}F]fluoride ion are the conditions that have been widely believed to be necessary for successful nucleophilic fluorinations. There are known examples of the deliberate addition of water to the synthesis as in the preparation of [^{18}F]*N*-methylspiroperidol (Shiue *et al.* 1989). Recently, Windhorst and colleagues (Windhorst *et al.* 2001) described the synthesis of [^{18}F]flumazenil using 'instant fluorination'. Target water (100 μL) was added directly to the reaction mixture with potassium carbonate and $K_{2.2.2}$ in 2,4,6-collidine/acetonitrile with no evaporation step. The [^{18}F] fluoro-for-nitro exchange produced 2–12% [^{18}F]flumazenil from starting [^{18}F]fluoride ion and the [^{18}F] fluoro-for-[^{19}F]fluoro gave 44% [^{18}F]flumazenil, albeit at a lower specific activity. This is an interesting approach to eliminating the evaporation step and decreasing the synthesis time; however, with the limited amount of target water that may be added, this reaction is not likely to be widely applicable without methods for concentrating the aqueous [^{18}F]fluoride ion.

Contrary to popular belief, ionic liquids and protic solvents have recently been shown to enhance nucleophilic [^{18}F]fluorination reactions. Ionic liquids consist of ionic species that are liquid at low temperatures. Room-temperature ionic liquids are comprised of a bulky organic cation coupled with either inorganic (BF_4, PF_6, SF_6) or organic (triflate, tosylate) counter-anions (see Figure 11.4). One ionic liquid, 1-butyl-3-methylimidazolium tetrafluoroborate ([bmim][BF_4]; Figure 11.4), has a melting point of −80°C and has been shown to enhance nucleophilic fluoride substitution of aliphatic mesylates and halides (Kim *et al.* 2003b). Initial reactions with [^{18}F]fluoride ion using

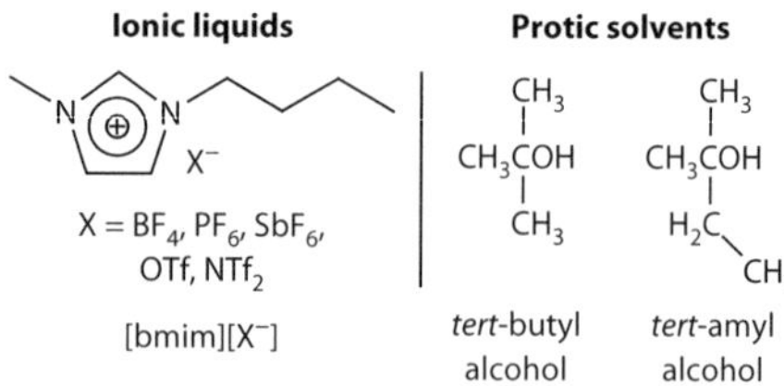

Figure 11.4 Alternative solvents for nucleophilic fluorination reactions.

[bmim][OTf] gave 80–93% [^{18}F]fluoro-for-mesylate substitution on an unactivated alkylmesylate with Cs_2CO_3 or K_2CO_3 as the base (Kim *et al.* 2003a). Cyclotron target water up to 250 μL was added directly to the reaction mixture. Reaction rates were dependent on the amount of target water added (50 μL was faster than 250 μL) and the base used (Cs_2CO_3 was faster than K_2CO_3). [^{18}F]FDG has been labelled with up to 75% and 3′-deoxy-3′-[^{18}F]fluorothymidine ([^{18}F]FLT) in 57–65% yield in ionic liquids.

Protic solvents have been avoided in nucleophilic [^{18}F]fluorination reactions as they are thought to solvate the fluoride ion and reduce its nucleophilic character. Contrary to this thinking, Chi and colleagues have demonstrated that protic solvents, especially the tertiary alcohols *tert*-butyl, *tert*-amyl and *tert*-hexyl, improve the nucleophilic substitution reactions of [^{18}F]fluoride ion for sulfonyl esters (mesylate, tosylate, triflate and nosylate), reducing radioactive by-products (Kim *et al.* 2006, 2008b; Lee *et al.* 2007a, b, 2008; Oh *et al.* 2007). This methodology has been applied to the synthesis of 2-[^{18}F]FDG (85.4 ± 7.8%), [^{18}F]FLT (65.5 ± 5.4%), [^{18}F]MISO (69.6 ± 1.8%), [^{18}F]FP-CIT (35.8 ± 5.2%; Figure 11.5, reaction b). Chi and colleagues are currently exploring the synergistic effect on nucleophilic fluorination by combining the ionic liquid with the protic solvent (Kim *et al.* 2008a; Shinde *et al.* 2008a,b). No radioactive [^{18}F] fluorinations have been reported. The initial results from these two solvent systems are encouraging and offer the potential to optimise fluorine-18 radiotracer production.

Nucleophilic aliphatic substitution

The widespread availability and the high specific activity (1–10 Ci/μmol) of [^{18}F]fluoride ion from modern cyclotron targets is attractive for the

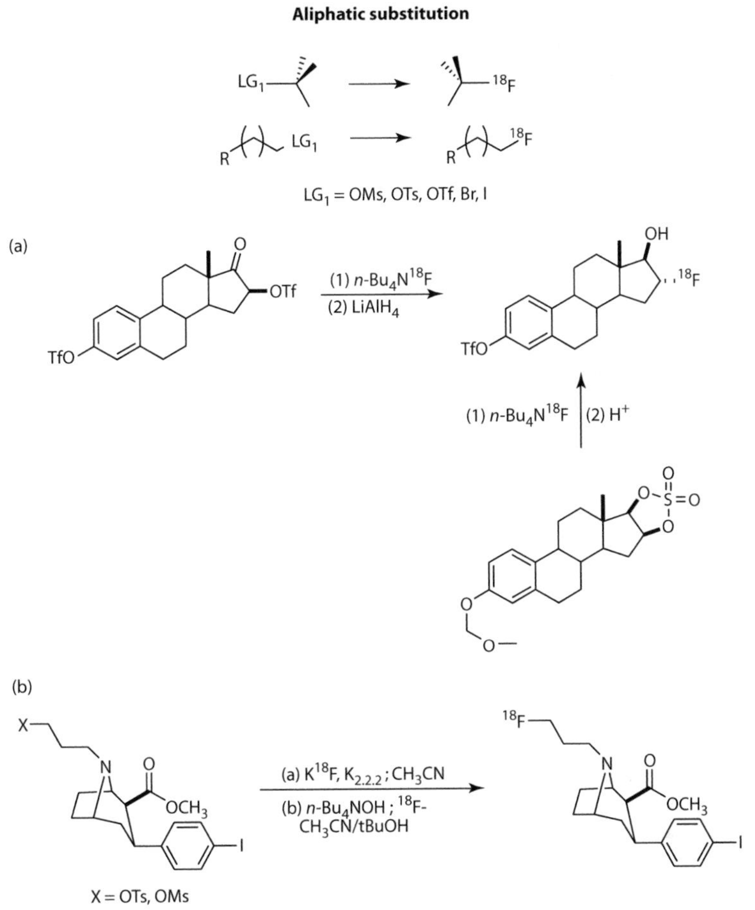

Aliphatic substitution

LG_1 = OMs, OTs, OTf, Br, I

(a) (1) $n\text{-}Bu_4N^{18}F$ (2) $LiAlH_4$; (1) $n\text{-}Bu_4N^{18}F$ (2) H^+

(b) (a) $K^{18}F$, $K_{2.2.2}$; CH_3CN (b) $n\text{-}Bu_4NOH$; ^{18}F-CH_3CN/tBuOH

X = OTs, OMs

Figure 11.5 Nucleophilic aliphatic substitution for FP-CIT. (Chaly *et al.* 1996.)

production of radiotracers with low associated mass. With these tracers one can visualise tissues with low concentrations of binding sites such as neurotransmitter receptors in the brain or cell surface proteins on tumour cells. Figure 11.5 shows the general schemes for the nucleophilic substitutions with fluoride ions followed by two radiotracer examples.

Nucleophilic substitutions on aliphatic substrates invoke an S_N2 mechanism whereby the [^{18}F]fluoride ion displaces leaving groups such as sulfonyl esters (mesylate, tosylate or triflate) or halogens (bromo or iodo). As shown at the top of Figure 11.5, if the leaving group is attached to a chiral carbon (with four different substituents) then the nucleophilic attack by [^{18}F] fluoride ion inverts the configuration of that carbon. This is seen in reaction a (Figure 11.5), where the triflate group in the 16β position of oestrone or the beta cyclic sulfate is displaced by the [^{18}F]fluoride ion to give the 16α-[^{18}F]fluoroestrone intermediate that is either reduced or hydrolysed under acidic conditions to give 16α-[^{18}F]fluoroestradiol (Kiesewetter *et al.* 1984; Lim *et al.* 1996). This same inversion of configuration takes place in the production of 2-FDG shown in Figure 11.2. The displacement of the mannose triflate gives the intermediate 2-[^{18}F]fluorodeoxyglucose tetraacetate that is hydrolysed by either acid or base to yield 2-FDG. The most common solvent for these [^{18}F] fluorination reactions is acetonitrile; however, as mentioned above, protic solvents and ionic liquids have been shown to be suitable solvents in the reaction with acetonitrile and in some cases enhance the production of the desired radiotracer. Reaction conditions for the application of ionic liquids are shown for the nucleophilic synthesis of 2-FDG in Figure 11.2 (Kim *et al.* 2004). The protic solvent *tert*-butanol is shown in the production of the tropane [^{18}F]FP-CIT, an imaging agent for the dopamine transporter (Figure 11.5 reaction b) (Lee *et al.* 2007a). Two production methods for reaction b are shown: (a) the conventional method with K^{18}F, $K_{2.2.2}$ in acetonitrile (Chaly *et al.* 1996) and (b) *tert*-butanol in addition to acetonitrile with tetrabutylammonium hydroxide as base (Lee *et al.* 2007a). Each reaction produces [^{18}F]FP-CIT in a single step. The yield for the conventional reaction is <5%, whereas the protic solvent reaction gave a 38% yield for an automated synthesis and 52% for a manual synthesis. The tosylate site on the propyl group is not activated towards nucleophilic substitution, yet the protic solvent enhances the reactivity of the nucleophile and improves the substitution reaction.

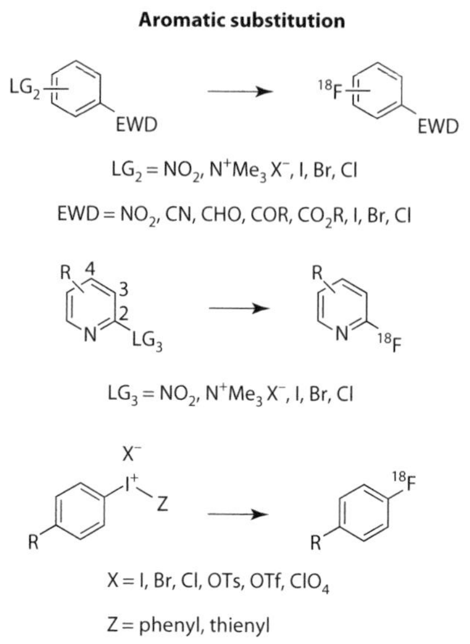

Aromatic substitution

LG_2 = NO_2, $N^+Me_3X^-$, I, Br, Cl

EWD = NO_2, CN, CHO, COR, CO_2R, I, Br, Cl

LG_3 = NO_2, $N^+Me_3X^-$, I, Br, Cl

X = I, Br, Cl, OTs, OTf, ClO_4

Z = phenyl, thienyl

Figure 11.6 Nucleophilic aromatic substitution.

Nucleophilic aromatic substitution

Fluorination of aromatic rings and heterocyclic aromatic rings (e.g. pyridine) with fluorine-18 provides a stable carbon–fluorine bond that demonstrates good metabolic stability. Introduction of [^{18}F]fluorine into the ring involves the substitution of a leaving group, generally nitro (NO_2), a trimethylammonium salt (NMe_3^+) or a halide (I, Br, Cl ion) in concert with an activating substituent that draws electrons away from the carbon with the leaving group to attract the [^{18}F]fluoride ion (Figure 11.6). The position of the substituent on the ring relative to the leaving group directs the site of attack. Strong electron-withdrawing groups such as nitro, nitrile, aldehyde, methylketone or ester direct nucleophilic attack at the *ortho* and *para* positions on the ring. Two example reactions are shown, one in Figure 11.3 and the other in Figure 11.7. The preparation of 6-[^{18}F]fluorodopa by the nucleophilic route involves four

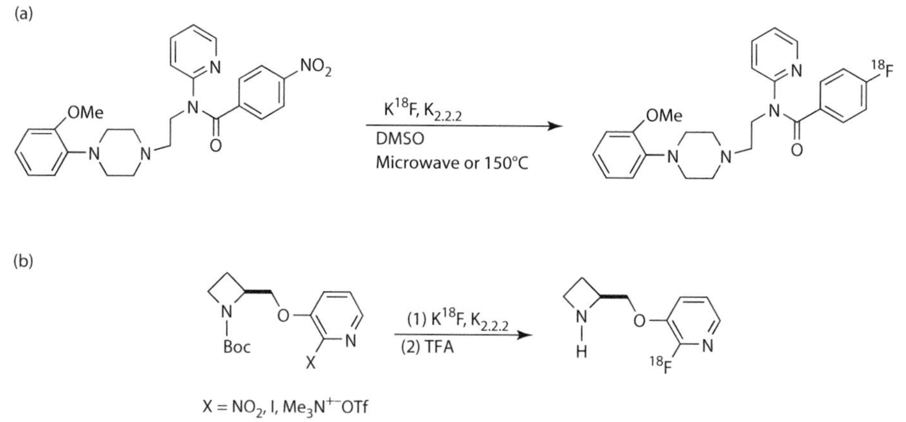

(a)

K^{18}F, $K_{2.2.2}$
DMSO
Microwave or 150°C

(b)

(1) K^{18}F, $K_{2.2.2}$
(2) TFA

X = NO_2, I, Me_3N^+ $^-$OTf

Figure 11.7 Examples of nucleophilic aromatic ^{18}F-fluorination. Reaction A: Preparation of 4-[^{18}F]fluoro-*N*-[2-[1-(2-methoxyphenyl)-1-piperazinyl]ethyl-*N*-2-pyridinyl-benzamide (*p*-[^{18}F]MPPF). Reaction B: Preparation of 2-[^{18}F]F-A85380, a nicotinic receptor imaging agent.

steps (Figure 11.3) (Lemaire *et al.* 1991, 1994). The first step is substitution of the trimethylammonium group, *ortho* to the aldehyde (CHO), by [^{18}F]fluoride on the phenyl ring that also has two methoxy groups in the 3- and 4-positions on the ring. The aldehyde directs the [^{18}F]fluoro-for-trimethylammonium exchange. Subsequent reductive iodination of the aldehyde gives the benzyl iodide followed by reaction with (*S*)-Boc-BMI to give the fully protected phenylalanine. Deprotection of the entire molecule gives the desired 6-[^{18}F]fluorodopa in 23% decay-corrected yield in 90 minutes reaction time. This synthesis is much more difficult to reproduce, which is why the preferred route to production of the regioselective 6-[^{18}F]fluorodopa is the electrophilic substitution reaction using [^{18}F]F_2 gas (Figure 11.3, B) (Dolle *et al.* 1998a; Fuchtner *et al.* 2002). The electrophilic synthesis provides comparable yields in 60 minutes, albeit at a lower specific activity.

Another illustrative reaction is shown in Figure 11.7. Le Bars and colleagues evaluated the synthesis of *ortho*-, *meta*- and *para*- [^{18}F]fluoro-for-nitro exchange using conventional and microwave heating (Le Bars *et al.* 1998). They found that only the *para*-nitro group was displaced by [^{18}F]fluoride ion and, furthermore, microwave heating gave a 40% yield versus 16% for conventional heating at 150°C. As higher temperatures are needed for these reactions, the most common solvent for these reactions is DMSO.

Nucleophilic aromatic substitution reactions offer high-yielding, strong carbon–fluorine bonds that can withstand varied subsequent reaction conditions. For this reason many of the labelled prosthetic groups that will be discussed below are produced in one step from [^{18}F]fluoride ion using nucleophilic aromatic substitution.

Heteroaromatic nucleophilic [^{18}F]fluorinations, especially with pyridines, have been studied extensively (Figure 11.6) (Dolle 2005, 2007). As in the aromatic substitution reactions, the leaving groups and the position of the leaving group relative to the ring nitrogen dictate the reactivity of the molecule to substitution. Good yields >60–70% have been reported for the 2- and 4-substituted pyridines. The fluoro-for-nitro or -bromo substitution in the 3-position is not favoured; thus, no product has been seen for these reactions under any conditions. One example of the direct labelling of a nicotinic receptor imaging agent, [^{18}F]fluoro-A85380, is shown in Figure 11.7, reaction b. The production of this compound has been performed with three leaving groups, nitro, iodo and trimethylammonium triflate (Dolle *et al.* 1998b, 1999; Horti *et al.* 1998). The yields for these three leaving groups were: nitro 49–64%, iodo 40% and trimethylammonium triflate 68–72%. Subsequent deprotection of the *N*-Boc group with TFA gives the labelled A85380 imaging agent.

The last approach to making fluorine-18-labelled benzenes and arenes (substituted phenyl compounds) is shown at the bottom of Figure 11.6. Phenyl arene iodonium salts or aryl-(2-thienyl) iodonium salts have been used to prepare substituted fluorophenyl compounds (Gail, Coenen 1994, 1997; Pike, Aigbirhio 1995; Ermert *et al.* 2004; Ross *et al.* 2007). The yields of arene decrease as the substituents (R) change as I > Br > Cl> CH_3> OCH_3. Concomitantly, the yield of [^{18}F] fluorobenzene increases as one goes from iodine to methoxy in the same series. This series of reactions offers another route to produce fluorine-18 labelled tracers.

Pyrimidine and acyloguanosine nucleosides for imaging gene therapy

Engineered cells that carry the gene for HSV thymidine kinase (HSV-tk) are being explored as gene therapy agents to treat cancer (Culver *et al.* 1992; Ram *et al.* 1993). Acyclovir, ganciclovir and penciclovir are potent drugs against HSV, acting as phosphorylating agents causing the inhibition of DNA polymerase (Martin 1986). [^{18}F]Fluorinated analogues of these drugs have been developed as a mechanism for imaging response to gene therapy. Such fluorinated compounds include 9-[(3-[^{18}F]fluoro-1-hydroxy-2-propoxy)methyl] guanine, [^{18}F]FHPG (Alauddin *et al.* 1996a,b; Gambhir *et al.* 1998) (Figure 11.8) the fluoro analogue of ganciclovir, and 9-(4-[^{18}F]fluoro-3-hydroxymethyl-butyl)guanine, [^{18}F]FHBG (Alauddin, Conti 1998; Hustinx *et al.* 2001) (Figure 11.8), the fluoro analogue of penciclovir. Both compounds were synthesised from the corresponding tosylate precursor via the no-carrier-added (n.c.a.) fluorination with

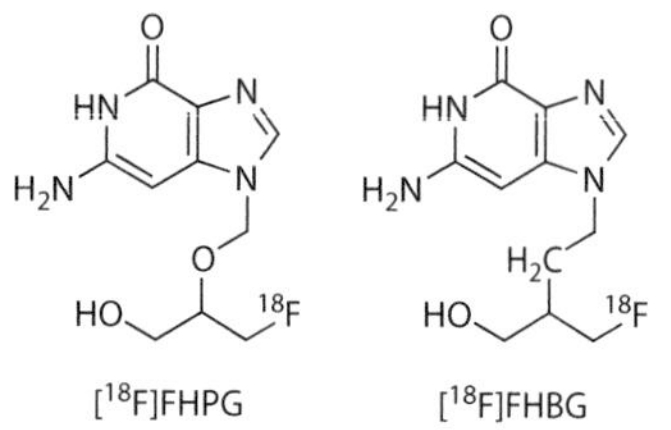

Figure 11.8 Structures of [^{18}F]FHPG and [^{18}F]FHBG.

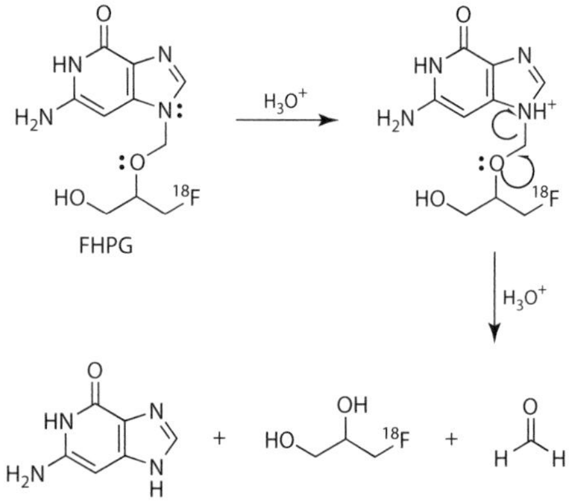

Figure 11.9 Instability of [^{18}F]FHPG in acidic medium.

[^{18}F]F/$K_{2.2.2}$, followed by a deprotection and HPLC purification. [^{18}F]FHBG has been the most widely used of the two as [^{18}F]FHPG is unstable in acidic medium (Figure 11.9).

A series of pyrimidine nucleoside derivatives have also been developed to monitor gene therapy. These include [^{18}F]FMAU, [^{18}F]FIAU, [^{18}F]FFAU, [^{18}F] FCAU, [^{18}F]FBAU, and [^{18}F]FEAU (Alauddin *et al.* 2002,2004a,b, 2007) (see Figure 11.11). These pyrimidine nucleosides are reported to be more sensitive than [^{18}F]FHBG and [^{18}F]FHPG, demonstrate much better pharmacokinetics, and are renally cleared. Overall, [^{18}F]FEAU is suggested as the most specific imaging agent for HSV1-tk. [^{18}F]FEAU is synthesised via the fluorination of 2-deoxy-2-trifluoromethanesulfonyl-1,3,5-tri-O-benzoyl-α-D;-ribofuranose, subsequently converted to the 1-bromo derivative and coupled to 5-ethyl uracil ((Soghomonyan *et al.* 2007) (Figure 11.12).

Enzymatic fluorination

A more recent novel approach to incorporating ^{18}F into biomolecules is the use of enzymes The enzyme fluorinase, isolated from the bacterium *Streptomyces cattleya* has been used to introduce ^{18}F into biomolecules (O'Hagan *et al.* 2002; Martarello *et al.* 2003). Examples of this approach include the synthesis of 5′-[^{18}F]fluoro-5′-deoxyadenosine ([^{18}F] F-5′-FDA), a potential tumour imaging agent. Improved reaction conditions (Deng *et al.* 2006) resulted in radiochemical yields of 45–75% within 4 hours. This approach does have limitations due to the specificity of fluorinase, but it is an attractive chemoselective approach to radiofluorination (Figure 11.10).

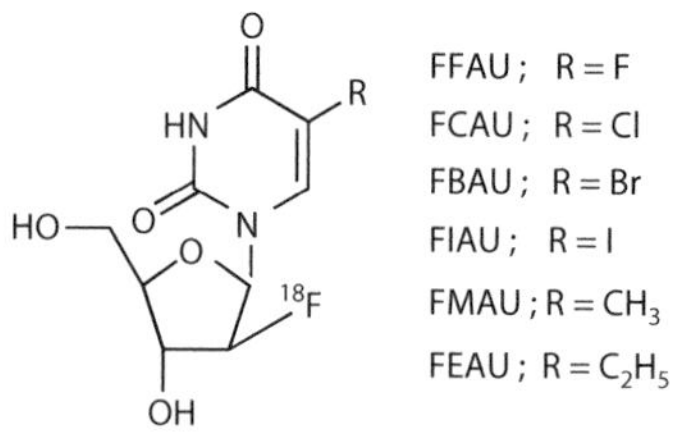

Figure 11.11 Structures of [^{18}F]pyrimidine nucleosides.

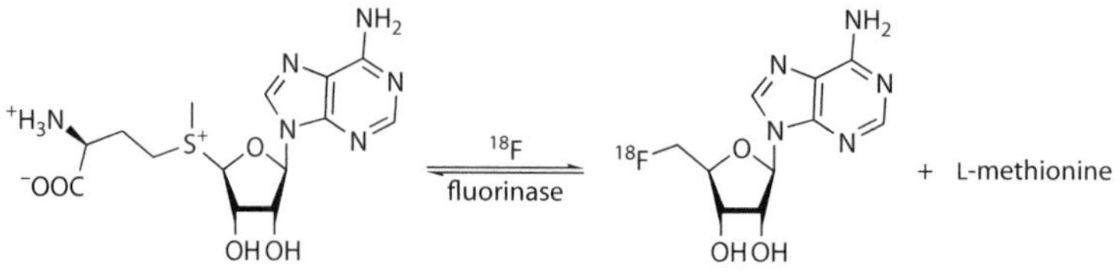

Figure 11.10 Synthesis of [^{18}F]F-5′-FDA via enzymatic fluorination.

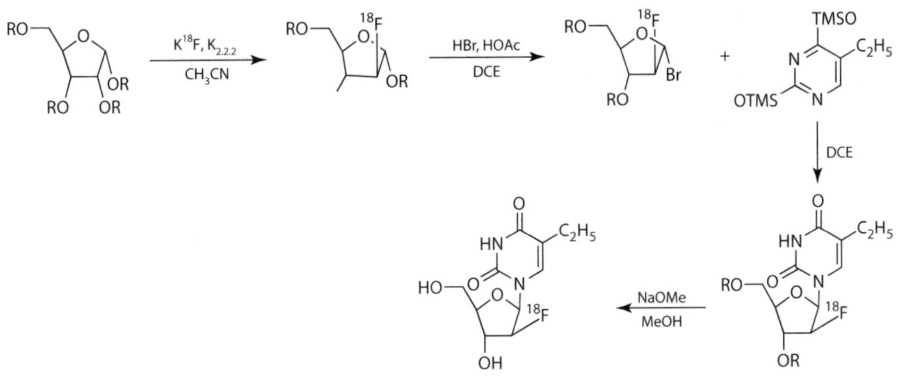

Figure 11.12 Synthesis of [^{18}F]FEAU.

Indirect labelling approaches

As the field of molecular imaging continues to evolve it is critical that rapid, reproducible radiolabelling approaches are developed and optimised for the labelling of biomolecules such as peptides, proteins and oligonucleotides. Unfortunately, direct labelling of such biomolecules is not possible owing to the often harsh conditions of pH, temperature and solvents that are necessary to perform direct fluorination. To circumvent these problems, numerous indirect approaches that utilise radiolabelled prosthetic groups have been developed (Okarvi 2001). Fluorinated prosthetic groups have been synthesised for the incorporation of ^{18}F into biomolecules either via alkylation using 4-[^{18}F]fluorophenacylbromide ([^{18}F]FPB) (Kilbourn *et al.* 1987), acylation using *N*-succinimidyl 4-[^{18}F]fluorobenzoate ([^{18}F]SFB) (Wester *et al.* 1996; Vaidyanathan, Zalutsky 2006), amidation using 4-([^{18}F]fluoromethyl)benzoylaminobutan-4-amine (Shai *et al.* 1989), photochemical conjugation using 4-azidophenacyl-[^{18}F]fluoride ([^{18}F]APF) (Wester *et al.* 1996) or chemoselective radiolabelling via oxime formation using 4-[^{18}F]fluorobenzaldehyde ([^{18}F]FBA), hydrazone bond formation and most recently utilisation of the 1,3-dipolar Huisgen cycloaddition reaction 'click chemistry' (Marik, Sutcliffe 2006). Unfortunately, it still appears that there is no universal prosthetic group and therefore labelling approaches and conditions need to be investigated on a peptide-to-peptide, protein-to-protein basis. This section will discuss the synthesis of the prosthetic groups and their applications in the synthesis of radiolabelled peptides and proteins.

Prosthetic groups

Numerous prosthetic groups have been developed for the radiolabelling of complex biomolecules. These include fluorinated aldehydes, acids, activated esters, pyridines, azides, alkynes and more. Examples of such prosthetic groups are illustrated in Figure 11.13.

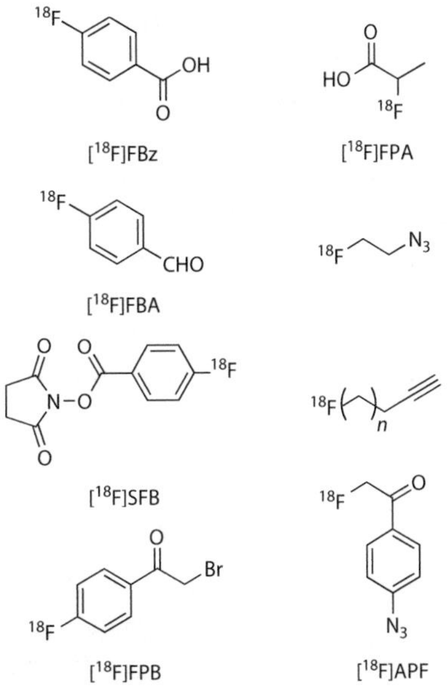

Figure 11.13 Widely used [^{18}F]F-prosthetic groups for radiolabelling of biomolecules.

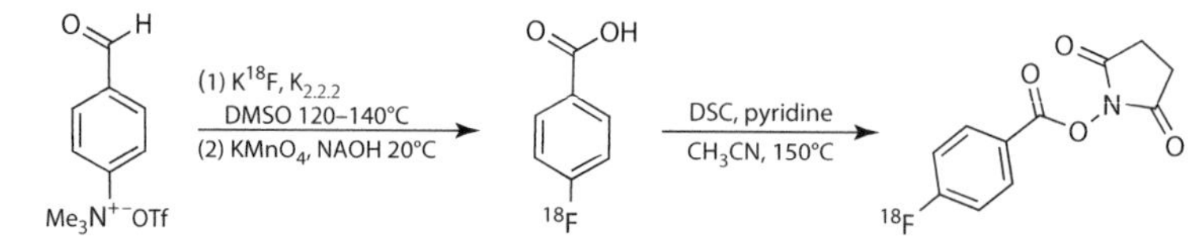

Figure 11.14 Synthesis of [^{18}F]SFB.

The most commonly used prosthetic group to date is [^{18}F]SFB. Several approaches for the synthesis of [^{18}F]SFB have been developed and optimised over the last decade.

Synthesis and optimisation of [^{18}F]SFB

[^{18}F]SFB has been synthesised via the oxidation of the 4-[^{18}F]fluorobenzaldehyde. Decay-corrected yields of 30–35% and a synthesis time of 80 minutes are reported. Using this approach the trimethylammonium group was substituted with ^{18}F to yield the 4-[^{18}F]fluorobenzaldehyde. This was then oxidised to 4-[^{18}F]fluorobenzoic acid ([^{18}F]FBA) using potassium permanganate and converted to [^{18}F]SFB using *N,N*-disuccinimidyl carbonate (Figure 11.14). The activated ester can subsequently be coupled to peptides and proteins in aqueous media.

Alternatively and most often used is the optimised three-step synthesis of [^{18}F]SFB as illustrated in Figure 11.15 (Wester *et al.* 1996). In this approach, the 4-trimethylammonium triflate precursor was fluorinated and a subsequent hydrolysis step yielded the [^{18}F]FBA. Activation of the [^{18}F]FBA to yield [^{18}F]SFB was achieved using *O*-(*N*-succinimidyl-*N,N,N′,N′*-tetramethyluronium tetrafluoroborate (TSTU). This approach eliminated the oxidation step that was difficult to automate as well as eliminating a HPLC purification step.

Solid-phase approach to radiolabelling of peptides

Most recently, a routine solid-phase approach has been utilised to radiolabel peptides attached to a solid phase using 4-[^{18}F]fluorobenzoic acid ([^{18}F]FBA). Rapid *in-situ* activation and coupling of [^{18}F]FBA to the peptide was achieved (2 minutes) using *O*-(7-azabenzotriazol-l-yl)-1,1,3,3-tetramethyluronium hexafluorophosphate and *N,N*-diisopropylethylamine (HATU/DIPEA) (Sutcliffe-Goulden *et al.* 2000, 2002). The 4-[^{18}F]benzoyl peptides were synthesised with a radiochemical purity of greater than 99 % and decay-corrected radiochemical yield (RCY) of greater than 90%. This approach is fast, efficient, site-specific and readily automatable.

This solid-phase approach was adapted for the synthesis of radiolabelled peptides using 2-[^{18}F]fluoropropionic acid ([^{18}F]FPA). [^{18}F]FPA was synthesised by the reaction of $K^{18}F/K_{222}$ with 9-methylanthranyl-2-bromopropionate (Guhlke *et al.* 1994). The [^{18}F]FPA was conjugated to the peptides attached to the solid-phase support. Coupling was achieved in 30 minutes at 30°C followed by a TFA cleavage. The ^{18}F-labelled peptides were

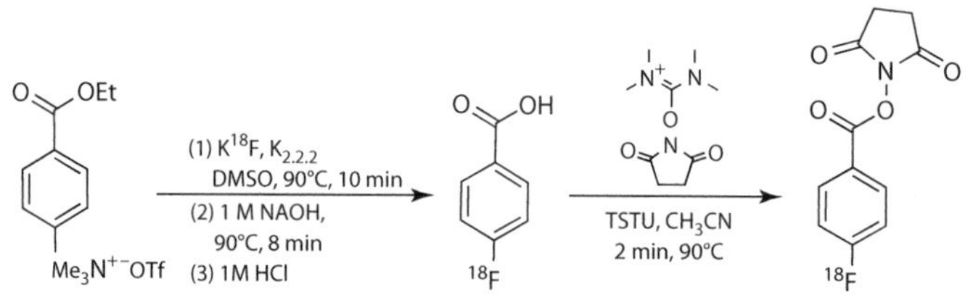

Figure 11.15 Optimised synthesis of [^{18}F]SFB.

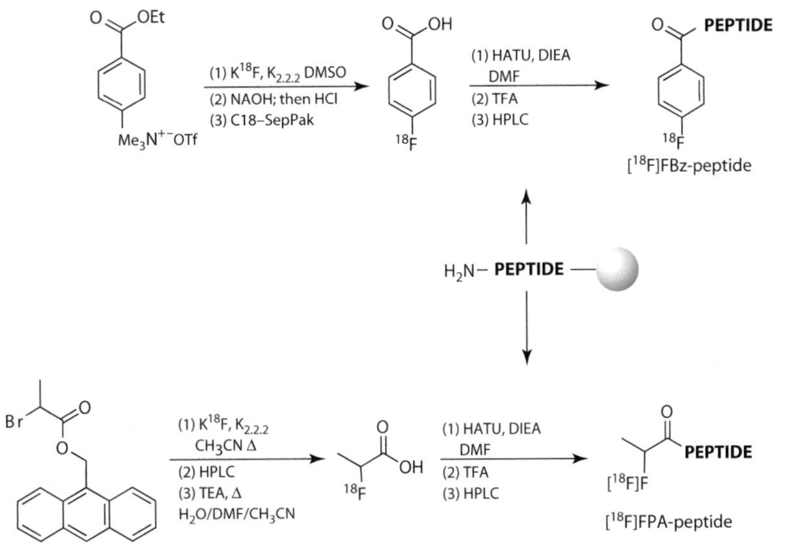

Figure 11.16 Solid-phase synthesis of ^{18}F-labelled peptide using [^{18}F]FBz and [^{18}F]FPA.

obtained in 175 minutes with decay-corrected yields of 6–16% and with a purity of 76–99% (Marik *et al.* 2006) (Figure 11.16).

Alkylation approaches

Alkylating agents include 4-[^{18}F]pentafluorobenzaldehyde (Herman *et al.* 1994) and 4-[^{18}F]fluorophenacyl bromide (Kilbourn *et al.* 1987). The synthesis of 4-[^{18}F]fluorophenacyl bromide was achieved by fluorination of 4-nitrobenzene using n.c.a [^{18}F]fluoride. The 4-[^{18}F]fluorobenzonitrile was converted into 4-[^{18}F] fluoroacetophenone followed by a bromination to yield 4-[^{18}F]fluorophenacyl bromide. Overall radiochemical yields of 28–40% were achieved in a synthesis time of 75 minutes. 4-[^{18}F]Fluorophenacyl bromide was subsequently used to label fibrinogen, with reported yields of 25–30% (Figure 11.17).

Photochemical conjugation

Photochemical conjugation was investigated as a method for fluorinating biomolecules in a one-step reaction. The prosthetic group used was 4-azidophenacyl [^{18}F]fluoride ([^{18}F]APF). The starting material, 4-azidophenacyl bromide, was reacted with n.c.a [^{18}F]fluoride at 90°C for 4 minutes to yield [^{18}F] APF; this was used to label proteins including HAS, transferrin, avidin and immunoglobulin using UV irradiation at 365 nm for 5–10 minutes. Radiolabelling efficiencies of 15–30% were observed and correlated with lysine content of the protein (Figure 11.18).

Chemoselective prosthetic approaches

Most prosthetic groups discussed so far have involved attachment of the prosthetic group (PG) to the

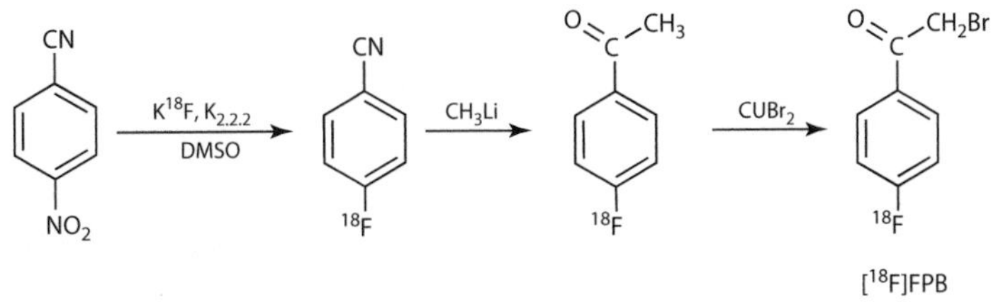

Figure 11.17 Synthesis of [^{18}F]FPB.

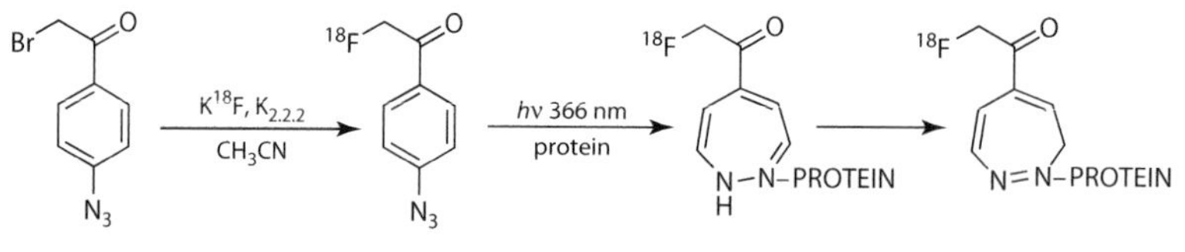

Figure 11.18 Photochemical conjugation of a protein using [^{18}F]APB.

N-terminus of a peptide or N-ε of a lysine residue. Chemoselective approaches to radiolabelling of biomolecules have been developed, including oxime and hydrazone bond formation as well as thiol reactive prosthetic groups. 'Click chemistry' approaches have most recently been exploited.

Oximes

Chemoselective radiofluorination of small peptides has been achieved using 4-[^{18}F]fluorobenzaldehyde ([^{18}F]FBA) and aminooxy functionalised peptides (Poethko *et al.* 2004a,b). 4-Formyl-*N,N,N*-trimethylanilium triflate was reacted with K^{18}F/K$_{222}$ in DMSO at 60°C for 15 minutes. [^{18}F]FBA was purified either by Sep-Pak C$_{18}$ cartridge or by RP-HPLC. [^{18}F]FBA was obtained in radiochemical yields of 50% within 30 minutes. Aminooxy functionalised peptides such as minigastrin, RGD and octreotate were radiolabelled with [^{18}F]FBA in a methanolic solution at pH 2.5 with overall radiochemical yields of 40% (Figure 11.19)

Hydrazones

Chemoselective fluorination has also been achieved with ^{18}F via hydrazone formation, for example between c(RGDyK)-hydrazinonicotinic acid (HYNIC) and 4-[^{18}F]fluorobenzaldehyde. Radiochemical purities of greater than 95% were reported with radiochemical yields greater than 90% within 30 minutes (Figure 11.20).

Thiol labelling agents

To date, the majority of prosthetic groups have been designed to label N-terminal amino functions, amino functions of lysine residues or carboxylic acids. Alternatively, thiol functions present only on cysteine residues are potential targets for chemoselective, site-specific modifications of peptides or proteins. Several maleimides have been developed to facilitate such reactions (de Bruin *et al.* 2005; Cai *et al.* 2006; Wuest *et al.* 2008a). Prosthetic groups include *N*-[2-(4-[^{18}F]-fluorobenzamido)ethyl]maleimide ([^{18}F]-FBEM), 1-[3-(2-[^{18}F]fluoropyridin-3-yloxy)propyl] pyrrole-2,5-dione ([^{18}F]FPyME) (Figure 11.21) and [^{18}F]-FDGmaleimidehexyloxime ([^{18}F]FDG-MHO).

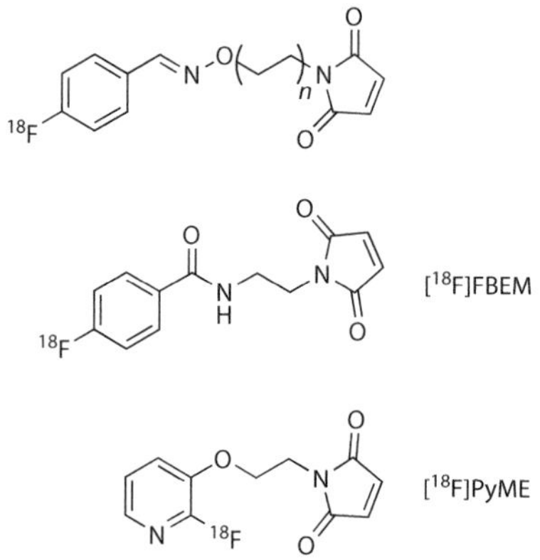

Figure 11.21 Structures of [^{18}F]FBAM, [^{18}F]FBEM and [^{18}F] FPyMe.

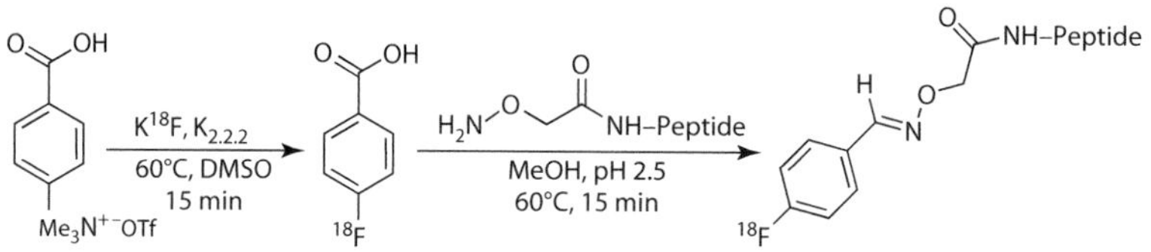

Figure 11.19 ^{18}F fluorination via oxime formation.

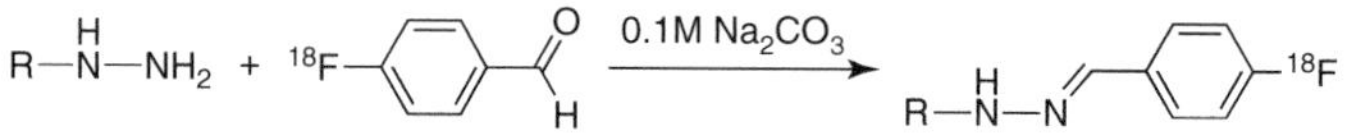

Figure 11.20 ^{18}F fluorination via hydrazone formation.

[^{18}F]FBEM

[^{18}F]FBEM was synthesised by the reaction of [^{18}F]SFB with *N*-(2-aminoethyl)maleimide at 40°C for 20 minutes. Radiochemical yields of 5% were achieved within 150 minutes. [^{18}F]FBEM was conjugated to a sulfhydryl-RGD peptide in DMSO. Radiolabelled peptides were obtained with radiochemical yields of 80% within 20 minutes.

[^{18}F]FPyME

The [^{18}F]fluoropyridine-based maleimide was synthesised as a thiol-reactive prosthetic group. This was a three-step procedure that involved the *ortho*-radiofluorination of [3-(3-*tert*-butoxycarbonylamino-propoxy)pyridine-2-yl]trimethylammonium trifluoromethanesulfonate precursor followed by *N*-Boc removal and maleimide formation using *N*-methoxycarbonylmaleimide. Radiochemical yields of 28–37% were obtained. [^{18}F]FPyME was conjugated to a model hexapeptide (N-Ac)KAAAAC with radiochemical yields of 60–70% in 10 minutes.

[^{18}F]FDG-MHO

FDG is the most widely used PET radiopharmaceutical and is now readily available worldwide. This site-specific radiolabelling approach (Wuest *et al.* 2008a) utilised FDG as a building block for radiolabelling peptides and proteins. The thiol-reactive prosthetic group [^{18}F]FDG-MHO was synthesised by the reaction of FDG with aminooxymaleimidehexyloxime. [^{18}F]FDG-MHO was tested with the tripeptide glutathione and with the protein annexin (Figure 11.22).

[^{18}F]FDG-MHO was obtained with radiochemical yields of 45–69% within 45 minutes; [^{18}F]FDG-MHO-glutathione demonstrated yields of greater than 90% (peptide concentration dependent) and [^{18}F]FDG-MHO-annexin was synthesised in radiochemical yields of 43–58%.

Click chemistry for fluorination

'Click' chemistry utilises chemical reactions to selectively provide high yields of products from a variety of easily accessible building blocks (Kolb 2001; Kolb, Sharpless 2003). The use of click chemistry, namely the Huisgen 1,3-dipolar cycloaddition reaction of terminal alkynes with organic azides to yield 1,4-disubstituted 1,2,3-triazoles under mild conditions, was first applied to PET radiochemistry by Sutcliffe and Marik in 2006. This report described the Cu(I)-catalysed 1,3-dipolar cycloaddition of ω-[^{18}F]fluoroalkynes ($n = 1$–3) with *N*-(3-azidopropionyl) peptides. Three different [^{18}F]fluoroalkynes were synthesised. Radiochemical yields of 54–99% were reported in 10 minutes.

This was soon followed by the reports of ^{18}F-fluorinated azides, namely 2-[^{18}F]fluorethylazide and the reaction with a small library of terminal alkynes (Glaser, Arstad 2007). This approach was also utilised to radiolabel a model peptide derivatised with propargylic acid. Radiochemical yields of 90% were achieved after HPLC purification (Figure 11.23)

Click chemistry has now been utilised to develop an [^{18}F]folic acid as a radiopharmaceutical for imaging folate receptor-positive tumours (Ross *et al.* 2008). This approach provided a regiospecific coupling to the γ-isomer. Radiochemical yields of 25–35% were achieved within 90 minutes. Click [^{18}F]folate demonstrated good tumour uptake *in vivo*; however, strong hepatobiliary clearance was observed, limiting the potential of this probe.

This is an important area of interest and *in-vivo* stability and toxicity of such approaches has now been reported (Li *et al.* 2007; Hausner *et al.* 2008).

Silicon and boron fluorination approaches

As described so far, current labelling approaches for the introduction of ^{18}F into biomolecules involve a multistep approach via a prosthetic group. The C–F bond formation often occurs in polar aprotic solvents at elevated temperatures using ^{18}F under dry conditions. A one-step approach is therefore highly desirable. Recent reports towards such efforts have

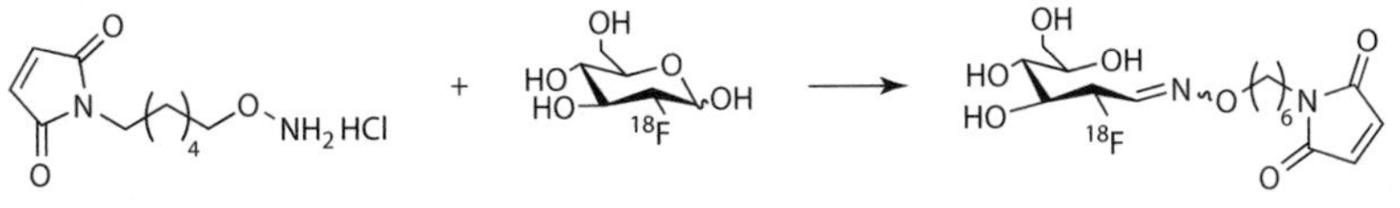

Figure 11.22 Synthesis of [^{18}F]FDG-MHO.

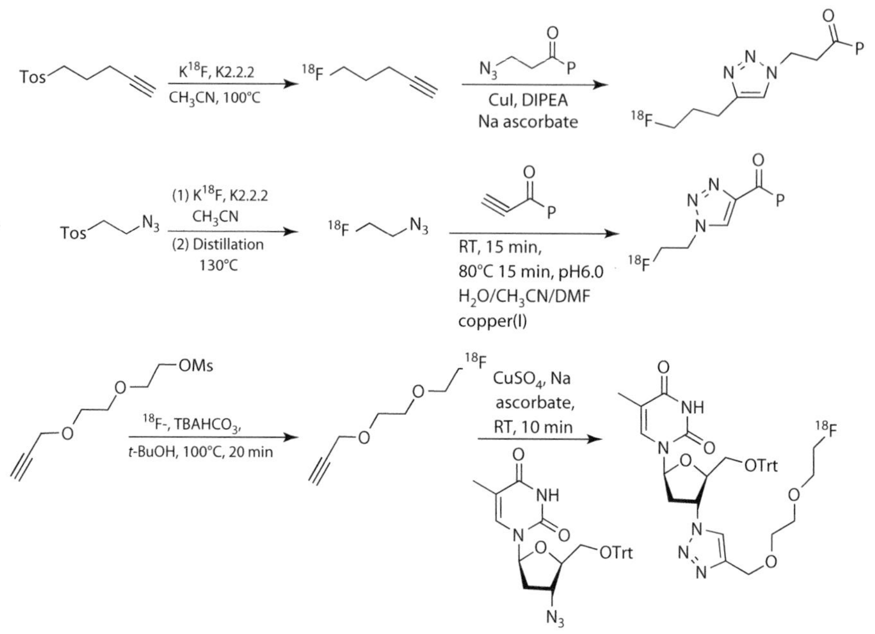

Figure 11.23 ^{18}F fluorination via the Huisgen 1,3 cycloaddition reaction. (P = peptide.)

included the one-step incorporation of ^{18}F into biomolecules via B–F and Si–F bond formation (Ting *et al.* 2005; Schirrmacher *et al.* 2006a). Aryl fluoroborate and alkyl fluorosilicates have been described as novel precursors for the radiolabelling of biotin molecules in aqueous media. Ting *et al.*(2005) reported a one-step synthesis of both a pinacol phenyl boronate diester and an alkyltriethoxysilane (Figures 11.24 and 11.25). Both compounds were chelated to biotin. Most recently the *in-vivo* stability of the B–F bond was demonstrated using an ^{18}F-labelled aryl triflurorborate; any free [^{18}F]fluoride would be deposited in the bone, but no bone uptake was observed.

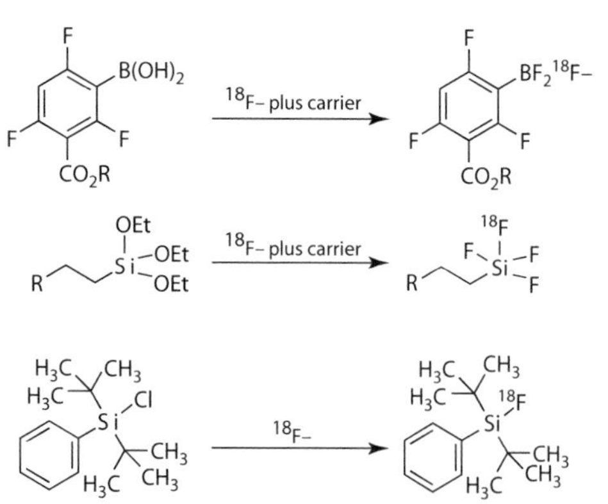

Figure 11.24 Structure of aryl fluoroborates and alkyl fluorosilicates.

Organofluorosilanes have also been proposed as a one-step approach for the introduction of ^{18}F into biomolecules. Schirrmacher (2006b) reported the fluorination of three organofluorosilanes, [^{18}F]fluorotriphenylsilane, [^{18}F]fluoro-*tert*-butyldiphenylsilane and [^{18}F]fluorodi-*tert*-butyldiphenylsilane Although almost quantitative yields were obtained in 15 minutes, unfortunately [^{18}F]fluorotriphenylsilane was not stable at pH 7.4–7.6 in human serum and [^{18}F]fluoro-*tert*-butyldiphenylsilane was hydrolysed in the liver to give free [^{18}F]fluoride. [^{18}F]Fluorodi-*tert*-butyldiphenylsilane proved to be the most stable of the three. To avoid the necessary purification by HPLC, an isotopic exchange reaction was proposed. [^{19}F]Fluorodi-*tert*-butyldiphenylsilane was reacted with n.c.a $K^{18}F/K_{222}$ in acetonitrile. Yields of 80–95% were obtained in 15 minutes and specific activities in the range of 194–230 GBq/µmol. To facilitate a one-step labelling of peptides and proteins an organosilicon-functionalised aldehyde was used to chemoselectively label an aminooxy derivative of octreotide via an oxime bond formation. Yields of 70–90% were achieved within 30 minutes; however, low specific activities of 3–5 GBq/µmol are reported.

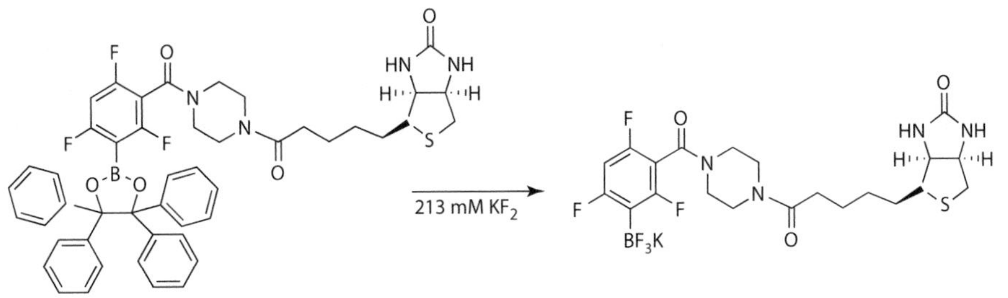

Figure 11.25 Synthesis of a biotin conjugate via the ^{18}F-labelled aryl trifluoroborate.

Although in their infancy, these approaches have interesting potential leading towards a 'kit-based' approach for the synthesis of ^{18}F-labelled radiopharmaceuticals, particularly peptides and proteins. The major hurdles will be to improve specific activity and assess the effect of these bioconjugates on the *in-vivo* efficacy of the compounds.

Summary of prosthetic groups for fluorine-18 radiolabelling of biomolecules

As peptides and proteins become important players in the field of molecular imaging, numerous approaches to routinely and reliably synthesising ^{18}F-labelled prosthetic groups for labelling biomolecules have emerged. The majority have focused on targeting amino and carboxy functions on peptides and proteins and most recently chemoselective conjugation of prosthetic group to thiol groups of cysteine residues has been exploited. Unfortunately, to date there is no universal approach that fits all. The design and synthesis of radiolabelled biomolecules is still a challenge and will continue to involve a trial-and-error approach on a peptide-to-peptide, protein-to-protein basis in order to assess the effect of the prosthetic group on the function of the biomolecule. Although we are a little way from the 'kit-based' approach for the reliable, reproducible and remotely controlled synthesis of the production of ^{18}F-labelled biomarkers, there has been great advancement over the last decade to at least 'simplify' approaches and make ^{18}F-biomolecules available to more than just the academic setting.

Radiolabelled peptides

Many cancers have demonstrated overexpression of a variety of receptors. These cell surface receptors have become of huge interest as molecular imaging targets. Their being cell surface receptors makes them relatively easy targets for radiolabelled biomolecules. Numerous radiolabelled peptides are under investigation as molecular probes to target receptor expression *in vivo* (Okarvi 2002; Reubi, Maecke 2008). As previously described, peptides cannot yet be labelled directly using [^{18}F]fluoride owing to the harsh reaction conditions required and therefore require the addition of appropriate prosthetic groups. Peptides are attractive molecular imaging probes as they are small in size and can penetrate tumours and are relatively easy to synthesise and, as described previously, there are numerous approaches to radiolabelling of peptides reliably, rapidly and reproducibly with ^{18}F.

Currently the best-studied peptide receptors include the somatostatin receptors, bombesin receptors and the integrin receptor $\alpha_v\beta_3$. Undoubtedly the somatostatin receptors, particularly the SSTR2 receptors, are the best-studied and best-characterised to date. Somatostatin receptors are overexpressed on many neuroendocrine tumours (Krenning *et al.* 1992a,b,c). Octreotide is an octapeptide analogue of somatostatin that has a high resistance towards peptidases and has a high *in-vivo* stability (Bauer *et al.* 1982). This peptide has been radiolabelled using numerous isotopes for both diagnostic imaging and therapy: ^{111}In (Kwekkeboom *et al.* 1999), ^{90}Y (Otte *et al.* 1997), ^{68}Ga (Hofmann *et al.* 2003) and ^{18}F (Guhlke *et al.* 1994; Wester *et al.* 1997).

Octreotide was radiolabelled with ^{18}F via the acylation reaction of n.c.a.2-[^{18}F]fluoropropionic acid 4-nitrophenyl ester with ε-Boc-Lys^5-octreotide. After acid deprotection, radiochemical yields for [^{18}F]fluoropropionylated octreotide were 65% based on the fluoroacylating agent. Full biological activity of octreotide was maintained (Figure 11.26).

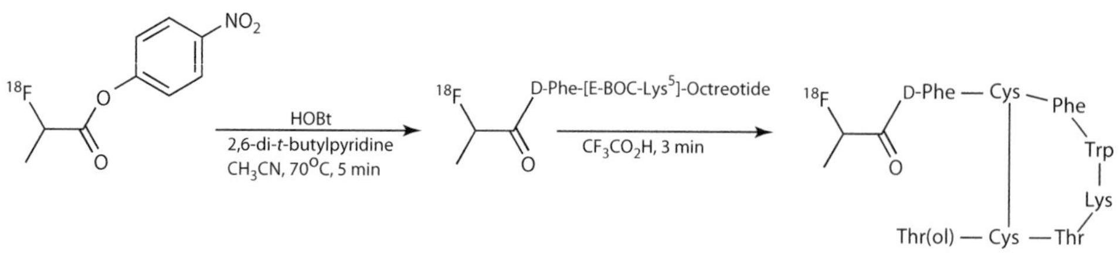

Figure 11.26 Synthesis of [^{18}F]FPA-octreotide.

Another receptor family of interest is that of the integrins. Integrins are a family of cell surface receptors involved in cell–cell and cell–extracellular matrix interactions. These receptors are heterodimers consisting of an α and a β subunit. To date, 24 integrins have been reported. Of these, the most widely researched integrin is $\alpha_v\beta_3$. This receptor is up-regulated on the surface of tumour cells and has been associated with tumour angiogenesis and metastasis (Brooks 1996). This receptor binds to proteins in the extracellular matrix via a three-amino-acid motif Arg-Gly-Asp (Pasqualini *et al.* 1997). Numerous small cyclic peptides have been developed to target this receptor. Over the past decade, optimisation of the small cyclic peptide by both multimerisation and pegylation has been widely reported (Haubner *et al.* 2001, 2005; Cai, Chen 2005; Wu *et al.* 2005). The pentapeptide, cyclic RGDfK has been radiolabelled using numerous isotopes for both PET and SPECT (Haubner *et al.* 2001; Liu *et al.* 2007). The [^{18}F]galactoRGD peptide has been used in clinical trials to image melanoma, sarcoma and breast cancer (Haubner *et al.* 2005; Beer 2007; Kenny *et al.* 2008).

This galacto-RGD peptide was radiolabelled via the acylation reaction of 4-nitrophenyl-2 [^{18}F] fluoropropionate with the glycosylated peptide. [^{18}F]Galacto-RGD was synthesised with a decay-corrected radiochemical yield of up to 85% and radiochemical purity >98%. The overall radiochemical yield was 29% with a total reaction time including final HPLC preparation of 200 minutes (Figure 11.27).

Other receptor targets include the gastrin-releasing peptide receptor GRP; these receptors have been shown to be overexpressed in prostate and breast cancer. The GRP receptors have been targeted using bombesin based ligands, particularly bombesin (7-14, TQAVGHLM). It was found that the C-terminus of bombesin is required for biological potency (Davis *et al.* 1992) and hence the N-terminus is often modified. Bombesin has been radiolabelled with numerous radioisotopes, ^{99m}Tc and ^{111}In for SPECT (Varvarigou *et al.* 2004), ^{90}Y, ^{177}Lu and ^{188}Re for therapy (Smith *et al.* 2003b; Zhang *et al.* 2004a,b) and ^{64}Cu, ^{68}Ga, ^{86}Y and ^{18}F for PET (Rogers *et al.* 2003; Schuhmacher *et al.* 2005; Zhang *et al.* 2006; Biddlecombe *et al.* 2007). Fluorine-18 was incorporated into two bombesin derivatives [Lys3]bombesin and amino-caproic acid bombesin (7-14) using [^{18}F]SFB at pH 8.5. Radiochemical yields of 30–40% were observed with a reaction time of 150 minutes.

It is anticipated, based on the success of receptor targeting peptides such as octreotide, RGD and bombesin, that over the next decade there will be a huge increase in the number of novel peptides with clinical relevance. The combination of library-based synthesis approaches with rapid radiolabelling techniques and high-throughput *in-vivo* screening will facilitate the rapid identification of novel radiopharmaceuticals. The optimisation of radiolabelling approaches will facility the shift of these compounds rapidly from the bench to the bedside. The next decade will prove an interesting and challenging time for the use of ^{18}F-labelled radiopharmaceuticals.

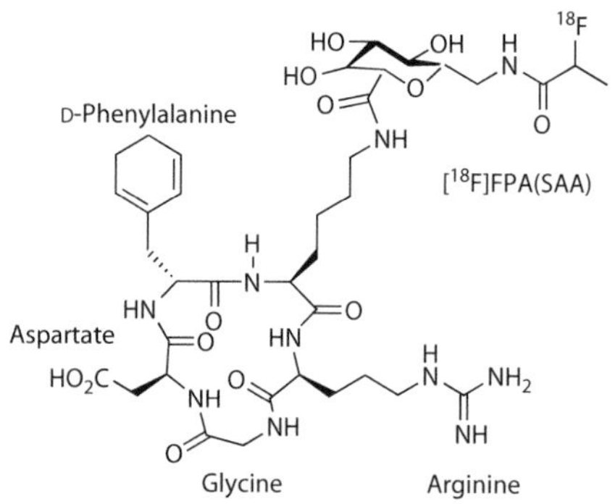

Figure 11.27 Synthesis of [^{18}F]galacto-RGD peptide.

References

Adam M (1982). A rapid, stereoselective, high yielding synthesis of 2-deoxy-2-fluoro-D-hexopyranoses: reaction of glycals with acetyl hypofluorite. *Chem Commun (Camb)* 13: 730–731.

Adam M *et al.* (1983). The cleavage of aryl-metal bonds by elemental fluorine – synthesis of aryl-fluorides. *Can J Chem* 61: 658–660.

Adam M *et al.* (1984). Fluorination aromatic compounds with F_2 and acetyl hypofluorite: synthesis of ^{18}F-aryl fluorides by cleavage of aryl-tin bonds. *J Fluor Chem* 25: 329–337.

Alauddin MM, Conti PS (1998). Synthesis and preliminary evaluation of 9-(4-[^{18}F]-fluoro-3-hydroxymethylbutyl) guanine ([^{18}F]FHBG): A new potential imaging agent for viral infection and gene therapy using PET. *Nucl Med Biol* 25: 175–180.

Alauddin MM *et al.* (1996a). Synthesis of [^{18}F] 9-[(3-fluoro-1-hydroxy-2-propoxy)-methyl]-guanine(FHPG) for in vivo imaging of viral infection and gene therapy with PET. *J Nucl Med* 37: 883.

Alauddin MM *et al.* (1996b). Synthesis of 9-[(3-[^{18}F]-fluoro-1-hydroxy-2-propoxy)methyl]guanine ([^{18}F]-FHPG): A potential imaging agent of viral infection and gene therapy using PET. *Nucl Med Biol* 23: 787–792.

Alauddin MM *et al.* (2002). Comparative evaluation of FMAU and acyclo-guanine derivatives, FHPG and FHBG in MDA-MB-468 breast cancer cells for gene therapy imaging. *J Nucl Med* 43: 275P.

Alauddin MM *et al.* (2004a). Synthesis of 2′-deoxy-2′-[^{18}F] fluoro-5-bromo-1-β-D-arabinofuranosyluracil ([^{18}F]-FBAU) and 2′-deoxy-2′-[^{18}F]fluoro-5-chloro-1-β-D-arabinofuranosyl-uracil ([^{18}F]-FCAU), and their biological evaluation as markers for gene expression. *Nucl Med Biol* 31: 399–405.

Alauddin MM *et al.* (2004b). Synthesis and evaluation of 2′-deoxy-2′-^{18}F-fluoro-5-fluoro-1-β-D-arabinofuranosyluracil as a potential PET imaging agent for suicide gene expression. *J Nucl Med* 45: 2063–2069.

Alauddin MM *et al.* (2007). In vivo evaluation of 2′-deoxy-2′-[^{18}F]fluoro-5-iodo-1-β-D-arabinofuranosyluracil ([^{18}F]FIAU) and 2′-deoxy-2′-[^{18}F]fluoro-5-ethyl-1-β-D-arabinofuranosyluracil ([^{18}F]FEAU) as markers for suicide gene expression. *Eur J Nucl Med Mol Imaging* 34: 822–829.

Attina M *et al.* (1983a). Displacement of a nitro-group by [^{18}F]-labeled fluoride-ion – a new route to aryl fluorides of high specific activity. *Chem Commun (Camb)*, 108–109.

Attina M *et al.* (1983b). Labeled aryl fluorides from the nucleophilic displacement of activated nitro-groups by [^{18}F]-F^-. *J Labelled Comp Radiopharm* 20: 501–514.

Bauer W *et al.* (1982). SMS 201-995: a very potent and selective octapeptide analogue of somatostatin with prolonged action. *Life Sci* 31(11): 1133–1140.

Bergman J, Solin O (1997). Fluorine-18-labeled fluorine gas for synthesis of tracer molecules. *Nucl Med Biol* 24: 677–683.

Bida GT *et al.* (1980). The effect of target-gas purity on the chemical form of F-18 during ^{18}F-F_2 production using the neon/fluorine target. *J Nucl Med* 21: 758–762.

Biddlecombe GB *et al.* (2007). Molecular imaging of gastrin-releasing peptide receptor-positive tumors in mice using ^{64}Cu- and ^{86}Y-DOTA-(Pro^1,Tyr^4)-bombesin (1-14). *Bioconjug Chem* 18: 724–730.

Blau M *et al.* (1962). Fluorine-18: a new isotope for bone scanning. *J Nucl Med* 3: 332–334.

Blessing G *et al.* (1986). Production of (^{18}F)F_2, H^{18}F and ^{18}Faq using the ^{20}Ne(d,alpha)^{18}F process. *Appl Radiat Isot* 37: 1135.

Block D *et al.* (1986). NCA [^{18}F] labeling of aliphatic-compounds in high yields via aminopolyether – supported nucleophilic-substitution. *J Labelled Comp Radiopharm* 23: 467–477.

Brodack JW *et al.* (1988). Robotic production of 2-deoxy-2-[^{18}F]fluoro-D-glucose – a routine method of synthesis using tetrabutylammonium [^{18}F] fluoride. *Appl Radiat Isot* 39: 699–703.

Brooks PC (1996). Cell adhesion molecules in angiogenesis. *Cancer Metastasis Rev* 15: 187–194.

Cai WB, Chen XY (2005). RGD-labeled quantum dot for imaging tumor cells overexpressing alpha V beta 3 integrin. *Biopolymers* 80: 565.

Cai WB *et al.* (2006). A thiol-reactive ^{18}F-labeling agent, *N*-[2-(4-^{18}F-fluorobenzamido)ethyl]maleimide, and synthesis of RGD peptide-based tracer for PET imaging of $\alpha_v\beta_3$ integrin expression. *J Nucl Med* 47: 1172–1180.

Casella V *et al.* (1980). Anhydrous F-18 labeled elemental fluorine for radiopharmaceutical preparation. *J Nucl Med* 21: 750.

Chaly T *et al.* (1996). Radiosynthesis of [^{18}F] *N*-3-fluoropropyl-2-β-carbomethoxy-3-β-(4-iodophenyl) nortropane and the first human study with positron emission tomography. *Nucl Med Biol* 23: 999–1004.

Chirakal R *et al.* (1984). The synthesis of [^{18}F]xenon difluoride from [^{18}F]fluorine gas. *Appl Radiat Isot* 35: 401–404.

Chirakal R *et al.* (1988). Sequential production of electrophilic and nucleophilic fluorinating agents from [^{18}F]fluorine gas. *Appl Radiat Isot* 39: 1099–1101.

Coenen HH, Moerlein S (1987). Regiospecific aromatic fluoroidemetallation of group IVb metalloarenes using elemental fluorine or acetyl hypofluorite. *J Fluor Chem* 36: 63–75.

Coenen HH *et al.* (1986). Preparation of N.C.A. [^{18}F]-CH_2BrF via aminopolyether supported nucleophilic-substitution. *J Labelled Comp Radiopharm* 23: 587–595.

Coenen HH *et al.* (1988). Direct electrophilic radiofluorination of phenylalanine, tyrosine and DOPA. *Appl Radiat Isot* 39: 1243–1250.

Culbert PA *et al.* (1995). Automated synthesis of [^{18}F]FDG using tetrabutylammonium bicarbonate. *Appl Radiat Isot* 46: 887–891.

Culver KW *et al.* (1992). In vivo gene-transfer with retroviral vector producer cells for treatment of experimental brain-tumors. *Science* 256(5063): 1550–1552.

Dahl JR *et al.* (1983). A new target system for the preparation of no-carrier-added ^{18}F-fluorinating compounds. *Int J Appl Radiat Isot* 34: 693–700.

Davis TP *et al.* (1992). Metabolic stability and tumor-inhibition of bombesin/GRP receptor antagonists. *Peptides* 13: 401–407.

de Bruin B *et al.* (2005). 1-[3-(2-[^{18}F]fluoropyridin-3-yloxy) propyl]pyrrole-2,5-dione: design, synthesis, and radiosynthesis of a new [^{18}F]fluoropyridine-based maleimide reagent for the labeling of peptides and proteins. *Bioconjug Chem* 16: 406–420.

de Visser M *et al.* (2004). In-111 versus Ga-68, in vivo comparison using new bombesin analogues. *Eur J Nucl Med Mol Imaging* 31: S257.

Deng H *et al.* (2006). Fluorinase mediated C-^{18}F bond formation, an enzymatic tool for PET labelling. *Chem Commun (Camb)* 6: 652–654.

Diksic M, Jolly D (1983). New high-yield synthesis of ^{18}F-labelled 2-deoxy-2-fluoro-D-glucose. *Int J Appl Radiat Isot* 34: 893–896.

Dolle F (2005). Fluorine-18-labelled fluoropyridines: advances in radiopharmaceutical design. *Cur Pharm Des* 11(25): 3221–3235.

Dolle F. (2007). [^{18}F]Fluoropyridines: from conventional radiotracers to the labeling of macromolecules such as proteins and oligonucleoides. In: Schubiger *et al.*, eds. *PET Chemistry – The Driving Force in Molecular Imaging.* Berlin, Heidelberg: Springer-Verlag, 114-157.

Dolle F *et al.* (1998a). 6- [^{18}F]fluoro-L-DOPA by radiofluorodestannylation: a short and simple synthesis of a new labelling precursor. *J Labelled Comp Radiopharm* 41: 105–114.

Dolle F *et al.* (1998b). Synthesis of 2-[^{18}F]fluoro-3-[2(*S*)-2-azetidinylmethoxy]pyridine, a highly potent radioligand for in vivo imaging central nicotinic acetylcholine receptors. *J Labelled Comp Radiopharm* 41: 451–463.

Dolle F *et al.* (1999). Synthesis and nicotinic acetylcholine receptor in vivo binding properties of 2-fluoro-3-[2(*S*)-2-azetidinylmethoxy]pyridine: a new positron emission tomography ligand for nicotinic receptors. *J Med Chem* 42: 2251–2259.

Ehrenkaufer RE, MacGregor RR (1983). Synthesis of [^{18}F] perchloro fluoride and its reaction with functionalized aryl lithiums. *Int J Appl Radiat Isot* 34: 613–615.

Ermert J *et al.* (2004). Comparison of pathways to the versatile synthon of no-carrier-added 1-bromo-4-[^{18}F]fluorobenzene. *J Labelled Comp Radiopharm* 47: 429–441.

Firnau G *et al.* (1984). Aromatic radiofluorination with [^{18}F] fluorine-gas: 6-[^{18}F]fluoro-D-dopa. *J Nucl Med* 25(11): 1228–1233.

Firnau G *et al.* (1986). Aromatic radiofluorination with [^{18}F] F_2 in anhydrous hydrogen fluoride. *J Labelled Comp Radiopharm* 23: 1106–1108.

Fowler JS *et al.* (1982). Synthesis of ^{18}F-labeled acetyl hypofluorite for radiotracer synthesis. *J Labelled Comp Radiopharm* 19: 1634–1636.

Fuchtner F *et al.* (2002). Aspects of 6-[^{18}F]fluoro-L-dopa preparation: precursor synthesis, preparative HPLC purification and determination of radiochemical purity. *Nucl Med Biol* 29: 477–481.

Gail R, Coenen HH (1994). A one step preparation of the n.c. a. fluorine-18 labelled synthons: 4-fluorobromobenzene and 4-fluoroiodobenzene. *Appl Radiat Isot* 45: 105–111.

Gail R, Coenen HH (1997). Direct n.c.a ^{18}F-fluorination of halo and alkylarenes via corresponding diphenyliodinium salts. *J Labelled Comp Radiopharm* 40: 50–52.

Gambhir SS *et al.* (1998). Imaging of adenoviral-directed herpes simplex virus type 1 thymidine kinase reporter gene expression in mice with radiolabeled ganciclovir. *J Nucl Med* 39: 2003–2011.

Glaser M, Arstad E (2007). Click labeling with 2- [^{18}F]]fluoroethylazide for positron emission tomography. *Bioconjug Chem* 8: 989–993.

Guhlke S *et al.* (1994). (2-[^{18}F]Fluoropropionyl-DPhe^{1})-octreotide, a potential radiopharmaceutical for quantitative somatostatin receptor imaging with PET – synthesis, radiolabeling, in-vitro validation and biodistribution in mice. *Nucl Med Biol* 21: 819–825.

Hamacher K *et al.* (1986). Efficient stereospecific synthesis of NCA 2-[^{18}F]-fluoro-deoxy-D-glucose using aminopolyether supported nucleophilic substitution. *J Nucl Med* 27: 235–238.

Haubner R *et al.* (2001). Glycosylated RGD-containing peptides, tracer for tumor targeting and angiogenesis imaging with improved biokinetics. *J Nucl Med* 42: 326–336.

Haubner R *et al.* (2005). Noninvasive visualization of the activated $\alpha v\beta 3$ integrin in cancer patients by positron emission tomography and [^{18}F]galacto-RGD. *PloS Medicine* 2(3): e70.

Hausner SH *et al.* (2008). In vivo positron emission tomography (PET) imaging with an $\alpha_v\beta_6$ specific peptide radiolabeled using ^{18}F-"click" chemistry: evaluation and comparison with the corresponding 4-[^{18}F]fluorobenzoyl- and 2-[^{18}F]fluoropropionyl-peptides. *J Med Chem* 51: 5901–5904.

Hefter GT, McLay PJ (1988). The solvation of fluoride ions. 1. Free-energies for transfer from water to aqueous alcohol and acetonitrile mixtures. *J Solution Chem* 17: 535–546.

Helus F *et al.* (1979). ^{18}F cyclotron production methods. *Radiochem Radioanal Lett* 38: 395–410.

Herman LW *et al.* (1994). The use of pentafluorophenyl derivatives for the ^{18}F 18 labeling of proteins. *Nucl Med Biol* 21: 1005–1010.

Herschied JDM *et al.* (1984). Is the addition of [^{18}F]-acetylhypofluorite to glucals really stereoselective? *J Labelled Comp Radiopharm* 21: 1192–1193.

Hoffman TJ *et al.* (2003). Novel series of ^{111}In-labeled bombesin analogs as potential radiopharmaceuticals for specific targeting of gastrin-releasing peptide receptors expressed on human prostate cancer cells. *J Nucl Med* 44: 823–831.

Horti A *et al.* (1998). Synthesis of radiotracer for studying nicotinic acetylcholine receptors: 2-[^{18}F]fluoro-3-(2(*S*)-azetidinylmethoxy)pyridine (2-[^{18}F]A-85380). *J Labelled Comp Radiopharm* 41: 309–318.

Hustinx R *et al.* (2001). Imaging in vivo herpes simplex virus thymidine kinase gene transfer to tumour-bearing rodents using positron emission tomography and [^{18}F]FHPG. *Eur J Nucl Med* 28: 5–12.

Ido T *et al.* (1978). Labeled 2-deoxy-2-fluoro-D-glucose analogs. ^{18}F-Labeled-2-deoxy-2-fluoro-D-glucose, 2-deoxy-2-fluoro-D-mannose and ^{14}C-2-deoxy-2-fluoro-D-glucose. *J Labelled Comp Radiopharm* 14: 175–183.

Irie T *et al.* (1982). ^{18}F-Fluorination by crown ether-metal fluoride. I: on labeling ^{18}F-21-fluoroprogesterone. *Int J Appl Radiat Isot* 33: 1449–1452.

Irie T *et al.* (1984). ^{18}F-Fluorination by crown ether metal fluoride. II. Non-carrier-added labeling method. *Int J Applied Radiat Isot* 35(6): 517–520.

Ismail FMD (2002). Important fluorinated drugs in experimental and clinical use. *J Fluor Chem* 118: 27–33.

Jewett DM *et al.* (1984). A gas-solid phase microchemical method for the synthesis of acetyl hypofluorite. *J Fluor Chem* 24: 477–481.

Kenny LM *et al.* (2008). Phase I trial of the positron-emitting Arg-Gly-Asp (RGD) peptide radioligand 18F-AH111585 in breast cancer patients. *J Nucl Med* 49(6): 879–86.

Kiesewetter DO *et al.* (1984). Preparation of four fluorine-18-labeled estrogens and their selective uptakes in target tissues of immature rats. *J Nucl Med* 25: 1212–1221.

Kiesewetter DO *et al.* (1986). Syntheses and D2 receptor affinities of derivatives of spiperone containing aliphatic halogens. *Appl Radiat Isot* 37: 1181–1186.

Kilbourn MR *et al.* (1987). ^{18}F- labeling of proteins. *J Nucl Med* 28: 462–470.

Kim DW *et al.* (2003a). A new nucleophilic fluorine-18 labeling method for aliphatic mesylates: reaction in ionic liquids shows tolerance for water. *Nucl Med Biol* 30: 345–350.

Kim DW *et al.* (2003b). Significantly enhanced reactivities of the nucleophilic substitution reactions in ionic liquid. *J Org Chem* 68: 4281–4285.

Kim DW *et al.* (2006). A new class of S_N2 reactions catalyzed by protic solvents: facile fluorination for isotopic labeling of diagnostic molecules. *J Am Chem Soc* 128: 16394–16397.

Kim DW *et al.* (2008a). Facile nucleophilic fluorination by synergistic effect between polymer-supported ionic liquid catalyst and tert-alcohol reaction media system. *Tetrahedron* 64: 4209–4214.

Kim DW *et al.* (2008b). Facile nucleophilic fluorination reactions using *tert*-alcohols as a reaction medium: Significantly enhanced reactivity of alkali metal fluorides and improved selectivity. *J Org Chem* 73: 957–962.

Kim HW *et al.* (2004). Rapid synthesis of [^{19}F]FDG without an evaporation step using an ionic liquid. *Appl Radiat Isot* 61: 1241–1246.

Kirk KL (2008). Fluorination in medicinal chemistry: methods, strategies, and recent developments. *Org Process Res Dev* 12: 305–321.

Kolb HC (2001). Application of click chemistry to the generation of new chemical libraries for drug discovery. *Abstracts of Papers of the American Chemical Society* 221: U174.

Kolb HC, Sharpless KB (2003). The growing impact of click chemistry on drug discovery. *Drug Discov Today* 8: 1128–1137.

Kolb HC *et al.* (2001). Click chemistry: diverse chemical function from a few good reactions. *Angew Chem Int Ed* 40(11): 2004–2021.

Korguth ML *et al.* (1988). Effects of reaction conditions on rates of incorporation of no-carrier added ^{18}F-Fluoride into several organic compounds. *J Labelled Comp Radiopharm* 25(4): 369–381.

Krenning EP *et al.* (1992a). Somatostatin receptor scintigraphy with indium-111-DTPA-D-Phe-1-octreotide in man – metabolism, dosimetry and comparison with iodine-123-Tyr-3-octreotide. *J Nucl Med* 33: 652–658.

Krenning EP *et al.* (1992b). Somatostatin receptor imaging of endocrine gastrointestinal tumors. *Schweiz Med Wochenschr* 122: 634–637.

Krenning EP *et al.* (1992c). ^{111}In-octreotide scintigraphy in oncology. *Metab Clin Exp* 41: 83–86.

Kwekkeboom DJ *et al.* (1992a). Somatostatin analog scintigraphy – a simple and sensitive method for the in-vivo visualization of merkel cell tumors and their metastases. *Arch Dermatol* 128: 818–821.

Kwekkeboom DJ *et al.* (1992b). Tumor-localization using ^{111}In-octreotide scintigraphy. *Eur J Nucl Med* 19: 599.

Kwekkeboom DJ *et al.* (1999). Comparison of ^{111}In-DOTA-Tyr^3-octreotide and ^{111}In-DTPA-octreotide in the same patients: Biodistribution, kinetics, organ and tumor uptake. *J Nucl Med* 40: 762–767.

Le Bars D *et al.* (1998). High-yield radiosynthesis and preliminary in vivo evaluation of *p*-[^{18}F]MPPF, a fluoro analog of WAY-100635. *Nucl Med Biol* 25: 343–350.

Lee SJ *et al.* (2007a). One-step high-radiochemical-yield synthesis of [^{18}F]FP-CIT using a protic solvent system. *Nucl Med Biol* 34: 345–351.

Lee SJ *et al.* (2007b). Simple and highly efficient synthesis of 3′-deoxy-3′-[^{18}F]fluorothymidine using nucleophilic fluorination catalyzed by protic solvent. *Eur J Nucl Med Mol Imaging* 34: 1406–1409.

Lee SJ *et al.* (2008). Comparison of synthesis yields of 3′-deoxy-3′-[^{18}F]fluorothymidine by nucleophilic fluorination in various alcohol solvents. *J Labelled Compd Radiopharm* 51: 80–82.

Lemaire C *et al.* (1991). An approach to the asymmetric synthesis of L-6-[^{18}F]fluorodopa via NCA nucleophilic fluorination. *Appl Radiat Isot* 42: 629–635.

Lemaire C *et al.* (1994). Enantioselective synthesis of 6-[fluorine-18]-fluoro-L-dopa from no-carrier-added fluorine-18-fluoride. *J Nucl Med* 35: 1996–2002.

Li ZB *et al.* (2007). Click chemistry for ^{18}F-labeling of RGD peptides and microPET imaging of tumor integrin $\alpha_v gb_3$ expression. *Bioconjug Chem* 18(6): 1987–1994.

Lim JL *et al.* (1996). The use of 3-methoxymethyl-16β, 17β-epiestriol-O-cyclic sulfone as the precursor in the synthesis of F-18 16α-fluoroestradiol. *Nucl Med Biol* 23: 911–915.

Liu S *et al.* (2007). Evaluation of a ^{99m}Tc-labeled cyclic RGD tetramer for noninvasive imaging integrin $\alpha_v\beta_3$-positive breast cancer. *Bioconjug Chem* 18: 438–446.

Maienfisch P, Hall RG (2004). The importance of fluorine in the life science industry. *Chimia* 58: 93–99.

Marik J, Sutcliffe JL (2006). Click for PET: rapid preparation of [^{18}F]fluoropeptides using Cu-I catalyzed 1,3-dipolar cycloaddition. *Tetrahedron Lett* 47: 6681–6684.

Marik J *et al.* (2006). Solid-phase synthesis of 2-[^{18}F]fluoropropionyl peptides. *Bioconjug Chem* 17: 1017–1021.

Martarello L *et al.* (2003). The first enzymatic method for C-^{18}F bond formation: the synthesis of 5′-[^{18}F]-fluoro-5′ deoxyadenosine for imaging with PET. *J Labelled Comp Radiopharm* 46: 1181–1189.

Martin JR (1986). The CNS in reactivated genital herpes-simplex virus type-2 (HSV-2) infection in mice. *J Neuropathol Exp Neurol* 45: 337.

Namavari M *et al.* (1992). Regioselective radiofluorodestannylation with [^{18}F]F_2 and [^{18}F]CH_3COOF: a high yield synthesis of 6-[^{18}F]fluoro-L-dopa. *Appl Radiat Isot* 43: 989–996.

Nickles RJ *et al.* (1982). Smaller, colder targets. *J Labelled Comp Radiopharm* 19: 1364–1365.

Nickles RJ *et al.* (1984). An $^{18}O_2$ target for the production of (^{18}F)F_2. *Int J Appl Radiat Isot* 35: 117–122.

Oberdorfer F *et al.* (1988a). Preparation of ^{18}F-labeled N-fluoropyridinium triflate. *J Labelled Comp Radiopharm* 25: 999–1005.

Oberdorfer F *et al.* (1988b). Preparation of a new ^{18}F-labelled precursor: 1-[^{18}F]fluoro-2-pyridone. *Appl Radiat Isot* 39: 685–688.

Oh YH *et al.* (2007). Facile S_N2 reaction in protic solvent: quantum chemical analysis. *J Phys Chem A* 111(40): 10152–10161.

O'Hagan D *et al.* (2002). Biosynthesis of an organofluorine molecule – a fluorinase enzyme has been discovered that catalyses carbon-fluorine bond formation. *Nature* 416: 279.

Okarvi SM (2001). Recent progress in fluorine-18 labelled peptide radiopharmaceuticals. *Eur J Nucl Med* 28: 929–938.

Okarvi SM (2002). Development of peptide-based radiopharmaceuticals as tumor imaging agents. *J Nucl Med* 43: 369P.

Otte A *et al.* (1997). DOTATOC: a powerful new tool for receptor-mediated radionuclide therapy. *Eur J Nucl Med* 24: 792–795.

Pasqualini R *et al.* (1997). α_v Integrins as receptors for tumor targeting by circulating ligands. *Nat Biotechnol* 15: 542–546.

Pike VW, Aigbirhio FI (1995). Reactions of [^{18}F]fluoride with aryliodonium salts – a novel route to no-carrier-added aryl [^{18}F]fluorides. *J Labelled Comp Radiopharm* 37: 120–122.

Poethko T *et al.* (2004a). Two-step methodology for high-yield routine radiohalogenation of peptides: ^{18}F-labeled RGD and octreotide analogs. *J Nucl Med* 45: 892–902.

Poethko T *et al.* (2004b). Chemoselective pre-conjugate radiohalogenation of unprotected mono- and multimeric peptides via oxime formation. *Radiochim Acta* 92: 317–327.

Qaim SM. *et al.* (1993). PET radionuclide production. In: Stocklin G, Pike VW, eds. *Radiopharmaceuticals for Positron Emission Tomography – Methodological Aspects*. Dordrecht: Kluwer, 1–43.

Ram Z *et al.* (1993). Toxicity studies of retroviral-mediated gene transfer for the treatment of brain tumors. *J Neurosurg* 79: 400–407.

Reubi JC, Maecke HR (2008). Peptide-based probes for cancer imaging. *J Nucl Med* 49: 1735–1738.

Rogers BE *et al.* (2003). MicroPET imaging of a gastrin-releasing peptide receptor-positive tumor in a mouse model of human prostate cancer using a 64Cu-labeled bombesin analogue. *Bioconjug Chem* 14(4): 756–63.

Ross TL *et al.* (2007). Nucleophilic ^{18}F-fluorination of heteroaromatic iodonium salts with no-carrier-added [^{18}F]fluoride. *J Am Chem Soc* 129: 8018–8025.

Ross TL *et al.* (2008). Fluorine-18 click radiosynthesis and preclinical evaluation of a new ^{18}F-labeled folic acid derivative. *Bioconjug Chem* 19(12): 2462–2470.

Ruth T, Wolf A (1979). Absolute cross sections for the production of ^{18}F via the ^{18}O(p,n)^{18}F reaction. *Radiochim Acta* 26: 21–24.

Ruth TJ *et al.* (2001). A proof of principle for targetry to produce ultra high quantities of ^{18}F-fluoride. *Appl Radiat Isot* 55: 457–461.

Satyamurthy N *et al.* (1990). N-[^{18}F]Fluoro-N-alkylsulfonamides – novel reagents for mild and regioselective radiofluorination. *Appl Radiat Isot* 41(8): 733–738.

Schirrmacher R *et al.* (2006a). Synthesis of ^{18}F-labelled peptides using a simple kit-procedure. *Eur J Nucl Med Mol Imaging* 33: S175.

Schirrmacher R *et al.* (2006b). F-18-labeling of peptides by means of an organosilicon-based fluoride acceptor. *Angew Chem Int Ed* 45: 6047–6050.

Schuhmacher J *et al.* (2005). GRP receptor-targeted PET of a rat pancreas carcinoma xenograft in nude mice with a ^{68}Ga-labeled bombesin(6-14) analog. *J Nucl Med* 46: 691–699.

Shai Y *et al.* (1989). ^{18}F-Labeled insulin – a prosthetic group methodology for incorporation of a positron emitter into peptides and proteins. *Biochemistry* 28: 4801–4806.

Shinde SS *et al.* (2008a). Polymer-supported protic functionalized ionic liquids for nucleophilic substitution reactions: superior catalytic activity compared to other ionic resins. *Tetrahedron Lett* 49(27): 4245–4248.

Shinde SS *et al.* (2008b). Synergistic effect of two solvents, *tert*-alcohol and ionic liquid, in one molecule in nucleophilic fluorination. *Org Lett* 10(5): 733–735.

Shiue CY *et al.* (1982). A new improved synthesis of 2-deoxy-2-[^{18}F]fluoro-D-glucose from ^{18}F-labeled acetyl hypofluorite. *J Nucl Med* 23(10): 899–903.

Shiue CY *et al.* (1985). Syntheses and specific activity determinations of no-carrier-added (NCA) fluorine-18-labeled butyrophenone neuroleptic drugs. *J Nucl Med* 26(2): 181–186.

Shiue CY *et al.* (1986). No-carrier-added fluorine-18-labeled N-methylspiroperidol: synthesis and biodistribution in mice. *J Nucl Med* 27(2): 226–234.

Shiue C-Y *et al.* (1989). Improvements in the production of [^{18}F]*N*-methylspiroperidol and (^{18}F)haloperidol. *J Labelled Comp Radiopharm* 26: 386–387.

Smart BE (2001). Fluorine substituent effects (on bioactivity). *J Fluor Chem* 109: 3–11.

Smith CJ *et al.* (2003a). Radiochemical investigations of ^{177}Lu-DOTA-8-Aoc-BBN[7-14]NH_2: an in vitro/in vivo assessment of the targeting ability of this new radiopharmaceutical for PC-3 human prostate cancer cells. *Nucl Med Biol* 30: 101–109.

Smith CJ *et al.* (2003b). Radiochemical investigations of [^{188}Re(H_2O)$(CO)_3$-diaminopropionic acid-SSS-bombesin(7-14)NH_2]: syntheses, radiolabeling and in vitro/in vivo GRP receptor targeting studies. *Anticancer Res* 23: 63–70.

Snell AH (1937). A new radioactive isotope of fluorine. *Phys Rev* 51: 143.

Soghomonyan S *et al.* (2007). Molecular PET imaging of HSV1-tk reporter gene expression using [18F]FEAU. *Nat Protoc* 2(2): 416–23.

Sutcliffe-Goulden JL *et al.* (2000). Solid phase synthesis of $[^{18}F]$labelled peptides for positron emission tomography. *Bioorg Med Chem Lett* 10: 1501–1503.

Sutcliffe-Goulden JL *et al.* (2002). Rapid solid phase synthesis and biodistribution of 18F-labelled linear peptides. *Eur J Nucl Med Mol Imaging* 29: 754–759.

Teare H *et al.* (2007). Synthesis and reactivity of $[^{18}F]$-N-fluorobenzenesulfonimide. *Chem Commun (Camb)*, 2330–2332.

Tewson TJ, Welch MJ (1980). Preparation and preliminary biodistribution of no carrier added fluorine-18 fluoroethanol. *J Nucl Med* 21: 559–564.

Ting R *et al.* (2005). Arylfluoroborates and alkylfluorosilicates as potential PET imaging agents: High-yielding aqueous biomolecular ^{18}F-labeling. *J Am Chem Soc* 127: 13094–13095.

Vaidyanathan G, Zalutsky MR (2006). Synthesis of N-succinimidyl 4-$[^{18}F]$fluorobenzoate, an agent for labeling proteins and peptides with ^{18}F. *Nat Protoc* 1(4): 1655–1661.

Varvarigou A *et al.* (2004). Gastrin-releasing peptide (GRP) analogues for cancer imaging. *Cancer Biother Radiopharm* 19: 219–229.

Wester HJ *et al.* (1996). A comparative study of NCA fluorine-18 labeling of proteins via acylation and photochemical conjugation. *Nucl Med Biol* 23: 365–372.

Wester HJ *et al.* (1997). PET-pharmacokinetics of ^{18}F-octreotide: a comparison with ^{67}Ga-DFO and ^{86}Y-DTPA-octreotide. *Nucl Med Biol* 24: 275–286.

Winchell HS *et al.* (1976). Process for preparing fluorine-18. US Patent 3,981,769.

Windhorst A *et al.* (2001). Labeling of $[^{18}F]$flumazenil via instant fluorination, a new nucleophilic fluorination method. *J Labelled Comp Radiopharm* 44(1): S930–S932.

Wu Y *et al.* (2005). MicroPET imaging of glioma integrin $\alpha_v\beta_3$ expression using ^{64}Cu-labeled tetrameric RGD peptide. *J Nucl Med* 46: 1707–1718.

Wuest F *et al.* (2008a). Synthesis and application of $[^{18}F]$FDG-maleimidehexyloxime ($[^{18}F]$FDG-MHO): a $[^{18}F]$FDG-based prosthetic group for the chemoselective ^{18}F-labeling of peptides and proteins. *Bioconjug Chem* 19: 1202–1210.

Wuest F *et al.* (2008b). Synthesis and evaluation in vitro and in vivo of a ^{11}C-labeled cyclooxygenase-2 (COX-2) inhibitor. *Bioorg Med Chem* 16: 7662–7670.

Zhang H *et al.* (2004a). Metabolically stabilised DOTA-bombesin based peptides by amino acid modification in position 11. *Eur J Nucl Med Mol Imaging* 31: S264.

Zhang HWC *et al.* (2004b). Synthesis and evaluation of bombesin derivatives on the basis of pan-bombesin peptides labeled with indium-111, lutetium-177, and yttrium-90 for targeting bombesin receptor-expressing tumors. *Cancer Res* 64: 6707–6715.

Zhang X *et al.* (2006). ^{18}F-labeled bombesin analogs for targeting GRP receptor-expressing prostate cancer. *J Nucl Med* 47(3): 492–501.

Further reading

Lasne M-C *et al.* (20023). Chemistry of β^+-emitting compounds based on fluorine-18. *Topics Curr Chem* 222: 201–258.

Miller PW *et al.* (2008). Synthesis of ^{11}C, ^{18}F, ^{15}O and ^{13}N radiolabels for positron emission tomography. *Angew Chem Intl Ed* 47: 8998–9033.

Schubiger PA. *et al.*, eds. (2007). *PET Chemistry – The Driving Force in Molecular Imaging.* Ernst Schering Research Foundation Workshop 62. Berlin, Heidelberg: Springer-Verlag.

Welch MJ, Redvanly CS, eds. (2003). *Handbook of Radiopharmaceuticals –Radiochemistry and Applications.* Chichester: Wiley.

12

Carbon-11

Tony Gee

Carbon-11 is a positron-emitting radionuclide, particularly valuable in labelling a wide variety of biologically relevant compounds for positron emission tomography (PET) imaging.

The half-life of carbon-11 is 20.4 minutes and it decays to stable boron-11 by the emission of a positron, the antimatter equivalent of an electron.

Cyclotron production of carbon-11

One of the great advantages of using the positron-emitting radionuclide carbon-11 as a labelling agent for a radiotracer is that almost any organic molecule can be labelled and studied, the tracer being chemically indistinguishable from its non-radioactive counterpart. This is of particular interest in the study of endogenous compounds and specific drug molecules. This contrasts with the use of fluorine-18, technetium-99m and iodine isotopes, for example, which are not well-represented elements in the biological chemistry of life. In these cases, analogues of the authentic compounds can have very different properties compared with their natural counterparts. Carbon-11 is typically produced by the bombardment of nitrogen gas with high-energy protons (typically 11–18 MeV) by the $^{14}N(p,\alpha)^{11}C$ reaction. The chemical form of carbon-11 obtained from the cyclotron can be dictated by adding a few parts per million of either oxygen or hydrogen to the nitrogen gas bombarded by the cyclotron's proton beam. In this way the starting materials [^{11}C]carbon dioxide or [^{11}C]methane, respectively, can be conveniently produced. Table 12.1 shows the radiological characteristics of carbon-11.

Synthesis

Synthesis using short-lived carbon-11 is a challenge to the chemist. In addition to the usual aspects of synthetic design used in organic chemistry, a number of additional criteria need to be considered:

- The availability of labelled starting materials is limited.
- The short half-life requires the use of rapid labelling techniques.
- Syntheses are typically performed on a nano/picomolar scale.

Table 12.1 Carbon-11 characteristics

Half-life	**20.4 min**
Mode of decay	Positron emission
Decay product	^{11}B
Mode of production	$^{14}N(p,\alpha)^{11}C$ (the bombardment of nitrogen gas with high-energy protons)
Chemical form from cyclotron	[^{11}C]Carbon dioxide, [^{11}C]methane
Theoretical specific activity	340 TBq/μmol
Practically achievable specific activity	50–500 GBq/μmol

- Confirmation of product identity requires rapid and sensitive analytical techniques.
- The radiation exposure to the chemist must be kept to a minimum.

The consequences of this are discussed here in greater detail, together with a description of various concepts, methods and strategies that are adopted in order to achieve rapid labelling syntheses with carbon-11.

Carbon-11 labelling precursors

The chemical form of carbon-11 obtained directly from a cyclotron is not in itself of great interest for medical imaging purposes. Thus the *primary precursors*, [^{11}C]carbon dioxide and [^{11}C]methane are generally converted into more reactive *secondary precursors* which can be further used to label a molecule of interest.

Some of the more commonly used labelling precursors are shown in Scheme 12.1.

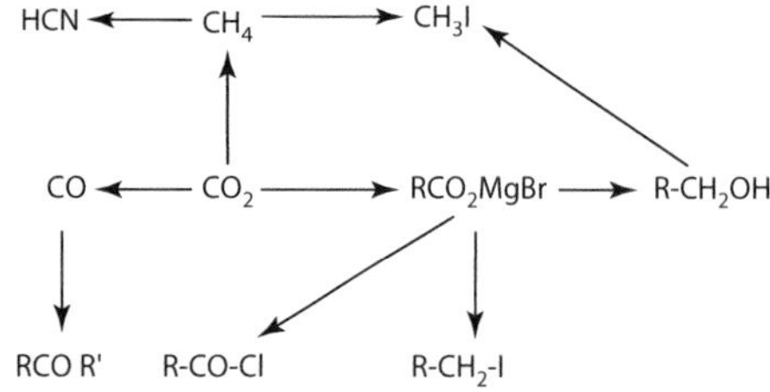

Scheme 12.1

To date, the majority of ^{11}C-labelled tracers have been synthesised by the alkylation of nitrogen, oxygen and sulfur nucleophiles using [^{11}C]methyl iodide, by nucleophilic substitution using cyanide, or by Grignard reactions using [^{11}C]carbon dioxide itself. These and other synthetic strategies will be covered in greater detail later in the chapter.

General considerations when working with carbon-11

Time constraints and rapid labelling synthesis

The 20.4-minute half-life of carbon-11 implies that in a labelling synthesis a radiochemical yield can reach a maximum even though a reaction has not formally reached completion.

For example, consider a theoretical reaction that requires 40 minutes to reach 100% *yield*, illustrated in Figure 12.1. If this reaction is performed with carbon-11, the radioactive decay of the product would have to be taken into account. After 40 minutes (with radioactive half-life of 20.4 minutes) the radioactivity would have decayed to approximately one-quarter of the original starting amount. Thus, even though the reaction reaches completion at 40 minutes, the *radiochemical yield* is only 25% at this time point. In this example a maximum radiochemical yield for the hypothetical reaction is reached between 10 and 15 minutes.

Taking into account the decay of radioactivity, the radiochemical yield reaches a maximum at around 12 minutes. Thus maximum radiochemical yields can often be maximised by stopping a reaction before completion. A basic principle of rapid labelling synthesis states that a synthesis (including precursor production, final purification, analysis and delivery to the PET scanner) should be performed within three radionuclide half-lives. Various strategies can be used so that these criteria can be met.

Incorporation of the label as late as possible in a synthetic pathway

Efficient design of non-labelled precursors can reduce the need for lengthy labelling procedures. When the use of protecting groups is required, they should be

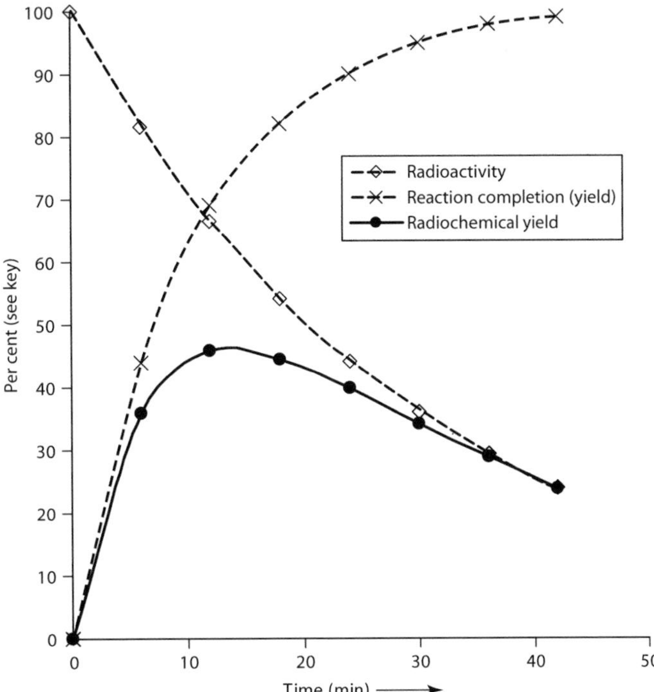

Figure 12.1 A hypothetical reaction that requires 40 minutes to reach 100% yield. With carbon-11 (radioactive half-life 20.4 minutes), even though the reaction reaches completion at 40 minutes, the *radiochemical yield* is only 25%. Maximum radiochemical yield for this reaction is reached between 10 and 15 minutes.

selected so that deprotection can be achieved quickly and efficiently after the labelling is complete.

Increasing reaction rates

Because syntheses using carbon-11 are usually performed on a nano/picomolar scale, reaction rates can be increased using a large stoichiometric excess of reagents. Thus a reaction that might proceed slowly or have an unfavourable equilibrium when performed on a 1 : 1 molar ratio, can be useful under carbon-11 labelling conditions. In addition to the use of high stoichiometric ratios of reagents, high temperatures and pressures can be used to speed up a reaction. Technological solutions to increasing reaction rates for carbon-11 labelling reactions include the use of microwaves and microfluidic devices.

One-pot reactions

The development of one-pot reactions, where possible, reduces the amount of technical handling required during a synthesis and so minimises reaction times and losses through intermediate work-up procedures.

Fast work-up procedures

In addition to the final purification of a labelled compound, often by preparative HPLC, work-up procedures may also be required during a synthesis to remove excess reagents and for changing solvents, etc. In this respect the use of solid-phase extractions can be advantageous.

Specific activity and isotopic dilution

Specific activity is defined as the amount of radioactivity measured per mole of material. As carbon is ubiquitous in our surroundings, dilution of radioactive ^{11}C with stable ^{12}C (so-called isotopic dilution) can cause a reduction in the specific activity of the labelled radiopharmaceutical. For example, cyclotron-produced $^{11}CO_2$ is easily contaminated with $^{12}CO_2$ from the atmosphere or other sources of stable carbon in reagents and instrumentation. It is usual therefore that the specific activity of carbon-11, although high, is many thousands of times lower than the theoretical maximum (i.e. every carbon-11-labelled molecule in a radiopharmaceutical is accompanied by several thousand carbon-12 homologues). If the radiopharmaceutical is a labelled counterpart of an endogenous compound that is present in the body in large amounts (glucose, amino acids, water, etc.), the production of a high-specific-activity radiopharmaceutical is not normally an overriding concern. High specific activities are important, however, if the radiopharmaceutical takes part in a saturable process in the body (e.g. if it is a receptor ligand or enzyme substrate), where the biological process of interest needs to be probed at a true tracer level (the mass of compound administered must not perturb the studied system), or if the compound to be administered could elicit a pharmacological or toxicological side-effect. Even under the above conditions, specific activities of around 50 GBq/μmol (typically corresponding to an administered mass of between 1 and 10 micrograms per human subject for a small molecule) are routinely achievable if sufficient precautions are taken. This can be further improved by an order of magnitude if great care is taken to minimise isotopic dilution. For the sake of comparison, tritium and carbon-14 have specific activities several orders of magnitude lower.

Radiolabelling reactions

The following section describes some of the more common labelling strategies employed for carbon-11 radiopharmaceuticals. The reader is directed to more detailed and exhaustive treatments of carbon-11 chemistry labelling agents and particular carbon-11 radiopharmaceuticals.

^{11}C-Methylating reagents

[^{11}C]Methyl iodide

There are two main methods for producing this labelling agent:

Method 1. Reduction with $LiAlH_4$. 'The wet method' (Scheme 12.2)

Carbon dioxide is bubbled in capillary tubing from the cyclotron to the chemistry laboratory in a stream of nitrogen or helium gas. The labelled carbon dioxide is bubbled through a solution of lithium aluminium hydride ($LiAlH_4$) in tetrahydrofuran (THF) where it

$$CO_2 \xrightarrow[\text{THF}]{\text{LiAlH}_4} CH_3O \xrightarrow{\text{HI}} CH_3I$$

Scheme 12.2

is instantaneously reduced to the methanolate salt. The THF is evaporated, and hydriodic acid (HI) is added and heated. The reaction vessel is purged with a stream of nitrogen or helium gas and the [^{11}C]methyl iodide is distilled off, through a drying agent (typically NaOH or ascarite) and bubbled through a solution of the precursor to be labelled.

Method 2. Radical gas-phase iodination of methane. 'The dry method' (Scheme 12.3)

$$CO_2 \xrightarrow[\text{Zn}]{\text{hydrogen}} CH_4 \xrightarrow{\text{Iodine}} CH_3I$$

Scheme 12.3

[^{11}C]Methane is obtained either directly from the cyclotron target (see above), or by a post-cyclotron conversion of [^{11}C]CO_2 by passage of the target gas over a heated zinc catalyst with a few per cent of hydrogen. In both cases the [^{11}C]methane is subsequently passed through a quartz tube with iodine crystals placed at the tube entrance. The iodine is heated to achieve a controlled iodine vapour which passes to the other end of the quartz tube in a stream of nitrogen or helium gas together with the [^{11}C]methane, where it is heated at higher temperatures to produce iodine radicals. These react with the [^{11}C]methane to produce the desired product. The yield of this method is typically lower than 50%, so the reactants are recirculated through the system a number of times to achieve a good conversion of the [^{11}C]methyl iodide. The product is trapped on a matrix of Porapack Q which, when heated, is released in a stream of inert gas to perform the alkylation reaction.

[^{11}C]Methyl triflate

In some cases, instead of using iodide as the leaving group, the use of the triflate leaving group can render a more reactive labelling agent with advantages over methyl iodide itself. Methyl triflate is simply formed by passage of [^{11}C]methyl iodide over a matrix of silver triflate in an inert gas stream to produce [^{11}C] methyl triflate.

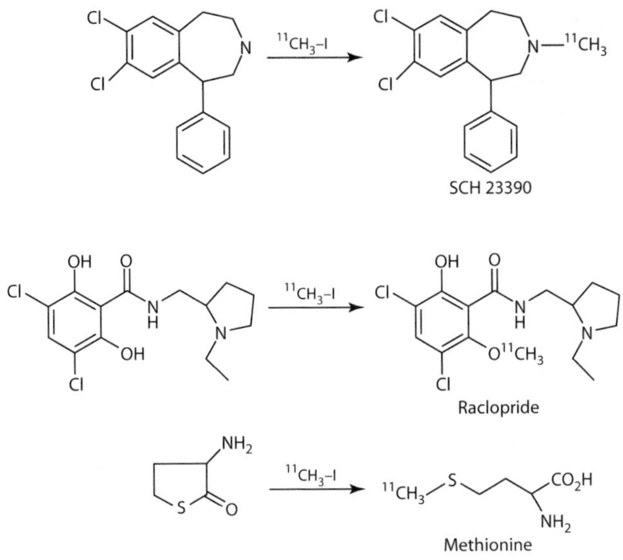

Scheme 12.4

^{11}C-Methylation reactions

Irrespective of the method of production, ^{11}C-methylation reactions can subsequently be performed in a number of ways

Traditionally, [^{11}C]methyl iodide is bubbled through a solution (typically a few hundred microlitres) of appropriate solvent (and base if required). The resulting solution is sealed and heated at an appropriate temperature and reaction time (typically 5 minutes or less). The crude product is typically purified by semi-preparative HPLC equipped with UV and radiation detectors. The fraction containing the product is collected and the HPLC solvent is evaporated, dissolved in an appropriate formulation and passed through a 0.22 μm filter into a sterile septum-sealed vial.

In some cases gas-phase [^{11}C]methyl iodide has been passed directly into an HPLC loop impregnated with a thin film of the labelling precursor and solvent/base. After being left to react for an appropriate time, the solution is directly injected onto the HPLC column and processed as described above. The method has the advantage that losses due to technical handling can be minimised in addition to reduced synthesis times.

A wide variety of PET radiotracers have been synthesised by alkylation of appropriate nucleophiles with [^{11}C]methyl iodide/triflate. These include amino acids, receptor, enzyme and transporter ligands, therapeutics, drugs of abuse and a wide variety of endogenous and exogenous substrates. A few examples are given below; however, a more comprehensive treatment can be found in the literature. Examples of PET radiotracers synthesised by the methylation of nitrogen, oxygen and sulfur nucleophiles are shown in Scheme 12.4.

Some other tracers labelled using [^{11}C]methyl iodide are listed in Table 12.2 (this list is not exhaustive).

Table 12.2 Some tracers labelled using [^{11}C] methyl iodide

Receptor ligands	
Dopamine receptors	
D1 receptors	[^{11}C]SCH 23390, [^{11}C]NNC 112
D2/3 receptors	[^{11}C]Raclopride, [^{11}C]FLB 457, [^{11}C]*N*-methyl spiperone
Serotonin receptors	
5-HT2a	[^{11}C]MDL100907
5-HT4	[^{11}C]SB 207145
5-HT6	[^{11}C]GSK 215083
Benzodiazepine receptors	[^{11}C]Flumazenil, [^{11}C]Ro-15453

(continued overleaf)

Table 12.2 *(continued)*

Histamine receptors	
H3	[^{11}C]GSK189254
Acetylcholine receptors	
Muscarinic	[^{11}C]methyl QNB
Nicotinic	[^{11}C]Epibatidine
Opioid receptors	
Mu	[^{11}C]Carfentanyl
Delta	[^{11}C]Methylnaltrindole
Non-selective	[^{11}C]Diprenorphine
Enzyme markers	
Monoamine oxidase A	[^{11}C]Harmine
Monoamine oxidase B	[^{11}C]Deprenyl
Phosphodiesterase 4	[^{11}C]Rolipram
Transporters	
Vesicular monoamine transporter	[^{11}C]DTBZ
Serotonin transporter	[^{11}C]DASB
Dopamine transporter	[^{11}C]PE2I, [^{11}C]beta-CFT
Endogenous compounds	[^{11}C]Methionine
	[^{11}C]Alanine
	[^{11}C]Dopa
	[^{11}C]Tyrosine
	[^{11}C]Chloline
Others	[^{11}C]Cocaine
	[^{11}C]Morphine

^{11}C-Labelling using Grignard chemistry

Aliphatic and aromatic magnesium halide reagents readily react with [^{11}C]carbon dioxide in a carbon–carbon bond-forming reaction to produce organic magnesium bromide salts of the corresponding acid.

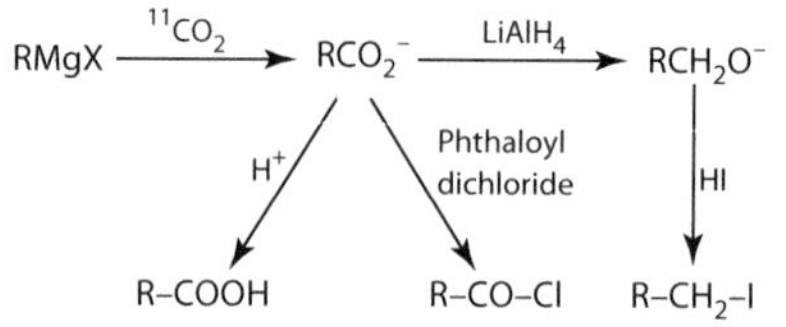

$$RMgX \xrightarrow{^{11}CO_2} RCO_2^- \xrightarrow{LiAlH_4} RCH_2O^-$$
$RCO_2^- \xrightarrow{H^+} R\text{–}COOH$; $RCO_2^- \xrightarrow{\text{Phthaloyl dichloride}} R\text{–}CO\text{–}Cl$; $RCH_2O^- \xrightarrow{HI} R\text{–}CH_2\text{–}I$

Scheme 12.5

This can be directly converted to the ^{11}C-labelled fatty acid by treatment with a proton source (e.g. acid/water). Alternatively some useful secondary precursors or labelling agents can be obtained if the MgBr salt is either reduced with $LiAlH_4$, followed by hydriodic acid to produce the corresponding ^{11}C-labelled organic iodide, or treated with phthaloyl dichloride or thionyl chloride to form the corresponding carbon-11 labelled acid chloride (Scheme 12.5).

Two examples of ^{11}C-labelled radiotracers labelled using Grignard chemistry are illustrated in Scheme 12.6.

Examples of other secondary labelling agents synthesised using Grignard chemistry include [^{11}C]benzyl iodide, [^{11}C]methoxybenzyliodide, [^{11}C]alkyl iodides (e.g. [^{11}C]ethyl, [^{11}C]butyl, [^{11}C]isopropyl iodide), [^{11}C]propionyl chloride, and [^{11}C]cyclohexyl acid chloride.

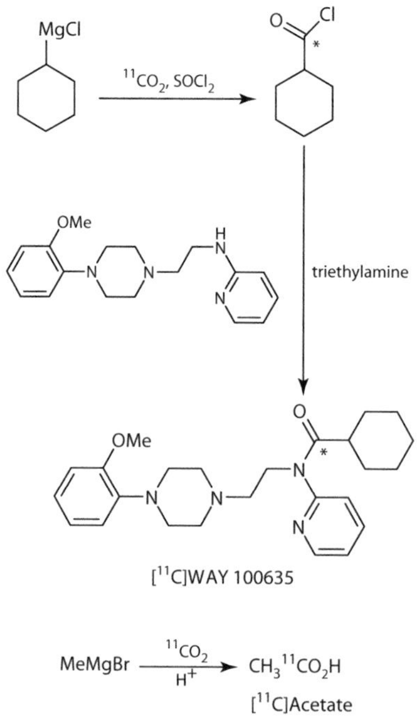

$$MeMgBr \xrightarrow[H^+]{^{11}CO_2} CH_3{}^{11}CO_2H$$
[^{11}C]Acetate

Scheme 12.6

Other labelling agents

Hydrogen [^{11}C]cyanide

The secondary precursor [^{11}C]cyanide is produced by the on-line conversion of [^{11}C]CH_4 with NH_3 in a stream of inert gas over a heated platinum catalyst (Scheme 12.7). The [^{11}C]cyanide is bubbled in a stream of inert gas into a solution to further react with a suitable substrate.

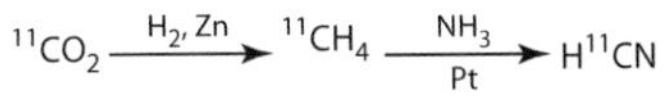

$$^{11}CO_2 \xrightarrow{H_2, Zn} {}^{11}CH_4 \xrightarrow[Pt]{NH_3} H^{11}CN$$

Scheme 12.7

[^{11}C]Cyanide has been used in a number of reaction types for labelling PET radiotracers.

Nucleophilic substitution reactions

Aliphatic halides readily react with [^{11}C]cyanide to produce the corresponding labelled nitrile. The nitrile group itself can be easily converted to the corresponding carboxylic acid or amide upon appropriate treatment. Aromatic nitriles can be prepared by a number of routes, including palladium-mediated insertion reactions and using copper cyanide.

Carbon monoxide

Recently carbon monoxide has emerged as a promising labelling agent for carbon-11 radiotracers. Carbon monoxide is produced from [^{11}C]carbon dioxide by reduction over a heated molybdenum or zinc catalyst in a stream of inert gas. Once formed, the carbon monoxide can be subjected to a number of palladium-mediated insertion reactions as a mild method to produce a wide variety of labelled carbonyl-containing compounds including ketones amines and amides (Scheme 12.8).

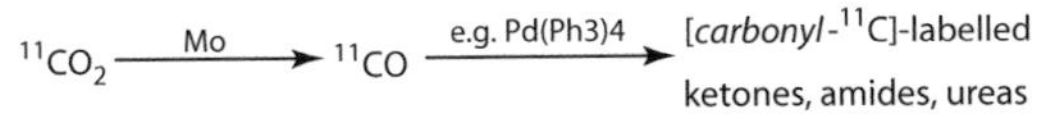

$$^{11}CO_2 \xrightarrow{Mo} {}^{11}CO \xrightarrow{\text{e.g. Pd(Ph3)4}} \text{[}\textit{carbonyl}\text{-}^{11}\text{C]-labelled ketones, amides, ureas}$$

Scheme 12.8

As carbon monoxide is poorly soluble in organic solvents, a number of techniques have been adopted to achieve useful radiolabelling procedures with [^{11}C]CO.

- Microautoclave reactions. The carbon monoxide is passed into a closed vessel (microautoclave) containing the appropriate solvent and reactants, pressurised, sealed and heated. This has been used successfully by a few laboratories, but the instrumentation required is complex and at the time of writing is not commercially available.
- Carbon monoxide complexing. Carbon monoxide is trapped in an organic solvent using a complexing agent. This has the advantage that reactions can be performed using relatively simple instrumentation and at normal pressures. An example of this is the use of [^{11}C]carbonyl borane. Labelled carbon monoxide is bubbled through a commercially available complex of THF-borane to produce [^{11}C]CO·BH_3, which is distilled into a reaction vial containing the reactants. Another example is the use of scorpionate ligands.
- Microfluidic reactors. Low-pressure palladium-mediated ^{11}C-carbonylation of aryl halides for [*carbonyl*-^{11}C]amide formation has also been effectively achieved using solid-supported palladium ‘micro-tube’ reactors by passing gaseous carbon monoxide through a capillary packed with palladium catalyst and flushing the product off the system after heating for a short period.

Carbon monoxide chemistry shows much promise for achieving labelling of compound classes that have thus far been intractable. However, as a more recent development in the field, its use has not yet become widespread.

Conclusion and outlook

With the carbon-11 half-life of 20.4 minutes, the availability of carbon-11-labelled starting reagents is limited. Carbon chemistry is, however, extremely versatile. In principle any organic molecule can be labelled with carbon-11 and studied in the human body, without recourse to studying biomimetic analogues that can behave very differently from their parent molecules. Since its use in the first PET neuroreceptor imaging studies in the 1970s, an incredible number of carbon-11-labelled radiopharmaceuticals have been produced. This versatility is the great strength of carbon-11 chemistry and carbon-11-labelled radiopharmaceuticals and the future of this area will be limited only by the creativity of the carbon-11 chemist and developing knowledge of *in-vivo* biochemistry.

Further reading

Elsinga P (2002). Radiopharmaceutical chemistry for positron emission tomography. *Methods* 27: 208–217.

Fowler J, Wolf A (1997). Working against time: rapid radiotracer synthesis and imaging the human brain. *Acc Chem Res* 30: 181–188.

Gee AD *et al.* (2008). Synthesis and evaluation of [^{11}C] SB207145 as the first in vivo serotonin 5-HT4 receptor radioligand for PET imaging in man. *Curr Radiopharm* 1: 110–114.

International Atomic Agency. (2008). *Cyclotron Produced Radionuclides: Principles and Practice.* Technical Reports Series No. 465. Vienna: IAEA. http://www.iaea.org/Publications/index.html (accessed 30 June 2010).

International Atomic Agency (2009). *Cyclotron Produced Radionuclides: Physical Characteristics and Production Methods.* Technical Reports Series No. 468. Vienna: IAEA. http://www.iaea.org/Publications/index.html (accessed 30 June 2010).

Langstrom B *et al.* (2007). [^{11}C]Carbon monoxide, a versatile and useful precursor in labelling chemistry for PET-ligand development. *J Labelled Comp Radiopharm* 50: 794–810.

Miller P *et al.* (2008). Synthesis of ^{11}C, ^{18}F, ^{15}O and ^{13}N radiolabels for positron emission tomography. *Angew Chem Int Ed* 47: 8998–9033.

13

Other radioelements

Philip J Blower

This chapter deals with miscellaneous radioelements that are not readily grouped with the radionuclides discussed in other sections. The review is not intended to be comprehensive either in radionuclide coverage or in detail, but rather to serve as an overview and entry into the literature. The elements are discussed in order of atomic number.

Phosphorus

Phosphorus-32 (^{32}P) is a pure high-energy beta emitter that was one of the earliest established for therapeutic applications. Its appeal is largely due to good availability and low cost. The main use has relied on its bone-targeting properties, offering palliative treatment of bone metastases in the form of phosphate or polyphosphates (Montebello, Hartsoneaton 1989; Bouchet *et al.* 2000; Pandit-Taskar *et al.* 2004; Silberstein 2005; Lechner *et al.* 2008) and for ablation of myeloprolferative disorders, especially polycythaemia vera rubra (Tefferi, Silverstein 1998; Berlin 2000; Tennvall, Brans 2007). This is probably due to incorporation of ^{32}P not only at bone surfaces but also into the DNA of rapidly proliferating haematopoietic cells. The myeloablative property is a major disadvantage in the treatment of bone metastases, as is clearly evident from the efforts that have been expended in developing marrow-sparing alternative bone-targeting therapeutic radionuclides. This perception has led to its replacement with other radionuclides such as ^{89}Sr, ^{153}Sm and $^{186/188}$Re for bone treatment. However, the evidence that marrow side-effects are significantly worse for ^{32}P is not universally seen as conclusive.

Phosphorus-32 emits β-particles with a mean energy of 0.695 MeV (max. 1.71 MeV) and no imageable photons. Its half-life is 14 days, which is reasonably well-suited to therapeutic applications if residence time in the target tissue is sufficiently long. Apart from the lack of imaging possibilities, these properties, combined with the low cost, are attractive for therapeutic applications and so it is surprising that almost all those applications investigated to date have been limited to use of phosphate as the targeting vector, even though phosphorus can in principle be incorporated into a variety of organic and inorganic molecule types. One avenue that has been explored is the enzymatic phosphorylation of protein vehicles by engineering the 'kemptide' peptide sequence into targeting proteins such as antibodies. Kemptide is an amino acid sequence, Leu-Arg-Arg-Ala-Ser-Gly that is phosphorylated by [γ-^{32}P]ATP under specific catalysis by bovine protein kinase A. Phosphorus-32 is thus site-specifically incorporated into the protein at the kemptide Ser residue and so may be selectively delivered to the target tissue (Patrick *et al.* 1998).

A potential alternative to ^{32}P, with a lower energy beta emission and a longer half-life (25 days), is phosphorus-33. With a mean β-energy of 77 keV (max. 0.249 MeV) its mean tissue penetration is 60 μm (compared with 1.7 mm for ^{32}P). This has led to the proposal that ^{33}P would be a useful radionuclide for palliative radionuclide therapy of bone metastases with reduced irradiation of bone marrow compared with ^{32}P (Goddu *et al.* 2000) and also that a combination or 'cocktail' of ^{32}P and ^{33}P would improve curability of tumours with a wider range of diameters than curable by ^{32}P alone (O'Donoghue *et al.* 1995; Lechner *et al.* 2008). However, there are no reports of therapeutic use of ^{33}P in humans to date.

Iron

Iron-52 (^{52}Fe; half-life 8.3 hours, γ 169 keV 100%, β^+ 56%) has found use as a positron emitter for *in-vivo* gamma or PET imaging, but it is not ideal for widespread general application in PET because interpretation of images is complicated by the positron-emitting daughter ^{52m}Mn (21 minutes half-life, 96% β^+ emission) and the need for a high-energy cyclotron for its production (by irradiating manganese-55 with 70 MeV protons via the reaction ^{55}Mn(p,4n)^{52}Fe) (Qaim 2007). Consequently, its use has been limited to imaging of iron metabolism in disease contexts such as anaemias (Beshara *et al.* 2003), Wilson disease (Bruehlmeier *et al.* 2000) and haematopoietic disorders (Shreeve 2006). However, the decay scheme can be exploited in the construction of a ^{52m}Mn generator, which may offer useful applications in its own right as a short-half-life generator-produced positron emitter (Qaim 2007).

Copper

Although radiopharmaceuticals based on copper radioisotopes have been under development for many years (Table 13.1) (Blower *et al.* 1996) for PET (^{60}Cu, ^{61}Cu, ^{62,64}Cu) and radionuclide therapy (^{67}Cu and to some extent ^{64}Cu), interest in this area has expanded greatly in the last few years. This has been driven partly by widespread interest in imaging hypoxia using [^{64}Cu]ATSM (Figure 13.1) (Vavere, Lewis 2007). coupled with development of relatively straightforward cyclotron-based production methods for ^{64}Cu (Sun, Anderson 2004), ^{61}Cu and ^{60}Cu, all of which can be easily produced by proton irradiation of the corresponding isotopically enriched metallic nickel target, from which the copper is readily separated by ion exchange (McQuade *et al.* 2005b). The recent growth in use of copper since the comprehensive 1996 review (Blower *et al.* 1996) justifies a more extensive discussion than presented herein, but various aspects of the subject have been reviewed in the intervening years (Smith 2004; Sun, Anderson *et al.* 2004; McQuade *et al.* 2005b; Williams *et al.* 2005; Rowshanfarzad *et al.* 2006; Vavere, Lewis 2007; Wadas *et al.* 2007; Wood *et al.* 2008) and so this section will be kept brief.

Because of its 12-hour half-life, and hence the possibility of long-distance transport, ^{64}Cu is popular for clinical use. Nevertheless, routine use in humans may

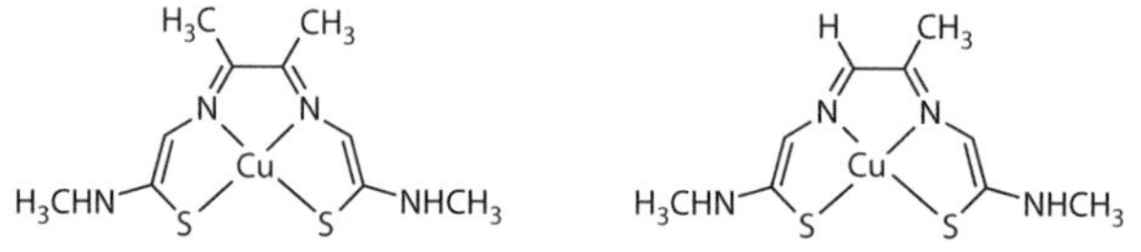

Figure 13.1 Structures of CuATSM and CuPTSM.

Table 13.1 Physical properties of useful copper radionuclides

Isotope	β^- (%), E_{ave}	β^+ (%), E_{ave}	Other	$t_{1/2}$
^{60}Cu		93%, 0.87 MeV	EC	24 minutes
^{61}Cu		62%, 0.53 MeV	EC	3.33 hours
^{62}Cu		98%, 1.32 MeV	EC	9.75 minutes
^{64}Cu	39%, 0.19 MeV	18%, 0.28 MeV	EC	12.7 hours
^{67}Cu	100%, 0.12 MeV		γ 93 keV, 52%	62 hours

be limited because, although its low-energy positron produces excellent PET images, the low positron yield and accompanying beta emissions and Auger electron emissions give rise to high radiation doses to patients. Indeed, it is viewed by some as a potentially useful therapeutic isotope that can be imaged with PET, rather than a PET imaging agent that can also be used for therapy. Copper-61 and ^{60}Cu, although potentially inferior in terms of image quality because of their high positron energy and accompanying high-energy gamma emissions (Williams *et al.* 2005) may be preferable on dosimetry grounds for purposes where the long half-life is not needed. Copper-64 remains a preferred isotope for labelling larger molecules, such as antibodies, that require delayed imaging to be performed. Copper-62 is attractive because it is generator-produced, although its applications are limited compared with some other generator systems because the parent zinc-62 has a rather short half-life (ca. 9 hours). Copper-62 has a very short half-life (ca. 10 minutes), offering the possibility of repeated administration and imaging on the same patient before and after intervention, but this requires very rapid chemistry to be developed. This has been demonstrated to be possible with the bis(thiosemicarbazone) complexes, particularly CuPTSM, which has been well-characterised as a blood flow imaging agent.

Hypoxia targeting with copper bis(thiosemicarbazones) has become established with CuATSM, but new derivatives based on this chemistry are now sought, involving different alkyl substitution patterns (Blower *et al.* 2007). Hydrophilic substituents (Bonnitcha *et al.* 2008) and different donor atoms (Dearling *et al.* 1998b; Castle *et al.* 2003; McQuade *et al.* 2005a) are being investigated in order to improve the pharmacokinetics, biodistribution and hypoxia-selectivity characteristics of the tracers, guided by early identification of structure–activity relationships (Dearling *et al.* 1998a; Mullen *et al.* 2000; Dearling *et al.* 2002; Maurer *et al.* 2002).

Aside from the copper(II) bis(thiosemicarbazone) complexes, which are useful because of their redox-related intracellular trapping, applications of copper isotopes have largely been focused on labelling of peptides and antibodies with Cu(II) using macrocyclic chelators such as cyclam, TETA, and DOTA (Figure 13.2) (Smith 2004). Although these chelates show good kinetic stability in serum, there is evidence that

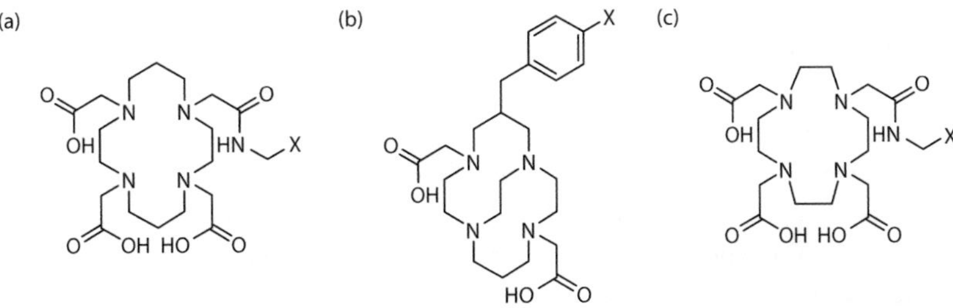

Figure 13.2 Structure of copper bifunctional chelators TETA (a), cross-bridged cyclam derivatives (b) and DOTA (c). X = targeting vehicle.

they undergo dissociation in tissues, especially the liver. This has led to efforts to improve the stability by employing more rigid ligands such as cross-bridged derivatives of TETA and cyclam (Figure 13.2) (Lewis *et al.* 2004; Sprague *et al.* 2004; Woodin *et al.* 2005; Wadas, Anderson 2006; Heroux *et al.* 2007; Silversides *et al.* 2007; Sprague *et al.* 2007; Wadas *et al.* 2008). Copper-64 and copper-67 are the most important isotopes for targeted radionuclide therapy using these biomolecule conjugates. Although ^{67}Cu in particular was shown to be a very effective therapeutic radionuclide in antibody conjugates (Frier 2004), it has not come into widespread use because it is not easy to manufacture and no large-scale, economic, reliable and widely available source of the isotope is available.

The chemistry of copper in oxidation state +1, especially with phosphine-containing ligands (Lewis *et al.* 1996; Lewis *et al.* 2000; Alidori *et al.* 2008) has also been explored to a limited extent because its kinetic lability offers the possibility of very rapid synthesis applicable to the short half-life isotope ^{62}Cu. This chemistry has not yet found its way into *in-vivo* imaging applications.

Arsenic

Arsenic has several potentially useful positron emitters having favourable characteristics for PET imaging: ^{71}As (half-life 64 hours, 30% β^+, average energy 2.49 MeV), ^{72}As (half-life 26 hours, 88% β^+, 1.024 keV), and ^{74}As (half-life 17.8 days, 29% β^+, 128 keV). It also has β-emitting isotopes that in principle could be used for radionuclide therapy, including: ^{77}As (half-life 38.8 hours) and ^{76}As (half-life 26.3 hours). All the positron emitters have relatively long half-lives compatible with use with antibody targeting. Arsenic-72 is particularly interesting because of the possibility of producing it from a generator (parent isotope selenium-72) (Jennewein *et al.* 2004a; Jennewein *et al.* 2004b). Methods have been developed for eluting it in the form of arsenic triiodide, AsI_3, which can be covalently attached to antibodies that have been modified to create thiol side-chains, by elimination of HI with formation of an arsenic–sulfur bond (Jennewein *et al.* 2008). Although use of ^{74}As for radionuclide imaging dates back to the 1950s (Sweet, Brownell 1955), use of arsenic radionuclides in nuclear medicine has been explored surprisingly little to date.

Krypton

Krypton is a noble gas and as such, ^{81m}Kr is useful only for imaging of the airways. It is produced from a generator loaded with ^{81}Rb, which itself has been produced in a cyclotron by a variety of nuclear reactions, e.g. ^{81}Br(α,4n)^{81}Rb, ^{79}Br(α,2n)^{81}Rb and ^{82}Kr(p,2n)^{81}Rb. The half-life of ^{81}Rb is 4.6 hours, so the generator has to be replaced daily, which is the main limitation of this ventilation imaging system. The ^{81m}Kr gas has been eluted by passage of air through a variety of media loaded with ^{81}Rb (resin, paper, aqueous solution, etc.). Krypton-81m has a half-life of 13.3 seconds and so must be directly inhaled from the generator. It emits 190 keV photons which are sufficiently separated from the 141 keV photons of technetium-99m to allow simultaneous dual-energy imaging of both radionuclides. The physical properties allow excellent imaging with very low radiation dose to patients, making ^{81m}Kr particularly suitable for lung ventilation in children (Lambrecht *et al.* 1997; Koyama *et al.* 1980).

Rubidium

Rubidium-82 (^{82}Rb, 96% positron emitter, half-life 75 seconds) in aqueous solution forms hydrated Rb^+, which mimics the potassium ion K^+ in being transported by transmembrane potassium transporters (e.g. the Na^+/K^+-ATPase pump that maintains potassium concentration and electrical potential gradients across cell membranes). Intravenously injected Rb^+ is accumulated quickly in cardiomyocytes of well-perfused myocardium via Na^+/K^+-ATPase. This property, together with its physical properties and its availability from the commercially available ^{82}Sr/^{82}Rb generator, make it particularly useful and convenient for myocardial perfusion imaging using PET in centres remote from a cyclotron (Machac 2005). The generator is replaced about once a month. The short half-life of ^{82}Rb leads to low radiation doses to the patient and the possibility of performing repeated PET imaging (every 5–10 minutes) before and after intervention or stress. The high positron energy (3.35 MeV, 2.6 mm mean path) places limitations upon the attainable imaging resolution, but there is a consensus among users that this is minor disadvantage compared with resolution limitations from other causes and does not adversely affect clinical utility. Overall, ^{82}Rb is a very efficient imaging agent for routine clinical use, and in a specialist centre with high throughput of scans (6–10 per day) its cost is comparable with that of SPECT perfusion imaging.

To form the ^{82}Rb generator, the parent isotope ^{82}Sr (half-life 25 days) is loaded as Sr^{2+} ($SrCl_2$) onto a stationary phase typically consisting of tin oxide (other materials such as alumina and zirconium oxide have been used also) which effectively operates as a cation exchange medium (Alvarez-Diez *et al.* 1999). Conversion of Sr^{2+} to Rb^+ diminishes its affinity for the cation exchanger and it is eluted with saline directly via an infusion set into the patient.

Strontium

Just as rubidium behaves biologically as an analogue of potassium, strontium behaves to a large extent as an analogue of calcium. This is manifested in accumulation in the skeleton, particularly at sites of mineralisation associated with metastatic bone cancer. This is most pronounced in cancers that lead to predominantly osteogenic metastases (e.g. prostate cancer) rather than osteolytic metastases (e.g. multiple myeloma). This bone affinity is put to use in the application of ^{89}Sr as a palliative radiopharmaceutical for patients with painful bone metastases, especially those whose metastases are too widespread for external beam radiotherapy to be safe (Bauman *et al.* 2005; Finlay *et al.* 2005; Silberstein 2005; James *et al.* 2006; Lin and Ray 2006; Lawrentschuk *et al.* 2007).

Strontium-89 is a pure beta emitter with a half-life of 53 days, decaying to stable ^{89}Y. The maximum β-particle energy is 1.46 MeV (average 0.58 MeV). It is produced and distributed as $SrCl_2$. Indeed, as discussed above, this is its only application because its chemistry does not lend itself to incorporation into more complex molecules. It is a reactor-produced isotope usually produced by neutron bombardment of highly enriched ^{88}Sr (>99.9%, to minimise formation of ^{85}Sr) by the reaction ^{88}Sr(n,γ)^{89}Sr.

Despite its lack of imageable photon emissions, ^{89}Sr is the most widely used palliative radionuclide therapy agent among several other beta-emitting isotopes (^{186}Re, ^{188}Re, ^{153}Sm, ^{32}P) that are available. Biodistribution data to support dosimetry estimates are obtained either by crude imaging of brehmsstralung radiation from ^{89}Sr or by PET imaging with the cyclotron-produced isotope ^{83}Sr (β^+, 24%, half-life 33 hours, max. positron energy 1.23 MeV), which is produced by proton irradiation of ^{85}Rb. The mechanism by which bone pain is relieved is unknown. Since the clinical activities administered are well below those at which tumour ablation typically might be expected, it is not thought to be due to tumoricidal effect. Nevertheless, many clinical trials agree that approximately 75% of patients experience some benefit in terms of quality of life and reduction in analgesic consumption, while 25% experience complete pain relief, at the expense of only minor side-effects, the most significant of which is transient bone marrow suppression.

Zirconium

The need for longer-lived PET tracer radionuclides for labelling targeting vehicles with long biodistribution and clearance times (e.g. antibodies and other large proteins) has identified a small number of potential candidates, of which ^{89}Zr is a leading example (others are ^{54}Cu, ^{72}As and ^{124}I). Like the others, it is not ideal because of low positron yield, but in the absence of better alternatives it is being adopted by some centres for use in 'immuno-PET' and related applications (Verel *et al.* 2003a; Brouwers *et al.* 2004; Perk *et al.* 2005, 2006). It has a half-life of 78 hours and decays by positron emission (23%, E_{max} 0.897 MeV) and electron capture (77%), with a high-energy gamma emission (909 keV) associated with almost all decompositions. It can potentially be produced in most biomedical cyclotrons by the ^{89}Y(p,n)^{89}Zr reaction, with 12 MeV proton irradiation (Meijs *et al.* 1994; Verel *et al.* 2003b; Kandil *et al.* 2007). A less widely available alternative route is via the ^{89}Y(d,2n)^{89}Zr reaction.

Zirconium is a hard (class a) metal with a favoured oxidation state under biological conditions of +4. The Zr^{4+} ion does not form kinetically inert chelates with DTPA derivatives, and the desferrioxamine iron-chelating ligand (Figure 13.3) has been used successfully instead (Meijs *et al.* 1992; Meijs *et al.* 1996).

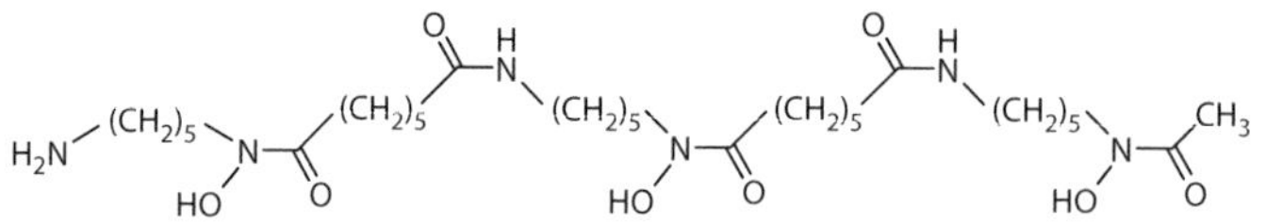

Figure 13.3 Structure of desferrioxamine (DFO).

Tin

Tin-117m, with a half-life of 13.6 days, emits a low-energy conversion electron with a mean energy of 135 keV, a mean range in bone of 0.15 mm and abundance of 1.14 per decay. It has been suggested that these properties are ideal for palliative radionuclide therapy of bone metastases, in particular because the short range of the low-energy electron emissions imparts a reduced bone marrow dose (Bishayee *et al.* 2000) compared with the more widely used, higher-energy beta emitters such as ^{89}Sr and ^{32}P. Selective delivery to bone metastases is very effectively achieved using the DTPA complex of Sn^{4+} (Swailem *et al.* 1998), as has been demonstrated by scintigraphy using the monoenergetic gamma photon of ^{117m}Sn at 159 keV in 86% abundance. Palliative benefit is similar to that achieved with the more conventional beta-emitting radionuclides, but bone marrow suppression is much less (Krishnamurthy *et al.* 1997).

Tin-117m is produced by neutron irradiation of tin-117 metal in a nuclear reactor, via the reaction ^{117}Sn(n,n,γ)^{117m}Sn. This route leads to limited activity and specific activity, which is one of the main factors limiting the widespread application of the isotope, and a carrier-free route would be preferable (Qaim *et al.* 1984). The initial success with the DTPA complex inhibited evaluation of alternative chelators, but more recently phosphonate derivatives have been revisited (Zeevaart *et al.* 2004).

Thallium

Thallium-201, in the form of thallium chloride (TlCl) was the first scintigraphic imaging agent in widespread routine use for myocardial perfusion imaging. It came into use in the 1970s after economic methods for its production emerged, involving irradiating a natural thallium target with high-energy protons (>30 MeV) giving the reaction ^{203}Tl(p,3n)^{201}Pb followed by decay of ^{201}Pb (half-life 9.4 hours) to ^{201}Tl (Lagunassolar *et al.* 1977; Malinin *et al.* 1984). Myocardial perfusion imaging with ^{210}Tl has since been largely superseded by technetium-99m complexes with improved dosimetry and imaging characteristics (Kailasnath, Sinusas 2001). The emissions properties of ^{201}Tl are less than ideal. It decays by electron capture with a 73-hour half-life and a complex photon emission spectrum including mercury K X-rays in high abundance (98%) but low energy (69, 83 keV) plus γ-rays of 135 and 167 keV that are very imageable but of low abundance (total 10%). However, the efficient myocardial extraction (>80% first pass) leads to excellent kinetics of uptake in the myocardium and clearance from blood. The uptake mechanism relies on the hydrated Tl^+ ion acting as a potassium analogue and being taken actively into cardiomyocytes via the Na^+/K^+-ATPase pump, analogous to that of ^{82}Rb described earlier. This mechanism is also exploited in wider applications of ^{201}Tl in tumour imaging, especially in brain tumours (Serrano *et al.* 2008) breast cancer and medullary thyroid carcinoma, and in parathyroid imaging.

The chemical nature of thallium in oxidation state +1 has precluded incorporation of ^{201}Tl into more complex molecules for alternative imaging applications, but recently attention has turned to investigation of the possibility that DTPA chelates of thallium in oxidation state +3 could be useful (Jalilian *et al.* 2006, 2007, 2008). Because radioisotopes with superior emission properties are more widely available nowadays, it is unlikely that new imaging applications of ^{201}Tl will emerge, although the possibility of using it as a therapeutic isotope should not be dismissed.

Lead

Lead-212 (half-life 10.6 hours) offers the possibility to serve as an '*in-vivo* generator' by administration of a targeted radiopharmaceutical such as a monoclonal antibody incorporating a lead-212 chelate (such as the NOTA, DOTA or TETA complex) (McDevitt *et al.* 1998; Hassfjell, Brechbeil 2001).

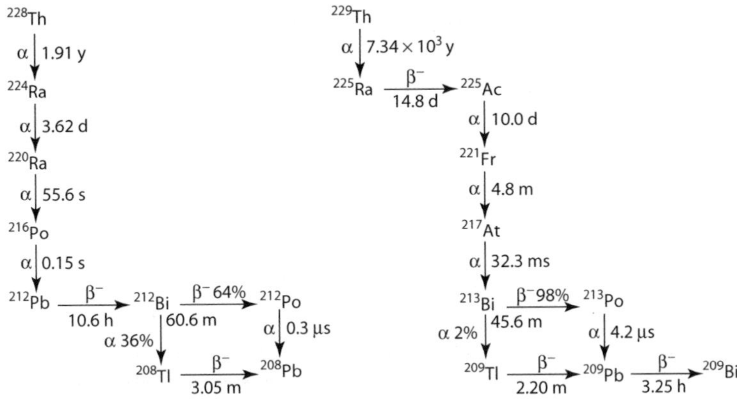

Figure 13.4 Decay schemes for thorium-228 (left) and thorium-229 (right).

It decays *in situ* by beta emission to ^{212}Bi, which is an alpha emitter (half-life 60 minutes). Provided it remains within the target tissue after the decay of ^{212}Pb (which is by no means certain because the accompanying Auger electron emissions induce a large charge-separation that destroys the chelator), this imparts a high localised dose of high-linear-energy-transfer (high LET) radiation to the target tissue. Lead-212 is produced as part of the thorium-228 decay scheme (Figure 13.4) by elution from a generator loaded with radon-224.

Bismuth

Bismuth is of potential value because of its alpha-emitting isotopes ^{212}Bi (most likely to be useful as the daughter of the '*in-vivo*' generator isotope ^{212}Pb discussed above) and generator-produced ^{213}B (Hassfjell, Brechbiel 2001). Bismuth-213 has a half-life of 45.6 minutes and is produced as a decay product of ^{225}Ac via the decay chain shown in Figure 13.4. A generator loaded with ^{225}Ac is available, with a shelf-life of 1–2 weeks, from which ^{213}Bi can be eluted with 0.1 mol/L hydriodic acid as the iodide complex BiI_5^{2-}. The bismuth is readily attached to targeting molecules using bifunctional derivatives of chelators such as the cyclohexyl-DTPA derivative CHX-A″-DTPA (Figure 13.5) (Wilbur *et al.* 2008) or DOTA (Yao *et al.* 2004). Radiobiological studies have shown that targeted alpha emitter therapy can overcome resistance to other modalities by inducing irreparable DNA damage (Friesen *et al.* 2007) and clinical trials of ^{213}Bi-labelled antibodies against the CD33 antigen are in progress in patients with acute myeloid leukaemia (Sgouros *et al.* 1999). The short half-life of ^{213}Bi may limit its application to diffuse cancers such as leukaemia rather than solid tumours because of the time required to penetrate the latter and clear from non-target tissues. Biodistribution and dosimetry data can be obtained by imaging the gamma photon at 440 keV (Sgouros *et al.* 1999). New inorganic materials are being developed to replace the organic cation-exchange resin-based stationary phases (McDevitt *et al.* 1999) used in generator construction, to overcome the problem of degradation due to the high radiation dose imparted by the ^{225}Ac alpha emissions (McDevitt *et al.* 1998).

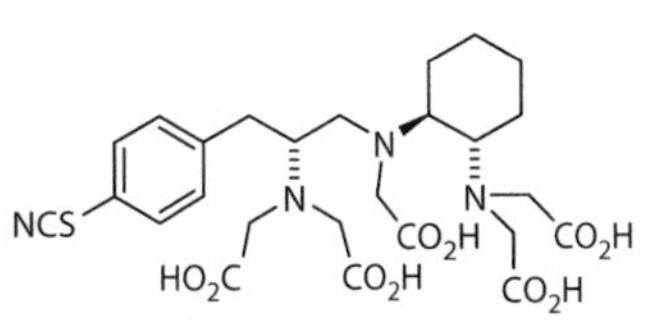

Figure 13.5 Structure of CHX-A″-DTPA (isothiocyanate derivative).

Radium

Like strontium, radium-223 is also a biological analogue of calcium with high affinity for bone metastases. It has a half-life of 11.4 days and was studied in preclinical animal models (Henriksen *et al.* 2002; Henriksen *et al.* 2003; Jonasdottir *et al.* 2006; Larsen *et al.* 2006) and has become notable as the first alpha-emitting radiopharmaceutical to enter extensive clinical trials. Although still at an early stage, these show promise in that palliative effects are observed with reduced bone marrow suppression compared with the conventional beta-emitting agents such as ^{89}Sr (Nilsson *et al.* 2005, 2007). This is attributable to the reduced tissue penetration of the high-LET α-particles. Radium-223 has a complex decay chain leading to the emission of a series of four α-particles in the series ^{223}Ra (α, $t_{1/2} = 11.4$ days), ^{219}Rn (α, $t_{1/2} = 3.96$ seconds), ^{215}Po (α, $t_{1/2} = 1.78$ milliseconds), ^{211}Pb (β, $t_{1/2} = 36.1$ minutes), ^{211}Bi (α, $t_{1/2} = 2.17$ minutes), ^{207}Tl (β, $t_{1/2} = 4.77$ minutes), ^{207}Pb (stable). It is fortunate that the radon formed in the first decomposition does not have time to escape from the vicinity of the adsorption site before undergoing the second decomposition, thus confining the dose to the site of deposition provided that the lead isotope formed in the chain remains localised in the bone matrix until the daughter bismuth isotope decays with alpha emission (this indeed appears to be the case experimentally). Thus the local high-LET dose is extremely high with great potential for cytotoxicity.

Besides the α-particles, there are various other types of radiation emitted from the radium-223 series, including radium X-rays at 81 and 84 keV, radium-223 γ-photons at 269 and 154 keV and radium-219 γ-photons at 271 keV, which can be used to image biodistribution. However, because of the low administered activities, long acquisition times are required.

Radium-223 is produced as a member of a natural radioactive family originating from uranium ($t_{1/2} = 7 \times 10^8$ years) via ^{231}Th ($t_{1/2} = 25.6$ years) in the sequence $^{231}\text{Th} \rightarrow {}^{231}\text{Pa}$ ($t_{1/2} = 3.3 \times 10^4$ years) $\rightarrow {}^{227}$Ac ($t_{1/2} = 21.7$ years) $\rightarrow {}^{227}$Th ($t_{1/2} = 18.7$ days) $\rightarrow {}^{223}$Ra (11.4 days). It can be purified from ^{227}Ac using a cation exchange system. A ^{226}Ra (n,γ)^{227}Ra nuclear reaction has also been used to produce ^{223}Ra. Radium-227 ($t_{1/2} = 42$ minutes) is rapidly transformed into ^{227}Ac ($t_{1/2} = 21.77$ years), which may be separated by different methods from the radium-226 target material.

Actinium

Actinium-225 offers a tantalising prospect of extremely high localised radiation dose delivery, per atom administered, because of the four alpha emissions and two beta emissions in the decay chain en route to stable Bi-209 (McDevitt *et al.* 1998). It has a half-life of 10 days and is available from the decay chain of thorium-229 (see Figure 13.4) by a number of methods including elution from a generator loaded with thorium-229 followed by a purification column to remove radium-225 and other decay products. For labelling biomolecules, the 12-coordination-site chelating ligand 1,4,7,10,13,16-hexaazacyclohexadecane-$N, N', N', N'', N''', N''''$-hexaacetic acid (HEHA) has been used as a bifunctional chelator to accommodate the large size and high charge of actinium-225. However, there are some major challenges to overcome because of this '*in-vivo* generator' scheme. The chemical nature of the elements formed in the decay chain varies widely (including group 1 metal, actinide, halogen, main group metal) and so the design of chelators or linkage chemistry to accommodate all these poses a problem. Moreover, chelate complexes able to withstand the recoil energy associated with the earlier α-decay processes in the series seem improbable. This is a formidable problem and causes major radiotoxicity in animal studies. Partial amelioration of the consequences has been achieved by demonstrating that accumulation of released bismuth-213 in kidney could be reduced by combined dithiol chelation therapy and diuresis, but major hurdles remain to be surmounted before application in humans can be contemplated.

References

Alidori S *et al.* (2008). Synthesis, in vitro and in vivo characterization of ^{64}Cu (I) complexes derived from hydrophilic tris(hydroxymethyl)phosphane and 1,3,5-triaza-7-phosphaadamantane ligands. *J Biol Inorg Chem* 13: 307–315.

Alvarez-Diez TM *et al.* (1999). Manufacture of strontium-82/rubidium-82 generators and quality control of rubidium-82 chloride for myocardial perfusion imaging in patients using positron emission tomography. *Appl Radiat Isot* 50: 1015–1023.

Bauman G *et al.* (2005). Radiopharmaceuticals for the palliation of painful bone metastases – a systematic review. *Radiother Oncol* 75: 258–270.

Berlin NI (2000). Treatment of the myeloproliferative disorders with ^{32}P. *Eur J Haematol* 65: 1–7.

Beshara S *et al.* (2003). Pharmacokinetics and red cell utilization of ^{52}Fe/^{59}Fe-labelled iron polymaltose in anaemic patients using positron emission tomography. *Br J Haematol* 120: 853–859.

Bishayee A *et al.* (2000). Marrow-sparing effects of ^{117m}Sn (4+)diethylenetriaminepentaacetic acid for radionuclide therapy of bone cancer. *J Nucl Med* 41: 2043–2050.

Blower PJ *et al.* (1996). Copper radionuclides and radiopharmaceuticals in nuclear medicine. *Nucl Med Biol* 23: 957–980.

Blower PJ *et al.* (2007). Imaging hypoxia in vivo by controlling the electrochemistry of copper radionuclide complexes. *J Labelled Comp Radiopharm* 50: 354–359.

Bonnitcha PD *et al.* (2008). In vitro and in vivo evaluation of bifunctional bisthiosemicarbazone ^{64}Cu-complexes for the positron emission tomography imaging of hypoxia. *J Med Chem* 51: 2985–2991.

Bouchet LG *et al.* (2000). Considerations in the selection of radiopharmaceuticals for palliation of bone pain from metastatic osseous lesions. *J Nucl Med* 41: 682–687.

Brouwers A *et al.* (2004). PET radioimmunoscintigraphy of renal cell cancer using ^{89}Zr-labeled cG250 monoclonal antibody in nude rats. *Cancer Biother Radiopharm* 19: 155–163.

Bruehlmeier M *et al.* (2000). Increased cerebral iron uptake in Wilson's disease: a ^{52}Fe-citrate PET study. *J Nucl Med* 41: 781–787.

Castle TC *et al.* (2003). Hypoxia-targeting copper bis (selenosemicarbazone) complexes: comparison with their sulfur analogues. *J Am Chem Soc* 125: 10040–10049.

Dearling JLJ *et al.* (1998a). Design of hypoxia-targeting radiopharmaceuticals: selective uptake of copper-64 complexes in hypoxic cells in vitro. *Eur J Nucl Med* 25: 788–792.

Dearling JLJ *et al.* (1998b). Redox-active metal complexes for imaging hypoxic tissues: structure–activity relationships in copper(II) bis(thiosemicarbazone) complexes. *Chem Commun*, 2531–2532.

Dearling JLJ *et al.* (2002). Copper bis(thiosemicarbazone) complexes as hypoxia imaging agents: structure–activity relationships. *J Biol Inorg Chem* 7: 249–259.

Finlay OG *et al.* (2005). Radioisotopes for the palliation of metastatic bone cancer: a systematic review. *Lancet Oncol* 6: 392–400.

Frier M (2004). Rhenium-188 and copper-67 radiopharmaceuticals for the treatment of bladder cancer. *Mini Rev Med Chem* 4: 61–68.

Friesen C *et al.* (2007). Breaking chemoresistance and radioresistance with [^{213}Bi]anti-CD45 antibodies in leukemia cells. *Cancer Res* 67: 1950–1958.

Goddu SM *et al.* (2000). Marrow toxicity of ^{33}P- versus ^{32}P-orthophosphate: implications for therapy of bone pain and bone metastases. *J Nucl Med* 41: 941–951.

Hassfjell S, Brechbiel MW (2001). The development of the alpha-particle emitting radionuclides ^{212}Bi and ^{213}Bi, and their decay chain related radionuclides, for therapeutic applications. *Chem Rev* 101: 2019–2036.

Henriksen G *et al.* (2002). Significant antitumor effect from bone-seeking, α-particle-emitting ^{223}Ra demonstrated in an experimental skeletal metastases model. *Cancer Res* 62: 3120–3125.

Henriksen G *et al.* (2003). Targeting of osseous sites with α-emitting ^{223}Ra: comparison with the β-emitter ^{89}Sr in mice. *J Nucl Med* 44: 252–259.

Heroux KJ *et al.* (2007). The long and short of it: the influence of *N*-carboxyethyl versus *N*-carboxymethyl pendant arms on in vitro and in vivo behavior of copper complexes of cross-bridged tetraamine macrocycles. *Dalton Trans*, 2150–2162.

Jalilian A R *et al.* (2006). Production and biological evaluation of [^{201}Tl (III)]bleomycin. *9th International Symposium on Synthesis and Application of Isotopes and Isotopically Labelled Compounds*, Edinburgh. New Jersey: International Isotope Society.

Jalilian AR *et al.* (2007). Development of [^{201}Tl](III)-DTPA-human polyclonal antibody complex for inflammation detection. *Radiochim Acta* 95: 669–675.

Jalilian AR *et al.* (2008). Preparation and evaluation of [^{201}Tl](III)-DTPA complex for cell labeling. *J Radioanal Nucl Chem* 275: 109–114.

James ND *et al.* (2006). The changing pattern of management for hormone-refractory, metastatic prostate cancer. *Prostate Cancer Prostatic Dis* 9: 221–229.

Jennewein M *et al.* (2004a). A no-carrier-added ^{72}Se/^{72}As radionuclide generator based on solid phase extraction. *6th International Conference on Nuclear and Radiochemistry* (NRC-6), Aachen. Forschungszentrum Jülich.

Jennewein M *et al.* (2004b). A no-carrier-added ^{72}Se/^{72}As radionuclide generator based on distillation. *Radiochim Acta* 92: 245–249.

Jennewein M *et al.* (2008). Vascular imaging of solid tumors in rats with a radioactive arsenic-labeled antibody that binds exposed phosphatidylserine. *Clin Cancer Res* 14: 1377–1385.

Jonasdottir TJ *et al.* (2006). First in vivo evaluation of liposome-encapsulated ^{223}Ra as a potential alpha-particle-emitting cancer therapeutic agent. *Anticancer Res* 26: 2841–2848.

Kailasnath P, Sinusas AJ (2001). Comparison of Tl-201 with Tc-99m-labeled myocardial perfusion agents: technical, physiologic, and clinical issues. *J Nucl Cardiol* 8: 482–498.

Kandil SA *et al.* (2007). A comparative study on the separation of radiozirconium via ion-exchange and solvent extraction techniques, with particular reference to the production of ^{88}Zr and ^{89}Zr in proton induced reactions on yttrium. *J Radioanal Nucl Chem* 274: 45–52.

Koyama *et al.* (1980). ^{81m}Kr gas generator for lung ventilation study. *Eur J Nucl Med* 5: 481–486.

Krishnamurthy GT *et al.* (1997). Tin-117m(4+)DTPA: pharmacokinetics and imaging characteristics in patients with metastatic bone pain. *J Nucl Med* 38: 230–237.

Lagunassolar MC *et al.* (1977). Cyclotron production of thallium-201 for myocardial imaging. *J Labelled Comp Radiopharm* 13: 189–189.

Lambrecht RM *et al.* (1997). Radionuclide generators. *Radiochim Acta* 77: 103–123.

Larsen RH *et al.* (2006). Radiotoxicity of the alpha-emitting bone-seeker ^{223}Ra injected intravenously into mice: histology, clinical chemistry and hematology. *In Vivo* 20: 325–331.

Lawrentschuk N *et al.* (2007). Diagnostic and therapeutic use of radioisotopes for bony disease in prostate cancer: current practice. *Int J Urol* 14: 89–95.

Lechner A *et al.* (2008). Targeted radionuclide therapy: theoretical study of the relationship between tumour control probability and tumour radius for a $^{32}P/^{33}P$ radionuclide cocktail. *Phys Med Biol* 53: 1961–1974.

Lewis JS *et al.* (1996). Copper(I) bis(diphosphine) complexes as a basis for radiopharmaceuticals for positron emission tomography and targeted radiotherapy. *Chem Commun*, 1093–1094.

Lewis JS *et al.* (2000). Copper bis(diphosphine) complexes: radiopharmaceuticals for the detection of multi-drug resistance in tumours by PET. *Eur J Nucl Med* 27: 638–646.

Lewis EA *et al.* (2004). Ultrastable complexes for in vivo use: a bifunctional chelator incorporating a cross-bridged macrocycle. *Chem Commun*, 2212–2213.

Lin A, Ray ME (2006). Targeted and systemic radiotherapy in the treatment of bone metastasis. *Cancer Metastasis Rev* 25: 669–675.

Machac J (2005). Cardiac positron emission tomography imaging. *Semin Nucl Med* 35: 17–36.

Malinin AB *et al.* (1984). Production of "no-carrier-added" ^{201}Tl. *Int J Appl Radiat Isot* 35: 685–687.

Maurer RI *et al.* (2002). Studies on the mechanism of hypoxic selectivity in copper bis(thiosemicarbazone) radiopharmaceuticals. *J Med Chem* 45: 1420–1431.

McDevitt MR *et al.* (1998). Radioimmunotherapy with alpha-emitting nuclides. *Eur J Nucl Med* 25: 1341–1351.

McDevitt MR *et al.* (1999). Preparation of α-emitting ^{213}Bi-labeled antibody constructs for clinical use. *J Nucl Med* 40: 1722–1727.

McQuade P *et al.* (2005a). Investigation into ^{64}Cu-labeled bis (selenosemicarbazone) and bis(thiosemicarbazone) complexes as hypoxia imaging agents. *Nucl Med Biol* 32: 147–156.

McQuade P *et al.* (2005b). Positron-emitting isotopes produced on biomedical cyclotrons. *Curr Med Chem* 12: 807–818.

Meijs WE *et al.* (1992). Evaluation of desferal as a bifunctional chelating agent for labeling antibodies with ^{89}Zr. *Appl Radiat Isot* 43: 1443–1447.

Meijs WE *et al.* (1994). Production of highly pure no-carrier added ^{89}Zr for the labeling of antibodies with a positron emitter. *Appl Radiat Isot* 45: 1143–1147.

Meijs WE *et al.* (1996). A facile method for the labeling of proteins with zirconium isotopes. *Nucl Med Biol* 23: 439–448.

Montebello JF, Hartsoneaton M (1989). The palliation of osseous metastasis with ^{32}P or ^{89}Sr compared with external beam and hemibody irradiation: a historical-perspective. *Cancer Invest* 7: 139–160.

Mullen GE *et al.* (2000). Computational and chemical insight into hypoxia selectivity of Cu(II)ATSM. *J Nucl Med* 41: 485.

Nilsson S *et al.* (2005). First clinical experience with alpha-emitting radium-223 in the treatment of skeletal metastases. *Clin Cancer Res* 11: 4451–4459.

Nilsson S *et al.* (2007). Bone-targeted radium-223 in symptomatic, hormone-refractory prostate cancer: a randomised, multicentre, placebo-controlled phase II study. *Lancet Oncol* 8: 587–594.

O'Donoghue JA *et al.* (1995). Relationships between tumor size and curability for uniformly targeted therapy with beta-emitting radionuclides. *J Nucl Med* 36: 1902–1909.

Pandit-Taskar N *et al.* (2004). Radiopharmaceutical therapy for palliation of bone pain from osseous metastases. *J Nucl Med* 45: 1358–1365.

Patrick MR *et al.* (1998). In vitro characterization of a recombinant ^{32}P-phosphorylated anti-(carcinoembryonic antigen) single-chain antibody. *Cancer Immunol Immunother* 46: 229–237.

Perk LR *et al.* (2005). ^{89}Zr as a PET surrogate radioisotope for scouting biodistribution of the therapeutic radiometals ^{90}Y and ^{117}Lu in tumor-bearing nude mice after coupling to the internalizing antibody cetuximab. *J Nucl Med* 46: 1898–1906.

Perk LR *et al.* (2006). Preparation and evaluation of ^{89}Zr-Zevalin for monitoring of ^{90}Y-Zevalin biodistribution with positron emission tomography. *Eur J Nucl Med Molec Imaging* 33: 1337–1345.

Qaim S M (2007). Decay data and production yields of some non-standard positron emitters used in PET. *17th International Symposium on Radiopharmaceutical Sciences*, Aachen. Forschungszentrum Jülich.

Qaim SM, Dohler H (1984). Production of carrier-free ^{117m}Sn. *Int J Appl Radiat Isot* 35: 645–650.

Rowshanfarzad P *et al.* (2006). An overview of copper radionuclides and production of ^{61}Cu by proton irradiation of Zn-nat at a medical cyclotron. *Appl Radiat Isot* 64: 1563–1573.

Serrano J *et al.* (2008). Radioguided surgery in brain tumors with thallium-201. *Clin Nucl Med* 33: 838–840.

Sgouros G *et al.* (1999). Pharmacokinetics and dosimetry of an α-particle emitter labeled antibody: ^{213}Bi-HuM195 (anti-CD33). in patients with leukemia. *J Nucl Med* 40: 1935–1946.

Shreeve W W (2006) Use of isotopes in the diagnosis of hematopoietic disorders. *International Symposium on Recent Advances in Radiation Effects, Hematopoiesis and Malignancy in honor of Eugene P Cronkite*, Upton, NY.

Silberstein EB (2005). Teletherapy and radiopharmaceutical therapy of painful bone metastases. *Semin Nucl Med* 35: 152–158.

Silversides JD *et al.* (2007). Copper(II) cyclam-based complexes for radiopharmaceutical applications: synthesis and structural analysis. *Dalton Trans*, 971–978.

Smith SV (2004). Molecular imaging with copper-64. *J Inorg Biochem* 98: 1874–1901.

Sprague JE *et al.* (2004). Preparation and biological evaluation of copper-64-labeled Tyr^{3}-octreotate using a cross-bridged macrocyclic chelator. *Clin Cancer Res* 10: 8674–8682.

Sprague JE *et al.* (2007). Synthesis, characterization and in vivo studies of Cu(II)-64-labeled cross-bridged tetraazamacrocycle-amide complexes as models of peptide conjugate imaging agents. *J Med Chem* 50: 2527–2535.

Sun X K, Anderson C J (2004). Production and applications of copper-64 radiopharmaceuticals. *Methods Enzymol* 386: 237–261 [*Imaging Biol Res B*].

Swailem FMC *et al.* (1998). In-vivo tissue uptake and retention of Sn-117m(4+)DTPA in a human subject with metastatic bone pain and in normal mice. *Nucl Med Biology* 25: 279–287.

Sweet WH, Brownell GL (1955). Localization of intracranial lesions by scanning with positron-emitting arsenic. *J Am Med Assoc* 157: 1183–1188.

Tefferi A, Silverstein MN (1998). Treatment of polycythaemia vera and essential thrombocythaemia. *Baillieres Clin Haematol* 11: 769–785.

Tennvall J, Brans B (2007). EANM procedure guideline for ^{32}P phosphate treatment of myeloproliferative diseases. *Eur J Nucl Med Mol Imaging* 34: 1324–1327.

Vavere AL, Lewis JS (2007). Cu-ATSM: A radiopharmaceutical for the PET imaging of hypoxia. *Dalton Trans*, 4893–4902.

Verel I *et al.* (2003a). Quantitative ^{89}Zr immuno-PET for in vivo scouting of ^{90}Y-labeled monoclonal antibodies in xenograft-bearing nude mice. *J Nucl Med* 44: 1663–1670.

Verel I *et al.* (2003b). ^{89}Zr immuno-PET: Comprehensive procedures for the production of ^{89}Zr-labeled monoclonal antibodies. *J Nucl Med* 44: 1271–1281.

Wadas TJ, Anderson CJ (2006). Radiolabeling of TETA- and CB-TE2A-conjugated peptides with copper-64. *Nature Protocols* 1: 3062–3068.

Wadas TJ *et al.* (2008). Preparation and biological evaluation of ^{64}Cu-CB-TE2A-sst$_2$-ANT, a somatostatin antagonist for PET imaging of somatostatin receptor-positive tumors. *J Nucl Med* 49: 1819–1827.

Wadas TJ *et al.* (2007). Copper chelation chemistry and its role in copper radiopharmaceuticals. *Curr Pharm Des* 13: 3–16.

Wilbur DS *et al.* (2008). Streptavidin in antibody pretargeting. 5. Chemical modification of recombinant streptavidin for labeling with the α-particle-emitting radionuclides ^{213}Bi and ^{211}At. *Bioconjug Chem* 19: 158–170.

Williams HA *et al.* (2005). A comparison of PET imaging characteristics of various copper radioisotopes. *Eur J Nucl Med Mol Imaging* 32: 1473–1480.

Wood KA *et al.* (2008). [^{64}Cu]Diacetyl-bis(N^4-methyl-thiosemicarbazone) – a radiotracer for tumor hypoxia. *Nucl Med Biol* 35: 393–400.

Woodin KS *et al.* (2005). Kinetic inertness and electrochemical behavior of copper(II) tetraazamacrocyclic complexes: Possible implications for in vivo stability. *Eur J Inorg Chem*, 4829–4833.

Yao ZS *et al.* (2004). Pretargeted alpha emitting radioimmunotherapy using ^{213}Bi 1,4,7,10-tetraazacyclododecane-*N*, *N*′,*N*″,*N*‴-tetraacetic acid-biotin. *Clin Cancer Res* 10: 3137–3146.

Zeevaart JR *et al.* (2004). Biodistribution and pharmacokinetics of variously molecular sized ^{117m}Sn(II)-polyethyleneiminomethyl phosphonate complexes in the normal primate model as potential selective therapeutic bone agents. *Arzneimittelforschung* 54: 340–347.

14

Radiolabelling of biomolecules

Stephen J Mather

The term 'biomolecule' might have many definitions, but for the purpose of this chapter it can be defined as a molecule made up of biomolecular building blocks such as amino acids, nucleotides/nucleosides or sugars. Examples would therefore be proteins, DNA, RNA and polysaccharides. This chapter will be confined to a description of the use of polypeptides since these represent by far the greatest number of applications in the field of radiopharmacy.

Introduction

Any biological structure that is present at increased levels in target tissues can potentially be pursued for radiopharmaceutical imaging or therapy Since there are thousands of pathways that are implicated in disease, a more discriminating selection can be made as follows: Ideally the target should be as specific as possible for the disease (i.e. not present in normal tissue and only present in the disease of particular interest) and should be present as abundantly as possible on diseased cells. In selecting a target, consideration should also be given to the value of the clinical information that would be gained from a diagnostic or therapeutic procedure that interacts with this pathway. Thus, the requirements for developing an imaging procedure that provides a sensitive and specific means for staging cancer on first presentation will be different from those required for assessing the response of a particular type of cancer to a particular therapeutic intervention. Targets of current interest in radiopharmaceutical development can be divided into two main (but overlapping) categories: (1) cell surface markers or receptors that show significantly increased levels of expression on diseased cells, and (2) intracellular metabolic pathways that either are up-regulated in disease or are implicated in the response to various types of treatment.

The requirements for biomolecules to bind to targets at the cell surface are less stringent than for those required to pass through the cell membrane and it is at such extracellular locations that most biomolecular radiopharmaceuticals interact.

Examples of ligands currently being pursued are those based on monoclonal antibodies, which bind to tumour-associated epitopes, and neuropeptide hormones that bind to a range of neuropeptide receptors.

Epitopes for monoclonal antibodies represent a good example of the type of target worthy of pursuit. These epitopes are often expressed at very high levels on tumour cells but at very low levels on normal tissues. The earliest exploitation of radiolabelled monoclonal antibodies occurred a few years after their initial development at the beginning of the 1980s. It was shown that these relatively large proteins could specifically interact with their complementary epitopes *in vivo*, but it also became apparent that they were far from ideal targeting vectors. Physical access to the tumour cells was limited by poor blood supply and a number of physical barriers due to their large size, which also resulted in a slow rate of clearance from the bloodstream. Normal organs such as the kidney and liver accumulated much larger amounts of radioactivity than most tumours and the xenogeneic origin of the antibodies (normally mice) resulted in their recognition as foreign proteins and production of neutralising antibodies by the recipient's immune system. In the intervening two decades, development has centred on the need to reduce the size and immunogenicity of these potentially useful molecules as described below.

To some extent this move towards size reduction has been driven by the success in tumour targeting of small radiolabelled peptide hormones, receptors for which are expressed on many tumours. The paradigm for this approach is the application of radiolabelled octreotide analogues for targeting somatostatin receptors, which show increased levels of expression by a number of tumour types (see Reubi 2003). These ligands lack many of the disadvantages of antibodies: they are small, typically 100 times smaller than IgG. This allows them to diffuse more easily into the tumour environment and clear more rapidly from the bloodstream and, because they are of human origin, they are not recognised by the patient's immune system. While peptides do possess disadvantages of their own, it is clear that, particularly as imaging radiopharmaceuticals, they represent a very useful class of compound.

Structure and production of proteins and peptides

All polypeptides consist of amino acids linked together by amide (peptide) bonds. They differ in the number and variety of amino acids they contain. Smaller oligomers are called peptides. Peptides larger than 5–6 amino acids are able to form secondary structures such as turns, folds, sheets and helices due to interactions between the side-chains of the constituent amino acids; and the greater the length of the peptide chain, the more complex the possible configurations. Eventually these secondary structures are themselves able to interact to form tertiary structures and at this stage the compounds are called proteins. These secondary and tertiary structures result in amino acid sequences being grouped together either on the surface or in the interior of the molecule. The former can form binding motifs (ligands) that are able to interact with other structures (receptors) on other molecules in order to elicit some sort of biological response. It is this interaction that forms the basis of the biomolecular targeting that can be exploited for radiopharmaceutical imaging and targeted therapy.

Two distinct methods of production are possible for these types of compounds. Small peptides – typically up to about 50 amino acids in size – are normally made by chemical synthesis, while larger proteins are produced by biosynthesis in cells.

Solid-phase peptide synthesis

Manual solid-phase peptide synthesis (SPPS) was originally developed by Merrifield but is now commonly performed using automated peptide synthesisers. However the basic principle remains the same. It consists of the sequential reaction of amino acid analogues in which the C-terminus is activated to form an active ester and the N-terminus and amino acid side-chain are blocked by different protecting groups as shown in Figure 14.1. The first protected amino acid (AA-1) in the chain (actually that at the C-terminus) is initially linked to a solid resin. The protection group on the N-terminus is released and a molar excess of the second activated amino acid (AA-2) added. The active ester of AA-2 reacts with the N-terminus of AA-1 to form a peptide bond. The protection group

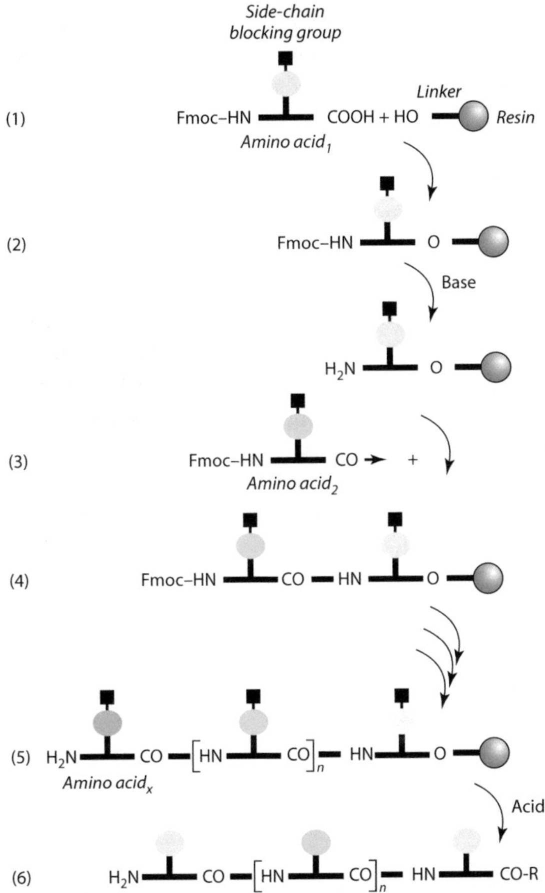

Figure 14.1 Typical solid-phase peptide synthesis (SPPS) using the Fmoc strategy. An analogue of the amino acid at the C-terminus of the desired peptide is first attached to an insoluble resin via hydroxyl groups to produce an acid labile bond (1). The amino group on this amino acid is blocked by Fmoc (fluorenylmethoxycarbonyl) and a reactive side-chain functionality is blocked by another appropriate blocking group to protect them during the linear peptide synthesis. The Fmoc protecting group is then removed by treatment with pyridine (2) to generate a free amino group and either a pre-formed activated ester of the second required (blocked) amino group is added to the resin or it is generated *in situ* (3). This active ester reacts with the exposed free amino-terminus of the first amino-acid to produce a dipeptide (4). This cycle of de-protection and peptide bond formation is repeated (5) until the full required sequence of the desired peptide is completed. The peptide is then released from the resin and the side-chain protecting groups are removed by treatment with acid (6).

on the N-terminus of AA-2 is then removed and unreacted components are washed away before the process is repeated with AA-3. In this way a linear peptide is gradually built up on the resin support. When the required peptide sequence is complete, the protection groups on the amino acid side-chains are removed and the peptide is cleaved from the resin into solution from where it can be isolated. One of the most important issues in SPPS is yield. Since the synthetic reactions are repetitive, even a relatively high yield for individual addition steps can lead to a low overall lead.

Protein biosynthesis

Biosynthesis in cells results from the natural process of ribosomal protein transcription. The principal task is therefore to transfect a suitable sequence of DNA into a host cell such that the resulting translation and transcription results in the expression of a protein of the desired sequence. Biosynthesis has a number of disadvantages compared with SPPS owing to the need for living cells. These require specialised production facilities and carry the risks of harbouring viruses and other microorganisms that could be transmitted to the ultimate human recipients.

Antibodies are relatively large, complex proteins in which the tertiary structures produced by association of peptide folding domains are further combined. Thus the IgG immunoglobulin subclass (the type most commonly used as pharmaceuticals) consist of two pairs of protein chains that are held together by disulfide bonds as well as non-covalent forces. Each protein chain consists of a number of domains that have different functions. The diversity of protein sequence that is the source of the antibodies' specificity for a particular target or 'epitope' resides in the highly 'variable' domains while the 'constant' domains or 'framework regions' vary little from one antibody to another and are responsible for initiating secondary immune systems such as complement activation. A diagram showing the various components and regions of IgG is shown in Figure 14.2.

The classical method of monoclonal antibody production is shown in Figure 14.3. A suitable animal, normally a mouse but alternatively any small mammal, is injected several times with the immunogen in order to boost the immune response. The animal is then killed and the spleen, which contains the majority of the lymphocytes responsible for antibody production, is dissected and separated into a cell suspension. The lymphocytes present in the cell suspension will grow and produce antibody for a short time in tissue culture, but after a few days will normally die. In order to immortalise the cells, they are fused with tumour cells – normally myeloma cells –using polyethylene glycol, which destabilises the cell membranes. The result of the fusion process is 'hybridoma' cells, which have both the antibody-producing properties of the lymphocyte and the immortality of the tumour cell. They can thus be grown indefinitely in tissue culture. At this stage, the cell population is still heterogeneous, consisting of a number of different hybridomas producing different antibodies. The cells can now be 'cloned' in order to separate them into 'monoclonal' populations of cells each producing a single antibody.

In recent years, at least for large-scale production such as is required for pharmaceutical application, this method has been supplemented or replaced by use of DNA recombinant methods. Thus the DNA is extracted from the lymphocytes and transfected into recipient cells for protein production. These recipient

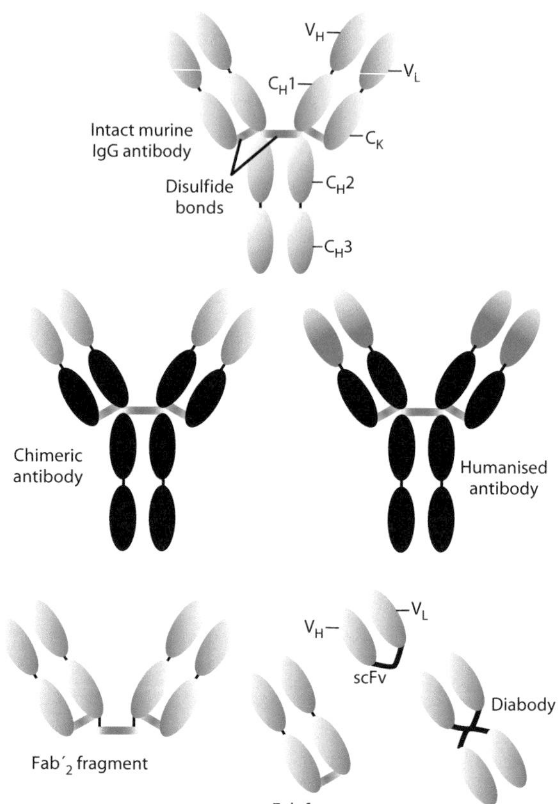

Figure 14.2 Structures of antibody-based biomolecules. Antibodies consist of two pairs of protein chains ('heavy' and 'light') joined together by disulfide bridges. The protein chains are composed of several 'domains' which have sequences that are either relatively constant (C_H1–3 and C_K or L) or highly variable V_H and V_L. The combination of the variable domains provides the unique binding sites of antibodies. Since most monoclonal antibodies are derived initially from mice, the protein sequences contain typical mouse-like sequences of amino acids. These are recognised as 'foreign' after administration to patients and can result in an anti-mouse immune response. In order to overcome this problem, more human-like antibodies can be produced using recombinant technology to graft mouse and human immunoglobulin sequences together. These are termed either 'chimeric' or 'humanised' antibodies depending on the proportion of mouse-derived protein remaining. Smaller antibody fragments can also be generated using either proteolytic enzymes (Fab′$_2$ and Fab) or recombinant approaches (e.g. scFv, diabody).

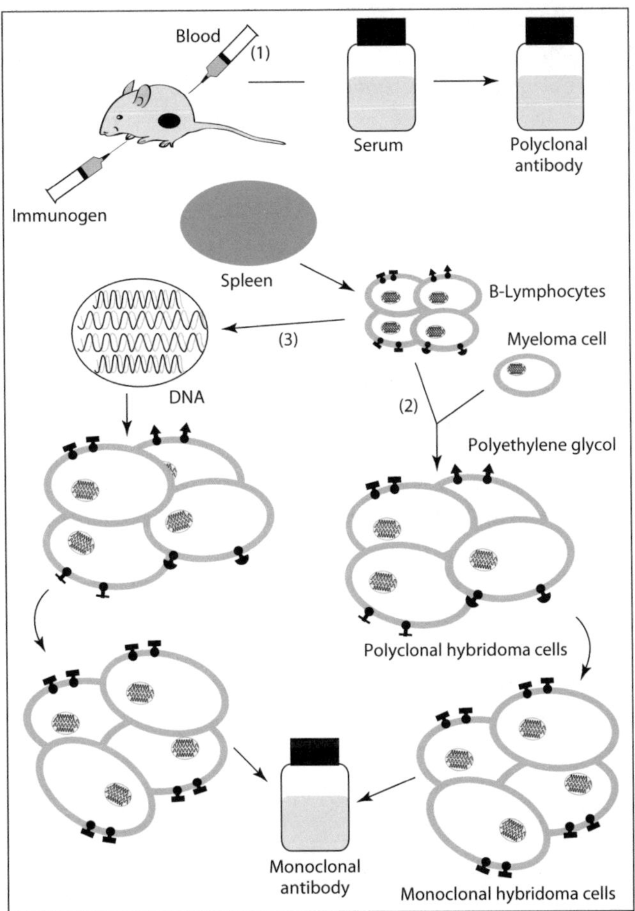

Figure 14.3 Methods for production of antibodies. The classical method of generating antibodies is by administration of an immunogen to a suitable animal, and purification of (polyclonal) antibodies from the harvested supernatant (route 1). Monoclonal antibodies may be generated by harvesting the spleen from the immunised animal and fusing the released B-lymphocytes with myeloma cells to produce hybridoma cells. After dilution cloning of these cells, a single population of hybridomas producing a homogeneous monoclonal antibody can be obtained (route 2). More commonly, especially for pharmaceutical applications, the DNA from the lymphocytes is cloned into recipient producer cells such as Chinese hamster ovary (CHO) cells to produce a library of antibody-producing cells from which the desired antibody can be selected (route 3).

cells are highly characterised, have optimal protein production systems, and are less likely to be infected by viruses than the hybridomas. A major disadvantage of antibodies produced by hybridoma technology is that the protein produced is essentially foreign, originating as it does from murine lymphocytes. When administered to patients, especially repeatedly, the recipient's immune system recognises them as foreign and mounts an immune response producing 'human anti-mouse-antibodies' (HAMA) that bind to and neutralise the administered antibody. This problem can be overcome by replacing those sequences responsible for the immune response by more human-like sequences using recombinant technology. Since the specificity of the antibody resides solely in the variable domains, it is possible to entirely replace the constant domains of murine origin by those of human origin to produce so called 'chimeric' antibodies that retain only around 30% of their mouse sequences and are considerably less immunogenic than entirely murine antibodies. A further reduction in immunogenicity can be achieved by transplanting the hypervariable regions of the original antibody – the complementarity determining regions (CDRs) into an entirely human framework to produce so-called 'humanised' antibodies as shown in Figure 14.2.

For the reasons outlined above, there are perceived advantages in producing smaller versions of antibodies for radiopharmaceutical use. The classical approach to such a problem was to generate so-called 'Fab fragments' (see Figure 14.2) by enzymatic degradation of intact immunoglobulins. However, recombinant approaches are now the preferred methods. In addition to generating Fab fragments, such methods can also be used to produce smaller antibody analogues such as single-chain variable fragments (ScFv), diabodies and minibodies (Figure 14.2). All of these antibody-derived constructs contain one or more epitope-binding sites but a smaller framework region.

A more recent approach to miniaturising of antibodies is to transplant the hypervariable regions into other smaller non-antibody-based frameworks. Some of the smallest of these constructs approach the size at which they can now be potentially synthesised by SPPS, although for large-scale preparation biosynthesis remains the preferred route of production. Antibody ligands are also increasingly being generated not via classical immunisation but by screening of libraries, for example by phage display. For more details of such screening approaches see Chapter 34.

Radiolabelling of proteins and peptides

While antibodies can be considered typical examples of 'receptor'-binding proteins, many other examples exist in mammalian biology such as growth factors, cytokines and peptide hormones and can potentially be exploited for *in-vivo* targeting. All of these compounds are composed of the same building blocks – amino acids – and can be radiolabelled in essentially the same way.

The choice of radionuclide will depend upon the ultimate application for the radiopharmaceutical. For imaging purposes the same radionuclides used for other SPECT or PET imaging applications will be employed. A list of those most commonly used is shown in Table 14.1. The general rule of thumb that

Table 14.1 Physical decay characteristics of radionuclides used for labelling biomolecules

Radionuclide	Type of decay	Energy (MeV)		Half-life
		$E_{\beta max}$ (abundance)	E_γ (abundance)	
^{125}I	EC		0.035(7%)	60 days
^{123}I	EC		0.159 (84%)	13 hours
^{111}In	EC		0.173(91%) 0.247(94%)	2.8 days
^{99m}Tc	IT		0.141(89%)	6.02 hours
^{68}Ga	β^+		0.511 (89%)	68 minutes
^{18}F	β^+		0.511 (100%)	110 minutes
^{131}I	β^-, γ	0.61(86%) 0.33(13%)	0.364(80%) 0.284(6%)	8.04 days
^{90}Y	β^-	2.27		64 hours
^{188}Re	β^-, γ	2.1	155(15%)	17 hours
^{186}Re	β^-, γ	1.08	137(9%)	89 hours
^{177}Lu	β^-, γ	0.5	0.208 (10%) 0.113(6%)	6.7 hours

the physical half-life of the radionuclide should match the biological half-life of the radiotracer remains true for biomolecular radiopharmaceuticals and therefore the radiolabel of choice for intact antibodies is usually indium-111 for SPECT and iodine-124 for PET, while technetium-99m, fluorine-18 and gallium-68 are preferred for smaller antibody fragments and peptides although, despite this generalisation, indium-111 is also widely employed for labelling neuropeptides.

Although a wide number of radionuclides have been explored in the past for experimental targeted therapy studies, a relatively small number remain in common use. To a large extent the choice of therapeutic radionuclide is determined by practical issues such as cost and availability, especially for clinical studies. It is also essential that the radionuclide is available in high specific activity.

Radiolabelling methods

Methods for radiolabelling biomolecules are often classified as either 'direct' or 'indirect'. In direct methods the radioactive atom forms either covalent or coordinate bonds directly with the constituent atoms of the amino acid side-chains, while indirect methods rely on an intervening prosthetic moiety which is first conjugated to the protein or peptide. Radiolabelling methods can also be categorised according to the chemistry of the radioactive element and the three main categories in general use are those used for halogens, in particular iodine, for trivalent metallic ions such as indium, gallium, lutetium and yttrium, and for group 7 elements such as technetium and rhenium. A detailed description of the chemistry of these labelling methods is contained elsewhere in this book (see Chapters 7–13) and details in this chapter are therefore confined to a description of the ways in which these methods have been employed for biomolecules.

Iodine

Iodine was the first isotope to be used for radiolabelling studies with antibodies. ^{125}I and ^{131}I have the advantages of cheapness and wide availability and, although neither is ideal for either diagnostic or therapeutic use, the same iodination methods can be used for ^{123}I.

Direct labelling by electrophilic substitution is by far the most widely practised method for labelling of proteins with iodine (see Chapter 10). The labelling is mediated by oxidation of the iodide ion to the positively charged iodous ion (H_2OI^+), which labels the phenolic ring of the tyrosine amino acid side-chain in the *ortho-* and *para-*positions. Many oxidising systems have been used for this purpose, but the most popular are chloramine-T and Iodogen. Chloramine-T is a powerful oxidant and if exposed to the fragile proteins for long periods may oxidise the side-chains of its constituent amino acids. For this reason, after a brief exposure to the chloramine-T, the reaction is stopped by the addition of sodium metabisulfite. For laboratory work, this method has the advantage of flexibility. The concentrations of the reagents can be adjusted in order to optimise the labelling for different proteins. When labelling for clinical application, however, the need to prepare fresh reagents for each labelling and the difficulties in ensuring sterility of the process argue against the use of this method. The Iodogen method is much more suitable for clinical application since sterile Iodogen tubes can be prepared, validated for clinical use, stored at reduced temperatures and used as required. Radiolabelling is performed by the addition of the protein and the radioiodine to the tube and incubation for 5–10 minutes. At the end of this time, a labelling efficiency of 70–80% will be achieved, and the unreacted 'free' iodine can be removed by either gel-filtration, ion exchange or reversed-phase chromatography.

These methods may need modification when used with iodine-123. This isotope has a much higher specific activity that either ^{125}I or ^{131}I and the chemical amounts of iodine present in the radioiodine solutions will be correspondingly much smaller. In the presence of very low iodide concentrations, these methods are not very efficient, but labelling efficiency can be improved by adding small amounts of carrier iodide in the form of 'cold' potassium iodide.

Radioiodination is much less commonly used for peptides than for proteins. One reason for this is that iodinated peptides are relatively hydrophobic and are excreted via the hepatobiliary tract (see below). Nevertheless, peptides containing tyrosine residues can also be labelled by the same methods. Peptides lacking tyrosine or larger proteins (in which electrophilic substitution results in a loss of biological activity) can also be labelled by indirect iodination methods, although these are rarely employed owing to their low labelling yields.

Trivalent metals

The radiochemistry of these elements is dominated by coordination chemistry (see Chapter 9), but such elements do not form stable complexes with amino acid side-chains. Accordingly a chelating group must first be inserted into the biomolecule in order to form a stable binding site for the radionuclide. This is normally achieved by the use of bifunctional chelating agents. These are compounds that contain a chelating group capable of forming a strong complex with the radionuclide of choice plus a chemically reactive group that allows the chelator to be attached to a functional group on the biomolecule – typically an amino group. Such bioconjugates can be prepared in two ways. For small peptides prepared by SPPS, the method of choice is to conjugate the chelating group while the peptide is on the resin; this improves reaction efficiency and simplifies purification, it also allows the conjugation to be placed at any desired point in the peptide sequence. This is essential to eliminate the possibility of inhibition of receptor binding by the chelate. For proteins prepared by biosynthesis, such a precise placement of the chelator is rarely possible. The conjugation is performed after production of the protein and the bifunctional chelator may react with any amino group present in the molecule. Thus the conjugation may occur at any lysine side-chain or the N-terminus of the protein. This results in a heterogeneous distribution of the chelating moieties throughout the bioconjugate, with the result that it is very difficult to predict effects on the receptor-binding properties of the molecule. It is, however, also possible to generate bifunctional chelating agents that react with other functionalities on amino acid side-chains, in particular carboxylic acids (e.g. glutamic acid) and thiols (cysteine). This latter chemistry often allows a more site-specific conjugation, especially if there is only a single free thiol group available in the molecule.

The chelating groups of choice are those based on DTPA (diethylenetriamine pentaacetic acid) and DOTA (1,4,7,10-tetraazacyclododecane-1,4,7,10-tetraacetic acid). The reader is referred to Chapter 9 for a detailed description of the use and radiolabelling of such chelating agents.

Group 7 elements: technetium and rhenium

Technetium-99m is a useful radionuclide for labelling small peptides and proteins and, although its relatively short half-life does not match the long blood clearance times of large proteins such as intact immunoglobulins, technetium-labelled antibodies have been used in clinical practice. Rhenium-labelled proteins and peptides have also been explored for targeted radionuclide therapy but their clinical use has so far been restricted to exploratory trials.

Biomolecules can be labelled with technetium-99m using either direct or indirect approaches. Technetium forms stable complexes with sulfur-containing compounds and can bind to free thiols in proteins. This method has been most widely exploited to label the thiol groups in the hinge region of immunoglobulins. Normally these thiol groups are in the oxidised, disulfide form and are unavailable for labelling. However, in the presence of mild reducing conditions, free thiols can be exposed in order to form a stable complex with technetium. The most effective reducing agents are either sulfur-containing compounds such as mercaptoethanol and dithiothreitol or phosphines such as tris(2-carboxyethyl) phosphine (TCEP). After a reduction in bulk, the reducing agent must be removed and the antibody divided into patient-sized aliquots. Disulfide reduction can also be achieved by irradiation with UV light and this provides a convenient method that removes the need for post reduction of the reduced antibody. After reduction by either means, the reduced thiols are prone to re-oxidation to disulfides and this must be prevented by removing oxygen from solvents and storing the reduced antibody either in frozen or in lyophilised form. The antibody is labelled by the addition of technetium, stannous ion and a weak complexing agent such as methylene diphosphonate. This ensures that any labelling of the protein occurs via the exposed thiol groups and not at other low-affinity binding sites in the protein. Labelling efficiencies of at least 95% can be routinely achieved without the need for any further purification of the radiopharmaceutical. Although this is a very simple and reliable method, its use is limited to disulfide-bridged proteins in which reduction of this bond does not compromise the biological function of the molecule. This is the case for very few types of protein since in many instances reduction of disulfide bridges results in a change in conformation that disturbs interaction with the receptor, also many proteins lack disulfide bridges completely. A further, somewhat academic, disadvantage is that the precise chemistry of the radiometal complex is unknown. Although the technetium is expected to bind to one or more of the exposed sulfur atoms, the remaining atoms contributing to the complex are unknown.

For most proteins and all small peptides, therefore, this direct labelling method is unsuitable and an indirect labelling method based on the use of bifunctional complexing agents must be used. Although similar in principle to the methods described above for trivalent metals, the chelating agents of choice for technetium will be different from those used for indium and yttrium. The most widely used chelating agents are those based on amino- or amido-thiol chelators such as mercaptoacetyltriglycine (MAG3) and hydrazinonicotinic acid (HYNIC). For further details see Chapter 8.

A further labelling method that falls somewhere in between the categories of direct and indirect is that based on the tricarbonyl Tc(I) precursor. In this complex the technetium or rhenium is bonded to three stable carbonyl bonds and three unstable bonds with water. These later unstable bonds can be replaced by coordinate bonds with suitable donors in the peptide side-chains. Pyridine nitrogen atoms in the side-chains of histidine amino acids have the potential to form strong complexes with this agent and it has been used for labelling recombinant proteins containing the hexahistidine tag. However, the conformation of histidine as presented in a normal amino acid sequence does not provide the most ideal binding site and 'artificial' binding sites are normally inserted into the peptide sequence during SPPS.

Analysis of radiolabelled biomolecules

Like all radiopharmaceuticals, radiolabelled biomolecules must be 'fit for purpose' and must comply with appropriate quality specifications. Many of these specifications such as radiochemical purity, sterility, and so on are shared with other simpler radiotracers, but in many cases the methods employed to analyse them are different.

Chemical and radiochemical purity

A simple assessment of labelling efficiency, suitable for routine quality control of the product, can be made using thin-layer chromatography (see Chapter 23). Cellulose-based papers or silica gel-coated plates or strips (e.g. ITLC) form a suitable solid phase and a variety of mobile phases can be used depending on the radiolabelling chemistry employed and the nature of the biomolecule. A list of potentially useful radio-TLC systems is shown in Table 14.2. Large proteins bind strongly to cellulose and silica gel and tend to remain at the site of application (together with insoluble impurities such as reduced hydrolysed technetium – 'colloid') unless the solid phase is first coated with a protecting agent such as albumin. However such methods are only able to separate protein- or peptide-bound radioactivity from unbound species and they are not able to detect the presence of undesired protein or peptide impurities. Detection of such contaminants requires a more powerful chromatographic separation such as liquid chromatography, normally in the form of HPLC (high performance liquid chromatography). Such methods have the advantage that they are able to detect the presence of both unlabelled compounds (normally by UV absorbance) and radioactive components (by on-line radioactivity detectors). The mode of HPLC employed depends on the physicochemical characteristics of the biomolecule. Larger proteins – those with molecular weights greater than around 20 000 Da are normally analysed by size-exclusion chromatography. TSK-based columns with pore-sizes appropriate for the particular protein studied are normally used in combination with simple salt buffers such as phosphate. However, the resolution of size-exclusion HPLC is not particularly high and differences in molecular weights of several thousands of daltons are required to achieve separation. Occasionally, therefore, other methods of separation will be used, in particular gel electrophoresis (GE). In SDS-PAGE the protein sample is loaded onto the top of a gel contained between glass plates.

Table 14.2 Thin-layer chromatographic systems for analysis of radiolabelled biomolecules

Stationary phase	Mobile phase	Component	R_f
Radiolabelled proteins			
ITLC-SG	85% methanol/water	Radiolabelled protein	0
		Iodide	0.8
ITLC-SG	0.9% sodium chloride	Radiolabelled protein	0
		Labelled chelates e.g. In-EDTA, Y-DOTA, Tc-MDP, etc.	1
ITLC-SG	0.1 mol/L sodium acetate pH 5 containing 2 mmol/L EDTA	Radiolabelled protein	0
		Labelled chelates, e.g. In-EDTA, Y-DOTA	1
		Indium chloride	1
ITLC-SG pre-soaked in 5% albumin and dried in air	ethanol : ammonia : water = 2 : 1 : 5	Insoluble 'colloids'	0
		Radiolabelled protein	0.3–1
		Labelled chelates	1
Radiolabelled peptides			
ITLC-SG	0.1 mol/L sodium acetate pH 5 containing 2 mmol/L EDTA	Radiolabelled peptide	0
		Insoluble indium colloids	0
		Labelled chelates, e.g. In-EDTA/DTPA	1
ITLC-SG	10% concentrated ammonia solution–methanol (1 : 1)	Radiolabelled peptide	1
		Insoluble indium colloids	0
		Labelled chelates, e.g. In-EDTA/DTPA	1

Under the influence of an electric potential difference, the protein passes into the gel and migrates at a rate determined by the size and shape of the molecule. Effects of the electric charge borne by the protein are nullified by the addition of a detergent – sodium dodecyl sulfate (SDS) – which gives everything an equal mass-to-charge ratio. The separation may be run in one of two modes: either reducing, in which the disulfide bonds holding the protein together are cleaved; or non-reducing, in which it migrates as a single molecule. After separation, the protein bands in the gel can be visualised by staining with a dye such as Coomassie Blue or, if radioactive, by autoradiography. An example of SDS-PAGE separation of an antibody is shown in Figure 14.4.

Smaller peptides and proteins without extensive tertiary structures are normally analysed using reversed-phase chromatography. For small peptides, ODS (octadecylsilane) columns with intermediate (100–300 Å) pore sizes are generally used in combination with moderately polar mobile phase combinations such as acetonitrile–water. Separation can also often be improved by protonation of basic side-chains using acidic additives such as trifluoroacetic acid (TFA). Larger, more hydrophilic peptides and small proteins use solid phases with shorter hydrocarbon chains (e.g. C_8, C_4) in combination with more polar solvents such as ethanol–water. The use of buffered mobile phases and ion-pairing agents may also improve peak shape and separation of components with similar properties.

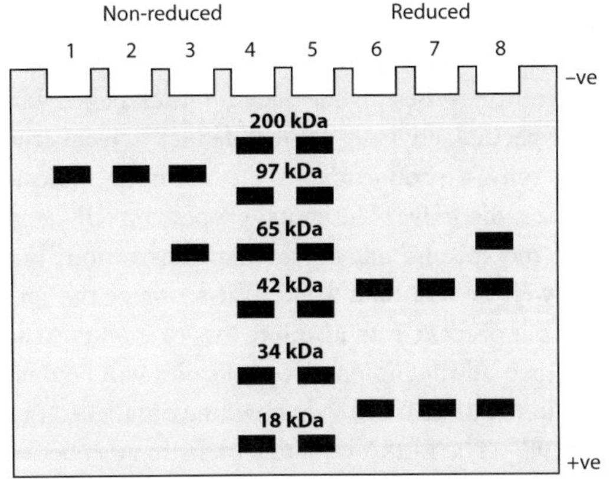

Figure 14.4 Example of a SDS-PAGE separation of a monoclonal antibody. Antibody-containing samples are first treated with a detergent sodium dodecyl sulfate (SDS) to unfold the protein chains and impose a net negative charge on the molecule. A reducing agent may also be included to cleave the intrachain disulfide bridges. The samples are then loaded into small wells in the top of a polyacrylamide (PA) gel contained between two glass plates and an electric potential difference is applied across the gel. The antibody molecules migrate into the gel at a speed determined by their molecular weight, after which their location can be determined by staining with a dye such as Coomassie blue. Typically the migration pattern of an unknown antibody sample will be compared with that of a standard antibody reference sample and with a mixture of proteins of defined molecular weight. The figure shows an example of a gel in which tracks 1 and 6 contain the reference antibody, tracks 2 and 7 a pure antibody preparation, tracks 3 and 8 an impure antibody, and tracks 4 and 5 the molecular weight markers. Tracks 1–4 contain no reducing agent, while tracks 5–8 are reduced. Tracks 1–3 show bands corresponding to the molecular weight of intact immunoglobulin, ~150 kDa, while tracks 6–8 show bands of 50 kDa and 25 kDa corresponding to heavy chain and light chain, respectively. Tracks 3 and 8 show an additional band caused by the presence of an unknown impurity.

Receptor binding

The functionality that distinguishes radiolabelled biomolecules from most simpler radiopharmaceuticals is their ability to bind to molecular targets such as receptors and antibody epitopes. It is essential that this property is maintained after the biomolecule has been through the extensive conjugation, radiolabelling and purification procedures that are often required. During the development of a new biomolecular radiopharmaceutical, therefore, it is essential to compare the binding functionality of the molecule before and after the conjugation and radiolabelling process. This is normally performed by measuring the ability of the compound to interact with its target in a suitable *in-vitro* binding assay.

Cells expressing the appropriate receptors or antibody epitopes are normally used for such assays but, when available, soluble receptors or proteins bearing the necessary epitopes are also used since they have the advantage that tissue culture of cell lines is not required.

The binding of antibody-based molecules is normally described in term of 'immunoreactivity'. This term, however, has two interpretations, either (a) the antigen binding ability of the radiolabelled antibody compared to the unlabelled starting material or (b) a measure of the proportion of the radiolabelled antibody preparation able to bind to antigen. More accurate descriptive terms might therefore be (a) relative immunoreactivity and (b) immunoreactive fraction. Both parameters are useful measures of the antibody's ability to bind to antigen, but it is important to appreciate that they are actually different and each has its own place in antibody targeting.

Relative immunoreactivity

This is a useful way of finding whether a particular process has damaged the antigen binding of an antibody preparation. It is effectively a 'before' and 'after' comparison normally performed as an enzyme linked immunosorbent assay (ELISA) on a multi-well plate. A source of the antigen, either in a purified form or as a tumour cell line, is first bound to the surface of the wells in a 96-well plate. Each well therefore contains a constant amount of antigen. Serial dilutions of the two antibody preparations to be compared are made, and a sample of each is added to separate wells and incubated for 1–2 hours to allow the antibodies to bind to the antigen. The amount of antibody that binds at any particular dilution will depend upon the affinity of that antibody preparation. Thereafter, any unbound antibody is removed by aspirating the solution from the wells and washing the plate. In order to measure the amount of antigen-bound antibody, a second antibody, capable of binding to the test antibodies, is used. This is normally an anti-species antibody such as, for example a 'rabbit anti-mouse' antibody that will bind to all immunoglobulins derived from mice. This second antibody is used in a form in which an enzyme such as horseradish peroxidase is conjugated to it. The enzyme-conjugated rabbit anti-mouse antibody is added at an appropriate dilution to each well on the plate, where it binds to the test antibodies bound to antigen. Any unbound second antibody is then, once again, washed away and an appropriate chromogenic peroxidase substitute is added. This substrate changes colour in the presence of the peroxidase and the intensity of the colour can be measured in a spectrophotometer. Thus the intensity of the colour produced is proportional to the amount of test monoclonal antibody binding to the plate.

A graph can be plotted of absorbance versus antibody dilution, giving a result similar to that shown in Figure 14.5. In this example curve 1 corresponds to the titration of a standard antibody reference sample; curve 2 corresponds to a second antibody or antibody-conjugate sample, which shows a slight but acceptable loss of immunoreactivity compared to the standard; while curve 3 corresponds to a third sample with a large and unacceptable loss of binding function.

An advantage of this technique is that the antibody does not have to be radiolabelled for the assay and the effect of any process on immunoreactivity can be determined. The assay has two disadvantages, however. The first is that the result is only relative; it does not give an absolute measure of the ability of the antibody preparation to bind to antigen. The other problem relates to heterogeneity within the antibody preparation. When an antibody is radiolabelled with a high-specific-activity radionuclide such as technetium-99m, only a proportion of the antibody molecules will be radioactive. The actual proportion will depend upon the specific activity of the preparation, but it may well be less than 10%. If a result of the radiolabelling process is an absolute loss of immunoreactivity, then all the radioactive molecules will be unable to bind to antigen, but the remaining unlabelled molecules will. The ELISA is unable to distinguish between 'hot' and 'cold' antibody and the binding of the 90% of unlabelled antibody will mask the effect of the radiolabelling.

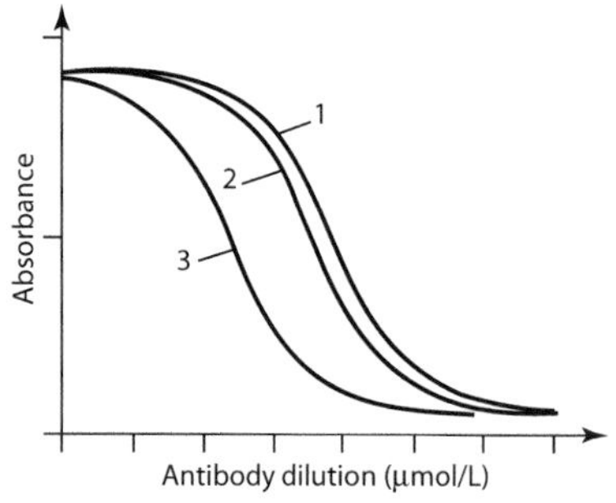

Figure 14.5 Example of an enzyme-linked immunosorbent assay (ELISA). Curve 1 corresponds to the titration of a standard antibody reference sample; curve 2 to a second antibody or antibody-conjugate sample, which shows a slight but acceptable loss of immunoreactivity compared with the standard; curve 3 corresponds to a third sample with a large and unacceptable loss of binding function.

Immunoreactive fraction

A 'direct' binding assay overcomes these disadvantages. Firstly, it measures only the binding ability of the radioactive antibody molecules, and secondly, it gives an absolute measure of immunoreactivity. This assay normally uses tumour cells as its source of antigen. A serial dilution of cells is prepared in test tubes and to each tube is added a constant small amount of radiolabelled antibody. The tubes are incubated for 1–2 hours to allow the antibody to bind, and unbound radioactivity is then removed by centrifuging and washing the cells. The amount of antibody binding to each cell preparation can then be calculated by counting the tubes and comparing the counts bound with the counts initially added. A graph is then plotted of [total counts added]/[counts bound] versus cell dilution and a straight line is obtained as shown in Figure 14.6. The reciprocal of the intercept of the line on the y-axis is a measure of the proportion of the radiolabelled antibody that would bind in the presence of an infinite amount of antigen; in other words, the proportion of radioactive antibody molecules that have the ability to bind to antigen, otherwise known as the immunoreactive fraction. Details of the methodology and mathematics of this and other direct binding techniques can be found in the paper by Lindmo and Bunn (1986).

The binding of radiolabelled peptide conjugates is normally expressed as a measure of the binding affinity of the peptide for its receptor. Two types of assay are commonly performed – so-called competition assays and saturation binding assays.

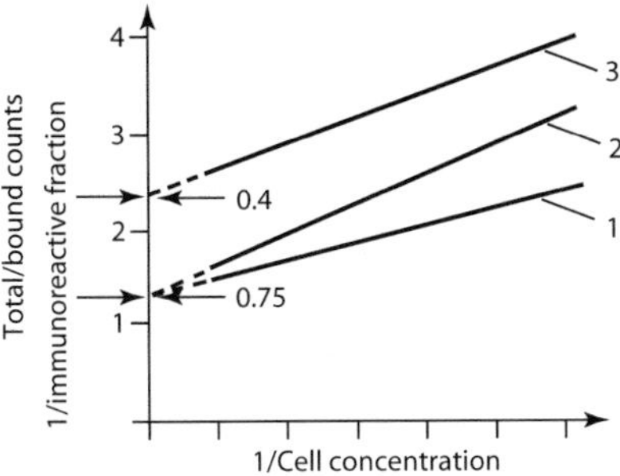

Figure 14.6 Example of an immunoreactive fraction assay. Lines 1 and 2 correspond to two antibody samples with different binding affinities but the same immunoreactive fraction of 0.75, while line 3 corresponds to an antibody with a lower immunoreactive fraction of 0.4.

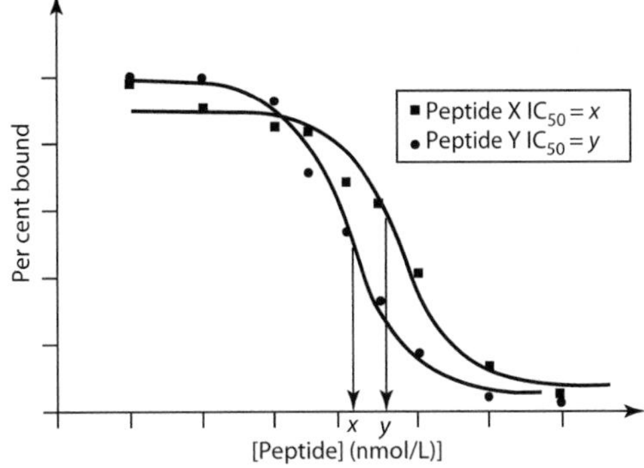

Figure 14.7 Example of a competition binding assay. Binding of a peptide radioligand in competition with two peptide analogues (X and Y) that bind to the same receptor. IC_{50} values are determined either by non-linear regression or by identification of the peptide concentration corresponding to a 50% reduction in radioligand binding.

Competition assays provide a measure of the binding affinity of unlabelled peptides. They are therefore useful for assessing the effect of chelator conjugation on peptide function and can be usefully employed to compare the binding of a series of related peptide conjugates. The assay measures the ability of the 'cold' peptides to compete with a radiolabelled peptide for a limited number of receptor sites – normally on whole cells or cell membranes. A series of dilutions of the peptides to be assayed are prepared and added, together with a constant amount of the radiolabelled peptide, to the cell preparation. After an incubation of a few hours the bound peptide is separated from the unbound by filtration, the cell-bound radioactivity is measured in a suitable counter, and the amount of cell-bound radioactivity is plotted against peptide concentration as shown in Figure 14.7. This assay describes the binding affinity in the form of a parameter called IC_{50}. This is the concentration of peptide required to inhibit the binding of the radiolabelled peptide by a factor of 50%. Thus the lower the IC_{50}, the higher the binding affinity of the peptide.

Such assays are relatively simple to perform but, similarly to the situation with antibodies described above, do not provide a measure of the binding performance of the radiolabelled form of the biomolecule. Such a measure is provided by saturation binding assays, which determine the dissociation constant K_d of the radiolabelled peptide. In such assays a series of increasing concentrations of the radiolabelled peptide are incubated with a fixed concentration of receptor-bearing cells or cell membranes and bound peptide determined as described above. Since such compounds are able to bind to cells in both a specific (i.e. saturable, receptor-mediated) and non-specific (non-saturable) manner, this provides a measure of total binding. Non-specific binding is determined by performing a parallel series of incubations in which a large excess concentration (around 1 µmol/L) of unlabelled peptide is added to saturate all the receptor binding sites on the cells. Subtraction of the non-specific component from total binding allows specific binding to be calculated and plotted against peptide concentration as shown in Figure 14.8. The value of K_d can be determined either by non-linear regression analysis or by

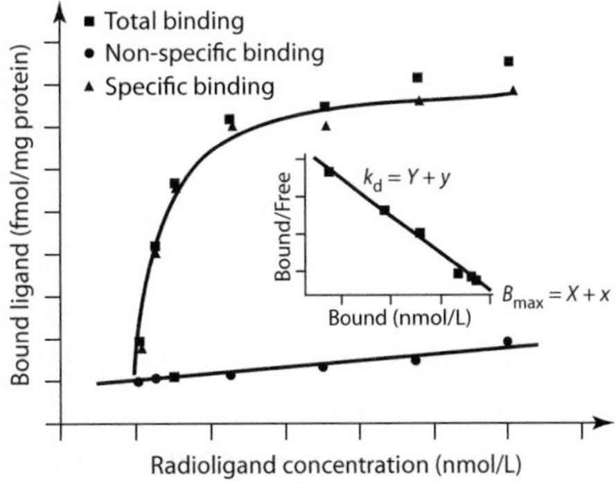

Figure 14.8 Example of a saturation binding assay. Binding of increasing concentrations of a peptide radioligand to a receptor preparation. The binding affinity of the peptide can be determined either by non-linear regression or by linear transformation (Scatchard analysis) as shown in the inset.

transformation of the data to perform a Scatchard analysis as shown Figure 14.8.

In-vivo performance of radiolabelled biomolecules

The *in-vivo* characteristics of these compounds are influenced by their physicochemical properties, in particular molecular size and hydrophilicity/lipophilicity. Proteins with a size that exceeds the molecular weight cut-off of the renal glomerular filtration system (around 50 000 Da) have long circulation times in the blood. This includes intact antibodies and many larger antibody fragments. As a result of this, blood background activity remains high with such agents for many hours or even days after administration. There is significant uptake into non-target organs such as liver, and metabolism in these organs results in the formation of radiolabelled metabolites. The fate of these metabolites depends on the radiolabelling method employed. Metabolism of radioiodinated proteins results in the formation of iodotyrosine and free iodide which are rapidly secreted out of the liver cells and then either excreted via the kidneys or (in the case of iodide) accumulated in thyroid and stomach. Metabolism of proteins labelled with metallic radionuclides results in labelled lysine adducts, which are trapped in the lysosomal compartments of the cells and are only slowly eliminated, while the metabolism of technetium-labelled antibodies follows a pattern somewhere between these two extremes. After administration, target uptake gradually increases, reaching a maximum (with intact antibodies) at about 24 hours after injection, although maximal target to non-target ratios may not be achieved until some time later. Target uptake in most tumours is limited by poor physical access of the labelled antibody to its cellular binding sites. Fluid flow within the tumour is limited by high intratumoral pressures and, since antibodies are relatively large, they leave the vasculature with difficulty and diffuse only slowly into the tumour. As a result, uptake into most solid tumours is low – of the order of 0.1% of the administered dose per gram of tumour tissue. The exception to this general observation is in haematological malignancies such as lymphoma. Such tumours have a much looser structure, allowing antibodies to gain access to their epitopes much more easily and resulting in a tumour uptake up to ten times that seen with solid tumours.

While antibody based-compounds show high stability in the blood, many naturally occurring neuropeptide hormones are unstable in the bloodstream and are rapidly degraded by serum proteases. This is a natural mechanism for limiting the duration of their normal pharmacological action. In addition, this pharmacological activity can lead to undesirable side-effects even at very low doses. To improve the stability, the sequence of the natural peptide can be modified by insertion of unnatural amino acids or modification of peptide bonds, provided that this does not disrupt their interaction with the receptor. The pharmacological activity can be viewed from both negative and positive angles. The fate of most pharmacological agonists after binding to the receptor is that the receptor–ligand complex is internalised and packed in intracytoplasmic vesicles from which the receptor is re-cycled to the cell surface but in which the ligand is degraded. Depending on the radionuclide being used, this can result in it being trapped within the cell for the duration of its physical decay. This long retention time can greatly enhance the imaging or therapeutic performance of the radiopharmaceutical. The downside of the pharmacological activity is that receptor binding also results in transmission of a secondary intracellular message that has some biological consequence. Depending on the nature of the biological effect, it may or may not be an acceptable side-effect of the nuclear medicine procedure. If it is considered unacceptable then either doses below the pharmacological limit must be used (if possible) or peptides with antagonist actions must be employed, even if these lack the desirable property of internalisation.

Peptides and proteins with a molecular weight below around 50 000 Da can be filtered through the glomerulus and show a much more rapid blood clearance. The behaviour of such conjugates is much more dependent on their relative hydrophilicity/lipophilicity than on their size. Lipophilic peptides show a mixed route of excretion – being eliminated by the hepatobiliary tract as well as the kidney. As a result, there is generalised accumulation of radioactivity in the gastrointestinal tract and this obscures any target tissue uptake in the abdomen. More hydrophilic peptides show little excretion through the hepatobiliary tract and are excreted solely by the renal tract. However, they also show a variable degree of retention in the kidneys. After filtration, many valuable substances in the primary urine such as vitamins, ions and peptides are reabsorbed in the proximal tubules. They are catabolised in the lysosomes and the constituent amino acids are trafficked back to the blood where they are reabsorbed and recycled. Radiometabolites show a variable pattern of behaviour depending on their characteristics. Radioiodinated compounds may be secreted out of the cells into the bloodstream, but radiometallated compounds are again trapped in the tubular cells, resulting in renal retention of radioactivity. The degree of renal retention varies considerably from compound to compound and can, to some extent, be reduced by co-administration of substances such as positively charged amino acids and gelofusine that compete for the renal reabsorption mechanisms.

Clinical use of radiolabelled biomolecules

Radiolabelled proteins and peptides have been widely explored in clinical studies but relatively few have received market authorisation by regulatory bodies for routine clinical use.

Two radiolabelled peptide conjugates have been approved. These are ^{111}In-DTPA–octreotide (Octreoscan) and ^{99m}Tc-depreotide (NeoSpect) both of which are use for imaging somatostatin receptors. Their structures are shown in Figure 14.9. Five different somatostatin receptor subtypes (SSTR) exist and these two peptides show different degrees of selectivity for the various subtypes. Octreoscan binds most strongly to the SST2R, which is highly expressed in neuroendocrine tumours, some types of brain tumours, and to a lesser extent in other tumours including lung, breast and lymphoma. NeoSpect, on the other hand, has relatively high binding on SST5R. While Octreoscan is excreted almost solely by the kidney, NeoSpect shows a significant degree of hepatobiliary excretion and this results in significant non-specific accumulation in the gastrointestinal tract a few hours after administration. As a result, NeoSpect is most useful for imaging lung adenocarcinoma, in which it has a negative predictive value of >90%.

Both of these peptides can be considered to be 'first-generation' radiopharmaceuticals and improvements on their design have been made since their original introduction, although these later-generation compounds have not been commercialised. The therapeutic use of these peptides represents a significant advance in the practice of targeted radionuclide therapy in recent years. DOTATOC and DOTATATE (see Figure 14.9) have structures similar to Octreoscan but the substitution of a phenylalanine residue in position 3 by tyrosine in both peptides and the replacement of the alcohol group at the C-terminus by a carboxylic acid group (in DOTATATE) results in a significant improvement in binding affinity to SST2R. At the same time, the replacement of DTPA as a chelator by DOTA allows the peptide to be labelled with high stability by therapeutic radionuclides such as yttrium-90 and lutetium-177.

Small-scale clinical studies have also been performed with neuropeptides binding to other receptor systems, of which the most promising are the gastrin-releasing peptide (bombesin) and gastrin/cholecystokinin receptors.

Because of the limitations described above, antibodies do not make ideal imaging agents and although a number of antibody-based bioconjugates were initially commercialised and approved for use,

Ala – Gly – Cys* – Lys – Asn – Phe – Phe – Trp – Lys – Thr – Phe – Thr – Ser – Cys*	**Somatostatin – 14**
(D)Phe – Cys* – Phe – (D)Trp – Lys – Thr – Cys* – Thr(ol)	**Octreotide (OC)**
(D)Phe – Cys* – Tyr – (D)Trp – Lys – Thr – Cys* – Thr(ol)	**Try-3-octreotide (TOC)**
(D)Phe – Cys* – Tyr – (D)Trp – Lys – Thr – Cys* – Thr – OH	**Try-3-octreotate (TATE)**
(D)Phe – Cys* – Nal – (D)Trp – Lys – Thr – Cys* – Thr(ol)	**Naphthyl-3-octreotide (NOC)**
(D)Phe – Cys* – Phe – (D)Trp – Lys – Val – Cys* – Thrv – NH_2	**Lanreotide**
(*N*-Me)Phe* – Tyr – (D)Trp – Lys – Val – Hcy*	**Depreotide**

Figure 14.9 Structures of radiopeptides binding to somatostatin receptors. The amino acid sequences of somatostatin-derived peptides used for imaging/therapy of somatostatin receptor-expressing tumours. All the peptides are cyclised through the residues shown by the asterisks.

they have now been withdrawn from the market. Only one radiolabelled antibody preparation is now licensed for clinical use and this is ^{99m}Tc-sulesomab (Leukoscan) a murine antibody fragment for imaging of activated granulocytes in infection.

Antibodies have also been extensively explored as vehicles for targeted radionuclide therapy but the long circulation times result in high radiation doses to non-target organs especially the bone marrow, and this, combined with the relatively low tumour uptake, has severely limited their clinical utility. However, as described above, haematological tumours represent an exception and in this indication bone marrow irradiation may actually be an advantage since much of the disease is actually located in this region. Two therapeutic radiolabelled antibodies have therefore been commercialised and approved for the treatment of non-Hodgkin lymphoma. Both are intact murine antibodies binding to the CD-20 receptor which is present both on normal mature B-cells and NHL tumour cells. Tositumomab (Bexxar) is labelled with iodine-131 and ibritumomab tiuxetan (Zevalin) with yttrium-90 via a DTPA chelator. Further details on these bioconjugates can be found in Chapter 9.

Conclusion

Radiolabelled biomolecules remain one of the most intensively explored fields in radiopharmaceutical development. Suitable methods for production and radiolabelling of these compounds are now well established and, as our ability to tailor their pharmacokinetics improves, it is likely that compounds of this class, especially those based on radiolabelled peptides, will continue to be the source of clinically useful diagnostic and therapeutic radiopharmaceuticals in the future.

References

Lindmo T, Bunn Jr PA (1986). Determination of the true immunoreactive fraction of monoclonal antibodies after radiolabelling. *Methods Enzymol* 121: 678–691.

Reubi JC (2003). Peptide receptors as molecular targets for cancer diagnosis and therapy. *Endocr Rev* 24(4): 389–427.

Further reading

Cooper MS *et al.* (2006). Conjugation of chelating agents to proteins and radiolabeling with trivalent metallic isotopes. *Nat Protoc* 1(1): 314–317.

Dillman RO (2006). Radioimmunotherapy of B-cell lymphoma with radiolabelled anti-CD20 monoclonal antibodies. *Clin Exp Med* 6(1): 1–12.

Ginj M, Maecke HR (2004). Radiometallo-labeled peptides in tumor diagnosis and therapy. *Met Ions Biol Syst* 42: 109–142.

Mather SJ (2005). Radioiodination of antibodies. In: Celis J, ed. *Cell Biology: A Laboratory Handbook*, 3rd edn. London: Academic Press.

Mather SJ (2007). Design of radiolabelled ligands for the imaging and treatment of cancer. *Mol Biosyst* 3(1): 30–35.

Reubi JC *et al.* (2005). Candidates for peptide receptor radiotherapy today and in the future. *J Nucl Med* 46(Suppl 1): 67S–75S.

Sosabowski JK, Mather SJ (2006). Conjugation of DOTA-like chelating agents to peptides and radiolabeling with trivalent metallic isotopes. *Nat Protoc* 1(2): 972–976.

Wu AM, Senter PD (2025). Arming antibodies: prospects and challenges for immunoconjugates. *Nat Biotechnol* 23(9): 1137–1146.

SECTION C

Radiopharmacokinetics

15

Radiopharmacokinetics

Roger D Pickett,

with the collaboration of colleagues at GE Healthcare

Introduction

In the pharma industry (Greek *pharmacon* = drug) the principal determinant of efficacy (and side-effects) is pharmacodynamics – or the effects that a drug has on physiological or pathological systems. With respect to diagnostic imaging radiopharmaceuticals, ideally there should be no pharmacodynamic effects. Efficacy is determined by the effects of physiological or pathological systems on the biodistribution of the drug (the radiopharmaceutical). This chapter deals with the effects that the body has on the radiopharmaceutical – which may be desired or undesired and are all covered by the general term 'radiopharmacokinetics'. Aspects to be covered include the mechanisms by which a radiolabelled entity gains access to its target, how it interacts with that target, and the mechanisms which serve to remove excess 'non-target' radioactivity. These processes are broken down into absorption, distribution, metabolism and excretion (ADME). Also discussed are the methods by which we can gain a better understanding of these mechanisms and how the pharmacokinetics of a radiopharmaceutical are used to provide diagnostic information to the nuclear medicine physician.

Mechanisms of localisation

Radiopharmaceuticals exhibit a large range of physical and chemical properties. Administration is usually by the intravenous route so absorption is not an issue. Mechanisms of (bio)distribution may depend on the physical form, as in the uptake of particulate material by phagocytosis, or may be brought about by the similarity of the radiopharmaceutical to a substrate or metabolite, as in the uptake of iodine isotopes by the thyroid gland. Some radiopharmaceuticals are distributed by well-understood mechanisms, while for others the processes are less well understood.

An important factor to bear in mind is that the observed biodistribution of a radiopharmaceutical cannot be explained in terms of a single mechanism but rather as the result of interactions between many different mechanisms involving initial dilution within the circulating blood, possible plasma protein binding, passive or active transmembrane transport, possible metabolic incorporation or catabolism and elimination and excretion. The molecule may also undergo non-biological degradation due to chemical or radiochemical instability, so it must also be borne in mind that the observed distribution is that of the radiolabel and not necessarily that of the intact molecule.

There are several key mechanisms through which radiopharmaceuticals become localised. These are summarised below with some examples.

Substrate non-specific

Diffusion

Xenon-133 and krypton-81m for lung ventilation

These gases simply diffuse into the air spaces within the lungs and are used to detect blockages by the absence of radioactivity in those areas. Krypton-81m is very short-lived and does not appear in other tissues. Xenon-133 gas diffuses across membranes in the lungs and circulates in the bloodstream, concentrating in fat (Alderson, Line 1980).

[^{15}O]Water

This short-lived agent is freely diffusible across membranes into all parts of the body permitting evaluation of tissue perfusion (Ter-Pogossian, Herscovitch 1985; Mullani *et al.* 2008).

Hypoxia

[^{18}F]Fluoromisonidazole

This agent localises in hypoxic regions, undergoing intracellular reduction and binding (Lee, Scott 2007).

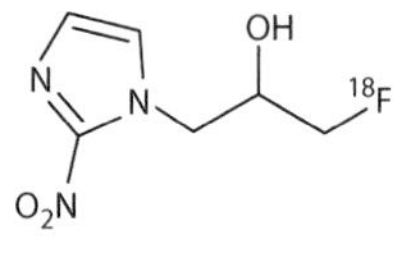

[^{18}F]Fluoromisonidazole

Isotope dilution

^{99m}Tc or ^{125}I human albumin for plasma volume determination; ^{99m}Tc or ^{51}Cr erythrocytes for red cell mass determination

An example of compartmental localisation is blood pool imaging using autologous ^{99m}Tc or ^{51}Cr-labelled red cells or ^{99m}Tc human serum albumin within the blood pool. The immediate distribution is within the blood pool; ultimately the ^{99m}Tc dissociates from these compounds and is cleared through the kidneys (Wang *et al.* 2007).

Capillary blockade and cell sequestration

^{99m}Tc macroaggregated albumin for regional lung perfusion studies

Intravenous injection of a particulate suspension results in trapping of the particles in the pulmonary bed if the particle size exceeds that of the pre-capillary diameter. There is a very large margin of safety since fewer than 1/1000 capillaries are blocked by the typical injection (Harding *et al.* 1973).

^{99m}Tc heat-denatured erythrocytes for splenic sequestration

Cell sequestration involves radiolabelling and then heat damaging a small volume of the patient's red cells (usually 10 mL) to take advantage of the spleen's normal function, i.e. removal of damaged red cells. If the cells are radiolabelled properly, this procedure permits visualisation of the spleen with minimal visualisation of the liver (Hagan *et al.* 2006).

^{111}In-oxine, ^{99m}Tc-HMPAO (exametazime, Ceretec)

Radiolabelled white blood cells (leukocytes) are used for SPECT imaging of inflammatory conditions (e.g. osteomyelitis, fever of unknown origin) (Kumar 2005).

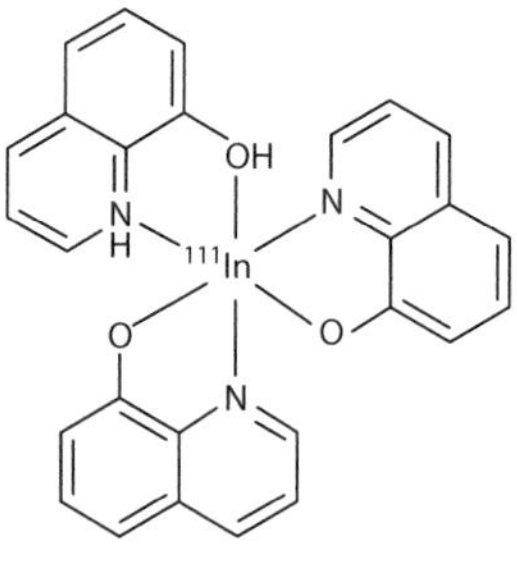

^{111}In-Oxine

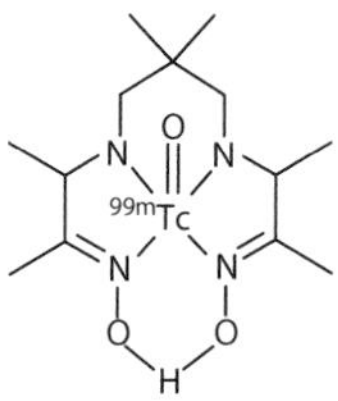

^{99m}Tc-HMPAO

Phagocytosis

^{99m}Tc tin and sulfur colloids for liver scanning

The technique uses phagocytic cells such as the Kupffer cells in the liver or macrophages in spleen or bone marrow. The most commonly used phagocytic agents, ^{99m}Tc-sulfur colloid and ^{99m}Tc-microaggregated albumin, typically have particle sizes ranging from approximately 0.1 to 2.0 μm. The smaller the particles, the greater the bone marrow uptake; larger particles tend to localise in the liver and spleen. Owing to the small size of the colloid compared with the diameter of the average capillary, which is 7 μm, capillary blockade does not occur. Distribution in the reticulo-endothelial system is typically 85% in the liver, 10% in the spleen, and 5% in marrow (Kuperus 1979).

Active or facilitated transport

Thallium-201

Myocardial perfusion imaging is routinely performed with ^{201}Tl in the form of the thallous ion (Tl^+). This involves use of the normally operative metabolic pathway for handling potassium since Tl^+ is a potassium analogue and is therefore handled efficiently by the well-documented ATPase-driven Na/K pump mechanism (Kailasnath, Sinusas 2001).

^{99m}Tc-Tetrofosmin (Myoview), ^{99m}Tc-sestamibi (Cardiolite)

^{99m}Tc-labelled tetrofosmin uptake by myocytes is reported to be a metabolism-dependent active process, not involving cation channel transport but more likely the diffusion of the lipophilic cation across the sarcolemmal and mitochondrial membranes (Platts *et al.* 1995; Younes *et al.* 1995).

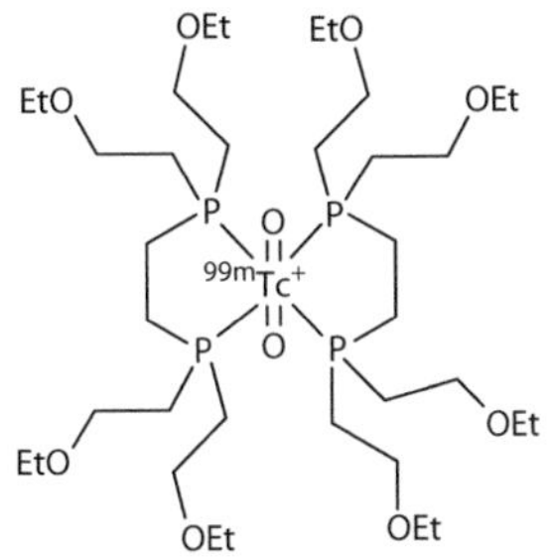

^{99m}Tc-Tetrofosmin

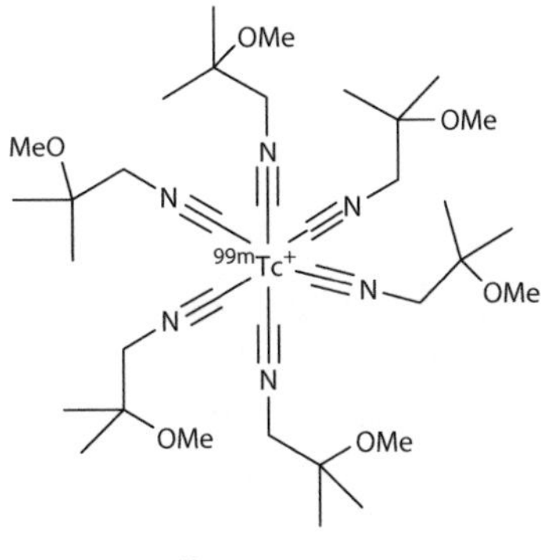

^{99m}Tc-Sestamibi

^{99m}Tc-HMPAO (Exametazime, Ceretec)

Diffusion of lipophilic complex across the blood–brain-barrier is followed by conversion to a less-lipophilic, non-diffusible complex, which is therefore trapped in proportion to regional cerebral perfusion (Neirinckx *et al.* 1988).

Substrate specific

Metabolic pathway/trapping

[^{18}F]Fludeoxyglucose

After facilitated diffusion via glucose transporters the compound is a substrate for hexokinase in glucose metabolism (Miles, Williams 2008).

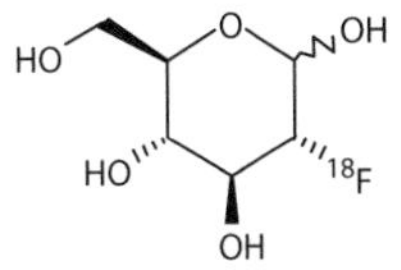

[^{18}F]Fludeoxyglucose

[^{123}I]Iodide for thyroid studies

The sodium–iodine symporter in the thyroid gland is responsible for uptake of iodine, which is then trapped by organification in thyroid hormones (Levy *et al.* 1998; Mattsson *et al.* 2006).

[^{123}I]Iodoheptadecanoic acid

Radiolabelled fatty acids are metabolic substrates and have been used for imaging the myocardium (Knapp *et al.* 1996).

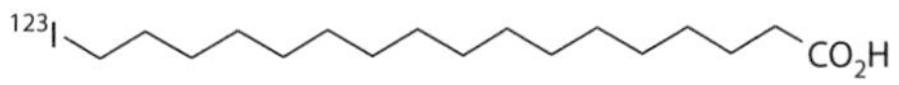

[^{123}I]Iodoheptadecanoic acid

Ion exchange/chemisorption

^{99m}Tc-MDP, ^{99m}Tc-HDP

The phosphonate groups bind avidly and essentially irreversibly to the hydroxyapatite structure of bone tissue. Typically, 40–50% of the injected dose localises in bone; the remainder is excreted through the kidneys (Weber *et al.* 1969).

[^{18}F]Fluoride

Fluoride ions are incorporated into hydroxyapatite crystals in bone (Blau *et al.* 1972).

Enzyme substrate

[^{75}Se]Selenomethionine

Selenomethionine is an analogue of the amino acid methionine. Its use in pancreas scanning is based on the fact that digestive enzymes produced by the pancreas require a very high rate of protein synthesis (Blau, Bender 1962).

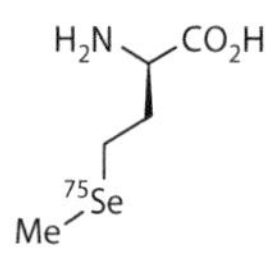

[^{75}Se]Selenomethionine

Receptor/transporter binding

^{111}In-DTPA-*d*-Phe-octreotide, ^{68}Ga-Edotreotide (DOTATOC)

These peptides bind specifically to the somatostatin receptor (SSTR-II) of many neuroendocrine tumours (Bakker *et al.* 1991a, b; Gabriel *et al.* 2007).

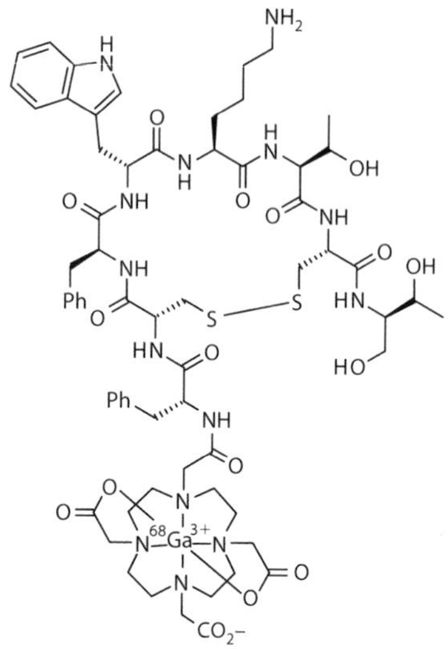

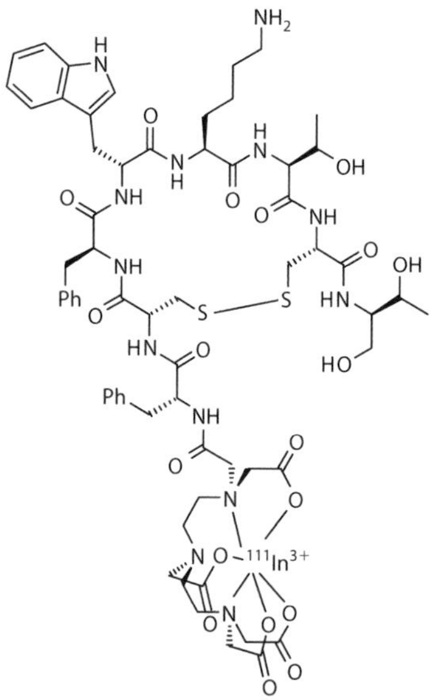

^{111}In-DTPA-D-Phe-octreotide

^{68}Ga-Edotreotide

[^{18}F]Fluoroestradiol (FES)

This radiolabelled steroid binds to oestrogen receptors in breast cancer (Mankoff *et al.* 2001; Sundararajan *et al.* 2007).

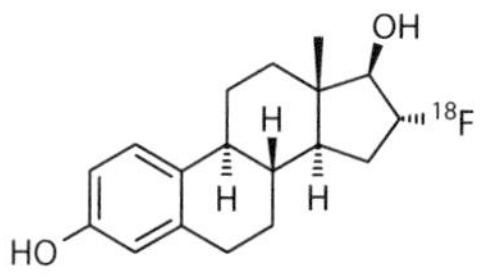

[^{18}F]Fluoroestradiol

^{64}Cu-DOTA-[Pro^1,Tyr^4]-bombesin, ^{64}Cu-MP2346

These peptide analogues of human gastrin-releasing peptide (GRP) conjugated with ^{64}Cu, have been developed for PET imaging of tumours with overexpressed GRP receptors (Biddlecombe *et al.* 2007). They have also been assessed with ^{99m}Tc and ^{111}In for SPECT imaging (de Visser *et al.* 2007).

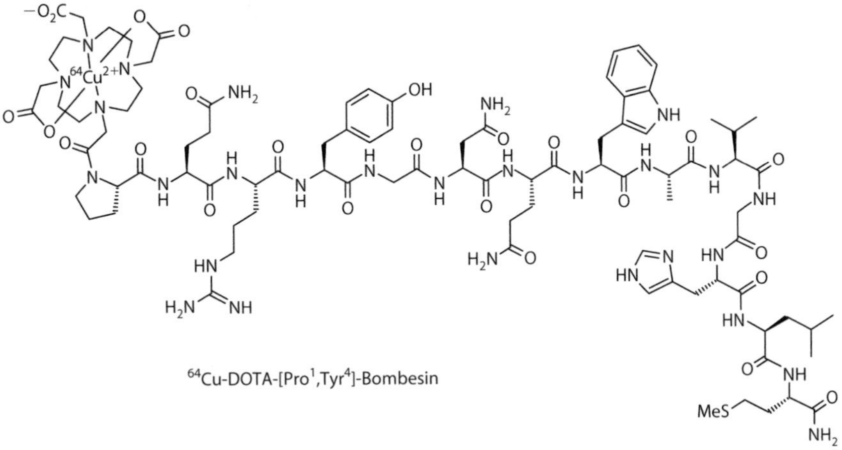

^{64}Cu-DOTA-[Pro^1,Tyr^4]-Bombesin

^{99m}Tc-NC100692 and [^{18}F]AH111585

Arginine-glycine-aspartic acid (RGD)-containing peptides conjugated with ^{99m}Tc or ^{18}F have been developed for SPECT or PET imaging of tumour-associated angiogenesis (Edwards *et al.* 2008; Glaser *et al.* 2008).

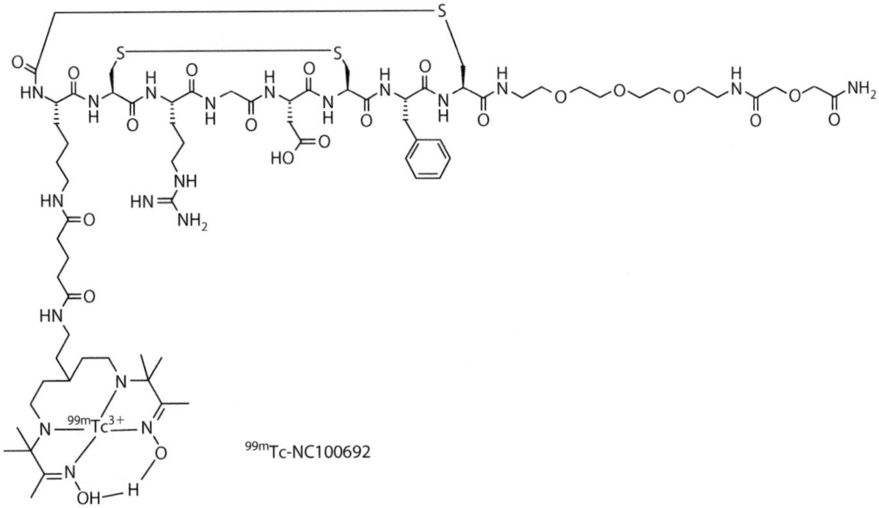

^{99m}Tc-NC100692

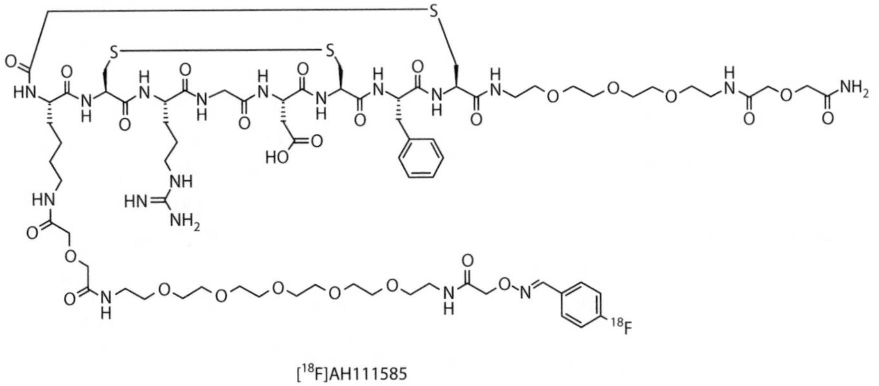

[^{18}F]AH111585

[^{11}C]PK11195

Specific binding to peripheral benzodiazepine receptors has been used to detect neuroinflammatory lesions (Banati *et al.* 1999).

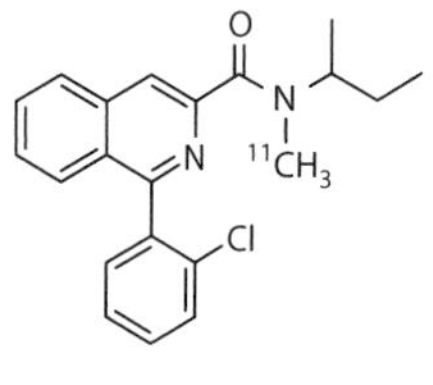

[^{11}C]PK-11195

[^{123}I]Ioflupane (DaTSCAN)

Cocaine analogues with selective affinity for the dopamine transporter are used to assess striatal dopaminergic deficits in movement disorders and dementias (Booij *et al.* 1998).

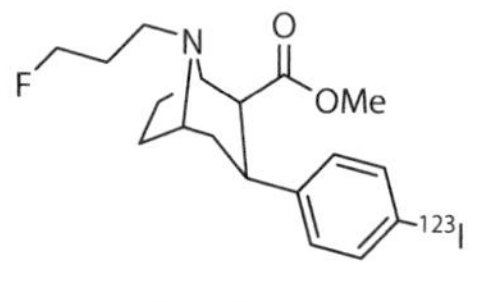

[^{123}I]Ioflupane

Antibodies

^{68}Ga-DOTA-F(ab′)$_2$-trastuzumab, ^{111}In-DTPA-trastuzumab

These labelled antibodies bind specifically to the HER2 tumour antigen (Perik *et al.* 2006).

^{64}Cu-DOTA-cetuxima

Specific binding to the epidermal growth-factor receptor antigen is used as a marker of cell proliferation (Smith-Jones *et al.* 2004).

^{111}In-Capromab pendetide (Prostascint)

Specific binding to PSMA (prostate-specific membrane antigen) allows localisation and staging of new or recurrent prostate cancer (Manyak 2008).

^{99m}Tc-Arcitumomab (CEA-Scan)

This radiolabelled antibody is used to visualise cancers expressing carcinoembryonic antigen (CEA) (Fuster *et al.* 2003).

^{99m}Tc-Sulesomab (LeukoScan)

This murine antibody fragment is used for nuclear imaging of activated granulocytes (Skehan *et al.* 2003).

Concluding remarks

The mechanisms through which radiopharmaceuticals become localised may be passive or active and may be substrate non-specific (not participating in a specific chemical reaction) or substrate specific (participating in a chemical reaction or interacting with a specific ligand). Understanding the mechanisms of biodistribution of a radiopharmaceutical requires not only a thorough knowledge of the pharmacokinetic and metabolic processes involved but also an understanding of the structure and fate of the radiopharmaceuticals themselves. Imaging shows the distribution and deposition of the radionuclide only, and not necessarily that of the intact radiopharmaceutical.

Principles of pharmacokinetics

Introduction

In general terms, the processes of absorption, distribution, metabolism and excretion (or elimination) can be described quantitatively by analysis of the concentrations of a drug in body tissues and fluids. Because most body tissues are not accessible for direct drug concentration analysis, systems have been devised whereby mathematical modelling of data that are readily available can enable inferences to be made about the behaviour of a drug in the whole body. This is particularly important for therapeutic drugs where the pharmacological responses (beneficial and/or undesired) are usually dependent upon the concentration of the drug at the locus of the effector site. A quantitative knowledge of uptake, distribution and elimination mechanisms is therefore important for determining the correct doses of drug to be administered and the frequency of dosing required to achieve an adequate concentration at the effector site. This may also be the case for therapeutic radiopharmaceuticals but for diagnostic (imaging) radiopharmaceuticals this is not absolutely essential, firstly because we are not striving to achieve a protracted pharmacologically effective concentration and secondly because of our ability to observe the processes non-invasively as they occur using the techniques described in this book. It is useful, however, to have a basic understanding of the concepts of clinical pharmacokinetics and how they may be applied to radiopharmaceuticals.

Pharmacokinetics of radiopharmaceuticals

The principles of pharmacokinetics are well established. Among the earliest authors on the subject, Teorell (1937a, b) was probably the first to introduce the concept that regards the distribution of a drug as the consequence of a series of consecutive processes or steps. These concepts were developed and extended by Wagner (1968, 1969), who described the main role of pharmacokinetics as the interpretation of data from studies of the time course of drug and metabolite levels in tissues and of the amounts excreted, and the construction of models mathematically describing the compartments into which and from which the drug appears and disappears. Models should enable the interpretation of the observed data, and the prediction of the effects of perturbations in the system. Current views on pharmacokinetics have moved away from rigid adherence to compartmental modelling to a non-compartmental approach. This recognises the fact that in many situations compartments have no physiological meaning. Gibaldi, Perrier (1982) described a non-parametric analysis that made estimates of integrals using the trapezoid rule. Bayesian analysis of non-linear models has been aided by advances in computational techniques that have broadened the class of models that can be analysed by this method (Racine *et al.* 1986). Many useful pharmacokinetic parameters can be derived from the coefficients and exponents of polyexponential equations fitted to biological data (Wagner 1976). Population pharmacokinetics will model data on a number of individuals to account for the fact that statistical variations in samples caused either by extended sampling intervals or by the presence of low levels of drug in the samples allow the data to be described by more than one model. A number of commercial pharmacokinetic analysis programmes are available.

The limitations of modelling do not apply to the same extent in nuclear medicine studies since uptake and removal of radioactivity in individual organs can be measured and described and the sampling can be almost continuous. However, it should be remembered that with diagnostic imaging radiopharmaceuticals it is the distribution of the radioactivity itself that is measured and provides the effectiveness of the product. Hence, unlike with therapeutics where pharmacokinetics relates to the parent drug compound or its active metabolite, the measured pharmacokinetics of a diagnostic imaging radiopharmaceutical may bear little relationship to the injected drug or its major metabolites. This is discussed later in this chapter.

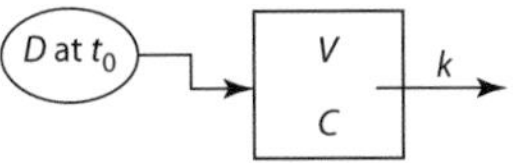

Figure 15.1 One-compartment open model with rapid intravenous injection.

One-compartment model

The simplest model is the one-compartment open model shown in Figure 15.1.

In the one-compartment open model, with rapid intravenous injection, a dose (D) of the drug is assumed to be administered at time zero (t_0) into a single compartment, with a volume of distribution V. The concentration (C) of the drug at time t, assuming first-order (concentration-dependent) kinetics, is given by the simple exponential relationship

$$C_t = C_0 e^{-kt}$$

where C_t is the concentration at time t after administration, C_0 is the concentration at time zero and k is the elimination rate constant. The relationship between the log of the concentration and time is linear. The elimination from a single compartment is shown graphically in Figure 15.2. This kind of elimination is exhibited by radiopharmaceuticals cleared from the blood by renal elimination.

This is a simple first-order process like radioactive decay, and the half-life concept can be applied here also, defined as the time required for the concentration to be halved. However, since we are dealing with radioactive materials, the effective half-life ($t_{1/2\,\mathrm{eff}}$) will be shorter than the true biological half-life ($t_{1/2\,\mathrm{biol}}$) because of simultaneous radioactive physical decay with half-life $t_{1/2\,\mathrm{phys}}$. Therefore, most radiopharmacokinetic studies make a correction for radioactive decay in order to arrive at the biological half-life. The relation between these three half-life concepts can be expressed as a sum of rate constants:

$$k_{\mathrm{eff}} = k_{\mathrm{phys}} + k_{\mathrm{biol}}$$

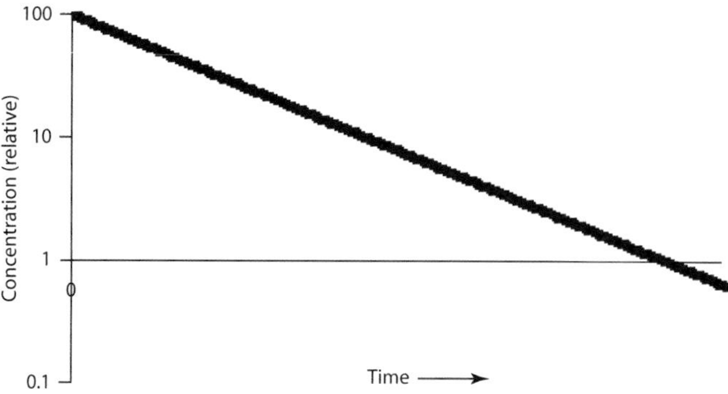

Figure 15.2 Elimination from a one-compartment open model.

and in terms of half-lives:

$$t_{1/2\ \mathrm{eff}} = \frac{t_{1/2\ \mathrm{biol}} t_{1/2\ \mathrm{phys}}}{t_{1/2\ \mathrm{biol}} + t_{1/2\ \mathrm{phys}}}$$

The effect is illustrated in Figure 15.3, where the effect of these half-lives is shown.

Two-compartment model

The two-compartment open model with rapid intravenous injection is shown in Figure 15.4.

In this model, the dose, D, equilibrates between the central compartment (volume V_1) and a peripheral compartment (V_2). Elimination is from the central compartment. In this situation the plasma activity concentration–time curve (after correction for physical decay) will look like that in Figure 15.5.

The rate of elimination from the central compartment can be expressed as

$$\frac{\mathrm{d}C_1}{\mathrm{d}t} = k_{\mathrm{el}} C_1 + k_{12} C_1 + k_{21} C_2$$

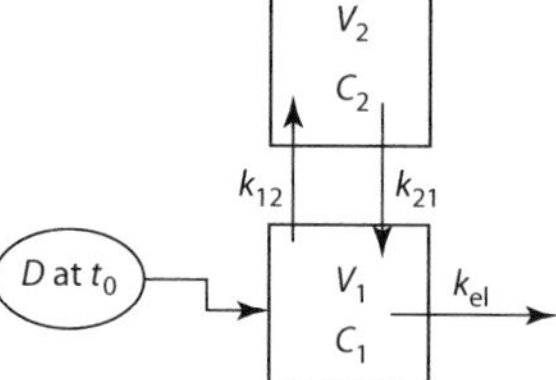

Figure 15.4 Two-compartment open model with rapid intravenous injection.

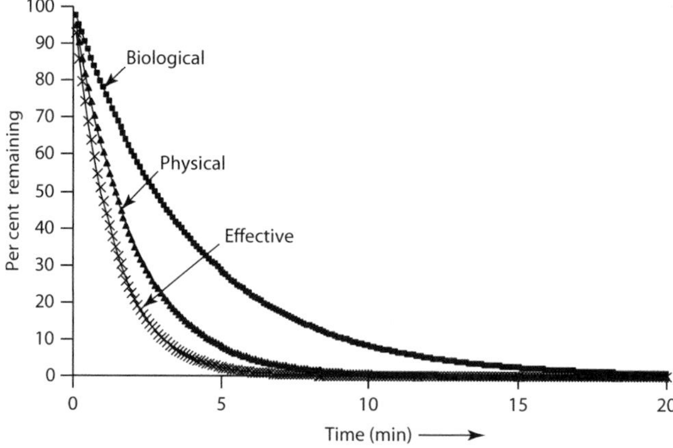

Figure 15.3 Physical, biological and effective half lives. (Physical = 0.25 min; biological = 0.5 min.)

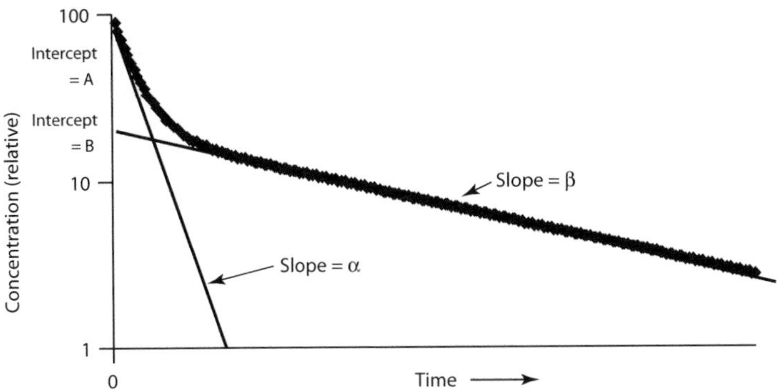

Figure 15.5 Elimination from a two-compartment open model.

and the elimination can be modelled with a biexponential equation of the form

$$C_t = Ae^{-\alpha t} + Be^{-\beta t}$$

The meaning of the constants can be seen from Figure 15.5, where the two linear components are shown. Determination of the constants can be made by least-squares fitting of the data to the model, or by manual fitting or deconvolution of the data plotted on a semilog graph.

Once the results of the pharmacokinetic modelling are known, it is possible to calculate a number of different derived parameters. Most are beyond the scope of this chapter and the interested reader is referred to the more specialised text books on pharmacokinetics that appear at the end of this chapter. It is useful, however, to understand one or two pharmacokinetic concepts that have applications in nuclear medicine and for which radiopharmaceuticals are used.

Volume of distribution

The volume of distribution, V_d, of a drug is the apparent volume into which it is distributed and is derived by dividing the administered dose (D) by the plasma concentration after the initial distribution throughout the body. In the case of the common two-compartment system described above, the value for the concentration (C) is given by the $t = 0$ intercept (B) of the elimination phase of the plasma activity concentration–time curve:

$$V_d = D/C_0$$

It should be noted that the volume of distribution is a notional concept and should not be conceived as an anatomically or physiologically defined compartment except in the cases of radiopharmaceuticals designed specifically for this purpose (see later). If a radiopharmaceutical concentrates highly in fat deposits for example, the resulting low concentration in the plasma will lead to an apparently high V_d (a value possibly in excess of the total body volume). It is for this reason that V_d is often referred to as the apparent volume of distribution.

Area under the curve

The area under the plasma activity concentration versus time curve from t_0 to infinity ($AUC_{0-\infty}$) can be derived, using the trapezoidal rule, by simple integration of the exponential function(s) describing the concentration–time relationship.

$$AUC_{0-\infty} = A/\alpha \text{ (for a monoexponential function)}$$

$$AUC_{0-\infty} = (A/\alpha) + (B/\beta) \text{ (for a bi-exponential function)}$$

In the field of toxicology the AUC for the plasma concentration of a drug, following intravenous injection, can be used as a means of extrapolating data from one species to another, being a measure of exposure. In the field of radiation dosimetry the AUC of tissue radioactivity versus time is known as the cumulative activity (MBq·h), or when divided by the injected radioactivity, as the residence time.

Clearance (CL) and elimination

Clearance of a drug occurs when it is removed irreversibly from the systemic circulation or body tissue by metabolism or excretion. Clearance occurs during the transit of drug in blood through an 'organ of elimination' such as the kidneys. During transit, a proportion of the drug is removed and so clearance may be defined as the notional volume of blood from which drug is totally removed per unit of time and has the units of millilitres per minute. Mathematically, total clearance of an intravenously administered drug can be calculated from the relationship:

$$\text{Clearance (CL)} = \text{Dose}/\text{AUC}$$

where AUC is the total area beneath the plot of plasma concentration against time after administration of the drug as described above.

The concept of clearance should not be confused with elimination. According to the equation above, if the same dose of two compounds is injected and the areas under their plasma concentration–time curves are the same, then the clearance of the two compounds is identical. Their elimination constants or biological half-lives may, however, be very different.

In the example shown in Figure 15.6, the areas under the two curves are equal, yet one curve (drug 2) falls at a substantially slower rate and starts with a much lower initial blood level (C_0) compared with the other curve (drug 1). This is because drug 2 is more widely distributed in tissue so that it has a larger apparent volume of distribution (V_d) than drug 1. The administered dose of both drugs was the same so their clearance is the same, but their elimination half-lives differ by a factor of 4. We shall see how some of these pharmacokinetic concepts are used in nuclear medicine later in this chapter.

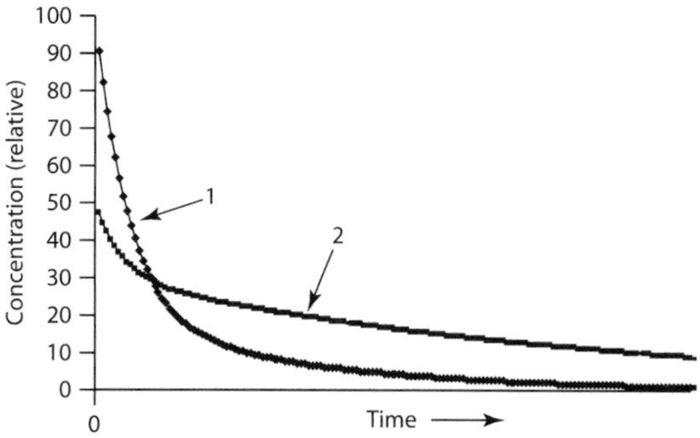

Figure 15.6 The relationship between clearance and elimination half-life.

As previously mentioned it should be recognised that most frequently we are observing the behaviour of only the radionuclide, regardless of its chemical or physical form within the body. For most purposes this is entirely acceptable. However, in certain circumstances it may be necessary to separate possible multiple species in plasma, for example, so that the more complex kinetics of receptor interactions can be modelled for the desired molecule in the absence of contaminating data from radiolabelled metabolites. It is also assumed that radiopharmacokinetic data are based on measurements of radioactivity that have first been corrected for radioactive physical decay.

Practical applications of radiopharmacokinetics in radiopharmaceutical R&D

Biodistribution

Preclinical biodistribution studies are used for determining the distribution of a radiolabelled compound within whole organs or specific organ regions, tissues and excreta. Biodistribution studies can be used to investigate a number of different factors such as imaging efficacy, including specific target-mediated tracer uptake or uptake in 'normal' versus 'disease' tissue, for estimating clinical absorbed radiation dosimetry or for the assessment of product quality (Ph. Eur. Physiological distribution tests). In research or development the overall aims of biodistribution studies depend on the stage of the project but can be broadly summarised as shown in Table 15.1.

The biodistribution of a radiolabelled compound can be studied using *ex-vivo* tissue sampling followed by direct or indirect counting methods (see Chapter 4), or via non-invasive *in-vivo* imaging studies (see 'Biodistribution by imaging' later). There are advantages and disadvantages to both dissection and non-invasive methods of determining the biodistribution of radiolabelled tracers, which are discussed in Table 15.2.

Table 15.1 Summary of the uses of biodistribution studies

R&D stage	Study	Aims
Research	Naive animal biodistribution	Determine initial distribution of tracer, elimination route and target-to-background ratios. Data from these studies can also be used to determine tracer stability (e.g. bone uptake due to defluorination of an ^{18}F-labelled tracer) and effects of impurities or metabolites on the tracer biodistribution
	Competition studies	Determine effect of administration of target blocking agent (e.g. excess unlabelled tracer) on the biodistribution of the radiolabelled tracer to confirm target binding specificity
	Model animal biodistribution	Confirm target tracer uptake is correlated with modulated target expression or disease state
Development	Detailed biodistribution for dosimetry	Tracer biodistribution typically studied in rats at a range of post-administration time points. Wide range of organs, tissues and excreta sampled. Clinical dosimetry estimates calculated according to the MIRD schema
	Formulation comparison	Comparative biodistribution studies performed to determine effect of changes in formulation of tracer on biodistribution during development

Biodistribution by dissection

The generation of biodistribution data by dissection can be performed in two ways: by direct determination of the amount of radioactivity in the collected samples using an appropriate counter (e.g. a scintillation counter such as a NaI detection crystal in a gamma-counter), or indirectly using autoradiographic techniques. Both of these require the initial administration of the radiolabelled tracer to the animal by the required administration route, typically via intravenous injection, followed by sacrifice of the animal at the specified time point. Following euthanasia of the animals, the required organs, tissue and excreta can be collected by dissection, or the whole animal can be fixed and sectioned for the quantitative determination of distribution of the radioactivity by quantitative whole body autoradiography (QWBA).

Table 15.2 Advantages and disadvantages of biodistribution techniques

Biodistribution technique	Advantages	Disadvantages
Dissection	Sensitivity – more sensitive than current imaging techniques Anaesthesia – studies can be performed in the absence of anaesthesia that may affect expression of or binding to the target Cost – equipment is generally less expensive than cameras required for imaging	Functional response assessment – tracer uptake during disease progression or after therapy response must be studied in individual animals which increases intra-animal variability during studies Many animals are required
Non-invasive imaging	Functional response assessment - repeat imaging of the same animal allows longitudinal imaging of tracer uptake during disease progression and/or response to therapy Fewer animals are required	Cost – higher equipment cost than typically required for dissection techniques Anaesthesia – required during imaging procedure may affect tracer uptake and biodistribution Sensitivity – currently lower than can be achieved with dissection techniques therefore higher doses of radioactivity are required to achieve adequate counting statistics for reconstruction of small volumes

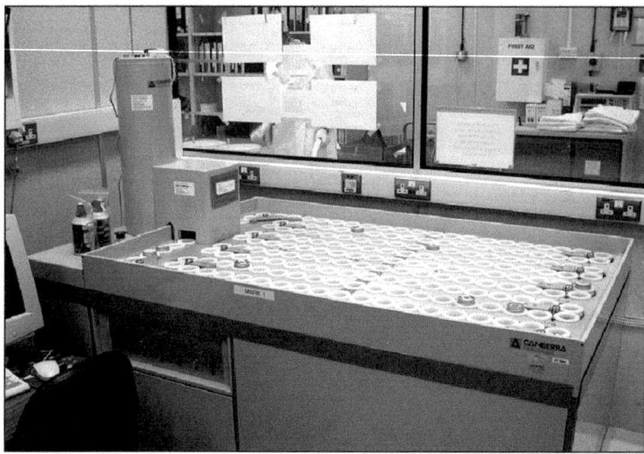

Figure 15.7 Large-sample automatic gamma counter with twin, vertically opposed detectors. Photograph courtesy of GE Healthcare Ltd.

Using a scintillation counter, the biodistribution data will be generated as the number of counts of radioactivity recorded by the detector in each sample over a specified period of time and converted to counts per second (cps). Uniformity of the counting geometry is important so that each sample is assayed with the same counting efficiency. To this end, a counter with horizontally or vertically opposed detectors can minimise the effects of differences between organ or tissue samples of varying size or geometry. (For an example, see Figure 15.7.) Alternatively a single-well crystal counter can be used, but for this to minimise counting geometry effects the crystal should ideally be large in comparison to the size of the sample and the sample should not be allowed to extend beyond the lower half of the well.

Typically the data are then expressed as a percentage of the injected dose (% id) present in each sample, or % id per gram of tissue (% id/g). Conversion of the raw cps data to % id requires either the total amount of radioactivity injected into each animal to be known, or, more accurately, that all the injected activity, whether remaining in the body or having been voided in the urine or faeces, be counted. The % id in a whole organ (e.g. brain) can then be calculated as shown in equation (15.1), following correction for background and radioactive decay:

% Injected dose (id) in whole organ

$$\%\ \text{id Organ} = \frac{A}{B} \times 100 \qquad (15.1)$$

where A = counts per second measured in the organ; B = total counts per second measured in all samples or total counts per second of injected activity (excluding the injection site if appropriate).

Conversion of whole organ % id values to % id/g data for that organ simply requires the % id value to be divided by the measured organ weight.

Calculation of the % id in incompletely sampled tissues (e.g. blood or muscle) requires the use of species-specific tissue composition factors as shown in equation (15.2). Tissue composition factors are the proportion of an animal's body weight that is due to muscle, bone or blood for example. Of a rat's total body weight, 43% is due to muscle. The tissue composition factors for bone, muscle, blood, skin and fat of rats and mice are shown in Table 15.3.

% Injected dose (id) in tissue or incompletely sampled organ

$$\%\ \text{id Tissue} = \frac{(Z_s \times W_b \times F)/B}{W_s} \times 100 \qquad (15.2)$$

where Z_s = counts per second in the sample; W_s = weight of the sample in grams; W_b = weight of the animal immediately after sacrifice, in grams; B = total counts per second measured in all samples or total counts per second of injected activity (excluding the injection site if appropriate); and F = tissue- or organ-specific composition factor representing the mass of the tissue as a proportion of the total body weight of the animal (see Table 15.3).

Table 15.3 Tissue composition factors (*F*) for rats and mice

Tissue	Composition factor	
	Rat	Mouse
Bone	0.05	0.05
Muscle	0.43	0.43
Blood	0.058	0.078
Skin	0.18	0.15
Fat	0.07	0.07

Conversion of tissue or incompletely sampled organ % id values to % id/g for that sample requires the % id value to be divided by the calculated total tissue or sample weight for that animal (i.e. tissue-specific composition factor multiplied by the body weight).

As a refinement to the above, and for more specialised applications, it is also possible to correct organ and tissue radioactivity values for the content of radioactivity in the residual blood within those organs and tissues. These values will depend on the mode of euthanasia and the individual laboratory's dissection techniques and so they would have to be determined locally using, for example, a tracer that was essentially retained within the blood pool to obtain laboratory-specific reference values. In general, however, for most radiopharmaceuticals, clearance from blood is quite rapid and hence correction for residual blood activity is not required.

In general the use of data in the form of % id provides a quantitative description of the biological behaviour of an administered radiopharmaceutical and can be applied across animals of different weight and even species. However, data in the form of % id/g provide a better description of potential imaging characteristics enabling a comparison of the different concentrations of radioactivity within the organs and tissues of a single animal. Without correction for an animal's body weight, % id/g data do not permit inter-animal comparisons unless used as a ratio. Consider Compound X, which is a lipophilic tracer, retained in the brain by a trapping mechanism producing images that reflect regional cerebral blood flow. In both rats and mice 2.5% of the injected dose is retained in the brain at 1 hour post injection. This could be reported as 1.6 % id/g in the rat but 6.3% id/g in the mouse. In both species, however, the brain-to-blood ratio would be similar (at approximately 1.5). Direct extrapolation of animal biodistribution data between species and indeed to humans is difficult without corrections for relative tissue or organ masses and compensation for relative metabolic rates. The latter is often done on the basis of relative body surface areas rather than a per-kilogram basis. Extrapolation of animal data to humans is the subject of numerous publications (Mordenti 1986; Lathrop *et al.* 1989; Ritschel *et al.* 1992; Mahmood, 1999).

Biodistribution by quantitative whole body autoradiography (QWBA)

Autoradiography is a high-resolution technique for imaging qualitatively the distribution of radioactivity in organs and tissues and is described in more detail later. The technique can be also used to study the quantitative whole body biodistribution of injected radioactivity. Sections of the whole animal are exposed to X-ray film, producing a photographic image or phosphor imaging plates which produce digital images of the distributed radioactivity. Using the digital phosphor imager method, the biodistribution data from autoradiography studies can be quantified using the appropriate calibration standards and software. Using similar methods to those above, the % id for the organs, tissue and excreta can be calculated.

The biodistribution of an RGD-integrin-binding ligand, NC100692, developed by GE Healthcare Ltd (Hua *et al.*, 2005; Bach-Gansmo *et al.* 2006; Bach-Gansmo *et al.* 2008; Edwards *et al.* 2008) has been studied in naive rats by dissection-scintillation counting (technetium-99m label) and by QWBA (carbon-14 label).

Biodistribution of ^{99m}Tc-NC100692

The biodistribution of the diagnostic radiopharmaceutical ^{99m}Tc-NC100692 was studied in male rats from 2 minutes to 24 hours after intravenous injection. The quantitative data are summarised in Table 15.4.

The biodistribution data show that this tracer is rapidly distributed around the body immediately following intravenous injection, and that subsequently the radioactivity is rapidly removed from the blood pool. The radioactivity is excreted predominantly via the urinary route (approximately 65% id by 24 hours post injection) but there is also some faecal excretion (approximately 15% id by 24 hours post injection). Excretion via the kidneys and urinary bladder is the predominant route for clearance of hydrophilic compounds from the body, while lipophilic compounds are excreted predominantly via the hepatobiliary route. There is no evidence of significant accumulation of radioactivity in the stomach or the thyroid gland, which would be indicative of metabolism or chemical degradation of the tracer resulting in the production of 'free pertechnetate' ($^{99m}TcO_4^-$), which preferentially accumulates in these organs. Similarly, for ^{18}F- or ^{123}I-labelled tracers, accumulation of radioactivity in the

Table 15.4 Biodistribution of ^{99m}Tc-NC100692 in male rats. Data are shown as % id ($n = 5–6$)

	Post-injection time point											
	2 min		**20 min**		**60 min**		**4 h**		**7 h**		**24 h**	
	Mean	**SD**	**Mean**	**SD**	**Mean**	**SD**	**Mean**	**SD**	**Mean**	**SD**	**Mean**	**SD**
Adrenal gland	0.06	0.01	0.04	0.01	0.03	0.01	0.02	0.00	0.01	0.01	0.01	0.01
Bladder and urine	0.25	0.16	23.70	3.37	39.65	1.26	52.94	3.59	57.35	4.93	62.06	6.40
Blood	11.15	1.61	3.24	0.36	1.69	0.18	0.42	0.02	0.32	0.04	0.19	0.03
Bone	7.31	0.44	5.01	0.17	3.95	0.14	2.59	0.25	2.15	0.16	1.28	0.22
Brain	0.07	0.02	0.03	0.01	0.02	0.00	0.02	0.01	0.01	0.00	0.01	0.01
Faeces	0.00	0.00	0.00	0.01	0.01	0.01	0.26	0.38	1.45	1.80	15.89	5.53
Fat	3.23	0.53	3.95	0.99	3.13	0.80	1.92	0.53	1.83	0.50	0.91	0.16
Heart	0.51	0.07	0.25	0.02	0.17	0.04	0.08	0.01	0.07	0.01	0.04	0.01
Injection site	2.41	0.30	2.69	0.35	2.26	0.13	1.38	0.12	1.12	0.22	0.82	0.18
Kidneys	13.80	2.06	5.15	0.96	4.77	0.85	8.44	1.88	7.62	0.74	5.64	0.87
Large intestines	2.23	0.15	1.78	0.04	1.35	0.10	0.91	0.12	0.79	0.11	0.38	0.08
Liver	6.68	0.28	5.68	0.44	4.97	0.82	2.83	0.40	2.21	0.30	1.32	0.20

Table 15.4 *(continued)*

	Post-injection time point											
	2 min		**20 min**		**60 min**		**4 h**		**7 h**		**24 h**	
	Mean	**SD**	**Mean**	**SD**	**Mean**	**SD**	**Mean**	**SD**	**Mean**	**SD**	**Mean**	**SD**
Lung	1.69	0.13	1.13	0.12	0.70	0.04	0.31	0.04	0.25	0.01	0.15	0.03
Muscle	23.92	1.25	17.66	1.03	12.74	0.57	6.96	0.56	5.41	0.45	3.04	0.47
Pancreas	0.54	0.10	0.34	0.08	0.34	0.11	0.17	0.02	0.12	0.05	0.08	0.04
Testes	0.25	0.06	0.27	0.03	0.22	0.05	0.12	0.01	0.10	0.01	0.07	0.01
Thyroid	0.12	0.05	0.09	0.02	0.06	0.02	0.03	0.01	0.03	0.01	0.01	0.01
Salivary gland	0.49	0.07	0.33	0.04	0.28	0.03	0.16	0.04	0.13	0.03	0.06	0.02
Skin	16.91	1.28	18.43	1.21	14.63	1.18	9.79	1.00	8.39	0.73	5.52	0.54
Small intestines	7.24	0.35	5.51	0.31	6.10	0.82	5.18	0.86	2.53	0.22	1.14	0.24
Spleen	0.86	0.07	0.71	0.09	0.56	0.12	0.40	0.05	0.33	0.09	0.15	0.03
Stomach and contents	1.51	0.05	1.23	0.07	1.04	0.07	0.71	0.14	0.43	0.06	0.39	0.23

bone or thyroid respectively would be indicative of metabolism or chemical instability *in vivo* of these tracers. Data of the type shown in Table 15.4 are not readily amenable to the derivation of values for traditional pharmacokinetic parameters but are more than adequate for the calculation or organ/tissue residence times for the first estimates of radiation absorbed doses.

Biodistribution of [^{14}C]NC100692

The biodistribution of [^{14}C]NC100692 has been studied by quantitative whole body autoradiography. For quantification, radioactivity standards of known radioactive concentration were prepared by the addition of known amounts of the tracer to samples of human blood, which were then placed into holes in the embedding medium for sectioning and exposure along with the whole body sections. These standards provide a calibration scale to allow conversion of the autoradiographic signal from the animal sections to % id/g data. An example of the autoradiograms at four different levels (and calibration standards) at 1 hour post injection is shown in Figure 15.8.

For quantification of organ or tissue distribution as a percentage of the total injected dose, all excreted urine and faeces were collected and assayed with appropriate injection standards by liquid scintillation counting. This enables assessment of whole body retention at the time of sacrifice; the activity (% id) per g data for each organ or tissue need to be multiplied by organ or tissue weight to body weight factors (see Table 15.3). The resulting data are shown in Table 15.5.

As with the ^{99m}Tc-labelled analogue, [^{14}C]-NC100692 was rapidly distributed throughout the body after intravenous injection, with the highest initial amounts of radioactivity being found in the blood and highly perfused organs such as the liver and lungs. At 7 days post dosing, as much as 30–35% of the injected radioactivity still remained in the body. The tracer was found to be mostly excreted via the kidneys and urinary bladder with approximately 45% id excreted in the urine between 4 and 24 hours post injection and no further renal elimination occurring from 24 hours to 7 days post dosing.

There are minor differences between the two sets of biodistribution data but these may be related to the different procedures used by two separate laboratories. The general pattern of biodistribution suggests, in this case, that the presence of the technetium atom has had some effect but not a major impact on the biological properties of the NC100692 molecule.

Biodistribution by imaging

The ability to quantify non-invasively the amount of the radioactive substance bound *in vivo* has led to the development of scintigraphy as an essential complementary imaging modality when coupled with structural imaging modalities such as X-ray (CT), ultrasound and magnetic resonance. The two commonly used imaging modalities that use radiopharmaceuticals are positron emission tomography (PET) and single-photon emission computed tomography (SPECT).

Both of these modalities use the properties of γ-rays that pass through the body to produce a three-dimensional image or map of functional processes in the body. PET detects pairs of γ-rays emitted indirectly by a positron-emitting radionuclide, whereas SPECT uses gamma radiation emitted directly from radionuclides.

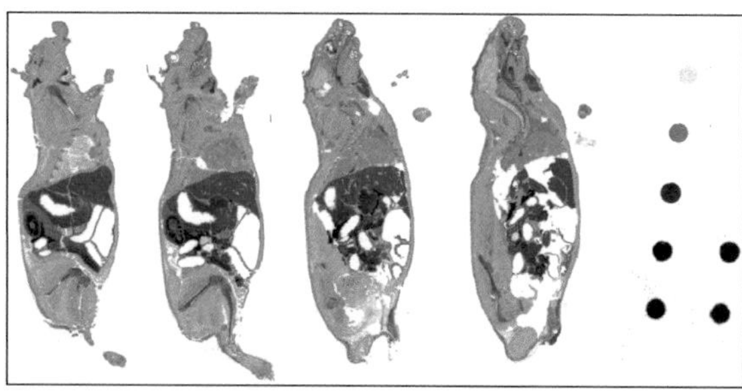

Figure 15.8 Whole-body autoradiograms of [^{14}C]NC100692 at 1 hour post injection in a male rat. Images courtesy of GE Healthcare Ltd.

Table 15.5 Biodistribution of [^{14}C]NC100692 in male rats. Data are shown as % injected dose ($n = 3$)

	Post-injection time point									
	5 min		1 h		4 h		24 h		7 days	
	Mean	SD	Mean	SD	Mean	SD	Mean	SD	Mean	SD
Adrenal gland	0.31	0.01	0.23	0.02	0.29	0.05	0.19	0.01	0.12	0.02
Blood	11.99	1.48	2.72	0.10	2.74	0.48	2.10	0.14	2.45	0.39
Bone	2.56	0.74	2.11	0.40	2.10	0.72	1.36	0.15	0.73	0.18
Brain	0.03	0.01	0.08	0.01	0.11	0.02	0.10	0.01	0.11	0.02
Fat	3.24	0.17	1.18	0.06	1.26	0.43	1.22	0.18	1.13	0.14
Heart	0.60	0.07	0.21	0.02	0.22	0.02	0.19	0.01	0.20	0.04
Kidneys	18.40	6.82	5.80	0.46	4.32	0.66	3.02	0.11	1.16	0.14
Large intestine	3.99	0.44	1.95	0.24	2.05	0.39	2.09	0.93	0.72	0.12
Liver	8.34	0.59	5.41	0.64	5.34	0.59	3.82	0.27	2.51	0.34
Lung	2.51	0.32	0.82	0.07	0.65	0.06	0.49	0.02	0.44	0.05
Muscle	24.50	1.83	12.06	0.36	13.99	0.99	13.03	1.09	17.16	2.10
Pancreas	0.49	0.02	2.22	0.28	1.54	0.19	0.32	0.03	0.19	0.03
Testes	0.25	0.04	0.27	0.04	0.26	0.03	0.24	0.01	0.22	0.03
Salivary gland	0.54	0.13	0.78	0.20	1.07	0.07	0.29	0.04	0.17	0.04
Skin	27.92	0.97	10.55	1.67	8.22	1.15	7.82	0.84	6.92	1.12
Small intestine	2.91	0.53	3.77	0.47	5.14	0.85	3.74	0.52	0.81	0.15
Spleen	0.39	0.02	0.37	0.07	0.50	0.02	0.30	0.02	0.14	0.02
Stomach and contents	0.67	0.02	1.23	0.23	1.04	0.26	0.53	0.07	0.19	0.03
Urine	–	–	–	–	8	–	45	–	45	–
Faeces	–	–	–	–	–	–	2	–	4	–

Positron emission tomography (PET)

In PET, a short lived positron-emitting radionuclide, the most commonly used being ^{11}C and ^{18}F, is attached to either a target-specific drug or a metabolic substrate. The radiotracers are injected into the animal and the compound is distributed and accumulates in those areas rich in the target. Emitted photons must travel through different tissues and are attenuated to different degrees depending on thickness and density of the tissue they are passing through. In order to correct for this, a scan to determine the attenuation of the subject is performed either with a rotating positron-emitting source or more recently using computed tomography of X-rays. Once the line of response and attenuation profile have been obtained, a tomographic algorithm is used to create a three-dimensional map of the radioactivity.

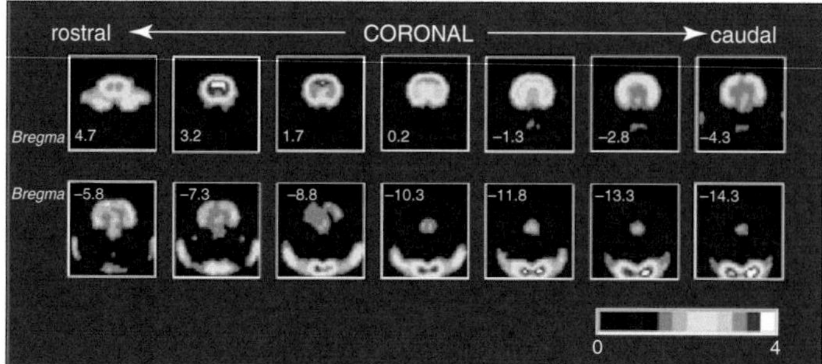

Figure 15.9 Images displaying the uptake of [^{11}C]MDL 100907 (5-HT_{2A} receptor antagonist) into the rat brain displaying uptake in the cortex. From Hirani E *et al.* (2003). © 2003 Wiley-Liss, Inc. Reprinted with permission of John Wiley & Sons, Inc.

Preclinical PET applications

Imaging metabolic and molecular function using PET has radically changed preclinical research. The main advantage of preclinical imaging is the ability to follow the course of a disease or therapy response longitudinally in the same subject thus facilitating the development of new drugs for both diagnosis and therapy. Owing to the quantitative nature of PET, this imaging modality is also useful for the study of receptor occupancy (see Figure 15.9) or the study of treatment efficacy.

In neurology, novel PET imaging compounds are being produced to diagnose degenerative diseases such as Alzheimer disease and psychiatric syndromes such as schizophrenia. With the advent of multimodality imaging, combined PET-CT or PET-MRI scanners allow very accurate delineation of anatomical regions, allowing the user to assess compound uptake in discrete regions over time.

Single-photon emission computed tomography (SPECT)

In SPECT, a gamma-emitting radionuclide is used; the most common are ^{99m}Tc and ^{123}I.

Preclinical SPECT applications

Until very recently SPECT has been a semi-quantitative methodology with relatively poor resolution, but with the advent of new technology, namely CZT (cadmium zinc telluride) detectors and the ability of CT imaging to allow attenuation corrections, the new multimodality SPECT cameras have similar resolution and sensitivity to those of current PET cameras (1–3 mm).

The radiolabelled cocaine analogue [^{123}I]ioflupane is taken up by the brain by diffusion and is selectively retained in regions containing a high density of the dopamine transporter. This is used clinically in the evaluation of diseases involving a dopaminergic deficit. Preclinically the molecule has been used to assess animal models of Parkinsonism (Alvarez-Fischer *et al.* 2007; Ashkan *et al.* 2007). In a study by Vastenhouw *et al.* (2007) its *in-vivo* selectivity for the dopamine transporter has been demonstrated by SPECT imaging in mice. Following injection of [^{123}I]ioflupane, a stable level of radioactivity was obtained in the striata. The mice then received an intraperitoneal injection of cocaine. From the reconstructed three-dimensional SPECT images of the brain, movies of the radioactivity displacement in the striata and associated regional time activity curves were generated. (The movie is available on-line at www.isi.uu.nl/People/Freek/.) This is an example of the 'longitudinal' capability of *in-vivo* imaging, gathering data from a single animal that would require the use of many if dissection techniques were to be used.

Autoradiography

Autoradiography is the technique by which the distribution of a radiopharmaceutical is imaged in two dimensions using a phosphor imaging plate or radiographic film or emulsion. The same pharmacokinetic principle applies as with the three-dimensional imaging techniques; the radionuclide is distributed around the body via the blood flow and accumulates in those areas rich in the target for the radiopharmaceutical. The method of detection in autoradiography is significantly different. In autoradiography the tissue of interest must be physically removed from the subject and prepared (either via fixative or by freezing). Once the tissue has been prepared it is sectioned using a microtome (or a cryotome if frozen tissue is used) and the resulting slices are exposed to either the imager plate or film or coated in radiographic emulsion. Film or plate autoradiography allows the user to visualise the location of the radionuclide with reasonable resolution (10–100 μm), but only in two dimensions, providing anatomical as well as radiological information, whereas emulsion autoradiography allows a quantitative estimate of the amount of radioactive substance in an area by counting silver grains in the section, but provides no anatomical data. The technique of micro-autoradiography is important, however, when trying to assess the radiation dosimetry of radionuclides with particle emissions (β-particles or Auger electrons) (Puncher, Blower 1994).

Autoradiography, as an imaging technique has several advantages and disadvantages when compared with PET or SPECT. PET has a spatial resolution in the region 1–2 mm and conventional SPECT 3–5 mm; while these imaging modalities are very useful they will only ever provide information at the tissue level. Autoradiography is able to reach resolutions of 10 μm or less and is able to provide information at the cellular or even subcellular level. Structures that are too small to be imaged accurately using the tomographic imaging techniques can be assessed using this method. Figure 15.10 shows binding of the PET tracer [^{11}C] MDL 100907 in slices of rat brain *in vitro*; the superior resolution available with autoradiography allows localisation of the tracer to discrete layers of the cortex, which is not possible using PET owing to the much lower resolution. This is important in non-clinical studies designed to confirm or demonstrate the mechanism of action of new radiopharmaceuticals.

Autoradiography, however, has two major drawbacks: the necessity for the tissue to be removed from the subject and the time taken for radio-transfer to the film, which for low-energy β-emitters such as tritium can be up to 6 months.

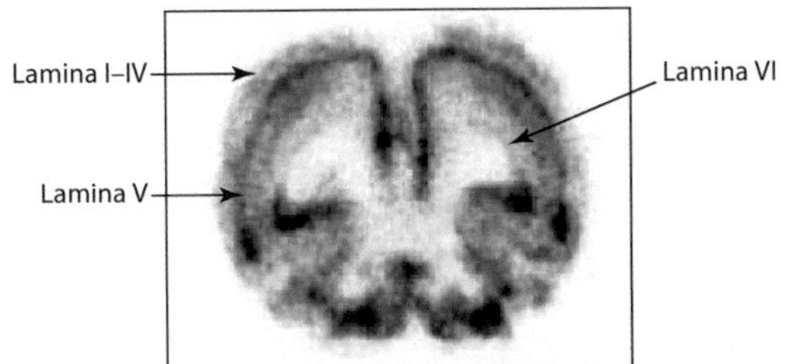

Figure 15.10 Specific binding of [^{11}C]MDL 100907 measured in fresh frozen rat frontal cortex sections using *in-vitro* digital autoradiography. Images courtesy of MRC Clinical Sciences Centre.

Practical application of radiopharmacokinetics in the clinical setting

Agents used to measure system functions

The different phases of radiopharmaceutical pharmacokinetics – absorption, distribution, metabolism and excretion – can be applied in a variety of ways in diagnostic nuclear medicine.

Absorption

[^{57}Co]Cyanocobalamin

Small quantities of [^{57}Co]cyanocobalamin (vitamin B_{12}) administered by mouth are retained within the intestinal mucosa for 2–3 hours before release into the bloodstream, where they circulate bound to plasma proteins. Peak plasma levels occur at 8–12 hours with peak redistribution to the liver around 24 hours. The dosing of a relatively large amount of unlabelled cyanocobalamin, just prior to intestinal release, alters the distribution of the radioactive species – flushing it via the kidneys into the urine as unbound [^{57}Co]cyanocobalamin. The concentration–time profile of urine samples for ^{57}Co is diagnostic for poor absorption due to ileal malabsorption. This may be due to local factors or the absence of gastric intrinsic factor (most commonly associated with pernicious

[^{57}Co]Cyanocobalamin

anaemia). The radioactivity in a 24-hour post-administration urine collection is assayed. Generally, 10–40% of the radioactive dose will be excreted into urine in 24 hours. In the event of a low value (less than 5%) a second stage of the test may be performed in which the [^{57}Co]cyanocobalamin is co-administered with intrinsic factor. A persistent low excretion is indicative of non-specific malabsorption.

[^{75}Se]Tauroselcholic (^{75}Se) acid (bile salt)

Tauroselcholic acid does not occur naturally but it is an analogue of the naturally occurring bile acid conjugate taurocholic acid. Endogenous bile acids are formed in the liver, secreted into bile and reabsorbed by an active transport mechanism across the ileal mucosa. [^{75}Se]Tauroselcholic acid can be considered to be specifically absorbed by the active mechanism of the ileum. After oral administration of a capsule, [^{75}Se] tauroselcholic acid becomes mixed with the endogenous bile acid pool and thus provides a means for measuring the rate of bile acid loss from the endogenous pool. This can be achieved by determining either the excretion of activity in faeces or the retention of activity in the body over a period of days – commonly using an uncollimated gamma camera. The results may be expressed as a rate of loss if several measurements are taken or, more simply, as a retained percentage after a fixed period such as 7 days. Since [^{75}Se] tauroselcholic acid is specifically absorbed by the ileum, the extent of loss of ileal bile acid absorptive function can be determined. This has proved useful in the investigation of inflammatory bowel disease and chronic diarrhoea (Wildt *et al.* 2003).

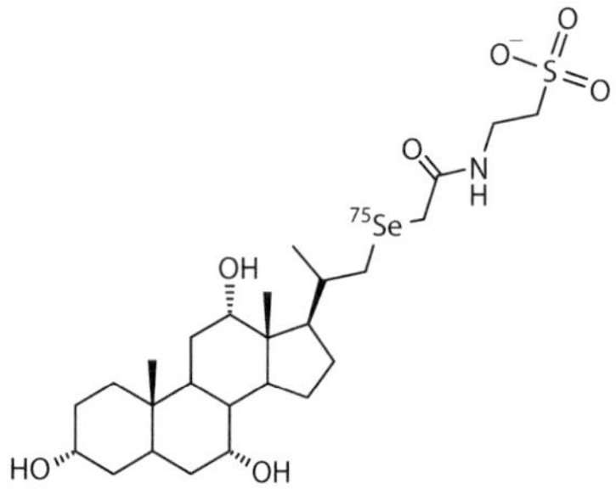

[^{75}Se]Tauroselcholic acid

The above two examples enable the assessment of absorption or absorption defects. Orally administered non-absorbable radiopharmaceuticals (there are a variety of recipes for the incorporation of ^{111}In or ^{99m}Tc into solid or liquid preparations) enable assessment of gastric emptying and gastrointestinal transit times (Urbain, Charkes 1995; Maurer, Parkman 2006).

Distribution

The plasma activity concentration–time curve referred to earlier can be used in conjunction with a variety of radiopharmaceuticals to derive diagnostically useful information. For example, radiopharmaceuticals that have a low apparent volume of distribution are retained essentially within the circulatory system, at least initially, and can be used to estimate the circulating plasma volume. Iodine-125-labelled human serum albumin may be injected and blood samples withdrawn at 10, 20 and 30 minutes. The zero-time plasma activity concentration is obtained by extrapolation from the clearance, which, initially, can be regarded as monoexponential. Division of the amount of activity administered by the zero-time plasma radioactivity concentration yields the plasma volume. Similarly, red blood cells can be labelled *in vitro* with ^{111}In (oxine, tropolone or acetylacetone) or ^{51}Cr (sodium [^{51}Cr] chromate) or using ^{99m}Tc in the form of [^{99m}Tc]pertechnetate following 'pre-tinning' of the cells with a stannous compound (*in vitro* or *in vivo*). After reinjection and allowing an adequate time for mixing, a blood sample is taken and assayed for radioactivity. This enables determination of the total red cell volume in the same way as the plasma volume, after correction by multiplying by the haematocrit.

For most other radiopharmaceuticals it is the 'distribution' and 'elimination' elements of pharmacokinetics that are responsible for the selective localisation of radioactivity that makes imaging possible. Of increasing importance is the retention mechanism involving binding of radiopharmaceuticals to receptors or transporters that are up-regulated as a consequence of a disease process and many examples of this are given in relation to neurology and oncology later in this chapter.

Metabolism

There are many examples where metabolism is the determinant of localisation. For example, many radiopharmaceuticals are distributed extensively throughout the body only to be subsequently redistributed and excreted. Use can be made of certain metabolic processes to reduce the molecule's ability to redistribute. Specific esterases in the brain are responsible for the conversion of the lipophilic and diffusible technetium (^{99m}Tc) bicisate (ECD, Neurolite) to a less lipophilic form that is trapped, thereby allowing visualisation of its initial distribution within the brain, that is, a reflection of regional perfusion. A similar conversion of a diffusible lipophilic species to a less-diffusible species under the influence of intracellular glutathione is postulated as the mechanism for the intracerebral trapping of technetium (^{99m}Tc) exametazime (Ceretec) (Neirinckx *et al.* 1988). On the other hand, the ability of [^{18}F]fludeoxyglucose (FDG) to visualise hypermetabolic regions, notably in oncology, is a result not only of up-regulated glucose transport into the cells but also of the fact that after phosphorylation by hexokinase the FDG molecule is not further metabolised to continue in the glycolytic pathway. This results in its retention within those hypermetabolic cells.

Excretion

An important use of radiopharmacokinetics is in the evaluation of renal function. The concept of 'clearance' (CL) has been described earlier. For a compound that is not metabolised or protein bound and is excreted exclusively via the kidneys the value of CL can be equated to kidney function. For example, for a compound that is excreted exclusively and quantitatively by glomerular filtration, the clearance equates to the glomerular filtration rate (GFR). For a compound that is completely removed from the plasma during transit through the kidneys (by a combination of glomerular filtration and active secretion without reabsorption), the clearance equates to the 'effective renal plasma flow'. Radiopharmaceuticals have been designed that fit the criteria necessary for the evaluation of these functions and a number of different protocols, with and without correction factors, have been developed.

Chromium (^{51}Cr) edetate (EDTA) and technetium (^{99m}Tc) pentetate (DTPA)

In each case, plasma samples collected post injection are counted for comparison with a counting standard to obtain an estimation of the per cent injected dose per litre of plasma. For an accurate estimate of the AUC, multiple samples (up to 10) from 5 minutes to 4 hours post injection are required. The process may be simplified by taking only 2, 3 or 4 samples of plasma between 2 and 4 hours post injection. From these it is possible to employ the 'slope–intercept' method whereby an approximate value for the AUC can be obtained by dividing the zero-time intercept of the monoexponential slow phase of the plasma clearance curve by its slope. This would be the equivalent of B/β in the example shown in Figure 15.5. If the units for the plasma concentration–time curve are % id/litre of plasma versus time in minutes, then the AUC will be calculated as minutes × % id/litre. When this is divided into the dose (100%), the units will be litres/minute, the glomerular filtration rate. If the radiopharmaceutical in question has an extraction fraction close to 1 for each pass through the kidneys, then a similar approach to that above will yield the value for the effective renal plasma flow. Radiopharmaceuticals for this application include *ortho*-iodohippurate injection ('Hippuran', radiolabelled with ^{123}I, ^{125}I or ^{131}I). An ideal ^{99m}Tc-radiolabelled alternative has yet to be developed.

Further information on relative renal function can be derived from imaging studies using the ^{99m}Tc- or ^{123}I-labelled radiopharmaceuticals. Regions of interest placed over each kidney in planar images during dynamic acquisitions enable the construction of renograms showing the movement of radioactivity into and out of each kidney separately. The technique can be further enhanced by the administration of a diuretic during the study to determine whether renal function is compromised as a result of mechanical outflow blockage.

The other principal route of excretion is via the liver, bile and gastrointestinal tract, and radiopharmaceuticals have been developed for the evaluation of hepatobiliary function. Lipophilic molecules tend to be excreted via the hepatobiliary route and, if they possess structural similarities to endogenous bilirubin, may be actively secreted via the anion clearance mechanism.

Following intravenous injection, technetium (^{99m}Tc) mebrofenin is bound to plasma proteins and carried to the liver. It is cleared rapidly from the plasma, less than 1% of administered radioactivity remaining 1 hour after injection. Technetium (^{99m}Tc) mebrofenin is taken up by active transport into hepatocytes in a manner similar to bilirubin, reaching peak activity in the liver in 12 minutes. The liver half-life is 25–30 minutes in health but this may be influenced by plasma albumin concentration, hepatic blood flow and hepatocyte function. The tracer can be excreted unchanged into bile or bound to bile salts either within the hepatocyte or immediately after excretion. Only small amounts are excreted in the urine unless there is a significant biliary obstruction. In healthy subjects, the biliary tree is visualised within 5–20 minutes of injection and the gall bladder within 10–40 minutes.

^{99m}Tc-Mebrofenin

Neurology

Positron emission tomography (PET) and single-photon emission computed tomography (SPECT) imaging use positron- and gamma-emitting radioisotopes that can easily be incorporated into biological molecules and thus allow the measurement of functional parameters (physiological and/or pharmacological interactions) of tissue rather than just providing the anatomical definition of structures. Both techniques are exceptionally sensitive (PET more than SPECT) and can detect picomolar or even femtomolar concentrations of the radiolabelled compound and enable the dynamic acquisition of relatively fast kinetics (of the order of seconds for PET). With these properties, PET/SPECT can facilitate the quantitative measurement of rapid physiological/pharmacological processes of biomolecules in the living brain, for example. The increase in neurological applications for PET/SPECT over the last decade has been greatly aided by the significant improvement in data acquisition (hardware technology), data quantification (model-based methodology) and the vastly growing number of available PET/SPECT metabolic radiotracers and receptor-specific radioligands. Table 15.6 lists the more common PET/SPECT radiotracers/ligands and their intended targets in clinical neurology; the structures of some of these are shown in Scheme 15.1. This section will briefly outline the potential applications of PET/SPECT imaging in clinical studies of neurology and/or neuropharmacology. A more detailed review can be found in Brooks (2005).

Table 15.6 Common radiotracers and radioligands available for neurology

Target	PET/SPECT radiotracer/ ligand
Cerebral blood flow	[^{15}O]water, ^{99m}Tc-HMPAO
Cerebral glucose metabolism	[^{18}F]fludeoxyglucose (FDG)
Dopamine synthesis	[^{18}F]fluorodopa (F-DOPA)
Dopamine D_1 receptors	[^{11}C]SCH23390
Dopamine $D_{2/3}$ receptors	[^{11}C]raclopride, [^{11}C]FLB457, [^{123}I]iodobenzamide, [^{123}I]epidepride
Dopamine reuptake (transporter) sites	[^{11}C]RTI-32, [^{11}C]CFT, [^{123}I]ioflupane
Serotonin (5-HT) 1A receptors	[^{11}C]WAY100635,
Serotonin (5-HT) 2A receptors	[^{11}C]MDL100907, [^{18}F]altanserin
Serotonin reuptake (transporter) sites	[^{11}C]DASB, [^{123}I]β-CIT
Peripheral benzodiazepine sites	[^{11}C]PK11195, [^{123}I]PK11195
Central benzodiazepine sites	[^{11}C]flumazenil
Amyloid	[^{11}C]PIB, [^{18}F]flutemetamol, [^{123}I]IMPY
Opioid receptors	[^{11}C]diprenorphine

Diagnosis and monitoring of disease progression

PET/SPECT imaging is increasingly being employed to aid in the diagnosis of neurodegenerative diseases. The short radioactive half-life of both PET/SPECT radiotracers and ligands enables subjects to be scanned periodically in order to study and monitor changes in signal as the disease progresses and/or after treatment.

In Alzheimer disease, [^{18}F]FDG PET studies have shown characteristic glucose hypometabolism in parietal and temporal cortices, which is possibly due to

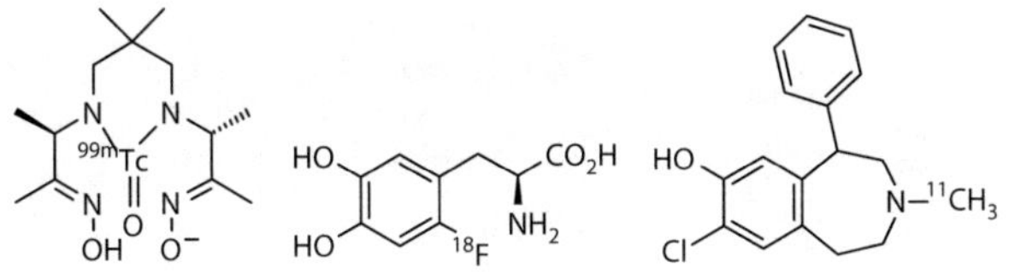

^{99m}Tc-HMPAO
[^{18}F]fluorodopa
[^{11}C]SCH 23390
[^{11}C]Raclopride 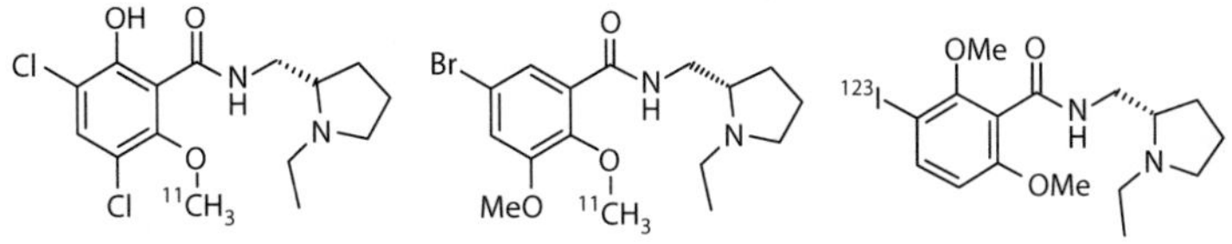
[^{11}C]FLB457
[^{123}I]Iodobenzamide (IBZM)
[^{123}I]Epidepride 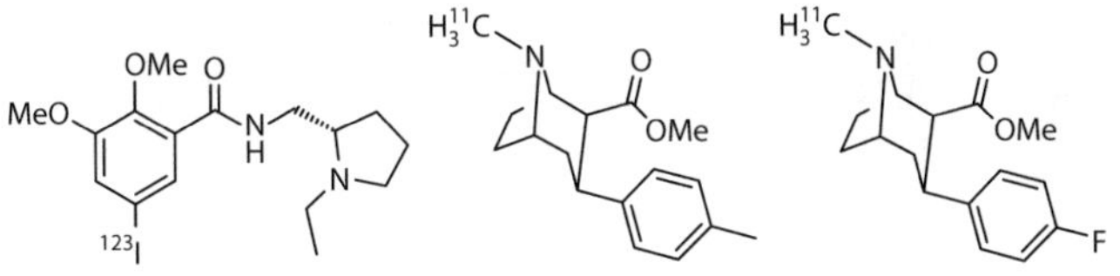
[^{11}C]RTI-32
[^{11}C]CFT
[^{11}C]WAY100635 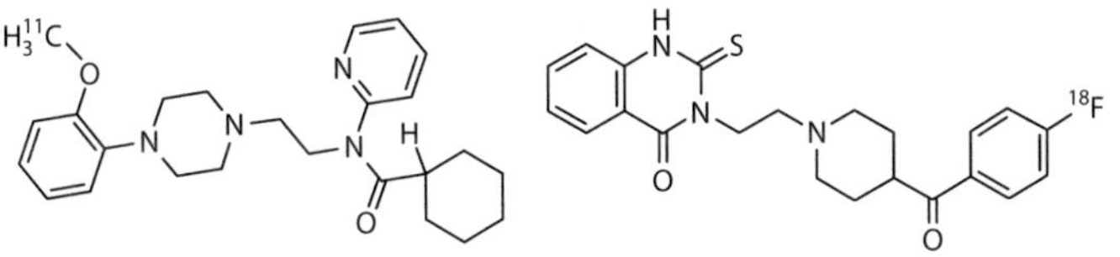
[^{18}F]Altanserin
[^{11}C]DASB 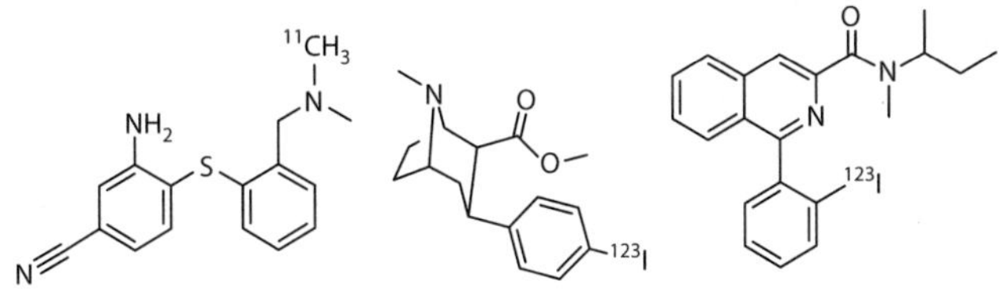
[^{123}I]-β–CIT
[^{123}I]PK11195
[^{11}C]flumazenil 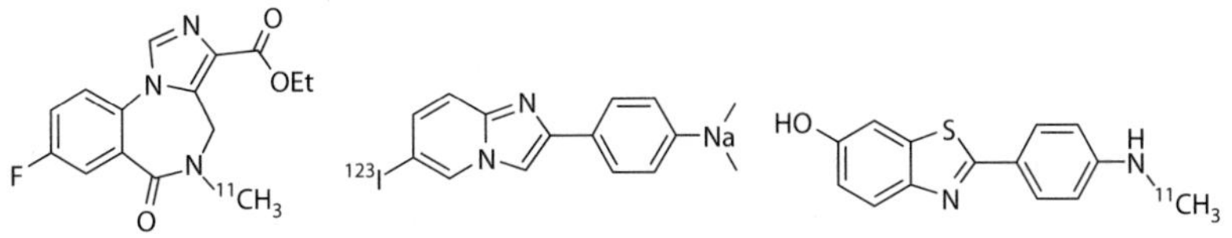
[^{123}I]IMPY
[^{11}C]PIB
[^{18}F]Flutemetamol 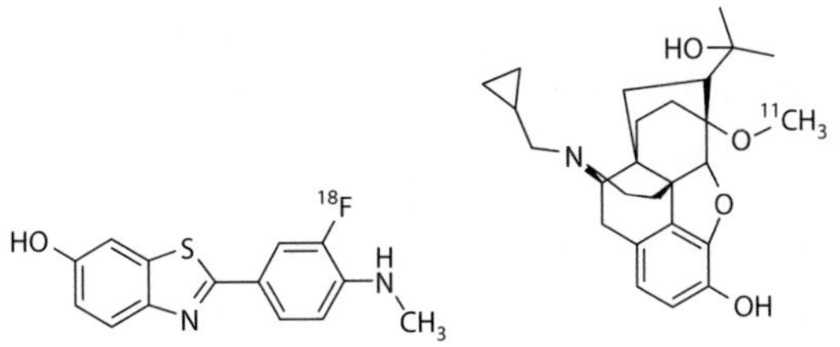
[^{11}C]Diprenorphine

Scheme 15.1

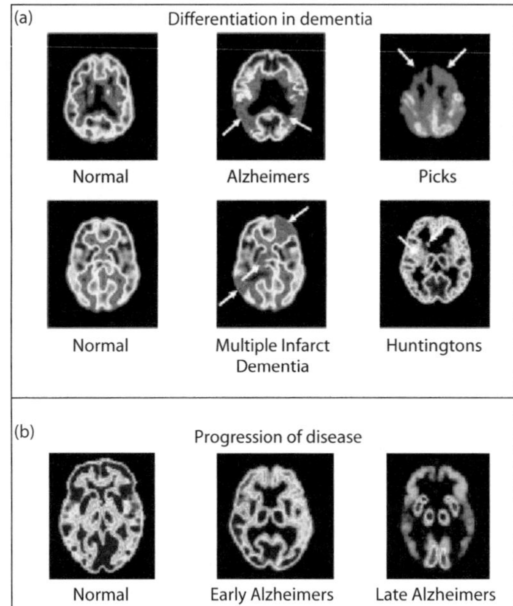

Figure 15.11 [^{18}F]FDG PET studies showing (a) glucose metabolism for differential diagnosis of dementia and (b) changes in glucose metabolism observed at early and late stage Alzheimer disease. Reprinted by permission of the Society of Nuclear Medicine from: Phelps (2000), Figures 2 and 3.

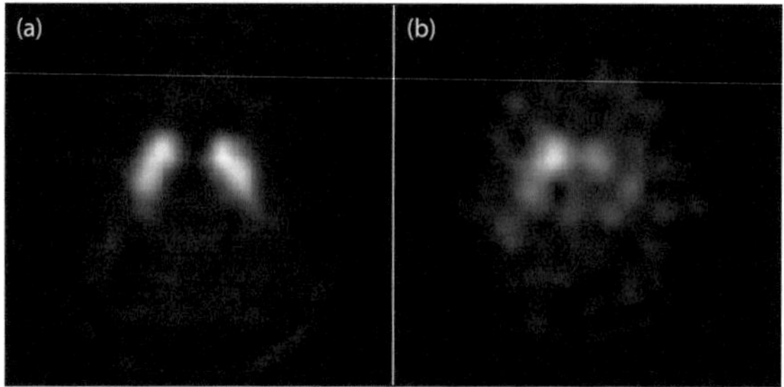

Figure 15.12 [^{123}I]ioflupane images of human striata. (a) Normal, (b) striatal dopaminergic deficit of Parkinson disease. Images courtesy of GE Healthcare Ltd.

neuronal cell loss and a decrease in synaptic activity (Salmon *et al.* 1996). The change in [^{18}F]FDG PET signal (i.e. glucose metabolism) from early to late stage Alzheimer disease can be correlated with the severity of dementia (Mazziotta *et al.* 1992). This type of study not only provides an early diagnosis of Alzheimer disease but is also able to differentiate between various types of dementias (see Figure 15.11). With [^{18}F]FDG PET improving diagnostic sensitivity to 93% (Silverman *et al.* 2001), this type of study can be used as a tool to detect subjects at risk of Alzheimer disease even before the onset of symptoms (Tai, Piccini 2004).

6-[^{18}F]Fluorolevodopa is a metabolic tracer that is taken up into dopaminergic nerve terminals and converted into [^{18}F]dopamine. The radiotracer can be used as a measure of dopamine synthesis and dopaminergic neuron density and, therefore, presynaptic dopaminergic function. In Parkinson disease conventional MRI is unable to identify any anatomical abnormalities. With [^{18}F]F-dopa PET, the loss of dopaminergic neurons is clearly detected in the striata and has been shown to be useful in early differentiation of Parkinson disease from other forms of movement disorders (Tai, Piccini 2004). In addition, [^{18}F]F-dopa can be used to detect a subclinical parkinsonian-like pattern (i.e. degeneration of dopaminergic neurones) in asymptomatic adult identical twins.

[^{123}I]Ioflupane (DaTSCAN) is a SPECT ligand that also binds to the presynaptic dopamine transporter to give images of the normal striata (Figure 15.12a). In cases of striatal dopaminergic deficit the characteristic symmetrical 'comma' shape of the two striata usually becomes asymmetric and/or degraded to the shape of a 'full stop' (Figure 15.12b).

Study of disease mechanisms

Amyloid plaques and neurofibrillary tangles are pathological markers found in Alzheimer disease postmortem brains. It is thought that these plaques are present as many as 10 years before any clinical symptoms of the disease appear (Teller *et al.* 1996). Recently, several PET tracers have been developed that bind to amyloid plaques and hence can be used as amyloid imaging agents. [^{11}C]PIB PET scans show a 2-fold increase in retention of signal in subjects with Alzheimer disease compared with controls. This increase in signal suggests widespread amyloid deposition in cortical areas and striata of Alzheimer disease subjects (Brooks 2005; Edison *et al.* 2007). Further analogues of this tracer such as [^{18}F]flutemetamol are currently under clinical investigation. Figure 15.13 shows images using this tracer in a normal subject (a) and a subject with Alzheimer disease (b).

Peripheral benzodiazepine binding sites (PBBS) are present at low levels in the normal brain. These sites are highly expressed *in vivo* by activated microglia,

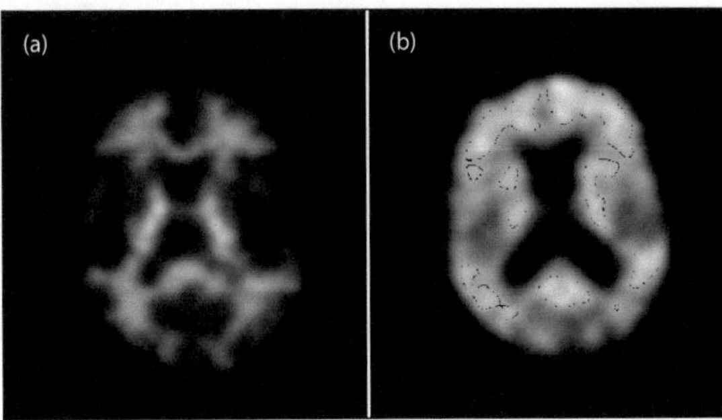

Figure 15.13 Coronal images obtained with the amyloid imaging agent [^{18}F]flutemetamol. (a) Normal, (b) Alzheimer disease. Images courtesy of GE Healthcare Ltd.

which are associated with CNS inflammation in a wide range of pathologies. In combination with MRI, to aid with anatomical definition, PET imaging using the PBBS-selective ligand (*R*)-[^{11}C]PK11195 provides a generic indicator of active disease in the brain and, to date, has been used in clinical studies of stroke, multiple sclerosis, dementia, Parkinson disease, Huntington chorea, epilepsy and schizophrenia (see review by Cagnin *et al.* 2002).

Receptor occupancy studies

Use of PET as a tool for neuroreceptor mapping can be very important for elucidation of basic mechanisms of disease and for investigating correlations with clinical parameters. For example, human PET studies with the antagonist radioligand, [^{11}C]WAY100635 to image presynaptic and postsynaptic 5-HT$_{1A}$ receptors is well established (e.g. Rabiner *et al.* 2000) and has been used extensively to study 5-HT$_{1A}$ receptor dysfunction in human disease states (e.g. Drevets *et al.* 2000; Sargent *et al.* 2000). The neuropharmacological data obtained from receptor-specific PET/SPECT studies can additionally help increase knowledge in potential therapeutic targets for novel pharmaceutical agents by determining their dose–occupancy profile. This can be done using the radiolabelled drug under investigation or by monitoring its effects on the binding of an established radioligand. With the former, regional brain pharmacokinetic data are obtained within a very short time-frame. With the latter case, by quantifying the reduction in specific binding of the labelled drug, the dose, plasma concentration and/or efficacy of the unlabelled drug can be related directly to receptor occupancy *in vivo*. In Figure 15.14 a reduction in [^{11}C]WAY100635 binding is seen following administration of 20 mg pindolol, a 5-HT$_{1A}$ antagonist used clinically as an adjunct to antidepressants (Artigas *et al.* 1996).

PET/SPECT can also be used non-invasively to indirectly monitor changes in neurotransmitter concentration, providing that (1), a PET radioligand specific and selective for the system of interest is available, and (2), the radioligand binds to the same site as the endogenous ligand, or neurotransmitter. Over the past 15 years, many studies have demonstrated the use of PET and SPECT to non-invasively measure acute changes in neurotransmitter levels *in vivo* (see review by Laruelle 2000), initially assuming a direct competition between the radioligand and the endogenous

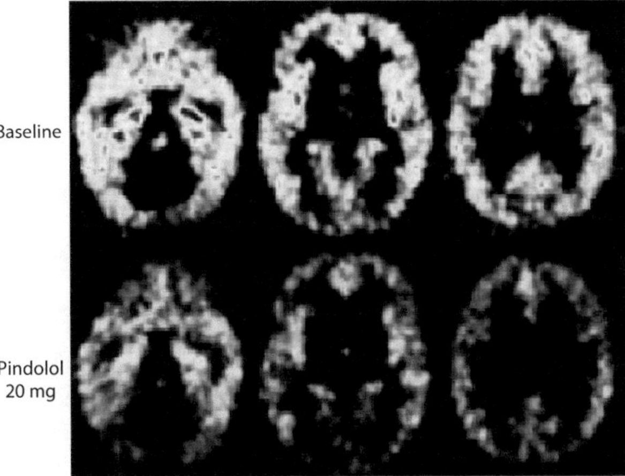

Figure 15.14 Reduction in [^{11}C]WAY100635 binding to 5-HT$_{1A}$ receptors following administration of the 5-HT$_{1A}$ antagonist pindolol. Images provided by D.J. Brooks; courtesy of MRC Clinical Sciences Centre.

neurotransmitter at the binding site. This is in part due to the successful discovery that the binding of D_2 receptor radioligands, [^{11}C]raclopride and [^{123}I]IBZM, is particularly sensitive to changes in dopamine levels (e.g. Farde *et al.* 1992; Laruelle *et al.* 1995). Although these types of studies are ideal for investigating the effect of a drug on neurotransmitter function, Koepp *et al.* (1998) have demonstrated the use of PET with [^{11}C]raclopride to measure endogenous dopamine release in human striatum during a goal-directed motor task (playing a video game).

As the number of PET/SPECT centres grows, applications of use in clinical neurology will increase for early and/or presymptomatic diagnosis of diseases. As more target-specific radiotracers and ligands are developed, the use of these in clinical research and drug development will help determine optimal drug dosing regimes and elucidate the downstream effect of drug actions.

Oncology

The range of radiopharmaceuticals already used in oncological PET studies is wide, and the list of tracers is continuously expanding.

2-[^{18}F]Fluoro-2-deoxyglucose ([^{18}F]FDG) is the most widely used tracer for tumour imaging with PET. [^{18}F]FDG is a structural analogue of glucose in which a hydroxyl group is replaced by ^{18}F. [^{18}F]FDG is transported into the cell like glucose, and is phosphorylated by hexokinase. This phosphorylation to [^{18}F]FDG 6-phosphate results in a polar intermediate, which is not further catabolised by the subsequent reactions of glycolysis or transported across the cell membranes in any substantial amount, i.e. it is metabolically trapped in the cell. Increased glucose metabolism is one of the basic biochemical characteristics of cancer cells. The enhanced glycolysis has been associated with an increase both in the amount of glucose membrane transporters and in the activity of the principal enzymes controlling the glycolytic pathway.

[^{18}F]FDG PET has been successfully used in an increasing number of clinical indications in oncology. A high uptake of [^{18}F]FDG has been recorded in a wide variety of different tumours and [^{18}F]FDG has an established role in the clinic. However, [^{18}F]FDG is not specific for malignant transformation. In particular, infections and inflammatory lesions accumulate [^{18}F]FDG as a result of uptake into macrophages and pose a significant differential diagnostic problem with using [^{18}F]FDG in clinical oncology. Furthermore, there is physiological accumulation of [^{18}F]FDG, for instance, in the brain, heart, kidney and urinary bladder, and these accumulations may interfere with the detection of malignancy. A high blood glucose concentration may also interfere with tumour imaging, since hyperglycaemia may considerably decrease the uptake of [^{18}F]FDG in human tumours.

In addition to activated glucose metabolism, increased amino acid utilisation is characteristic of cancer, and several amino acids have been labelled for PET imaging. These include L-[*methyl*-^{11}C]methionine and 1-amino-[3-^{18}F]fluorocyclobutane-1-carboxylic acid.

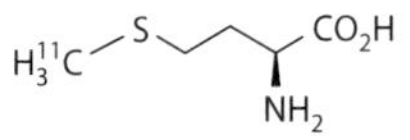

$H_3^{11}C$ S CO_2H NH_2

L-[*Methyl*-^{11}C]methionine

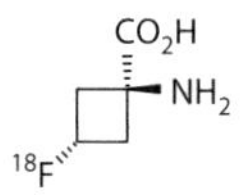

CO_2H NH_2 ^{18}F

1-Amino-[3-^{18}F]fluorocyclobutane-1-carboxylic acid

Carcinogenesis is characterised by enhanced cell membrane synthesis and changes in phospholipid metabolism. Choline, a precursor in the biosynthesis of phospholipids, has been labelled with positron emitters, and has also been used for cancer imaging (Hara *et al.* 1997).

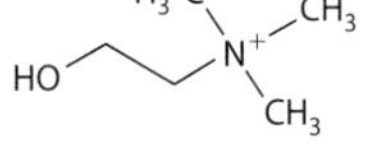

$H_3^{11}C$ CH_3 HO N^+ CH_3 | H_3C ^{18}F HO N^+ CH_3

[^{11}C]Choline 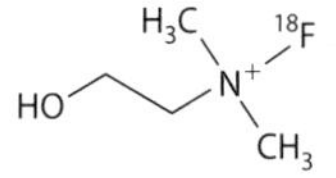 | [^{18}F]Fluorocholine

Uncontrolled proliferation is one of the characteristic features of the biology of malignant tissue. Since thymidine is incorporated into newly synthesised DNA and is the only base that is not also incorporated into RNA, thymidine has been a logical choice as a tracer of cell growth. Thymidine labelled with long-lived tracers such as ^{3}H has been used in *in-vitro* studies to assess cell growth (Hall, Levison 1990). Results of clinical studies with [^{11}C]thymidine PET in patients with a range of tumours have demonstrated its potential to image tumours and to monitor tumour proliferation and response to therapy (e.g. Wells *et al.* 2002). The complex metabolism of [^{11}C]thymidine led to the development of thymidine analogues such as [^{124}I]iododeoxyuridine (IudR) and [^{76}Br]bromodeoxyuridine (BrudR) for tumour imaging (Blasberg *et al.* 2000; Gudjonssona *et al.* 2001). Both of these analogues are incorporated into DNA but share the problem of rapid dehalogenation, which liberates the label as a free halide, thus reducing the fraction of radioactivity incorporated into the DNA.

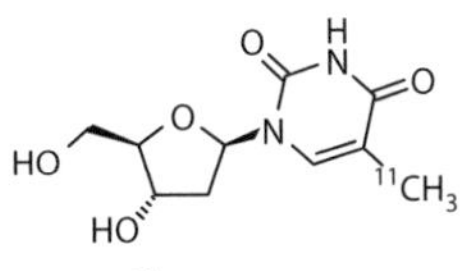

[^{11}C]Thymidine

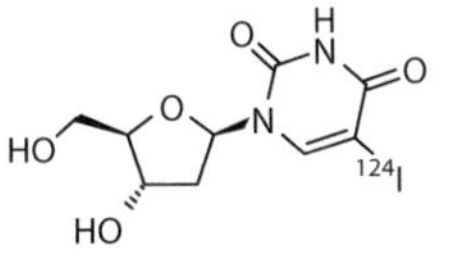

[^{124}I]Iododeoxyuridine

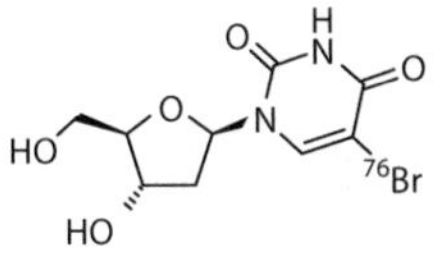

[^{76}Br]Bromodeoxyuridine

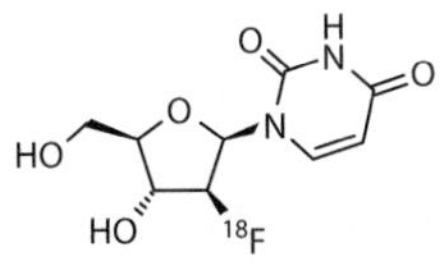

[^{18}F]FAU

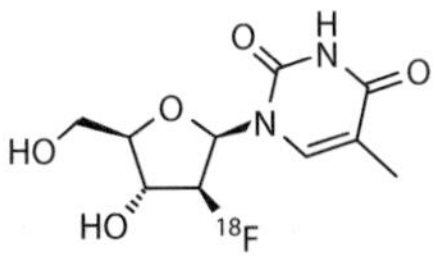

[^{18}F]FMAU

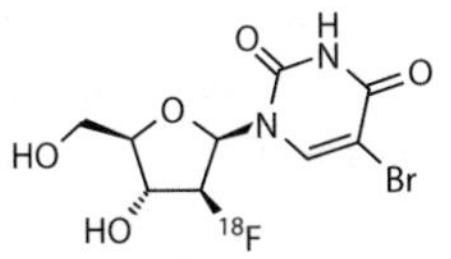

[^{18}F]FBAU

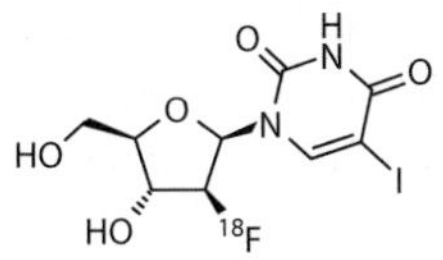

[^{18}F]FIAU

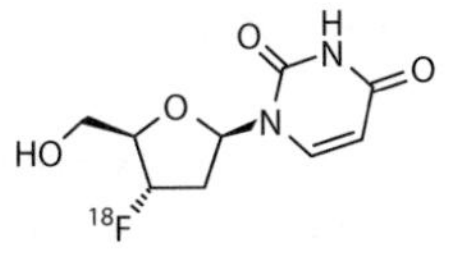

[^{18}F]FLT

Several ^{18}F-labelled thymidine analogues resistant to metabolism, such as 1-(2′-deoxy-2′-[^{18}F]fluoro-β-D-arabinofuranosyl)uracil (FAU), 1-(2′-deoxy-2′-[^{18}F]-fluoro-β-D-arabinofuranosyl)-5-methyluracil (FMAU), 1-(2′-deoxy-2′-[^{18}F]fluoro-β-D-arabinofuranosyl)-5-bromouracil (FBAU) and 1-(2′-deoxy-2′-[^{18}F]fluoro-β-D-arabinofuranosyl)-5-iodouracil (FIAU), have been synthesised (Mangner *et al.* 2003). Shields *et al.* (1998) introduced 3′-deoxy-3′-[^{18}F]fluorothymidine ([^{18}F]FLT or [^{18}F]alovudine), which is retained in proliferating tissues by the action of thymidine kinase-1 and is resistant to degradation. [^{18}F]FLT has shown promise as an imaging agent in patients with lung tumours, colorectal cancer and lymphoma. A positive correlation has been reported between uptake of [^{18}F]FLT and cellular proliferation markers (Vesselle *et al.* 2002).

Regional blood flow, tissue oxygenation and nutrient supply influence the response of malignant tumours to both radiotherapy and chemotherapy and also affect the proliferative activity of tumours. Accurate non-invasive measurement of blood flow to tumours may assist in monitoring the effect of therapies such as the efficiency of novel anti-angiogenic agents, and in assessment of drug delivery.

Most solid tumours have hypoxic cells, which may induce angiogenesis and enhance the invasive potential of neoplastic cells. Hypoxic cells in solid tumours reduce the sensitivity of tumours to radiotherapy and chemotherapy, and thus it would be valuable to assess the oxygenation status of tumours before treatment and for the selection of patients for different types of therapy. Hypoxic cells can be imaged non-invasively with PET using radiolabelled hypoxia-avid compounds, such as nitroimidazole compounds.

Fluorine-18-labelled fluoromisonidazole ([^{18}F]-FMISO), the most widely studied hypoxia marker in clinical PET, has been used to study patients with several types of cancer, including head and neck, lung, prostate, and brain tumours. [^{18}F]FMISO accumulates in viable hypoxic cells that contain nitroreductase enzymes. However, [^{18}F]FMISO is not optimal because of its relatively poor uptake into cells and slow clearance from the surrounding healthy tissues. ^{18}F-labelled fluoroerythronitroimidazole ([^{18}F]FETNIM) is another nitroimidazole compound that has recently been used in clinical studies in patients with head and neck cancer (Lehtio *et al.* 2003). [^{18}F]FETNIM is more hydrophilic than [^{18}F]FMISO and it is eliminated rapidly from well-oxygenated tissues and thus results, in rat mammary cancer, in a higher tumour-to-liver and tumour-to-blood ratio than [^{18}F]FMISO. Cu-ATSM is a copper-bisthiosemicarbazone complex that can be labelled with three positron-emitting isotopes (^{64}Cu, ^{62}Cu, ^{60}Cu). ^{64}Cu-ATSM PET has successfully been used in hypoxia studies on patients with lung cancer, cervical cancer, and head and neck cancer (Chao *et al.* 2001; Dehdashti *et al.* 2003).

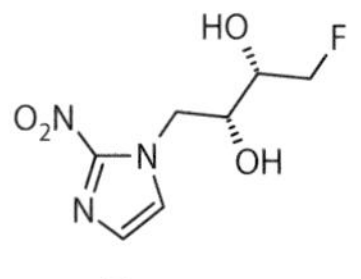

[^{18}F]FETNIM

Proliferation of some types of cancer cells such as breast and prostate cancer is regulated by steroid hormones, which bind to intracellular receptors. The oestrogen receptor imaging agent 16α-[^{18}F]fluoroestradiol-17β ([^{18}F]FES) is so far the most commonly used sex hormone receptor-imaging compound for PET. Many other cell membrane and intracellular receptors are up-regulated in cancer cells and these receptors are potential targets for PET tracers. Examples of other receptor tracers that have been introduced for PET are ^{64}Cu- or ^{68}Ga-labelled octreotide and edotreotide for targeting somatostatin receptor-positive tumours. Radioligands targeting tumour growth factors such as the vascular endothelial growth factor (VEGF) and epidermal growth factor (EGF) have recently been labelled and tested for PET imaging (Collingridge *et al.* 2002; Ben-David *et al.* 2003). The development of anticancer drugs that target tumour growth factors is a growing area in oncology, and *in-vivo* imaging with PET serves as a valuable tool in both the preclinical and clinical assessment of drugs.

Many tumour-associated antigens, including antigens that are products of oncogenes or proto-oncogenes such as the c-erb B2 protein, in addition to other growth factors, can serve as *in-vivo* targets for radiolabelled monoclonal antibodies (Bakir *et al.* 1992). There are human studies with monoclonal antibodies labelled with positron emitters targeted at breast cancer, neuroblastoma and colorectal cancer. Because monoclonal antibodies have a relatively low clearance from the blood, engineered antibody fragments that have a more rapid blood clearance owing to their smaller size may be more useful. A fragment of an antibody against carcinoembryonic antigen has been successfully labelled with ^{64}Cu (Wu *et al.* 2000).

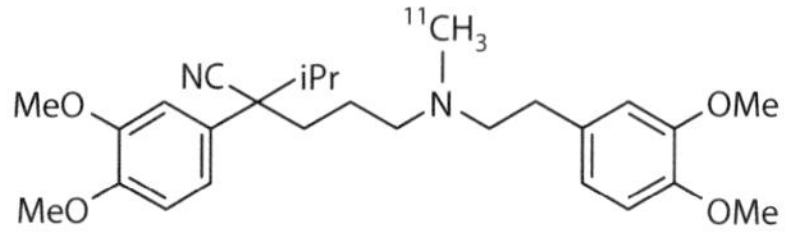

[^{11}C]Verapamil

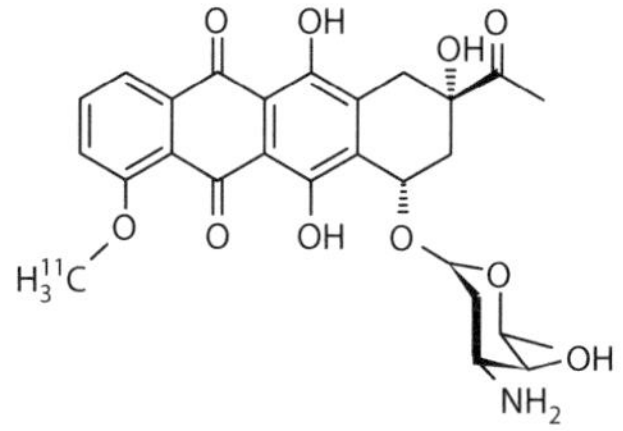

[^{11}C]Daunorubicin

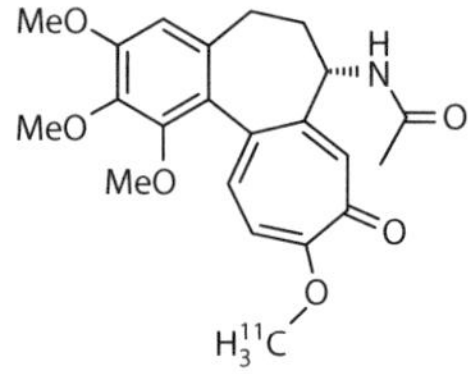

[^{11}C]Colchicine

PET can also be used to monitor components involved in apoptosis and drug resistance. Annexin V is an endogenous human protein with a high affinity for phosphatidylserine exposed on the surface of apoptotic cells. Annexin V can be labelled with SPECT radionuclides such as iodine-123 or technetium-99m to detect apoptotic cells *in vivo*, and has also been labelled with ^{124}I for PET imaging (Glaser *et al.* 2003). Overexpression of P-glycoprotein, a plasma membrane transporter encoded for by the multi-drug resistance (MDR) gene, is one of the mechanisms that cause MDR in human tumours. So far, *in-vivo* PET studies involved in evaluation of MDR have mostly been confined to experimentation in animals. [^{11}C]Verapamil, [^{11}C]daunorubicin and [^{11}C]colchicine have been studied as *in-vivo* probes for P-glycoprotein.

Concluding remarks

The essence of the mechanism of action of radiopharmaceuticals is embodied in radiopharmacokinetics – absorption, distribution, metabolism and excretion. One or more of these dictate whether a radiopharmaceutical will be efficacious or not. Assessment of the radiopharmacokinetics of new radiotracers, using a variety of techniques described in this chapter, is vital to their ultimate introduction to clinical practice. The utility of a radiopharmaceutical is a reflection of our ability to detect altered radiopharmacokinetics in disease states.

Acknowledgments

The author gratefully acknowledges the contributions and critique of the following colleagues from GE Healthcare, Medical Diagnostics: Lucy Allen, Julian Goggi, Brian Higley, Ella Hirani, Matthew Morrison, James Nairne and Ian Wilson

References

Alderson PO, Line BR (1980). Scintigraphic evaluation of regional pulmonary ventilation. *Semin Nucl Med* 10: 218–242.

Alvarez-Fischer D *et al.* (2007). Quantitative [^{123}I]FP-CIT pinhole SPECT imaging predicts striatal dopamine levels, but not number of nigral neurons in different mouse models of Parkinson's disease. *NeuroImage* 38: 5–12.

Artigas F *et al.* (1996). Acceleration of the effect of selected antidepressant drugs in major depression by 5-HT$_{1A}$ antagonists. *Trends Neurosci* 19: 378–383.

Ashkan K *et al.* (2007). SPECT imaging, immunohistochemical and behavioural correlations in the primate models of Parkinson's disease. *Parkinsonism Rel Disord* 13: 266–275.

Bach-Gansmo T *et al.* (2006). Integrin receptor imaging of breast cancer: a proof-of-concept study to evaluate 99mTc-NC100692. *J Nucl Med* 47: 1434–1439.

Bach-Gansmo T *et al.* (2008). Integrin scintimammography using a dedicated breast imaging, solid-state gamma-camera and (99m)Tc-labelled NC100692. *Clin Physiol Funct Imaging* 28: 235–239.

Bakir MA *et al.* (1992). C-erb2 protein expression in breast cancer as a target for PET using iodine-124-labeled monoclonal antibodies. *J Nucl Med* 33: 2154–2160.

Bakker WH *et al.* (1991a). [^{111}In-DTPA-D-Phe^{1}]-octreotide, a potential radiopharmaceutical for imaging of somatostatin receptor-positive tumors: synthesis, radiolabeling and in vitro validation. *Life Sci* 49: 1583–1591.

Bakker WH *et al.* (1991b). In vivo application of [^{111}In-DTPA-D-Phe^{1}]-octreotide for detection of somatostatin receptor-positive tumors in rats. *Life Sci* 49: 1593–1601.

Banati RB *et al.* (1999). [^{11}C](*R*)-PK11195 positron emission tomography imaging of activated microglia in vivo in Rasmussen's encephalitis. *Neurology* 53: 2199–2203.

Ben-David I *et al.* (2003). Radiosynthesis of ML03, a novel positron emission tomography biomarker for targeting epidermal growth factor receptor via the labelling of synthin [^{11}C] acryloyl chloride. *Appl Radiat Isot* 58: 209–217.

Biddlecombe GB *et al.* (2007). Molecular imaging of gastrin-releasing peptide receptor-positive tumors in mice using ^{64}Cu- and ^{86}Y-DOTA-(Pro1,Tyr^{4})-bombesin(1–14). *Bioconjug Chem* 18: 724–730.

Blasberg RG *et al.* (2000). Imaging brain tumour proliferative activity with [^{124}I]iododeoxyuridine. *Cancer Res* 60: 624–635.

Blau M, Bender MA (1962). Se 75-selenomethionine for visualization of the pancreas by isotope scanning. *Radiology* 78: 974.

Blau M *et al.* (1972). ^{18}F-Fluoride for bone imaging. *Semin Nucl Med* 2: 31–37.

Booij J *et al.* (1998). Human biodistribution and dosimetry of [^{123}I]FP-CIT: a potent radioligand for imaging of dopamine transporters. *Eur J Nucl Med* 25: 24–30.

Brooks DJ (2005). Positron emission tomography and single photon emission computed tomography in central nervous system drug development. *NeuroRx* 2: 226–236.

Cagnin A *et al.* (2002). In vivo imaging of neuroinflammation. *Eur Neuropsychopharmacol* 12: 581–586.

Chao KS *et al.* (2001). A novel approach to overcome hypoxic tumour resistance: Cu-ATSM-guided intensity-modulated radiation therapy. *Int J Radiat Oncol Biol Phys* 49: 1171–1182.

Collingridge DR *et al.* (2002). The development of [^{124}I] iodinated-VGT6e: a novel tracer for imaging of vascular endothelial growth factor in vivo using positron emission tomography. *Cancer Res* 62: 5912–5919.

Dehdashti F *et al.* (2003). Assessing tumor hypoxia in cervical cancer by positron emission tomography with ^{60}Cu-ATSM: relationship to therapeutic response – a preliminary report. *Int J Radiat Oncol Biol Phys* 55: 1233–1238.

de Visser M *et al.* (2007). Novel ^{111}In-labelled bombesin analogues for molecular imaging of prostate tumours. *Eur J Nucl Med Mol Imaging* 34: 1228–1238.

Drevets WC *et al.* (2000). Serotonin type-1A receptor imaging in depression. *Nucl Med Biol* 27: 499–507.

Edison P *et al.* (2007). Amyloid, hypometabolism, and cognition in Alzheimer disease: an [^{11}C]PIB and [^{18}F]FDG PET study. *Neurology* 68: 501–508.

Edwards D *et al.* (2008). ^{99m}Tc-NC100692 – a tracer for imaging vitronectin receptors associated with angiogenesis: a preclinical investigation. *Nucl Med Biol* 35: 365–375.

Farde L *et al.* (1992). Positron emission tomographic analysis of central D1 and D2 dopamine receptor occupancy in patients treated with classical neuroleptics and clozapine. Relation to extrapyramidal side effects. *Arch Gen Psychiatry* 49: 538–544.

Fuster D *et al.* (2003). Is there a role for ^{99m}Tc-anti-CEA monoclonal antibody imaging in the diagnosis of recurrent colorectal carcinoma? *Q J Nucl Med* 47: 109–115.

Gabriel M *et al.* (2007). 68Ga-DOTA-Tyr3-octreotide PET in neuroendocrine tumors: comparison with somatostatin receptor scintigraphy and CT. *J Nucl Med* 48: 508–518.

Gibaldi M, Perrier D (1982). *Drugs and the Pharmaceutical Sciences 15: Pharmacokinetics*, 2nd edn. New York: Marcel Dekker.

Glaser M *et al.* (2003). Iodine-124 labeled Annexin V as a potential radiotracer to study apoptosis using positron emission tomography. *App Radiat Isot* 58: 55–62.

Glaser M *et al.* (2008). Radiosynthesis and biodistribution of cyclic RGD peptides conjugated with novel [^{18}F]fluorinated aldehyde-containing prosthetic groups. *Bioconjug Chemistry* 19: 951–957.

Gudjonssona O *et al.* (2001). Analysis of [^{76}Br]bromodeoxyuridine in DNA of brain tumors after PET study does not support its use as a proliferation marker. *Nucl Med Biol* 28: 59–65.

Hagan I *et al.* (2006). Superior demonstration of splenosis by heat-denatured Tc-99m red blood cell scintigraphy compared with Tc-99m sulfur colloid scintigraphy. *Clin Nucl Med* 31: 463–466.

Hall PA, Levison DA (1990). Review: Assessment of cell proliferation in histological material. *J Clin Pathol* 45: 184–192.

Hara T *et al.* (1997). PET imaging of brain tumour with [methyl-^{11}[C]choline. *J Nucl Med* 38: 842–847.

Harding LK *et al.* (1973). The proportion of lung vessels blocked by albumin microspheres. *J Nucl Med* 14: 579–581.

Hirani E *et al.* (2003). Fenfluramine evokes 5-HT2A receptor-mediated responses but does not displace [^{11}C]MDL 100907: small animal PET and gene expression studies. *Synapse* 50: 251–260.

Hua J *et al.* (2005). Noninvasive imaging of angiogenesis with a ^{99m}Tc-labeled peptide targeted at $\alpha_v\beta_3$ integrin after murine hindlimb ischemia. *Circulation* 111: 3255–3260.

Kailasnath P, Sinusas AJ (2001). Comparison of Tl-201 with Tc-99m-labeled myocardial perfusion agents: technical, physiologic, and clinical issues. *J Nucl Cardiol* 8: 482–498.

Knapp FF Jr *et al.* (1996). Pharmacokinetics of radioiodinated fatty acid myocardial imaging agents in animal models and human studies. *Q J Nucl Med* 40: 252–269.

Koepp MJ *et al.* (1998). Evidence for striatal dopamine release during a video game. *Nature* 393: 266–268.

Kumar V (2005). Radiolabeled white blood cells and direct targeting of micro-organisms for infection imaging. *Q J Nucl Med Mol Imaging* 49: 325–338.

Kuperus J (1979). The role of phagocytosis and pinocytosis in the localisation of radiotracers. In: *Principles of Radiopharmacology*, Vol. III. Boca Raton: CRC Press, 267–276.

Laruelle M (2000). Imaging synaptic neurotransmission with in vivo binding competition techniques: a critical review. *J Cereb Blood Flow Metab* 20: 423–451.

Laruelle M *et al.* (1995). SPECT imaging of striatal dopamine release after amphetamine challenge. *J Nucl Med* 36: 1182–1190.

Lathrop KA *et al.* (1989). Multiparameter extrapolation of biodistribution data between species. *Health Phys* 57 (Suppl 1): 121–126.

Lee ST, Scott AM (2007). Hypoxia positron emission tomography imaging with ^{18}F-fluoromisonidazole. *Semin Nucl Med* 37: 451–461.

Lehtio K *et al.* (2003). Quantifying tumour hypoxia with fluorine-18 fluoroerythronitroimidazole ([^{18}F]FETNIM) and PET using the tumour to plasma ratios. *Eur J Nucl Med* 30: 101–108.

Levy O *et al.* (1998). The Na^+/I^- symporter (NIS): recent advances. *J Bioenerg Biomembr* 30: 195–206.

Mahmood I (1999). Prediction of clearance, volume of distribution and half-life by allometric scaling and by use of plasma concentrations predicted from pharmacokinetic constants: a comparative study. *J Pharm Pharmacol* 51: 905–910.

Mangner TJ *et al.* (2003). Synthesis of 2′-deoxy-2′-[^{18}F]-fluoro-β-D-arabinofuranosyl nucleosides, [^{18}F]FAU, [^{18}F]-FMAU, [^{18}F]FBAU and [^{18}F]FIAU, as potential PET agents for imaging cellular proliferation. Synthesis of [^{18}F]labelled FAU, FMAU, FBAU, FIAU. *Nucl Med Biol* 30: 215–224.

Mankoff DA *et al.* (2001). [^{18}F]Fluoroestradiol radiation dosimetry in human PET studies. *J Nucl Med* 42: 679–684.

Manyak MJ (2008). Indium-111 capromab pendetide in the management of recurrent prostate cancer. *Expert Rev Anticancer Ther* 8: 175–181.

Mattsson S *et al.* (2006). Radioactive iodine in thyroid medicine – how it started in Sweden and some of today's challenges. *Acta Ocol* 45: 1031–1036.

Maurer AH, Parkman HP (2006). Update on gastrointestinal scintigraphy. *Semin Nucl Med* 36: 110–118.

Mazziotta JC *et al.* (1992). The use of positron emission tomography in the clinical assessment of dementia. *Semin Nucl Med* 4: 233–246.

Miles KA, Williams RE (2008). Warburg revisited: imaging tumour blood flow and metabolism. *Cancer Imaging* 8: 81–86.

Mordenti Y (1986). Man versus beast: pharmacokinetic scaling in mammals. *J Pharm Sci* 75: 1028–1040.

Mullani NA *et al.* (2008). Tumor blood flow measured by PET dynamic imaging of first-pass ^{18}F-FDG uptake: a comparison with ^{15}O-labeled water-measured blood flow. *J Nucl Med* 49: 517–523.

Neirinckx RD *et al.* (1988). The retention mechanism of technetium-99m-HM-PAO: intracellular reaction with glutathione. *J Cereb Blood Flow Metab* 8: S4–12.

Perik PJ *et al.* (2006). Indium-111-labeled trastuzumab scintigraphy in patients with human epidermal growth factor receptor 2-positive metastatic breast cancer. *J Clin Oncol* 24: 2276–2282.

Phelps ME (2000). PET: the merging of biology and imaging into molecular imaging. *J Nucl Med* 41: 661–681.

Platts EA *et al.* (1995). Mechanism of uptake of technetium-tetrofosmin. I: Uptake into isolated adult rat ventricular myocytes and subcellular localization. *J Nucl Cardiol* 2: 317–326.

Puncher MR, Blower PJ (1994). Radionuclide targeting and dosimetry at the microscopic level: the role of microautoradiography [Review]. *Eur J Nucl Med* 21: 1347–1365.

Rabiner EA *et al.* (2000). Drug action at the 5-HT_{1A} receptor *in vivo*: autoreceptor and postsynaptic receptor occupancy examined with PET and [carbonyl-^{11}C]WAY-100635. *Nucl Med Biol* 27: 509–513.

Racine A *et al.* (1986). Bayesean models in practice: experience in the pharmaceutical industry. *Appl Stat* 35: 93–150.

Ritschel WA *et al.* (1992). The allometric approach for interspecies scaling of pharmacokinetic parameters. *Comp Biochem Physiol C* 103: 249–253.

Salmon E *et al.* (1996). Combined study of cerebral glucose metabolism and [^{11}C]methionine accumulation in probable Alzheimer's disease using positron emission tomography. *Cereb Blood Flow Metab* 16: 399–408.

Sargent PA *et al.* (2000). Brain serotonin$_{1A}$ receptor binding measured by positron emission tomography with [^{11}C] WAY-100635: effects of depression and antidepressant treatment. *Arch Gen Psychiatry* 57: 174–180.

Shields AF *et al.* (1998). Imaging of proliferation in vivo with [F-18]FLT and positron emission tomography. *Nature Med* 4: 1334–1336.

Silverman DH *et al.* (2001). Positron emission tomography in evaluation of dementia: regional brain metabolism and long-term outcome. *JAMA* 286: 2120–2127.

Skehan SJ *et al.* (2003). Mechanism of accumulation of ^{99m}Tc-sulesomab in inflammation. *J Nucl Med* 44: 11–18.

Smith-Jones PM *et al.* (2004). Imaging the pharmacodynamics of HER2 degradation in response to Hsp90 inhibitors. *Nat Biotechnol* 22: 701–706.

Sundararajan L *et al.* (2007). ^{18}F-Fluoroestradiol. *Semin Nucl Med* 37: 470–476.

Tai YF, Piccini P (2004). Applications of positron emission tomography (PET) in neurology [Review]. *J Neurol Neurosurg Psychiatry* 75: 669–676.

Teller JK *et al.* (1996). Presence of soluble amyloid beta-peptide precedes amyloid plaque formation in Down's syndrome. *Nat Med* 2: 93–95.

Teorell T (1937a). Kinetics and distribution of substances administered to the body I. The extravascular modes of distribution. *Arch Intern Pharmacodynam* 57: 205–225.

Teorell T (1937b). Kinetics and distribution of substances administered to the body II. The intravascular modes of distribution. *Arch Intern Pharmacodynam* 57: 226–240.

Ter-Pogossian MM, Herscovitch P (1985). Radioactive oxygen-15 in the study of cerebral blood flow, blood volume, and oxygen metabolism. *Semin Nucl Med* 15: 377–394.

Urbain JL, Charkes ND (1995). Recent advances in gastric emptying scintigraphy. *Semin Nucl Med* 25: 318–325.

Vastenhouw B *et al.* (2007). Movie of dopamine transporter occupancy with ultra-high resolution focusing pinhole SPECT. *Mol Psychiatry* 12: 984–987.

Vessell H *et al.* (2002). In vivo validation of introduced 3′-deoxy-3′-[^{18}F]fluorothymidine ([^{18}F]FLT) as a proliferation imaging tracer in humans; correlation of [^{18}F]FLT uptake by positron emission tomography with ki-67 immunohistochemistry and flow cytometry in human lung tumors. *Clin Cancer Res* 8: 3315–3323.

Wagner JG (1968). Pharmacokinetics 1. Definitions, Modeling and reasons for measuring blood levels and urinary excretion. *Drug Intell* 2: 38–42.

Wagner JG (1969). Pharmacokinetics 2. Introduction to compartment models. *Drug Intell* 3: 250–257.

Wagner JG (1976). Linear pharmacokinetic equations allowing direct calculation of many needed pharmacokinetic parameters from the coefficients and exponents which have been fitted to the data. *J Pharmacokinet Biopharm* 4: 443–467.

Wang YF *et al.* (2007). On-site preparation of technetium-99m labeled human serum albumin for clinical application. *Tohoku J Exp Med* 211: 379–385.

Weber DA *et al.* (1969). Kinetics of radionuclides used for bone studies. *J Nucl Med* 10: 8–17.

Wells P *et al.* (2002). Assessment of proliferation in vivo using 2-[^{11}C]thymidine positron emission tomography in advanced intra-abdominal malignancies. *Cancer Res* 62: 5698–5702.

Wildt S *et al.* (2003). Bile acid malabsorption in patients with chronic diarrhoea: clinical value of SeHCAT test. *Scand J Gastroenterol* 38: 826–830.

Wu AM *et al.* (2000). High-resolution microPET imaging of carcinoembryonic antigen-positive xenografts by using a copper-64-labeled engineered antibody fragment. *Proc Natl Acad Sci USA* 97: 8495–8500.

Younes A *et al.* (1995). Mechanism of uptake of technetium-tetrofosmin. II: Uptake into isolated adult rat heart mitochondria. *J Nucl Cardiol* 2: 327–333.

Further reading

Beekman F, van der Have F (2007). The pinhole: gateway to ultra-high-resolution three-dimensional radionuclide imaging [Review]. *Eur J Nucl Med Mol Imaging* 34: 151–161.

Bundy DC (2001). Autoradiography. *Curr Protoc Protein Sci* Chapter 10: Unit 10.11.

Kötter R *et al.* (2007). Databasing receptor distributions in the brain [Review]. *Methods Mol Biol* 401: 267–284.

Myers R, Hume S (2002). Small animal PET [Review]. *Eur Neuropsychopharmacol* 12: 545–555.

Owunwanne A *et al.*, eds (1995). *Handbook of Radiopharmaceuticals*. London: Chapman & Hall Medical.

Parker RP *et al.*, eds (1984). *Basic Science of Nuclear Medicine*, 2nd edn. Edinburgh: Churchill Livingstone.

Theobald AE, ed. (1985). *Radiopharmacy and Radiopharmaceuticals*. London: Taylor and Francis.

Vallabhajosula S (2007). ^{18}F-Labeled positron emission tomographic radiopharmaceuticals in oncology: an overview of radiochemistry and mechanisms of tumor localization. *Semin Nucl Med* 37: 400–419.

Vaska P *et al.* (2006). Quantitative imaging with the microPET small-animal PET tomograph. *Int Rev Neurobiol* 73: 191–218.

16

Receptors and transporters

James M Stone and Erik Årstad

Introduction

One of the great strengths of positron emission tomography (PET) and single-photon emission computed tomography (SPECT) imaging, from both clinical and research perspectives, is the ability to image the molecular components of endogenous ligand interactions with receptors and transporters in living humans. The sensitivity of these methods means that they are able to detect relatively small but clinically meaningful changes in receptor or transporter binding. Thus PET and SPECT imaging have been used in assessing underlying differences in receptor availability in illness states, estimating endogenous ligand concentration and measuring drug–receptor binding, as well as being used in diagnosis and in the monitoring of treatment response. Although receptors and transporters are present in diverse tissues throughout the body, they share the same general principles in terms of endogenous ligand binding and signal transduction, regardless of their site of expression. This chapter will deal primarily with neurotransmitters in the brain, but the concepts discussed may equally well be applied to receptors and transporters in other tissues.

The machinery of neurotransmission

In the brain, unidirectional electrical impulses are carried by neurons, which form connections with each other through synapses. Synapses compose a close alignment of the (presynaptic) cell membrane of the neuron from which the impulse originates (synaptic bouton) with the (postsynaptic) cell membrane of the adjacent neuron. Neurotransmitters are chemical messengers that are stored in vesicles within the synaptic bouton. With the arrival of an electrical impulse, these vesicles fuse with the presynaptic membrane and the neurotransmitter is released into the synaptic cleft, where it diffuses to bind to neuroreceptors expressed on both the pre- and postsynaptic membranes. After binding, the neurotransmitter molecules dissociate and diffuse back into the synaptic cleft. In some cases they are then actively transported back inside the cell via transporters.

Receptor subtypes

Receptors are membrane-bound proteins that act as signal transducers in the cell. Most are expressed on the cell surface, but some are present inside the cell. All receptors have one or more specific binding sites (active sites) for interaction with their specific endogenous ligand. This may be a neurotransmitter, a hormone or another chemical depending upon the receptor type.

Following receptor–ligand binding, receptors change their physical conformation and, depending upon their type, transmit a signal by altering ion channel permeability (leading to changes in cell membrane potential or increasing entry of calcium ions which then affect intracellular mechanisms), or by activating second messenger systems, which in turn lead to changes in intracellular enzyme activity.

Receptors are classified by their endogenous ligand, and given subtypes according to their behaviour. Thus, for example, dopamine receptors are divided into two main subgroups D1-like (D_1 and D_5), which activate adenylate cyclase and D2-like (D_2, D_3 and D_4), which inhibit adenylate cyclase (for examples see Table 16.1).

Receptor and transporter binding

Neuroreceptors and transporters are highly selective, binding only to a particular neurotransmitter at specific binding sites. Drugs and radioligands can bind at the same binding sites as the neurotransmitter (endogenous ligand), in which case they compete for binding to the site (active binding site), or they can bind at other sites on the receptor, exerting a conformational change on the receptor regardless of the concentration of endogenous ligand.

Drugs that bind to receptors can be agonists (having the same intrinsic action as the endogenous ligand (e.g. bromocriptine, a dopamine receptor agonist), antagonists (blocking the effect of endogenous ligand binding without any intrinsic activity), or inverse agonists (having an opposing action to the endogenous ligand, e.g. haloperidol, a dopamine receptor inverse agonist). Drugs may bind to several different types of receptors, having different effects at each receptor subtype. They may also have different affinities for binding. Drugs that bind to transporters can be substrates or inhibitors. Substrates are actively transported across the cell membrane and accumulate in the cell over time (e.g. L-dopa, a dopamine substrate), whereas inhibitors block active transport of substrates when they bind to their transporter binding site (e.g. cocaine, a dopamine reuptake inhibitor).

Radioligands for specific receptors/transporters are radiolabelled drugs. When used as tracers in imaging studies, they are administered in very small doses (in the nanomolar range) and so do not have any pharmacological effect. Most receptor radioligands are either antagonists or inverse agonists, as these have higher affinity and so bind more avidly. Some receptor radioligands are agonists, however, and these are more sensitive to levels of endogenous ligand (competitive binding).

Relevance of receptors/transporters to disease and drug development

Receptors and transporters, being the molecular machinery of neurotransmission, are of key interest to understanding the basis of central nervous system illnesses. In some cases they can be used for diagnostic purposes. For example, dopamine transporter binding can be used to differentiate between different diseases presenting with parkinsonian symptoms (Scherfler *et al.* 2007), and receptor expression on the surface of cancer cells can be used for diagnosis and for the monitoring of treatment response (Van Den Bossche, Van de Wiele 2004).

Changes in receptor binding measured with SPECT or PET imaging reflect underlying changes in receptor availability through up- or down-regulation. In the case of ligands that bind to the active binding site, changes may also be due to alteration in the level of endogenous ligand. Thus disease-specific changes can be investigated using these methods, shedding light on the abnormalities that are present in living subjects. It is also possible to relate changes in receptor and transmitter binding to the levels of particular symptoms, giving insight into their molecular basis.

Table 16.1 A small example selection of receptors with different mechanisms of signal transduction. The endogenous ligand and downstream (intracellular) effect on activation are shown for each receptor subtype

Endogenous ligand	Group	Receptor subtype	Receptor type	Downstream effect
Dopamine	D1-like	$D_{1/5}$	G-protein linked	Stimulate cAMP formation
	D2-like	$D_{2/3/4}$	G-protein linked	Inhibit cAMP formation
Glutamate	Group I metabotropic	$mGluR_{1/5}$	G-protein linked	Modulate Na^+ and K^+ channels
	Group II metabotropic	$mGluR_{2/3}$	G-protein linked	Inhibit cAMP formation
	Group III metabotropic	$mGluR_{4/6/7/8}$	G-protein linked	Inhibit cAMP formation
	Ionotropic	NMDA	Ion channel	Increase cell membrane Ca^{2+} permeability
	Ionotropic	AMPA	Ion channel	Increase cell membrane Na+ K+ (and Ca++ if GluR2 subunit is not present) permeability
	Ionotropic	Kainate	Ion channel	Increase cell membrane Na^+ and K^+ permeablilty
GABA	Ionotropic	$GABA_{A/C}$	Ion channel	Increase cell membrane Cl- permeability
	Metabotropic	$GAB_{A\text{-}B}$	G-protein linked	Modulate adenylate cyclase activity
Insulin	Metabotropic	Insulin receptor	Tyrosine kinase	Insulin receptor substrate 1 phosphorylation leading to increase in high affinity glucose transporter expression
Acetylcholine	Ionotropic	Nicotinic (I–IV)	Ion channel	Increase Na^+ and K^+ conductance
	Metabotropic	Muscarinic $M_{1/3}$	G-protein linked	Increase inositol triphosphate formation
		Muscarinic $M_{2/4}$	G-protein linked	Decrease cAMP formation

PET and SPECT receptor and transporter imaging can also be a useful tool in the process of developing new drug treatments. Firstly they can help to identify receptors or transporters that are altered in particular illnesses as potential therapeutic targets for novel drugs. Secondly, they can be used to assess the pharmacokinetic and pharmacodynamic profile of drugs – whether a given dose leads to adequate receptor occupancy, and whether a given degree of receptor occupancy leads to a reduction in symptoms. They can also be used to relate drug-receptor occupancy to side-effects.

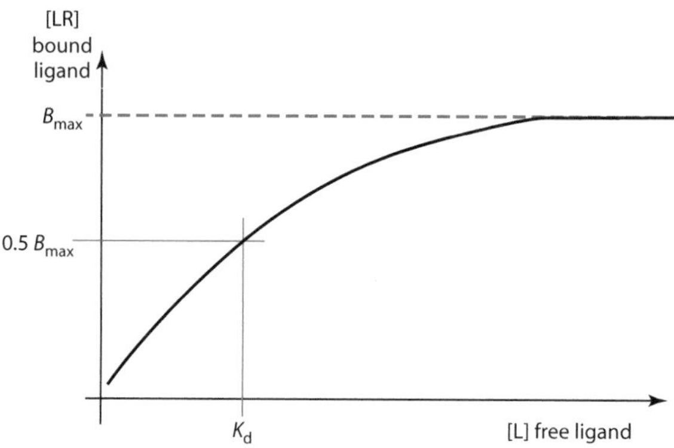

Figure 16.1 Graph of bound versus free ligand showing relationship between K_d and B_{max}.

Binding equations

Radioligand–receptor binding theory assumes that each receptor has a single active site, with the ligand free to bind. This is not always true as some receptors have multiple binding sites, and binding regions are inaccessible in certain receptor states (e.g. the intra-channel MK-801 binding site of NMDA receptors when the ion channel is closed). It also assumes that the law of mass action applies.

The association between free ligand L and free receptor R to bound ligand/receptor LR can be summarised with the equation:

$$L + R \underset{k_{off}}{\overset{k_{on}}{\rightleftharpoons}} LR$$

The rate of association is equivalent to $[L][R]k_{on}$ and the rate of dissociation to $[LR]k_{off}$. The rate of accumulation of LR can be summarised by the following equation:

$$\frac{d[LR]}{dt} = k_{on}[L][R] - k_{off}[LR]$$

At steady state equilibrium, there is no net change in [LR], so:

$$k_{on}[L][R] = k_{off}[LR]$$

The dissociation constant at equilibrium, K_d, is defined as

$$\frac{k_{off}}{k_{on}} = \frac{[L][R]}{[LR]} = K_d$$

where the lower the value of K_d, the higher the affinity of the ligand for binding the receptor. At equilibrium, in the presence of excess free ligand, it is possible to estimate $[LR]_{max}$, also termed B_{max} (see Figure 16.1). Binding potential, BP, is defined as:

$$BP = \frac{B_{max}}{K_d}$$

and is proportional to the total number of receptors in the region of interest.

Radioligand development

Ideal radioligand properties for imaging receptors and transporters

Effective radioligands must approach a number of different ideal physical, chemical and biological properties:

1. The radiosynthesis must be rapid, high yielding and suitable for automation or kit labelling under GMP conditions. The process may involve multiple chemical steps, however, intermediate HPLC purification of prosthetic labelling groups may be difficult to implement for routine production.
2. The labelled compound should be obtained in high specific activity and free of toxic side-products. Once labelled, the compound should be stable and resistant to radiolysis. The radioligand should also be readily soluble in water to facilitate formulation. A common problem with lipophilic radioligands is their ‘stickiness’ to surfaces and filters. This can result in substantial losses during formulation, sterile filtration and administration of the radiotracer.

3. The radioligand must have high affinity and specificity for the target of interest.
4. The tracer must be available for binding at the receptor or transporter, i.e. it must be transported to the target tissue with limited binding to plasma proteins. For imaging of targets within the brain the radioligand has to penetrate the blood–brain barrier (BBB). Radioligands can penetrate the BBB through passive diffusion or by active transport. A moderate lipophilicity of log $P = 1.0–3.5$ is considered to be optimal for passive diffusion (Waterhouse 2003).
5. Radioligands that bind reversibly to their target should have a rapid association rate to ensure that equilibrium between free and bound ligand is reached within the time-frame of the scan. For radioligands that bind irreversibly or act as substrates for transporters, it is preferable that the association rate is rate limiting to avoid blood flow dependency of the signal.
6. As the image obtained will depend on the uptake and retention of the radioligand in the target tissue, as well as clearance of background activity, the radioligand should ideally clear rapidly from non-target tissues.
7. The ideal radioligand should be metabolically inert, as metabolic breakdown of radioligands *in vivo* reduces the amount of radioactivity available for binding and creates radioactive metabolites that complicates image interpretation. In practice, however, most radioligands are metabolised *in vivo*. To minimise the impact of radioactive metabolites radioligands are usually designed to form polar radioactive metabolites without biological activity. This is a particularly attractive strategy for brain imaging as polar metabolites are less likely to cross the BBB. Although no radioligands are perfect, those that approach these ideal characteristics permit the semi-quantitative determination of receptor properties such as receptor density and affinity *in vivo* (Kerwin, Pilowsky 1995).

Choice of radionuclide and ligand

The choice of radionuclide for tracer development depends on the intended application, the local capabilities for production and handling of radionuclides, and the chemical and pharmacological properties of the candidate ligand. Ligands for imaging of neuroreceptors and transporters tend to be small molecules (molecular weight <500), whereas larger biomolecules such as peptides are often used for imaging of receptors expressed on cancer cells.

Small molecules for receptor and transporter imaging are most often labelled with ^{11}C and ^{18}F for PET and ^{123}I for SPECT. Carbon-11 has a half-life of 20.4 minutes and is therefore limited to specialised centres with an in-house cyclotron. While ^{11}C radiolabelling is technically challenging to establish and only allows imaging to be undertaken locally, it is often preferred for development of radioligands for imaging of neuroreceptors and transporters. There are several factors that make ^{11}C attractive for PET imaging. The half-life is sufficiently short to allow repeated PET studies in the same subject within a short time; ^{11}C can be introduced into natural compounds such as neurotransmitters without changing their chemical structure; and the chemistry of carbon is exceptionally rich enabling a wide range of labelling strategies. The most common route for labelling with ^{11}C is alkylation of nucleophiles, such as phenols, with [^{11}C]iodomethane.

Fluorine-18 has a half-life of 109.8 minutes and low positron energy (maximum of 0.635 MeV), making it ideal for PET imaging. As opposed to ^{11}C, the half-life of ^{18}F is sufficient to allow transport to centres without cyclotron facilities and it is therefore considered to be the most viable radionuclide for widespread routine imaging with PET. Fluorine also has very attractive chemical properties for radioligand development; it is small and extremely electronegative and it forms hydrogen bonds. As a consequence, ^{18}F can often replace hydrogen or hydroxyl groups while retaining the biological activity of ligands. However, the labelling chemistry of ^{18}F can be challenging. Electrophilic fluorination requires addition of carrier F_2 gas, leading to low specific activity; the reactivity is often difficult to control; and the maximum theoretical yield for incorporation of one fluorine atom is 50%. For these reasons, nucleophilic fluorination with [^{18}F]fluoride, which can be obtained in high specific activity, is preferred. When carried out under vigorous anhydrous conditions, nucleophilic fluorination of alkyls and electron-poor aryls can proceed in high yields. Electron-rich aromatic groups are usually labelled by formation of an alkylating reagent such as [^{18}F]fluoroethyltosylate, which is subsequently reacted with a nucleophilic group such as phenol.

Iodine-123 is a gamma emitter with a half-life of 13.3 hours. It can readily be introduced into small molecules by electrophilic aromatic substitution of electron-rich aryls, or by iododemetallation of trialkyltin aryls and alkenes. Iodinated alkyls are usually too unstable for *in-vivo* imaging. A great advantage for radioligand development is the availability of the longer-lived ^{125}I (half-life 60.14 days). The long half-life makes it ideal for development of labelling chemistry and for biological evaluation. ^{125}I decays by electron capture and emits low-energy γ-rays that are highly suited for autoradiography. Iodine is relatively large and can be difficult to incorporate into a ligand without impairing its biological activity. Another complication is enzymatic deiodination *in vivo*, which results in circulation of free [^{123}I]iodide. Iodide rapidly accumulates in the thyroid, and to a lesser extent in the stomach and intestines. Iodine preparations (potassium iodide tablets and oral solution, Lugol's solution, potassium iodate tablets) or potassium perchlorate tablets are therefore usually administrated to patients before imaging with ^{123}I-labelled radioligands to block uptake of free [^{123}I]iodide in the thyroid. The polarity and size of radiometal–chelate complexes make them difficult to incorporate into small molecules without impairing the biological activity. Neuroreceptor imaging with SPECT is therefore performed almost exclusively with ^{123}I. However, considerable progress has been made in recent years with development of neuroreceptor ligands labelled with ^{99m}Tc-chelates, suggesting that ^{99m}Tc may play a significant role in neuroreceptor imaging in the future.

Peptides offer more flexibility than small molecules for incorporation of radionuclides and can readily be labelled with metal-chelates. Currently ^{18}F and ^{68}Ga are the most promising radionuclides for PET imaging with peptide tracers, whereas ^{99m}Tc is generally preferred for SPECT. Extensive efforts have been made to develop automated processes for peptide labelling with ^{18}F. A number of new methods have emerged in recent years, most notably oxime formation of aminooxy precursors with [^{18}F]fluorobenzaldehyde, and 'click labelling' by copper-catalysed cycloaddition of azides and terminal alkynes. However, it remains to be demonstrated that these methods are suitable for large-scale routine production. Gallium-68 is attractive as it is generator produced and therefore avoids the complications of central radionuclide production in a cyclotron facility and the requirement for a transport network. Labelling of peptides with ^{68}Ga is typically achieved by chelation with DOTA (1,4,7,10-tetraazacyclododecane-1,4,7,10-tetraacetic acid). Technetium-99m is the most widely used radionuclide in nuclear imaging. It is generator produced, has a convenient half-life (6.01 hours), and emits 140.5 keV γ-rays, which are close to ideal for SPECT imaging. Peptides are usually labelled with ^{99m}Tc by complexation with a chelator such as HYNIC (hydrazinonicotinic acid).

The availability of suitable ligands is usually a limiting factor for development of PET and SPECT tracers. The need for high affinity, typically in the range of $K_d = 100$ pmol/L to 5 nmol/L depending on the density of the target, is particularly difficult to achieve. A common approach is therefore to select compound classes with sufficiently high affinity and devise strategies for radiolabelling that retain the biological activity. It is often difficult to find information on the *in-vivo* properties of ligands and, in many cases, preliminary biological studies are required to assess the suitability of a ligand for tracer development. Within these restrictions a fruitful approach is to select compounds that can be synthesised by fusing smaller fragments (convergent synthesis) as opposed to compounds prepared by linear syntheses. This makes it easier to modify the functional groups in the molecule and investigate the optimal position for labelling. It is also worth bearing in mind that increased lipophilicity generally leads to increased metabolism, and that electron-rich aromatic groups (such as phenols, ethers and anilines) are more prone to metabolic breakdown *in vivo* than electron-poor aromatic groups (such as fluoro-, trifluoromethyl- or sulfonamide-substituted aryls). Anionic groups such as carboxylates are usually avoided for development of brain tracers as they tend to reduce brain uptake.

Biological evaluation of neuroreceptor radioligands

Once a ligand has been identified for tracer development, the compound is evaluated in a sequence of biological studies aimed at supporting the structural design, and in later stages to validate its properties for *in-vivo* imaging. Typically the ligand and derivatives modified for labelling are screened for affinity in binding studies *in vitro*. As this often can be achieved by displacement of established ^{3}H-labelled radioligands (competitive binding experiments), it is possible to evaluate the suitability of selected labelling positions with non-radioactive derivatives. Once a lead compound has been identified, the specific binding of the labelled compound is usually assessed by comparing its uptake in tissue preparations with and without addition of excess of the non-radioactive reference compound (blocking studies). The non-radioactive reference compound should be added in a sufficient concentration to bind to essentially all the target receptors. With the receptor population blocked by the non-radioactive reference compound, binding of the radioligand in the sample can only be non-specific. The specific binding is calculated as the difference between total binding of the radioligand in the sample and the non-specific binding measured as described above. Blocking experiments can also be carried out with unlabelled drugs that compete for the same receptor binding site as the radioligand. The advantage of this approach is that blocking of the radioligand by a known drug confirms the binding site of the radioligand (or at least that the binding site is shared with the known drug). In addition, the use of a structurally different drug to block the radioligand is more likely to reveal any cross activity (binding to other receptors). If possible, blocking should be carried out with both the non-radioactive reference compound and a structurally different unlabelled drug to provide independent measurements of the specific binding. The selectivity of the radioligand can be further evaluated by broad receptor screen assays using *in-vitro* binding studies.

Biodistribution studies are carried out to evaluate the *in-vivo* properties of the radioligand. Initial studies typically aim at identifying the uptake in target tissues and background over time. In addition, the *in-vivo* stability of the radiotracer is evaluated by taking blood samples as selected time points and analysing the percentage of intact parent compound in plasma by radio-HPLC. Radioligands that have sufficient metabolic stability for *in-vivo* imaging and that accumulate in target tissues are evaluated further in a series of experiments designed to reveal the extent of specific binding *in vivo*.

This typically involves the use of blocking studies where the pharmacokinetic profile of the radioligand is compared in untreated animals and animals treated with a blocking agent (reference compound or an unlabelled drug). The difference in uptake in target tissues is attributed to specific binding. In addition, radioligands are often evaluated in animal models with altered expression or activity of the target receptor/transporter. Combined, such experiments help to demonstrate the suitability of a radioligand for imaging and its ability to detect changes in receptor or transporter expression levels in disease states.

Quantification of neuroreceptor density using PET or SPECT imaging: kinetic analysis

Data obtained by a PET or SPECT camera allow measurement of gamma photons emitted in a given brain region (corrected for scatter and attenuation). The number of detected γ-rays will be affected by the amount of radioligand and labelled metabolites in the region of interest and the decay of the radionuclide. In order to convert the data recorded during a PET or SPECT scan into an outcome measure proportional to neuroreceptor density, a simplified mathematical model of the process of delivery and uptake of the ligand must be applied to these data (Lammertsma 2003). As it is not possible to fully model the complex physiological processes involved in ligand distribution *in vivo*, the outcome measure depends upon a number of assumptions and can therefore only provide at best an estimate of the true value of biological parameters. It is not possible to estimate K_d or B_{max} individually in a single session. With two scanning sessions, one at high, and the other at low specific activity, a Scatchard plot can be generated (a plot of [LR] on the x-axis against [LR]/[L] on the y-axis), which will permit separate measurement of these parameters, with a reasonable estimate of B_{max} (intercept of the line with the x-axis), and a less accurate estimate of K_d (the slope of the line approximates to $-1/K_d$) (Holden *et al.* 2002; Slifstein *et al.* 2004), but this method may be impractical or unethical in human studies. Furthermore,

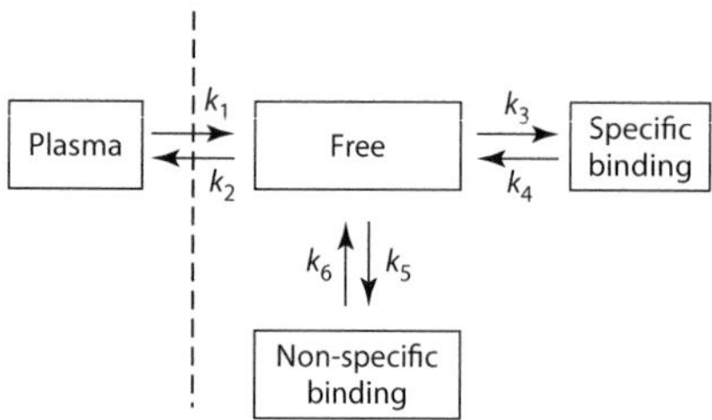

Figure 16.2 A three tissue compartment model representing the exchange of ligand between plasma, free, non-specific and specific binding within the region of interest. Constants are shown that define the rate of ligand distribution between the different compartments.

because there are only two data points on the plot, the accuracy of this method is far from ideal.

The usual outcome measures in single-session SPECT or PET studies are measures proportional to binding potential, BP (B_{max}/K_d). The standard model to describe the kinetic data from SPECT and PET imaging is shown in Figure 16.2. This model has three main compartments for ligand distribution: free, specifically bound, and non-specifically bound. Distribution between the compartments is dependent upon rate constants, which define the rate of association or dissociation for each compartment. Often the three-compartment model is simplified further depending upon experimental studies of a specific ligand behaviour *in vivo* and two- or even one-compartment models may provide an adequate description of the kinetic data. Because SPECT and PET have no way of distinguishing between bound and free ligand in a given region, in regions of specific binding, the measured concentration of the ligand (C_{tot}) at time t can be defined as

$$C_{tot}(t) = C_f(t) + C_b(t) + C_{ns}(t)$$

comprising free, specifically bound and non-specifically bound ligand (C_f, C_b and C_{ns}, respectively). Concentration of unbound or free ligand (C_f) is increased by ligand entering from arterial blood or from the bound compartments and reduced by ligand leaving into the other compartments, or back into the plasma:

$$\frac{dC_f(t)}{dt} = K_1 \cdot C_a(t) - (k_2 + k_3 + k_5)C_f(t) + k_4 \cdot C_b(t) + k_6 \cdot C_{ns}(t)$$

where $C_a(t)$ is metabolite-corrected activity concentration in arterial plasma at a given time point. As SPECT or PET regions of interest will also contain a vascular component, total concentration recorded from a given region of interest in a SPECT or PET time–activity curve, C_{SPECT}. $C_{SPECT}(t)$ (Bq/mL) is defined as

$$C_{SPECT}(t) = (1 - V_b)C_{tot}(t) + V_b C_{wb}(t)$$

where V_b is the vascular volume in the region of interest and C_{wb} is the activity concentration of whole blood uncorrected for metabolites. In order to estimate concentration of ligand in the specific binding compartment using standard kinetic analysis of SPECT or PET data, it is therefore necessary to measure the time course of ligand concentration in whole blood and in metabolite-corrected arterial plasma (input function) as well as the time–activity data from the region of interest. Non-linear regression can then be used to find the best fit for the data points, resulting in best estimates for the rate constants and V_b. Although it is not possible to estimate individual constants with any degree of certainty, ratios between rate constants usually show more stability. The rate constants k_3 and k_4 are defined as

$$k_3 = k_{on} \cdot f_2\left(B_{max} - \frac{C_b(t)}{SA}\right)$$

and

$$k_4 = k_{off}$$

where B_{max} is the receptor concentration, f_2 is the free fraction of ligand in tissue, and SA is the specific activity of injected ligand. Because, under tracer conditions, C_b is small compared with SA, k_3 may be simplified to

$$k_3 = k_{on} \cdot f_2 \cdot B_{max}$$

Therefore, k_3/k_4 is often used as a measure proportional to BP including free fraction of ligand in tissue:

$$\frac{k_3}{k_4} = f_2 \frac{B_{max}}{K_d} = f_2 \cdot BP = BP_2$$

In some circumstances, it is not possible to derive k_3/k_4 with adequate certainty. In these cases, volume of distribution in the tissue compartment (V_T), which is still proportional to B_{max}/K_d but includes free and non-specific binding, is used. At equilibrium, volume of distribution is given by

$$V_{\mathrm{T}} = \frac{C_{\mathrm{tot}}}{C_{\mathrm{a}}}$$

For a single-compartment model,

$$\frac{\mathrm{d}C_{\mathrm{tot}}}{\mathrm{d}t} = K_1 \cdot C_{\mathrm{a}} - k_2 \cdot C_{\mathrm{tot}}$$

At equilibrium,

$$K_1 \cdot C_a = k_2 \cdot C_{\mathrm{tot}}$$

Therefore,

$$V_{\mathrm{T}} = \frac{K_1}{k_2}$$

and for a two-tissue compartment,

$$V_{\mathrm{T}} = \left(\frac{K_1}{k_2}\right)\left(1 + \frac{k_3}{k_4}\right)$$

Even if it is only possible to derive volume of distribution, it is still possible to calculate two measures proportional to BP if there is a reference region containing no receptors. In this case,

$$\mathrm{BP}_1 = V_{\mathrm{T}} - V_{\mathrm{Tref}} = \mathrm{BP} \cdot f_1$$

$$\mathrm{BP}_2 = \frac{V_{\mathrm{T}} - V_{\mathrm{Tref}}}{V_{\mathrm{Tref}}} = \mathrm{BP} \cdot f_2$$

where f_1 is the free fraction of unchanged ligand in plasma and V_{T} is the volume of distribution in the reference region. If such a reference region exists, it is possible to derive the input function from the activity curve of the reference region rather than from metabolite-corrected plasma, obviating the need for arterial blood sampling. This technique is used by the reference tissue model and the simplified reference tissue model (Lammertsma, Hume 1996; Lammertsma 2003).

Research and future clinical uses

Imaging studies in schizophrenia research

Research into mental illness is one field that clearly benefits from tools that allow measurement of clinically meaningful variables in living subjects. Unlike other illnesses, which can be diagnosed with blood tests or other physical investigations, mental illnesses are identified almost entirely from the history that the patient gives – the description of their internal experiences. PET and SPECT imaging have allowed the study of receptor and transporter imaging in living patients with mental illness, permitting the relationship of receptor availability with symptoms to be directly tested.

Schizophrenia is a severe mental illness that affects individuals in their late teens and early twenties. Antipsychotic medications had been available since the 1950s, and it was known that these drugs all had their primary action through dopamine D2 receptor blockade (Seeman, Lee 1975; Creese *et al.* 1976). Because of this discovery, it was hypothesised that patients with schizophrenia might have increased dopamine D2 receptors in the brain. Postmortem studies seemed to support this, but the effect of chronic medication on D2 receptor up-regulation could not be ruled out (Owen *et al.* 1978; Clow *et al.* 1980; Mackay *et al.* 1980; Seeman *et al.* 1984). SPECT studies used a specific ligand for the D2 receptor ([^{123}I]IBZM, Figure 16.3) but found no difference in D2 receptor availability in unmedicated first-episode patients compared with healthy controls (Farde *et al.* 1990; Pilowsky *et al.* 1994), suggesting that if there is excessive dopamine sensitivity in the illness, it is not caused by overexpressed D2 receptors.

Following these findings, [^{123}I]IBZM scans were performed before and after amphetamine administration in patients with schizophrenia and in healthy controls. It emerged that patients showed a much greater reduction in [^{123}I]IBZM binding following amphetamine administration. This was interpreted as showing that patients with schizophrenia have greater stores of dopamine, and increased dopamine turnover in the brain (Laruelle *et al.* 1996). Subsequent work supported this hypothesis, finding that patients

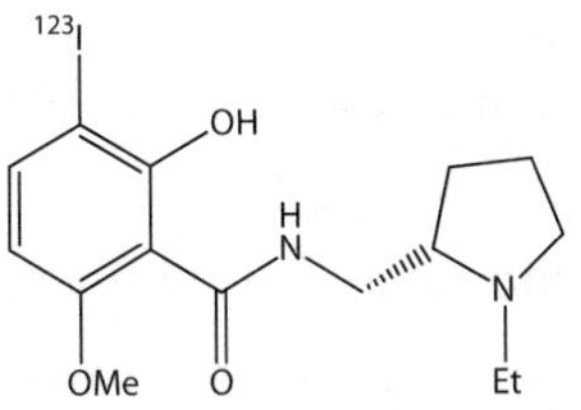

Figure 16.3 The molecular structure of [^{123}I]IBZM.

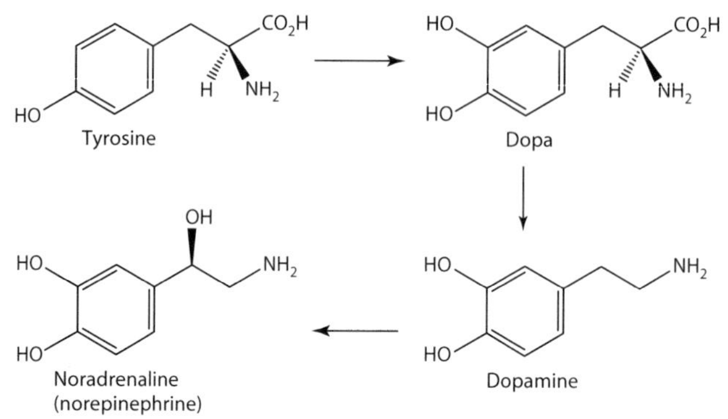

Figure 16.4 The biosynthesis of noradrenaline (norepinephrine) from tyrosine.

with schizophrenia have increased [^{18}F]DOPA uptake (a marker of dopamine metabolism) (Hietala *et al.* 1995; Hietala *et al.* 1999; McGowan *et al.* 2004), and that following dopamine depletion, patients with schizophrenia had higher D2 receptor binding than healthy controls, implying that synaptic dopamine concentrations were higher in patients (Abi-Dargham *et al.* 2000).

Approximately 1/3 of patients with schizophrenia fail to respond to antipsychotic medication. It was thought that this could be due to pharmacokinetic issues – that these patients might not be taking sufficient dose to fully occupy dopamine D2 receptors. This led to the use of 'mega doses' of antipsychotic drugs, which induced severe side-effects. SPECT imaging using [^{123}I]IBZM was used to test the hypothesis that D2 receptors were not fully occupied in patients who did not respond well to antipsychotic treatment. Good and poor responders underwent SPECT scanning with [^{123}I]IBZM while they were still taking medication. It emerged that at standard doses of haloperidol there was no difference in striatal D2 receptor occupancy (greater than 90% in both cases) (Pilowsky *et al.* 1993). This study proved that there was no advantage to be conferred by using antipsychotic doses greater than the normal treatment dose, and implied that non-responders might be different from other patients with schizophrenia in terms of the underlying neurochemical basis of the illness.

Imaging the cardiac nervous system

Heart disease is a major killer in Western countries with approximately 300 000 sudden cardiac deaths in the United States each year (Carrio 2001). Dysfunction of the cardiac nervous system is implicated in a significant proportion of these cases (about 20% of cardiac deaths occur without evidence of coronary artery disease).

The function of the heart is regulated by sympathetic and parasympathetic nerves. The sympathetic branch exerts cardiac stimulation and is mainly mediated by activation of β-adrenergic receptors by norepinephrine, whereas the parasympathetic branch causes cardiac slowing by acetylcholine activation of M_2 muscarinic receptors (Langer, Halldin 2002). PET and SPECT imaging allows detailed studies of the involvement of the cardiac nervous system in heart diseases. While a wide range of radioligands have been developed for imaging of receptor populations in the heart (Bengel, Schwaiger 2004; Kopka *et al.* 2008), clinical studies have mainly focused on imaging of the norepinephrine transporter.

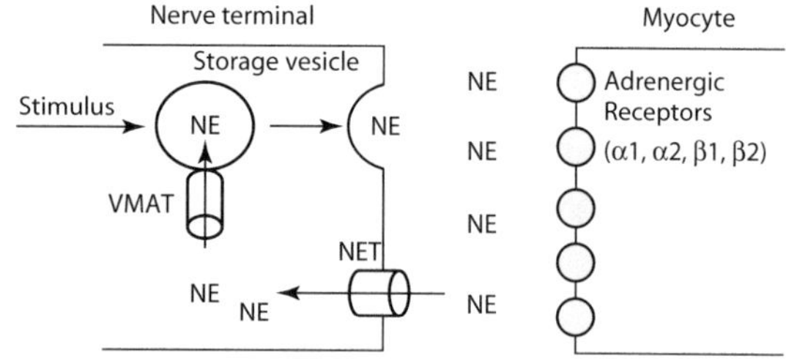

Figure 16.5 Illustration of a sympathetic nerve terminal. Norepinephrine (NE; noradrenaline) is stored in vesicles, but is released following a stimulus. In the synaptic cleft NE stimulates adrenergic receptors. The norepinephrine transporter (NET) rapidly transports NE back to the cytoplasm where another transporter, known as VMAT, transports NE into storage vesicles. Modified from Bengel and Schwaiger (2004).

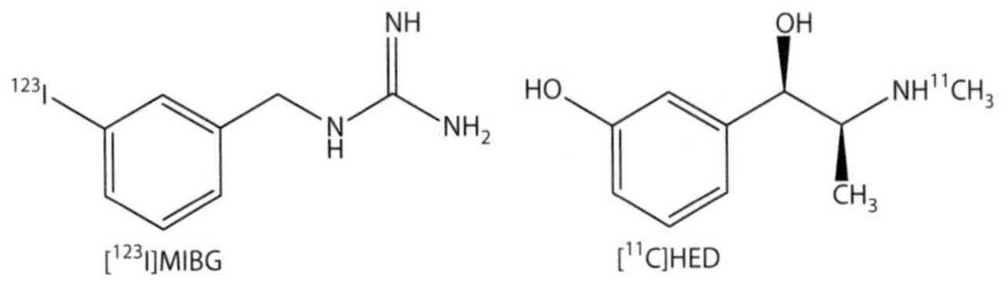

Figure 16.6 The molecular structures of [^{123}I]MIBG and [^{11}C]HED.

Norepinephrine is synthesised by cardiac neurons via an enzymatic cascade (Figure 16.4). Tyrosine is converted to dopa, which subsequently is decarboxylated to form dopamine. Hydroxylation of dopamine finally provides norepinephrine (Bengel, Schwaiger 2004). Neural stimulation leads to release of norepinephrine into the synaptic cleft where it stimulates β-adrenorecepetors. The stimulus is rapidly terminated by the norepinephrine transporter (NET) located on the nerve terminals. NET removes norepinephrine from the synaptic cleft and circulates it back into the cytoplasm (Figure 16.5).

The most widely used radioligand for imaging of the norepinephrine transporter is ^{123}I-labelled *meta*-iodobenzylguanidine ([^{123}I]MIBG) (Figure 16.6) (Flotats, Carrio 2004). [^{123}I]MIBG is a high-affinity substrate for NET, and following binding it is rapidly transported into neurons. The transport of [^{123}I]MIBG by NET is so fast that the uptake is partially blood-flow-dependent. Still, [^{123}I]MIBG allows semi-quantification of NET density, which is a good indicator of cardiac innervation. The most extensively used PET tracer for imaging of NET is ^{11}C-labelled *meta*-hydroxyephedrine (HED). [^{11}C]HED is a high-affinity substrate for NET with high specific binding. A number of ^{18}F-labelled NET tracers have been evaluated, but their practical use has so far been hampered by low radiochemical yields and poor specific activity.

In the early phase of heart failure, enhanced sympathetic nervous system activity has a protective effect on the heart. However, long-term increased activity can lead to elevated energy and oxygen consumption, myocardial wall stress, arrhythmias and myocyte death (Flotats, Carrio 2004). Several clinical studies have demonstrated decreased myocardial uptake of [^{123}I]MIBG in patients with heart failure (Agostini *et al.* 2008). Importantly, the uptake of [^{123}I]MIBG provides a powerful prognostic value, with indications of a quantitative threshold predicting low versus high risk of major cardiac events. Studies with [^{11}C]HED has provided similarly encouraging results (Bengel, Schwaiger 2004). Imaging of NET can therefore play an important role in guiding treatment for patients with heart failure, and may find use for treatment monitoring and evaluation of new therapeutic approaches. However, there is still a need for large-scale clinical studies to further evaluate the clinical value of imaging NET in patients with heart failure.

Conclusions

Nuclear medicine PET and SPECT imaging of receptors and transporters are the only methods available to directly image the molecular mechanisms underlying neurotransmission in living patients. As such they are powerful tools in research as well as in drug development and in clinical diagnostic application. It is likely that the coming years will see an explosion in the number of receptor subtypes that can be imaged as pharmaceutical companies move to employ these methods in the process of developing and screening new compounds. Further expansion of their use in clinical practice in oncology, neurology and psychiatry is also anticipated.

References

Abi-Dargham A *et al.* (2000). Increased baseline occupancy of D2 receptors by dopamine in schizophrenia. *Proc Natl Acad Sci U S A* 97(14): 8104–8109.

Agostini D *et al.* (2008). I-123-mIBG myocardial imaging for assessment of risk for a major cardiac event in heart failure patients: insights from a retrospective European multicenter study. *Eur J Nucl Med Mol Imaging* 35(3): 535–546.

Bengel FM, Schwaiger M (2004). Assessment of cardiac sympathetic neuronal function using PET imaging. *J Nucl Cardiol* 11(5): 603–616.

Carrio I (2001). Cardiac neurotransmission imaging. *J Nucl Med* 42(7): 1062–1076.

Clow A *et al.* (1980). Changes in rat striatal dopamine turnover and receptor activity during one years neuroleptic administration. *Eur J Pharmacol* 63(2–3): 135–144.

Creese I *et al.* (1976). Dopamine receptor binding predicts clinical and pharmacological potencies of antischizophrenic drugs. *Science* 192: 481–483.

Farde L *et al.* (1990). D2 dopamine receptors in neuroleptic-naive schizophrenic patients. A positron emission tomography study with [^{11}C]raclopride. *Arch Gen Psychiatry* 47: 213–219.

Flotats A, Carrio I (2004). Cardiac neurotransmission SPECT imaging. *J Nucl Cardiol* 11(5): 587–602.

Hietala J *et al.* (1995). Presynaptic dopamine function in striatum of neuroleptic-naive schizophrenic patients. *Lancet* 346: 1130–1131.

Hietala J *et al.* (1999). Depressive symptoms and presynaptic dopamine function in neuroleptic-naive schizophrenia. *Schizophr Res* 35: 41–50.

Holden J *et al.* (2002). In vivo assay with multiple ligand concentrations: an equilibrium approach. *J Cereb Blood Flow Metab* 22(9): 1132–1141.

Kerwin RW, Pilowsky LS (1995). Traditional receptor theory and its application to neuroreceptor measurements in functional imaging. *Eur J Nucl Med* 22(7): 699–710.

Kopka K *et al.* (2008). ^{18}F-labelled cardiac PET tracers: selected probes for the molecular imaging of transporters, receptors and proteases. *Basic Res Cardiol* 103(2): 131–143.

Lammertsma, A. (2003). *PET Pharmacokinetic Course Manual*. Groningen: University of Groningen; Montreal: McGill University.

Lammertsma A, Hume S (1996). Simplified reference tissue model for PET receptor studies. *Neuroimage* 4(3Pt1): 153–158.

Langer O, Halldin C (2002). PET and SPECT tracers for mapping the cardiac nervous system. *Eur J Nucl Med Mol Imaging* 29(3): 416–434.

Laruelle M *et al.* (1996). Single photon emission computerized tomography imaging of amphetamine-induced dopamine release in drug-free schizophrenic subjects. *Proc Natl Acad Sci U S A* 93: 9235–9240.

Mackay AV *et al.* (1980). Dopamine receptors and schizophrenia: drug effect or illness? *Lancet* 2: 915–916.

McGowan S *et al.* (2004). Presynaptic dopaminergic dysfunction in schizophrenia: a positron emission tomographic [^{18}F]fluorodopa study. *Arch Gen Psychiatry* 61: 134–142.

Owen F *et al.* (1978). Increased dopamine-receptor sensitivity in schizophrenia. *Lancet* 2: 223–226.

Pilowsky LS *et al.* (1993). Antipsychotic medication, D2 dopamine receptor blockade and clinical response: a ^{123}I IBZM SPECT (single photon emission tomography) study. *Psychol Med* 23: 791–797.

Pilowsky LS *et al.* (1994). D2 dopamine receptor binding in the basal ganglia of antipsychotic-free schizophrenic patients. An ^{123}I-IBZM single photon emission computerised tomography study. *Br J Psychiatry* 164: 16–26.

Scherfler C *et al.* (2007). Role of DAT-SPECT in the diagnostic work up of parkinsonism. *Mov Disord* 22(9): 1229–1238.

Seeman P, Lee T (1975). Antipsychotic drugs: direct correlation between clinical potency and presynaptic action on dopamine neurons. *Science* 188(4194): 1217–1219.

Seeman P *et al.* (1984). Bimodal distribution of dopamine receptor densities in brains of schizophrenics. *Science* 225: 728–731.

Slifstein M *et al.* (2004). In vivo affinity of [^{18}F]fallypride for striatal and extrastriatal dopamine D2 receptors in non-human primates. *Psychopharmacology (Berl)* 175 (3): 274–286.

Van Den Bossche B, Van de Wiele C (2004). Receptor imaging in oncology by means of nuclear medicine: current status. *J Clin Oncol* 22(17): 3593–3607.

Waterhouse RN (2003). Determination of lipophilicity and its use as a predictor of blood-brain barrier penetration of molecular imaging agents. *Mol Imaging Biol* 5(6): 376–389.

Further reading

Bergström M *et al.* (2003). Autoradiography with positron emitting isotopes in positron emission tomography tracer discovery. *Mol Imaging Biol* 5: 390–396.

Miller PW *et al.* (2008). Synthesis of ^{11}C, ^{18}F, ^{15}O, and ^{13}N radiolabels for positron emission tomography. *Angew Chem Int Ed* 47: 8998–9033.

Motulsky, H. (2001). *The GraphPad Guide to Analyzing Radioligand Binding Data*. http://www.graphpad.com/www/radiolig/radiolig.htm (accessed 30 June 2010).

Stahl, S.M. (2000). *Essential Psychopharmacology*, 2nd edn. New York: Cambridge University Press.

17

Radiation dosimetry for targeted radionuclide therapy

Glenn Flux

Introduction

Internal dosimetry for targeted radionuclide therapy (TRT) has been developed for over 60 years (Marinelli *et al.* 1948). Substantial progress was made in the 1960s and the basic formalism has been widely agreed and adopted. Significant improvements continue to be made in the accuracy with which absorbed doses can be calculated and this has had increasing impact on the clinical implementation of existing and emerging radiopharmaceuticals.

The MIRD dosimetry formalism

The most widely used formalism for performing internal dosimetry was developed by the Medical Internal Radiation Dosimetry (MIRD) Committee of the Society of Nuclear Medicine in the 1960s (Loevinger *et al.* 1988). This system presented a reasonably accessible approach that encouraged clinical and research centres to adopt the methods formulated. The schema require the identification and delineation of two regions. The source volume is that which contains radioactive uptake and the target volume is defined as that which receives an absorbed dose from the activity in the source organ (Figure 17.1). A full dosimetry calculation will account for multiple sources irradiating a given target and frequently includes self-irradiation of a volume containing activity.

The basic equation used by the MIRD formalism to calculate the total mean absorbed dose to a target organ from activity in a source organ $\left(\overline{D}_{(\mathrm{t}\leftarrow\mathrm{s})}\right)$ is given by

$$\overline{D}_{(\mathrm{t}\leftarrow\mathrm{s})} = \frac{k\ \tilde{A}_{\mathrm{s}} \sum_i n_i\ E_i\ \phi_{i(\mathrm{t}\leftarrow\mathrm{s})}}{m_{\mathrm{t}}}$$

where k = a conversion factor to account for different systems of units; $\tilde{A}_{\mathrm{s}}$ = the cumulated activity in the source organ; n_i = the number of particles of energy E_i emitted per nuclear transition in the source organ; $\phi_{i(\mathrm{t}\leftarrow\mathrm{s})}$ fraction of energy emitted in the source organ that is deposited in the target organ; m_{t} = the mass of the target organ.

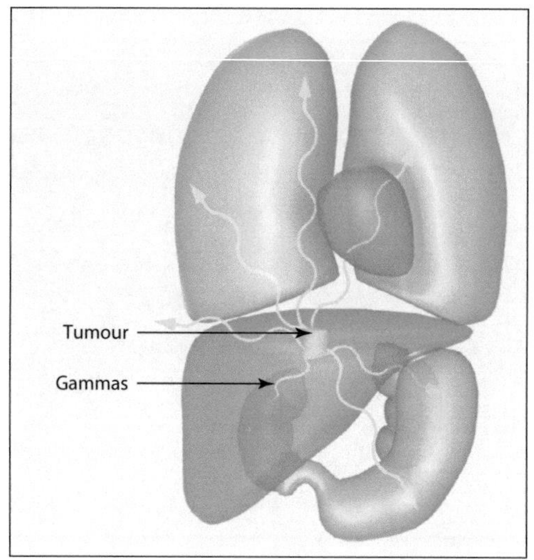

Figure 17.1 Source and target regions for absorbed dose calculations. Both the source and target may be either normal organs or a tumour. Irradiation at a distance is caused by gamma rays, while self-irradiation is mainly due to local energy deposition from beta or alpha particles. Image courtesy of Maria Holstensson.

The cumulated activity is simply the area under the activity–time curve and effectively gives the total number of disintegrations in the source organ. This is usually considered over all time, i.e.

$$\tilde{A}_s = \int_0^\infty A(t)\mathrm{d}t$$

where $A(t)$ is the activity at time t. For multiexponential decay, consisting of n phases this is given by

$$A(t) = \sum_n A_n \ \mathrm{e}^{-\lambda_n t}$$

Here A_n = the activity at time $t = 0$ and λ_n is the effective decay constant for the nth phase.

Thus, if there is a single decay phase the cumulated activity is given by

$$\tilde{A}_s = \frac{A_0}{\lambda}$$

The MIRD S value enables all physical parameters to be grouped for easy tabulation:

$$S_{(t \leftarrow s)} = \frac{\sum_i n_i \ E_i \ \phi_{i(t \leftarrow s)}}{m_t}$$

The simplified MIRD equation is then given by

$$\overline{D}_{(t \leftarrow s)} = \tilde{A}_s S_{(t \leftarrow s)}$$

A key element of this scheme is that organ geometries were standardised (initially constituting an entity referred to as 'reference man', but later joined by anthropomorphic phantoms for a female, child and newborn infant). This allowed the tabulation of S values for all organs defined and for all radionuclides (Snyder *et al.* 1975).

A comprehensive software package, MIRDOSE (Stabin 1996) (now superseded by Olinda EXM (Stabin *et al.* 2005)), was produced independently to aid calculation of absorbed doses for all clinically relevant radionuclides and for all relevant organs.

The elegance of the system may be seen from the distinction between the patient-specific factor (i.e. the cumulated activity) and the physical factor (the S value). The only information required to compute absorbed doses is therefore the uptake and retention of the radiopharmaceutical in the individual patient. One unavoidable outcome of an absorbed dose calculation based on this system is that only a uniform distribution of activity can be assumed in a source organ and only a mean absorbed dose can be calculated for target organs. In practice, further simplifications have included an assumption of an effective half-life obtained from a single uptake scan. Whilst these applications have sometimes led the schema to be criticised as being inaccurate and simplistic, it is important to note that the basic MIRD formalism, which essentially states that the absorbed dose to a target is equal to the absorbed dose delivered by a single radioactive decay in a source, multiplied by the total number of decays, is well founded. The clinical application of this system must be considered and adapted as required, dependent on the required accuracy of the absorbed dose calculations. A basic calculation will often be sufficient to ensure that normal organs receive a low absorbed dose from a diagnostic test. A higher degree of accuracy will be required if calculations are performed to ascertain whether a tumour is likely to receive an absorbed dose that may produce a beneficial effect.

Further advances in dosimetry

Internal dosimetry has been the subject of intensive research since the initial formulation of the MIRD schema. Improvements have been sought for both the methods by which individual cumulated activities can be determined and the accuracy with which absorbed doses can be calculated from any given source distribution. Particular emphasis is increasingly being placed on patient-specific dosimetry, whereby individual patient source and target organ geometries are taken into account, and on the development of methods to account for non-homogeneous distributions of source activity.

Three-dimensional dosimetry

The application of radiopharmaceuticals for therapeutic purposes raises issues that are less relevant for diagnostic examinations. In many cases target organs, which may be tumours or normal organs-at-risk, are also source organs. Frequently the distribution of activity is heterogeneous, which will result in a similarly heterogeneous absorbed dose distribution (Giap *et al.* 1995; Sgouros *et al.* 2004; Dewaraja *et al.* 2005). This can have dramatic effects on the results of a therapy procedure. It can be also argued that the calculation of mean absorbed doses based on standardised geometries (and of course tumours cannot be considered as standard organs) are not sufficient to obtain accurate results (Divoli *et al.* 2009). However the basic MIRD formalism can still be applied to these cases. MIRD pamphlet 17 (Bolch *et al.* 1999) lists tabulated S values for voxels of 3 mm and 6 mm and states that S values for voxel sizes between these can be interpolated. This enables absorbed doses to be calculated for individual voxels within a region of interest, taking into account both the self-dose to the voxel and the absorbed dose contributions from neighbouring voxels.

A three-dimensional absorbed dose distribution can be obtained from digital image data by calculating the contribution to the absorbed dose in a given voxel (D_i) from all other source voxels and from the activity in the voxel itself (Figure 17.2). This is

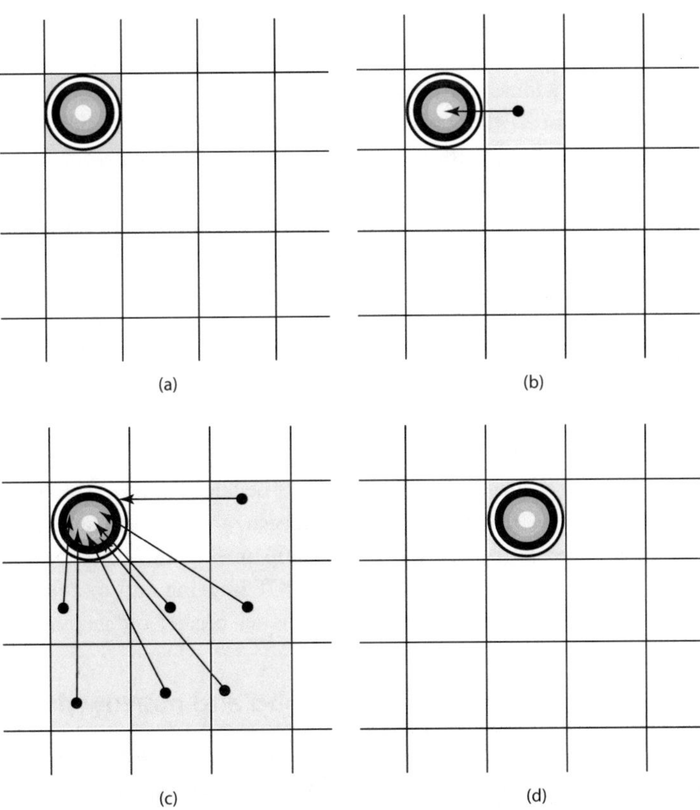

Figure 17.2 Convolution dosimetry. These steps are required for convolution dosimetry. (a) The self-absorbed dose to the first voxel (initially the target voxel) is calculated. (b) The absorbed dose to the target voxel from activity in an adjacent source voxel is performed, and this is repeated for all other source voxels (c). Finally, the process is repeated for a second target voxel (d) and subsequently for all target voxels.

performed by a convolution of the activity distribution with a point-source dose kernel, which is effectively a look-up table of the absorbed dose deposited as a function of distance from a point source. The convolution is given by:

$$D_i = \sum_j [\tilde{A}_j \times K(r_{ij})]$$

where

$\tilde{A}_j$ = the cumulated activity in voxel j, and $K(r_{ij})$ = the absorbed dose deposited in voxel i from voxel j.

Monte Carlo dosimetry

The most accurate method of computing an absorbed dose distribution from a given source activity distribution is the use of Monte Carlo simulations, by which the energy deposition from each individual decay is tracked and scored (Furhang *et al.* 1996; Clairand *et al.* 1999). A number of codes are available for this purpose, including EGSnrc, MCNP and PENELOPE. This can be regarded as the logical extension to the initial MIRD schema, which uses Monte Carlo methods to compute S values for standardised organs, and to the process of convolution dosimetry for which Monte Carlo is used to compute the dose kernels. This methodology requires significant computing resources and expertise.

Applications of dosimetry

Internal dosimetry may be applied in a range of circumstances. Methods for data collection and calculations, along with the degree of accuracy required, can vary according to the purpose for which it is intended. Broadly, dosimetry may be considered in four categories:

Whole body dosimetry

Possibly the simplest application of dosimetry is to consider the absorbed dose received by the whole body. There are a number of advantages and drawbacks to this approach. The process of calculating whole body absorbed doses is relatively easy and can be performed in any centre that offers targeted radionuclide therapy (TRT). The basic principles of the MIRD schema apply and the initial aim is to determine the cumulated activity in the whole body. The activity at time $t = 0$ is the known administered activity and if counts are acquired immediately after administration using a compensated Geiger counter these will provide a baseline for future measurements. The ratio of subsequent readings to the initial measurement can then be applied to the injected activity (Chittenden *et al.* 2007). Whole body dosimetry has been used as a surrogate for bone marrow dosimetry for both ^{131}I-tositumomab therapy of non-Hodgkin lymphoma (Jacene *et al.* 2007), and for iodine-131 mIBG therapy of neuroblastoma (Gaze *et al.* 2005; Buckley *et al.* 2007).

Normal organ dosimetry

The aim of radiotherapy is to maximise the absorbed doses delivered to target tissues while minimising the absorbed doses received by normal organs. Organs at risk for any radiotherapeutic procedure using TRT depend largely on the treatment administered and on the radiopharmaceutical used. For some treatments (e.g. radiolabelled peptide therapy) the dose limiting organ is the kidney (Bodei *et al.* 2008). Several models exist to help determine kidney dosimetry, and these are becoming increasingly refined (Bouchet *et al.* 2003). Cumulated activity can be obtained from quantitative imaging or can be extrapolated from activity concentrations measured directly from urine samples. Uptake in a tumour within a normal organ will cause irradiation of that organ, which may be problematic when treating liver metastases, for example. The aim of internal dosimetry in these cases is to ensure that absorbed doses fall well below levels that would cause concern, and in practice it is usually sufficient to calculate mean absorbed doses from serial planar or SPECT imaging and to apply S values calculated for reference organs and geometries.

Blood and marrow dosimetry

Frequently, the circulation of activity in blood following a therapeutic administration results in a delivered absorbed dose to the red marrow, which is the most radiosensitive organ. Marrow dosimetry is particularly challenging and a number of approaches have been made to address this issue. An obvious technique is to apply similar methodology to that described above, i.e. to acquire and quantify sequential images following administration and to use suitable S values (Siegel *et al.* 1989). However, accurate quantification of red marrow uptake is particularly challenging owing to scatter and attenuation of photons by bone. It is therefore not uncommon to consider surrogate targets. Absorbed doses calculated for the blood have also been used as an indication of the absorbed dose to the red marrow, and have been used clinically to personalise treatment (Benua *et al.* 1962). This approach is motivated by the observation that the concentration of activity in the blood is proportional to that in the red marrow (Sgouros 1993). This is valid where there is no specific uptake in bone marrow, bone or components of blood. The mean absorbed dose to blood (D_{blood}) per unit administered activity (A_{adm}) is considered to be delivered from both the circulating activity and from the rest of the body (Lassmann *et al.* 2008), i.e.

$$\frac{\overline{D}_{\text{blood}}}{A_{\text{adm}}} = (S_{\text{bloodblood}} \times \tau_{\text{millilitre of blood}}) + (S_{\text{blood} \gets \text{total body}} \times \tau_{\text{total body}})$$

where τ is the residence time, calculated from dividing the cumulated activity by the administered activity.

Cumulated activities in the whole body can be obtained either from whole body measurements as described above or from conjugate view planar imaging.

Direct measurements of activity within bone marrow can be obtained from biopsy samples, although this invasive procedure is difficult to justify for dosimetry alone and does not account for heterogeneous distribution of activity within the marrow and the diffuse distribution of active marrow throughout the body (Sgouros 1993).

Tumour dosimetry

As discussed above, the requirement for accurate tumour dosimetry is generally greater than that for normal organs and ideally should take into account the heterogeneity of uptake where this occurs. The techniques employed should be dependent on the geometry and location of the tumour. Thus, for example, 3D dosimetry should be applied to a large neuroendocrine tumour exhibiting heterogeneous uptake, whereas mean or maximum tumour dosimetry could be sufficient for a smaller tumour in which heterogeneity of uptake cannot be distinguished due to the partial volume effect.

Data acquisition and processing for internal dosimetry

Of the factors required for an absorbed dose calculation, the cumulated activity most concerns the physicist or technician. This parameter is obtained from integration of time–activity data and the accuracy of the final calculation is dependent on the quality of the data and on subsequent analysis. A particular problem inherent in imaging for radionuclide therapy is that gamma cameras are primarily designed for qualitative imaging of radionuclides with low-energy photon emissions. Quantitative imaging, particularly for higher-energy radionuclides such as iodine-131, which has a primary photon emission of 364 keV, or for pure beta emitters such as yttrium-90, is arguably the single most challenging factor involved in internal dosimetry.

Pre-acquisition procedures

Camera settings must be optimised for the radionuclide imaged. In particular it is important that the collimator and energy window settings should be chosen to optimise the spatial resolution and sensitivity and to enable dual- or triple-energy window scatter correction. Individual cameras should be characterised for dead time, particularly in the case of imaging ^{131}I following a therapeutic procedure.

Number and timing of scans

Insufficient numbers of scans can lead to substantial errors in the calculation of cumulated activities and consequently in absorbed doses. Ideally, three data points should be acquired for each uptake or decay phase so that errors may be calculated. In practice, tumour or normal organ dosimetry tends to exhibit a monoexponential decay, whilst whole body decay can vary from one phase only (for example thyroid

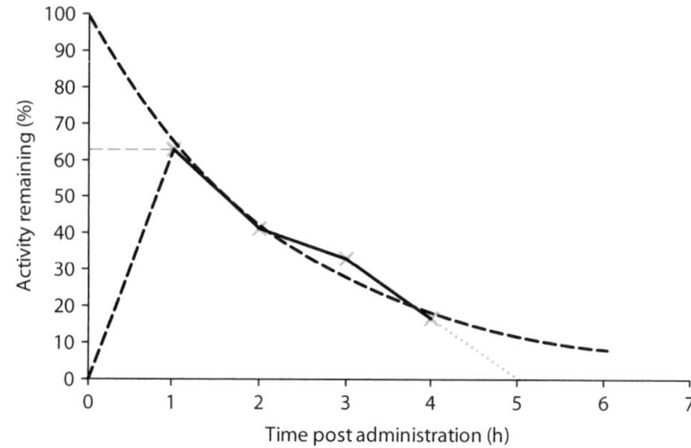

Figure 17.3 Illustration of the effect of data acquisition and integration. Assumed data points on the activity–time curve are denoted by crosses. The accuracy of calculating the area under the curve (i.e. the cumulated activity) is dependent on the number and timing of points. Here a curve fit has been performed both with trapezoidal integration (—) and with an exponential fit (– – –). Extrapolation beyond the final acquired data point can either be made according to the exponential fit or from the final two data points (··········). Assumptions regarding initial uptake can include continuous uptake until the time of the first data point (diagonal – – –) and a static uptake from time $t = 0$ (horizontal – – –), which would fall between continuous uptake and the exponential fit.

ablation following successful surgery) to five phases or more (as is frequently seen for iodine-131 mIBG therapy) (Buckley *et al.* 2009).

Image quantification

Image quantification is widely regarded as the single largest potential source of error in dosimetry calculations. Attenuation and scatter corrections are essential procedures to achieve accurate quantification. Factors to convert counts to activity can be obtained from calibration phantoms scanned separately to the patient (Koral, Dewaraja 1999; Buckley *et al.* 2007) and are sometimes acquired from sources placed next to the patient during the scan (Monsieurs *et al.* 2002; Delpon *et al.* 2003; Lassmann *et al.* 2004).

Integration of activity–time curve

A number of methods may be employed to integrate the activity–time data. Commonly, phase fitting is performed under the assumption that uptake or decay is exponential. Phase fitting may be performed by eye or by using an automatic method such as spectral analysis (Divoli *et al.* 2005). An advantage of this technique is that the error in the final dose calculation can be determined directly as a function of the goodness of fit (Flux *et al.* 2002). Alternatively, numerical integration techniques can be employed. It is necessary to extrapolate acquired data to account for uptake and retention of activity prior to or following data acquisition (Figure 17.3).

Radiobiology for targeted radionuclide therapy

Introduction

Treatment procedures for external beam radiotherapy (EBRT), particularly including fractionation, are largely founded on radiobiological principles. In contrast, radiobiology for TRT is less advanced and clinical implementation is currently sparse. Nevertheless, principles and concepts developed for EBRT provide an initial framework that is applicable to TRT.

Basic LQ model

Traditionally, the radiobiology is largely based on the linear-quadratic (LQ) model, which deals directly with radiation damage to the DNA. It is assumed that lethal radiation damage can be caused either by a single ionising event (type A damage) or by two separate events that combine to cause cell death (type B damage) (Dale 1996). This is usually interpreted as either a DNA double-strand break (DSB) or as two DNA single-strand breaks (SSB). Repair of a SSB prior to further breaks is more likely than repair of a DSB. This indicates the importance of dose rate.

The basic LQ model is given by

$$SF = e^{-\alpha D - \beta G D^2}$$

where D = the absorbed dose; SF = the surviving fraction of cells; α and β are radiosensitivity parameters; and G = the Lea Catcheside dose protraction factor (Millar 1991; Sachs *et al.* 1997), which takes into account cellular repair.

While this model has demonstrated good agreement when applied to *in-vitro* studies, it has been shown that other cellular targets, for example in the membrane, may also be linked to lethal damage (Gillies 1997). This is potentially of more importance to TRT than to EBRT owing to the varying localisation of radiopharmaceuticals consistent with different therapies.

The 4 Rs

The main parameters pertinent to radiobiology are often summarised as the so-called 'four Rs'. Each of these parameters can be considered in the light of TRT.

Repair

As already stated, repair of DNA damage is a prime factor affecting the efficacy of radiation. This is of particular importance to TRT which is administered as a continuous low dose-rate (CLDR) treatment. The consequences of this can be both advantageous and disadvantageous and have yet to be fully explored.

Redistribution

The cell cycle undergoes distinct phases, consisting of:

1. G_0 phase, in which the cell is effectively resting
2. G_1 phase, in which the cell grows
3. S phase, in which the cell prepares for replication
4. G_2 phase, in which the cell continues to grow, and
5. Mitosis, when the cell divides.

Cells are relatively radiosensitive during the G_1 and mitotic phase, so that irradiation will tend to result in surviving cells residing in the same phase. A potential advantage of TRT is that cells will be irradiated continually during these phases, so that dose rate (rather than absolute absorbed dose) may be a determining factor in effecting cell kill.

Reoxygenation

Cells are more radiosensitive when exposed to oxygen. This again has particular relevance to TRT. Radiation delivery of an injected radiopharmaceutical is dependent on the blood supply to the tumour. Targeting of large solid tumours is recognised as problematic, partly due the frequent lack of supply to the inner hypoxic part of the mass. However, an outer rim of the tumour can be targeted, which may in turn allow reoxygenation. This could form the basis of a fractionation schedule based on optimal delivery times.

Repopulation

Reoxygenation of hypoxic cells will occur when a blood supply is returned, thereby increasing the number of clonogenic cells. Ideally, the timing of successive administrations should take this into account.

Application of radiobiology to targeted radionuclide therapy

Issues pertinent to EBRT have a similar importance for TRT, where it is conceivable that dose-rates, fractionation and linear energy transfer (LET) will have a significant effect on therapeutic efficacy. An issue debated heavily in the 1920s in EBRT concerned the relative merits of concentrated and fractionated treatments, with two opposed schools of thought. The main argument in favour of concentrated treatments was that growing cells were more able to recover from the effects of radiation, while the proponents of fractionation maintained that dividing cells were more radiosensitive (Thames, Hendry 1987). This issue remains a debate in TRT where advocates of both approaches can be found (O'Donoghue *et al.* 2000). An interesting example is iodine-131 NaI therapy for thyroid cancer, which relies on a single administration for remnant ablation but will typically administer fixed activities at fixed intervals to treat metastatic disease. Practicalities and local procedures concerning radiation protection can prevent large single administrations, although tumours subject to multiple fractions of radiotherapy can become less radiosensitive and prone to de-differentiation. However, multiple administrations can counter potential saturation of target sites from a single large administration and re-vascularisation following an initial treatment may allow subsequent irradiation of hypoxic regions.

Models developed for EBRT to describe the effects of radiation on tissue may not be entirely applicable to TRT. The tumour control probability (TCP), used to determine the possibility of eradicating a tumour formed of a number (N_c) of clonogenic cells is given by

$$\mathrm{TCP}(N_c, D) = e^{-N_c \mathrm{SF(D)}} = e^{-N_c\, e^{-\alpha D - G \beta D^2}}$$

If the distribution of absorbed dose is heterogeneous, it has been shown that the TCP is the product of the values of the TCPs of groups of clonogenic cells receiving the same absorbed dose (Webb, Nahum 1993).

$$\mathrm{TCP}(N, D) = \prod_{i=1}^{n_d} \mathrm{TCP}(N_i, D_i) = \prod_{i=1}^{n_d} e^{-N_i\, e^{-\alpha\alpha D_i - G \beta D_i^2}}$$

This of course is of particular relevance to TRT, where extreme heterogeneities of uptake can be observed. Similar arguments apply to normal tissue complication probability (NTCP) and information is still being accrued to determine maximum tolerated absorbed doses to normal organs receiving CLDR, as has been done for EBRT (Emami *et al.* 1991).

Non-uniformity of uptake and consequently of absorbed dose distribution may be addressed by concepts such as the equivalent uniform dose (EUD) (Niemierko 1997), which calculates the mean absorbed dose to produce the same radiobiological effect that will be achieved by a heterogeneous distribution of absorbed dose. Correspondence between the biological effect of an absorbed dose delivered by an administration of a radiopharmaceutical and one delivered from external beam irradiation is found from calculation of the biologically equivalent dose (BED) (Dale, Carabe-Fernandez 2005). This approach has been shown to successfully predict renal toxicity in a study of ^{90}Y-DOTATOC treatment (Barone *et al.* 2002) and is increasingly being applied to internal dose calculations (Bodey *et al.* 2004; Chiesa *et al.* 2007). These considerations imply that mean absorbed doses calculated for TRT can only give an approximation to the biological effect, and that the distribution of absorbed dose should ideally be taken into account, possibly aided by the depiction of dose–volume histograms.

Further issues currently being explored include the radiation induced biological bystander effect whereby it has been shown that unirradiated cells can undergo apoptosis if they are in sufficient proximity to irradiated cells (Boyd *et al.* 2006), and also hyper-radiosensitivity, which implies that cells may respond more readily to a smaller amount of radiation than to a larger one (Marples, Collis 2008).

Conclusion

Radiobiology is a complex issue for TRT. Uptake mechanisms, localisation, the cellular effects of irradiation with particles of different range and LET, and the response of different tissues to radiation are all factors to be considered. Nevertheless, the understanding of radiobiological effects is essential to the further development of TRT. Further possibilities may then be explored, such as the use of cocktails of radionuclides (Cremonesi *et al.* 2006) and the use of radiosensitisers.

Clinical applications of dosimetry

The range of radiopharmaceuticals and malignancies treated with TRT require different approaches to dosimetric evaluation. Although at present dosimetry is seldom applied in routine clinical practice, there is increasing need to calculate absorbed doses for new radiopharmaceuticals and to improve the efficacy of existing products. Internal dosimetry has been applied to a wide range of treatments, the most common of which are listed below.

Iodine-131 NaI for thyroid cancer

Thyroid cancer and hyperthyroidism have been treated with iodine-131 NaI (radioiodine) since the 1940s. This treatment has a high degree of success relative to other radionuclide treatments, although recurrence of thyroid cancer following ablation can be as high as 75% in high risk patients, including the young and the elderly, and can be fatal. There are conflicting guidelines regarding the administration of radioiodine and measurement of response. Despite the difficulties inherent in imaging and quantifying iodine-131 uptake, numerous studies have calculated absorbed doses from fixed administrations of activity and evidence exists to indicate that response is proportional to the absorbed dose delivered (O'Connell *et al.* 1993; Maxon 1999; Dorn *et al.* 2003; Flux *et al.* 2010). Methods for calculating absorbed doses have varied widely, although it is clear that superior results can be obtained from careful consideration of the imaging parameters (Lassmann *et al.* 2004) and that fixed activities can deliver absorbed doses differing by up to two orders of magnitude (Maxon 1999; Sgouros *et al.* 2004). Patient-specific treatments have been carried out by Benua *et al.* (1962), who aimed to administer an activity that would deliver a 2 Gy absorbed dose to the blood, and by Dorn *et al.* (2003), who administered up to 38 500 MBq to deliver a 3 Gy marrow absorbed dose.

Iodine-131 mIBG for neuroendocrine tumours

In terms of imaging and dosimetry, the administration of iodine-131 mIBG for adult and paediatric neuroendocrine tumours extends the requirements associated with the treatment of thyroid disease. The relatively high levels of activity often administered place greater emphasis on the absorbed doses delivered to the red marrow, which can be difficult to calculate accurately because of potential marrow involvement. Whole body dosimetry has been used successfully to administer maximum tolerated activities on a patient-specific basis (Gaze *et al.* 2005; Buckley *et al.* 2007, 2009). Patients often present with large solid tumours that exhibit a heterogeneous degree of uptake, so that tomographic imaging is essential to accurately calculate the resulting absorbed dose distributions. Treatment is usually palliative, although complete responses have been observed and the introduction of new initiatives such as carrier-free mIBG and the concomitant use of radiosensitisers such as topotecan (McCluskey *et al.* 2002) offer a strong potential for a significant improvement in this therapy.

Radiolabelled peptides for neuroendocrine tumours

An increasing number of radiopharmaceuticals are currently being developed for this treatment. Yttrium-90-labelled peptides offer the potential to target solid masses with long-range beta emitters that can help to overcome the problem of non-homogeneous uptake. However, imaging, and consequently dosimetry, is problematic owing the lack of gamma emissions, so that it is necessary either to perform bremsstrahlung imaging or to administer a tracer activity of indium-111. This may be given either prior to therapy or concomitantly with the therapeutic administration. Studies have shown a wide range of absorbed doses resulting from fixed administrations of activity, although the biokinetics of an individual patient tend to be sufficiently consistent that individualised treatment planning is feasible where multiple administrations are performed (Hindorf *et al.* 2007). PET dosimetry using yttrium-86 has demonstrated clear dose–response correlations in terms of renal toxicity and tumour shrinkage (Barone *et al.* 2002). Lutetium-177 octreotate is currently emerging as a promising candidate for radionuclide therapy of neuroendocrine tumours. This emits a 208 keV gamma photon that permits imaging and consequently dosimetry (Turner 2009).

Radioimmunotherapy for NHL

Various antibodies have been radiolabelled with either iodine-131 or yttrium-90 for radioimmunotherapy (De Nardo *et al.* 1999; Kletting *et al.* 2009). Two products (^{90}Y-ibritumomab tiuxitan (Zevalin) and ^{131}I-tositumomab (Bexxar)) have received FDA approval. Biodistribution studies have been performed for Zevalin using a pre-therapy administration of indium-111 and have demonstrated a wide range of absorbed doses delivered to normal organs and to tumours from an administration of 15 MBq/kg (Wiseman *et al.* 2001). Bexxar is administered according to a predicted 0.75 Gy whole body absorbed dose.

Intra-arterial treatments for HCC

Hepatocellular carcinoma and liver metastases from colorectal cancer may be treated with radioembolisation, whereby an intra-arterial administration of embolic particles is used to selectively target these lesions. Radiopharmaceuticals used for this purpose include iodine-131 lipiodol and rhenium-188 lipiodol. Yttrium-90 microspheres, bound to resin (SIR-Spheres, Sirtex Medical, Lane Cove, NSW, Australia) or embedded in a glass matrix (TheraSphere, MDS Nordion, Kanata, ON, Canada) are also in routine use. A strong advantage of this technique is that the tumour-to-background uptake ratio is significantly higher than for an intravenous infusion, resulting in lower absorbed doses to normal organs. Absorbed doses have been calculated for an administration of 3.7 GBq ^{188}Re-HDD lipiodol to be < 8 Gy to the liver and < 5 Gy to lungs (Lambert *et al.* 2006). Nevertheless, lung shunting remains a concern of this treatment, and the standard protocol for yttrium-90 microspheres is to assess potential lung uptake from a tracer administration of ^{99m}Tc-MAA prior to therapy. If significant lung uptake is seen, administered activities are decreased accordingly.

Conclusion

Internal dosimetry is increasingly being performed to calculate absorbed doses to target tissues and to normal organs from established treatments and is becoming mandatory for the initial clinical implementation of new radiopharmaceuticals. Routine application can ensure the optimal use of a radiopharmaceutical that has been developed at significant cost over an extended period of time. As the need for evidence-based medicine becomes more widespread, quantitative imaging and dosimetry will enable radionuclide therapies to be performed on a patient-specific basis, as is mandatory for external beam radiotherapy. It is likely that significant developments will be seen in this area in the coming years.

References

Barone R *et al.* (2002). Correlation between acute red marrow (RM) toxicity and RM exposure during Y-90-SMT487 therapy. *J Nucl Med* 43(5): 1267.

Benua RS *et al.* (1962). The relation of radioiodine dosimetry to results and complications in the treatment of metastatic thyroid carcinoma. *Am J Roentgenol Radium Ther Nucl Med* 87: 171–182.

Bodei L *et al.* (2008). Long-term evaluation of renal toxicity after peptide receptor radionuclide therapy with ^{90}Y-DOTATOC and ^{177}Lu-DOTATATE: the role of associated risk factors. *Eur J Nucl Med Mol Imaging* 35(10): 1847–1856.

Bodey RK *et al.* (2004). Application of the linear-quadratic model to combined modality radiotherapy. *Int J Radiat Oncol Biol Phys* 59(1): 228–41.

Bolch WE *et al.* (1999). MIRD Pamphlet No. 17: The dosimetry of nonuniform activity distributions – Radionuclide *S* values at the voxel level. *J Nucl Med* 40(1): 11S–36S.

Bouchet LG *et al.* (2003). MIRD Pamphlet No. 19: Absorbed fractions and radionuclide *S* values for six age-dependent multiregion models of the kidney. *J Nucl Med* 44(7): 1113–1147.

Boyd M *et al.* (2006). Radiation-induced biologic bystander effect elicited in vitro by targeted radiopharmaceuticals labeled with alpha-, beta-, and Auger electron-emitting radionuclides. *J Nucl Med* 47(6): 1007–1015.

Buckley SE *et al.* (2007). Dosimetry for fractionated ^{131}I-mIBG therapies in patients with primary resistant high-risk neuroblastoma: preliminary results. *Cancer Biother Radiopharm* 22(1): 105–112.

Buckley SE *et al.* (2009). Whole-body dosimetry for individualised treatment planning of ^{131}I-mIBG radionuclide therapy for neuroblastoma. *J Nucl Med* 50(9): 1518–1524.

Chiesa C *et al.* (2007). Dosimetry in myeloablative ^{90}Y-labeled ibritumomab tiuxetan therapy: possibility of increasing administered activity on the base of biological effective dose evaluation. Preliminary results. *Cancer Biother Radiopharm* 22(1): 113–120.

Chittenden SJ *et al.* (2007). Optimization of equipment and methodology for whole-body activity retention measurements in children undergoing targeted radionuclide therapy. *Cancer Biother Radiopharm* 22(2): 243–249.

Clairand I *et al.* (1999). DOSE3D: EGS4 Monte Carlo code-based software for internal radionuclide dosimetry. *J Nucl Med* 40(9): 1517–1523.

Cremonesi M *et al.* (2006). Dosimetry in peptide radionuclide receptor therapy: a review. *J Nucl Med* 47(9): 1467–1475.

Dale R, Carabe-Fernandez A (2005). The radiobiology of conventional radiotherapy and its application to radionuclide therapy. *Cancer Biother Radiopharm* 20(1): 47–51.

Dale RG (1996). Dose-rate effects in targeted radiotherapy. *Phys Med Biol* 41(10): 1871–1884.

Delpon G *et al.* (2003). Impact of scatter and attenuation corrections for iodine-131 two-dimensional quantitative imaging in patients. *Cancer Biother Radiopharm* 18(2): 191–199.

DeNardo GL *et al.* (1999). Factors affecting ^{131}I-Lym-1 pharmacokinetics and radiation dosimetry in patients with non-Hodgkin's lymphoma and chronic lymphocytic leukemia. *J Nucl Med* 40(8): 1317–1326.

Dewaraja YK *et al.* (2005). Accurate dosimetry in I-131 radionuclide therapy using patient-specific, 3-dimensional methods for SPECT reconstruction and absorbed dose calculation. *J Nucl Med* 46(5): 840–849.

Divoli A *et al.* (2005). Whole-body dosimetry for targeted radionuclide therapy using spectral analysis. *Cancer Biother Radiopharm* 20(1): 66–71.

Divoli A *et al.* (2009). Effect of patient morphology on dosimetric calculations for internal irradiation as assessed by comparisons of monte carlo versus conventional methodologies. *J Nucl Med* 50(2): 316–323.

Dorn R *et al.* (2003). Dosimetry-guided radioactive iodine treatment in patients with metastatic differentiated thyroid cancer: largest safe dose using a risk-adapted approach. *J Nucl Med* 44(3): 451–456.

Emami B *et al.* (1991). Tolerance of normal tissue to therapeutic irradiation. *Int J Radiat Oncol Biol Phys* 21(1): 109–122.

Flux GD *et al.* (2002). Estimation and implications of random errors in whole-body dosimetry for targeted radionuclide therapy. *Phys Med Biol* 47(17): 3211–3223.

Flux *et al.* (2010). A dose–effect correlation for radioiodine ablation in differentiated thyroid cancer. *Eur J Nucl Med Mol Imaging* 37(2): 270–275.

Furhang EE *et al.* (1996). A Monte Carlo approach to patient-specific dosimetry. *Med Phys* 23(9): 1523–1529.

Gaze MN *et al.* (2005). Feasibility of dosimetry-based high-dose ^{131}I-meta-iodobenzylguanidine with topotecan as a radiosensitizer in children with metastatic neuroblastoma. *Cancer Biother Radiopharm* 20(2): 195–199.

Giap HB *et al.* (1995). Validation of a dose-point kernel convolution technique for internal dosimetry. *Phys Med Biol* 40(3): 365–381.

Gillies NE (1997). Radiation damage to cell membranes: insights from the oxygen effect. *Int J Radiat Biol* 71(6): 643–648.

Hindorf C *et al.* (2007). Dosimetry for ^{90}Y-DOTATOC therapies in patients with neuroendocrine tumors. *Cancer Biother Radiopharm* 22(1): 130–135.

Jacene HA *et al.* (2007). Comparison of ^{90}Y-ibritumomab tiuxetan and ^{131}I-tositumomab in clinical practice. *J Nucl Med* 48(11): 1767–1776.

Kletting P *et al.* (2009). Improving anti-CD45 antibody radioimmunotherapy using a physiologically based pharmacokinetic model. *J Nucl Med* 50(2): 296–302.

Koral KF, Dewaraja Y (1999). I-131 SPECT activity recovery coefficients with implicit or triple-energy-window scatter correction. *Nucl Instrum Methods Phys Res, Sect A – Accelerators Spectrometers Detectors and Associated Equipment* 422(13): 688–692.

Lambert B *et al.* (2006). ^{188}Re-HDD/Lipiodol for hepatocellular carcinoma: our experience with the first 100 treatments. *Eur J Nucl Med Mol Imaging* 33: S215–S216.

Lassmann M *et al.* (2004). Impact of ^{131}I diagnostic activities on the biokinetics of thyroid remnants. *J Nucl Med* 45(4): 619–625.

Lassmann M *et al.* (2008). EANM Dosimetry Committee series on standard operational procedures for pre-therapeutic dosimetry I: Blood and bone marrow dosimetry in differentiated thyroid cancer therapy. *Eur J Nucl Med Mol Imaging* 35(7): 1405–1412.

Loevinger R *et al.* (1988). *MIRD Primer for Absorbed Dose Calculations*. New York: Society of Nuclear Medicine.

Marinelli L *et al.* (1948). Dosage determination with radioactive isotopes. II Practical considerations in therapy and protection. *Am J Roent Radium Ther* 59: 260–280.

Marples B, Collis SJ (2008). Low-dose hyper-radiosensitivity: past, present, and future. *Int J Radiat Oncol Biol Phys* 70 (5): 1310–1318.

Maxon HR (1999). Quantitative radioiodine therapy in the treatment of differentiated thyroid cancer. *Q J Nucl Med* 43(4): 313–323.

McCluskey AG *et al.* (2002). Experimental determination of the optimum means of combining topotecan and mIBG therapy in the treatment of neuroblastoma. *Br J Cancer* 86: S57.

Millar WT (1991). Application of the linear-quadratic model with incomplete repair to radionuclide directed therapy. *Br J Radiol* 64(759): 242–251.

Monsieurs M *et al.* (2002). Patient dosimetry for ^{131}I-MIBG therapy for neuroendocrine tumours based on ^{123}I-MIBG scans. *Eur J Nucl Med Mol Imaging* 29(12): 1581–1587.

Niemierko A (1997). Reporting and analyzing dose distributions: a concept of equivalent uniform dose. *Med Phys* 24 (1): 103–110.

O'Connell MEA *et al.* (1993). Radiation-dose assessment in radioiodine therapy – dose–response relationships in differentiated thyroid-carcinoma using quantitative scanning and PET. *Radiother Oncol* 28(1): 16–26.

O'Donoghue JA *et al.* (2000). Single-dose versus fractionated radioimmunotherapy: model comparisons for uniform tumor dosimetry. *J Nucl Med* 41(3): 538–547.

Sachs RK *et al.* (1997). The link between low-LET dose–response relations and the underlying kinetics of damage production/repair/misrepair. *Int J Radiat Biol* 72(4): 351–374.

Sgouros G (1993). Bone-marrow dosimetry for radioimmunotherapy – theoretical considerations. *J Nucl Med* 34(4): 689–694.

Sgouros G *et al.* (2004). Patient-specific dosimetry for ^{131}I thyroid cancer therapy using ^{124}I PET and 3-dimensional-internal dosimetry (3D-ID) software. *J Nucl Med* 45(8): 1366–1372.

Siegel JA *et al.* (1989). Sacral scintigraphy for bone-marrow dosimetry in radioimmunotherapy. *Nucl Med Biol* 16(6): 553.

Snyder W S *et al.* (1975). Absorbed dose per unit cumulated activity for selected radionuclides and organs (Part 1). Reston, VA: Society of Nuclear Medicine.

Stabin MG *et al.* (2005). OLINDA/EXM: The second-generation personal computer software for internal dose assessment in nuclear medicine. *J Nucl Med* 46(6): 1023–1027.

Stabin MG (1996). MIRDOSE: Personal computer software for internal dose assessment in nuclear medicine. *J Nucl Med* 37(3): 538–546.

Thames HD, Hendry JH (1987). *Fractionation in Radiotherapy*. London: Taylor & Francis.

Turner JH (2009). Defining pharmacokinetics for individual patient dosimetry in routine radiopeptide and radioimmunotherapy of cancer: Australian experience. *Curr Pharm Des* 15(9): 966–982.

Webb S, Nahum AE (1993). A model for calculating tumor-control probability in radiotherapy including the effects of inhomogeneous distributions of dose and clonogenic cell-density. *Phys Med Biol* 38(6): 653–666.

Wiseman GA *et al.* (2001). Biodistribution and dosimetry results from a phase III prospectively randomized controlled trial of Zevalin (TM) radioimmunotherapy for low-grade, follicular, or transformed B-cell non-Hodgkin's lymphoma. *Crit Rev Oncol Hemat* 39(12): 181–194.

SECTION D

Radiopharmaceutics

18

Survey of current diagnostic radiopharmaceuticals

Paul Maltby, Tony Theobald and members of the UK Radiopharmacy Group

Introduction

This survey of radiopharmaceuticals in nuclear medicine practice is designed to inform the reader to a limited degree about the specifications and uses of the products in regular use in the specialty. Where taken from official monographs, the information provided should be taken as the starting point prior to proceeding to the complete text in the relevant pharmacopoeias.

The previous edition of this textbook noted that while a product may be the subject of an official monograph it may not necessarily be available on the open market, and may have to be prepared 'in house'. This is especially true today where PET tracers are concerned, and where the number of large radiopharmaceutical companies has contracted as a result of business rationalisation and mergers in 'big pharma'.

A radiopharmaceutical may have been granted marketing authorisation or a product licence in one or more countries, but may not have been made the subject of an official monograph. The reverse situation may also be true; thus the legal status of any radiopharmaceutical must be checked by the radiopharmacist prior to its use to ensure that the clinician prescribing the product is aware of any personal legal liabilities that may arise should an adverse event occur in the patient.

In the UK the Medicines and Healthcare products Regulatory Agency maintains a list of radiopharmaceuticals granted UK marketing authorisations; likewise, the EMEA maintains a list of those granted marketing authorisations in the European Union.

Pharmacopoeias and monographs

There are two pharmacopoeias that have legal status within the UK – the British Pharmacopoeia (BP) and the European Pharmacopoeia (Ph Eur).

The British Pharmacopoeia, which is now published annually, is the only comprehensive collection of standards for UK medicinal substances. It contributes to the overall control of the quality of medicinal products by providing an authoritative statement of the standard that a product is expected to meet at any time during its period of use. The publicly available and legally enforceable pharmacopoeial standards are designed to complement and assist the licensing and inspection processes, and are part of the system for safeguarding public health.

The European Pharmacopoeia derives from the Council of Europe Convention on the elaboration of a European Pharmacopoeia, an international treaty signed by member states. There were eight founder countries in 1964 and currently 34 countries are parties to the Convention as individual states together with the European Union. A further 17 European and non-European countries plus the World Health Organization have observer status at the European Pharmacopoeia Commission (EPC). Monographs of the European Pharmacopoeia are legally enforced in the countries which are signatories to the Convention, and they are enforced in the EU through Directive EC 2001/83. Preparation of the European Pharmacopoeia is the responsibility of the EPC. The technical secretariat of the EPC is part of the Council of Europe's European Directorate for the Quality of Medicines and Healthcare, which is located in Strasbourg. The UK participates at all stages of European Pharmacopoeia monograph development and revision via UK membership of the Groups of Experts (radiopharmaceuticals are amended or added by Group 14), and through the UK delegation to the EPC.

The European Pharmacopoeia contains monographs for pharmaceutical substances, general monographs for formulated dosage forms, and individual monographs for vaccines, immunosera and radiopharmaceutical preparations. The monographs of the European Pharmacopoeia apply to substances used in either human or veterinary medicines, or in both. The European Pharmacopoeia also contains individual monographs of vaccines for veterinary use. Other than vaccines and immunosera and radiopharmaceuticals, there are no monographs for individual dosage forms in the European Pharmacopoeia.

Future work of the Group of Experts of European Pharmacopoeia

A new monograph is introduced by a process called elaboration, and once adopted by the European Pharmacopoeia Commission (EPC), the text is continually adapted to keep pace with regulatory needs in public health, with industrial constraints and technological or scientific advances. The text is also updated taking into account changes in marketed products, scientific progress and comments from users and authorities. Text revision can be seen as systematic revisions where obsolete monographs are updated or removed, minor revisions of monographs on similar substances for harmonisation, and individual revision following requests received by the EPC either when the monograph has been found to be unsatisfactory or the manufacturing method has changed. The European Pharmacopoeia will thus be producing monographs on non-radioactive precursors for radiopharmaceuticals, e.g. mannose triflate and medronic acid, and radioactive precursors for radiopharmaceuticals, e.g. Sodium Molybdate [^{99}Mo] Solution (Fission), as well as revising existing monographs.

The British Pharmacopoeia

The monographs of the British Pharmacopoeia (BP) are legally enforced by the Medicines Act 1968. Where a pharmacopoeial monograph exists, medicinal products sold or supplied in the UK must comply with that monograph. All the monographs and texts of the European Pharmacopoeia are reproduced in the British Pharmacopoeia. These include the monographs for pharmaceutical substances, general monographs, and individual monographs. The BP Commission is responsible for preparing new editions of the British Pharmacopoeia and the British Pharmacopoeia (Veterinary) and for keeping them up to date. Under Section 100 of the Medicines Act, the BP Commission is also responsible for selecting and devising British Approved Names. The BP Commission is comprised of experts from the pharmaceutical industry, academia, regulators and hospital pharmacy and, in addition, there are two lay members. There are also seven expert advisory groups that advise on and finalise the BP texts (three of these advise on medicinal chemicals and the remainder on antibiotics, pharmacy, herbal and complementary medicine, nomenclature and unlicensed medicines) and four panels of experts on inorganic chemistry, biological products (including blood products and immunological products), microbiology and radiopharmaceuticals that provide advice in these fields when necessary.

In contrast to the European Pharmacopoeia, the British Pharmacopoeia contains monographs for individual dosage forms. This allows the BP to define standards for individual medicinal products on the UK market. Since its first publication in 1864, the distribution of the British Pharmacopoeia has grown throughout the world. Now used in over 100 countries with exposure in most continents of the world, the British Pharmacopoeia is setting the standard for pharmaceutical compliance across the globe. In Australia and Canada it is still a legally enforced national standard and it is used by competent authorities throughout Europe and the Commonwealth to advise and complement the licensing and regulation of medicines.

BP Supplementary Chapter on Unlicensed Medicines

Specifically to suit UK legislation, in the latest edition (2009), guidance is now provided to prescribers, manufacturers and suppliers of unlicensed medicines on the legal and ethical considerations of such medicines. Further guidance on the standards for the preparation and manufacture of unlicensed medicines is also given.

Finished products and labelled kit products

A list of currently available UK radiopharmaceuticals is shown in Table 18.1.

Survey of diagnostic radiopharmaceuticals

The following sections describe some of the most commonly used diagnostic radiopharmaceuticals. The information is taken from public documents such as the statement of product characteristics (SPC) and manufacturer's literature and re-presented in an abridged form. These entries should be regarded as examples only, and the current SPC or manufacturer's literature should be consulted for current information. More information on the composition of ^{99m}Tc agents is given in Chapter 20 on formulation of radiopharmaceuticals

Bone

Disodium medronate: kit for the preparation of Technetium (^{99m}Tc) Medronate Injection

Pharmaceutics

Chemical formula: $CH_4Na_2O_6P_2$.

Composition and pH: Supplied as a multidose vial containing the following sterile, pyrogen-free, freeze-dried products under nitrogen. Each vial contains: methylene diphosphonic acid 6.25 mg (as the sodium salt), stannous fluoride and sodium *p*-aminobenzoate. It contains no antimicrobial agent. Following reconstitution with a pyrogen-free, isotonic Sodium Pertechnetate [^{99m}Tc] Injection it forms Technetium [^{99m}Tc] Medronate Injection ([^{99m}Tc]MDP) with a pH of 5.0–7.0.

Expiry (after reconstitution): 8 hours

Indication: After reconstitution with sodium pertechnetate, it is used for bone scintigraphy as it delineates areas of altered osteogenesis. Imaging can start 2–4 hours post injection.

Administered dose (MBq): The ARSAC recommended adult dose is 600 MBq or 800 MBq for SPECT. The activity administered to children should be a fraction of the adult dose calculated on body weight using the factors recommended by ARSAC. For paediatric doses, a minimum activity of 40 MBq is necessary to obtain images of sufficient quality.

Radiopharmacology

Mode of localisation: [^{99m}Tc]MDP accumulates in the mineral phase of bone, nearly two-thirds by adsorption onto the hydroxyapatite crystals and one-third in calcium phosphate.

Pharmacokinetics: Initially within 3 minutes of injection there is soft tissue uptake and renal accumulation. As clearance starts from these areas there is a progressive increase in accumulation in the skeleton. About 50% of the dose injected accumulates in the skeleton. Maximum bone accumulation is reached about one hour after injection and remains constant for up to 72 hours. Excretion of unbound complex is via the kidneys

Radiation dosimetry

Critical organs: Normal bone uptake: bladder wall 35 mGy. High bone uptake and/or severe renal impairment: bone marrow 12.6 mGy.

Whole body dose: For an average adult (70 kg): 5.6 mSv.

Adverse reactions and drug interactions

Adverse reactions to ^{99m}Tc-medronate injection are rare with reports suggesting an incidence of not more

Table 18.1 Currently available UK radiopharmaceuticals

Official name (where appropriate according to EP, BP)	Alternative and trade names™	Existing monograph	Method of preparation
Choline ([^{11}C]-methyl)	Choline	Yes (draft)	In house
Flumazenil (*N*-[^{11}C]-methyl)	Flumazenil	Yes	In house
L-Methionine ([^{11}C]-methyl)	Methionine	Yes	In house
Sodium [^{11}C] Acetate		Yes	In house
Ammonia [^{13}N]		Yes	In house
Carbon monoxide [^{15}O]		Yes	In house
Water [^{15}O]		Yes	Generator produced
Fludeoxyglucose [^{18}F]	FDG, Flucis™,	Yes	Finished product
Fludeoxythymidine [^{18}F]	FLT	Yes (draft)	In house
Fluorethyltyrosine [^{18}F]	FET	Yes (draft)	In house
Fluoromisonidazole [^{18}F]	FMISO	Yes (draft)	In house
Sodium [^{18}F] Fluoride		Yes	In house
Chromium [^{51}Cr] Edetate	EDTA	Yes	Finished product
Sodium Chromate [^{51}Cr]		Yes	Finished product
Gallium [^{67}Ga] Citrate		Yes	Finished product
Gallium [^{68}Ga] chloride		Yes (draft)	Generator produced
Tauroselcholic acid [^{75}Se]	SeHCAT	No	Finished product
Krypton [^{81m}Kr] Gas		Yes	Generator produced
Technetium [^{99m}Tc] Albumin		Yes	Labelling kit
Technetium [^{99m}Tc] Albumin Colloid (nanosized)	Nanocolloid, Nanocoll™	No	Labelling kit
Technetium [^{99m}Tc] Bicisate	ECD, Neurolite™	Yes	Labelling kit
Technetium [^{99m}Tc] Colloidal Rhenium Sulphide	Rhenium Sulfide Colloid	Yes	Labelling kit
Technetium [^{99m}Tc] Colloidal Tin	Tin Colloid	Yes	Labelling kit
Technetium [^{99m}Tc] Depreotide	NeoSpect™	No	Labelling kit
Technetium [^{99m}Tc] Exametazime	HMPAO, Ceretec™	Yes	Labelling kit
Technetium [^{99m}Tc] Human Immunoglobulin G	HIG	Yes	Labelling kit
Technetium [^{99m}Tc] Human Serum Albumin	HSA, Vasculocis™	Yes	Labelling kit
Technetium [^{99m}Tc] Colloidal Rhenium Sulphide (Nanocolloid)	Rhenium sulfide colloid, Nanocis™	Yes	Labelling kit
Technetium [^{99m}Tc] Phytate	Phytacis™	No	Labelling kit

(continued overleaf)

Table 18.1 *(continued)*

Official name (where appropriate according to EP, BP)	Alternative and trade names™	Existing monograph	Method of preparation
Technetium [^{99m}Tc] diphosphonopropanedicarboxylic acid	DPD, Teceos™	No	Labelling KIt
Technetium [^{99m}Tc] Macrosalb	MAA	Yes	Labelling kit
Technetium [^{99m}Tc] Mebrofenin	TrimethylbromoHida, Choledіam™	No	Labelling kit
Technetium [^{99m}Tc] Medronate	MDP	Yes	Labelling kit
Technetium [^{99m}Tc] Mertiatide	MAG3	Yes	Labelling kit
Technetium [^{99m}Tc] Monoclonal Antibody BW250/183	MAb 250/183, Scintimun™, Granulocyte™	No	Labelling kit
Technetium [^{99m}Tc] Oxidronate	HMDP	No	Labelling kit
Technetium [^{99m}Tc] Pentetate	DTPA	Yes	Labelling kit
Technetium [^{99m}Tc] Sestamibi	MIBI, Cardiolite™	Yes	Labelling kit
Technetium [^{99m}Tc] sodium pertechnetate		Yes (fission & non-fission)	Generator produced
Technetium [^{99m}Tc] Succimer	DMSA	Yes	Labelling kit
Technetium [^{99m}Tc] Sulesomab	Leukoscan™	No	Labelling kit
Technetium [^{99m}Tc] Tetrofosmin	Myoview™	Yes	Labelling kit
Technetium [^{99m}Tc] Tin Pyrophosphate	PYP	Yes	Labelling kit
Indium [^{111}In] Chloride		Yes	Finished product
Indium [^{111}In] Oxine		Yes	Finished product
Indium [^{111}In] Pentetate	DTPA	Yes	Finished product
Indium [^{111}In] Pentreotide	Octreotide, Octreoscan™	No	
Iobenguane [^{123}I]	MIBG	Yes	Finished product
Ioflupane [^{123}I]	FP-β-CIT, DATSCAN™	No	Finished product
Sodium [^{123}I] Iodide		Yes	Finished product
Sodium [^{123}I] Iodohippurate	Hippuran™	Yes	Finished product
Iodinated [^{125}I] Albumin		Yes	Finished product
Sodium [^{131}I] Iodide		Yes	Finished product
Iobenguane [^{131}I]	MIBG	Yes	Finished product
Iodinated [^{131}I] Norcholesterol		Yes	Finished product
Sodium [^{131}I] Iodohippurate	Hippuran™	No	Finished product
Thallous [^{201}Tl] Chloride		Yes	Finished product

than 1 in 200 000 administrations. These reactions are of an anaphylactoid type and symptoms can include rash, nausea, hypotension and occasionally arthralgia. Symptoms may manifest themselves up to 24 hours post injection. Decreased uptake in the skeleton may occur in patients taking diphosphonates, iron-containing drugs, tetracycline and medication containing chelates. Aluminium-containing drugs such as antacids, when taken regularly, may lead to an abnormally high accumulation of technetium-99m in the liver, thought to be caused by the formation of labelled colloids.

Sodium oxidronate: kit for the preparation of Technetium [^{99m}Tc] Oxidronate Injection

Pharmaceutics

Chemical formula: $CH_4Na_2O_7P_2$.

Composition and pH: Supplied as a multidose vial containing the following sterile, pyrogen-free, freeze-dried products under nitrogen: sodium oxidronate (INN) 3.0 mg, stannous chloride dihydrate 0.45 mg, ascorbic acid 0.75 mg, sodium chloride 10.0 mg. It contains no antimicrobial agent. Following reconstitution with a pyrogen-free, isotonic sodium pertechnetate [^{99m}Tc] injection it forms Technetium (^{99m}Tc) Oxidronate Injection ([^{99m}Tc]HMDP) with a pH of 5.0–7.0.

Expiry (after reconstitution): 8 hours.

Indication: After reconstitution with sodium pertechnetate, it is used for bone scintigraphy as it delineates areas of altered osteogenesis. Imaging can start 2–4 hours post injection.

Administered dose (MBq): The ARSAC recommended adult dose is 600 MBq or 800 MBq for SPECT. The activity administered to children should be a fraction of the adult dose calculated on body weight using the factors recommended by ARSAC. For paediatric doses, a minimum activity of 40 MBq is necessary to obtain images of sufficient quality.

Radiopharmacology

Mode of localisation: [^{99m}Tc]Oxidronate accumulates in the mineral phase of bone, nearly two-thirds by adsorption onto the hydroxyapatite crystals and one-third in calcium phosphate.

Pharmacokinetics: After intravenous injection, [^{99m}Tc]oxidronate is distributed rapidly throughout the extracellular space. Uptake in the skeleton begins almost immediately and proceeds quickly. At 30 minutes post injection, 10% of the initial activity is still present in whole blood, falling to 5%, 3%, 1.5% and 1% after 1 hour, 2 hours, 3 hours and 4 hours, respectively. The mechanism of excretion is via the kidneys, with 30% of the administered activity cleared within the first hour, 48% within 2 hours and 60% within 6 hours.

Radiation dosimetry

Critical organs: Normal bone uptake: bladder wall 35 mGy. High bone uptake and/or severe renal impairment: bone marrow 12.6 mGy.

Whole body dose: For an average adult: 5.6 mSv.

Adverse reactions and drug interactions

Adverse drug reactions to Technetium [^{99m}Tc] Oxidronate Injection are rare, with reports suggesting an incidence of not more than 1 in 200 000 administrations. These reactions are of an anaphylactoid type and symptoms can include rash, nausea, hypotension and occasionally arthralgia. Symptoms may manifest themselves up to 24 hours post injection. Decreased uptake in the skeleton may occur in patients taking diphosphonates, iron containing drugs, tetracycline and medication containing chelates. Aluminium containing drugs such as antacids, when taken regularly, may lead to an abnormally high accumulation of technetium-99m in the liver, thought to be caused by the formation of labelled colloids.

Brain

Technetium [^{99m}Tc] Bicisate Injection (Neurolite; Du Pont Merck Pharmaceutical Company)

Pharmaceutics

Chemical structure: *N,N′*-1,2-ethylenedi(bis-L-cysteine diethyl ester dihydochloride) which forms [*N,N′*-ethylenedi-L-cysteinato(3-)]oxo [^{99m}Tc]technetium (V), diethyl ester on reaction with reduced pertechnetate.

Composition and pH: A two-vial preparation. Vial 1 contains bicisate dihydrochloride (ECD·2HCl) 0.9 mg, stannous chloride dihydrate 0.072 mg (maximum), sodium EDTA dihydrate 0.36 mg, mannitol

24 mg as a freeze dried mixture sealed under nitrogen. Vial 2 contains dibasic sodium phosphate heptahydrate 4.1 mg, monobasic sodium phosphate monohydrate 0.46 mg. Water for Injection to 1 ml. The reconstitution of vial 1 with Sodium Pertechnetate [^{99m}Tc] Injection, previously buffered by adding it to vial 2, yields Technetium [^{99m}Tc] Bicisate Injection. The pH of the stabilised injection is 7.2–8.

Expiry (after reconstitution): 8 hours.

Indications: Technetium [^{99m}Tc] Bicisate Injection is indicated for brain scintigraphy to be used in the diagnosis of stroke.

Administered dose (MBq): Adult dose: 370–1110 MBq.

Radiopharmacology

Mode of localisation: Technetium [^{99m}Tc] Bicisate forms a stable, lipophilic complex that crosses the blood–brain barrier by passive diffusion. Localisation in the brain depends upon both perfusion of the region and uptake of the tracer by the cells. Once in the brain cell the parent compound is metabolised to polar, less diffusible compounds. After background clearance, brain images may be obtained from 10 minutes to 6 hours after injection (optimum 30–60 minutes).

Pharmacokinetics: The primary route of excretion is through the kidneys with 73% of the injected dose being cleared through the bladder during the first 24 hours (up to 50% cleared in the first 2 hours). Approximately 11% of the injected dose is cleared through the GI tract over 48 hours.

Radiation dosimetry

For cerebral scintigraphy based on a dose of 370 MBq with a 2 hour void.

Critical organs: Bladder, 11.1 mGy; gallbladder, 9.25 mGy; small intestine, 3.48 mGy; upper large intestine, 5.92 mGy; lower large intestine, 4.81 mGy; kidneys, 2.70 mGy; liver, 1.96 mGy; brain, 2.04 mGy.

Whole body dose: 0.89 mGy.

Adverse reactions and drug interactions

Fewer than 1% of patients reported headache, dizziness, seizure, agitation/anxiety, malaise/somnolence, parosmia, hallucinations, rash, nausea, syncope or faintness, cardiac failure, hypertension, angina and apnoea/cyanosis.

Technetium [^{99m}Tc] Exametazime Injection (hexamethylpropylene amine oxine; HM-PAO) (Stabilised Ceretec N199; GE Healthcare)

Pharmaceutics

Chemical structure: [*RR*,*SS*]-4,8-Diaza-3,6,9-tetramethylundecane-2,10-dione bisoxime, for labelling with reduced ^{99m}Tc.

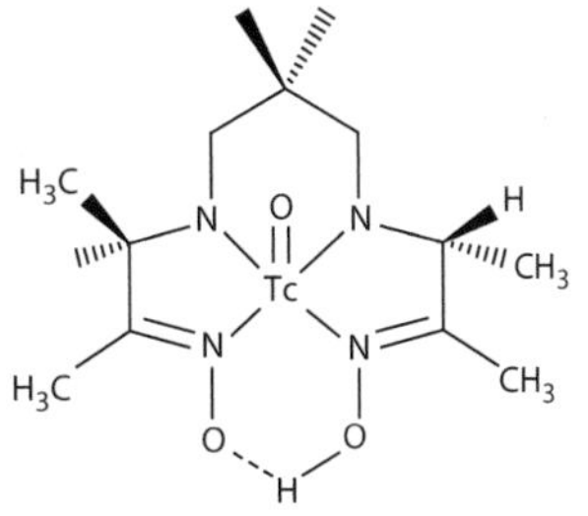

H_3C N O N H Tc CH_3 H_3C N N CH_3 O O H

Composition and pH: Vial 1 contains [*RR*,*SS*]-4,8-diaza-3,6,9-tetramethylundecane-2,10-dione bisoxime 0.5 mg, stannous chloride dihydrate 0.0076 mg, sodium chloride 4.5 mg as a freeze-dried mixture sealed under nitrogen. Vial 2 contains cobalt(II) chloride 6-hydrate in 2.5 mL water for injection. The reconstitution of vial 1 with 5 mL of sodium pertechnetate [^{99m}Tc] at a radioactive concentration of 74–222 MBq/mL) yields [^{99m}Tc]exametazime, which is subsequently stabilised by the addition of 2 mL of cobalt chloride from vial 2. The pH of the stabilised injection is 5–8.

Expiry (after reconstitution): The shelf-life of the ^{99m}Tc-exametazime with addition of the cobalt stabiliser is between 30 minutes and 5 hours, otherwise without the stabiliser only 30 minutes.

Indication: Technetium [^{99m}Tc] Exametazime Injection is indicated for brain scintigraphy to be used in the diagnosis of abnormalities of regional cerebral blood flow.

Administered dose (MBq): Adult dose: 350–500 MBq.

Radiopharmacology

Mode of localisation: The ^{99m}Tc-exametazime primary complex is uncharged, lipophilic and of sufficiently low molecular weight to readily cross the blood–brain barrier. However, it converts, at approximately 12% per hour, to a less lipophilic secondary complex which does not cross the blood–brain barrier and which limits the useful shelf-life of the product to 30 minutes. The *in-vitro* addition of the cobalt stabiliser, after 30 minutes of incubation, lengthens this shelf-life to 5 hours.

Pharmacokinetics: The primary complex rapidly clears from the blood after intravenous injection. Uptake in the brain reaches a maximum of 3.5–7% of the injected dose within one minute of injection. Up to 15% of the cerebral activity washes out of the brain after 2 minutes post injection, after which there is little loss of activity for the following 24 hours, reducing due to the physical decay of ^{99m}Tc.

Activity not associated with the brain is distributed widely throughout the body, especially in the muscle and soft tissue. Approximately 30% of the injected dose is found in the GI tract immediately after injection, with about 50% of this being excreted through the GI tract over 48 hours. In addition, over the 48-hour period 40% of the injection dose is excreted through the kidneys and urine.

Radiation dosimetry

For cerebral scintigraphy based on a dose of 500 MBq.

Critical organs: Bladder, 11.5 mGy; gallbladder, 9 mGy; stomach, 3.2 mGy; small intestine, 6 mGy; upper large intestine, 9 mGy; lower large intestine, 7.5 mGy; kidneys, 17 mGy; lungs 5.5 mGy; thyroid, 13 mGy.

Whole body dose: 1.8 mGy.

Adverse reactions and drug interactions

Rash with generalised erythema, facial oedema and fever has been reported in less than 1% of patients. A transient increase in blood pressure was seen in 8% of patients. There have been reports of fever, erythema, flushing, diffuse rash, hypertension, hypotension, respiratory reaction, seizures, diaphoresis, cyanosis, anaphylaxis, facial swelling, abdominal pain, dyspnoea with myoclonus (labelled WBC).

[^{123}I]Ioflupane Injection (DaTSCAN; CYI8; GE Healthcare)

Pharmaceutics

Chemical structure: *N*-ω-fluoropropyl-2β-carbomethoxy-3β-(4-[^{123}I]iodophenyl) nortropane.

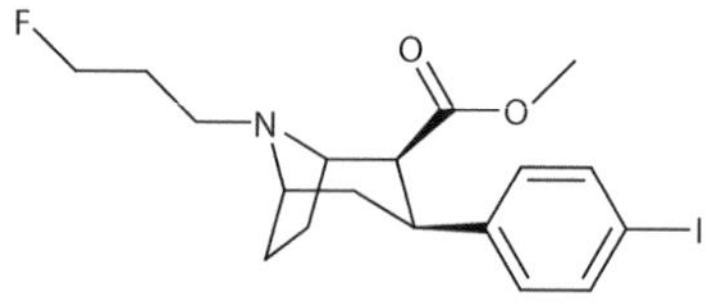

Composition. [^{123}I]Ioflupane 74 MBq/mL at reference in a 5% ethanolic solution (excipients: acetic acid, sodium acetate, ethanol, water for injection) presented in a 2.5 mL solution containing 185 MBq and a 5 mL solution containing 370 MBq.

Expiry: The shelf life of [^{123}I]ioflupane is 7 hours from the activity reference time stated on the label (31 hours from end of manufacture) for 2.5 mL presentations and 20 hours from the activity reference time stated on the label (44 hours from end of manufacture) for 5 mL presentations.

Indications: [^{123}I]Ioflupane is indicated for detecting loss of dopaminergic neuron terminals in the striatum of patients with clinically uncertain parkinsonian syndromes in order to help differentiate essential tremor from parkinsonian syndromes. It is also useful in helping to differentiate dementia with Lewy bodies from Alzheimer disease.

Administered dose (MBq): Adult dose: 111–185 MBq.

Radiopharmacology

Mode of localisation: [^{123}I]Ioflupane is a cocaine analogue which binds to the presynaptic dopamine transporter mechanism and so this agent can be used to examine the integrity of the dopaminergic nigrostriatal neurons.

Pharmacokinetics: [^{123}I]Ioflupane is cleared rapidly from the blood with only 5% remaining at 5 minutes after intravenous injection. Uptake in the brain is rapid, with 7% of the injected activity being present in the brain after 10 minutes, decreasing to 3% after 5 hours. The primary route of excretion is through the kidneys with 60% of the injected dose being excreted in the urine at 48 hours post injection with faecal excretion calculated at approximately 14%.

Radiation dosimetry

Critical organs: Based on a dose of 185 MBq: bladder, 9.90 mGy; gallbladder, 4.75 mGy; small intestine, 3.81 mGy; upper large intestine, 7.05 mGy; lower large intestine, 7.84 mGy; kidneys, 2.05 mGy; liver, 5.24 mGy; lungs, 7.86 mGy. Thyroid blocking via oral administration of potassium iodate is recommended to minimise unnecessary excessive uptake of radioiodine.

Whole body dose: 2.13 mGy.

Adverse reactions and drug interactions

Common side-effect are headache, vertigo, increased appetite and formication (paraesthesia).

Drugs that bind to the dopamine transporter can interfere with [^{123}I]ioflupane. These include amphetamine, benzatropine, buproprion, cocaine, mazindol, methylphenidate, phentermine and sertraline.

Endocrine

Sodium Iodide [^{131}I] Solution and Injection

Pharmaceutics

Chemical formula: Na^+I^-.

Composition and pH: Prepared as an oral solution or as sterile non-pyrogenic solution for injection. May contain sodium iodide, acetic acid, sodium hydroxide, sodium thiosulfate, sodium bicarbonate. The pH may range from 7.0 to 10.0 for oral solution.

Expiry (after date of manufacture): Up to 29 days.

Indications: Sodium [^{131}I]iodide is used as a diagnostic agent in the functional or morphological study of the thyroid gland by means of scintigraphy or radioactive uptake measurements. It is used therapeutically to treat thyroid disease.

Administered dose (MBq): 0.2 MBq for thyroid uptake, 80 MBq for thyroid imaging (for ablation planning), 400 MBq for thyroid metastases imaging (following ablation), 500-9250 MBq for treatment of thyroid disease and ablation therapy of residual thyroid tissue (and metastases) following total thyroidectomy.

Radiopharmacology

Mode of localisation: Orally or intravenously administered iodide is taken up by the thyroid.

Pharmacokinetics: About 20% of the available radioactivity enters the thyroid in one pass of the blood volume. Normal thyroid clearance of blood iodide is 20–50 mL/min with an increase to 100 mL/min in thyroid deficiency. Peak levels of iodide occur in thyroid gland within a few hours so that diagnostic imaging can take place from one hour after dosing. The half-time of iodide elimination from the thyroid is estimated at 80 days so that the physical half-life of ^{131}I governs the temporal opportunity for imaging. Without considering the thyroid uptake, the iodide leaves the body stream chiefly by urinary excretion (37–75%), while faecal excretion is low (about 1%).

Normal biodistribution: Iodide is predominantly taken up by the thyroid, but small amounts are taken up by salivary glands, gastric mucosa, placenta and choroids plexus. It is excreted in breast milk.

Radiation dosimetry

See Table 18.2.

Whole body dose: In the adult, the effective dose resulting from an administered activity of 0.2 MBq is 6 mSv. This is dependent on the uptake in the thyroid gland. Other isotopes e.g. ^{99m}Tc or ^{123}I must be used for imaging benign disease.

Adverse reactions and drug interactions

Adverse reactions to sodium [^{131}I]iodide have only been reported at therapeutic levels of administered activities. Many medicines and dietary products affect the uptake of iodine by the thyroid gland. The time taken for thyroid uptake to return to normal following

Table 18.2 Sodium [^{131}I]iodide. Critical organs

Organ	Absorbed dose (mGy/MBq)			
	Thyroid blocked	15% uptake	35% uptake	55% uptake
Kidneys	0.065	0.06	0.56	0.051
Bladder wall	0.61	0.52	0.40	0.29
Adrenals	0.037	0.036	0.042	0.049
Liver	0.033	0.032	0.037	0.043
Uterus	0.054	0.054	0.050	0.046
Red marrow	0.035	0.054	0.086	0.12
Thyroid	0.029	210	500	790
Pancreas	0.035	0.052	0.054	0.058

medication withdrawal varies from weeks to years (see Table 18.3).

Sodium Iodide [^{123}I] Solution and Injection

Pharmaceutics

Chemical formula: $Na^{+}I^{-}$.

Table 18.3 The time taken for thyroid uptake to return to normal following medication with iodide

Medication	Time for thyroid to return to normal function
Amiodarone	4 weeks
Antithyroid (propylthiouracil, methimazol)	1 week
Lithium	4 weeks
Natural or synthetic thyroid preparations (thyroxine sodium, liothyronine sodium thyroid)	2–3 weeks
Expectorants, vitamins	2 weeks
Perchlorate	1 week
Phenylbutazone	1-2 weeks
Salicylates	1 week
Steroids	1 week
Sodium nitroprusside	1 week
Sulfobromophthalein sodium	1 week
Miscellaneous agents: anticoagulants, antihistamines, antiparasitics, penicillins, sulfonamides, tolbutamide, thiopental	1 week
Benzodiazepines	4 weeks
Topical iodides	1–9 months
Intravenous contrast agents	1–2 months
Oral cholecystographic agents	6–9 months
Oil-based iodinated contrast agents:	
Bronchographic	6–12 months
Myelographic	2–10 years

Composition and pH: Prepared as a sterile non-pyrogenic solution in 0.9% NaCl or water for injection. May contain sodium iodide, acetic acid, sodium hydroxide, sodium thiosulfate, sodium bicarbonate. Radioactive concentration ranges from 18.5 to 185 MBq/mL.

Expiry (after calibration): 36 hours.

Indications: Sodium [^{123}I]iodide is used as a diagnostic agent in the functional or morphological study of the thyroid gland by means of scintigraphy or radioactive uptake measurements

Administered dose (MBq): 2 MBq for thyroid uptake, 20 MBq for thyroid imaging, 400 MBq for thyroid metastases imaging (following ablation)

Radiopharmacology

Mode of localisation: Intravenously administered iodide is taken up by the thyroid gland.

Pharmacokinetics: About 20% of the available radioactivity enters the thyroid in one pass of the blood volume. Normal thyroid clearance of blood iodide is 20–50 mL/min with an increase to 100 mL/min in thyroid deficiency. Peak levels of iodide occur in thyroid gland within a few hours so that diagnostic imaging can take place from one hour after dosing. The half-time of iodide elimination from the thyroid is estimated at 80 days so that the physical half-life of ^{123}I governs the temporal opportunity for imaging. Without considering the thyroid uptake, the iodide leaves the body stream chiefly by urinary excretion (37–75%), while faecal excretion is low (about 1%).

Normal biodistribution: Iodide is predominantly taken up by the thyroid, but small amounts are taken up by salivary glands, gastric mucosa, placenta and choroids plexus. It is excreted in breast milk.

Radiation dosimetry

Depending on the production procedure of iodine-123, impurities like iodine-125 and/or iodine-124 may be present as longer-lived contaminants, increasing the radiation dose to the different organs. The ICRP model refers to intravenous administration. See Table 18.4.

Whole body dose: In the adult, the effective dose resulting from an administered activity of 20 MBq is 4 mSv. This is dependent on the uptake in the thyroid gland.

Table 18.4 Sodium [^{123}I]iodide. Critical organs

Organ	Absorbed dose (mGy/MBq)			
	Thyroid blocked	15% uptake	35% uptake	55% uptake
Kidneys	0.011	0.010	0.0091	0.0093
Bladder wall	0.090	0.076	0.060	0.043
Adrenals	0.007	0.0063	0.0065	0.0065
Liver	0.0067	0.0062	0.0063	0.0064
Uterus	0.014	0.015	0.014	0.012
Red warrow	0.0094	0.0094	0.010	0.011
Thyroid	0.0051	1.9	4.5	7.0
Pancreas	0.0076	0.014	0.014	0.014

Adverse reactions and drug interactions

Adverse reactions have not been reported to sodium [^{123}I]iodide. Many medicines and dietary products affect the uptake of iodine by the thyroid gland. The time taken for thyroid uptake to return to normal following medication withdrawal varies from weeks to years (see Table 18.3).

[^{131}I]Iodomethyl norcholesterol

Pharmaceutics

Chemical formula: 6-Iodomethyl norcholesterol

Composition and pH: Prepared as a sterile non-pyrogenic solution in water for injection, pH 3.5–7.0, containing up to 0.1% ethanol and 0.01% polysorbate 80 as an aid to solubility of the cold norcholesterol carrier. Radioactive concentration ranges from 8 to 30 MBq/mL.

Expiry (after reference date): Up to 14 days if stored at −20°C.

Indications: Diagnostic evaluation of the functional state of adrenal cortical tissue. Differentiation between metastatic disease to the adrenals and non-malignant adrenal enlargement in cancer patients. Detection of remnants of functioning tissue in hypercortisonism after adrenalectomy or ectopic tissue.

Administered dose (MBq): 20 MBq.

Radiopharmacology

Mode of localisation: [^{131}I]Iodomethyl norcholesterol is an analogue of cholesterol that follows the pathway of cholesterol up to active accumulation in the adrenal gland, but does not take part in hormone synthesis. A considerable part of this synthesis takes place in the adrenal cortex.

Pharmacokinetics and biodistribution: Less than 1% of a dose of [^{131}I]iodomethyl norcholesterol accumulates in the adrenals. The majority of this uptake takes place in the first 48 hours following administration. Part of the fraction that accumulates in the adrenals does so after one or more enterohepatic circulation cycles. It is eliminated in the urine and faeces (30% in each after 9 days), with 30% retained in the body, mainly diffusely distributed, but with approximately 2% in the liver. Varying degrees of thyroid uptake occur even with adequate blockade. It may be excreted in breast milk.

Radiation dosimetry

For administered activity of 20 MBq.

Critical organs: Kidneys, 8.2 mGy; adrenals, 80 mGy; bladder wall, 7.8 mGy; liver, 24 mGy; pancreas, 8.6 mGy; thyroid (blocked), 6.0 mGy; lungs, 7.6 mGy.

Whole body effective dose: 30 mSv for 20 MBq administered activity.

Adverse reactions and drug interactions

Anaphylactoid reactions have been reported immediately following injection. However several more severe reports of intense chest and back pain with early onset and of long duration (>24 hours) have also been reported. The following medicines are known to or may be expected to prolong or to reduce the uptake of [^{131}I]iodomethyl norcholesterol in the adrenal cortex: oral contraceptives; inhibitors of the biosynthesis of adrenocortical steroids (milotane, ketoconazole, metyrapone, aminglutethimide); adrenocortical steroids, including their synthetic analogues, e.g. dexamethasone; diuretics active at the adrenal cortex, e.g. spironolactone.

Sodium Pertechnetate [^{99m}Tc] Injection

Pharmaceutics

Chemical formula: $Na^+TcO_4^-$.

Composition and pH: Prepared as a sterile non-pyrogenic solution in 0.9% NaCl directly from a $^{99}Mo/^{99m}Tc$ generator. pH 4.0–8.0.

Expiry (after elution from generator): 12 hours.

Indications: Sodium Pertechnetate [^{99m}Tc] Injection may be used as a diagnostic agent in the functional or morphological study of the thyroid gland by means of scintigraphy or radioactive uptake measurements using probes.

Administered dose (MBq): 80 MBq for thyroid imaging.

Radiopharmacology

Mode of localisation: Owing to their common ionic characteristics, iodide and pertechnetate ions behave similarly following IV injection. Pertechnetate ions, TcO_4^-, become partly protein bound in plasma but clear rapidly from this compartment depending on the diffusion equilibrium with interstitial fluid. Pertechnetate is trapped by glandular tissues possessing an ionic pump mechanism; thus it is trapped but not organified in the thyroid. It is concentrated temporarily by the salivary glands, choroid plexus and stomach. Pertechnetate is then secreted by gastric mucosa and the intestine. Finally, it is slowly cleared by glomerular filtration in the kidneys.

Pharmacokinetics: Plasma clearance has a half-life of about 3 hours. Excretion during the first 24 hours after administration is mainly urinary (~ 25%) with faecal excretion occurring over the next 48 hours. Approximately 50% of the administered activity is excreted within the first 50 hours.

Normal biodistribution: Pertechnetate is predominantly taken up by the thyroid, but small amounts are taken up by salivary glands, gastric mucosa, placenta and choroids plexus. Pertechnetate has been shown to cross the placenta and is excreted in breast milk.

Radiation dosimetry

Critical organs (main ones only): See Table 18.5.

Whole body dose: In the (unblocked thyroid) adult, the effective dose resulting from an administered activity of 80 MBq is 1 mSv. This is reduced to 0.35 mSv if blocked.

Table 18.5 Sodium [^{99m}Tc]pertechnetate. Critical organs

Organ	Absorbed dose mGy/MBq	
	Thyroid blocked	Thyroid unblocked
Kidneys	0.0047	0.005
Bladder wall	0.032	0.019
Adrenals	0.0033	0.0036
Liver	0.0031	0.0039
Uterus	0.0066	0.0081
Red marrow	0.0045	0.0061
Thyroid	0.0021	0.023
Pancreas	0.0035	0.0059

Adverse reactions and drug interactions

In a very small number of patients an allergic type reaction has occurred with symptoms such as rash, facial swelling and itching. Extremely rarely, cardiac events and coma have been noted.

In abdominal imaging: atropine, isoprenaline and analgesics can result in delay in gastric emptying and redistribution of pertechnetate

Heart

Fludeoxyglucose [^{18}F] Injection

Pharmaceutics

Chemical structure: 2-[^{18}F]Fluoro-2-deoxy-D-glucose ($C_6H_{11}O_5{}^{18}F$).

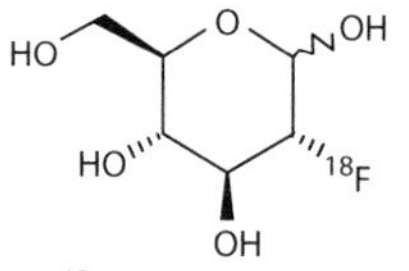

HO, O, OH, HO, ^{18}F, OH

[^{18}F]Fludeoxyglucose

Composition and pH: Sterile pyrogen free aqueous solution of fluorine-18 in the form of 2-[^{18}F]fluoro-2-deoxy-D-glucose containing sufficient sodium chloride to make the solution isotonic with blood.

Expiry (after reconstitution): 12 hours after production time and following the first use.

Indication: Diagnostic radiopharmaceutical in positron emission tomography (PET): glucose utilisation in brain, cardiac, and neoplastic disease.

Administered dose (MBq): 100–400 MBq.

Radiopharmacology

Mode of localisation: Fludeoxyglucose (FDG) is a glucose analogue and therefore taken up by cells in part by glucose transporters and is then phosphorylated by hexokinase into FDG 6-phosphate which cannot be metabolised (unlike glucose) and is consequently trapped in the cell.

Pharmacokinetics: Following IV administration the pharmacokinetic profile of [^{18}F]FDG in the vascular compartment is biexponential. It has a distribution half-life of 1 minute and an elimination half-life of approximately 12 minutes without being metabolised. Elimination is mainly renal. Approximately 20% of the injected dose is excreted in urine during the first 2 hours. After IV administration of [^{18}F]FDG, most of the dose is rapidly distributed throughout the body with a plasma half-life of 0.2–0.3 minutes with a large volume of distribution. The product is then cleared from the blood compartment with a half-life of 11.5 minutes. It is distributed mainly to the brain and heart. Approximately 7% of injected dose is accumulated in the brain within 80–100 minutes after injection. Approximately 3% of the injected activity is taken up by the myocardium within 40 minutes. Approximately 0.3% and 0.9%–2.4% of the injected activity is accumulated in the pancreas and lungs, respectively.

Radiation dosimetry

For administered dose of 400 MBq (individual weighing 70 kg).

Critical organs: Bladder, 64 mGy; heart, 25 mGy; brain, 11 mGy.

Whole body dose: Effective dose is about 7.6 mSv.

Adverse reactions and drug interactions

All medicinal products that modify blood glucose levels can affect the sensitivity of the examination, such as corticosteroids, valproate, carbamazepine, phenytoin, phenobarbital, and catecholamines. Diabetics should have blood glucose levels controlled before injection and closely monitored after administration.

Ammonia [^{13}N] Injection

Pharmaceutics

Chemical formula: NH_3.

Composition and pH: Ammonia [^{13}N] Injection is provided as a ready to use sterile, pyrogen free, clear and colourless solution in 0.9% NaCl with a pH of 4.5–7.5.

Expiry (after reconstitution): 8 hours.

Use of Ammonia [^{13}N] Injection requires an on-site cyclotron since the half-life of the radionuclide is 10 minutes. Ammonia [^{13}N] Injection must be used within 30 minutes of the end-of-synthesis (EOS) calibration.

Indication: [^{13}N]Ammonia has been proven to be one of the most effective myocardial perfusion tracers in PET and can be used for both rest and stress scans.

Administered dose: 370–740 MBq (10–20 mCi).

Radiopharmacology

Mode of localisation: Once [^{13}N]ammonia is given by intravenous injection, imaging is started 5 minutes later to allow clearance of excess tracer and allow the agent to be taken up by the myocytes. Ammonia is then fixed as [^{13}N]glutamine by enzymatic conversion of glutamic acid by glutamine synthetase.

Pharmacokinetics: [^{13}N]Ammonia has a high first pass extraction of >90% due to the rapid diffusion of uncharged lipophilic ammonia across the capillary endothelium and sarcolemma of myocytes. However, back diffusion of the unfixed tracer occurs and the amount retained decreases due to the high coronary blood flow. Coronary blood flows of 1 and 3 mL/min/g produce average first pass retention of 83% and 60%, respectively.

Radiation dosimetry

Critical organs (mGy/MBq): Urinary bladder wall, 6.9×10^{-3}; brain, 4.7×10^{-3}; liver, 3.8×10^{-3}.

Whole body dose: 2.2×10^{-3} mSv/MBq.

Adverse reactions and drug interactions

No adverse reactions have been reported so far for Ammonia [^{13}N] Injection. Drug interactions for Ammonia [^{13}N] Injection have not yet been studied.

Thallous [^{201}Tl] Chloride Injection

Pharmaceutics

Composition and pH: Thallous [^{201}Tl] Chloride Injection is prepared as a sterile, isotonic, non-pyrogenic solution in 0.9% NaCl and water for injection with a pH of 5–7.

Expiry (after reconstitution): 7 days after activity reference date and time (3 days is typically the maximum useful life).

Indications: Myocardial perfusion (ischaemia and infarct) imaging:

Ischaemia: treadmill exercise tolerance test. The patient is exercised to a defined end point (e.g. ECG pattern, chest pain, 85% maximum heart rate). The tracer is administered intravenously then exercise is continued for a further 90 seconds. Initial imaging is started immediately and completed within 30 minutes since later images will show redistribution out of normal tissue. Redistribution images are obtained 2–4 hours after injection.

Infarct: resting studies. Have the patient fast for 4 hours and do some mild exercise (walking) before injection. Allow 20 minutes before imaging to allow blood clearance.

Muscle perfusion imaging in peripheral vascular disorders.

Non-specific tumour imaging (thyroid, brain, and metastases).

Parathyroid imaging.

Administered dose (MBq): 50–150 MBq (average dose is around 80 MBq).

Radiopharmacology

Mode of localisation: Uptake in myocytes via potassium-uptake mechanisms such as activating the Na^+/K^+-ATPase system and intracellular binding. Uptake is blocked by ouabain and NaF since these are known blockers of Na^+/K^+-ATPase. Thallium binds 10 times more firmly to Na^+/K^+-ATPase than does potassium.

Pharmacokinetics: After IV injection, approximately 90% is cleared by the first pass. The myocardial extraction is 85% during first pass and the peak activity is 4–5% of the injected dose, which remains constant for 20–25 minutes. Muscle uptake depends on workload and during stress imaging can increase 2–3-fold in the skeletal muscle and the myocardium, which leads to reduced levels of activity in other organs. Thallium-201 is excreted 80% in the faeces and 20% in the urine and has a biological half-life of about 10 days.

Radiation dosimetry

Critical organs (mGy/MBq): Testes, 5.6×10^{-1}; bone, 3.4×10^{-1}; kidney, 5.4×10^{-1}; thyroid, 2.5×10^{-1}; descending colon, 3.6×10^{-1}; heart 2.3×10^{-1}.

Whole body dose: 2.3×10^{-1} mSv/MBq.

Adverse reactions and drug interactions

Altered biodistributions have been reported with beta-adrenergic blockers and nitrates; discontinue therapy 24 hours before imaging. Digitalis analogues and insulin reduce heart uptake, but there is not much literature to support this. Other adverse reactions include hypotension, pruritus, flushing, rash, nausea, vomiting, diarrhoea, tremor, shortness of breath, fever, chills, conjunctivitis, sweating, and blurred vision.

[^{99m}Tc]Pyrophosphate Injection (TechneScan PYP kit for the preparation of Technetium (^{99m}Tc) Pyrophosphate (PYP) Injection)

Pharmaceutics

Chemical structure: The exact formula and structure of the stannous-PYP and ^{99m}Tc-stannous-PYP complexes are currently unknown at this time.

Composition and pH: TechneScan PYP is a sterile, non-pyrogenic, radiopharmaceutical for intravenous administration after reconstitution with either sterile sodium [^{99m}Tc]pertechnetate or sterile 0.9% NaCl. Each 10 mL vial contains 11.93 mg of sodium pyrophosphate, 3.2 mg minimum of stannous chloride, 4.4 mg maximum of tin, and nitrogen. TechneScan PYP contains no preservatives. The final pH when reconstituted is 4.5–7.5.

Expiry (after reconstitution): 4 hours.

Indications: *In-vivo* or *in-vivo/in-vitro* labelling of red blood cells for multigated acquisition (MUGA) scans or blood pool scintigraphy. Some of these indications may include angiocardioscintigraphy for the evaluation of ventricular ejection fraction, global and regional cardiac wall motion, or myocardial phase imaging; perfusion of organs and imaging of vascular abnormalities; diagnosis and localisation of occult gastrointestinal bleeding; determination of blood volume; scintigraphy of the spleen.

Administered dose (MBq): Multigated acquisition (MUGA) scan or blood pool scintigraphy: 740–925 MBq (average 890 MBq). Optimal amount of nonradioactive stannous tin is 0.05–1.25 μg/mL of total blood volume (approximately 5000 mL in a 70 kg man) and should not be exceeded.

Determination of blood volume: 1–5 MBq (average 3 MBq).

Scintigraphy of the spleen: 20–70 MBq (average 50 MBq).

Radiopharmacology

Mode of localisation: Intravenous injection of stannous salts induces a 'stannous loading' of erythrocytes. Injection of sodium [^{99m}Tc]pertechnetate results in an accumulation and retention of the ^{99m}Tc in the choroid plexus and erythrocytes. The use of 10–20 μg/kg of stannous PYP followed by 370–740 MBq of technetium-99m 30 minutes later yields an efficiently labelled blood pool.

Pharmacokinetics: Normally, technetium-99m freely diffuses into and out of the erythrocytes; however, when the erythrocytes have been preloaded with stannous PYP the technetium-99m is reduced inside the cells and then becomes bound to the chains of globin. This mechanism is not clearly understood.

Normal biodistribution: 20% of technetium-99m enters the erythrocytes and binds to the chains of globin. The remaining 70–80% is located in the cytoplasm or on the erythrocyte membrane. It has been noted that reducing the surface charge of erythrocytes decreases the efficacy of labelling to 20%.

Radiation dosimetry

Critical organs: Heart, 2.3×10^{-2}; lungs, 1.4×10^{-2}; kidney, 1.0×10^{-2}; spleen, 1.5×10^{-2} mGy/MBq.

Whole body dose: 8.5×10^{-3} mSv/MBq.

Adverse reactions and drug interactions

Adverse reactions: After administration of both the unlabelled and the ^{99m}Tc complexes, the following adverse reactions occurred in 1–8 per 100 000 cases: nausea, vomiting, vasodilatation, flushing, headache, dizziness, erythema/itching/swelling at the injection site, diaphoresis, tinnitus, urticaria, and generalised pruritus. Cardiac arrhythmia, facial oedema, and coma are not as common but have been reported.

Drug interactions: Use of other medicinal agents that will decrease the yield of red blood cell labelling: heparin, tin overload, aluminium, methyldopa, prazosin, hydralazine, digitalin-related compounds, quinidine, calcium channel blockers, β-adrenergic blockers, nitrates, anthracycline, iodinated contrast agents, and Teflon catheters.

Technetium [^{99m}Tc] Tetrofosmin Injection

Pharmaceutics

Chemical structure: Tetrofosmin is 6,9-bis(2-ethoxyethyl)-3,12-dioxa-6,9-diphosphatetradecane.

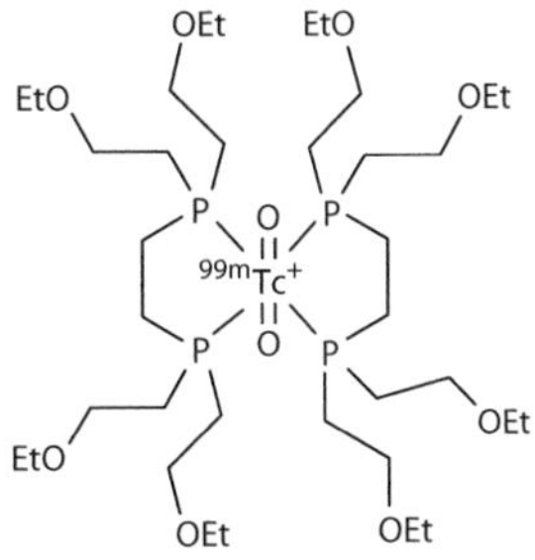

[^{99m}Tc-(tetrofosmin)$_2$O$_2$$^+$]

Composition and pH: The kit contains: tetrofosmin, stannous chloride dihydrate, disodium sulfosalicylate, sodium D-gluconate, and sodium hydrogencarbonate. When sterile, pyrogen-free sodium [^{99m}Tc]pertechnetate in isotonic saline is added to the vial, a ^{99m}Tc complex of tetrofosmin is formed. The pH of the reconstituted vial is 7.5–9.0.

Expiry (after reconstitution): 12 hours after reconstitution.

Indications: Myocardial perfusion agent for use as an adjunct in the diagnosis and localisation of myocardial ischaemia and/or infarction.

In patients undergoing myocardial perfusion scintigraphy, ECG-gated SPECT can be used for assessment of left ventricular function (left ventricular ejection fraction and wall motion).

As an adjunct to the initial assessments in the characterisation of malignancy of suspected breast lesions where other tests are inconclusive.

Administered dose (MBq): *Myocardial infarction:* same day: 250–400 MBq first dose followed by 600–800 MBq second dose. Other days: 400–600 MBq per dose per day. Maximum dose: not to exceed 1200 MBq (over the period of 1 or 2 days). *Breast imaging:* 500–750 MBq.

Radiopharmacology

Mode of localisation: Potential-driven diffusion of the lipophilic cation across the sarcolemmal and mitochondrial membranes (cytosol). The normal biodistribution is linearly related to coronary blood flow. Less than 4.5% of the dose appears after 60 minutes in the liver and less than 2% after 30 minutes in the lung.

Pharmacokinetics: The agent is rapidly cleared from the blood after intravenous injection; less than 5% of the administered dose remains in the whole blood at 10 minutes post injection. Approximately 66% of the injected activity is excreted in 48 hours, about 40% in urine and 26% in faeces, the slow washout indicating insignificant redistribution over time.

Radiation dosimetry

Critical organs: Gallbladder wall, 48.6 μGy/MBq (stress) and 33.2 μGy/MBq (rest).

Whole body dose: At rest, 11.2 μSv/MBq; in stress, 86.1 μSv/MBq.

Adverse reactions and drug interactions

Adverse interactions are very rare (<0.01%). Beta-adrenergic blockers, calcium channel blockers, and nitrates may lead to false negative results in the diagnosis of coronary artery disease.

Rubidium [^{82}Rb] Chloride

Pharmaceutics

Chemical formula: [^{82}Rb]Cl.

Composition and pH: The agent is eluted from the generator with additive free 0.9% sodium chloride injection that has a pH of 5–7.

Expiry (after reconstitution): Usually provided with the label on the generator. Owing to the very short half-life (1.27 minutes), most of the product decays away within 15 minutes after elution.

Indications: Rubidium-82 is a myocardial perfusion agent that is useful in distinguishing normal from abnormal myocardium in patients with suspected myocardial infarction.

Administered dose (MBq): 1110–2220 MBq per dose at the rate of 50 mL/min, with maximum of 4400 MBq cumulative dose at the rate of 50 mL/min.

Radiopharmacology

Mode of localisation: Following administration, rubidium-82 rapidly clears from the blood and is extracted by myocardial tissue in a manner analogous to potassium. The rubidium cation is taken up across the sarcolemmal membrane via the Na^+/K^+-ATPase pump within a few minutes after the injection.

Pharmacokinetics: In animal models, the first-pass extraction fraction is 50–60% at rest and decreases to 25–30% at peak flow. The radiotracer is retained in the myocardium and equilibrates with the potassium pool.

Normal biodistribution: Uptake is also observed in kidney, liver, spleen, and lung over time.

Radiation dosimetry

Critical organs: Kidneys 19.1 mGy/2220 MBq; heart wall, 4.22 mGy/2220 MBq; lungs, 3.77 mGy/2220 MBq; small intestine, 3.11 mGy/2220 MBq; adrenals, 2.15 mGy/2220 MBq.

Whole body dose: 0.95 mGy/2220 MBq.

Adverse reactions and drug interactions

Beta-blockers, calcium channel blockers, nitrates and other medications may alter the results. Diabetes mellitus may affect the results.

Technetium [^{99m}Tc] Sestamibi Injection

Pharmaceutics

Chemical structure:

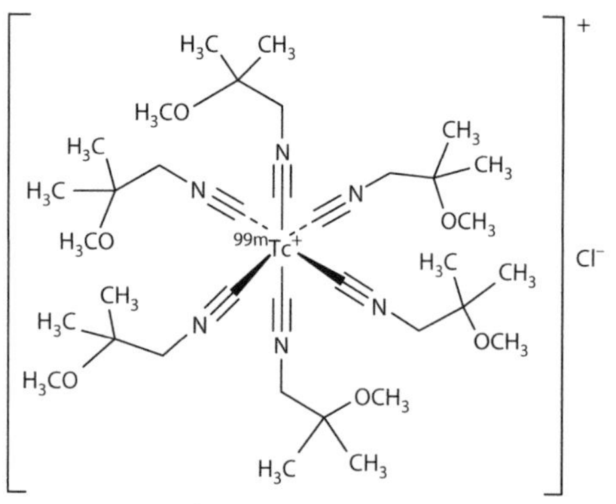

^{99m}Tc-Sestamibi

Composition and pH: One vial contains tetrakis(2-methoxyisobutylisonitrile) copper(I) tetrafluoroborate, stannous chloride dihydrate, L-cysteine hydrochloride monohydrate, sodium citrate dihydrate, mannitol. The vial is reconstituted with a maximum of 11.1 GBq (300 mCi) of Sodium Pertechnetate [^{99m}Tc] Injection] 1–3 mL.

Expiry (after reconstitution): 10 hours.

Indications: Adjunct for diagnosis of ischaemic heart disease, myocardial infarction, assessment of global ventricular function. Second-line diagnostic aid in the investigation of patients with suspected breast cancer. Investigation of patients with recurrent or persistent hyper-parathyroidism.

Administered dose (MBq): Suggested dose range for intravenous administration to a 70-kg patient: in reduced coronary perfusion and myocardial infarction, 185–740 MBq; for global ventricular function, 600–800 MBq injected as bolus. For diagnosis of ischaemic heart disease, two injections (rest and stress) are required in order to differentiate transiently from persistently reduced myocardial uptake. Not more than a total of 925 MBq should be administered in these two injections, which should be done at least 6 hours apart but may be performed in either order. Breast imaging: 740–925 MBq injected as bolus. Parathyroid imaging: 185–740 injected as bolus.

Radiopharmacology

Mode of localisation: ^{99m}Tc-Sestamibi is a lipophilic monovalent cation that is taken up into myocytes by passive diffusion associated with negative plasma and mitochondrial membrane potentials. Retention is dependent on maintenance of these membrane potentials.

Pharmacokinetics: The biological myocardial half-life is approximately 7 hours at rest and stress. The effective half-life is approximately 3 hours. The major metabolic pathway for clearance is the hepatobiliary system. Activity from the gallbladder appears in the intestine within 1 hour of injection. About 27% of the injected dose is cleared through renal elimination after 24 hours and 33% through faeces in 48 hours. At 5 minutes post injection about 8% of the injected dose remains in circulation.

Normal biodistribution: The agent accumulates in the viable myocardial tissue proportional to the circulation. Myocardial uptake is 1.5% of the injected dose at stress and 1.2% of the injected dose at rest.

Table 18.6 ^{99m}Tc-Sestamibi. Radiation dosimetry

	Absorbed dose per unit administered activity (mGy/MBq) for adults (70 kg),	
Organ	Rest	Stress
Gallbladder	3.9×10^{-2}	3.3×10^{-2}
Kidneys	3.6×10^{-2}	2.6×10^{-2}
Upper large intestine	2.7×10^{-2}	2.2×10^{-2}

Radiation dosimetry

Absorbed dose per unit administered activity (mGy/MBq) for adults (70 kg), see Table 18.6.

Whole body dose: 7.9 mSv at rest and 6.9 mSv at stress from administration of a 925 MBq dose.

Adverse reactions and drug interactions

Metallic and bitter taste, transient headache, flushing, non-itching rash, injection site inflammation, oedema, dyspepsia, nausea, vomiting, pruritus, urticaria, dry mouth, fever dizziness, fatigue, dyspnoea, hypotension. No drug interactions have been described to date.

Liver and the reticuloendothelial system

Technetium [^{99m}Tc] Colloidal Rhenium Sulfide Injection

Pharmaceutics

Chemical structure: A colloidal dispersion of rhenium sulfide labelled with technetium-99m.

Composition and pH: Supplied as a kit containing two vials. Vial A contains 1 mL of a sterile, pyrogen-free solution of 0.24 mg rhenium sulfide, gelatin, ascorbic acid, sodium hydroxide and hydrochloric acid in a nitrogen atmosphere. Vial B contains a freeze-dried powder of sodium pyrophosphate, stannous chloride and sodium hydroxide in a nitrogen atmosphere. Neither vial contains an antimicrobial. To prepare the radiopharmaceutical, 2 mL water for injections is introduced into vial B and 0.5 mL of the resulting solution is transferred to vial A. Sodium Pertechnetate [Tc^{99m}] Injection 370–5550 MBq/1–2 mL is added to vial A, which is then incubated in a boiling water-bath for 15–30 minutes. The vial is cooled to room temperature. The mean diameter of the colloidal particles is around 100 nm and the pH is 4–7.

Expiry (after reconstitution): 4 hours.

Indication: Lymphoscintigraphy and sentinel node localisation.

Administered activity (MBq): Bone marrow imaging: intravenous injection of 400 MBq. Lymphoscintigraphy and sentinel node localisation: subcutaneous injection of 20 MBq.

Radiopharmacology

Mode of localisation: Phagocytosis by Kupffer cells.

After subcutaneous injection into the interstitial space of the region to be investigated, the colloidal particles cross the lymphatic capillary pores and migrate into the lymph where they are phagocytosed in the lymph nodes by the bordering cells of the reticuloendothelial system. The phenomenon is repeated from one lymph node to the next. Lymph nodes bind approximately 3% in the first hour and approximately 4% by the third hour.

Radiation dosimetry

Critical organs: Injection site 190 mGy from a subcutaneous injection of 20 MBq.

Effective dose: 0.05 mSv from a subcutaneous injection of 20 MBq.

Adverse reactions and drug interactions (if known)

Occasional hypersensitivity reactions and pain at the site of injection. The use of local anaesthetic agents or hyaluronidase prior to administering ^{99m}Tc colloidal rhenium sulfide has been shown to disturb lymphatic uptake.

Technetium [^{99m}Tc] Albumin Nanocolloid Injection

Pharmaceutics

Chemical structure: A pre-formed colloid of human albumin.

Composition and pH: Supplied as a multidose vial containing the following sterile, pyrogen-free, freeze-dried products under nitrogen. Each vial contains: human albumin colloidal particles 0.5 mg, stannous chloride, dihydrate 0.2 mg, glucose, poloxamer 238, disodium hydrogenphosphate and sodium phytate. It contains no antimicrobial agent. At least 95% of the colloidal particles have a diameter $\leq$ 80 nm. Following reconstitution with a pyrogen-free, isotonic Sodium Pertechnetate [Tc^{99m}] Injection, it forms Technetium (Tc^{99m}) Albumin Nanocolloid Injection.

Expiry (after reconstitution): 6 hours.

Indication: Bone marrow imaging, lymphoscintigraphy and sentinel node localisation.

Administered activity (MBq): Bone marrow imaging: intravenous injection of 400 MBq. Lymphoscintigraphy and sentinel node localisation: subcutaneous injection of 20 MBq.

Radiopharmacology

Mode of localisation: Phagocytosis by Kupffer cells.

Pharmacokinetics: After intravenous injection, the agent is cleared rapidly by the liver, spleen and bone marrow. A small fraction passes through the kidneys and is eliminated in the urine. The maximum activity in the liver and spleen is reached after approximately 30 minutes, but in the bone marrow after only 6 minutes. After subcutaneous injection, 30–40% of the particles are filtered into lymphatic capillaries. The particles are then transported along the lymphatic vessels to lymph nodes where they are trapped by reticular cells.

Radiation dosimetry

Critical organs: Liver 31 mGy from an intravenous injection of 400 MBq. Injection site 240 mGy from a subcutaneous injection of 20 MBq.

Effective dose: 4 mSv from an intravenous injection of 400 MBq; 0.05 mSv from a subcutaneous injection of 20 MBq.

Adverse reactions and drug interactions

Occasional hypersensitivity reactions. Iodinated contrast media used in lymphangiography may interfere with lymphatic imaging with Technetium [^{99m}Tc] Albumin Nanocolloid.

Lung

KryptoScan generator [^{81}Rb/^{81m}Kr] for Krypton [^{81m}Kr] Inhalation Gas

Pharmaceutics

Description/formulation: The radionuclide generator contains the mother radionuclide ^{81}Rb immobilised on a membrane. The daughter radionuclide ^{81m}Kr is eluted by passing environmental air over the membrane. The produced gas from the generator contains the radionuclide ^{81m}Kr mixed with environmental air. The generator containing krypton-81m is placed in a lexan housing and then in shielding which is fixed within a synthetic housing. Rubidium-81 is bound as the ion to a cation-exchange resin and is in equilibrium with the daughter-product ^{81m}Kr and serves as a generator for krypton-81m gas. The generator is available with activities ranging between 75 and 740 MBq. Rubidium-81 decays with a physical half-life of 4.58 hours to its metastable daughter-product krypton-81, thus generating this short lived radionuclide with a half-life of 13 seconds. Krypton-81m decays by isomeric transition to ^{81}Kr, emitting pure gamma radiation of 0.190 MeV which is internally converted. Krypton-81m decays to stable bromine-81.

Expiry: The shelf-life of the product is 20 hours after activity reference date. The expiry date is stated on the generator label. Do not store the generator above 25°C.

Indications: Investigation of pulmonary ventilation; because of the low radiation dose, this product is especially recommended for paediatric patients. Combined with a pulmonary perfusion scintigraphy for diagnosis of pulmonary embolism. Pulmonary ventilation (^{81m}Kr)/perfusion (^{99m}Tc-macroaggregates) studies are possible because of the different spectrometric windows of ^{81m}Kr and ^{99m}Tc.

Administered dose (MBq): *Adults*: Krypton images are acquired during the continuous inhalation of the short-lived and otherwise inert radioactive gas krypton-81m. This is eluted with humidified air from a rubidium generator and administered to the patient through a face mask or airway. In general, adequate imaging is achieved when 200 000–350 000 counts are accumulated per gamma camera image. This corresponds to ~18 MBq/kg body weight. Most investigations require a number of views, between 4 and 6. The activities for children may be calculated to the following equation:

$$\text{Activity} - \text{child (MBq)} = \text{Activity} - \text{adult(MBq)} \times \text{body weight (kg)}/70 \text{ kg}$$

Continuous inhalation is stopped upon acquisition of ~300 000 counts per gamma camera image.

Radiopharmacology

Pharmacokinetics: Krypton-81m is an inert gas with a short biological half-life. Owing to its rapid decay the effective half-life of lung elimination is equal to the physical half-life of 13 seconds. Peripheral krypton-81m activity is exhaled after the first passage.

Radiation dosimetry

For this product the effective dose equivalent resulting from an administered activity of 3000–9000 MBq (the range of actual exposure) in adults is 0.08–0.24 mSv.

Owing to differences in half-lives, the amount of ^{81}Kr per 37 MBq ^{81m}Kr is about 2 nCi (2 μBq/MBq). Thus the contribution of the total radiation burden of the patient is negligible.

Technetium [^{99m}Tc] Macrosalb Injection (^{99m}Tc-MAA)

Pharmaceutics

Description/formulation: Each vial contains macroaggregates of human serum albumin 2.0 mg. The product is prepared from batches of human albumin but has been screened for hepatitis B surface antigen (HBsAg), antibodies for human immunodeficiency virus (anti-HIV) and antibodies for hepatitis C virus (anti-HCV). After reconstitution of the vial contents and after labelling with the eluate from a ^{99m}Tc-generator (usually 0.9% sodium chloride), the solution will in addition to sodium chloride also contain sodium acetate, tin(II) chloride and human serum albumin.

Pharmaceutical particulars: In the labelled product the distribution of particle size (largest dimension) is as follows: 95% of the particles are between 10 and 100 μm, of which the large majority are between 10 and 90 μm. No particles are larger than 150 μm. The number of particles is 4.5×10^6.

Properties of the medicinal product after reconstitution and labelling: Technetium [^{99m}Tc] Macrosalb Injection is a white liquid suspension of particles which may separate on standing.

Shelf-life and storage: The lyophilisate should be stored at 2–8°C. The labelled product should be stored at 15–25°C.

Expiry after reconstitution: The product may be used for 12 hours after preparation.

Indications: The product is designed for diagnostic use only. Pulmonary perfusion scintigraphy.

As a secondary indication ^{99m}Tc-albumin macroaggregates may be used for venoscintigraphy.

Administered dose (MBq): *Adults*: Varies between 37 and 185 MBq. The number of particles per administered dose must be in the range of 60×10^3 to 700×10^3. The number of albumin macroaggregate (MAA) particles per adult dose should never exceed 1.5×10^6. Special care should be exercised when administering ^{99m}Tc-MAA to patients with significant right-to-left cardiac shunt. In order to minimise the possibility of microembolism to the cerebral and renal circulations, ^{99m}Tc-MAA should be given by slow intravenous injection and the number of particles reduced by up to 50%. Such precautions are also advised in patients with respiratory failure complicating pulmonary hypertension.

Radiopharmacology

Mode of localisation: Following injection into the superficial vein of the systemic venous circulation, the macroaggregates are carried at speed of this circulation to the first capillary filter, i.e. the capillary tree of the pulmonary artery system. The albumin macroaggregate particles do not penetrate the lung parenchyma (interstitial) or the wall of the capillary. When pulmonary flow distribution is normal, the compound distributes over the entire pulmonary area following physiologic gradients: when district flow is altered the areas of reduced flow are reached by a proportionally smaller amount of particles.

Pharmacokinetics/normal biodistribution: The technetium-labelled macroaggregates remain in the lungs for variable periods of time, depending on the structure, size and number of particles.

The disappearance of activity from the particles in the lungs is governed by an exponential law; the larger aggregates have a longer biological half-life, whereas particles between 5 and 90 µm in diameter have a half-life ranging from 2 to 8 hours. The decrease in pulmonary concentration is caused by the mechanical breakdown of the particles occluding the capillaries, stemming from the systo-diastolic pressure pulsations within the capillary itself. The products of macroaggregate breakdown, once recirculated as albumin microcolloid, are quickly removed by the macrophages of the reticuloendothelial system, i.e. the liver and spleen. The microcolloid is metabolised with introduction of the radioactive label (^{99m}Tc) into the systemic circulation from which it is removed and excreted in urine.

Radiation dosimetry

For this product the effective equivalent resulting from an administered activity of 185 MBq is typically 2.2 mSv (per 70 kg individual). For an administered activity of 185 MBq the typical radiation dose to the target organ (lung) is 12.3 mGy and the typical radiation doses to the critical organs, adrenals, bladder wall, liver, pancreas, spleen, are 1.07, 1.85, 2.96, 1.07 and 0.81 mGy, respectively.

Adverse reactions and drug interactions

Single or repeated doses of 99mTc-MAA may be associated with hypersensitive-type reactions, with chest pain, rigor and collapse. Local allergic reactions have been seen at the injection site. Changes in the biological distribution of ^{99m}Tc-MAA are induced by different drugs. Pharmacological interactions are caused by chemotherapeutic agents, heparin and bronchodilators. Toxicological interactions are caused by heroin, nitrofurantoin, busulfan, cyclophosphamide, bleomycin, methotrexate, methysergide. Pharmaceutical interactions are caused by magnesium sulfate.

Renal

Chromium [^{51}Cr] Edetate Injection

Pharmaceutics

Composition and pH: Vials containing 10 mL sterile aqueous solution comprising 0.64 mg/mL chromium edetate, disodium edetate, benzyl alcohol (1%), having a radioactivity of 3.7 MBq/mL at the activity reference date.

Expiry: The shelf-life is not more than 90 days after the date of release.

Indication: Determination of glomerular filtration rate in the assessment of renal function.

Administered dose (MBq): Between 1.1 and 6 MBq by intravenous injection or continuous infusion.

Radiopharmacology

Mode of localisation: After intravenous administration the chromium [^{51}Cr]edetate equilibrates between the intra- and extravascular spaces within 30–90 minutes. Beyond this period the kidneys excrete a constant percentage present in the extracellular fluid in unit time. Total body retention is described by a double exponential function.

Pharmacokinetics: Following intravenous administration the chromium complex is excreted almost exclusively by the kidneys via the glomerular membrane. Less than 0.5% plasma protein binding occurs. Less than 1% faecal excretion in 24 hours has been reported for an anuric patient.

Radiation dosimetry

Critical organs: Bladder wall: 0.024 mGy/MBq in the adult; more in children, rising to 0.66 mGy/MBq in a 12-month-old child.

Whole body dose: Effective dose 0.002 mGy/MBq for adult; 0.007 in a 12-month-old child.

Adverse reactions and drug interactions

Mild allergenic phenomena have been reported. Benzyl alcohol may cause toxic and allergenic reactions in infants and children up to 3 years old.

Technetium [^{99m}Tc] Succimer Injection

Pharmaceutics

Composition and pH: A sterile freeze-dried product containing dimercaptosuccinic acid 1 mg, stannous chloride dihydrate 0.36 mg, inositol 50 mg, ascorbic acid 0.7 mg. Reconstitution with sterile pyrogen-free sodium [^{99m}Tc]pertechnetate gives a clear colourless product with a pH ranging from 2.3 to 3.5.

Expiry (after reconstitution): 8 hours.

Indications: By static (planar or tomographic) renal imaging: morphological studies of renal cortex, kidney function, location of ectopic kidney.

Administered dose (MBq): In adults, from 30 to 120 MBq (0.8–3.2 mCi). In children the dose is adjusted according to body weight, or to body surface area in some circumstances.

Radiopharmacology

Mode of localisation: [^{99m}Tc]Technetium succimer localises in high concentration in the renal cortex.

Pharmacokinetics: After intravenous administration [^{99m}Tc]technetium succimer is eliminated from the blood with a triphasic pattern in patients with normal renal function. The effective half-life of this tracer is about 1 hour. Maximum localisation occurs within 3–6 hours of intravenous injection, with about 40–50% of the dose retained in the kidneys. Less than 3% of the administered dose localises in the liver, but this amount can be increased significantly and renal distribution decreased in patients with impaired renal function.

Radiation dosimetry

Critical organs: Kidney: 0.17 mGy/MBq, proportionally greater in children and up to 0.73 mGy/MBq in a 12-month-old child.

Whole body dose: Effective dose equivalent is 0.016 mGy/MBq in the adult, rising to 0.069 mGy/MBq in a 12-month-old child.

Adverse reactions and drug interactions

Allergic reactions have been reported in the literature, although to date these have been inadequately described. Some chemical compounds or drugs may affect the function of the tested organs and influence the uptake of the tracer: ammonium chloride may substantially reduce renal and increase hepatic uptake; sodium bicarbonate and mannitol will reduce the renal uptake. In patients with unilateral renal artery stenosis taking captopril, uptake of this tracer is impaired in the affected kidney but the effect is reversible after discontinuation of the drug.

Technetium [^{99m}Tc] Pentetate Injection

Pharmaceutics

Composition and pH: One vial contains 37.5 mg of lyophylate comprising calcium trisodium diethylenetriamine pentaacetate 25 mg, gentisic acid, tin(II) chloride and sodium chloride. After reconstitution and labelling with sodium [^{99m}Tc]pertechnetate solution eluted from a generator, the final solution is clear to slightly opalescent with a pH of 4.0–5.0.

Expiry (after reconstitution): 8 hours.

Indications: Dynamic renal scintigraphy for perfusion, function and urinary tract studies; measurement of glomerular filtration rate; cerebral angiography and brain scanning when CT and MRI are not available; lung ventilation imaging, gastro-oesophageal reflux and gastric emptying.

Administered dose (MBq): Measurement of glomerular filtration rate from plasma, 1.8–3.7 MBq; with sequential dynamic renal scanning, 37–370 MBq. Brain scanning, 185–740 MBq. Lung ventilation, 500–1000 MBq in nebuliser to give 50–100 MBq in lung. Gastro-oesophageal reflux and gastric emptying 10–20 MBq.

Radiopharmacology

Mode of localisation: Following intravenous injection [^{99m}Tc]technetium pentetate rapidly distributes throughout the extracellular fluid. Less than 5% of the injected dose is bound to plasma proteins, and a negligible amount to red blood cells. The agent does not cross the normal blood–brain barrier but diffuses weakly in breast milk. Following oral administration the agent does not pass through the digestive barrier

Pharmacokinetics: Plasma clearance is multiexponential with an extremely fast component. The complex is extremely stable with more than 98% of urine radioactivity in the form of a chelate. Approximately 90% of the injected dose is eliminated in the urine within the first 24 hours mainly by glomerular filtration. Plasma clearance may be delayed in patients with renal disease. In lung ventilation studies, after inhalation the agent diffuses rapidly from the pulmonary alveoli towards the vascular space where it is diluted. The half-life in the lungs is slightly less than 1 hour. Many factors are likely to modify the permeability of the pulmonary epithelium, such as cigarette smoking.

Radiation dosimetry

Critical organs: For adults: bladder wall, 0.065 mGy/MBq in normal renal function, 0.022 mGy/MBq in abnormal renal function. For aerosol administration: bladder wall, 0.047 mGy/MBq. For oral administration: stomach, 0.086 mGy/MBq; small intestine, 0.07 mGy/MBq.

Whole body dose: 0.0063 mGy/MBq (normal kidney); 0.0053 mGy/MBq (abnormal kidney).

Adverse reactions and drug interactions

Mild allergic reactions have been reported such as skin reactions, nausea, vomiting, tissue swelling, reduced blood pressure and other allergic responses. Many drugs may affect the function of the tested organ and modify the uptake of this agent. The diagnostic use of captopril may reveal haemodynamic changes in a kidney affected by renal artery stenosis. Administration of intravenous frusemide during dynamic renal scanning increases the elimination of the agent. Psychotropic drugs increase blood flow in the territory of the external carotid artery which may lead to rapid uptake of this agent in the nasopharyngeal area.

Technetium [^{99m}Tc] Mertiatide Injection (Technescan, MAG3)

Pharmaceutics

Chemical structure:

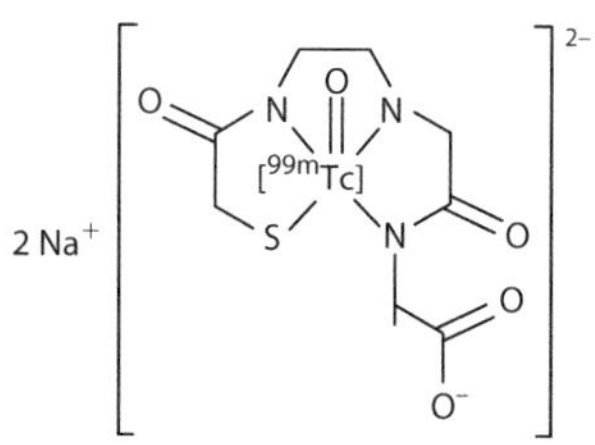

2 Na$^+$ [^{99m}Tc] complex, charge 2−

Composition and pH: Individual vials containing 1 mg betiatide, 16.9 mg disodium tartrate and 0.04 mg tin(II) chloride. Reconstitution and labelling with the eluate of ^{99m}Tc generator produce a clear to slightly opalescent solution with pH 5.0–6.0. Use of eluates with the highest radioactive concentration is recommended, to a maximum of 1110 MBq (30 mCi). The vial does not contain a preservative.

Expiry (after reconstitution): Store at 2–8°C; expires after 4 hours when labelled with an end volume of 10 mL, 1 hour when labelled with an end volume of 4 mL.

Administered dose (MBq): Adults and the elderly: 37–185 MBq (1–5 mCi) depending on the pathology to be studied and the method to be used. Children: adjust the dose according to the recommendations of The Paediatric task Group, EANM.

Indication: Evaluation of nephrological and urological disorders in particular for the study of morphology, perfusion, function of the kidney and characterisation of urinary outflow.

Radiopharmacology

Mode of localisation: The method of excretion is predominantly based on tubular secretion. Glomerular secretion accounts for 11% of the total clearance.

Pharmacokinetics: After intravenous injection, [^{99m}Tc]technetium tiatide has a relatively high binding to plasma proteins. In normal renal function 70% of the administered dose has been excreted after 30 minutes and more than 95% after 3 hours. These latter percentages are dependent on the pathology of the kidneys and the urogenital system.

Radiation dosimetry

Critical organs: Bladder wall: 0.127 mGy/MBq (4-hour void); 0.057 mGy/MBq (2-hour void).

Whole body dose: Effective dose equivalent is 0.11 mSv/MBq.

Adverse reactions and drug interactions

Anaphylactoid reactions have been reported (urticaria, swelling of eyelids, itching, nausea and headache). Mild vasovagal reactions have been reported.

Tumour

Indium [^{111}In] Pentetreotide (Octreotide; Octreoscan)

Pharmaceutics

Chemical structure:

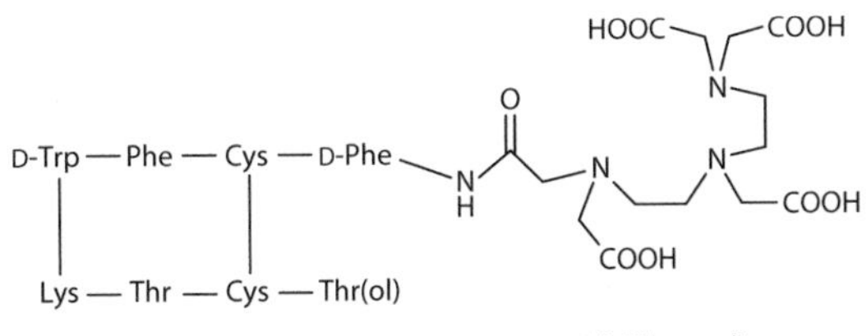

[*N*-(diethylenetriamine-*N,N,N′,N″*-tetraacetic acid-*N″*-acetyl]-D-phenylalanyl-L-hemicystyl-L-phenylalanyl-D-tryptophyl-L-lysyl-L-threonyl-L-hemicystyl-L-threoninol cyclic disulfide.

Composition and pH: Contains gentisic acid, citrate buffer, inositol; ^{111}In chloride is supplied in separate vial.

Expiry (after reconstitution): 6 hours.

Indications: Localisation of primary and metastatic neuroendocrine tumours bearing somatostatin receptors.

Administered dose (MBq): 110 MBq for planar imaging; 220 MBq for SPECT.

Radiopharmacology

Mode of localisation: Binding to somatostatin receptors on the surface of tumours.

Pharmacokinetics: Radioactivity leaves the plasma rapidly; one-third of the radioactive injected dose remains in the blood pool at 10 minutes after administration. Plasma levels continue to decline so that by 20 hours post injection, about 1% of the radioactive dose is found in the blood pool. The biological half-life is 6 hours. Half of the injected dose is recoverable in urine within 6 hours after injection, 85% is recovered in the first 24 hours, and over 90% is recovered in urine by 2 days.

Normal biodistribution: In addition to somatostatin receptor-rich tumours, the normal pituitary gland, thyroid gland, liver, spleen and urinary bladder also are visualised in most patients, as is the bowel to a lesser extent.

Radiation dosimetry

Critical organs: Spleen, 148 mGy; kidney, 108 mGy per 220 MBq.

Whole body dose: 12 mSv per 220 MBq.

Adverse reactions and drug interactions: Rare and mild. Sensitivity may be reduced in patients concurrently receiving therapeutic doses of octreotide; discontinuation of therapy should be considered but is not essential.

Gallium [^{67}Ga] Citrate Injection

Pharmaceutics

Chemical formula: $Ga[HOOCC(OH)(CH_2COOH)_2]$.

Composition and pH: Sterile solution containing benzyl alcohol 0.9% v/v; pH 5–8.

Expiry: 7 days post reference.

Indications: Used in a variety of tumours, particularly lymphoma and bronchogenic carcinoma; also for chronic infection.

Administered dose (MBq): Maximum 150 MBq.

Radiopharmacology

Mode of localisation: In tumours it is believed to be taken up via the transferrin transporter; in infection/inflammation there is non-specific leakage of ^{67}Ga-transferrin through inflamed vessels.

Pharmacokinetics: After intravenous injection, the highest tissue concentration of radiotracer – other than tumours and sites of infection – is in the renal cortex. After the first day, the maximum concentration shifts to bone and lymph nodes, and after the first week, to liver and spleen. Gallium is excreted relatively slowly from the body. The average whole body retention is 65% after 7 days with 26% having been excreted in the urine and 9% in the faeces.

Normal biodistribution: Excreted into the bowel; use of laxatives is required to reduce radiation dose and improve image quality.

Radiation dosimetry

Critical organs: Lower large intestine, 40 mGy; bone marrow, 25 mGy per 150 MBq administered.

Whole body dose: 15 mSv per 150 MBq.

Adverse reactions and drug interactions: Rare.

Fludeoxyglucose [^{18}F] Injection (^{18}F-Fluorodeoxyglucose, FDG)

Pharmaceutics

Chemical structure:

[^{18}F]Fludeoxyglucose

Composition and pH: An isotonic solution; may contain buffer; pH 4.5–7.5.

Expiry (after reconstitution: 12 hours.

Administered dose (MBq): 400 MBq.

Indications: Imaging of enhanced glucose metabolism in tumours, normal glucose metabolism in brain and heart.

Radiopharmacology

Mode of localisation: Substrate for the GLUT-1 glucose transporter and phosphorylated by hexokinase, then trapped as fluorodeoxyglucose 6-phosphate.

Pharmacokinetics: Twenty per cent is excreted via kidneys in the first 2 hours after administration. Radioactivity in brain and heart accumulates over 1 hour. Radioactivity in other organs and tissues follows triexponential kinetics with half-lives of 25 seconds, 3.4 minutes, and 47 minutes.

Normal biodistribution: Heart, brain, active skeletal muscle (including shivering and chewing); excretion through renal system. FDG can also accumulate in sites of inflammation/infection.

Radiation dosimetry

Critical organs: Urinary bladder wall, 70 mGy; heart, 30 mGy per 400 MBq.

Whole body dose: 8 mSv per 400 MBq.

Adverse reactions and drug interactions: Adverse reactions are extremely rare.

Technetium [^{99m}Tc] Depreotide Injection (Neospect; Neotect)

Pharmaceutics

Chemical formula: The precursor is:

Cyclo (L-homocysteinyl-*N*-methyl-L-phenylalanyl-L-tyrosyl- D-tryptophyl-L-lysyl-L-valyl), (1→1′)-sulfide with 3-[(mercaptoacetyl)amino]- L-alanyl-L-lysyl-L-cysteinyl-L-lysinamide.

Composition and pH: Sodium glucoheptonate, stannous chloride dihydrate, sodium edentate, sodium iodide; pH 7.4.

Expiry (after reconstitution): 6 hours.

Indications: Identification of somatostatin receptor-bearing pulmonary masses in patients presenting with pulmonary lesions on computed tomography and/or chest radiography who have known malignancy or who are highly suspect for malignancy.

Administered dose (MBq): 600 MBq.

Radiopharmacology

Mode of localisation: Binds to somatostatin receptor.

Pharmacokinetics: The time course of radioactivity in blood follows a three-compartment model with half-lives of 4 minutes, 44 minutes, and 22 hours. Twelve per cent of the injected dose is recovered in urine within 4 hours of administration.

Normal biodistribution: Serial scintigraphic body images indicated the highest activities (% injected dose) in the kidneys (13%), liver (10%), pelvic area (6.3%), and lungs (6.12%) at 10 minutes post injection, and during the first 24 hours relative activity in these regions remained nearly constant.

Radiation dosimetry

Critical organs: Kidneys, 54 mGy; spleen, 24 mGy per 600 MBq.

Whole body dose: 6 mSv per 600 MBq.

Adverse reactions and drug interactions

Headache, dizziness, and/or nausea were observed in 1% of patients in clinical trials.

19

Survey of current therapeutic radiopharmaceuticals

Pei-san Chan and Jilly Croasdale

Targeted therapy using radiopharmaceuticals, in which particle-emitting radionuclides are administered to the patient to deliver a cytotoxic radiation dose to selected tissues, is by no means a new concept. Iodine-131 in the form of sodium [^{131}I]iodide has routinely been used for therapeutic purposes for over 60 years. Not only can it be used to treat hyperthyroidism, it could arguably be considered the original 'magic bullet' in the treatment of thyroid carcinoma.

Many radiopharmaceuticals utilising different radionuclides have since been developed for a variety of other clinical indications, including the treatment or palliation of oncological and haematological malignancies, notably metastatic bone pain, hepatocellular cancer and neuroendocrine tumours, as well as non-oncological applications such as synovectomy for inflammatory joint diseases. In the last 20 years, the focus of research has been with radiolabelled antibodies and peptides; biomolecules provide the specific targeting approach, leading to their increasing use, e.g. ^{90}Y-ibritumomab tiuxetan (Zevalin) and ^{131}I-tositumomab (Bexxar), licensed for the treatment of non-Hodgkin lymphoma.

Many therapeutic radiopharmaceuticals are sufficiently stable with suitable half-lives to be obtained as ready-to-inject solutions but some, primarily the antibody and peptide preparations, require in-house radiolabelling. While not all nuclear medicine and radiopharmacy departments undertake the manufacture of such therapeutic doses, many are likely to be involved in the dispensing of doses and providing advice for those more commonly used.

The aim of this chapter is to give an overview of the general principles of using therapeutic radiopharmaceuticals and examples of those currently in use and some under development, categorised under the radionuclide, with the exception of radiolabelled peptides and antibodies which now form an increasingly important area of radionuclide therapy.

Targeted therapy concept

For the targeted therapy to be successful:

- The target must be sufficiently radiosensitive.
- The target must be specific to the disease and not present in normal tissues or involved in other disease such as infection or inflammation.
- The radiopharmaceutical must reach the target in adequate concentration to be cytotoxic and remain stable during biodistribution.
- The radiopharmaceutical must be selectively taken up with minimal non-specific uptake and retained by the target (e.g. physiological conditions, cell surface markers or receptors, metabolic pathways) and be sufficiently stable to remain intact at the target for the required effect.
- The radiopharmaceutical must have a good and rapid clearance from non-target tissue and achieve an adequate target to background ratio.
- The radiopharmaceutical must not cause unnecessary radiation dose to normal tissues.
- The radionuclide must have an appropriate type of radioactive emission, energy and physical half-life (matched with the *in-vivo* pharmacokinetics of the pharmaceutical, if applicable) for the size and type of target.

Compared to external beam radiotherapy, for example, the more specific targeted radiopharmaceutical therapy advantageously offers a lower incidence of side-effects associated with less irradiation of normal tissues and the ability to treat widespread metastases in the body from a single administration. If the administered radionuclide emits sufficiently high levels of penetrating gamma radiation (e.g. ^{131}I), the patient disadvantageously becomes an external radioactive source. Precautions are then often required, including limitation of contact with people in terms of time and distance, admission into a hospital shielded room or holding medical declaration letters if intending to travel abroad because of airport radiation detectors, until the surface dose rate of the patient falls sufficiently.

While the most desirable treatment outcome is clearly a complete response (i.e. no remaining evidence of disease), this is not always achievable. However, a partial response is still a valuable outcome, resulting in an improved quality of life and sometimes survival rates as well as enabling the patient to benefit from previously unsuitable treatment options (e.g. bone marrow transplantation, surgery).

Handling therapeutic radiopharmaceuticals

When considering using a new therapeutic radiopharmaceutical, a radiological risk assessment must be undertaken before introducing the service to demonstrate all possible precautions have been taken to minimise the radiation dose to the operator. The dose rates associated with handling the radionuclide must be estimated initially and the handling process reviewed to ensure all possible measures are taken to comply with the ALARA ('as low as reasonably achievable') principle. New shielding equipment may be required, particularly if using beta emitters or high-dose iodine-131.

A trial run must be performed, particularly if manufacturing a therapeutic dose from its raw materials, to determine any necessary personal protective equipment and method amendments to reduce operator radiation doses. The actual operator dose involved can be measured at this point. The use of automated equipment can be considered to decrease the operator dose – syringe drivers, modification of PET radiopharmaceutical synthesis units.

Since the procedure may be more complex than the manufacture of standard diagnostic kit radiopharmaceuticals, staff training must be carried out with appropriate records being kept.

Radionuclides

Physical and chemical characteristics

Particulate radiation is the most effective type of radiation to elicit a cytotoxic effect (i.e. killing cells) for therapy. The cytotoxic mechanism is believed to be DNA double-strand breaks. The radiation is absorbed by tissue over a wide range (μm to mm) depending on the radiation type and radionuclide energy. Radiation types include beta (β) emitters (the most extensively used), alpha (α) emitters and Auger electron emitters, some of which may also have gamma emissions. While

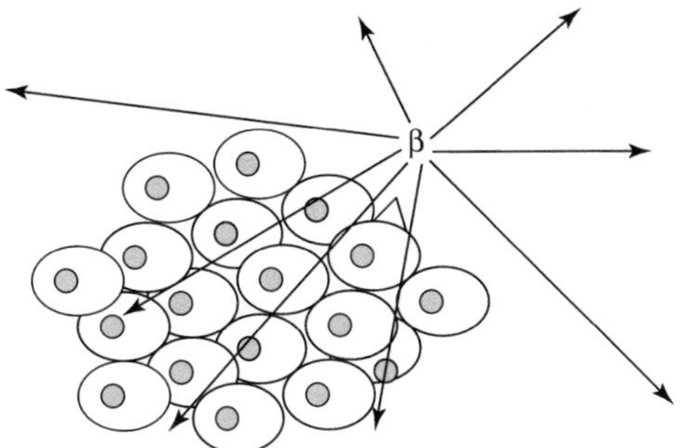

Figure 19.1 Cross-fire effect of beta-emitting radionuclides.

some gamma (γ) emissions (e.g. 10%) may be useful for imaging for biodistribution studies, higher levels irradiate non-target tissue and other people (see section above). In the absence of gamma emissions, imaging bremsstrahlung from high beta emitters, may be used.

Compared with alpha and Auger-electron emitters, beta emitters are less densely ionising and have a longer tissue range but lower LET (linear energy transfer) (typically 0.2 keV/μm) compared with alpha and Auger-electron emitters. They exert a crossfire effect (Figure 19.1) whereby emissions pass through and kill a number of cells adjacent to the targeted cell (e.g. 100–300 cell diameters, dependent upon the energy of the radioisotope), so that homogeneous irradiation of tumour cells occurs despite heterogeneous radiopharmaceutical distribution. They are therefore useful for bulky disease and poorly vascularised tumours. The availability of a number of radioisotopes emitting different β-particle energies (low, medium, high), in particular those in the lanthanide chemistry group, provide short- to long-range tissue penetration paths of 0.1 to 10 mm so that treatment can be tailored to the size of the tumour. Higher-energy beta emitters (e.g. ^{90}Y, ^{188}Re) are used for treating large tumours (≤ 1 cm diameter), as small clusters of tumour cells will not be treated efficiently because energy deposition will be predominantly in the normal surrounding tissue rather than in the target tumour cells. Medium-energy emitters such as ^{131}I, ^{186}Re, ^{177}Lu, are used for treating smaller tumours (~1 mm). In radiation synovectomy, high-energy emitters are used for thicker, inflamed synovium, with lower energies for thinner synovium to minimise irradiation of the bone. Radionuclides with shorter half-lives may be employed for quicker therapeutic effects. Table 19.1 contains a summary of the physical characteristics of the beta-emitting radionuclides most commonly in use.

Alpha emitters (see Table 19.6) and Auger-electron emitters (Table 19.7) are also suitable as therapeutic agents but their use is presently limited by difficulties in achieving specific targeting due to their respective short range in tissue. With Auger-electron emitters, the range (<1–10 μm) and very low energy (a few electronvolts to 1 keV) result in a high linear energy transfer (LET) (16 keV/μm) but necessitate targeting to the cell nucleus. Alpha emitters produce

Table 19.1 Physical properties of beta-emitting radionuclides commonly used for current therapy

Radionuclide		Half-life (days)	Max. beta energy (MeV)	Max. range in tissue (mm)	Suitable gamma emission (MeV) for imaging (% abundance)
Iodine-131	^{131}I	8	0.61	2.3	0.364 (81%)
Lutetium-177	^{177}Lu	6.7	0.50	1.8	0.208 (11%)
Phosphorus-32	^{32}P	14.3	1.71	8.2	–
Rhenium-186	^{186}Re	3.8	1.077	4.8	0.137 (9%)
Samarium-153	^{153}Sm	1.9	0.81	4.0	0.103 (29%)
Strontium-89	^{89}Sr	50.5	1.46	8.0	–
Yttrium-90	^{90}Y	2.7	2.28	11.3	–

particles (5–9 MeV) giving very high densities of ionisation energy over a short path length (40–100 μm) corresponding to 5–10 cell diameters, resulting in a high LET (80–100 keV/μm). This renders them highly toxic to non-target as well as to target tissue.

Useful and useable chemistry is often required to enable binding between the ligand and radionuclide, though some radionuclides can be used without any further chemical manipulation. e.g. sodium [^{131}I] iodide, colloidal preparations for intracavity use. Iodine can radiolabel biomolecules directly, whereas other radionuclides require a bifunctional chelating agent (a linker group that binds the radionuclide and the targeting molecule at either end).

Iodine-131

Iodine-131 is the oldest and most widely known radionuclide for therapy. When used in the sodium iodide form, ^{131}I becomes incorporated into the iodine metabolic pathway (Figure 19.2) via the sodium/iodide (Na/I) symporter (NIS) to treat both hyperthyroidism and cancer of the thyroid. As well as thyroid uptake, ^{131}I it will also be taken up into any other tissue in the body expressing the NIS, effectively targeting any secondary tumours. However, the emission of 364 keV γ-rays gives rise to significant radiation protection challenges.

Iodine-131 can be used to radiolabel antibodies and peptides. ^{131}I remains popular for labelling antibodies owing to its well-understood chemistry, low cost and availability. See Chapters 10 and 14. ^{131}I-tositumomab (Bexxar) for treatment of non-Hodgkin lymphoma is detailed below in the section on radiolabelled antibodies. ^{131}I is also available in the pharmaceutical form of *meta*-[^{131}I]iodobenzylguanidine (mIBG) to treat neuroendocrine tumours and [^{131}I]lipiodol to treat hepatocellular carcinoma and liver metastases.

Sodium [^{131}I]iodide

Treatment of hyperthyroidism

At lower doses (200–600 MBq), ^{131}I is an effective treatment for hyperthyroidism due to Graves disease or toxic nodular goitre and has been used in the treatment of subclinical hyperthyroidism in the USA (Surks *et al.* 2004; RCP 2007). It has the advantage over surgery of being non-invasive and requiring only an out-patient appointment. An initial thyroid scan may be performed using either sodium [^{123}I]iodide or sodium [^{99m}Tc]pertechnetate to assess and estimate the likely uptake of radioiodine. However, performing

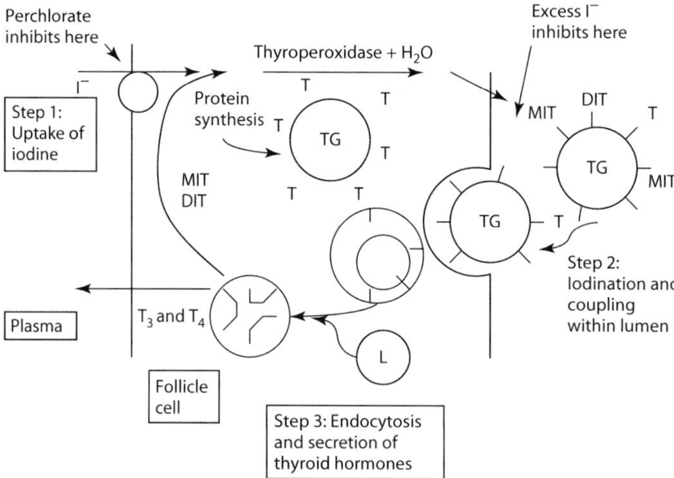

Figure 19.2 Mechanism of uptake of iodide. TG = thyroglobulin; T = tyrosine; MIT = monoiodotyrosine; DIT = diiodotyrosine; T_4 = thyroxine; T_3 = triiodothyronine; L = lysosome. With permission from Rang HP *et al.* (1990) *Rang & Dale's Pharmacology* 1st edn. Elsevier.

the uptake scan does not necessarily result in lower remission or hypothyroid rates as the individual response to administered radioiodine varies (Jarløv *et al.* 1995; Leslie *et al.* 2003; RCP 2007).

Practical considerations

It is important the patient receives counselling prior to therapy. This should include the following:

- Avoiding pregnancy for 6 months, or fathering any children for a 4-month period post therapy.
- Discontinuing breastfeeding permanently (ARSAC 2006).
- Maintaining time limits for avoiding contact with adults and children, and for returning to work. The recommended limits are found in Table 19.2. It is important to convey this information in a manner that does not result in an already anxious patient leaving the department before having their treatment!
- Confirming that any antithyroid medication has been stopped and whether and when to re-start it. Carbimazole should be withdrawn a minimum of 2 days prior to treatment. Many departments stop propylthiouracil 2–7 days before treatment. Data on the cessation duration are conflicting, and there is some evidence that medication continues to exert an effect for up to two weeks (Ming-der, Shaw 2003) and it is thought to have a radioprotective action on the thyroid (RCP 2007). A larger dose of radioiodine may be used to counteract this. Propranolol may be given at a dose of 20–40 mg three times a day for the alleviation of cardiac symptoms. This does not need to be stopped prior to radioiodine treatment.
- Warning of the possibility of thyroid storm (a transient worsening of the hyperthyroid symptoms).
- Checking whether the patient has taken any other medication or eaten any food that could interfere with the uptake of the radioiodine, such as certain types of fish. Compounds containing iodine, such as amiodarone and some radiographic contrast agents, may block uptake for up to one year after cessation of treatment.
- Explaining how the treatment works and the possibility of the necessity for a repeat radioiodine dose or of becoming hypothyroid (50–75% of patients would be rendered euthyroid within 6–8 weeks) (RCP 2007). Therefore, there may be a need for repeat radioiodine treatment. Again, some reassurance may be required.
- Explaining the treatment for hypothyroidism (i.e. thyroxine).
- Explaining that there is some evidence of worsening thyroid eye disease after treatment (Sridamma, DeGroot 1989; RCP 2007), though there are other risk factors that can affect this such as smoking or early treatment with thyroxine. Treatment with prednisolone may prevent this.
- Requirement for good hygiene as urine and faeces will be radioactive. The length of time depends upon the administered dose and the individual patient.

The patient must be given an information sheet containing a summary of the precautions to be taken after receiving treatment, as well as a contact number should they have any problems. The patient must sign

Table 19.2 Time limits to be applied for patients after receiving radioiodine

Behaviour restriction (1 mSv dose constraint)	Period of restriction (days) for activity of ^{131}I administered (MBq):			
	200	400	600	800
Stay at least 1 m away from children under 3 years of age	15	21	25	27
As above but for children of 3–5 years	11	16	20	22
As above for children of over 5 years and for adults not comforters or carers	5	11	14	16
Sleep separately from comforters and carers	–	–	4	8
Avoid prolonged close contact of more than 3 hours at >1m with other adults (one-off exposure)	–	–	–	1

Taken from *Medical and Dental Guidance Notes 2002*, prepared by the Institute of Physics and Engineering in Medicine.

a consent form to state they understand all the advice provided and that they are not pregnant or breastfeeding.

If the patient is happy to proceed, the dose is administered in capsule or liquid form. There is less likelihood of spillage and subsequent radiation decontamination and protection problems with a capsule. However, there are no means of adjusting the dose with a capsule, so this would not be suitable for a 'one-stop' clinic where the patient has a ^{123}I uptake scan and subsequent dose calculation and administration on the same day.

Any member of staff involved in the explanation of the procedure, calibration of the activity or the equipment used to measure the activity, confirming that the patient is a suitable candidate for treatment, prescribing, or administering the capsule is considered an 'operator' under Ionising Radiation (Medical Exposure) Regulations 2000 (IRMER) and must therefore receive appropriate recorded training.

Treatment of thyroid carcinoma

Sodium [^{131}I]iodide can also be used as an ablative agent for the treatment of thyroid carcinoma. In this case, the radioiodine is given after surgery to target any residual disease.

Practical points

- The administered dose in adults is usually 3.7–7.4 GBq (Luster *et al.* 2008), although higher doses have been used. Care in handling is paramount when using such high activities.
- The dose is given as a liquid or liquid-filled capsules: operator protection must be given careful consideration.
- For some time after administration, the patient will emit a high surface radiation dose, requiring treatment to be performed as an in-patient, requiring a shielded room with en-suite bathroom.
- The patient's surface dose must be monitored while they are in hospital. They can be discharged when the surface dose rate drops to limits compatible with those laid down in the Ionising Radiation Regulations. This can be measured directly and would be expected to decrease to approximately 20 mSv/h before the patient is discharged, especially if having contact with children. An alternative method would be to calculate the activity remaining in the patient. This limit used may vary depending on personal circumstances. For example, a patient living alone may be allowed home earlier than someone looking after a baby (Allisy-Roberts 2002).
- The room must be monitored after vacating and any contaminated items must be stored until the activity has decayed.
- Up to six treatment doses may be required in advanced or resistant cases. Several large studies have shown good tolerance in terms of side-effects and long-term complications (Clarke 1991; Hoefnagel 1991; Hall *et al.* 1992).

meta-[^{131}I]iodobenzylguanidine ([^{131}I]MIBG)

This therapeutic agent is a catecholamine analogue, similar in structure to the adrenergic neuron blocker guanethidine and the neurotransmitter adrenaline (epinephrine). It is taken up by the adrenal medulla and other tissues rich in sympathetic innervation by catecholamine receptors via the noradrenaline (norepinephrine) receptor. It has been used as a palliative treatment in a number of neuroendocrine diseases; commonly phaeochromocytoma (a tumour of the adrenal medulla), neuroblastoma (particularly paediatric) and carcinoid tumours, for many years. However, there are few controlled trials. In a review of cumulated experience from several major centres, an objective response was seen in 56% of patients with malignant phaeochromocytoma, and in 35% of patients with neuroblastoma. Objective responses ranging from 19% to 38% have been seen in patients with other neuroendocrine tumours (Hoefnagel *et al.* 1994). [^{131}I]mIBG can also be used as first-line treatment in high risk neuroblastoma patients (Hoefnagel 1994), and may be given in combination with chemotherapy and whole-body irradiation (Gaze *et al.* 1995).

Practical points

- A prior diagnostic [^{123}I]mIBG scan is required to show uptake.
- Note: occasionally uptake may be seen after therapeutic dosing that was not visible on the diagnostic scan. This is thought to be due to the increased count rates with the therapeutic dose.

- Admission to a therapy ward with a shielded room is required owing to the high surface dose rate of the patient after administration.
- The patient's drug history must be checked, as drugs which interfere with uptake of mIBG diagnostic studies could adversely affect the therapy outcome. More information can be found in Chapter 32.
- The treatment is toxic to bone marrow and platelets. The levels of these must be checked before treatment can go ahead. The limiting factor for treatment is the effect on the bone marrow (Fielding *et al.* 1991).
- The patient must be well hydrated to maximise clearance of radiopharmaceutical not taken up by the tumour.
- The patient's renal function must be checked to ensure it has not been affected by previous chemotherapy as this will affect clearance and subsequently radiation dose.
- The administered intravenous dose of [^{131}I]mIBG ranges from 3.7 to 11.1 GBq.
- After administration, the excreta will be radioactive. The patient must have adequate bowel function to prevent accumulation within the bowels. Some centres administer a laxative to assist with this.
- Thyroid blockade with cold iodine (e.g. potassium iodide, Lugol's solution) is required, commencing one day before treatment and continuing for 3 weeks afterwards.
- The high injected radioactive doses mean that operator protection must be carefully considered. A slow infusion over 60 minutes is required to minimise the occurrence of any side-effects. The main radiation dose to the operator is not, therefore, associated with preparation, but with administration. The manufacturer should be contacted for advice on specialist shielding and handling equipment to minimise this.
- There is the possibility of a rise in the patient's blood pressure during mIBG infusion and for up to 2 hours afterwards due to the displacement of noradrenaline. Monitoring is therefore required.
- Once the therapy has been administered, the patient becomes a radioactive source, and contact from medical and nursing staff must be limited where possible without adversely affecting the patient's care.
- Almost 50% of the activity will clear within the first 10 hours, with the remainder clearing more slowly. The dose rate from the patient must be measured (as described above for sodium [^{131}I]iodide). The patient will generally be discharged after a week, with instructions to limit contact with other members of the public in the same manner.

[^{131}I]Lipiodol

Iodine-131-labelled lipiodol (an iodised poppy seed oil also used as an X-ray contrast medium) has been used with some success in hepatocellular carcinoma (HCC) and liver metastases. Response rates of 40–70% and median survival times of 6–9 months have been demonstrated with [^{131}I]lipiodol. When used alongside a curative resection, the 3-year survival rate increased to 86% compared with 46% in control group (Keng, Sundram 2003).

Agents are administered by intra-arterial administration into the tumour, with the catheter positioned into the hepatic artery under fluoroscopy. The [^{131}I] lipiodol deposits in the arterioles or capillaries of the tumour, leading to selective retention in the tumour vessels as well as the tumour cells (Yumoto *et al.* 2005).

Practical points

- The radiolabelled agent is available ready-prepared. In the case of lipiodol, the injection volume may be increased by dilution with up to 10 mL of 'cold' lipiodol. This must be done in a contained or ventilated work-station to prevent aerosol inhalation.
- The agents are administered via a catheter (inserted using contrast). A good relationship with interventional radiology is important since the procedure will be performed in the X-ray department.
- The EANM guidelines recommend an administered dose of 2.22 GBq for [^{131}I]lipiodol (Lewandowski *et al.* 2005). Administered activities for the other agents may vary according to published safety and efficacy data.
- Lipiodol is excreted in urine. The patient must be advised to follow rigorous hygiene precautions,

particularly in the first two days following administration. If the patient is an in-patient, staff on the ward must be advised appropriately.

- Some patients may experience side-effects, early and/or delayed. The most common of the early side-effects are pyrexia and liver pain upon injection. A later side-effect is reversible leukopenia.
- Care must be taken to use Luer lock syringes and taps that do not dissolve with lipiodol (Lewandowski *et al.* 2005).

Yttrium-90

^{90}Y-Resin or glass microspheres

More recently ^{90}Y-resin microspheres (SIR-Spheres) and ^{90}Y-glass microspheres (TherSphere), have been used in hepatocellular carcinoma and liver metastases (see also [^{131}I]lipiodol). Responses to treatment have been demonstrated using [^{18}F]FDG (Goin *et al.* 2005) and median survival rates of 9–13 months have been demonstrated for patients receiving ^{90}Y-microspheres (Keng and Sundram 2003).

A variety of parameters can have an effect on the 3-month survival rates. The absence of other contributing factors, such as raised liver enzymes or bulky disease, resulted in an improved 3-month survival rate after administration of the radiopharmaceutical (EANM 2002). This should be taken into consideration when making the decision to treat.

Practical points

- Prior imaging with ^{99m}Tc-MAA (administered via the hepatic catheter) may be required to check for arteriovenous shunting to the lung. For example, for SIR-Spheres, if lung shunt is >20%, the therapy should not be administered and a reduced dose is recommended in the event of 10–20% shunting.

^{90}Y-Colloid

Synovectomy treatment

Radiopharmaceuticals are injected directly into a joint, into the synovium (inflamed joint tissue), for inflammatory joint diseases (e.g. rheumatoid arthritis) and arthropathy, to control and abate inflammation by destroying the synovium; a procedure known as radiation synovectomy. A suitable energy and half-life are selected for the thickness of the synovium and allow it to remain in place long enough to effectively destroy the synovium. The colloid size must also be small enough to facilitate phagocytosis and eventual removal from the joint, but large enough to be retained in the joint (Ugur *et al.* 2008).

The first radioisotope used for synovectomy was colloidal gold (^{198}Au), but its gamma emission (see Table 19.4) and small colloidal size, leading to 48% leakage, made it unfavourable (Fellinger *et al.* 1952). In colloidal form, yttrium-90 silicate (no longer available in the UK) or citrate has been used in the UK for many years for synovectomy (mainly knee and shoulder joints) and is the main agent still used. Other radionuclides have also been used for radiation synovectomy such as rhenium-186 sulfide in mid-sized joints and erbium-169 for interdigital administration (see Table 19.5).

Practical points

- A calibration factor for the dose calibrator should be determined for the type of container and volume being measured as the pure beta emission of ^{90}Y activity is difficult to measure accurately. The dose may be checked by subtraction of the activity remaining in the vial after withdrawal of the dose from the initial measured activity.
- The preparation pH is important in maintaining the colloidal nature of the preparation. pH-adjusted diluents may be used; alternatively, the time between dilution and administration must be kept very short.
- After treatment administration, the area must be monitored carefully for any beta contamination.
- The treatment is often administered by a rheumatologist, who may drain the joint first.

Radiolabelled antibodies

Antibodies form part of the body's immune response system. They are immunoglobulins and have two roles:

1. To 'recognise' and interact with specific antigens.
2. To activate one or more of the host's defence systems – e.g. complement sequence.

By radiolabelling antibodies, targeting is achieved primarily via utilisation of the first role. However, Zevalin treatment utilises both roles: the patient is pre-treated with non-labelled rituximab antibody to activate the host defence system, and then given ^{90}Y-ibritumomab antibody which recognises the target CD20 antigen on tumour cells. Although not tumour-specific, the CD20 antigen is restricted to B-cells, which are present in 95% of B-cell non-Hodgkin lymphoma (NHL).

The main developments in radiolabelled antibodies are currently for the treatment of B-cell lymphomas, which are well known to be radiosensitive. Other radiolabelled antibodies are being investigated in areas such as myeloma (CD66 antigen) and acute myeloid leukaemia (CD33 antigen). Therapy with radiolabelled antibodies is often referred to as radioimmunotherapy (RIT).

Iodine-131 tositumomab (Bexxar)

Iodine-131 tositumomab is licensed in the United States for the treatment of NHL. There are currently no data showing a direct comparison between Bexxar and Zevalin. However, Bexxar has been shown to produce overall response rates of 57% and 65%, with complete responses in 32% and 20% respectively and a time to progression of up to 9.9 months (Vose *et al.* 2000; Kaminski *et al.* 2001).

Practical points

- It is ready-prepared, so does not required manufacture in a radiopharmacy.
- Manipulation is still required. The emission of a 360 keV gamma photon means that the operator dose has to be assessed and managed.
- A dosimetry study is required before the therapeutic dose can be administered.
- The higher patient surface dose of ^{131}I results in increased radiation exposure to family members. However, admission to a hospital for administration is not required in most US states so long as the patient takes precautions to minimise the radiation dose including avoiding close contact with adults and children, and observing stringent hygiene rules.
- The radiopharmaceutical is excreted in urine.
- Thyroid blockade is required as Bexxar is less stable than Zevalin, resulting in the release of free ^{131}I.

^{90}Y-Ibritumomab tiuxetan (Zevalin)

^{90}Y-labelled Zevalin (^{90}Y-ibritumomab tiuxetan) was first licensed in the UK in 2004 and was indicated for the treatment of adult patients with relapsed or refractory CD20 positive follicular B-cell NHL. Its use in the UK has not been as widespread as in the USA. The cost of the preparation – which is high compared with other radiopharmaceuticals, although not when compared to a course of chemotherapy – and the initial limited indications may have contributed to this.

Zevalin is composed of ibritumomab, a murine anti-CD20 monoclonal antibody and the chelating agent, tiuxetan. It can be radiolabelled with ^{90}Y or ^{111}In (for optional dosimetric and biodistribution studies before administration of the therapeutic dose).

The administered dose is dependent on the patient's body weight and platelet count. If platelets are above 150 000/mm^3, the administered dose is 15 MBq/kg, up to a maximum of 1200 MBq. If the platelet count is between 100 000 and 150 000/mm^3 the dose is reduced to 11 MBq/kg, up to a maximum of 1200 MBq. A scheme of the dosing schedule is shown in Figure 19.3.

Witzig *et al.* published the first data comparing responses of 73 patients receiving ^{90}Y-ibritumomab tiuxetan (pre-treated with two doses of rituximab to improve biodistribution) with 70 receiving rituximab alone (Witzig *et al.* 2002a). The number of patients with a complete response rose from 16% to 30%, while the number of overall responders rose from 56% to 80%. The time to progression increased in patients with follicular histology and in those who had a complete response to the treatment, although this was not shown to be statistically significant in this study.

Although myelosuppression can occur (Witzig *et al.* 2002b), its onset is gradual and is seen later than that resulting from chemotherapy. Thrombocytopenia continues in a number of patients, and platelets must be monitored closely. However, Zevalin can still be administered in patients who have pre-existing mild thrombocytopenia, at a reduced dose, and overall response rates of 83% (with 37% complete responses)

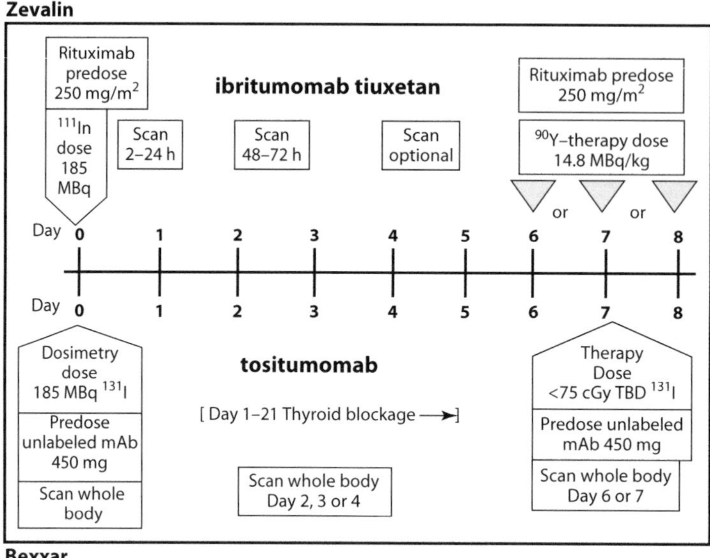

Figure 19.3 Schematic of dosing schedule. Comparison of administration conditions for ^{131}I-tositumomab and ^{90}Y-ibritumomab tiuxetan. Reprinted with permission from Goldenberg DM (2004). Therapeutic use of radiolabelled antibodies: haematopoietic tumours. In: Ell PJ, Gambhir SS, eds. *Nuclear Medicine in Clinical Diagnosis and Treatment*, 3rd edn. London: Churchill Livingstone, 428-434.

have been demonstrated, even in patients with poor prognostic factors such as large tumours of more than 5 cm, more than one site of extranodal disease, chemoresistant disease or bone marrow involvement (Wiseman *et al.* 2002).

In 2008, an additional indication was granted for the use of Zevalin as consolidation therapy after remission induction in previously untreated patients with follicular lymphoma. Of patients who had shown a partial response to first-line chemotherapy, 77% converted to a complete response after consolidation with ^{90}Y-ibritumomab tiuxetan with a high overall complete response rate of 87% and prolonged progression-free survival (Hagenbeek *et al.* 2007). This expansion in the indications for Zevalin is likely to lead to its increased use in the UK.

Practical points

- Radiopharmacy is required to undertake the radiolabelling. Preparation of the dose is relatively complex compared with other radiopharmaceuticals (see kit preparation below).
- The ^{90}Y setting on the dose calibrator must be determined for the different vials and syringes used for the preparation. A calibration dose can be bought for this purpose.
- Radiopharmacy and nuclear medicine staff must undergo a training programme from other established centres in order to be granted an ARSAC certificate.
- The low surface dose from the patient after administration and minimal urinary excretion means that it can be given as an out-patient procedure. Good laboratory practice and use of appropriate shielding and devices are required (Cremonesi *et al.* 2006; Jodal 2009).
- Immediate adverse events to the rituximab dose are predictable and manageable using antihistamines, antipyretics or, rarely, steroids. Reduction of the infusion rate can also reduce side-effects. Although it is rare to have an adverse event following the Zevalin infusion, it is important to have the appropriate drug treatment available when administering the dose and to monitor the patient.
- The Zevalin dose should be administered intravenously over 10 minutes via a 0.22 μm low protein binding filter, within 4 hours of completion of the prior rituximab infusion.

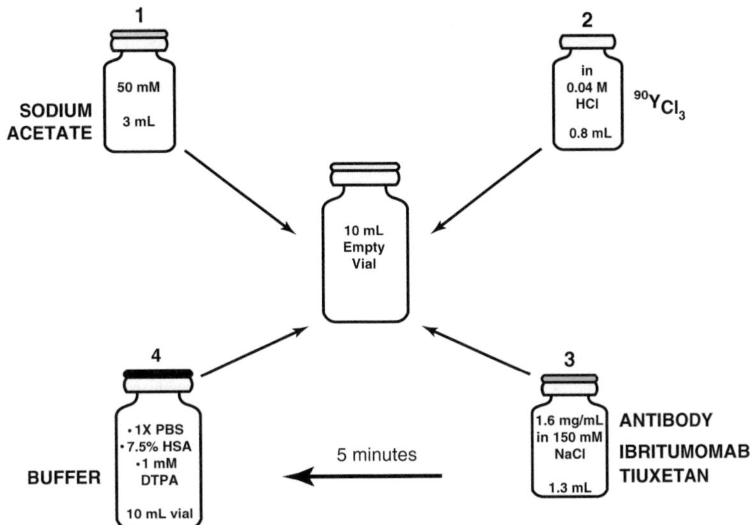

Figure 19.4 Schematic of Zevalin dose preparation.

Kit preparation The kit consists of four vials (Figure 19.4):

- Empty reaction vial
- Sodium acetate buffer vial
- Ibritumomab tiuxetan vial
- Formulation buffer.

Radiolabelled peptides

Peptides play an important role in the regulation of many physiological processes. Peptide receptors are overexpressed in numerous cancers, providing a specific target for radiolabelled peptides for therapy; referred to as peptide receptor radiation therapy (PRRT).

For PRRT, the cancer must express the corresponding peptide receptor in high density and ideally homogeneously; determined by prior *in vivo* receptor diagnostic scintigraphy. Since many peptides act through multiple peptide receptor subtypes, the radiolabelled peptide subtype must match the subtype expressed by the tumour.

Generally, PRRT is administered intravenously. However, peptides do not usually cross the blood–brain barrier and PRRT has been applied locally for the treatment of glioma and medulloblastomas. Owing to their smaller size, peptides diffuse more easily into the tumour environment, clear more rapidly from the bloodstream and have relatively lower immunogenicity compared to antibodies. The *in-vivo* binding affinity, biodistribution and pharmacokinetics of the radiolabelled peptide are determined not only by the peptide molecule but also by the bifunctional chelator used with the radionuclide as this contributes significantly to the overall size and molecular weight of the final product.

The key established PRRT is for the palliative treatment of neuroendocrine tumours (NETs), performed primarily by targeting tumours expressing the neuropeptide receptors, somatostatin (SST) and cholecystokinin (CCK2). The SST receptors, particularly sst2 subtype are expressed in a variety of cancers, especially gastroenterohepatic (GEP) NETs such as carcinoids and gastrinomas. Radiolabelled CCK2 analogues such as minigastrin are also being investigated in medullary thyroid cancer (MTC) (Béhé, Behr 2002; Mather *et al.* 2007).

The main radiolabelled peptides in clinical use are the SST analogues, resulting in a better quality of life by symptomatic improvements and a high overall response rate (for an average duration of 30 months) with a mean 50% tumour regression in 25% of patients (Waldherr *et al.* 2001; Teunissen *et al.* 2004; Van Essen *et al.* 2007). The main SST analogues used are; Tyr^3-octreotide (TOC), Tyr^3-Thr^3-octreotide (TATE) and lanreotide (LAN) (Kwekkeboom *et al.* 2005). For radiolabelling purposes, they are coupled to a bifunctional chelator, usually DOTA, and are thus referred to as DOTATOC, DOTATATE and DOTALAN (also known as 'MAURITIUS'), respectively.

These SST analogues have differing SST receptor subtype binding affinities, for example DOTATATE has 9 times higher affinity for type 2 (sst2) than DOTATOC, DOTALAN has more sst5 affinity (Reubi *et al.* 2000). They have been radiolabelled mainly with ^{90}Y and ^{177}Lu (depending on the required path length properties in relation to the tumour size, see Table 19.1) A radionuclide combination has been proposed for enhanced therapeutic effects (de Jong *et al.* 2005) or the use of ^{177}Lu for relapsed disease (after previous ^{90}Y therapy) because of less associated nephrotoxicity (Forrer *et al.* 2005).

^{111}In-DTPA-octreotide has been suggested for therapy, demonstrating favourable symptom control but with only partial remissions reported (Anthony *et al.* 2002; Valkema *et al.* 2002; Virgolini *et al.* 2002) and SST analogues radiolabelled with alpha emitters have also been explored (Norenberg *et al.* 2006; Nayak *et al.* 2007).

No SST analogues are currently available as licensed products but some are in commercial development; for example Onalta (edotreotide) (previously known as Octreother (SMT-487)), a SST analogue for radiolabelling with ^{90}Y product, is presently being developed for marketing by Molecular Insight Pharmaceuticals Inc., and a ^{177}Lu SST analogue by Covidean. New SST analogues with different affinities are also being investigated.

Practical points

- The radionuclide and the peptide (pre-conjugated to DOTA) are usually purchased separately and the preparation requires radiolabelling by radiopharmacy.
- The specific activity of the radionuclide is important in determining the amount of peptide to use.
- ^{90}Y dose ranges between 1 GBq for intra-arterial administration to 3–7.4 GBq for intravenous administration labelled with 100–250 micrograms of SST analogue. Three administrations are routinely given before assessment.
- ^{177}Lu dose ranges between 1.85 and 7.4 GBq with 100–400 micrograms of SST analogue. Four administrations are routinely given before assessment.
- Administrations (up to 12) are given at 4- to 8-week intervals.
- Renal toxicity is a dose-limiting factor of radiolabelled SST analogues. Before administration of radiolabelled SST analogues, patients must receive 1–2 litres of amino acid solution (e.g. Vamin) infused over 2–4 hours, starting a minimum of 30 minutes before therapy, to prevent renal toxicity by inhibiting renal tubular reabsorption (Behr *et al.* 1998; Jamar *et al.* 2003; Rolleman *et al.* 2003).
- Imaging after administration (using bremsstrahlung) may be used to check for localisation.

Several other peptide receptors overexpressed specifically on tumours have also been discovered with the corresponding peptide radiopharmaceuticals being developed. These include neurotensin, neurokinin (NK)1, substance P, vasoactive intestinal peptide (VIP), bombesin/gastrin releasing peptide (GRP), glucagon-like peptide (GLP), alpha-melanocyte-stimulating hormone (α-MSH), integrin α(v)β3, and neuropeptide Y (NPY). Preclinical studies and some clinical studies show a great potential for PRRT in the future by using a range of beta-emitting radioisotopes to embrace the wide range of tumour types expressing receptors, such as brain tumours, breast, prostate, ovary, thyroid, gut, renal cell, pancreatic and small cell lung cancers (de Jong *et al.* 2003; Reubi *et al.* 2005; de Visser *et al.* 2008).

Some cancers (e.g. breast, gastrointestinal stromal tumours (GISTs)) may also express multiple peptide receptors, forming the basis of multireceptor targeting radiotherapy using two or more radiolabelled peptides. This approach could lead to an increased therapeutic dose to the tumour and possibly overcome receptor heterogeneity.

Phosphorus-32

Phosphorus-32 (as sodium orthophosphate or sodium phosphate) has been used as a therapeutic radiopharmaceutical since the 1960s but is now seldom used within the UK, particularly as there is currently no

UK licensed product (Vinjamuri, Ray 2008). It is a pure beta emitter, is presented as a solution ready for injection, and may be administered orally or intravenously with similar bioavailability.

The main use of ^{32}P is for the treatment of myeloproliferative disorders (i.e. polycythaemia rubra vera, chronic leukaemias, essential thrombocythaemia) as ^{32}P concentrates highly in rapidly proliferating cells such as bone marrow. It can be used when failure or significant side-effects are experienced with standard management, though not widely due to the reported incidence of leukaemia (10–15%) (Berlin 2000). Depending on the disease type, stage and body surface area, 37–555 MBq is administered with repeated administrations and dose increments at 3-month intervals if required.

Phosphorus-32 can also be used for the palliation of metastatic bone pain due to being incorporated into the bone matrix by direct substitution for stable phosphates but its use has been succeeded by newer agents as it is commonly associated with a higher incidence and degree of myelotoxicity (due to uptake in bone marrow cells), although no significantly higher incidence has been demonstrated (Baumann *et al.* 2005; Silberstein 2000, 2005).

Local administration of ^{32}P (in colloidal/chromic form, now unavailable) has been employed via the intra-articular route for radionuclide synovectomy (Dunn *et al.* 2005) and the intracavity/interstitial route for the treatment of craniopharyngiomas, astrocytomas, lung, uterine and ovarian cancers (dose 370–740 MBq) (Tulchinsky, Eggli 1994).

Strontium-89 and samarium-153

A number of radiopharmaceuticals have a role in the palliation of metastatic bone pain (commonly associated with advanced carcinomas of the prostate, breast and lung) after the failure of conventional chemotherapy or hormonal therapy and there are a number of metastatic bone sites. Such radiopharmaceuticals directly target the bone to irradiate the tumour–bone microenvironment, resulting in a cytotoxic effect. Compared to external beam radiotherapy, they are associated with lower gastrointestinal toxicity and less irradiation of normal tissues (Bolger *et al.* 1993). Analgesic effects also occur by allowing the re-calcification of osteolytic lesions and inhibiting the release of pain mediators.

For unknown reasons, bone-targeted radiopharmaceuticals are retained by bone surrounding osteoblastic metastases for a longer period than by normal bone, providing an enhanced target-to-non-target ratio and enhancing therapeutic efficacy. Owing to biochemical methods of localisation, a prophylactic role occurs with these radiopharmaceuticals by treatment of previously non-detected sites. A delay in the onset of action occurs after intravenous administration that is dependent upon the half-life of the radionuclide. Therefore, radionuclide therapy should not be used when bone pain is caused by spinal cord compression or if there is a risk of fracture. Multiple doses of either radiopharmaceutical can be given without significant toxicity, but repeated use may have reduced efficacy. Treatment should not be repeated within 90 days depending on the previous response and haematological status.

Strontium-89 as ^{89}Sr chloride (Metastron) behaves metabolically as a calcium analogue, being incorporated preferentially in increased sites of hydroxyapatite bone mineral turnover as associated with bone metastases. Samarium-153 as ^{153}Sm-lexidronam pentasodium (Quadramet), also known as ^{153}Sm-EDTMP (ethylenediaminetetramethylene phosphonic acid), binds to the surface of hydroxyapatite by chemisorption.

Because of the differing half-lives, energies and associated tissue range of the particular radioisotope, the radiopharmaceutical used can be tailored to the number and size of metastases and expected survival of the patient. Therefore, patients with a short life expectancy would receive a short-half-life therapy. The energy of the particle is an important factor because the dose to the bone marrow depends on the range of penetration of particles into the bone marrow from the radioactivity deposited on the bone surface. Other reasons for choice include availability and cost.

Few randomised trials have compared the different available radiopharmaceuticals. Comparisons are difficult because of the unpredictable individual response to therapy, but comparative reviews have found no substantial difference between them in the palliative efficacy with regard to overall (45–92%) and complete response (10–30%) or myelotoxicity

Table 19.3 Comparison of physical characteristics and response of radiopharmaceuticals used for the palliation of bone pain

Radiopharmaceutical[a]	Dose	Half-life (days)	Max. energy (MeV)[b]	Max. range in tissue (mm)	Mean range in tissue (mm)	Time to response	Duration of response
^{32}P-Phosphate	185–450 MBq	14.3	1.71 β	8.5	3.0	5–14 days	2–4 months
^{89}Sr chloride	150 MBq	50.5	1.46 β	7.0	2.4	2–4 weeks	3–6 months
^{153}Sm-EDTMP	37M Bq/kg	1.9	0.81 β	4.0	0.6	2–7 days	2–4 months
^{186}Re-HEDP	1.4 GBq	3.8	1.07 β	5.0	1.1	2–7 days	2–4 months
^{188}Re-HEDP	2.5–3.3 GBq	0.7	2.12 β	10.0	2.7–3.1	2–7 days	2–6 months
^{117m}Sn-DTPA	2–10 MBq/kg	13.6	0.16 (EC)	0.3	–	2–8 days to 2–4 weeks	NA
^{223}Ra chloride	50 kBq/kg	11.4	5.78 α	100 μm	–	NA	NA

[a] EDTMP = ethylenediaminetetramethylene phosphonic acid; HEDP = hydroxyethylidene diphosphonate; DTPA = diethylenetriamine pentaacetic acid.
[b] β = beta particle emitter, EC= conversion electron emitters, α =alpha particle emitter.
Compiled from IAEA-TECDOC-1549, April 2007.

(Bauman *et al.* 2005; Baczyk *et al.* 2007; IAEA 2007; Liepe, Kotzerke 2007). See Table 19.3.

^{153}Sm-particulate hydroxyapatite (PHYP) has demonstrated clinical benefit as a synovectomy agent (O'Duffy *et al.* 1999).

Practical points

- The nuclides are available as ready-to-inject solutions.
- They can be administered in an out-patient setting.
- Prior diagnostic ^{99m}Tc-bone scintigraphy is required to demonstrate uptake and confirm bone pain sites correspond to uptake.
- Haematological toxicity is expected following administration. Blood counts should be monitored, 2 weeks after administration, for at least 8 weeks.
- Calcium therapy should be discontinued at least 2 weeks before administration of ^{89}Sr chloride.
- If not incorporated into bone, ^{89}Sr chloride is predominantly excreted via the kidneys in urine with some biliary excretion into excreta. The patient must be advised to follow rigorous hygiene precautions, particularly in the first 5 days following administration.
- Initial bone pain flare may occur for 2–3 days after administration, treatable with analgesics.
- Imaging after administration (using bremsstrahlung) may be used to check for localisation.

Other beta-emitting therapeutic radiopharmaceuticals

Many other radiopharmaceuticals are available for clinical use or are currently in the development or assessment stage with a number of the wide range of beta-emitting radioisotopes. This will enable a better choice of therapy agent for the patient by having alternative options with different energies and thus path lengths to suit the type and extent of disease. The more prominent radionuclides with an ever-increasing clinical role are rhenium-Re, rhenium-188 and lutetium-177, with rising applications with holmium-166 and, in time, copper-67 and copper-Cu (see Tables 19.4 and 19.5).

Table 19.4 Physical properties of less commonly used beta particle-emitting radionuclides for therapy

Radionuclide		Half life	Max. β energy (MeV)	Max. range in tissue (mm)	Suitable gamma emission (MeV) for imaging (% abundance)
Rhenium-188	^{188}Re	17.0 hours	2.12	10.4	0.155 (15%)
Holmium-166	^{166}Ho	1.1 days	1.85	9.0	0.081 (6.7%)
Copper-67	^{67}Cu	2.58 days	0.58	2.1	0.185 (42%)
Copper-64	^{64}Cu	12.7 hours	0.57	<1.0	β^+ (656KeV)[a]
Dysprosium-165	^{165}Dy	2.3 hours	1.29	5.9	0.095(3.6%)
Erbium-169	^{169}Er	9.5 days	0.34	1.0	–
Gold-198	^{198}Au	2.7 days	0.96	3.6	0.41 (96%)

[a] β^+ = positron for PET imaging.

Table 19.5 Examples of other beta-emitting radiopharmaceuticals for radionuclide therapy (in various stages of development and assessment)

Radionuclide	Ligand[a]	Clinical indication	References
^{186}Re	Etidronate	Metastatic bone pain	Siberstein (2000)
	HEDP	Metastatic bone pain	Liepe, Kotzerke (2007)
	Lipid nanoparticles	Head and neck tumours, ovarian	Wang *et al.* (2008), Zavaleta *et al.* (2008)
	Sulfide	Synovectomy (medium-sized joints)	Kavakli *et al.* (2008)
^{188}Re	HEDP	Metastatic bone pain	Liepe, Kotzerke (2007)
	DMSA(V)	Medullary thyroid cancer	Blower *et al.* (1998)
	Lipiodol	Hepatocellular cancer	Bernal *et al.* (2008)
	Tin colloid	Synovectomy	Shukla *et al.* (2007)
	Antibodies (various)	e.g. Leukaemia, melanoma	De Decker *et al.* (2008), Dadachova *et al.* (2008), Koenecke *et al.* (2008)
^{177}Lu	EDTMP	Metastatic bone pain	Ando *et al.* (1998)
	Hydroxyapatite	Synovectomy	Chakraborty *et al.* (2006)
		Metastatic liver cancer	Chakraborty *et al.* (2008)
^{166}Ho	Macroaggregates	Synovectomy	Kraft *et al.* (2007)
	Chitosan antibodies (various)	Hepatocellular cancer	Sohn *et al.* (2009)
		Multiple myeloma	Giralt *et al.* (2003)

(continued overleaf)

Table 19.5 *(continued)*

Radionuclide	Ligand[a]	Clinical indication	References
^{64}Cu	ATSM	Hypoxic tumours	Lewis (2000)
^{169}Er	Citrate	Synovectomy (interdigital)	Gumpel *et al.* (1979)
^{117m}Sn	DTPA	Metastatic bone pain	Srivastava *et al.* (1998)
^{165}Dy	FHMA	Synovectomy	Barnes *et al.* (1994)

[a] HEDP = hydroxyethylidenebisphosphonate; DMSA(V) = dimercaptosuccinic acid, pentavalent; EDTMP = ethylenediaminetetramethylene phosphonic acid; ATSM = diacetyl-bis(N^4-methylthiosemicarbazone; DTPA = diethylenetriamine pentaacetic acid; FHMA = ferric hydroxide macroaggregates

Alpha emitters

Alpha emitters are attractive for therapeutic applications because they have a potential to effect a complete cure. The high LETs of alpha-emitting radionuclides make them highly toxic with a high relative biological effectiveness (RBE) while also being effective in killing radioresistant hypoxic cells (oxygen independent) resulting in a lower likelihood of treatment failure.

For optimal therapeutic efficacy, alpha emitters need to be targeted to the cell by direct administration or indirectly via a carrier (e.g. liposomes) in order to deposit energy close to the cell nucleus owing to the short range but, as a result, less administered activity is required. As there is little cross-fire, distribution must be highly homogeneous with respect to tumour volume in order to uniformly irradiate all tumour cells. The short half-lives of alpha emitters also impose restrictions on clinical use based on the biological half-life of the radiolabelled complex and for localisation time. The use of ligands radiolabelled with alpha emitters is therefore best suited for the treatment of rapidly accessible cancer cells, haematological disorders such as leukaemia or specific target structures in body cavities/compartments, small-volume tumours or minimal residual disease. Despite minimal irradiation of surrounding normal healthy tissue, regulatory concerns and stringent precautions required for safe handling and administration both contribute to the limitations on the use alpha emitters.

The main alpha emitters with therapeutic applications are listed in Table 19.6. To date, only a few clinical studies have been undertaken with alpha emitters, with many in the pre-clinical stage. Examples include ^{213}Bi, ^{212}Bi (possibly administered as ^{212}Pb), ^{211}At and ^{225}Ac radiolabelled monoclonal

Table 19.6 Physical properties of alpha-emitting radionuclides suitable for therapy

Radionuclide		Half-life	Mean alpha energy (MeV)	Mean range in tissue (μm)	Suitable gamma emission (MeV) for imaging
Bismuth-212	^{212}Bi	60.5 minutes	7.8	75	–
Astatine-211	^{211}At	7.2 hours	6.76	60	–
Bismuth-213	^{213}Bi	46 minutes	8.32	84	–
Actinium-225	^{225}Ac	10 days	6.83	61	–
Terbium-149	^{149}Tb	4.15 hours	3.97	27	–
Radium-223	^{223}Ra	11.4 days	27.4	50	0.154

antibodies and peptides (Behr *et al.* 1999; McDevitt *et al.* 2000; Wesley *et al.* 2004; Andersson *et al.* 2005; Brechbiel 2007; Zalutsky *et al.* 2008). Radium-223 chloride (Alpharadin) has been used for the palliation of bone metastases (Table 19.3) (Nilsson *et al.* 2007).

Auger and Internal conversion electrons

Currently, no Auger or internal conversion electron emitters are employed in routine clinical use but the feasibility of a number of agents is being assessed in a few clinical studies.

Auger electron emitters have a high LET, resulting in a high radiotoxicity and high relative biological efficacy (RBE) similar to that of alpha particles when targeted into the tumour cell and incorporated into the cell nucleus, in close proximity to DNA. For optimal efficacy, tight binding to DNA is required as the highest energy deposition occurs in a 1–2 nm sphere (the diameter of a double-strand DNA helix is 2 nm). Besides the direct effect of Auger electrons on DNA double strands, further DNA damage occurs by indirect irradiation from targeted neighbouring cells – a 'bystander effect'.

The use of Auger emitters is suited for small tumours such as individual cells, micrometastases or small clusters of tumour cells. However, in contrast to alpha emitters, Auger emitters or internal conversion electron emitters have low toxicity outside the cell nucleus.

The main radionuclides of clinical interest, with a significant percentage of Auger emissions and suitable half-lives, are listed in Table 19.7. Other low-energy electron emitters with potential include rhodium-103m, cobalt-58, antimony-119, holmium-161, osmium-189m, thulium-167 and platinum-195m.

Tin-117m [^{117m}Sn] has been investigated for metastatic bone pain (Table 19.3). Iodine-125 has been explored for therapy of hyperthyroidism and thyroid cancer and [^{125}I]mIBG for adrenergic tumours, but with demonstration of only modest therapeutic efficacy and no significant advantage compared with iodine-^{131} therapy (Roa *et al.* 1998). One promising approach employs radiolabelled DNA intercalators such as the thymidine analogue, 5-[$^{125/123}$I]iodo-2′-deoxyuridine (IUdR/IdUrd). Therapeutic efficacy has been demonstrated when administered during the synthesis phase of the cell cycle, infused over several days (to cover 2–3 cell cycles and overcome rapid *in-vivo* degradation) and in conjunction with endogenous thymidine inhibition. The direct, intratumoral or locoregional application of [$^{125/123}$I]IUdR has been used for brain tumours and intra-arterial injection in liver metastases from colorectal cancer (Kassis *et al.* 1996; Mariani *et al.* 1996). ^{111}In-DTPA-trastuzumab (modified with peptides harbouring the nuclear localisation sequence) (Costantini *et al.* 2007) and ^{111}In-octreotide (20–160 GBq) are also being evaluated (Virgolini *et al.* 2002). Auger-radiolabelled internalising radiopharmaceuticals have been explored, such as monoclonal antibodies that are directed against a tumour-associated antigen to elicit antigen internalisation upon binding; for example

Table 19.7 Physical properties of Auger electron or conversion electron emitters suitable for therapy

Radionuclide		Half-life	Max. particle energy (keV) and type	Max. range in tissue	Suitable gamma emission (MeV) for imaging (% abundance)
Iodine-125	^{125}I	60.5 days	0.7–30 Auger	10 nm	36 (7%)
Iodine-123	^{123}I	13.3 hours	0.7–30 Auger	10 nm	159 (83%)
Indium-111	^{111}In	3.0 days	0.5–25 c.e.	0.6 mm	171 (90%) 245 (89%)
Tin-117m	^{117m}Sn	13.6 days	127, 152 c.e.	0.3 mm	159 (83%)

c.e. = internal conversion electron.

^{125}I-radiolabelled humanised CC49 monoclonal antibody (HuCC49deltaC(H)2) in recurrent and metastatic colorectal cancer patients (Xiao *et al.* 2005). Other DNA or mRNA targeting approaches include use of radiolabelled steroid hormones, growth factors, and oligonucleotides including aptamers and antisense oligonucleotides.

The future

The availability (and large-scale production feasibility) of radionuclides with suitable therapeutic properties based on their physical and chemical characteristics, biological factors, methods for their selective targeting and *in-vivo* distribution and, importantly, economics, have remained the main obstacles to radiopharmaceutical therapy assuming a wider role. Huge progress has been made in all these areas, providing an impetus for further research to develop more licensed, simple to prepare radiopharmaceuticals.

The effectiveness of therapeutic radiopharmaceuticals may be maximised in the future. This could involve using a 'cocktail' of different energies or types of emitters, using a 'cocktail' of antibodies or peptides that target different antigens or receptors within the same tumour, using as part of integrated therapy with other treatment modalities such as chemotherapy, external beam radiotherapy or administration of higher amounts of activity.

The use of Auger and alpha-emitting radionuclides for therapy is hopeful for the future but the main challenge is their ability to target DNA directly. Future progress will be aided with developments in transfection of non-thyroid tumours with the sodium/iodide symporter, providing a selective therapy approach with ^{125}I, ^{123}I or ^{211}At. Alternatively, by the use of radio-targeted gene therapy to promote cellular uptake, any radiopharmaceutical may be developed further (Willhauck *et al.* 2007).

The discovery of new targets and the development of pre-targeting approaches (to overcome low target abundance and slow pharmacokinetics of large radiolabelled molecules) and new immunoconjugates (e.g. antibodies, diabodies (di-ScFv), aptamers) with the ability to attach to any suitable radionuclide, using existing or new radiolabelling strategies, will contribute greatly to the advancing role of therapy using radiopharmaceuticals, bringing a resurgence of interest and enormous clinical benefit.

Acknowledgments

The authors would like to acknowledge the kind help of the following people: Dr. John Buscombe, Consultant in Nuclear Medicine, Royal Free Hospital, London; Dr. Gopinath Gnanasegaran, Consultant in Nuclear Medicine, Guy's and St. Thomas' Hospital, London; Dr. Tom Wheldon, Department of Radiation Oncology, CRC Beatson Laboratories, Glasgow; Dr. Thomas Murray, Radiopharmacist, Western Infirmary in Glasgow; and Thomas Erskine Hilditch.

References

Allisy-Roberts P, ed. (2002). *Medical and Dental Guidance Notes*. York: Institute of Physics and Engineering in Medicine, 129.

Andersson H *et al.* (2005). ^{211}At radioimmunotherapy of subcutaneous human ovarian cancer xenografts: evaluation of relative biologic effectiveness of an alpha-emitter in vivo. *J Nucl Med* 46(12): 2061–2067.

Ando A *et al.* (1998). ^{177}Lu-EDTMP: a potential therapeutic bone agent. *Nucl Med Commun* 19(6): 587–591.

Anthony LB *et al.* (2002). Indium-111-pentetreotide prolongs survival in gastroenteropancreatic malignancies. *Semin Nucl Med* 2: 123–132.

ARSAC (2006) Notes for Guidance, section 7, Conception, Pregnancy and Breastfeeding. Didcot: ARSAC.

Baczyk M *et al.* (2007). ^{89}Sr versus ^{153}Sm-EDTMP: comparison of treatment efficacy of painful bone metastases in prostate and breast carcinoma. *Nucl Med Commun* 28 (4): 245–250.

Barnes CL *et al.* (1994). Intra-articular radiation treatment of rheumatoid synovitis of the ankle with dysprosium-165 ferric hydroxide macroaggregates. *Foot Ankle Int* 15(6): 306–310.

Bauman G *et al.* (2005). Radiopharmaceuticals for the palliation of painful bone metastasis – a systemic review. *Radiother Oncol* 75(3): 258–270.

Béhé M, Behr TM (2002). Cholecystokinin-B (CCK-B)/gastrin receptor targeting peptides for staging and therapy of medullary thyroid cancer and other CCK-B receptor expressing malignancies. *Biopolymers* 66(6): 399–418.

Behr TM *et al.* (1998). Reducing the renal uptake of radiolabelled antibody fragments and peptides for diagnosis and therapy: present status, future prospects and limitations. *Eur J Nucl Med* 25: 201–212.

Behr TM *et al.* (1999). High-linear energy transfer (LET) alpha versus low-LET beta emitters in radioimmunotherapy of solid tumors: therapeutic efficacy and dose-limiting toxicity of ^{213}Bi- versus ^{90}Y-labeled CO17-1A Fab′ fragments in a human colonic cancer model. *Cancer Res* 59 (11): 2635–2643.

Berlin NI (2000). Treatment of the myeloproliferative disorders with ^{32}P. *Eur J Haematol* 65(1): 1–7.

Bernal P *et al.* (2008). International Atomic Energy Agency-sponsored multination study of intra-arterial rhenium-188-labeled lipiodol in the treatment of inoperable hepatocellular carcinoma: results with special emphasis on prognostic value of dosimetric study. *Semin Nucl Med* 38 (2): S40–45.

Blower PJ *et al.* (1998). Pentavalent rhenium-188 dimercaptosuccinic acid for targeted radiotherapy: synthesis and preliminary animal and human studies. *Eur J Nucl Med* 25(6): 613–621.

Bolger JJ *et al.* (1993). Strontium-89 (Metastron) versus external beam radiotherapy in patients with painful bone metastases secondary to prostatic cancer: preliminary report of a multicenter trial. UK Metastron Investigators Group. *Semin Oncol* 20(3 Suppl 2): 32–33.

Brechbiel MW (2007). Targeted alpha-therapy: past, present, future? *Dalton Trans* 43: 4918–4928.

Chakraborty S *et al.* (2006). Preparation and preliminary biological evaluation of ^{177}Lu-labelled hydroxyapatite as a promising agent for radiation synovectomy of small joints. *Nucl Med Commun* 27(8): 661–668.

Chakraborty S *et al.* (2008). Preparation and preliminary studies on ^{177}Lu-labeled hydroxyapatite particles for possible use in the therapy of liver cancer. *Nucl Med Biol* 35 (5): 589–597.

Clarke SEM (1991). Radionuclide therapy of the thyroid. *Eur J Nucl Med* 18: 984–991.

Costantini DL *et al.* (2007). ^{111}In-Labeled trastuzumab (Herceptin) modified with nuclear localization sequences (NLS): an Auger electron-emitting radiotherapeutic agent for HER2/neu-amplified breast cancer. *J Nucl Med* 48(8): 1357–1368.

Cremonesi M *et al.* (2006). Radiation protection in radionuclide therapies with ^{90}Y-conjugates: risks and safety. *Eur J Nucl Med Mol Imaging* 33(11): 1321–1327.

Dadachova E *et al.* (2008). Pre-clinical evaluation and efficacy studies of a melanin-binding IgM antibody labeled with ^{188}Re against experimental human metastatic melanoma in nude mice. *Cancer Biol Ther* 7(7): 1116–1127.

De Decker M *et al.* (2008). In vitro and in vivo evaluation of direct rhenium-188-labeled anti-CD52 monoclonal antibody alemtuzumab for radioimmunotherapy of B-cell chronic lymphocytic leukemia. *Nucl Med Biol* 35(5): 599–604.

de Jong M *et al.* (2003). Radiolabelled peptides for tumour therapy: current status and future directions. Plenary lecture at the EANM 2002. *Eur J Nucl Med Mol Imaging* 30(3): 463–469.

de Jong M *et al.* (2005). Combination radionuclide therapy using ^{177}Lu- and ^{90}Y-labeled somatostatin analogs. *J Nucl Med* 46(Suppl 1): 13S–17S.

de Visser M *et al.* (2008). Update: improvement strategies for peptide receptor scintigraphy and radionuclide therapy. *Cancer Biother Radiopharm* 23(2): 137–157.

Dunn AL *et al.* (2005). Leukemia and P32 radionuclide synovectomy for hemophilic arthropathy. *J Thromb Haemost* 3 (7): 1541–1542.

EANM (2002). *Guidelines for I-131 Ethiodised Oil (Lipiodol) Therapy*. Vienna: European Association of Nucear Medicine.

Fellinger K *et al.* (1952). Local therapy of rheumatic disease. *Wien Z Inn Med* 33: 351–363.

Fielding SL *et al.* (1991). Dosimetry of [^{131}I] metaiodobenzylguanidine for treatment of resistant neuroblastoma: results of a UK study. *Eur J Nucl Med* 18: 308–316.

Forrer F *et al.* (2005). Treatment with ^{177}Lu-DOTATOC of patients with relapse of neuroendocrine tumors after treatment with ^{90}Y-DOTATOC. *J Nucl Med* 46(8): 1310–1316.

Gaze MN *et al.* (1995). Multi-modality megatherapy with [^{131}I] meta-iodobenzylguanidine, high dose melphalan and total body irradiation with bone marrow rescue: feasibility study of an innovative strategy for advanced neuroblastoma. *Eur J Cancer* 31A: 252–256.

Giralt S *et al.* (2003). ^{166}Ho-DOTMP plus melphalan followed by peripheral blood stem cell transplantation in patients with multiple myeloma: results of two phase 1/2 trials. *Blood* 102(7): 2684–2691.

Goin *et al.* (2005). Treatment of unresectable hepatocellular carcinoma with intrahepatic yttrium 90 microspheres: a risk stratification analysis. *J Vasc Interv Radiol* 16(2Pt1): 195–203.

Goldenberg DM (2004). Therapeutic use of radiolabelled antibodies: haematopoietic tumours. In: Ell PJ, Gambhir SS, eds. *Nuclear Medicine in Clinical Diagnosis and Treatment*, 3rd edn. London: Churchill Livingstone, 428-434.

Gumpel JM *et al.* (1979). Synoviorthesis with erbium-169: a double-blind controlled comparison of erbium-169 with corticosteroid. *Ann Rheum Dis* 38(4): 341–343.

Hagenbeek A *et al.* (2007). ^{90}Y Ibritumomab tiuxetan (Zevalin) consolidation of first remission in advanced stage follicular non-Hodgkin's lymphoma: first results of the international randomized phase 3 First-line Indolent Trial (FIT) in 414 patients. *Blood* 110 [Abstract 643].

Hall P *et al.* (1992). Leukaemia incidence after iodine-131 exposure. *Lancet* 340: 1–4.

Hoefnagel CA (1991). Radionuclide therapy revisited. *Eur J Nucl Med* 18: 408–431.

Hoefnagel CA (1994). Metaiodobenzylguanidine and somatostatin in oncology: role in the management of neural crest tumours [Review]. *Eur J Nucl Med* 21(6): 561–581.

Hoefnagel CA *et al.* (1994). [^{131}I]MIBG as a first-line treatment in high-risk neuroblastoma patients. *Nucl Med Commun* 15: 712–717.

IAEA (2007). *Criteria for Palliation of Bone Metastases – Clinical Applications*. TecDoc-1549. Vienna: International Atomic Energy Agency. ISSBN 92-0-104507-7.

Jamar F *et al.* (2003). ^{86}Y-DOTA^{0}-D-Phe^{1}-Tyr^{3}-octreotide (SMT487): a phase 1 clinical study – pharmacokinetics, biodistribution and renal protective effect of different regimens of amino acid co-infusion. *Eur J Nucl Med Mol Imaging* 30: 510–518.

Jarløv AE *et al.* (1995). Is calculation of the dose in radioiodine therapy of hyperthyroidism worthwhile? *Clin Endocrinol (Oxf)* 43(3): 325–329.

Jodal L (2009). Beta emitters and radiation protection. *Acta Oncol* 48(2): 308–313.

Kaminski MS *et al.* (2001). Pivotal study of iodine I 131 tositumomab for chemotherapy-refractory low-grade or transformed low-grade B-cell non-Hodgkin's lymphoma. *J Clin Oncol* 19: 3918–3928.

Kassis AI *et al.* (1996). Intratumoral administration of 5-[^{123}I]iodo-2′-deoxyuridine in a patient with a brain tumor. *J Nucl Med* 37(4 Suppl): 19S–22S.

Kavakli K *et al.* (2008). Radioisotope synovectomy with rhenium186 in haemophilic synovitis for elbows, ankles and shoulders. *Haemophilia* 14(3): 518–523.

Keng GH, Sundram FX (2003). Radionuclide therapy of hepatocellular carcinoma. *Ann Acad Med Sing* 32(4): 518–534.

Koenecke C *et al.* (2008). Radioimmunotherapy with [^{188}Re]-labelled anti-CD66 antibody in the conditioning for allogeneic stem cell transplantation for high-risk acute myeloid leukemia. *Int J Hematol* 87(4): 414–421.

Kraft O *et al.* (2007). Radiosynoviorthesis of knees by means of ^{166}Ho-holmium-boro-macroaggregates. *Cancer Biother Radiopharm* 22(2): 296–302.

Kwekkeboom DJ *et al.* (2005). Overview of results of peptide receptor radionuclide therapy with 3 radiolabeled somatostatin analogs. *J Nucl Med* 46(Suppl 1): 62S–66S.

Leslie WD *et al.* (2003). A randomised comparison of radioiodine doses in Graves' hyperthyroidism. *J Clin Endocrinol Metab* 88: 978–983.

Lewandowski RJ *et al.* (2005). ^{90}Y microsphere (Therasphere) treatment for unresectable colorectal cancer metastases of the liver: response to treatment at targeted doses of 135-150 Gy as measured by [^{18}F] fluorodeoxyglucose positron emission tomography and computed tomographic imaging. *J Vasc Interv Radiol* 16 (12): 1641–1651.

Lewis JS (2000). Copper-64-diacetyl-bis(N^4-methylthiosemicarbazone): an agent for radiotherapy. *Proc Natl Acad Sci USA* 98(3): 1206–1211.

Liepe K, Kotzerke J (2007). A comparative study of ^{188}Re-HEDP, ^{186}Re-HEDP, ^{153}Sm-EDTMP and ^{89}Sr in the treatment of painful skeletal metastases. *Nucl Med Commun* 28(8): 623–630.

Luster M *et al.* (2008). Guidelines for radioiodine therapy of differentiated thyroid cancer. *Eur J Nucl Med Mol Imaging* 35(10): 1941–1959.

Mariani G *et al.* (1996). Tumor targeting by intra-arterial infusion of 5-[^{123}I]iodo-2′-deoxyuridine in patients with liver metastases from colorectal cancer. *J Nucl Med* 37 (4 Suppl): 22S–25S.

Mather SJ *et al.* (2007). Selection of radiolabeled gastrin analogs for peptide receptor-targeted radionuclide therapy. *J Nucl Med* 48(4): 615–622.

McDevitt MR *et al.* (2000). An alpha-particle emitting antibody ([^{213}Bi]J591) for radioimmunotherapy of prostate cancer. *Cancer Res* 60(21): 6095–6100.

Ming-der Y, Shaw SM (2003). Potential interference of agents on radioiodine thyroid uptake in the euthyroid rat. *J Nucl Med* 44(5): 832–838.

Nayak TK *et al.* (2007). Somatostatin-receptor-targeted α-emitting ^{213}Bi is therapeutically more effective than β^--emitting ^{177}Lu in human pancreatic adenocarcinoma cells. *Nucl Med Biol* 34(2): 185–193.

Nilsson S *et al.* (2007). Bone-targeted radium-223 in symptomatic, hormone-refractory prostate cancer: a randomised, multicentre, placebo-controlled phase II study. *Lancet Oncol* 8(7): 587–594.

Norenberg JP *et al.* (2006). ^{213}Bi-[DOTA^0, Tyr^3]octreotide peptide receptor radionuclide therapy of pancreatic tumors in a preclinical animal model. *Clin Cancer Res* 12(3Pt1): 897–903.

O'Duffy EK *et al.* (1999). Double blind glucocorticoid controlled trial of samarium-153 particulate hydroxyapatite radiation synovectomy for chronic knee synovitis. *Ann Rheum Dis* 58(9): 554–558.

Rang HP *et al.* (1990). *Rang and Dale's pharmacology.* Elsevier.

RCP (2007). Radioiodine in the management of benign thyroid disease; Clinical guidelines; Report of a Working Party 2007. London: Royal College of Physicians.

Reubi JC *et al.* (2000). Affinity profiles for human somatostatin receptor subtypes SST1-SST5 of somatostatin radiotracers selected for scintigraphic and radiotherapeutic use. *Eur J Nucl Med* 27: 273–282.

Reubi JC *et al.* (2005). Candidates for peptide receptor radiotherapy today and in the future. *J Nucl Med* 46(Suppl 1): 67S–75S.

Roa WH *et al.* (1998). Targeted radiotherapy of multicell neuroblastoma spheroids with high specific activity [^{125}I] meta-iodobenzylguanidine. *Int J Radiat Oncol Biol Phys* 41(2): 425–432.

Rolleman EJ *et al.* (2003). Safe and effective inhibition of renal uptake of radiolabelled octreotide by a combination of lysine and arginine. *EurJ Nucl Med Mol Imaging* 30: 9–15.

Shukla J *et al.* (2007). Characterization of Re-188-Sn microparticles used for synovitis treatment. *Int J Pharm* 338(1-2): 43–47.

Silberstein EB (2000). Systemic radiopharmaceutical therapy of painful osteoblastic metastases [Review]. *Semin Radiat Oncol* 10(3): 240–249.

Silberstein EB (2005). Teletherapy and radiopharmaceutical therapy of painful bone metastases. *Semin Nucl Med* 35(2): 152–158.

Sohn JH *et al.* (2009). Phase II study of transarterial holmium-166-chitosan complex treatment in patients with a single, large hepatocellular carcinoma. *Oncology* 76(1): 1–9.

Sridama V, DeGroot LJ (1989). Treatment of Graves disease and the course of ophthalmopathy. *Am J Med* 87: 70–73.

Srivastava SC *et al.* (1998). Treatment of metastatic bone pain with tin-117m stannic diethylenetriaminepentaacetic acid: a phase I/II clinical study. *Clin Cancer Res* 4(1): 61–68.

Surks MI *et al.* (2004). Subclinical thyroid disease: scientific review and guidelines for diagnosis and management. *JAMA* 291: 228–238.

Teunissen J *et al.* (2004). Quality of life in patients with gastro-entero-pancreatic tumors treated with [^{177}Lu-DOTA^0,Tyr^3]octreotate. *J Clin Oncol* 22: 2724–2729.

Tulchinsky M, Eggli DF (1994). Intraperitoneal distribution imaging prior to chromic phosphate (P-32) therapy in ovarian cancer patients. *Clin Nucl Med* 19(1): 43–48.

Uğur O *et al.* (2008). Radiosynovectomy: current status in the management of arthritic conditions [Editorial]. *Nucl Med Commun* 29(9): 755–758.

Valkema R *et al.* (2002). Phase I study of peptide receptor radionuclide therapy with [In-DTPA]octreotide: the Rotterdam experience. *Semin Nucl Med* 32(2): 110–122.

Van Essen M *et al.* (2007). Peptide receptor radionuclide therapy with radiolabelled somatostatin analogues in patients with somatostatin receptor positive tumours. *Acta Oncol* 46(6): 723–734.

Vinjamuri S, Ray S (2008). Phosphorus-32: the forgotten radiopharmaceutical? *Nucl Med Commun* 29(2): 95–97.

Virgolini I *et al.* (2002). Experience with indium-111 and yttrium-90-labeled somatostatin analogs [Review]. *Curr Pharm Des* 8(20): 1781–1807.

Vose JM *et al.* (2000). Multicenter phase II study of iodine-131 tositumomab for chemotherapy-relapsed/refractory low-grade and transformed low-grade B-cell non-Hodgkin's lymphomas. *J Clin Oncol* 18: 1316–1323.

Waldherr C *et al.* (2001). The clinical value of [^{90}Y-DOTA]-DPhe^{1}-Tyr^{3}-octreotide (^{90}Y-DOTATOC) in the treatment of neuroendocrine tumours: a clinical phase II study. *Ann Oncol* 12: 941–945.

Wang SX *et al.* (2008). Intraoperative ^{186}Re-liposome radionuclide therapy in a head and neck squamous cell carcinoma xenograft positive surgical margin model. *Clin Cancer Res* 14(12): 3975–3983.

Wesley JN *et al.* (2004). Systemic radioimmunotherapy using a monoclonal antibody, anti-Tac directed toward the alpha subunit of the IL-2 receptor armed with the alpha-emitting radionuclides ^{212}Bi or ^{211}At. *Nucl Med Biol* 31(3): 357–364.

Willhauck MJ *et al.* (2007). Application of ^{188}rhenium as an alternative radionuclide for treatment of prostate cancer after tumor-specific sodium iodide symporter gene expression. *J Clin Endocrinol Metab* 92(11): 4451–4458.

Wiseman GA *et al.* (2002). Ibritumomab tiuxetan radioimmunotherapy for patient with relapsed or refractory non-Hodgkin lymphoma and mild thrombocytompenia: a phase II multicenter trial. *Blood* 99: 4336–4342.

Witzig TE *et al.* (2002a). Randomised controlled trial of yttrium-90-labelled ibritumomab tiuxetan radiotherapy versus rituximab immunotherapy for patients with relapsed or refractory low-grade, follicular, or transformed B-cell non-Hodgkin's lymphoma. *J Clin Oncol* 20: 2453–2463.

Witzig TE *et al.* (2002b). Treatment with ibritumomab tiuxetan radioimmunotherapy in patients with rituximab-refractory follicular non-Hodgkin's lymphoma. *J Clin Oncol* 20: 3262–3269.

Xiao J *et al.* (2005). Pharmacokinetics and clinical evaluation of ^{125}I-radiolabeled humanized CC49 monoclonal antibody (HuCC49deltaC(H)2) in recurrent and metastatic colorectal cancer patients. *Cancer Biother Radiopharm* 20(1): 16–26.

Yumoto Y *et al.* (1985). Hepatocellular carcinoma detected by iodized oil. *Radiology* 154: 19–24.

Zalutsky MR *et al.* (2008). Clinical experience with alpha-particle emitting ^{211}At: treatment of recurrent brain tumor patients with ^{211}At-labeled chimeric antitenascin monoclonal antibody 81C6. *J Nucl Med* 49 (1): 30–38.

Zavaleta CL *et al.* (2008). Imaging of ^{186}Re-liposome therapy in ovarian cancer xenograft model of peritoneal carcinomatosis. *J Drug Target* 16(7): 626–637.

Further reading

ARSAC (2006). *Notes for Guidance on the Clinical Administration of Radiopharmaceuticals and Use of Sealed Radioactive Sources*. Didcot: ARSAC. http://www.arsac.org.uk/notes_for_guidance/index.htm (accessed 30 June 2010).

Bodei L *et al.* (2008). EANM procedure guideline for treatment of refractory metastatic bone pain. *Eur J Nucl Med Mol Imaging* 35(10): 1934–1940.

Brechbiel MW (2007). Targeted alpha-therapy: past, present, future? *Dalton Trans* 43: 4918–4928.

Forrer F *et al.* (2007). Neuroendocrine tumors. Peptide receptor radionuclide therapy [Review]. *Best Pract Res Clin Endocrinol Metab* 21(1): 111–129.

Giammarile F *et al.* (2008). EANM procedure guidelines for 131I-meta-iodobenzylguanidine (131I-mIBG) therapy. *Eur J Nucl Med Mol Imaging* 35(5): 1039–1047.

International Commission on Radiological Protection. (2004). Release of patients after therapy with unsealed radionuclides. *Ann ICRP* 34(2):v–vi, 1–79.

Kassis AI, Adelstein SJ (2005). Radiobiologic principles in radionuclide therapy [Review]. *J Nucl Med* 46(Suppl 1): 4S–12S.

Luster M *et al.* (2008). Guidelines for radioiodine therapy of differentiated thyroid cancer. *Eur J Nucl Med Mol Imaging* 35(10): 1941–1959.

Otte A *et al.* (2009). Radiolabeled immunotherapy in non-Hodgkin's lymphoma treatment: the next step. *Nucl Med Commun* 30(1): 5–15.

Royal College of Physicians. (2007). *Radioiodine in the Management of Benign Thyroid Disease; Clinical Guidelines*. Report of a Working Party 2007 for the Royal College of Physicians. London: Royal College of Physicians.

Tennvall J, Brans B (2007). EANM procedure guideline for 32P phosphate treatment of myeloproliferative diseases. *Eur J Nucl Med Mol Imaging* 34(8):1324–1327. Erratum in: *Eur J Nucl Med Mol Imaging* 2007 Aug; 34(8):1328.

20

Formulation of radiopharmaceuticals

James R Ballinger

Introduction

Most radiopharmaceuticals are administered by intravenous injection and so must be sterile and apyrogenic. The challenge is to prepare them in this state while working against the physical half-life of the radionuclide and dealing with radiation protection issues. In this chapter we will first consider ^{99m}Tc products and other radiometals prepared in a similar manner, then other products.

Many of these products are prepared from 'kits'. A kit is a vial that contains all the non-radioactive components necessary for formation of a radiometal complex in high yield upon the addition of the radiotracer. There have been efforts made to develop kits for ^{123}I labelling, but all currently available kits are for radiometals. The kit contents, which are manufactured in bulk, are usually lyophilised and kept in quarantine by the manufacturer until all testing, including sterility and apyrogenicity, has been completed and the batch is released for use. As long as the radiotracer is sterile and is added under aseptic conditions, the resultant product can be used clinically without further sterilisation or sterility testing. This process is ideal for use with short lived radiolabels.

It is a general principle of pharmaceutical formulations, particularly for intravenous use, that every component should be both necessary and present in the optimal quantity. However, commercial considerations sometimes conflict with this ideal. The first generation of ^{99m}Tc kits introduced in the 1970s contained only the active ingredient and reducing agent in a nitrogen atmosphere. As stability problems were recognised and addressed, many kits were reformulated with antioxidant stabilisers in the 1980s. However, there have been relatively few changes in formulation since then, largely due to the cost of relicensing the product. Adding an antioxidant or changing the size of the vial will only be done if absolutely necessary or if it is commercially favourable. For example, there are different formulations of mertiatide (MAG3) in Europe and the USA (Hung 1992). The US formulation, which was introduced later, is much more robust (higher activity limit, longer shelf-life, less restrictive preparation parameters), but it has not been introduced in Europe.

Most kits consist of a lyophilised mixture of all the non radioactive ingredients. Preparation of a ^{99m}Tc radiopharmaceutical involves addition of the required activity of ^{99m}Tc pertechnetate in an appropriate volume of saline to the kit. Although this looks like simple reconstitution, it is classified as manufacturing since it involves the formation of a new chemical species (albeit not in quantities measurable by standard techniques of chemical analysis), not merely a change in physical state.

Kit formulations: technetium

The objective of a kit for labelling with ^{99m}Tc is to produce the desired complex quickly and in high yield while minimising side reactions as shown in Figure 20.1.

The properties of an ideal kit for labelling with ^{99m}Tc include: single-vial formulation; >95% radiochemical purity achieved within 10 minutes at room temperature; the complex is stable for 12 hours post labelling; both the kit and labelled product can be stored at room temperature; and the shelf-life of the kit is at least 1 year. It is evident that many kits do not meet this ideal.

The Summary of Product Characteristics (SPC or SmPC, also known as product monograph, technical leaflet, or package insert) will list the components of the kit. However, under current regulations the quantities need only be stated for the active ingredient, making it difficult to compare formulations directly.

Components

Active ingredient

The active ingredient, which is to be labelled with ^{99m}Tc, is also called the ligand, targeting agent, or final intermediate. It must be synthesised to current Good Manufacturing Practices (cGMP) standards because it remains in solution in the final product and is administered to the patient. Changes in European legislation requiring GMP synthesis led to several products being discontinued by their manufacturers as no longer financially viable. The active ingredient is generally present in a large excess over the stoichiometric amount of radioactive complex formed.

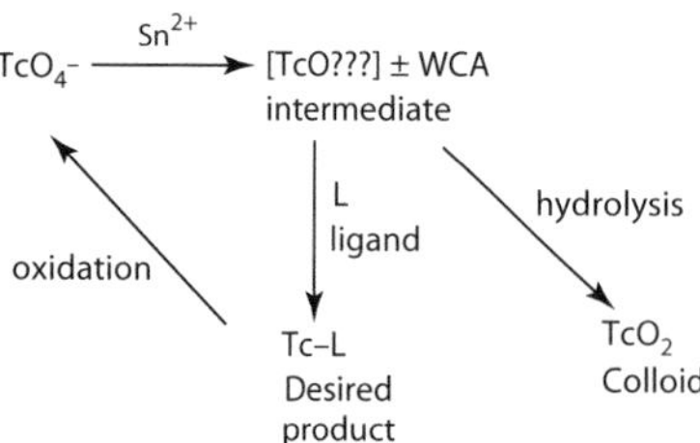

Figure 20.1 Schematic representation of the chemistry taking place following the addition of [^{99m}Tc]pertechnetate to a kit. L, ligand; WCA, weak chelating agent.

The stability of the active ingredient is one factor in the shelf-life of the kit prior to labelling. Thiols, which are susceptible to oxidation, can be protected as a benzoyl ester, as in the MAG3 kit; the ester is cleaved by heat during the labelling process. Similarly, the sestamibi kit contains 2-methoxyisobutyl isonitrile (MIBI) as a crystalline copper tetrafluoroborate salt for reasons of stability, ease of handling, and aesthetics (free isonitriles have a pungent odour).

Reducing agent

Pertechnetate, the chemical form of ^{99m}Tc eluted from the generator, is very stable and unreactive, and can only form salts. Technetium-99m must be reduced from its +7 oxidation state in order to form a complex with the active ingredient. Stannous chloride is the most common reducing agent, though some manufacturers use stannous fluoride or stannous tartrate. Tin is popular because it is water soluble, effective at room temperature, and has low toxicity. However, the stannous ion is quite easily oxidised and correct formulation of the kit is critical to maintain the tin in its active, reduced state.

The quantity of Sn(II) must be sufficient to reduce ^{99m}Tc for labelling but should not be entirely consumed as residual Sn(II) contributes to stability post labelling. Conversely, an excess of Sn(II) can lead to the formation of reduced-hydrolysed ^{99m}Tc colloid as an impurity (Figure 20.1). Kits that contain low quantities of Sn(II) tend to be sensitive to the quantity and 'quality' of pertechnetate added (see below). Typically, kits contain 10–500 μg stannous chloride (0.05–2.5 μmol). Since the maximum activity of ^{99m}Tc added to a kit is ~20 GBq (1 nmol), it can be seen that there is a vast excess of reductant (50 : 1 in the worst case).

Antioxidant stabiliser

Many kits contain an antioxidant stabiliser to maintain reducing conditions and mop up oxidants and free radicals to stabilise the complex post labelling. The presence of an antioxidant also enhances the shelf-life of the kit prior to labelling (Ballinger *et al.* 1988). Commonly used antioxidants include ascorbic acid, gentisic acid, and *para*-aminobenzoic acid (PABA) (Tofe *et al.* 1980).

^{99m}Tc-HMPAO is a special case in which an additional stabiliser is required due to the instability of the complex (expiry 30 minutes post labelling), though the agent used varies in different countries. In the UK, ^{99m}Tc-HMPAO is stabilised by addition of cobalt chloride after formation of the complex (GE Healthcare 2006a) whereas in the USA it is stabilised with methylene blue (GE Healthcare 2006b). These stabilisers lengthen the shelf-life from 30 minutes to 4–5 hours. Neither of these stabilised formulations is licensed for use in leukocyte labelling. Another special case is ^{99m}Tc-tetrofosmin, in which, counter intuitively, air is added to the vial immediately after reconstitution to stabilise the complex (Murray *et al.* 2000).

Inert atmosphere

An inert atmosphere of nitrogen or argon gas also helps maintain reducing conditions to stabilise the kit both before and after labelling. It is important to minimise the entry of air into the vial during the labelling process and withdrawal of doses. Tofe and Francis (1976) compared the relative effectiveness of antioxidants and inert atmosphere in stabilising ^{99m}Tc-diphosphonate complexes (Figure 20.2).

Weak chelating agent

Some kits contain a weak chelating agent (WCA) that stabilises the reduced ^{99m}Tc as an intermediate prior to formation of the final complex. Some textbooks refer to the WCA as a catalyst since it is not consumed. The presence of a WCA is particularly important if the formation of the final complex is slow. The WCA can also minimise the formation of reduced hydrolysed ^{99m}Tc colloid at alkaline pH. The quantity of the active ingredient can be minimised, reducing both the risk of toxicity and the expense of manufacturing the kit. Examples of WCAs include gluconate and sulfosalicylate in the tetrofosmin kit, citrate in the sestamibi kit, and tartrate in the MAG3 kit.

Buffer

The pH is critical for formation of the desired complex. An extreme example of this is dimercaptosuccinic acid (DMSA), which forms a trivalent complex at acidic pH and pentavalent complex under alkaline conditions. These complexes have completely different biological characteristics and clinical applications (Blower *et al.* 1991).

Most kits are adjusted to the correct pH during the manufacturing process by addition of acid or base prior to lyophilisation, although some contain a buffer. Some active ingredients are not stable at labelling pH. For example, bicisate (ECD) is supplied as a two-vial kit, the second vial containing a phosphate buffer to bring the ligand to neutral pH immediately prior to labelling. Similarly, sulfide colloid kits

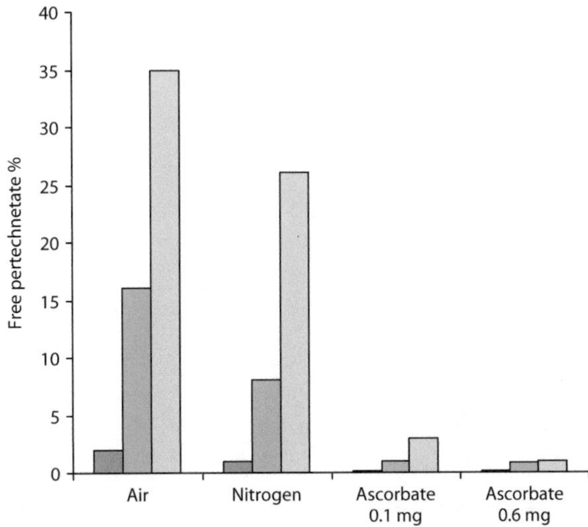

Figure 20.2 Comparison of the effects of inert atmosphere and antioxidants on release of free pertechnetate from ^{99m}Tc-HEDP as a function of time. Key to bars: dark blue bars, 0 hours; medium blue, 6 hours; pale blue, 24 hours. Adapted from Tofe and Francis (1976).

generally involve two additional vials or prefilled syringes, first to lower the pH for the labelling reaction then to raise the pH to make it suitable for injection and stop further growth of the colloidal particles.

Solubiliser/surface active agent

Some kits, particularly those based on colloids or particles, may require a surfactant to maintain the particulate dispersion. Examples include poloxamer 238 in the albumin nanocolloid kit, native albumin in the macroaggregated albumin kit, and gelatin in the rhenium sulfide colloid kit.

Some active ingredients are poorly soluble in water and a surfactant is required to solubilise the ligand, such as cyclodextrin in the teboroxime kit. In some cases the need for a surfactant can be avoided by choice of a salt of the active ingredient or by using extremely small quantities.

Bulking agent

The presence of an inert chemical bulking agent such as mannitol, inositol, lactose, or dextrose preserves pharmaceutical elegance during the lyophilisation process and results in a reproducible and visible plug. This agent is not involved in the labelling reaction. However, poor choice of bulking agent can be detrimental to the stability of the product, as in the case of the HMPAO formulation where sodium chloride was used as a bulking agent, only to be found later to destabilise the complex (Ballinger, Gulenchyn 1991).

Bacteriostat

Bacteriostats are rarely present in ^{99m}Tc kits, both because they are not necessary for products with a shelf-life of <12 hours and because most bacteriostats would interfere with the labelling chemistry. Indeed, the residue from peroxide-containing alcohols used to sanitise the exterior of kit vials has been found to destroy the ^{99m}Tc MAG3 complex (Stringer *et al.* 1997). One formulation of mebrofenin contains methyl and propyl parabens as bacteriostats and the kit has an expiry of 18 hours (Bracco Diagnostics 2007).

The formulations of some common radiopharmaceuticals are presented in Table 20.1 together with the roles of the individual components.

Table 20.1 Composition of selected commercially available kits for labelling with ^{99m}Tc

Product (alternative name, trade name; manufacturer)	Component	Quantity (mg)	Quantity (μmol)	Role[a]	Activity limit; nmol range
Albumin nanocolloid (Nanocoll; GEHC)[b]	Albumin nanocolloid	0.5	N/A	AI	5.5 GBq; 0.6–2.3 nmol
	Stannous chloride dihydrate	0.2	0.9	Red	
	Poloxamer 238	2.0	–	Susp	
	Disodium phosphate	0.5	–	Buf	
	Sodium phytate	0.25			
	Glucose	15.0	–	Bulk	
Albumin nanocolloid (SentiScint; Medi-Radiopharma)	Albumin nanocolloid	1.0	N/A	AI	2.2 GBq; 0.2–0.8 nmol
	Stannous chloride dihydrate	0.2	0.9	Red	
	Sodium/disodium phosphate	1.0	–	Buf	
	Glucose	15.0	–	Bulk	

(continued)

Table 20.1 *(continued)*

Product (alternative name, trade name; manufacturer)	Component	Quantity (mg)	Quantity (μmol)	Role[a]	Activity limit; nmol range
Bicisate (ECD, Neurolite; Lantheus, IBA)[c]	Ethyl cysteinate dimer dihydrochloride	0.3	0.8	AI	3.7 GBq; 0.4–1.5 nmol
	Stannous chloride dihydrate	0.024	0.1	Red	
	Disodium EDTA dihydrate	0.12	0.32	WCA	
	Disodium phosphate heptahydrate	4.1	–	Buf	
	Monosodium phosphate monohydrate	0.46	–	Buf	
	Mannitol	8.0	–	Bulk	
Depreotide (Neospect; IBA)	Depreotide trifluoroacetate	0.047	0.035	AI	1.8 G Bq; 0.2–0.7 nmol
	Stannous chloride dihydrate	0.05	0.22	Red	
	Sodium glucoheptonate dihydrate	75.0	280	WCA	
	Disodium EDTA dihydrate	0.1	0.27	WCA	
	Sodium iodide	10.0	–		
Exametazime (HMPAO, Ceretec; GEHC, ROTOP, Polatom)	HMPAO	0.5	1.9	AI	1.1 GBq; 0.1–0.4 nmol
	Stannous chloride dihydrate	0.0076	0.034	Red	
	Sodium chloride	4.5	–	Bulk	
Hynic-TOC (Tektroyd; Polatom)[c]	Hynic-Tyr-octreotide	0.02	0.017	AI	2.2 GBq; 0.2–0.8 nmol
	Stannous chloride	0.04	0.18	Red	
	Tricine	50.0	280	Colig	
	EDDA	5.0	28	Colig	
	Disodium phosphate	12.5	–	Buf	
	Mannitol	10.0	–	Bulk	
Macroaggregated albumin (MAA, Covidien)	Macroaggregated albumin	2.0	N/A	AI	3.7 GBq; 0.4–1.5 nmol
	Stannous chloride	0.17	0.8	Red	
	Sodium acetate	1.27	–	Buf	
	Sodium chloride	13.5	–		

(continued overleaf)

Table 20.1 *(continued)*

Product (alternative name, trade name; manufacturer)	Component	Quantity (mg)	Quantity (μmol)	Role[a]	Activity limit; nmol range
Macroaggregated albumin (IBA)	Macroaggregated albumin	2.0	N/A	AI	3.7 GBq; 0.4–1.5 nmol
	Stannous chloride dihydrate	0.2	0.9	Red	
	Albumin	7.0	–	Susp	
	Sodium chloride	8.7	–		
Macroaggregated albumin (Draximage)	Macroaggregated albumin	2.5	N/A	AI	5.2 GBq; 0.5–2.0 nmol
	Stannous chloride dihydrate	0.1	0.4	Red	
	Albumin	5.0	–	Susp	
	Sodium chloride	1.2	–		
Mebrofenin (Cholediam; Mediam)	Mebrofenin	40.0	100	AI	3.7 GBq; 0.4–1.5 nmol
	Stannous chloride dihydrate	0.6	2.7	Red	
Mertiatide (MAG3; Covidien-EU)	Betiatide	1.0	2.7	AI	1.1 GBq; 0.1–0.4 nmol
	Stannous chloride dehydrate	0.04	0.2	Red	
	Disodium tartrate dihydrate	16.9	75	WCA	
Mertiatide (MAG3; Covidien-USA)	Betiatide	1.0	2.7	AI	3.7 GBq; 0.4–1.5 nmol
	Stannous chloride dihydrate	0.2	0.9	Red	
	Disodium tartrate dihydrate	40.0	180	WCA	
	Lactose monohydrate	20.0	–	Bulk	
Medronate (MDP; GEHC)	Sodium medronate	6.25	28	AI	18.5 GBq 1.9–7.2 nmol
	Stannous fluoride	0.34	2.2	Red	
	Sodium p-aminobenzoate	2.0	–	Stab	
Medronate (MDP; Draximage)	Sodium medronate	10.0	44	AI	18.5 GBq 1.9–7.2 nmol
	Stannous chloride	1.1	4.9	Red	
	p-Aminobenzoic acid	2.0	–	Stab	

(continued)

Table 20.1 *(continued)*

Product (alternative name, trade name; manufacturer)	Component	Quantity (mg)	Quantity (μmol)	Role[a]	Activity limit; nmol range
Oxidronate (HDP; Covidien)	Sodium oxidronate	3.0	14	AI	7.4 GBq; 0.7–2.8 nmol
	Stannous chloride	0.24	1.1	Red	
	Gentisic acid	0.84	–	Stab	
	Sodium chloride	30.0	–	Bulk	
Pentetate (DTPA; Covidien)	Calcium trisodium DTPA	25.0	50	AI	11.1 GBq 1.1–4.2 nmol
	Stannous chloride	0.3	1.3	Red	
	Gentisic acid		–	Stab	
	Sodium chloride		–	Bulk	
Pentetate (DTPA; Draximage)	DTPA (free acid)	20.0	50	AI	18.5 GBq 1.9–7.2 nmol
	Calcium chloride dihydrate	3.73	25	AI	
	Stannous chloride dihydrate	0.35	1.5	Red	
	p-Aminobenzoic acid	5.0	–	Stab	
Rhenium sulphide colloid (Nanocis; IBA)[c]	Rhenium sulfide	0.24	N/A	AI	5.5 GBq; 0.6–2.3 nmol
	Stannous chloride dihydrate	0.125	0.6	Red	
	Gelatin	9.6	–	Susp	
	Ascorbic acid	7.0	–	Stab	
	Sodium pyrophosphate decahydrate	0.75	1.7	WCA	
Sestamibi (Cardiolit; Lantheus, IBA, Covidien, Polatom)	$Cu(MIBI)_4BF_4$	1.0	1.7	AI	11 GBq; 1.1–4.2 nmol
	Stannous chloride dihydrate	0.075	0.33	Red	
	Sodium citrate dihydrate	2.6	8.8	WCA	
	L-Cysteine HCl monohydrate	1.0	5.7	Red	
	Mannitol	20.0	–	Bulk	
Stannous agent (GEHC)	Sodium medronate	6.8	30	AI	N/A
	Stannous fluoride	4.0	25	AI, Red	
Stannous pyrophosphate (Covidien)	Sodium pyrophosphate	11.9	45	AI	N/A
	Stannous chloride dihydrate	4.4	20	AI, Red	

(continued overleaf)

Table 20.1 *(continued)*

Product (alternative name, trade name; manufacturer)	Component	Quantity (mg)	Quantity (μmol)	Role[a]	Activity limit; nmol range
Succimer (DMSA, Renocis; IBA)	DMSA	1.0	5.5	AI	3.7 GBq; 0.4–1.5 nmol
	Stannous chloride dihydrate	0.36	1.6	Red	
	Ascorbic acid	0.7	–	Stab	
	Inositol	50.0	–	Bulk	
Succimer (DMSA; Polatom)	DMSA	1.0	5.5	AI	3.7 GBq; 0.4–1.5 nmol
	Stannous chloride dihydrate	0.34	1.5	Red	
	Ascorbic acid	0.5	–	Stab	
	Mannitol	20.0	–	Bulk	
Sulesomab (Leukoscan; Immunomedix)	Sulesomab	0.31	N/A	AI	1.1 GBq; 0.1–0.4 nmol
	Stannous chloride dihydrate	0.22	1.0	Red	
	Potassium sodium tartrate tetrahydrate	3.2	11.3	WCA	
	Sodium chloride	5.5	–	Bulk	
	Sodium acetate trihydrate	7.4	–	Buf	
	Sucrose	37.8	–	Bulk	
Tetrofosmin (Myoview; GEHC)	Tetrofosmin	0.23	0.6	AI	12 GBq; 1.2–4.6 nmol
	Stannous chloride dihydrate	0.03	0.13	Red	
	Disodium sulfosalicylate	0.32	1.2	WCA	
	Sodium D-gluconate	1.0	4.6	WCA	
	Sodium hydrogen carbonate	1.8	–	Buf	
Tin colloid (Hepatate; GEHC, Polatom)	Sodium fluoride	1.0	24	AI	3.7 GBq; 0.4–1.5 nmol
	Stannous chloride	0.15	0.8	AI, Red	
	Polyvinyl pyrrolidone	0.5	–	Susp	
	Sodium chloride	0.32	–		

[a] Component roles: AI, active ingredient; Buf, buffer; Bulk, bulking agent; Colig, coligand; Red, reducing agent; Stab, antioxidant stabiliser; Susp, suspending agent/surfactant; WCA, intermediate weak chelating agent.

[b] GEHC – GE Healthcare.

[c] Supplied as multivial kit; quantities are as in final formulation

Table 20.2 Effect of generator history on ^{99m}Tc and ^{99}Tc content of eluates

	Hours between elutions		
	2	24	72
Mole fraction of ^{99m}Tc	0.77	0.28	0.08
Ratio $^{99}Tc/^{99m}Tc$	0.3/1	2.6/1	12/1
Total atoms per GBq ^{99m}Tc	40×10^{12}	110×10^{12}	375×10^{12}
nmoles ($^{99m}Tc + ^{99}Tc$) per GBq	0.04	0.10	0.38

Stability, shelf-life; technetium 'quality' effects

A number of factors affect the stability of a ^{99m}Tc complex and thus the shelf-life of the preparation. General factors are discussed later but the two most important here are autoradiolysis and quantity of ^{99}Tc (technetium 'quality').

Autoradiolysis

Most ^{99m}Tc complexes are only moderately stable and are subject to decomposition by radiolytic species in solution. Two manoeuvres which minimise radiolysis are the presence of an antioxidant and an inert atmosphere (Tofe, Francis 1976). The production of radiolytic species is dependent upon radioactivity concentration and many kits specify a maximum concentration (Billinghurst *et al.* 1979).

Technetium quality

As discussed elsewhere, ^{99m}Tc is never totally free of 'carrier' ^{99}Tc. There is a minimum of 14% ^{99}Tc present due to branching in decay of ^{99}Mo. Thus, the theoretical maximum mole fraction of ^{99m}Tc is 0.86. This fraction continues to decrease over time after elution as ^{99m}Tc decays to ^{99}Tc (eluate history). However, the mole fraction is also affected by the time since the previous elution of the generator, as the eluate will contain all the ^{99}Tc produced by decay of ^{99m}Tc while sitting on the column (generator history). When the generator is eluted daily (i.e. with 24 hours in-growth) the mole fraction of ^{99m}Tc is 0.277 immediately after elution. In contrast, the mole fraction of ^{99m}Tc from a generator eluted on a Monday, not having been eluted since Friday, is 0.077 (Lamson *et al.* 1975). The role of generator history is illustrated in Table 20.2.

The problem is that ^{99m}Tc and ^{99}Tc are chemically identical and both will consume reducing equivalents of Sn(II) (Ballinger 2002). That is one reason for the huge excess of tin in most kits, as mentioned earlier. Most kit formulations are designed to withstand the insult of 'Monday pertechnetate', though a few do specify a maximum period of in-growth. The problem will be most evident in kits that contain a small quantity of tin. The HMPAO kit contains 7.6 μg $SnCl_2$ and it is specified that the pertechnetate used for reconstitution must be no more than 2 hours old from a generator eluted no more than 24 hours previously (GE Healthcare 2006b). The problem of Monday pertechnetate resulting in poorer labelling has also been noted with *in-vivo* red blood cell labelling used in cardiac blood pool studies.

Alternative practices

In most of the world, ^{99m}Tc kits are supplied as 10 mL vials, usually in packs of five vials. However, in some countries the more heavily used products are sold in packs of 30 vials. With the popularity of central radiopharmacies, a few products are made in larger vials for preparation of more doses at one time.

'Kit bashing' is a term applied to the practice of adding excessive quantities of ^{99m}Tc pertechnetate to a kit, much higher than the manufacturer's specification. This practice originated in the late 1980s with the introduction of the second generation of ^{99m}Tc kits, such as HMPAO, MAG3, sestamibi, and tetrofosmin, which were much more expensive than the earlier, generic kits. As we saw above, the quantity of Sn(II) in the kit far exceeds the stoichiometric requirement. In part, this is to render the kit less sensitive to pertechnetate quality. However, largely for economic reasons, some radiopharmacies have taken advantage of this in order to obtain more doses from a vial. This practice is frowned upon by the manufacturers, for obvious reasons, and by the regulatory authorities. All liability in the case of a product failure falls upon the radiopharmacy rather than the manufacturer. The physician who is responsible for the radiopharmaceutical being administered to patients must be informed of this practice.

A related practice is 'kit splitting', in which the kit contents are dissolved in saline and split into several fractions, and ^{99m}Tc pertechnetate is added to only one fraction. The other fractions are saved for labelling at a later time. This may or may not involve obtaining more doses than the manufacturer specified. For example, if the maximum activity allowed by the manufacturer would allow five doses but only one is needed, it can be argued that it would be a waste to use the entire vial for one dose. However, this practice results in two additional problems. First, the stability of the subsequent fractions might be impaired; precautions to minimise this problem include the use of saline that has been purged with nitrogen to remove dissolved oxygen, flushing the headspace of the splitting vial with nitrogen to displace air, and storing the fractions in a freezer (Ballinger 1990). Second, there is concern about the sterility of the fractions since the kit does not contain a bacteriostat.

In summary, any deviation from the manufacturer's instructions must be undertaken with caution. Some deviations are less controversial, such as extension of the shelf-life of a product post labelling, as there will be logistical as well as economic benefits. However, even something as simple as this must be validated on site rather than depending on literature data and there must be an ongoing quality assurance programme to monitor for the emergence of problems.

Kit formulations: other metals (^{111}In, $^{67/68}$Ga, ^{90}Y, ^{177}Lu)

As noted earlier, the goal is to develop a kit formulation that will result in a high level of radiochemical purity (generally >90% or >95%) without the need for purification, though this is not always achievable. In a true kit preparation, the excess ingredients remain in the final dosage form and thus must be manufactured to GMP, whereas if there is purification of the labelled product there may be some relaxation of this requirement.

Components

Active ingredient

These trivalent metals require a bifunctional macrocyclic or acyclic chelator for attachment to the targeting agent. Commonly used chelators include DTPA, DOTA, and variations thereof. These are stable and do not require protection as do thiols in some chelators for ^{99m}Tc. The choice of chelator affects the stability of the labelled product but also determines the harshness of the labelling conditions required. Furthermore, there are subtle differences between the radiometals. For example, DTPA will complex ^{90}Y within 5 minutes but requires 30 minutes to achieve a similar degree of labelling with ^{111}In. DOTA forms stronger chelates with these metals but generally requires heating for these complexes to form (Breeman *et al.* 2003; Cooper *et al.* 2006).

Buffer/weak chelating agent

Most of these radiometals are supplied in dilute HCl solution. Labelling generally takes place under mildly acidic conditions, which are achieved by addition of sodium acetate or sodium citrate acting as both buffer and weak chelating agent to prevent precipitation of the metal. If the radiometal is transferred out of its stock vial into the buffer, it is important to minimise the contact time in the syringe to avoid leaching of iron from the stainless steel needle by the acid; iron can compete for radiometal binding (Breeman *et al.* 2003). When labelling proteins it is particularly important that the buffer be added to the acidic radionuclide solution before the protein is added, to prevent denaturation of the protein. Only gentle heat can be used with proteins (up to 45°C), whereas peptides can be heated to 100°C.

Quenching/stabilising agent

Following the labelling reaction, a buffer containing EDTA is often added to chelate any unbound radiometal and direct it out of the body via the kidneys, thus reducing the radiation dose to the patient. The ^{90}Y labelling reaction with the monoclonal antibody ibritumomab tiuxetan (Zevalin) specifies a reaction time of 5 ± 1 minutes. The reaction is terminated at this point by addition of a buffer that minimises radiolysis both by dilution of the radioactivity concentration and by the presence of albumin. Some kits for labelling with radiometals contain an antioxidant to protect the complex against autoradiolysis. For example, the pentetreotide (Octreoscan) kit contains gentisic acid, and ascorbate can be added to [^{18}F]FDG, [^{123}I]IBF, and ^{64}Cu-ATSM preparations.

Stability and shelf-life

As with ^{99m}Tc, radioactivity concentration and autoradiolysis are factors in the stability and shelf-life with other radiometals, particularly with the high quantities of beta-emitters used for therapy (Salako *et al.* 1998).

General aspects

Vehicle

Most radiopharmaceuticals are formulated in an aqueous vehicle, most commonly physiological saline (0.9% w/v sodium chloride). If there are enough salts present in the formulation to render the solution near isotonic, water for injection may be used in place of saline. For ^{99m}Tc kits, bacteriostatic saline cannot be used. The MAG3 kit has been shown to be sensitive to an unknown component formed upon the exposure to light of saline in plastic ampoules (Beattie *et al.* 2008). Occasionally a co-solvent such as ethanol is required, either to increase the solubility of a lipophilic compound or as the residue from a purification method (Serdons *et al.* 2008).

Sterilisation

The most widely accepted methods of sterilisation are heat sterilisation in an autoclave and gamma irradiation. However, many products are heat labile and cannot be autoclaved. Some manufacturers autoclave [^{18}F]FDG but the formulation is critical to avoid decomposition of the product (Fawdry 2007). Although it has been commonly used for many years, sterilisation by filtration through a 0.22 μm membrane filter is less acceptable to regulatory authorities.

Bacteriostat

The most commonly used bacteriostat in long-lived radiopharmaceuticals is benzyl alcohol 10 mg/mL. However, there are concerns about the effectiveness of this bacteriostat. In addition, it can be toxic to neonates if given in quantities greater than 10 mg/kg per day (Rabiu *et al.* 2004). As mentioned earlier, bacteriostats and surface sanitising agents can be detrimental to many ^{99m}Tc complexes. Bacteriostatic saline must not be used. Furthermore, ^{111}In-oxine and other blood cell labelling reagents cannot contain a bacteriostat as it would be toxic to the cells.

Isotonicity

Isotonicity is important to avoid hypotonic lysis of red blood cells or burning upon injection due to hypertonicity. However, most radiopharmaceuticals are given as small-volume injections, so isotonicity is not critical.

pH

The pH of the product must be suitable for injection yet also maintain the stability of the product. Buffering will occur in the circulatory system, but any residue at the injection site can cause pain if the pH is extreme. It is essential that ^{123}I and ^{131}I iodide solutions be maintained at alkaline pH to avoid the release of volatile molecular iodine.

Storage temperature

Some unlabelled kits are shipped on ice and must be stored in a refrigerator for stability. Indeed, clinical trials materials may come with a data logger to prove that the cold chain was maintained. The first generation of ^{99m}Tc kits required refrigeration after labelling for reasons of stability. Although manufacturers recommend that most labelled kits be stored in the refrigerator, this is less important now since most kits contain antioxidant stabilisers that are more effective than refrigeration. However, refrigeration also helps suppress microbial growth, which can be important in multidose vials that do not contain a bacteriostat.

Some therapeutic radiopharmaceuticals containing beta-emitters are shipped frozen for stability to minimise radiolysis and dehalogenation. For example, [^{131}I]MIBG is shipped on dry ice and in its frozen state remains stable for at least 2 days post reference date;

however, once thawed it must be used within 2 hours (GE Healthcare, 2006c).

Factors that determine shelf-life

Prior to labelling, the main limitation is the stability of Sn(II) in ^{99m}Tc kits, although some other chemical components can be unstable. Storage temperature and maintenance of the inert gas atmosphere within the kit vial are important. With labelled products, a variety of factors determine shelf-life; these are detailed below.

Microbiological

Since ^{99m}Tc kits do not (indeed, usually cannot) contain a bacteriostat, their use is generally limited to 12 hours. Refrigeration is recommended to inhibit the growth of microorganisms in multidose vials. Generators must be stored in a clean environment and eluted under aseptic conditions. There is particular concern about maintaining sterility in long-lived generators such as ^{68}Ge/^{68}Ga (^{68}Ge half-life is 271 days).

Chemical stability

There can be chemical or physical alterations in the product over time, such as clumping of MAA particles and colloids or radiolytic damage to antibodies with loss of immunoreactivity (Salako *et al.* 1998).

Radiochemical purity (RCP)

The most common determinant of shelf-life is radiochemical stability, maintaining >95% or >90% labelling efficiency of the product. Radiochemical stability is affected by radioactivity concentration and pertechnetate quality, as discussed earlier. Some complexes are inherently unstable, such as ^{99m}Tc-HMPAO in its original form with an expiry time of 30 minutes, although stabilised formulations have been developed. With most products RCP gradually declines with time, eventually reaching a point where the contribution of radiochemical impurities could influence the interpretation of the study.

Radionuclidic purity

As the primary radionuclide decays, trace contamination with longer-lived radionuclides becomes significant. Examples of this include ^{125}I in ^{123}I and ^{202}Tl in ^{201}Tl.

Specific activity

As the primary radionuclide decays and the specific activity declines, the quantity of the vial contents that must be administered in order to deliver the required activity increases and at some point this quantity would produce pharmacological or toxic effects. This can be important for short-lived PET labels (e.g. ^{11}C), particularly with receptor-binding radiopharmaceuticals. In contrast, [^{18}F]FDG is relatively stable and insensitive to specific activity; with a shelf-life of 12 hours the quantity of material injected at expiry is 93 times greater than that immediately after production.

Vials and closures

Vials and closures must be of pharmaceutical quality for safety and consistency. Generally, borosilicate glass is used, though occasionally products will stick to glass. Rubber closures can also show problems of incompatibility with products. Another issue to be aware of is the potential for coring of the closure through the use of wide-bore needles, though caution must be exercised in visual inspection of products owing to the radiation exposure, particularly to the lens of the eye.

Research formulations

Although most commercial products are lyophilised, it is quite practical to prepare research formulations that are liquid or frozen. One approach is to use individual solutions of each component, which are mixed freshly and labelled. Equally, in many instances a multicomponent kit can be prepared analogously to commercial kits. The individual components are dissolved and mixed, the pH may be adjusted, then the solution is purged with nitrogen gas for a few minutes to drive out the dissolved oxygen, and aliquots are transferred into vials through a 0.22 μm membrane filter. The headspace of the vial is purged with nitrogen to displace air, then the vial is frozen and kept in that form until it is needed, when it is thawed and labelled. Early radiopharmacists did this routinely, but it is becoming a lost art.

References

Ballinger JR (1990). Preparation of [^{99m}Tc]HM–PAO. *J Nucl Med* 31: 1892.

Ballinger JR (2002). The effect of carrier on technetium-99m radiopharmaceuticals. *Q J Nucl Med* 46: 224–232.

Ballinger JR, Gulenchyn KY (1991). Alternative formulations of technetium-99m HMPAO. *Appl Radiat Isot* 42: 315–316.

Ballinger JR *et al.* (1988). Stabilization of stannous pyrophosphate kits with gentisic acid. *Nucl Med Biol* 15: 391–393.

Beattie LA *et al.* (2008). Preparation of ^{99m}Tc-MAG3: the effect on radiochemical purity of using sodium chloride injection from plastic ampoules that have been exposed to light. *Nucl Med Commun* 29: 649–653.

Billinghurst MW *et al.* (1979). Radiation decomposition of technetium-99m radiopharmaceuticals. *J Nucl Med* 20: 138–143.

Blower PJ *et al.* (1991). The chemical identity of pentavalent technetium-99m-dimercaptosuccinic acid. *J Nucl Med* 32: 845–849.

Bracco Diagnostics (2007). *CHOLETEC® Kit for the Preparation of Technetium Tc 99m Mebrofenin.* Princeton, NJ: Bracco Diagnostics Inc.

Breeman WA *et al.* (2003). Optimising conditions for radiolabelling of DOTA-peptides with ^{90}Y, ^{111}In and ^{177}Lu at high specific activities. *Eur J Nucl Med Mol Imaging* 30: 917–920.

Cooper MS *et al.* (2006). Conjugation of chelating agents to proteins and radiolabeling with trivalent metallic isotopes. *Nature Protoc* 1: 314–317.

Fawdry RM (2007). Radiolysis of 2-[^{18}F]fluoro-2-deoxy-D-glucose (FDG) and the role of reductant stabilisers. *Appl Radiat Isot* 65: 1193–1201.

GE Healthcare (2006a). *Stabilised Ceretec Kit for the preparation of Technetium [^{99m}Tc] Exametazime Injection.* Little Chalfont: GE Healthcare.

GE Healthcare (2006b). *CERETEC™ Kit for the Preparation of Technetium Tc99m Exametazime Injection.* Arlington Heights, IL: GE Healthcare.

GE Healthcare (2006c). *[^{131}I]Metaiodobenzylguanidine for Therapeutic Use.* Little Chalfont: GE Healthcare.

Hung JC (1992). Comparison of technetium-99m MAG3 kit formulations in Europe and the USA. *Eur J Nucl Med* 19: 990–992.

Lamson ML *et al.* (1975). Generator-produced ^{99m}TcO4$^-$: carrier free? *J Nucl Med* 16: 639–641.

Murray T *et al.* (2000). Technetium-99m-tetrofosmin: retention of nitrogen atmosphere in kit vial as a cause of poor quality material. *Nucl Med Commun* 21: 845–849.

Rabiu O *et al.* (2004). Preservatives can produce harmful effects in paediatric drug preparations. *Pharm Pract* 14: 101–110.

Salako QA *et al.* (1998). Effects of radiolysis on yttrium-90-labeled Lym-1 antibody preparations. *J Nucl Med* 39: 667–670.

Serdons K *et al.* (2008). The presence of ethanol in radiopharmaceutical injections. *J Nucl Med* 49: 2071.

Stringer RE *et al.* (1997). MAG3 failure due to inadvertent oxidant contamination. *Nucl Med Commun* 18: 294.

Tofe AJ, Francis MD (1976). In vitro stabilization of a low-tin bone-imaging agent (^{99m}Tc-Sn-HEDP) by ascorbic acid. *J Nucl Med* 17: 820–825.

Tofe AJ *et al.* (1980). Gentisic acid: a new stabilizer for low tin skeletal imaging agents. *J Nucl Med* 21: 366–370.

21

Principles and operation of radionuclide generators

Joao Osso and Russ Knapp

Introduction

The dependable on-demand availability of radioisotopes is a key requirement for their use in nuclear medicine. Radionuclide generators are important in-house production systems that can economically provide both diagnostic and therapeutic radioisotopes on demand in hospital-based and central radiopharmacy settings. A significant number of radionuclide generators have been developed, evaluated and discussed over the past four decades. Since there are a large number of publications on most of the generators described in this chapter, key references are provided rather then an exhaustive review of the literature. More detailed references can be found in a number of reviews on radionuclide generators (Brucer 1965; Yano, Anger 1968; Stang 1969; Lebowitz, Richards 1974; Boyd *et al.* 1984; Knapp, Butler 1984; Paras, Thiessen 1985; Boyd 1986; Mani 1987; Lambrecht, Sajjad 1988; Ruth *et al.* 1989; Knapp *et al.* 1992; Knapp, Mirzadeh 1994; Mirzadeh, Knapp 1996; Lambrecht *et al.* 1997; Mirzadeh 1998; Roesch, Knapp 2003). This chapter focuses on those radionuclide generator systems that are relevant to current clinical use or whose introduction into clinical practice is expected. In addition to generator systems that have regulatory approval for routine clinical use, many of the generators and generator radioisotope products of current interest are provided as radiochemical and used in clinical trials under physician-sponsored protocols. The regulatory issues required for approval for clinical use of radionuclide generators are also discussed. This chapter provides an overview of the well-established physical laws that govern parent–daughter relationships, the chemical processes that are used for effective separation of daughter from parent species, and a brief discussion of generator-derived radioisotopes for diagnostic and therapeutic applications.

Radionuclide generator systems provide both diagnostic and therapeutic radioisotopes, primarily for various applications in nuclear medicine and oncology. Although many parent–daughter pairs have been evaluated as radionuclide generator systems, a relatively small number of generators are currently used in routine clinical and research applications. Essentially every conceivable strategy has been explored for separation of the desired daughter radioisotopes from the parent, including sublimation, thermo chromatographic separation, solvent extraction and adsorptive column chromatography. The most widely used radionuclide generator for clinical applications is the ^{99}Mo/^{99m}Tc generator system. It is estimated that in the USA alone, over 13 million diagnostic applications are conducted with technetium-99m-labelled radiopharmaceuticals annually (National Academy Report 2009). Parallel with increasing use of unsealed therapeutic radioisotopes, primarily in nuclear medicine and oncology, recent years have witnessed an enormous increase in the development, refinement and use of generators to provide therapeutic radioisotopes. The development of therapeutic agents has paralleled the development of complementary technologies for targeting agents for therapy and in the general increased interest in the use of unsealed therapeutic radioactive sources. Key advantages in the use of radionuclide generators include reasonable costs, the convenience of obtaining the desired daughter radionuclide on demand, and availability of the daughter radionuclide in high specific activity, no-carrier-added form.

A radionuclide generator is defined as a separation system for the effective radiochemical separation of a generally much shorter-lived daughter radioisotope (i.e. from secular equilibrium) formed by continuous decay of the parent radionuclide. Use of a radionuclide generator does not require the clinical proximity to either a reactor or an accelerator production site. The desired daughter is separated from the parent radionuclide, which then generates a fresh supply of the daughter by radioactive decay. The goal is to obtain the daughter in a pure and chemically suitable form, generally for further post-separation radiolabelling of the desired radiopharmaceutical agent. Compared with the use of accelerator or nuclear reactor production facilities, radionuclide generators provide inexpensive and convenient in-house and on-demand sources for many useful radioisotopes. Generator systems have traditionally been installed in hospital-based radiopharmacies, but are now installed commonly in some countries in centralised radiopharmacies for preparation and dispensing for delivery to local or regional clinical facilities. Those generator systems which provide therapeutic radionuclides (i.e. ^{90}Y from the ^{90}Sr/^{90}Y generator) are generally installed in a central manufacturing facility or centralised radiopharmacy, because of radiation safety issues, expense and effective unit dose distribution.

Development of generators has been primarily motivated by the widening spectrum of applications of radioisotopes and radiolabelled compounds in the life sciences, in particular for diagnostic applications in nuclear medicine. More recently, however, promising applications of generator-derived therapeutic radioisotope have developed in the fields of nuclear medicine, oncology and interventional cardiology/radiology. This increasing importance of radioisotope generators has initiated an increasing resurgence of interest for production of the generator parent radioisotope, for sophisticated radiochemical separations as well as reliable technical design of the generator systems.

The tellurium-132 ($t_{1/2} = 3.26$ days)/iodine-132 ($t_{1/2} = 1.39$ hours) generator was the first practical system (Winsche *et al.* 1951) and subsequent development of the molybdenum-99/technetium-99m generator was a major breakthrough which provided a practical source of a diagnostic radioisotope with attractive availability and radionculidic properties (Stang 1969). This key advance represented an important opportunity to provide a useful diagnostic radioisotope in a clinical setting, although the usefulness for clinical use was not realised and demonstrated until some time later (Richards 1960). Since those early days of generator development, the availability of this generator has provided the radiopharmaceutical basis for diagnostic nuclear medicine. In addition, other generator systems provide a variety of single-photon-emitting radioisotope daughters for tissue imaging by single photon and PET imaging, first-pass ventriculography, etc. A variety of useful generators that are used in routine clinical practice for therapy have been developed, including those which provide beta- and alpha-emitting daughters. In general, these developments have paralleled developments and progress in radiopharmaceutical targeting, methods for chemical attachment and progress in instrumentation.

The wide use of the ^{99}Mo/^{99m}Tc generator system in nuclear medicine is a key example that has been crucial for more than two decades for the hospital or central radiopharmacy preparation of a wide variety of diagnostic agents for applications in nuclear medicine and oncology. It is estimated that over 35 000 diagnostic procedures (>13 million studies per year) are currently conducted daily in the USA with ^{99m}Tc-labelled radiopharmaceuticals. This reliance on the availability of ^{99m}Tc clearly underscores the crucial importance of reliable ^{99}Mo production (see IAEA 2008; National Academy Report 2009; Ruth 2009) and processing facilities to ensure the uninterrupted supply of the generator parent radioisotope required for fabrication of these generator systems.

In addition to the reviews published on radionuclide generators mentioned earlier, other authors have addressed a variety of technical issue including parent–daughter half-lives (Finn *et al.* 1983), reactor-produced generators (Mani 1987), accelerator-produced generators (Lambrecht 1983), ultra short-lived generator-produced radioisotopes (Guillaume, Brihaye 1986), generator-derived positron-emitting radionuclides (Knapp *et al.* 1994), and clinical applications (Knapp, Butler 1984; Knapp, Mirzadeh 1994). In addition to the generators discussed here in a clinical context, it should be noted that a significant number of additional generator pairs exist. Other parent–daughter radionuclide pairs continued to be identified and discussed whose potential feasibility for generators has not yet been previously considered, such as the ^{230}U/^{226}Th system (Morgenstern *et al.* 2008)) and ^{227}Ac/^{227}Th/^{223}Ra (Bruland *et al.* 2006) generator systems which provide useful daughter radionuclides for therapeutic applications.

Principles

Equations of radioactive decay and growth

The exponential laws of radioactive-series decay and growth of radionuclides were first formulated by Rutherford and Soddy in 1902 (Rutherford, Soddy 1902) to explain the thorium series of radionuclides. Equations were first derived (Bateman 1910) to describe the decay and growth of naturally occurring actinium, uranium and thorium series. The main equations that describe the radioactive decay and growth of radionuclides are described here. The activity A of a given radioactive isotope is related to the number of atoms N at a time t, where λ represents the radionuclide decay constant:

$$A = \lambda N \qquad (21.1)$$

The decay of the radionuclide follows the exponential law:

$$N = N_0 e^{-\lambda t} \qquad (21.2)$$

$$A = A_0 e^{-\lambda t} \qquad (21.3)$$

where N and A represent respectively the number of atoms and the activity at time t, and N_0 and A_0 are the quantities when $t = 0$. The half-life, $t_{1/2}$, is the time required to reduce the activity of a radionuclide to 50% of its initial value, and is related to λ according to:

$$t_{1/2} = \frac{\ln 2}{\lambda} = \frac{0.6935}{\lambda} \qquad (21.4)$$

Considering the generation of a second radioisotope (daughter, denoted by subscript 2) from the decay of a first radioisotope (parent, denoted by subscript 1), the equations that describe the decay of the parent and growth and decay of the daughter are:

$$-\left(\frac{\partial N_1}{\partial t}\right) = \lambda_1 N_1 \qquad (21.5)$$

$$N_1 = N_1^0 e^{-\lambda_1 t} \qquad (21.6)$$

$$-\left(\frac{\partial N_2}{\partial t}\right) = \lambda_1 N_1 - \lambda_2 N_2 \qquad (21.7)$$

$$\left(\frac{\partial N_2}{\partial t}\right) = \lambda_2 N_2 - \lambda_1 N_1^0 e^{-\lambda_1 t} \qquad (21.8)$$

Solving the equations above and assuming that when $t = 0$, $N_2^0 = 0$ (i.e. no second radioisotope present), the result will be:

$$N_2 = \frac{\lambda_1}{\lambda_2 - \lambda_1} N_1^0 (e^{-\lambda_1 t} - e^{-\lambda_2 t}) \qquad (21.9)$$

or

$$A_2 = \frac{\lambda_2}{\lambda_2 - \lambda_1} A_1^0 (e^{-\lambda_1 t} - e^{-\lambda_2 t}) \qquad (21.10)$$

Equation (21.10) allows calculation of the activity of the daughter radionuclide at any time t knowing the initial activity of the parent, and is used to estimate the daughter activity in growth curves illustrated for a variety of daughter radionuclides beginning with Figure 21.2, illustrated for the ^{99}Mo/^{99m}Tc generator.

Depending on the relation of the half-lives between the parent and the daughter radionuclides, three types of equilibria can arise.

Transient equilibrium

In this case, the half-life of the parent is longer than the daughter half-life, i.e., $t_{1/2(1)} > t_{1/2(2)}$ or $\lambda_1 < \lambda_2$. Equation (21.9) can be simplified when $t \gg t_{1/2(2)}$, i.e. the decay time is much longer than the daughter half-life:

$$N_2 = \frac{\lambda_1}{\lambda_2 - \lambda_1} N_1^0 (e^{-\lambda_1 t}) = \frac{\lambda_1}{\lambda_2 - \lambda_1} N_1 \quad (21.11)$$

or

$$\frac{A_1}{A_2} = 1 - \frac{\lambda_1}{\lambda_2} \quad (21.12)$$

After reaching the equilibrium, the daughter decays with the half-life of the parent and the activity of the daughter will be higher than the parent activity. A typical example of a radioactive pair that forms a transient equilibrium is ^{99}Mo ($t_{1/2} = 66.0$ h)/^{99m}Tc ($t_{1/2} = 6.0$ h), which is of utmost importance in nuclear medicine.

Secular equilibrium

In this case, the half-life of the parent is much longer than the daughter half-life, i.e. $t_{1/2(1)} \gg t_{1/2(2)}$ or $\lambda_1 \ll \lambda_2$. When the radioactive equilibrium is achieved, equation (21.9) can be simplified to:

$$N_2 \lambda_2 = N_1 \lambda_1 \quad (21.13)$$

or

$$A_2 = A_1 \quad (21.14)$$

In this equilibrium, the daughter activity is the same as the parent activity. A classical example of secular equilibrium is the ^{90}Sr ($t_{1/2} = 30.0$ y)/^{90}Y ($t_{1/2} = 64.0$ h) radioactive pair, which is the route for the preparation of a very useful no-carrier-added (n.c. a.) radionuclide, ^{90}Y, for use in therapy.

No equilibrium

In this case, the half-life of the parent is shorter than the daughter half-life, i.e. $t_{1/2(1)} < t_{1/2(2)}$ or $\lambda_1 > \lambda_2$. There is no application of this equilibrium for preparing an applicable radionuclide generator system. The time (t_{max}) required for reaching the maximum activity of the daughter nuclide is given by:

$$t_{max} = \frac{1}{\lambda_2 - \lambda_1} \ln \frac{\lambda_2}{\lambda_1} \quad (21.15)$$

A practical graphical representation of these concepts illustrating, for example, daughter activity levels for four successive repeated generator elution/in-growth cycles, is shown in Figure 21.1. Such curves can be constructed for any parent/daughter radionuclide pair using standard software, and several such curves are subsequently included in this chapter,

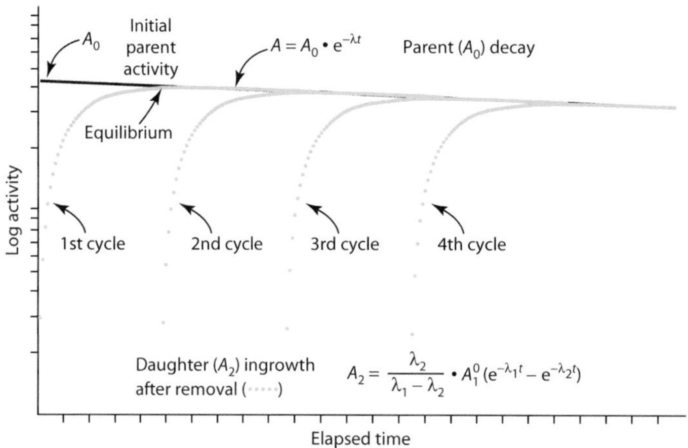

Figure 21.1 Graphical illustration of the activity levels during four repeated daughter radionuclide elution/in-growth cycles of a radionuclide generator system.

which include elution of: ^{99m}Tc (Figure 21.2), the short-lived ^{81m}Kr daughter (Figure 21.3), and ^{68}Ga from the long-lived ^{68}Ge parent (Figure 21.4).

Radionuclide separation techniques

One of the main concepts behind the preparation of a suitable radionuclide generator system is the selection of a proper and adequate separation method between the parent and daughter radionuclides. To assemble a feasible generator, there must be important differences in chemical and/or physical properties between these two elements, in order to allow the isolation of the desired daughter radionuclide with a high separation yield and a low contamination from the parent radionuclide. Several methods have been employed, such as chemical (chromatographic system: ion exchange (IE) and extraction column (EC); solvent extraction (SE); membrane extraction (ME); electrochemical deposition (ED); precipitation (PT) and physical (sublimation (SB); distillation (DT); gas evolution (GE); thermochromatography (TC)). Table 21.1 summarises the radionuclide separation techniques that being employed in the main generator systems.

Chromatographic systems

This is the most commonly used technique for manufacturing generators because of its simplicity and easy-to-use design. Basically, the generator contains one or more columns loaded with a chromatographic material that can perform the chemical separation between the parent and daughter radionuclide. This material is usually an ion-exchange (IE) or a modified inert support material that is treated with an organic solvent, bringing to the material a solvent extraction property (EC).

The early ion-exchange materials were natural zeolites, but currently used materials are synthetic, and can be either inorganic or organic. The most commonly used inorganic ion-exchange material is alumina (Al_2O_3), which has a defined capacity for several anions, such as molybdate, and the best example of this application is the $^{99}Mo/^{99m}Tc$ generator. At acidic pH, $^{99}MoO_4{}^{2-}$ (Mo(VI)) is strongly adsorbed into a small column containing few grams of acidic alumina, ^{99}Mo decays to ^{99m}Tc, while the daughter $^{99m}TcO_4{}^-$ (Tc(VII)) can be easily eluted with Cl^--containing solution, such as isotonic saline solution (0.9% NaCl). The retention order for these anions in alumina is molybdate > chloride > pertechnetate. Commercial ion-exchange resins are also employed in the assembling of radionuclide generators. An example is the use of cation exchange

Table 21.1 Examples of parent/daughter radionuclide separation techniques used for key radionuclide generator systems

Radionuclide generator	Separation techniques[a]
$^{99}Mo/^{99m}Tc$ (high specific activity ^{99}Mo)	Alumina-based IE
$^{99}Mo/^{99m}Tc$ (low to medium specific activity ^{99}Mo)	Gel type IE; SB; SE
$^{44}Ti/^{44}Sc$	IE, EC, SE
$^{113}Sn/^{113m}In$	EC
$^{81}Rb/^{81m}Kr$	IE, GE
$^{195}Hg/^{195m}Au$	IE, EC
$^{178}W/^{178}Ta$	IE
$^{191}Os/^{191}mIr$	IE
$^{52}Fe/^{52m}Mn$	IE
$^{82}Sr/^{82}Rb$	IE, EC
$^{62}Zn/^{62}Cu$	IE
$^{68}Ge/^{68}Ga$	IE
$^{72}Se/^{72}As$	PT, DT
$^{90}Sr/^{90}Y$	IE, SE, ME, ED
$^{188}W/^{188}Re$	Alumina IE, gel IE, TC
$^{166}Dy/^{166}Ho$	IE
$^{225}Ac/^{213}Bi$	IE, EC
$^{224}Ra/^{212}Pb/^{212}Bi$	IE, GE
$^{230}U/^{226}Th$	SE
$^{103}Ru/^{103m}Rh$	IE

[a] Ion exchange (IE); extraction column (EC); solvent extraction (SE); membrane extraction (ME); electrochemical deposition (ED); precipitation (PT); sublimation (SB); distillation (DT); gas evolution (GE); thermochromatography (TC).

resins, such as Dowex 50W X4, commonly used for the $^{90}Sr/^{90}Y$ generators. While the $^{90}Sr^{2+}$ is strongly adsorbed in the resin, the ^{90}Y daughter is readily eluted with a complexing agent solution, such as EDTA.

The main disadvantage of this kind of generator is the effect of radiolysis on the exchanger material, particularly with organic resins, or the organic solvent used to prepare the extraction column. These effects can be minimised if the parent is removed from the column following elution of the daughter, and stored before loading onto another batch of exchanger. An alternative approach is the use of an exchanger where the daughter is adsorbed and the parent eluted. The daughter can then be subsequently eluted from the exchanger.

Solvent extraction

Solvent extraction uses the difference in the distribution coefficients of the two elements towards the two immiscible solvents used in the technique. Shaking the two solvents with the radionuclide pair helps the migration of the species by providing a larger interfacial surface. The phases are separated and the phase containing the daughter is then treated to convert the desirable radionuclide into the appropriate chemical form. For example, [^{99m}Tc]pertechnetate can be separated from the parent [^{99}Mo]molybdate using methyl ethyl ketone as the solvent of choice (Robinson 1972). The organic phase containing ^{99m}Tc is heated to dryness and then dissolved in saline solution. This kind of generator is selective but not easy to assemble, making it necessary for the user to deal with organic solvents, extraction and heating devices.

Membrane extraction

Membrane extraction separations are based on the affinity of one of the species of the radionuclide pair for an organic solvent present in a porous membrane. The principle is similar to that of solvent extraction and it is being employed for the preparation of low-activity $^{90}Sr/^{90}Y$ generators (Chakravarty *et al.* 2008; Pandey *et al.* 2008). These investigators used a polytetrafluoroethylene (PTFE) membrane incorporating the chelating agent 2-ethylhexyl 2-ethylhexyl phosphoric acid (KSM-17) that divided two chambers. In this configuration, ^{90}Y migrates from the chamber containing the feed solution in HNO_3 pH 1–2 to the chamber containing 1 mol/L HCl. A three-stage chamber design was also tested.

Electrochemical deposition

In this kind of generator, the difference between the electrochemical potentials of the parent and daughter radionuclides is employed for the chemical separation, allowing the selective deposition of the daughter activity. This principle was applied with success for the $^{90}Sr/^{90}Y$ generator (Chakravarty *et al.* 2008). Y^{3+} and Sr^{2+} have different electrochemical potentials that allowed a clean and quick separation of ^{90}Y from ^{90}Sr.

Precipitation

Although a very simple technique for chemical separation, precipitation is rarely used for assembling radionuclide generators. The parent or the daughter must be quantitatively precipitated in order to give good yields and purity. If the daughter element is to be precipitated, some carrier amount must be added, thus decreasing the specific activity of the radionuclide. This technique can only be employed in a production centre or a centralised radiopharmacy due to difficulties in handling and assembling.

Sublimation

Sublimation requires volatility of one of the radionuclides – preferably the daughter. This method is still used at some institutions, such as for the separation of ^{131}I from Te targets. The use of high-temperature sublimation methods developed to obtain ^{99m}Tc as TcO_7 from low-specific-activity ^{99}Mo has been recently reviewed (Christian *et al.* 2000). This technique is conducted in a central processing facility, and involves difficult handling and special devices, which are generally not available in the day-to-day routine in nuclear medicine departments.

Gas evolution

This technique requires the evolution of the daughter as a gas or vapour and it is suitable for only a few generator systems, in particular the $^{81}Rb/^{81m}Kr$, where the daughter can be eluted by a gas stream for direct inhalation.

Thermochromatography

This is another interesting but not often used technique that can be used to obtain the daughter radionuclide via thermal separation from the radionuclide parent, but which evidently has not yet been demonstrated on the large, commercial scale (Novgorodov *et al.* 2000).

Table 21.2 Examples of strategies for production of radionuclides used for generator parents

Production method/target	Generator parent	Generator system	Daughter application
Fission produced (n, fission)			
Uranium-235	Molybdenum-99	Mo-99/Technetium-99*m*	Diagnosis
	Strontium-90	Sr-90/Yttrium-90	Therapy
Accelerator produced			
Gallium (p,2n)	Germanium-68	Ge-68/Gallium-68	PET imaging
Gold(p,3n)	Mercury-195m	Hg-195m/Gold-195m	First pass
Rubidium(p,4n) Rb, Mo, Y Spallation	Strontium-92	Sr-92/Rubidium-82	PET imaging
Nickel-63 (p,2n)	Zinc-62	Zn-62/Copper-62	PET imaging
Krypton-82 (p,2n)	Rubidium-81	Rb-81/Krypton-81*m*	Perfusion
Tantalum-181 (p,4n)	Tungsten-178	W-178/Tantalum-178	First pass
Radium-226 (p,2n)	Actinium-225	Ac-225/Bismuth-213	Alpha therapy
Reactor produced			
Tungsten-186 (2n,γ)	Tungsten-188	W-188/Rhenium-188	Beta therapy
Dysprosium-164	Dysprosium-166	Dy-166/Holmium-166	Beta therapy
Osmium-190 (n,γ)	Osmium-191	Os-191/Iridium-191*m*	First pass
Radium-226 (3n→)	Thorium-229 → Actinium-225	Ac-225/Bismuth-213	Alpha therapy
Decay of long-lived progenitor			
U-233 → Thorium-229 → Actinium-225	Actinium-225	Ac-225/Bismuth-213	Alpha therapy
U-230 → Th-226	Uranium-230	U-230/Thorium-226	Alpha therapy
Ac-227 → Th-227 → Ra-223	Actinium-227	Ac-227 → Th-227 → Ra-223	Alpha therapy

Production and availability of radionuclide parents

An important consideration for the development and fabrication of radionuclide generators is the predictable and readily available source of the parent radionuclide species. Although a discussion of parent radionuclide production and processing strategies is beyond the scope of this chapter, there are several excellent articles that discuss the issues associated with production of these parents (Knapp, Mirzadeh 1994), including separation and purification from fission products, or production in research reactors or accelerators (Table 21.2).

Generators providing diagnostic radionuclides

Single-photon-emitting radionuclides

Molybdenum-99/technetium-99m generator

The use of this generator system and the ready availability of technetium-99m is the basis of modern day

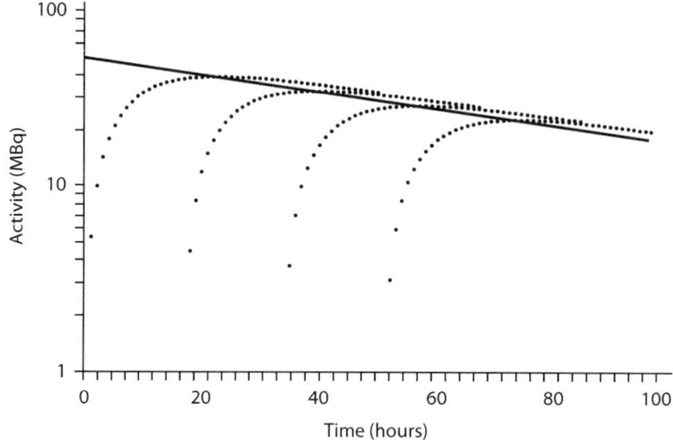

Figure 21.2 Illustration of sequential in-growth/elution cycles for the ^{99}Mo/^{99m}Tc generator system. ——, ^{99}Mo; ······, ^{999m}Tc.

diagnostic nuclear medicine. The ^{99}Mo/^{99m}Tc generator has been described in previous reviews (Boyd *et al.* 1982, 1984; Boyd 1986). Technetium-99m continues to be the most widely used diagnostic radioisotope in nuclear medicine, and ^{99m}Tc-labeled tissue-specific radiopharmaceuticals are available for diagnostic studies of essentially all major organs, and comprise an estimated 90% of all diagnostic procedures. The widely used chromatographic-type ^{99}Mo/^{99m}Tc generator system provides sodium pertechnetate (Na^{99m}TcO$_4$) by elution with saline and uses very high specific activity no-carrier-added ^{99}Mo, produced by the ^{235}U(n, fission)^{99}Mo process, which is adsorbed on aluminium oxide.

In this case, aluminium oxide acts as an anion exchanger having the following adsorption order for these anions: $MoO_4^- > Cl^- > TcO_4^-$. When the generator is first loaded onto the column, MoO_4^- is strongly adsorbed, ^{99}Mo decays to ^{99m}Tc in the form of TcO_4^-, and when saline is percolated through the column, the chloride ions replace TcO_4^- ions, assuring the total elution of the desired radioisotope. The elution process is fast, with high elution yield (>98%) and high elution efficiency (>95%) and usually the elution volume is 6 mL providing ^{99m}Tc with high radioactivity concentration. Glass flasks in vacuum are used for the elution of ^{99m}Tc in this generator. The ^{99}Mo breakthrough values must be <0.5 kBq/MBq ^{99m}Tc (<0.5 μCi/mCi) (USP/NF 1995). The elution yield is related to the amount of ^{99m}Tc eluted in 6 mL compared with the total level of ^{99m}Tc that can be eluted from the generator. Elution efficiency is related to the amount of ^{99m}Tc eluted in 6 mL compared with the theoretical amount of ^{99m}Tc coming from the decay of ^{99}Mo in the generator. These parameters are very useful for comparison between different kinds of generators.

Figure 21.2 illustrates the in-growth and well-known possible repeated recovery of ^{99m}Tc from saline elution of the alumina-based chromatographic type generator. In addition to the chromatographic-type generators, 'batch' preparation of ^{99m}Tc involves solvent extraction (Evans *et al.* 1982), for instance with methyl ethyl ketone, or sublimation of the low specific activity ^{99}Mo, which can be reactor-produced by neutron activation of enriched ^{98}Mo. The latter approach may become more attractive in the future as radioactive waste disposal issues become more crucial.

In addition to the well-established use of high-specific-activity ^{99}Mo obtained from fission of ^{235}U, there are two principal approaches for use of low-specific-activity ^{99}Mo (produced by the ^{98}Mo(n,γ)^{99}Mo) reaction for generator fabrication, which involve the 'gel-type' generator or post-elution concentration strategies. The 'gel-type' generator approach (Boyd *et al.* 1982) involves preparation of a molybdenum–zirconium gel. The use of preformed and post-formed gels are two strategies for preparation of the gel generator. In the preformed technique, the gel is prepared before being irradiated in the reactor, while in the post-formed technique ^{99}Mo is produced by neutron activation of Mo in the trioxide or metal form and the gel is then prepared. The preformed technique provides easier generator assembly and involves less handling of radioactivity but has the disadvantages of producing more chemical and radionuclidic impurities, resulting from radiolysis of the gel during irradiation. The post-formed technique provides a generator with better performance quality and the generator can be assembled either wet or dry. With elution in about 12 mL of saline, the wet generator has a higher ^{99m}Tc elution efficiency (>85%) than the dry system (<80%). It is more difficult to load reproducible levels of ^{99}Mo during fabrication of the wet generator, however, since the wet gel cannot be weighed. In the dry technique the gel can be loaded by weight. Based on the ^{99}Mo specific activity, even if the 'gel type' generator system is used, the specific concentration (i.e. mCi/mL) of the ^{99m}Tc may be too low for practical use. A useful alternative involves post-elution concentration of ^{99m}Tc on an anion-exchange column in tandem with the Al_2O_3 generator column, similar to that developed for the ^{188}W/^{188}Re generator (Knapp *et al.* 1998; Guhlke *et al.* 2000; Sarkar *et al.* 2001). Although the chromatographic alumina generator is generally considered impractical for use with low-specific-activity ^{99}Mo because of the significantly larger amounts of alumina adsorbent that are required, the post-elution concentration of the initial low radioactive concentration of ^{99m}Tc provides solutions of sufficient activity for labelling (Blower 1993). This latter approach can be very useful to provide ^{99}Mo/^{99m}Tc generators in countries that can use locally produced ^{99}Mo, to assure the national demand, especially when there is a worldwide crisis of production of ^{99}Mo owing to several setbacks from the major manufacturers, a reality dating from 2007.

Rubidium-81/krypton-81m generator

Following its initial introduction in the late 1960s (Yano, Anger 1968; Jones, Clark 1969; Clark *et al.* 1976), this generator system became available for clinical applications for continuous inhalation or intravenous infusion for evaluation of regional pulmonary ventilation and perfusion (Clark *et al.* 1976; Guillaume *et al.* 1983). Because of the short 13-second half-life of ^{81m}Kr, high-count-rate imaging with low patient radiation dose is possible with continuous administration of this radionuclide. The rubidum-81 parent is usually adsorbed on cation exchange resins, including AG 50W-X8 and BioRad AG MP50. For ventilation studies, the ^{81m}Kr is isolated by purging the generator with either air or oxygen. Elution of the generator with normal saline or 5% glucose solution is used for perfusion studies. Typical generators consist of glass or metal columns filled with resin. The in-growth/separation of the very short-lived ^{81m}Kr daughter from ^{81}Rb is shown in Figure 21.3, and illustrates that repeat studies are possible in just a few minutes' time.

A study by Rizzo-Padoin *et al.* (2001) described the use of ^{81m}Kr from a commercially available Kryptoscan generator for localisation of pulmonary emboli. Use of this system is cost effective, and cost varies based on the number of patients evaluated with each generator from \$104/study (6 patients) to \$266/patient (2 patients). A different strategy using a 'bubble type' generator for parallel gas and solution separation and an alternative generator approach implanting Mylar foils with ^{81}Rb atoms following

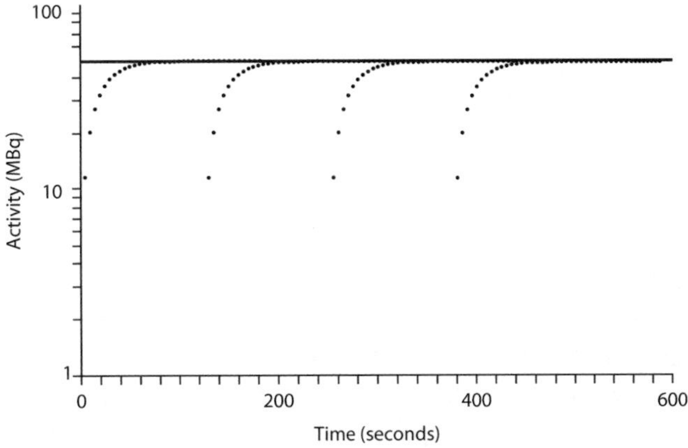

Figure 21.3 Illustration of sequential in-growth/elution cycles for the ^{81}Rb/^{81m}Kr generator system. ——, ^{81}Rb; ·······, ^{81}Kr.

Table 21.3 Examples of generator-produced single-photon emitters used for first-pass ventriculography/perfusion imaging

Parent	$t_{1/2}$	Daughter	$t_{1/2}$	Principal gamma E_{max}		Clinical application
				(keV)	(%)	
Mercury-195m	1.73 d	Gold-195m	30.5 s	181	23.5	Left ventriculography
Osmium-191	15.4 d	Iridium-191m	4.96 s	129.4	67.0	Left ventriculography
Rubidium-81	4.58 h	Krypton-81m	13 s	190.4	25.7	Right ventriculography
Tungsten-178	21.5 d	Tantalum-178	9.31 s	93.2	6.1	Left ventriculography

s, second(s); h, hour(s); d, day(s).

separation with a mass separator after spallation production have been discussed (Beyer and Raun 1991).

Mercury-195m/gold-195m generator

As one of the first successful ultra-short-lived radioisotopes for angiography, ^{195m}Au (Table 21.3) was identified as an important candidate for first-pass radionuclide angiography (Bett *et al.* 1983; Panek *et al.* 1985; Paras, Thiessen 1985). Following accelerator production (Table 21.2), the ^{195m}Hg is separated either by solvent extraction or by distillation methods and several chemical concepts had been evaluated for separation of n.c.a. ^{195m}Au using adsorption-type column-type generators. Since gold ions can be strongly complexed by sulfur moieties, dithiocellulose adsorbents were evaluated and demonstrated 1–2% breakthrough of ^{195m}Hg and 10–20% elution yield of ^{195m}Ag using 10 mmol/L NaCN solution (Bett *et al.* 1983). The subsequent use of silica gel coated with ZnS showed better retention of the ^{195m}Hg parent and demonstrated higher elution yield of 28–30% using $Na_2S_2O_3$/$NaNO_3$ solutions (Panek *et al.* 1984, 1985). In another strategy, ^{195m}Hg was loaded onto a Chelex 100 column and ^{195m}Au was eluted with 5% glucose solutions. The ^{195m}Hg was obtained in primarily an ionic form in ~20% yield with about 10^{-3}% ^{195}Hg parent breakthrough/bolus (Brihaye *et al.* 1982). Formation of ^{195}Au by isomeric transition of ^{195m}Au results in increasing absorbed radiation dose. Although both cardiac metabolism and function studies have been performed comparing ^{195m}Au with ^{201}Tl (Mena 1985), the use of ultra short-lived generator-derived radioisotopes is not pursued in current clinical practice because of the availability of competing technologies.

Tungsten-178/tantalum-178 generator

For first-pass studies, this generator is a convenient source of ^{178}Ta (Table 21.3). Early studies (Neirinckx *et al.* 1978) evaluated AGI-X8 as the support and demonstrated satisfactory operation by elution with 0.1–0.15 mol/L HCl containing 0.1% H_2O_2. Although initial ^{178}Ta breakthrough levels were about 10^{-3}%/bolus, these values increased with subsequent elutions. In addition to the early demonstration of the use of ^{178}Ta-labelled myocardial perfusion agents (Holman *et al.* 1978), the use ^{178}Ta for lung and liver imaging had also been reported (Neirinckx *et al.* 1979). The most recently reported system uses a Dowex AG 1-X8 anion exchange column eluted with 0.03 mol/L HCl and provides reproducible ^{178}Ta yields with consistently low ^{178}W parent breakthrough (Lacy *et al.* 1991). Rapid, repeat elution of ^{178}Ta is possible for sequential studies. First-pass radionuclide nuclear analysis (FPRNA) studies of ventricular performance were demonstrated in a group of 38 patients and demonstrated high resolution and good statistical quality in comparison with the traditional ^{99m}Tc methods (Lacy *et al.* 1991). For cardiology applications, the usefulness of this system for evaluation of systolic and diastolic left ventricular function was studied in 46 patients undergoing coronary balloon angioplasty (Verani *et al.* 1992). This generator has been demonstrated in combination with a portable multiwire proportional counter gamma camera as an excellent source of ^{178}Ta for the evaluation of ventricular performance (Lacy *et al.* 1988b, 2001). The $^{178}W/^{178}Ta$ generator is the only current system providing a short-lived daughter for evaluation of FPRNA which has recently been reported in the literature.

Osmium-191/iridium-191m generator

This generator is another system that had been developed for perfusion and FPRNA and provides the ultra-short-lived ^{191m}Ir from the reactor-produced ^{191}Os parent (Table 21.2). Iridium-191m was initially proposed for evaluation of intracardiac shunts and ventricular ejection and wall motion by rapid bolus injection, and for measurement of blood flow for various organs by continuous infusion. The first generator provided ^{191m}Ir for intravenous administration. Early generator systems were based on ion-exchange chromatography, and a later system from which ^{191m}Ir was obtained for primarily paediatric intracardiac shunt evaluation used absorption of $K_2[^{191}OsO_2Cl_4]$ or $K_2[^{191}OsO_2(OH)_2Cl_2]$ on AGMP-1 anion exchange resin from which ^{191m}Ir was obtained in relatively low yield (<10%) (Cheng *et al.* 1980). Because of the importance of minimising any ^{191}Os parent breakthrough, post-elution passage through a second column assured ^{191}Os breakthrough of $<10^{-2}\%$. Iridium-191m in isotonic saline buffered with Na_2HPO_4 from this prototype generator was used in about 100 patients (Treves *et al.* 1980). Another system using an Os(VI) species bound to silica gel impregnated with tridodecylmethylammonium chloride (SG-TDMAC) provided ^{191m}Ir in 21–33% yield by elution with HCl-acidified saline at pH 1 with the final eluate buffered with 1 mol/L succinate solution to pH 9 (Issacher *et al.* 1989). An activated carbon 'scavenger' column was used in tandem with the SG-TDMAC column to remove ^{191}Os parent breakthrough before the eluent is rapidly buffered.

Another system was specifically used for quantification of intracardiac shunts in children (Treves *et al.* 1976, 1980) and for evaluation of ventricular function in adults. Use of ^{191m}Ir for renal radionuclide angiograms and continuous infusion for the rapid renal single-photon emission tomographic evaluation of renal blood flow has also been described (Treves *et al.* 1999).

Another generator system that did not require a post-elution 'scavenger' column was also developed for angiocardiography in children which utilised a potassium Os(VI) oxalate species adsorbed on AGMP-1 anion-exchange resin (Cheng *et al.* 1980). Elution with pH 1 0.9% saline solution provided ^{191m}Ir in good yields (20%/mL) with low ^{191}Os parent breakthrough ($<5 \times 10^{-5}\%$).

The use of $^{191}Os(IV)$ species bound on heat-activated carbon and eluted with 0.9% saline containing 0.025% KI at pH 2 was also developed and was an excellent generator system, providing the daughter isotope in 16–18% yields with correspondingly low ^{191}Os parent breakthrough ($2\text{–}3 \times 10^{-4}\%$/bolus). For patient studies, the low-pH bolus was neutralised by simultaneous buffering of the generator eluent with 0.13 mol/L Tris buffer (Brihaye *et al.* 1986a,b). With this system, the neutralised bolus was then rapidly administered intravenously mixed with physiological saline using a microprocessor-controlled automated elution/injection system. Using this activated carbon adsorbent-based generator system, rapid sequential first-pass multiple views in over 600 patient studies were conducted for the evaluation of left ventricular ejection fraction and regional wall motion (Franken *et al.* 1989, 1991).

Generator systems providing positron-emitting radioisotopes for positron emission tomography (PET)

Radionuclide generators that provide position-emitting daughters for PET use are fabricated using neutron-deficient parent radioisotopes that are accelerator produced and can be categorised according to the daughter radioisotope half-lives (Table 21.4). The useful generator daughter radioisotopes have significant positron branching and decay may also be accompanied by emission of high-energy photons. The short-lived daughters have half-lives of a few minutes to hours. Rubidium-82 is an example that is exclusively used after intravenous bolus administration for perfusion studies. In contrast, longer-lived daughters, such as ^{68}Ga, can be incorporated into targeting agents via efficient, rapid radiochemical synthesis. The ^{68}Ga-labelled DOTATAT/DOTATOC/DOTANOC ligands are important examples that exhibit rapid *in-vivo* targeting and are of current widespread use for PET. The benefit for radiopharmacy in using the $^{68}Ge/^{68}Ga$ is the large number of PET studies

Table 21.4 Examples of key generator-produced positron-emitters used for clinical positron emission tomographic (PET) imaging

Parent	$t_{1/2}$	Daughter	$t_{/2}$	Per cent β^+ branch	$E_{\beta+}$ (MeV)	Clinical application
Short-lived generator daughters						
Iron-52	8.28 d	Manganese-52*m*	21.1 m	97.0	1.13	Perfusion
Strontium-62	25.6 d	Rubidium-82	1.27 m	95.0	1.41	Perfusion Rb^+ cation
Zinc-62	9.26 h	Copper-62	9.74 m	97.0	1.28	Radiolabelling perfusion
Longer-lived generator daughters						
Germanium-68	270.8 d	Gallium-68	1.135 h	89.0	0.74	Targeted imaging; Radiolabelling DOTATOC, EDTMP
Selenium-72	8.4 d	Arsenic-72	1.083 d	88.0	1.02	Radiolabelling

possible per generator, which would be expected to result in lower costs per patient study.

Zinc-62/copper-62 generator

The ^{62}Zn parent radionuclide is accelerator produced (Table 21.2) and the use of anion-exchange column chromatography provides effective generator systems. Such systems include adsorption of the n.c.a. $^{62}Zn^{2+}$ on Dowex 1 and elution of $^{62}Cu^{2+}$ with hydrochloric acid (Fujibayashi *et al.* 1989; Green *et al.* 1990). Use of CG-120 Amberlite resin provides ~70% ^{62}Cu elution yield with a glycine solution or HCl/ethanol from which subsequent ligand radiolabelling is possible (Fujibayashi *et al.* 1989).

Copper-62 can be used for a variety of PET imaging applications; for instance, chelation to human serum albumin (HSA) and benzyl-TETA-chelated HSA have been used for blood pool imaging (Mathias *et al.* 1991). Major research and clinical applications of ^{62}Cu are as radiolabelled agents for hypoxia imaging and organ perfusion by PET. Key examples include ^{62}Cu-ATSM (diacetyl-bis(N^4-methylthiosemicarbazone) (Fujibayashi *et al.* 1997) and ^{62}Cu-PTSM (pyruvaldehyde bis(N^4-methylthiosemicarbazone) (Green *et al.* 1990; Taniuchi *et al.* 1995). Clinical evaluation of ^{62}Cu-PTSM has demonstrated that this tracer is a good candidate for sequential myocardial imaging (Wallhaus *et al.* 1998) and also for quantification of the cerebral blood flow (Okazawa *et al.* 1994).

Initial evaluation of ^{62}Cu-PTSM in conjunction with the performance of the $^{62}Zn/^{62}Cu$ generator and results of studies in 68 patients have demonstrated that this generator system is easily manufactured and transported, and is an inexpensive source of the ^{62}Cu positron emitter for in-house radiopharmaceutical preparation (Haynes *et al.* 2000). The detection of coronary artery disease with ^{62}Cu-PTSM was reported in 47 patients (Wallhaus *et al.* 2001) and the use of ^{62}Cu liquid-filled angioplasty balloons for the inhibition of coronary restenosis has also been reported.

Germanium-68/gallium-68 generator

Because of the broad interest and increasing clinical relevance of PET imaging, the availability of radionuclide generator systems that provide positron emitters continues to stimulate significant interest (Velikyan *et al.* 2008). The $^{68}Ge/^{68}Ga$ generator has been expected to offer great advantages, because the long 270-day physical half-life of the ^{68}Ge parent would provide generators that would be expected to having a very long operational shelf-life, and would provide useful levels of ^{68}Ga on a daily basis for PET studies (Figure 21.4).

The accelerator production of germanium-68 has been summarised (Mirzadeh, Lambrecht 1996).

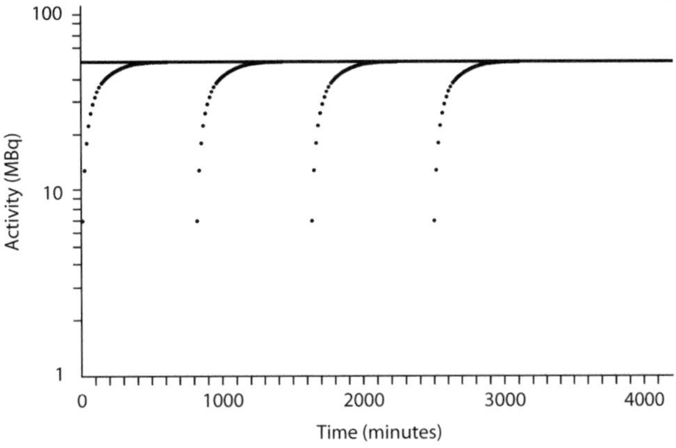

Figure 21.4 Illustration of sequential in-growth/elution cycles for the $^{68}Ge/^{68}Ga$ generator system. ——, ^{68}Ge; ·······, ^{68}Ga.

Although the first $^{68}Ge/^{68}Ga$ generator was described many years ago, the non-ionic ^{68}Ga was obtained as the EDTA complex from ^{68}Ge absorbed on aluminium or zirconium. The neutral ^{68}Ga-EDTA solution was used directly in attempts at tumour imaging. Other systems provided ^{68}Ga by oxalate elution of ^{68}Ge bound to antimony oxide Sb_2O_5. Elution of anion-exchange resins with dilute hydrofluoric acid solutions permitted separation of high-purity ^{68}Ge owing to the significant differences in the Ge/Ga distribution coefficients (Neirinckx, Davis 1980). These generators provided ^{68}Ga yields of >90% and ^{68}Ge breakthrough levels of $<10^{-4}\%$ for up to 600 elutions. The non-ionic chemical forms of ^{68}Ga obtained from these generators, however, limited the chemical strategies available for preparation of targeted radiopharmaceuticals

For this reason, recent development of $^{68}Ge/^{68}Ga$ generator prototypes has focused on providing ^{68}Ga as free ionic Ga^{3+} species. The adsorption of ^{68}Ge on a variety of adsorbents has been evaluated, including use of 1,2,3-trihydroxybenzene (pyrogallol)–formaldehyde resin, with ^{68}Ga elution yields of ~75%, and ^{68}Ge breakthrough values of <0.5 ppm. Radiolytic by-products were not detected using a 370 MBq (10 mCi) generator over a 250-day period (Schumacher, Maier-Borst 1981), indicating that the pyrogallol–formaldehyde resin may be resistant to radiolysis at these activity levels. Most studies have evaluated the use of a variety of inorganic matrix materials for the adsorption of ^{68}Ge, which include alumina, $Al(OH)_3$ and $Fe(OH)_3$, and metallic oxides such as SnO_2, ZrO_2, TiO_2 and CeO_2. Tin(II) oxide has been most widely evaluated and is used in current $^{68}Ge/^{68}Ga$ generators (Roesch, Knapp 2003). On elution with 1 mol/L hydrochloric acid, these generators exhibit low ^{68}Ge parent breakthrough (10^{-6}–$10^{-5}\%$ per bolus) and good $^{68}Ga^{3+}$ elution yields of 70–80% (Loc'h *et al.* 1980). Although the ^{68}Ga-BAT-TECH agent for instance, was evaluated for myocardial perfusion (Mathias *et al.* 1991), this application has not been further studied, and most current studies focus on the preparation of ^{68}Ga-labelled targeted peptides.

Most recently, because of the advances that have been made with the tumour targeting of DOTA-linked neuroendocrine tumour (NE)-targeting agents, development, *in vitro* and animal studies have rapidly progressed to clinical trials of ^{68}Ga-DOTA-DPhe^1-Tyr^3-octreotide (^{68}Ga-DOTATOC) for PET imaging of NE tumours. For instance, DPhe^1-Tyr^3-octreotide shows high affinity to the sstr2 subtype of somatostatin receptor expressed on NE and other tumours, and the conjugated macrocylic bifunctional chelator DOTA binds the trivalent $^{68}Ga^{3+}$ with high thermodynamic and kinetic stability. Although ^{68}Ga has a relatively short half-life of 1.1 hours, rapid *in-vivo* targeting of ^{68}Ga-DOTATOC allows excellent visualisation of tumours and small metastases (Hoffman *et al.* 2001). More recently, a $^{68}Ge/^{68}Ga$ generator prototype system using acetone for elution of the lipophilic $^{68}Ga^{3+}$ cation has been described for clinical use (Zhernosekov *et al.* 2007).

Strontium-82/rubidium-82 generator

The ^{82}Rb positron emitter was recognised as a potential PET isotope by analogy with the physiological monovalent potassium cation, which is transported across the cell membrane via the sodium-potassium ATP ion exchange pathway. Rubidium-82 is partially extracted by the myocardium during a single capillary pass. The development of this generator has taken place over the past 25 years and has been intensively discussed in numerous reviews (Waters, Coursey 1987). Strontium-82 for use in the $^{82}Sr/^{82}Rb$ generator is usually obtained from 600–800 MeV high-energy proton spallation of molybdenum targets (Table 21.2). Pharmaceutical and operational requirements for the generator are crucial since the ^{82}Rb cation must be obtained by generator elution in a sterile pyrogen-free physiological medium for direct intravenous injection (www.cardiogen.com, Bracco Diagnostics, Inc.). A number of resins have been evaluated for elution of ^{82}Rb with 2% NaCl solution (Roesch, Knapp 2003), including BioRex-70 and Chelex and inorganic oxide ion exchangers such as ZrO_2 and Al_2O_3, and SnO_2 has been evaluated as an adsorbent for ^{82}Rb elution with physiological saline for bolus or continuous infusion.

FDA-approved generators are commercially available from Bracco, Inc. (www.cardiogen.com, Bracco Diagnostics, Inc.), with activity levels up to 3.7 GBq (100 mCi) at calibration and are used for routine clinical evaluation of myocardial perfusion. The generators are provided with an automated infusion system. The ^{82}Rb perfusion PET images are used to identify regional normal versus abnormal myocardium perfusion in patients with suspected myocardial infarction, as well as for the assessment of coronary blood flow, degree of stenosis, and viability, and to monitor recovery and maintenance. Since the generator yields are a function of eluent flow rate, the ^{82}Rb yields range from 10% to 40%, while the ^{82}Sr breakthrough is in the order of 10^{-6}%/mL (Brihaye *et al.* 1987). One study assessed myocardial flow with two-dimensional versus three-dimensional imaging in myocardial regions smaller than 1 cm^3, which is within the accuracy achieved with $H_2{}^{15}O$ (Lin *et al.* 2001). The automated elution system provides ^{82}Rb for direct intravenous bolus injection, with an average dose of about 180 MBq (5 mCi) for cardiac PET and sequential rest versus stress studies.

Generators providing therapeutic radionuclides

During the past two decades there has been a tremendous increase in the development and use of therapeutic radiopharmaceuticals radiolabelled with radionuclides available from generator systems (see Tables 21.5 and 21.7). The availability of generator-derived therapeutic radioisotopes is necessary for the development, testing and commercialisation of agents with potential for endoradiotherapy (ERT), which includes both unsealed (radiopharmaceuticals) and sealed sources (devices). Just as availability of ^{99m}Tc from the $^{99}Mo/^{99m}Tc$ generator has played such a key role in the development of a wide variety of ^{99m}Tc-labelled radiopharmaceuticals, the availability of generator-derived radionuclides has stimulated the development of a widening spectrum of therapeutic tracers. It is important to note that in most cases, increased need and further development of generators which provide therapeutic radionuclides has been driven by the successful development of the complementary targeting agents or vectors.

Generator-derived therapeutic radionuclides are convenient in-house production systems providing radioisotopes for a large variety of therapeutic applications. As discussed in this section, generators are available that provide both beta- and alpha-emitting

Table 21.5 Examples of key generator-produced beta-emitting radioisotopes for therapy

Parent	$t_{1/2}$	Daughter	$t_{1/2}$	E_{max} (MeV)	Clinical application
Strontium-90	28.6 y	Yttrium-90	64.1 h	2.32	Targeted Therapy
Tungsten-188	69 d	Rhenium-188	16.9 h	2.12	
Dysprosium-166	3.4 d	Holmium-166	1.117 h	1.90	

radioisotopes, and there may also be opportunities in limited cases for systems that can provide Auger emitters. Many therapeutic radioisotope parent radionuclides provide the desired beta-emitting daughters by beta decay, and are thus often produced in research reactors (Table 21.2). Key examples of n.c.a. therapeutic radioisotopes obtained directly from reactor-produced parent radionuclides (i.e. neutron activation of target atoms) include ^{166}Ho and ^{90}Y (Table 21.5). In addition, nuclear fission of ^{235}U can also provide important radionuclides, and the ^{90}Sr parent for the ^{90}Sr/^{90}Y generator system is isolated from fission products. The availability of the ^{90}Y-labelled murine anti-CD20 antibody Zevalin (ibritumomab tiuxetan) as an approved product for the treatment of patients with low-grade, follicular or transformed non-Hodgkin lymphoma is the first antibody radiolabelled with a therapeutic, generator-derived radionuclide, and would be expected to be the first of many new therapeutic radiopharmaceuticals for oncological applications. In addition to direct reactor production and recovery from fission products, another source of parent radionuclides for fabrication of generator systems is the recovery of radioactive parents from 'extinct' radioactive decay processes. Thorium-229 (see Table 21.7) is a key example of an important long-lived progenitor ($t_{1/2}$ = 7340 years), which is recovered from ^{233}U decay products and from which ^{225}Ac is extracted as the parent for the ^{225}Ac/^{213}Bi generator system.

Generators providing beta-emitting radioisotopes

Strontium-90/yttrium-90 generator

Yttrium-90 decays with the emission of a high-energy β-particle (E_{max} = 2.3 MeV) and is employed for therapy of solid tumours where deep penetration of radiation is important for cross-fire (see Table 21.5). Although various forms of the ^{90}Sr/^{90}Y generator have been available for a number of years, broad interest in clinical therapeutic applications of ^{90}Y was stimulated by development of methods of radiation synovectomy of large synovial joints. An inventory of the ^{90}Sr parent can be maintained for a very long period because of the long 28-year physical half-life, without the reliance for routine production and processing. A variety of bifunctional chelating groups that strongly bind the tripositive yttrium cation have been developed, since the skeletal localisation of free trivalent yttrium species would result in significant marrow suppression (see Chapter 9). The availability of DOTA and the CHX-substituted DTPA chelates provides an opportunity to use ^{90}Y in a predictably safe manner. The availability of good chelates in conjunction with effective targeting agents – such as the DOTATOC octreotide agent binding with high specificity for the somatostatin receptors – offers important agents for the treatment of a wide variety of tumours. Because of the safety issues associated with the use and handling of ^{90}Y and ^{90}Sr, these high-level generators are typically installed in a centralised processing area for preparation of the n.c.a. ^{90}Y by batch solvent extraction techniques and distribution of the highly purified ^{90}Y product.

The use of freshly purified 1-hydroxyethylidene-1,1-phosphonic acid (HDEHP) extraction of ^{90}Y from a nitric acid solution of the purified ^{90}Sr/^{90}Y mixture is one primary current strategy used for production (http://las.perkinelmer.com/Catalog/FamilyPage.htm?CategoryID=Yttrium-90; Bray *et al.* 1996), which provides a product in which the ^{90}Y/^{90}Sr ratio of the purified ^{90}Y is $<10^{-7}$ with a concentration of metal impurities of $<$10 ppm/Ci (37 GBq) ^{90}Y. A generator system has also been described for the separation of ^{90}Y from ^{90}Sr using the strongly acidic Dowex exchange resin (Chinol, Hnatowich 1987). Because of potential skeletal localisation of the tripositive ^{90}Y and ^{90}Sr cations, there are stringent quality controls required for handling clinical radiolabelling grade ^{90}Y. The generator is usually installed and eluted in a central manufacturing setting, and the ^{90}Y commercially provided after batch extraction and separation. A comparison of solvent extraction, ion exchange and other radiochemical separation techniques for this generator has been reported (Chuang, Lo 1996). Ion exchange-based generators utilise various organic cation exchange resins, but also inorganic compounds, with a particular focus on high radiation resistance. Because of the limited availability and significant costs of high-purity ^{90}Sr and the potential dangers in handling this isotope, installation of this generator in a hospital-based nuclear pharmacy or a central radiopharmacy is unusual, and high-purity ^{90}Y is generally obtained from a GMP-approved central processing facility providing both research-grade and sterile, pyrogen-free ^{90}Y for human studies (Pandey *et al.* 2008).

Tungsten-188/rhenium-188 generator

Rhenium-188 is currently of broad interest for the development of new therapeutic approaches in nuclear medicine, oncology and even interventional cardiology/radiology, because of its excellent radionuclidic properties (Knapp *et al.* 1997). The emission of a primary gamma photon with an energy of 155 keV (15%), a useful half-life of 16.9 hours, and the similarity in chemistry of rhenium and technetium, make this radioisotope an important candidate for many therapeutic applications. There are a number of benefits, advantages and significantly reduced expense of using ^{188}Re in comparison with many other therapeutic radioisotopes (Knapp *et al.* 1997; Knapp 1998). A large number of physician-sponsored clinical protocols are in progress (Knapp *et al.* 1997, 1998; Jeong, Chung 2003; Lambert, deKlerk 2006).

The tungsten-188 parent radionuclide ($t_{1/2}$ 69 days) is reactor-produced by double neutron capture of enriched ^{186}W by the ^{186}W(n,γ)^{187}W(n,γ)^{188}W route (Table 21.5), capture cross sections and burn-up of the ^{188}W product (Mirzadeh *et al.* 1997). Early ^{188}W/^{188}Re generators for experimental purposes using zirconium oxide and aluminium oxide were described in the 1960s and 1970s. Practical use of this therapeutic radioisotope was not demonstrated until the 1980s and 1990s, after new therapeutic strategies were explored and appropriate carrier molecules and targeting agents became available (Knapp *et al.* 1998, 1999; Jeong, Chung 2003; Lambert, deKlerk 2006).

The ^{188}W/^{188}Re generator systems available today are mainly based on a separation chemistry similar to that used for the ^{99}Mo/^{99m}Tc generator by the adsorption of tungstic acid using a chromatographic-type alumina-based generator (Callahan *et al.* 1989; Knapp *et al.* 1994). Zirconium oxide and gel-type generators as well as 'batch' separation of ^{188}Re by a thermochromatographic technique have also been described (Novgorodov *et al.* 2000). The adsorption-type generator is the most practical, since it is easy to prepare, has long-term stability, high ^{188}Re yields and consistently low ^{188}W breakthrough (Knapp *et al.* 1997). The availability of effective and inexpensive post-elution tandem column-based concentration systems (Knapp *et al.* 1997,1998; Guhlke *et al.* 2000) provides a useful method for ^{188}Re concentration to very high radioactive concentrations (<1 mL total volume).

Currently these generators are available from several sources as radiochemicals to provide ingredients for radiopharmaceutical preparations (Table 21.6), and are expected to be provided as cGMP products in the near future.

Because the tungsten-188 is reactor produced and involves a double neutron capture, the specific activity of the tungsten-188 is a function of the square of the thermal neutron flux. For this reason, reactors that have very high thermal neutron flux are required for the production of ^{188}W. However, ^{188}W with only low specific activity (i.e. 4–5 Ci ^{188}W/mg ^{186}W) can be produced in even the high-flux reactors. Thus, much larger amounts of alumina generator bed are required to bind the tungsten, requiring much higher elution volumes of saline, and resulting in low radioactive concentration. Although dependent on the subsequent

Table 21.6 Availability of tungsten-188/rhenium-188 generators and rhenium-188, currently in clinical trials under physician-sponsored protocols

Institution/company providing generator	Adsorbent	cGMP availability	Comment/web info.
Oak Ridge National Laboratory (ORNL), Oak Ridge, TN	Alumina	Yes – As BPI	Up to 3 Ci activity Level – detailed information for bolus concentration provided
Polatom, Swierk, Poland	Alumina	Yes	500 mCi – bolus concentration not required
ITM, Munich, Germany	Alumina	Pending	Central Radiopharmacy Setting – Ci levels of ^{188}Re provided
IRE, Fleurus, Belgium	Alumina	Pending	Provided with integral ^{188}Re concentration unit

post-elution radiolabelling method, the low radioactive concentration is often adequate in the early time periods following ^{188}W processing and generator fabrication. But for practical radiopharmacy use – especially for prolonging the generator shelf-life – post-elution concentration of ^{188}Re is required.

Post-elution concentration after saline elution of the alumina-based $^{188}W/^{188}Re$ generator system provides ^{188}Re perrhenate solutions of high radioactive concentration (Knapp 1998). The generator is eluted with physiological saline (for instance, 25–50 mL) at a flow-rate of 1–2 mL/min through the disposable, one-time-use tandem cation/anion exchange system. After generator elution, the ^{188}Re perrhenate is trapped on a small disposable anion column, such as the silica-based hydrophilic strong anion exchanger QMA SepPak column (Waters, Inc.), which is then eluted with a small volume (1–2 mL) of saline.

A large number of physician-sponsored clinical trials are in progress using the ORNL alumina-based tungsten-188/rhenium-188 generator system (Knapp *et al.* 1997; Jeong, Chung 2003; Lambert, deKlerk 2006). Rhenium-188-labelled HEDP (Palmedo *et al.* 2000; Savio *et al.* 2001) and DMSA (Blower *et al.* 2000) have proven to be effective agents for the palliative relief of bone pain from skeletal metastases in patients with prostatic carcinoma, and may represent a more cost-effective alternative for this application. The HEDP agent has also been successfully demonstrated as an effective tool for palliative treatment of metastases from lung cancer. In addition, the use of angioplasty balloons filled with ^{188}Re-perrhenate was shown as one of the first effective radionuclide techniques for the inhibition of hyperplastic re-stenosis after coronary balloon angioplasty (Knapp *et al.* 2001; Reynen *et al.* 2006), ^{188}Re-MAG3 (Weinberger, Knapp 1999; Weinberger *et al.* 1999; Park *et al.* 2001) and ^{188}Re-DTPA (Hong *et al.* 2002). The ^{188}Re-labelled anti-CD66 antibody (anti-NCA95) has been found to be useful for marrow ablation using combinational pre-conditioning in leukaemia patients (Buchman *et al.* 2002).

The use of the tungsten-188/rhenium-188 generator in developing regions is of particular value because of its cost effectiveness, and multicentre trials supported by the International Atomic Energy Agency (IAEA) are in progress for re-stenosis therapy with ^{188}Re-perrhenate and for the treatment of liver cancer (Sundram *et al.* 2002; Padhy and Dondi 2008) with ^{188}Re-labelled Lipiodol analogues (Jeong, Knapp 2008). Other applications include use of ^{188}Re-labelled antibody for treatment of bladder cancer, the ^{188}Re-labelled P2045 sstr-targeting peptide for the treatment of lung cancer, and the recent Phase II studies with the ^{188}Re-PTI-6D2 antibody targeted to melanoma, in progress at the Hadassah Medical Center (ClinicalTrials.gov 2008).

Dysprosium-166/holmium-166 generator

Holmium-166 continues to be of interest as a useful therapeutic radioisotope for therapy (Table 21.5), with a half-life of 1.1 hours and beta emission with an average energy of 1.9 MeV. It is traditionally 'directly' produced in a high-thermal-flux reactor with a relatively high specific activity of 8–9 Ci/mg (300–330 GBq/mg) ^{165}Ho by the $^{165}Ho(n,\gamma)^{166}Ho$ reaction. In contrast, no-carrier-added ^{166}Ho with a very high theoretical specific activity about 700 Ci/mg (26T Bq/mg) can be obtained by decay of ^{166}Dy, which is reactor-produced by the $^{164}Dy(n,\gamma)$ $^{165}Dy(n,\gamma)^{166}Dy$-($\beta^- \rightarrow$) ^{166}Ho pathway. Although separation of ^{166}Ho from ^{166}Dy in a true generator system is difficult, column separation is possible, where the ^{166}Ho and ^{166}Dy are well separated, but are removed from the adsorption column during elution (Dadachova *et al.* 1995a,b). Such a scenario then requires reloading of the column for subsequent separation of ^{166}Ho. This method has been described for successful $^{166}Ho/^{166}Dy$ separation that uses an HPLC reversed-phase ion-exchange chromatographic method with Dowex AG 50WX12 or Aminex A5 cation exchangers by elution with α-hydroxyisobutyric acid (HIBA; 0.085 mol/L, pH 4.3), providing a Dy/Ho separation factor of approximately 10^3. Following subsequent acid decomposition of the Ho-HIBA complex, the $^{166}Ho^{3+}$ is subsequently purified by cation-exchange column chromatography (Dadachova *et al.* 1995a,b). Another method has been described involving Dy/Ho separation on the Eichrome LN resin by elution with dilute nitric acid (Ketring *et al.* 2002).

Although ^{166}Ho has attractive radionuclidic properties as a lanthanide for various vector labelling and therapeutic strategies, it has not yet been widely used. An example is the study of protein labelling with the CHX-B-DTPA ligand system. Animal studies demonstrated that no translocation of the ^{166}Ho daughter radionuclide occurred when the ^{166}Ho-DTPA complex was administered to rats (Smith *et al.* 1995). The results of these studies suggest that the ^{166}Ho/^{166}Dy system may have some promise as an *in-vivo* generator. Clinical applications that have been reported recently include radiation synovectomy with ^{166}Ho-ferric hydroxide (Ofluoglu *et al.* 2002), the use of ^{166}Ho-DTPA liquid-filled balloons for the inhibition of re-stenosis following coronary angioplasty (Hong *et al.* 2002), and use of ^{166}Ho-DOTMP for myeloablative therapy of multiple myeloma (Rajendran *et al.* 2002). If the availability of n.c.a. ^{166}Ho becomes a reality, improvements will be required before the use of such a generator system could be a source of ^{166}Ho for these applications.

Generator systems providing alpha-emitting radioisotopes

It is interesting that in 1920 the separation of ^{222}Rn from ^{226}Ra represented the first generator developed for medical use and provided the ^{222}Rn for preparation of therapeutic seed implants. Until the 1980s there was little interest in the availability of generator-derived alpha-emitting radioisotopes, but in the past 10–20 years or so interest in this area has blossomed and clinical research and evaluation of these high-LET radioisotopes is an area of major radiochemical and clinical research (Table 21.7).

Actinium-225/bismuth-213 generator

Because of the very high linear energy transfer (LET) in the 50–90 μm range, α-particles have many advantages for therapy of microscopic or subclinical disease. The attachment of alpha emitters to cellular-targeted carrier molecules such as antibodies or peptides is the most common approach. For this reason, interest in the ^{225}Ac/^{213}Bi generator system has increased in the past few years.

The ^{225}Ac is generally obtained as a decay product of ^{229}Th, which is extracted as a radioactive decay product of ^{233}U, a member of the 'extinct' ^{237}Np decay chain. The ^{229}Th can be obtained from processing of the ^{233}U stockpile, which had originally been produced in a proposed molten salt breeder reactor programme at the Oak Ridge National Laboratory (ORNL).

Studies directed at optimising production of ^{225}Ac using accelerators by the ^{226}Ra(p,2n)^{225}Ac reaction are also in progress (Apostolidis *et al.* 2005). From a complex series of ion-exchange and extraction chromatographic steps for recycling of ^{229}Th(IV), the Ra(II) decay product is separated at optimal timing, and the ^{225}Ac then separated. A variety of chromatographic-type ^{225}Ac/^{213}Bi generators have been described (Mirzadeh 1998; Hassfjell, Brechbiel 2001; Boll *et al.* 2005). At ORNL, the ^{225}Ac/1 mol/L HNO_3 solution is generally provided to investigators together with generator components for on-site generator loading, to minimise the effects of radiolysis. This solution is loaded onto a small AG 50W-X4 strong cation-exchange resin with elution of the ^{213}Bi daughter by 0.15 mol/L HI solution.

Other ^{225}Ac/^{213}Bi generator systems that have been described include the use of two successive Dowex 50W-X8 cation exchange columns, with initial separation of ^{225}Ac from $^{224/225}$Ra and subsequent separation of the desired ^{213}Bi from the ^{225}Ac formed from radon decay (Geerlings *et al.* 1993). The ^{213}Bi is under evaluation for the clinical treatment of acute myeloid leukaemia (AML) under physician-sponsored protocols (Jurcic *et al.* 2002). In another variation,

Table 21.7 Examples of key generator-produced alpha-emitting radioisotopes for therapy

Parent	$t_{1/2}$	Daughter	$t_{1/2}$	Major γ (keV, [%])	α, E_{max} (MeV)	Clinical application
Actinium-225 (from Th-229)	10 d	Bismuth-213	45.6 m	440 [28]	5.87	Targeted therapy; palliation
Lead-212 (from Th-228 → Ra-224)	10.6 h	Bismuth-212	60.55 m	727 [11.8]	6.05	
Uranium-230	20.8 d	Thorium-226	30.9 m	111 [3.29]	6.3	
Actinium-227 → Thorium-227	27.7 y	Radium-223	11.4 d	171 [9]	5.7	

^{213}Bi is bound to a disc containing a thin film of the Anex strong anion-exchange resin (3M Company) by passage of the ^{225}Ac solution. The ^{213}Bi is subsequently eluted with 1.0 mol/L NaOAc buffered at pH 5.5 (Bray *et al.* 2000).

Radium-224/lead-212/bismuth-212 generator

Bismuth-212 has been of interest for some time and is available from the decay of ^{212}Pb. The traditional generator involves loading a cation-exchange resin with ^{224}Ra and subsequent elution of the ^{212}Bi with HCl or HI (Atcher *et al.* 1988), and requires replacement of the generator every 3–6 days. More recently, a generator based on gaseous ^{222}Ra emanating from thin films of ^{228}Th barium stearate has been described (Hassfjell, Brechbiel 2001) that involves collecting the gaseous ^{224}Ra in a trap containing an organic solvent such as methanol or hexane or a methanol–hexane mixture, at temperatures lower than −72°C. The ^{212}Pb decay product can be obtained in about 70% yield and this system has the advantage of the indefinite shelf-life of the long-lived ^{228}Th source ($t_{1/2} = 1.913$ years).

Actinium-227/thorium-227/radium-223 generator

Radium specifically targets the skeleton after intravenous administration, and for this reason the use of ^{223}Ra for palliation of cancer metastasised to the skeleton has been reported (Nilsson *et al.* 2005).

Uranium-230/thorium-226 generator

This system was recently described as an avenue for routine recovery of ^{226}Th for therapy. The routine production of ^{230}U from ^{241}Pr (Morgenstern *et al.* 2008) and therapeutic use of ^{226}Th rather than ^{213}Bi, would preclude the evidently difficult problem of identifying significantly increased levels of ^{229}Th. As described above, decay of ^{229}Th is a very favourable route to obtain significant levels of ^{225}Ac required for fabrication of the ^{225}Ac/^{213}Bi generator.

Generator systems providing Auger electron-emitting daughters

Ruthenium-103/rhodium-103m generator

Although not yet explored beyond the evaluation of separation chemistry and discussions of its possible benefits, the potential availability of ^{103m}Rh ($t_{1/2}$ 56.1 minutes) from decay of reactor-produced ^{103}Ru represents a unique availability of this Auger electron emitter for therapeutic applications. The ^{103}Ru parent ($t_{1/2}$ 39.3 days) is a fission product, and separation of Rh/Ru by solvent extraction was established sometime earlier (Chiu *et al.* 1978). More recently, this separation has seen renewed interest (Bartos *et al.* 2009), where the ^{103m}Rh has been obtained by acidic extraction from carbon tetrachloride treated with chlorine gas (CCl_4/Cl_2 solution) of low-specific-activity ^{103}Ru obtained by neutron activation of ruthenium. Repeated organic back extraction of the acid solution then provided the radiochemically pure ^{103m}Rh. It remains to be seen whether such a strategy is practical using high activity levels produced by fission. Another strategy under discussion is the reactor production of ^{103}Ru by neutron irradiation of enriched ^{102}Ru, and development/assessment of a chromatographic-type generator for the simple repeated availability of ^{103m}Rh. Because of the relatively short physical half-life of 56.1 minutes, rapid *in-vivo* targeting of ^{103m}Rh-labelled agents would be required. If a ^{103}Ru/^{103m}Rh generator were routinely available, the potential therapeutic effectiveness of ^{103m}Rh could be explored

The concept of in-vivo radionuclide generators

A relatively recent and potentially useful approach is based on the concept of an *in vivo* generator (Mausner 1992). The concept involves labelling of various molecular carriers (complexes, peptides, mcAb, mcAb-fragments, etc.) with generator parents of intermediate half-life, which after accumulation in the desired tissue generate much shorter half-life daughter radioisotopes (Table 21.8). These *in-vivo* generated daughter radioisotopes can act either as imaging agent (if decaying via single-photon or positron emission) or as therapeutic agent (if decaying via α, β^- or Auger electron emission). In particular for therapy, since the daughter will be in equilibrium *in vivo* with the parent, formation of the particle-emitting daughter will add *in situ* a significant radiation dose. This concept of targeting the parent radioisotope will help increase the radiation dose delivered to the target, which is of particular importance since the usefulness of radiotherapy is often limited by the irradiation of sensitive non-target tissues. The *in-vivo* generator is thus an alternative that could minimise exposure. However, the

Table 21.8 Examples of *in-vivo* generator-type systems

Parent	$t_{1/2}$	Daughter	$T_{1/2}$	Major γ (KeV [%])	E_{max} (MeV)
Actinium-225 (From Th-229)	10 d	Bismuth-213	45.6 m	440 [28]	5.87
Dysprosium-166	81.6 d	Holmium-166	26.8 h	80.5 [6.2]	1.85
Lead-212	10.6 h	Bismuth-212	60.55 m	727 [11.8]	6.05
Palladium-103	16.9 d	Rhodium-103m	56.1 m	20.2 [4.18]	2.39

concept implies that the chemical binding of the daughter isotope is analogous to that of the parent one and the daughter radioisotope is thus retained at the original position. If it is released from the targeted tracer because of various factors that are well known from hot-atom chemistry processes, the decay product will either be bound in the near surrounding environment of the parent owing to other chemical or biochemical binding (such as intracellular trapping effects) or be released from the target site.

The '*in-vivo*' generator is a useful strategy for initial *in-vivo* localisation of the generator parent radionuclide, which then provides localised continued formation of the desired daughter by radioactive decay. Several generator pairs could be used as *in-vivo* systems, providing the parent isotope offers adequate chemical properties for synthesis of labelled compounds and a half-life sufficient for the biochemical or physiological processes in which the labelled compound is involved. In this context, stable labelling with ^{66}Ni and ^{112}Pd, for instance, is not yet established, whereas there are reliable bifunctional chelators available to bind trivalent parent isotopes such as ^{166}Ho and ^{213}Bi.

The pair most intensively studied as *in-vivo* generator is $^{166}Ho/^{166}Dy$ (Smith *et al.* 1995). Following intravenous administration of ^{166}Dy-DTPA and subsequent osseous accumulation, no translocation of the daughter ^{166}Ho was observed subsequent to the β^- decay of ^{166}Dy. Although the clinical utility of such an *in-vivo* system has not yet been realised, studies using ^{213}Bi-labelled targeted agents may already be considered as a version of this concept, since the radioisotopes formed during the $^{213}Bi—\alpha \rightarrow {}^{209}Tl$ ($t_{1/2}$ 2.20 min)—$\beta^- \rightarrow {}^{209}Pb$ ($t_{1/2}$ 3.253 h)—$\beta^- \rightarrow$ and $^{213}Bi—\beta^- \rightarrow {}^{213}Po$ ($t_{1/2}$ 4.2 μs)—$\alpha \rightarrow {}^{209}Pb$ decay chain probably remain in the vicinity of the parent isotope cellular environment and significantly contribute to an enhanced radiation dose in the target tissue. The use of complexed ^{225}Ac as an *in-vivo* generator was described as a 'nano generator' (McDevitt *et al.* 2001). Other studies with ^{225}Ac have demonstrated that some carboxylate-derived calixarene agents have an ionophore cavity capable of highly selective complexation of Ac^{3+} in weak acid and neutral solution (McDevitt *et al.* 2001). Successful functionalisation of these molecules may provide other candidate chelate approaches for use of ^{225}Ac for the *in-vivo* generator approach. The use of *in-vivo* generators has been discussed in the context of radiation therapy seeds and of diagnostic tests with ultra-short-lived daughters (Lambrecht *et al.* 1997). Another suggested system is the formation of the ^{103m}Rh Auger emitter via decay of ^{103}Pd (Van Rooyen *et al.* 2008).

Practical issues for use of radionuclide generators

Quality control

Any radionuclide to be used in nuclear medicine must comply with rigorous pharmaceutical quality standards, which include radionuclidic purity, radiochemical purity, chemical purity, pH, sterility, and apyrogenicity. Of course, except in a research setting, the manufacturer must be responsible for the quality of the generator, and in particular sterility and apyrogenicity are not discussed in this chapter. All the components of the generator in contact with the solution containing the daughter and the final solution must be sterilised by gamma irradiation or autoclaving, depending on the materials. Good Manufacturing Practice (GMP) guidelines must be followed to assure the product quality.

The pH value cannot always be measured with pH meter owing to the small volumes that are handled; pH indicator strips are an alternative. The normal accepted pH range for parenteral solutions is 5–7 but it will depend on the further use of the daughter radionuclide solution, whether it will be directly injected into the patient or if it is to be used for a radiolabelling procedure.

Radionuclidic impurities are in most cases gamma emitters and gamma spectroscopy is the recommended technique using a high-purity Ge (HPGe) detector. This detector has the proper resolution for the gamma spectral analysis, both qualitative and quantitative. Beta and alpha spectroscopy can be used depending on the impurities that can be produced. The radionuclidic purity is related to the amount of radionuclidic impurities present in the daughter nuclide solution. Special care must be taken to ensure detection of breakthrough of the parent in column chromatography procedures or its presence due to any type of chemical or physical separation procedures. Other radionuclidic impurities may originate from the nuclear reactions employed for the production of the parent radionuclide, the presence of chemical impurities in the irradiated targets, or – in the case of the parent being produced by a fission reaction – the presence of fission products. Special care must be taken when ^{99}Mo is produced by ^{235}U fission, since the radionuclidic purity of ^{99}Mo is critical before assembling the alumina-based ^{99}Mo/^{99m}Tc generator. In addition to possible presence of ^{99}Mo breakthrough, the possible presence of fission products must be evaluated in ^{99m}Tc samples, a task for the commercial manufacturer.

A particular generator product that requires rigorous and careful analysis is ^{90}Y obtained from the ^{90}Sr/^{90}Y generator. In addition to being a pure beta emitter obtained from uranium fission products, very pure ^{90}Sr must be used to prepare the generators. The radionuclidic quality control of ^{90}Sr is very difficult because the ^{90}Y daughter is also a pure beta emitter. Since ionic ^{90}Sr is a bone-seeking agent, the levels of ^{90}Sr allowed in the ^{90}Y product must be very low. The current quality control guidelines allow only ^{90}Sr levels less than 74 kBq (2 μCi) per 37 MBq. Since even very low levels ^{90}Sr cannot be detected in the beta spectra of ^{90}Sr/^{90}Y mixtures, the current method of beta spectroscopy requires adequate time for the complete decay of ^{90}Y before the possible levels on contaminating ^{90}Sr can be assessed. Some new methods are being studied for a rapid estimated analysis, such as the use of Eichrom resins and chromatography paper impregnated with KSM-17 chromatography (Pandey *et al.* 2008).

Radiochemical purity measures the amount of the daughter radionuclide in the specified radiochemical form. The methods are all well known, most of them described in the pharmacopoeias, and the main techniques employed are paper chromatography (PC), thin-layer chromatography (TLC), instant thin layer chromatography (ITLC) and high performance liquid chromatography (HPLC). One factor that can increase the radiochemical level of impurities is radiolysis within the generator system. It is well known that the alumina-based ^{99}Mo/^{99m}Tc generator must be dried after the ^{99m}Tc elution, because the radiolysis of water can lead to low elution yields and the presence of $^{99m}TcO_2$. The same post-elution drying procedure has also been recommended for use of the ^{188}W/^{188}Re generator system.

The chemical purity control measures the level of chemical impurities that can be toxic when injected into the patient or can interfere in the labelling procedures performed with the daughter radionuclide. These chemical impurities can arise from the generator system employed; an example is Al^{3+}, which can be released from alumina-based chromatographic generators. In addition, impurities arising from the target materials during the production of the parent radionuclide and chemical impurities can also be introduced from reagents, solutions and glassware. The level of chemical impurities allowed is very low and can be determined by several techniques, such as atomic absorption spectrometry, inductively coupled plasma (ICO)–optical spectrometry (ICP-OES) or ICP–mass spectrometry (ICP-MS), gas chromatography (solvents coming from solvent extraction generators), HPLC and even spot tests.

Radiation protection and generator automation/semiautomation

Radiation protection when handling radionuclide generators in the radiopharmacy is of central importance and the need for limiting the doses to the extremities (hands) in particular cannot be overstated. High-level doses can result from routine/repeated handling of high levels of generator-derived and other therapeutic and diagnostic radioisotopes that are now being used at increasing activity levels. Although ALARA and GLP practices must be followed, adequate radiation protection measures to minimise doses encountered during the routine handling of high-energy beta-emitting and positron-emitting radioisotopes is a relatively new challenge for routine radiopharmacy practice. This area often does not receive adequate attention and vigilance and continued implementation of improved methods and engineering controls is important. In this regard, the development and use of automated elution and synthesis modules is important, and good practice in this area is important both for standardising generator elution, concentration, and radiolabelling procedures, and for significantly reducing radiation dose to radiopharmacy staff.

An example of such a generator that provides a therapeutic radioisotope is the development and operation of an automated system for elution of the tungsten-188/rhenium-188 generator and subsequent use of the high-specific-activity rhenium-188 (McKillop *et al.* 2007). Modular components make up an automated system for saline elution and concentration of the rhenium-188 bolus, and a microprocessor-controlled system for preparation of the rhenium-188-labelled *N,N*-diethyldithiocarbamate (DEDC) agent for treatment of hepatocellular hepatoma.

In addition to the well-known automation required for routine use of the $^{82}Sr/^{82}Rb$ generator system (Gennaro *et al.* 1984), another example is the recent development of an automated system to provide the gallium-68 positron emitter obtained from the $^{68}Ge/^{68}Ga$ generator (Asti *et al.* 2008). This automated system elutes the $^{68}Ge/^{68}Ga$ generator and prepares the ^{68}Ga-(DOTA-Tyr^{3})-octreotide (DOTATOC) agent for cancer therapy. Gallium-68-labelled DOTATOC and analogous peptides are increasingly used for PET imaging of receptor-mediated targets, the availability of such a system helps to reduce radiation exposure during radiopharmaceutical preparation. The development of these two automated systems is an important example of effective collaboration between academia and industry. More recently, a semiautomated system for operation of the $^{188}W/^{188}Re$ generator for on-line concentration of the ^{188}Re bolus has also been described (Wunderlich *et al.* 2008).

Challenges and expected developments

Key operational challenges for the practical use of new and improved radionuclide generator systems include optimal yields and purity of the daughter, optimised operational shelf-life, use of the highest parent loading capacity adsorbents in the case of adsorbent-type systems and optimisation of the daughter eluent activity concentration. Radiation protection is paramount for the safe handling, especially in the use of higher-activity generators that provide positron-emitting and therapeutic radioisotopes. In many cases, the installation and use of these high-activity generators in centralised radiopharmacy facilities will be an effective strategy for the their cost-effective utilisation and the efficient distribution of unit doses under well-established quality systems.

Acknowledgments

ORNL is managed by UT Battelle, LLC, for the US Department of Energy, under contract No. DE-AC05-00OR22725. The authors thank their colleagues and collaborators who have helped review this chapter.

References

Apostolidis C *et al.* (2005). Cyclotron production of Ac-225 for targeted alpha therapy. *Appl Radiat Isot* 62: 383–387.

Asti M *et al.* (2008). Validation of $^{68}Ge/^{68}Ga$ generator processing by chemical purification for routine clinical application of ^{68}Ga-DOTATOC. *Nucl Med Biol* 35: 721–724.

Atcher RW *et al.* (1988). An improved generator for the production of ^{212}Pb and ^{212}Bi from ^{224}Ra. *Int J Rad Appl Instrum [A]* 39: 283–286.

Bateman H (1910). The solution of a system of differential equations occurring in the theory of radioactive transformations. *Proc Cambridge Philos Soc* 15: 423–427.

Bartos B *et al.* (2009). $^{103}Ru/^{103m}Rh$ generator. *J Radioanalyt Nucl Chem* 279(2): 655–657.

Bett R *et al.* (1983). Development and use of the $^{195m}Hg/^{195m}Au$ generator for first pass radionuclide angiography of the heart. *Int J Appl Radiat Isot* 34: 959–963.

Beyer GH, Raun HL (1991). A $^{81}Rb/^{81m}Kr$ generator made from ion implantation. *Appl Radiat Isot* 42: 141–142.

Blower PJ (1993). Extending the life of a ^{99m}Tc generator: a simple and convenient method for concentrating generator eluate for clinical use. *Nucl Med Commun* 14: 995–997.

Blower PJ *et al.* (2000). $^{99m}Tc(V)$DMSA quantitatively predicts $^{188}Re(V)$DMSA distribution in patients with prostate cancer metastatic to bone. *Eur J Nucl Med* 27: 1405–1409.

Bokhari TH *et al.* (2009). Concentration of ^{68}Ga via solvent extraction. *Appl Radiat Isot* 67: 100–102.

Boll RA *et al.* (2005). Production of actinium-225 for alpha particle mediated radioimmunotherapy. *Appl Radiat Isot* 62: 667–679.

Boyd ELR *et al.* (1984). Radionuclide generator technology. Status and prospects. In: *Proceedings International Conference on Radiopharmaceuticals and Labeled Compounds*, Tokyo, October 1984. CN 45/102. Vienna: IAEA.

Boyd RE (1986). In: *Seminar on Radionuclide Generator Technology*, Paper 21, IAEA-Sr.131. Vienna: IAEA

Boyd RE *et al.* (1982). In: Raynaud C, ed. *Proceedings of the 3rd World Congress of Nuclear Medicine and Biology*, 29 August–2 September, Paris. Vol. II. New York: Pergamon Press, 1592.

Bray LA, Wester DW (30 April 1996). *Method of Preparation of Yttirum-90 from Strontium-90*. US Patent 5,512,256

Bray LA *et al.* (2000). Development of a unique bismuth (Bi-213) automated generator for use in cancer therapy. *Ind Eng Chem Res* 39: 3189–3194.

Brihaye C *et al.* (1982). Development of a reliable Hg-195m→Au-195m generator for the production of Au-195m, a short-lived nuclide for vascular imaging. *J Nucl Med* 23: 1114–1120.

Brihaye C *et al.* (1986a). A new osmium-191/iridium-191m radionuclide generator system using activated carbon. *J Nucl Med* 27: 380–387.

Brihaye C *et al.* (1986b). In: Seminar on Radionuclide Generators, Vienna, Austria, 13–17 October 1986. IAEA Symposium IAEA-Sr-131/08. Vienna: IAEA.

Brihaye C *et al.* (1987). Preparation and evaluation of a hydrous tin (IV) oxide $^{82}Sr/^{82}Rb$ medical generator system for continuous elution. *Int J Appl Radiat Isot* 38: 213–217.

Brucer M (1965). Medical radioisotope cows. *Isot Radiat Tech* 3: 1–12.

Bruland OS *et al.* (2006). High-linear energy transfer irradiation targeted to skeletal metastases by the α-emitter ^{223}Ra: adjuvant or alternative to conventional modalities? *Clin Can Res* 12(Suppl. 20): 6250s–6257s.

Buchmann I *et al.* (2002). Myeloablative radioimmunotherapy with Re-188-anti-CD66-antibody for conditioning of high-risk leukemia patients prior to stem cell transplantation: biodistribution, biokinetics and immediate toxicities. *Can Biother Radiopharm* 17: 151–163.

Callahan AP *et al.* (1989). Rhenium-188 for therapeutic applications from alumina-based tungsten-188/rhenium-188 radionuclide generator. *Nucl Compact Eur/Am Commun Nucl Med* 20: 3–6.

Chakravarty R *et al.* (2008). Development of an electrochemical $^{90}Sr/^{90}Y$ generator for separation of ^{90}Y suitable for targeted therapy. *Nucl Med Biol* 35: 245–253.

Cheng C *et al.* (1980). A new osmium-191/iridium-191m generator. *J Nucl Med* 21: 1169–1176.

Chinol M, Hnatowich DJ (1987). Generator-produced yttrium-90 for radioimmunotherapy. *J Nucl Med* 28: 1465–1470.

Chiu J-H *et al.* (1978). Separation of Rhodium-103 by volvent extraction. *Anal Chem* 50: 670–671.

Christian JD *et al.* (2000). Advances in sublimation separation of technetium-99m low-specific-activity molybdenum-99. *Ind Eng Chem Res* 39: 3157–3168.

Chuang JT, Lo JG (1996). Extraction chromatographic separation of carrier-free ^{90}Y from $^{90}Sr/^{90}Y$ generator by crown ether coated silica gels. *J Radioanal Nucl Chem* 204: 83–93.

Clark JC *et al.* (1976). Krypton-81m generators. *Radiochem Radioanal Lett* 25: 245–253.

Clinical Trials.gov (2008) [Dose escalation and safety study of ^{188}Re-PTI-6D2 in patients with metatstatic melanoma]. http://clinicaltrials.gov/ct2/results?term=rhenium-188 (accessed 30 June 2010).

Dadachova E *et al.* (1994). An improved tungsten-188/rhenium-188 gel generatopr based on zirconium tungstate. *J Radioanal Nucl Chem Lett* 188: 267–278.

Dadachova E *et al.* (1995a). Separation of carrier-free holmium-166 from neutron-irradiated dysprosium targets. *Anal Chem* 66: 4272–4277.

Dadachova E *et al.* (1995b). Separation of carrier-free holmium-166 from dysprosium oxide targets by partition chromatography and electrophoresis. *J Radioanal Nucl Chem Lett* 199: 115–123.

Evans JV *et al.* (1982). A new generator for ^{99m}Tc. In: Raynaud C, ed. *Proceedings of the 3rd World Congress of Nuclear Medicine and Biology*, 29 August–2 September, Paris. Vol. II. New York: Pergamon Press, 1592–1595.

Finn RD *et al.* (1983). *NAS-NS-3202 (De83016360).* Nuclear Science Series – Nuclear Medicine. Washington DC: US DOE.

Franken PR *et al.* (1989). Clinical usefulness of a ultra-short-lived iridium-191m from a carbon-based generator system for the evaluation of left ventricular ejection fraction. *J Nucl Med* 30: 1025–1031.

Franken PR *et al.* (1991). Comparison between exercise myocardial perfusion and wall motion using ^{201}Tl and ^{191m}Ir simultaneously. *Nucl Med Commun* 12: 473–484.

Fujibayashi F *et al.* (1989). A new zinc-62/copper-62 generator as a copper-62 source for PET radiopharmaceuticals. *J Nucl Med* 30: 1838–1842.

Fujibayashi Y *et al.* (1997). Copper-62-ATSM: a new hypoxia imaging agent with high membrane permeability and low redox potential. *J Nucl Med* 38: 1155–1160.

Geerlings MW *et al.* (1993). The feasibility of ^{225}Ac as a source of alpha-particles in radioimmunotherapy. *Nucl Med Commun* 14: 121–125.

Gennaro GP *et al.* (1984). In: Knapp Jr FF, Butler TA, eds. *Radionuclide Generators – New Systems for Nuclear Medicine Applications.* ACS Symposium Series No. 241. Washington, DC: American Chemical Society 135.

Green MA *et al.* (1990). Copper-62-labeled pyruvaldehyde bis (N^4-methylthiosemicarbazonato)copper(II): synthesis and evaluation as a positron emission tomography tracer for cerebral and myocardial perfusion. *J Nucl Med* 31: 1989–1996.

Guhlke S *et al.* (2000). Tandem cation/anion column treatment of ammonium acetate eluants of the alumina-based tungsten-188/rhenium-188 generator: a new simple method for effective concentration of rhenium-188 perrhenate solutions. *J Nucl Med* 41: 1271–1278.

Guillaume M, Brihaye C (1986). Generator for short-lived gamma and positron-emitting radionuclides: current state and perspectives. *Int J Appl Radiat Isot* 13: 89–100.

Guillaume M *et al.* (1983). Krypton-81m generator for ventilation and perfusion. *Bull Soc Roy Liège* LII: 213–281.

Hassfjell S, Brechbiel MW (2001). The development of the alpha-particle emitting radionuclides ^{212}Bi and ^{213}Bi, and their decay chain related radionuclides, for therapeutic applications. *Chem Rev* 101: 2019–2036.

Haynes NE *et al.* (2000). Performance of a ^{62}Zn/^{62}Cu generator in clinical trials of PET perfusion agent ^{62}Cu-PTSM. *J Nucl Med* 41: 309–314.

Hoffman M *et al.* (2001). Biokinetics and imaging with the somatostatin receptor PET radioligand ^{68}Ga-DOTATOC: preliminary data. *Eur J Nucl Med* 28: 1751–1577.

Holman BL *et al.* (1978). Tantalum-178 – a short-lived nuclide for nuclear medicine: production of the parent W-178. *J Nucl Med* 19: 510–513.

Hong YD *et al.* (2002). Holmium-166-DTPA as a liquid source for endovascular brachytherapy. *Nucl Med Biol* 29: 833–839.

IAEA (2008). Homogeneous Aqueous Solution Nuclear Reactors for the Production of Mo-99 and Other Short Lived Radioisotopes. TECDOC-1601. Vienna: IAEA. ISSN 1011-4289

Issacher D *et al.* (1989). Osmium-191/iridium-191m generator based on silica gel impregnated with tridecylmethylammonium chloride. *J Nucl Med* 30: 538–541.

Jeong JM, Chung J-K (2003). Update: therapy with ^{188}Re-labeled radiopharmaceuticals: an overview of promising results from initial clinical studies. *Can Biother Radiopharm* 18: 707–718.

Jeong JM, Knapp FF Jr (2008). Use of the Oak Ridge National Laboratory tungsten-188/rhenium-188 generator for preparation of the rhenium-188 HDD/lipiodol complex for trans-arterial liver cancer therapy. *Semin Nucl Med* 38: S19–29.

Jones T, Clark JC (1969). A cyclotron produced ^{81}Rb-^{81m}Kr generator and its uses in gamma-camera studies. *Br J Radiol* 42: 237.

Jurcic JG *et al.* (2002). Targeted alpha particle immunotherapy for myeloid leukemia. *Blood* 100: 1233–1239.

Ketring AR *et al.* (2002). Production and supply of high specific activity radioisotopes for radiotherapy. *Rev Med Nucl Alasbimn J* 5: 1.

Knapp FF Jr (1998). Use of rhenium-188 for cancer treatment. *Cancer Biother Radiopharm* 13: 337–349.

Knapp Jr FF, Butler TA, eds. (1984). *Radionuclide Generators: New Systems for Nuclear Medicine Applications*. ACS Advances, Chemistry Series No. 241. Washington DC: American Chemical Society.

Knapp Jr FF, Mirzadeh S (1994). The continuing important role of radionuclide generator systems for nuclear medicine. *Eur J Nucl Med* 21: 1151–1166.

Knapp Jr FF *et al.*, eds. (1992). Symposium on Radionuclide Generator Systems for Nuclear Medicine Applications, American Chemical Society, Washington, D.C., August 1992. *Radioact Radiochem (Special Issue)* 3.

Knapp Jr FF *et al.* (1994). Processing of reactor-produced tungsten-188 for fabrication of clinical scale alumina-based tungsten-188/rhenium-188 generators. *Appl Radiat Isot* 45: 1123–1128.

Knapp Jr FF *et al.* (1997). Development of the alumina-based tungsten-188/rhenium-188 generator and use of rhenium-188-labeled radiopharmaceuticals for cancer treatment. *Anticancer Res* 17: 1783–1796.

Knapp Jr FF *et al.* (1998). Rhenium-188 liquid-filled balloons effectively inhibit restenosis in a swine coronary overstretch model – a simple new method bridging nuclear medicine and interventional cardiology. *J Nucl Med* 39: 48P.

Knapp Jr FF *et al.* (1999). Endovascular beta irradiation for prevention of restenosis using solution radioisotopes: pharmacologic and dosimetric properties of rhenium-188 compounds. *Cardiovasc Rad Med* 1: 1–9.

Knapp Jr FF *et al.* (2001). Intravascular radiation therapy with radioactive liquid-filled balloons for inhibition of restenosis after angioplasty – a new opportunity for nuclear medicine? *J Nucl Med* 42: 1384–1387.

Lacy JL *et al.* (1988a). An improved tungsten-178/tantalum-178 generator system for high volume clinical applications. *J Nucl Med* 29: 1526–1538.

Lacy JL *et al.* (1988b). First-pass radionuclide angiography using a multiwire gamma camera and tantalum-178. *J Nucl Med* 29: 293–301.

Lacy JL *et al.* (1991). Development and clinical performance of an automated portable tungsten-178/tantalum-178 generator. *J Nucl Med* 32: 2158–2161.

Lacy JL *et al.* (2001). Development and validation of a novel technique for murine first-pass radionuclide angiography with a fast multiwire camera and tantalum 178. *J Nucl Card* 8: 171–181.

Lambert B, de Klerk JMH (2006). Clinical applications of ^{188}Re-labelled radionuclides for radionuclide therapy. *Nucl Med Commun* 27: 223–230.

Lambrecht RM (1983). Radionuclide generators. *Radiochim Acta* 34: 9–24.

Lambrecht RM, Sajjad M (1988). Accelerator-derived radionuclide generators. *Radiochim Acta* 43: 171–179.

Lambrecht RM *et al.* (1997). Radionuclide generators. *Radiochim Acta* 77: 103–123.

Lebowitz E, Richards P (1974). Radionuclide generators. *Semin Nucl Med* 4: 257–268.

Lin JW *et al.* (2001). Quantification of myocardial perfusion in human subjects using ^{82}Rb and wavelet-based noise reduction. *J Nucl Med* 42: 201–208.

Loc'h C *et al.* (1980). A new generator for ionic gallium-68. *J Nucl Med* 21: 171–173.

Mani RS (1987). Reactor production of radionuclides for generators. *Radiochim Acta* 41: 103–110.

Mathias CJ *et al.* (1991). In vivo comparison of copper blood-pool agents: potential radiopharmaceuticals for use with copper-62. *J Nucl Med* 32: 475–480.

Mausner LF (1992). The in vivo generator. Presented at the Division of Nuclear Chemistry and Technology, 204th Annual Meeting, American Chemical Society National Meeting, Washington DC, 24–28 August 1992.

McDevitt MR *et al.* (2001). Tumor therapy with targeted atomic nanogenerators. *Science* 294: 1537–1540.

McKillop JH *et al.* (2007). Highlights of the European Association of Nuclear Medicine Congress, Athens, Greece, September 30th – October 4th, 2006. *Eur J Nucl Med* 34: 274–293.

Mena I (1985). In: Paras P, Thiessen JW, eds. *Single-Photon Ultrashort-Lived Radionuclides.* Proceedings of the Symposium Held in Washington, DC, 9–10 May 1983. *Nat Tech Inform Service, Conf-830504* (De 83017017). Washington DC: US DOE, 19.

Mirzadeh S (1998). Generator produced alpha emitters. *Appl Radiat Isot* 49: 345–349.

Mirzadeh S, Knapp FF Jr (1996). Biomedical radionuclide generator systems. *J Radioanal Nucl Chem* 203: 471–486.

Mirzadeh S, Lambrecht RM (1996). Radiochemistry of germanium. *J Radioanal Nucl Chem* 202: 7–102.

Mirzadeh S *et al.* (1997). Burn-up cross section of tungsten-188. *Radiochim Acta* 77: 99–102.

Morgenstern A *et al.* (2008). Production of $^{230}U/^{226}Th$ for targeted alpha therapy via proton irradiation of ^{231}Pa. *Anal Chem* 80: 8763–8770.

National Academy Report (2009). *Medical Isotope Production without Highly Enriched Uranium.* Washington DC: National Academy Press.

Neirinckx RD, Davis MA (1980). Potential column chromatography for ionic Ga-68. II: Organic ion exchangers as chromatographic supports. *J Nucl Med* 21: 81–83.

Neirinckx RD *et al.* (1978). Tantalum-178 – a short-lived nuclide for nuclear medicine: development of a potential generator system. *J Nucl Med* 19: 514–519.

Neirinckx RD *et al.* (1979). Production and purification of tungsten-178. *Int J Appl Radiat Isot* 30: 341–344.

Nilsson S *et al.* (2005). First clinical experience with α-emitting radium-223 in the treatment of skeletal metastases. *Clin Can Res* 11: 4451–4459.

Novgorodov AF *et al.* (2000). Thermochromatographic separation of no-carrier-added ^{186}Re or ^{188}Re from tungsten targets relevant to nuclear medical applications. *Radiochim Acta* 88: 163–167.

Ofluoglu S *et al.* (2002). Radiation synovectomy with ^{166}Ho-ferric hydroxide: a first experience. *J Nucl Med* 43: 1489–1494.

Okazawa H *et al.* (1994). Clinical application and quantitative evaluation of generator-produced copper-62-PTSM as a brain perfusion tracer for PET. *J Nucl Med* 35: 1910–1915.

Padhy AK, Dondi MA (2008). Management of liver cancer using radionuclide methods with special emphasis on trans-arterial radio-conjugate therapy and internal dosimetry. Report on the Implementation Aspects of the International Atomic Energy Agency's First Doctoral Coordinated Research Project. *Semin Nucl Med* 38: S5–S12.

Palmedo H *et al.* (2000). Dose escalation study with rhenium-188-HEDP in prostate cancer patients with osseous metastases. *Eur J Nucl Med* 27: 123–130.

Pandey U *et al.* (2008). Extraction paper chromatography technique for the radionuclide purity evaluation of ^{90}Y for clinical use. *Anal Chem* 80: 801–807.

Panek KJ *et al.* (1984). In: Knapp Jr FF, Butler TA, eds. *Radionuclide Generators – New Systems for Nuclear Medicine Applications.* ACS Symposium Series No. 241. Washington, DC: American Chemical Society 3.

Panek KJ *et al.* (1985). In: Paras P, Thiessen JW, eds. Single-*Photon Ultrashort-Lived Radionuclides.* Proceedings of the Symposium held in Washington, DC, 9–10 May 1983. Nat Tech Inform Service, Conf-830504 (De 83017017). Washington DC: US DOE, 202.

Paras P, Thiessen, eds. (1985). Single-*Photon Ultrashort-Lived Radionuclides.* Proceedings of the Symposium held in Washington, DC, 9–10 May 1983. Nat Tech Inform Service, Conf-830504 (De 83017017). Washington DC: US DOE.

Park SW *et al.* (2001). Treatment of diffuse in-stent restenosis with rotational atherectomy followed by radiation therapy with a rhenium-188-mercaptoacetyltriglycine-filled balloon. *J Am Coll Cardiol* 38: 631–637.

Rajendran JG *et al.* (2002). High-dose ^{166}Ho-DOTMP in myeloablative treatment of multiple myeloma: pharmacokinetics, biodistribution, and absorbed dose estimation. *J Nucl Med* 43: 1383–1390.

Reynen K *et al.* (2006). Intracoronary radiotherapy with a rhenium-188 liquid-filled angioplasty balloon system in in-stent restenosis: a single center, prospective, randomized, placebo-controlled, double-blind evaluation. *Coron Artery Dis* 17: 371–377.

Richards P (1960). A survey of the production at BNL of isotopes for medical research. *V Congresso Nucleare, Rome* 2: 225–244.

Rizzo-Padoin N *et al.* (2001). A comparison of the radiopharmaceutical agents used for the diagnosis of pulmonary embolism. *Nucl Med Commun* 22: 375–381.

Robinson DG (1972). Impurities in ^{99m}Tc-sodium pertechnetate produced by methyl-ethyl ketone extraction. *J Nucl Med* 13(5): 318–320.

Roesch F, Knapp Jr FF (2003). Radionuclide generators. In: Vertes A, Klencsar NS, eds. *Handbook of Nuclear Chemistry*, Vol. 4, Chapter 3. Amsterdam: Kluwer Academic Publishers, 81–118.

Ruth T (2009). Accelerating production of medical radioisotopes. *Science* 457: 536–537.

Ruth TJ *et al.* (1989). Radionuclide production for the biosciences. *Nucl Med Biol* 16: 323–336.

Rutherford E, Soddy F (1902). The course and nature of radioactivity. *Phil Mag* 4: 370–396.

Sarkar SK *et al.* (2001). Post-elution concentration of $^{99m}TcO4^-$ by a single anion exchange column. I. Feasibility of extending the useful shelf life of column chromatographic ^{99m}Tc generator. *Appl Radiat Isot* 55: 561–567.

Savio E *et al.* (2001). Rhenium-188-HEDP: pharmacokinetic characterization in osseous metastatic patients with two levels of radiopharmaceutial dose. *BMC Nucl Med* 1: 1471–1485.

Schumacher J, Maier-Borst W (1981). A new $^{68}Ge/^{68}Ga$ radioisotope generator system for production of ^{68}Ga in dilute HCl. *Int J Appl Radiat Isot* 32: 31–36.

Smith SV *et al.* (1995). Dysprosium-166/holmium-166 *in vivo* generator. *Appl Radiat Isot* 46: 759–764.

Stang L. (1969). *Radionuclide Generators: Past, Present and Future.* BNL 50186, T-541. Upton, NY: Brookhaven National Laboratory.

Sundram FX *et al.* (2002). Phase I Study of transarterial rhenium-188-HDD lipiodol in treatment of inoperable primary hepatocellular carcinoma – a multicentre evaluation. *World J Nucl Med* 1: 5–11.

Taniuchi H *et al.* (1995). Cu-pyruvaldehyde-bis(N^4-methylthiosemicarbazone) (Cu-PTSM), a metal complex with selective NADH-dependent reduction by complex I in brain mitochondria: a potential radiopharmaceutical for mitochondria-functional imaging with positron emission tomography (PET). *Biol Pharm Bull* 18: 1126–1129.

Treves S *et al.* (1976). Angiocardiography with iridium-191m. An ultrashort-lived radionuclide ($T^1/_2$ 4. 9 sec). *Circulation* 54: 275–279.

Treves S *et al.* (1980). Iridium-191m angiocardiography for the detection and quantification of left-to-right shunting. *J Nucl Med* 21: 1151–1157.

Treves ST *et al.* (1999). Rapid single-photon emission tomography by continuous infusion of iridium-191m. *Eur J Nucl Med* 26: 489–493.

USP/NF (1995). *U.S. Pharmacopeia/National Formulary*, USP 23, NF 18.

Velikyan I *et al.* (2008). Convenient preparation of ^{68}Ga-based PET-radiopharmaceuticals at room temperature. *Bioconjug Chem* 19: 569–573.

Verani MS *et al.* (1992). Quantification of left ventricular performance during transient coronary occlusion at various anatomic sites in humans: a study using tantaloum-178 and a multi-wire gamma camera. *J Am Coll Card* 19: 297.

Van Rooyen J *et al.* (2008). A possible in vivo generator – $^{103}Pd/^{103m}Rh$ – recoil considerations. *Appl Radiat Isot* 66: 1346–1349.

Wallhaus TR *et al.* (1998). Human biodistribution and dosimetry of the PET perfusion agent copper-62-PTSM. *J Nucl Med* 39: 1958–1964.

Wallhaus TR *et al.* (2001). Copper-62-pyruvaldehyde bis(N-methyl-thiosemicarbazone) PET imaging in the detection of coronary artery disease in humans. *J Nucl Card* 8: 67–74.

Waters SL, Coursey BM, eds. (1987). *Appl Radiat Isot (Special Issue)* vol. 38.

Weinberger J, Knapp Jr FF (1999). Use of liquid-filled balloons for coronary irradiation. In: Waksman R, ed. *Vascular Brachytherapy*, 2nd edn, Chapter 45. Armonk, NY: Futura Publishing Co., Inc., 521–535. ISBN 0-87993-4131.

Weinberger J *et al.* (1999). Radioactive beta-emitting solution-filled balloon treatment prevents porcine coronary restenosis. *Cardiovasc Rad Med* 1: 252–256.

Winsche WE, Stang LG, Jr Tucker WD (1951). Production of iodine-132. *Nucleonics* 8: 14–18.

Wunderlich G *et al.* (2008). A semi-automated system for concentration of rhenium-188 for radiopharmaceutical applications. *Appl Radiat Isot* 66: 1876–1880.

Yano Y, Anger HO (1968). Visualization of the heart and kidneys in animals with ultra-short-lived ^{82}Rb and the positron scintillation camera. *J Nucl Med* 9: 412–415.

Zhernosekov KP *et al.* (2007). Processing of generator-produced ^{68}Ga for medical application. *J Nucl Med* 48: 1741–1748.

22

Quality assurance requirements

Alison Beaney

The EU Rules and Guidance for Pharmaceutical Manufacturers and Distributors (MHRA 2007), commonly referred to as the 'Orange Guide', states that Quality Assurance is a wide-ranging concept that covers all matters that individually or collectively influence the quality of a product. It is the total sum of the organised arrangements made with the object of ensuring that medicinal products are of the quality required for their intended use. Quality Assurance (QA) incorporates Good Manufacturing Practice (GMP) plus other factors outside the scope of the Orange Guide (such as product design).

GMP is that part of QA that ensures that products are consistently produced and controlled to the quality standards appropriate to their intended use. GMP is concerned with both production and quality control (QC).

Quality control is the part of GMP that is concerned with sampling, specifications and testing, and with the organisation, documentation and release procedures that ensure that the necessary and relevant tests are actually carried out and that materials are not released for use, nor products released for sale or supply, until their quality has been judged to be satisfactory.

It can therefore be appreciated that QA is a much wider concept than QC (which is only concerned with sampling, testing and release). One of the fundamental principles of GMP is that there must be independence of production and QC. This can sometimes be difficult to achieve in practice in a radiopharmacy with few staff, but independent checks should be carried out wherever possible and release should be carried out by someone not directly involved in the preparation of the particular product. When this is not possible, for example in an out-of-hours emergency situation, there should be a mental break between the processes of production and release, and a rigorous self-check should be carried out.

The EU GMP guide (MHRA 2007)) acknowledges that, because of their short shelf-life, some radiopharmaceuticals must be released before completion of certain QC tests. In this case, it stresses, the continuous assessment of the effectiveness of the quality assurance system becomes very important, and self-inspection plays a vital role.

Where some aspects of QC testing are subcontracted, for example sterility testing, the responsibility for auditing the off-site service lies with the purchaser. It is essential that any testing laboratory is fully conversant with the technical background and requirements of aseptic preparation of radiopharmaceuticals and must have validated methodology for testing. Its personnel must also have a comprehensive knowledge of pharmaceutical microbiology. A current technical agreement between the purchaser and provider of the service must be in place. An example of a technical agreement is available in the Quality Assurance of Aseptic Preparation Services standards (Beaney 2006).

Good documentation constitutes an essential part of any quality assurance system. It prevents errors from verbal communication and allows the history of products to be traced. All documentation – procedures, master worksheets, logs, etc. – must be clear and detailed, and approved by an appropriate senior person. Documents should be regularly reviewed at defined intervals.

Operation, cleaning, maintenance, and fault logs should be maintained for all equipment, including air-handling units. All planned preventative and breakdown maintenance must be clearly documented for the facility in which radiopharmaceuticals are prepared, and also for key equipment. Calibration records should be kept and should include regular external calibration to traceable standards.

Pharmaceutical parameters

Preparation of radiopharmaceuticals will be undertaken in an EU Grade A zone (refer to EU guide). This will be provided by a pharmaceutical isolator, generally negative pressure, sited in a minimum EU GMP Grade D background. Alternatively, a laminar flow workstation, offering both operator and product protection, sited in a Grade B background with three-stage change, can be used. These situations are described in more detail in Chapter 27.

It is now normal practice for blood labelling processes to be carried out in separate Grade A zones from the preparation of routine radiopharmaceutical products. Blood labelling is discussed in Chapter 25 Detailed guidance on facilities for radiopharmaceutical preparation, including blood labelling, is also available in Health Building Note 14-01 (Department of Health 2009).

A comprehensive monitoring programme should be in place to demonstrate on-going compliance with the design criteria for the unit. Validation of the facility, staff and processes is required at commissioning (performance qualification – see Chapter 27) but should be regularly repeated to give continued assurance that these criteria are met. In reality, a routine monitoring schedule has been well described in Chapter 11 of the Quality Assurance of Aseptic Preparation Services text (Beaney 2006). Detailed guidance on procedures that can be used to demonstrate that processes and operators are capable of maintaining the sterility of the product is also available in Appendices 2.1 and 2.2 of the same text.

The microbiological monitoring programme for viable organisms is based on sessional finger dabs and settle plates, weekly surface sampling and quarterly active air sampling. Limits for these tests and for the physical monitoring programme are based on EU GMP. The two programmes complement each other and need to be considered together in the light of any excursions.

It is essential that any out-of-specification monitoring results are investigated, not merely filed. The investigation should be documented (even briefly) and closed out. Any significant or sustained deviations should undergo root cause analysis as these are an indication of loss of control of the environment and therefore are a potential patient risk. Under certain circumstances it may be advisable to increase the frequency of monitoring until confidence in control is restored.

For example, investigation of a problem with finger dab results could include the following:

- Observation of operator aseptic techniques
- Observation of spray/wiping transfer technique
- Isolator integrity (gloves, filters)
- Investigation of portable equipment contamination with swabs (e.g. lead pots).

This list is not comprehensive but gives an indication of suitable topics for investigation.

All units are recommended to carry out routine trend analysis of microbiological results. This may be by use of bar charts, graphs or performance of rolling average calculations. Some units use computer-based software to provide trend analysis electronically. The importance of trend analysis is that it gives an early indication of loss of environmental control. It also provides assurance that this control has been regained after an intervention or problem.

Sterility testing of the final product, as described in Chapter 23 is of questionable value as an indication of quality since a false result could be due to:

- Poor operator technique
- Non-validated positive and negative controls
- The bacteriostatic effect of the chemical environment of the radiopharmaceutical
- The inoculation technique adopted.

Although routine sterility testing is one factor that may be used, it should not give a false sense of security about control of the overall process.

British Pharmacopoeia (BP) monographs (British Pharmacopoeia Commission Secretariat) for individual radiopharmaceutical preparations have the general format of defining the product and setting limits for content of the active ingredient. After describing production methods, the monograph then gives the characteristics of the product and several identification tests. Other tests generally include pH, sterility and tests to control bacterial endotoxins. The monograph will then describe tests for chemical, radionuclidic, and radiochemical purity (often by liquid chromatography) before requiring a measurement of radioactivity. Specific impurities are usually listed, along with their limits and test methodology.

Consequences of impurities/QC failures

Impurities can be classified on the bases of chemical, radiological, physical or microbiological imperfections in a radioactive medicinal product. The consequences to the patients of these imperfections vary from minimal to catastrophic (in diagnostic terms this equates to complete patient mismanagement, i.e. wrong diagnosis; on a therapeutic level, a catastrophic consequence could lead to death).

Chemical impurities

In BP monographs on radiopharmaceutical preparations, chemical purity is controlled by specifying limits on chemical impurities. Chemical purity determination requires the identification and quantification of individual chemical constituents or impurities in a radiopharmaceutical preparation. Assurance of the absence of chemical impurities cannot rely on chemical testing and must be met by means of an assurance of the production process itself along with process design and monitoring. In a normal hospital radiopharmacy, the majority of products are prepared from licensed kits in accordance with their Summary of Product Characteristics (SPC). So long as there is no cross-contamination due to poor process flow in the radiopharmacy, chemical impurities in these types of products should not be an issue. However, use of radiochemical starting materials that are not prepared as active pharmaceutical ingredients (APIs), for example in PET tracer production, presents a much greater risk of impurity excess.

Chemical impurity assessment may be undertaken routinely in the radiopharmacy whereby qualitative assessment of aluminium Al^{3+} ions is made on the first and last elution of each technetium generator and on days when products sensitive to this ion are being prepared. This is usually performed with a commercial test kit that depends upon a visual comparison in colour intensity between a sample of eluate and an Al^{3+} standard. Filter paper is impregnated with a colour complexing agent. A standard solution of aluminium Al^{3+} (10 μg/mL) is supplied. A spot of the standard solution causes a colour change in the paper. A spot of generator eluate is compared to the standard spot. If the colour is more intense in the eluate spot, then the eluate contains more than 10 μg/mL aluminium Al^{3+} and implies a lack of stability in the column; consequently the eluate should be discarded.

The consequences of chemical impurities are minimal. At tracer level, the mass of substance present is often of the order of picomoles or less and is therefore insufficient to saturate the binding sites on any tissue or substrate, and cannot be regarded as an issue for toxicity in the same way as 'classical' pharmaceutical impurities.

Radiochemical impurities

Radiochemical purity has been defined (BP 2009) as the ratio, expressed as a percentage, of the radioactivity of the radionuclide concerned that is present in the radiopharmaceutical preparation in the stated chemical form, to the total radioactivity of that radionuclide present in the radiopharmaceutical preparation. The relevant radiochemical impurities are listed with their limits in the individual BP monographs.

A product failure due to radiochemical impurities occurs when free pertechnetate or unexpected complexes are formed that are present in quantities greater than that defined in the monograph for the particular radiopharmaceutical. Where the level of the impurities (as defined by the monograph or SPC) is above the limits, unforeseen consequences may result, in both diagnosis and therapy. For example, owing to its wide biodistribution, free pertechnetate may mask or reduce the expected uptake, subsequently leading to incorrect diagnosis.

There are consequences for the patient of radiochemical impurities in therapeutic products, e.g. peptide labelling with yttrium-90 could be catastrophic, with free yttrium chloride ablating bone marrow. The quality control of these products is hence of paramount importance to protect patients and is described later in this chapter.

Intermediate levels of, for example, free pertechnetate may result in images that are unreportable. The consequences are two-fold:

- The scan will have to be repeated and thus will result in a needless radiation dose to the patient with associated unnecessary patient distress and inconvenience.
- There is a waste of resources in terms of materials, staff and equipment time.

Physical impurities

The main physical impurity in a radiopharmaceutical is a non-viable particle. This may be a foreign body or may be due to the creation of particles of an incorrect particle size for the correct agent (for example, if particles of a lung scanning agent are 'clumped', there will be central deposition in the lung capillaries only).

The pharmacokinetics of colloids in lymphatics depend on particle size. Different batches from the same manufacturer of albumin colloids have shown markedly different clearance rates during sentinel node investigations. This could lead to a false negative report for identification of a sentinel node from a tumour.

With regard to the presence of non-viable foreign particulate impurities, the BP monograph states that injectable products of volume greater than 100 mL should be 'practically free' (meaning free in practice) from visible particles. The authors would, however, not recommend that radiopharmaceuticals are examined with the same degree of scrutiny as other aseptically prepared non-radioactive products. The radiation dose to the operator, specifically to the cornea, precludes this. However, the absence of gross particulate contamination should be verified by a quick visual examination in order to prevent damage to veins and capillaries on subsequent injection of the radiopharmaceutical.

Microbiological impurities

These arise mainly from the following five sources:

- Airborne contamination
- Contamination by touch
- Surface contamination of components
- Contamination during storage
- Contamination during administration.

Minimising the risk of microbiological contamination is vitally dependent on the aseptic technique of the operator, which should be regularly confirmed by broth transfer operator validation.

The risk is also mitigated by performing aseptic manipulations in a validated EU GMP Grade A environment, generally using closed procedures. The allocation of a short expiry period (often less than 6 hours) coupled with storage at 2–8 °C, which restricts multiplication of any microbiological contamination, is likely to reduce the chance of infection of patients as a consequence of contamination. It must be borne in mind, however, that this risk remains considerable for immunocompromised patients if microbiological impurities are present in their radiopharmaceutical injections.

Types of defects and consequences

Problems reported with radiopharmaceuticals are collated nationally by the UK Radiopharmacy Group (UKRG). Problems generally fall into one of two categories: adverse reactions or quality defects. When reporting, the information required is the name of the manufacturer, the name of the product, its batch number, along with a description of the problem and any action taken.

An adverse reaction is any untoward and unintended response in a patient to whom a medicine has been administered; for example development of a rash, or nausea. This is different from a quality defect, which is defined as a shortcoming in the product when it does not conform to its specification (MHRA 2004). Quality defects are categorised as hazardous, major, or minor, as defined in Table 22.1.

Hazardous or major defects should be reported immediately to the Defective Medicines Report Centre (DMRC) of the MHRA, and there should be a procedure in each radiopharmacy giving details of how to do this based on the MHRA Guidance (MHRA 2004).

Where a defect is considered to be a risk to public health, the holder of the marketing authorisation must withdraw the affected medicine from the market and the DMRC will issue a 'Drug Alert', classified from 1 to 4 depending upon the risk from the defective product. Class 1 (the most critical) requires immediate recall, including out of hours, although this is rare with radiopharmaceuticals. Examples would include serious mislabelling, microbial contamination, or incorrect ingredients.

Table 22.1 Categorisation of quality defects[a]

Adverse drug reaction	Any untoward and unintended response in a subject to whom a medicinal product has been administered, including occurrences which are not necessarily caused by or related to that product.
Defect/defective	Not conforming to specification. A shortcoming.
Hazardous/critical defect	A defect, which has the capability to adversely affect the health of the patient.
Major defect	A defect, which impairs the therapeutic activity of the product. It may not be hazardous.
Minor defect	A defect, which has no important effect upon the therapeutic activity of the product, and does not otherwise produce a hazard.

[a] Taken from *A Guide to Defective Medicinal Products*, Appendix 1 (Glossary), MHRA, 2004, available at http://www.mhra.gov.uk/home/groups/is-lic/documents/publication/con007572.pdf.

In addition to the reporting of minor defects via the UKRPG system, they should also be reported to the manufacturer so that their quality systems can be improved. These defects are also reported to the MHRA, but less urgently and not directly via DMRC, as they have no important effect on the therapeutic activity of the product and do not compromise patient safety; for example, a batch number missing from a label.

Radiopharmacies holding MHRA 'Specials' manufacturing licences are obliged to report any quality defect in a medicine they have produced to the DMRC as part of the terms of their licence. As distribution of radiopharmaceuticals from NHS 'Specials' units is generally restricted, often to within the NHS Trust in which the radiopharmacy is situated, this is unlikely to result in the issue of a Drug Alert.

Audit

Audit is an essential requirement to maintain and update the quality system in a radiopharmacy. Put simply, it is 'taking note of what we do, learning from it, and changing if necessary' (University of Dundee 1993). Several terms are used in relation to audit, and useful guidance is available in the NHS Pharmaceutical Quality Control Committee document 'Quality Audits and Their Application to Hospital Pharmacy Technical Services'(NHS 1999). For example, audit may be either external (where the auditor is from outside the organisation) or internal (from within the organisation). The term self-inspection is often used in licensed units as being equivalent to internal audit.

In all cases, audit forms a cycle (Figure 22.1) wherein data are collected and then performance is evaluated against recognised standards. Changes are then made, in response to an action plan, and the effects of these changes are monitored. To complete the audit cycle, the standards should then be reviewed to ensure they are still relevant and up to date.

Radiopharmacies legally must operate in one of two ways. The first can be under Section 10, Exemption to the 1968 Medicines Act, which allows preparation of medicines to be undertaken without a MHRA Manufacturing Licence if preparation is in response to a prescription and is supervised by a

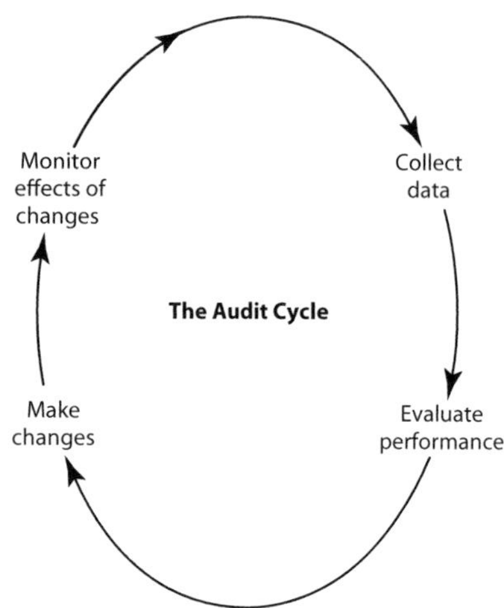

Figure 22.1 The audit cycle.

pharmacist. In this situation a radiopharmacy in the UK NHS will be subject to external audit by Regional Quality Assurance every 12–18 months under the auspices of Executive Letter (97) 52.

Alternatively, a radiopharmacy may hold a MHRA manufacturing licence (ML) (generally a 'Specials' ML, where products are made to the order of a clinician). In this case external audit will be carried out by the MHRA Inspectorate with a frequency determined on a risk basis dependent on performance and the critical nature of the products.

In either case, internal audit (self-inspection) programmes are essential to maintain the quality management system. A comprehensive standard operating procedure (SOP) should be available giving details of personnel involved in leading audits, which aspects will be audited and at what frequency, and how observations will be recorded. The inclusion of a pro-forma action plan and details of the reporting mechanism for the results of the audit is also recommended. Highlighting audit deficiencies as a regular agenda item at quality management meetings is a helpful way of stressing the importance of audit to managers.

The UKRG audit is a useful tool to assist with the audit process (UKRPG 2009). It is wide-ranging in that it covers a number of different aspects of the radiopharmacy service – not merely those relating to GMP.

The workload of the unit should be regularly reviewed, and related to the capacity plan. This is discussed elsewhere in the text (see Chapter 26), but is often considered as part of the audit process as it can impact on quality performance indicators, such as error rates.

References

Beaney AM ed. On behalf of NHS Pharmaceutical Quality Assurance Committee (2006). *Quality Assurance of Aseptic Preparation Services*, 4th edn. London: Pharmaceutical Press.

Department of Health (2009). *Health Building Note 14-01: Pharmacy and Radiopharmacy Facilities*, 2nd edn. Available at http://195.92.246.148/knowledge_network/documents/HBN_14_01_Exec_summ_20070823130817.pdf (accessed April 2009).

MHRA (2004). *A Guide to Defective Medicinal Products*. London: Medicines and Healthcare products Regulatory Agency. Available at www.mhra.gov.uk) (accessed 30 June 2010).

MHRA (2007). *Rules and Guidance for Pharmaceutical Manufacturers and Distributors 2007*. London: Pharmaceutical Press.

NHS (NHS Pharmaceutical Quality Control Committee) (1999). *Quality Audits and Their Application to Hospital Pharmacy Technical Services*. Available at http://www.ukqainfozone.nhs.uk (accessed 30 June 2010).

UKRPG (UK Radiopharmacy Group) (2009). *Radiopharmacy Audit*. Available at http://www.ukrg.org.uk (accessed 30 June 2010).

University of Dundee (1993). *Moving to Audit. An Educational Package for Professions Allied to Medicine*. Centre for Medical Education, University of Dundee.

23

Quality control methods for radiopharmaceuticals

Tony Theobald and Paul Maltby

Introduction

Radiopharmaceuticals are mainly formulated as sterile, apyrogenic injections and are administered to patients for diagnostic or therapeutic purposes. In this respect they are no different from conventional parenteral medicines in their requirements of purity or efficacy. Standards of quality and purity must be specified for these materials and dispensed products should be tested to ensure compliance with those standards. The main difference between radiopharmaceuticals and conventional medicines lies in the very short usable lives of the radioactive product (often measured in hours) compared with those of conventional injectable pharmaceuticals (measured in months or years). Unlike standard parenteral pharmaceuticals, radiopharmaceuticals cannot be manufactured, tested and quarantined until the test results (e.g. sterility) are available as the radioactivity will have decayed to non-useful levels. In contrast to ordinary pharmaceuticals, many radiopharmaceuticals have to be manufactured, quality tested, and then administered to the patient within a short period of time, often within the same working day.

Under these circumstances the radiopharmacist has adopted a set of quick, efficient discriminative tests that can be applied to the dispensed materials before they are released for use in the clinic. These quality control tests are the subject of this chapter. By themselves they do not, and cannot, guarantee the quality of the radiopharmaceutical. Alongside these tests lies another set of controls, such as operator training and performance testing, environmental monitoring, etc., which are the subjects of other chapters in this volume. Radiopharmaceutical quality control testing involves the application of a set of well-defined and validated test procedures to samples of the dispensed or manufactured product. All quality control laboratories will apply the principles of Good Laboratory Practice (GLP), among which are the provision and use of Standard Operating Procedures (SOPs). Test methods are illustrated in this chapter by the inclusion of SOPs in the hope that the reader can adopt similar procedures, suitably modified for local conditions and equipment. However, these SOPs do not indicate the actions to be taken in the event of a product failure as this will depend on local conditions.

There are a number of useful sources of information on the quality control of radiopharmaceuticals. The Pharmacopoeias (European Pharmacopoeia (EP), British Pharmacopoeia (BP), and Unites States Pharmacopeia (USP)) give full specifications for official preparations. Several books and monographs, although now quite dated, still provide detailed descriptions of techniques and applications. Among these may be cited *Quality Control in Nuclear Medicine* (Rhodes 1978), *Guidelines for the Preparation of Radiopharmaceuticals in Hospitals* (British Institute of Radiology 1979), *Quality Assurance of Radiopharmaceuticals – A Guide to Hospital Practice* (Frier, Hesslewood 1980), and *Analytical and Chromatographic Techniques in Radiopharmaceutical Chemistry* (Wieland *et al.* 1986). The European Association for Nuclear Medicine has issued guidelines on current good radiopharmaceutical practices (cGRPP) for both kit-based and PET-radiopharmaceuticals which address some aspects of quality control, and a recent book on technetium radiopharmaceuticals edited by Zolle (2007) is a very useful source of information on the quality control, among much other detail, of these agents. The UK Radiopharmacy Group website has a number of radiochemical purity (RCP) methods described in the Handbook, and several of these are quoted in this chapter.

All radiopharmacies that prepare radiopharmaceuticals for clinical use are required to have a prospective quality assurance programme in place as part of Good Pharmaceutical Manufacturing Practice. The ability to determine radiochemical purity is crucial to check the quality of an approved formulation or kit, or to establish standards for in-house preparations. Every batch of manufactured PET radiopharmaceuticals has to have the results of such testing prior to clinical use. For 'traditional single-photon' tracers, it is accepted that some methods of determination of their radiochemical purity may take longer to achieve a result than the shelf-life of the product itself, thus the result is necessarily retrospective. However, this does not diminish the importance of undertaking these tests.

Several methods for determining the radiochemical purity of an individual radiopharmaceutical may be described in the literature. If the product has a monograph in a pharmacopoeia, then the official method will allow its purity to be determined. In a hospital radiopharmacy it would be more accurate to say that radiochemical purity determinations show the level of impurities rather than describe the purity of a product.

Quality control parameters

There are a number of parameters that are routinely measured as indicators of quality.

Radioactivity

Radioactivity is defined in the BP as 'the number of nuclear transformations per unit time in a given amount of the [radioactive] preparation'. Radioactivity is measured in units of the becquerel (Bq), equivalent to an average transformation rate of one per second. The becquerel is an inconveniently small unit for radiopharmaceutical work and the multiples kBq (10^3 Bq), MBq (10^6 Bq), and GBq (10^9 Bq) are used in practice. The older units of the Curie (Ci, equivalent to 37 GBq), and its submultiples mCi (37 MBq) and μCi (37 kBq) are still used in the USA and in many other countries.

Absolute measurement of radioactivity is difficult and time consuming: it requires equipment and techniques available only in specialist laboratories such as the UK's National Physical Laboratory. The BP sets limits of ±10% (or ±15% in a few cases) for the radioactivity of official radiopharmaceuticals and in the radiopharmacy there is a requirement to measure the radioactivity of dispensed radiopharmaceuticals to a precision of about 2–5%.

Specific radioactivity

Specific radioactivity is defined as the radioactivity of a radionuclide per unit mass of the element or of the chemical form concerned. It is usually calculated taking into account the radioactive concentration (radioactivity per unit volume) and the concentration of the chemical substance being studied, after verification that the radioactivity is attributable only to the radionuclide (radionuclidic purity) and the chemical species (radiochemical purity) concerned. Specific radioactivity changes with time. The statement of the specific radioactivity therefore includes reference to a date and, if necessary, time. The requirement of the specific radioactivity must be fulfilled throughout the period of validity.

Radioactive concentration refers to the radioactivity per unit volume of the preparation, expressed in MBq/mL, for example. As the radioactivity decays with time, so the radioactive concentration decreases and a statement of radioactive concentration must include reference to the date and time, as for specific radioactivity.

Ionisation chambers

Radioactivities in the high kBq and MBq range (i.e. the normal radioactive doses given to patients) are measured with ionisation chambers or radionuclide calibrators. In these instruments the current flowing between a charged cylindrical electrode and ground depends on the radioactivity of a sample placed in a re-entrant chamber. Although the magnitude of this current is small, about 1–10 pA (10^{-12} A), it is easily measured with modern electrometric instruments. The ionisation current (i) depends on the radioactivity (A) and ionising ability (k) of a particular radionuclide:

$$i(\text{pA}) = k(\text{pA/MBq}) \times A(\text{MBq})$$

Different radionuclides have specific ionising factors (k), and commercial ionisation chambers have built-in scaling factors for commonly used radionuclides that give a direct readout in appropriate units (kBq or MBq, or mCi). More advanced instruments can print the measurements on a label or a quality control record sheet.

These instruments will give measurements of adequate precision for the radiopharmacy as long as they are regularly checked with standard calibrated radioactive sources.

Calibration

Checking the calibration of an ionisation chamber or radionuclide calibrators involves three separate measurements.

1. *The calibration factor*: Calibration factors are checked by using standard sources, either sealed solid, or liquid, obtained from a national testing and calibration agency such as the National Physical Laboratory in the UK, or by comparing measurements on samples previously measured in a Secondary Standard Radionuclide Calibrator. In either case a correction for radioactive decay is essential to compensate for the loss of radioactivity in the time between initial standard calibration and local calibration measurements.

   Standardised sources of short-lived radionuclides are expensive, of limited availability, and impracticable. Radiopharmacies use secondary standards containing long-lived radionuclides of similar gamma energy. For example, ^{57}Co ($t_{1/2} = 270$ days, $E_\gamma = 0.122$ MeV) is used as a standard for ^{99m}Tc ($t_{1/2} = 6.02$ hours, $E_\gamma = 0.140$ MeV).
2. *The sample geometry factor*: All ionisation chambers are sensitive to changes in the geometry of the radioactive sample and for reliable measurements the calibration standard sources

should have the same geometry as the radioactive sample (i.e. same volume in the same size injection vial).

Calibration problems can arise when measurements are made on small volumes (less than 5 mL) contained in 20 mL vials, and with single doses pre-packed in disposable syringes, because the calibration factor will vary according to sample volume and shape. It is good practice to recalibrate the instrument for use with syringes preloaded with radiopharmaceuticals and especially with small-volume, high-radioactivity bolus injections. The effect of variations in sample geometry should be assessed initially, then at yearly intervals over a range of sample volumes, vial sizes, and radionuclides expected to be used.

3 *The dynamic range accuracy*: All measuring and readout devices used with ionisation chambers have a number of different ranges or scales, and it is essential to check that the range factors are correct and provide a continuous linear scale over the full measuring range of the instrument.

The simplest method of checking is to take a high-activity sample of a short-lived radionuclide and to measure its radioactivity frequently and repeatedly over the full range of the instrument. Assuming the initial reading is correct, a semilogarithmic plot of measured and calculated radioactivities against time will quickly show any errors in the range factors and linearity of instrument response. A detailed procedure is given in Hauser and Cavallo (1977) and a typical operating procedure is illustrated in SOP 1 (Calibration of Ionisation Chamber). A quicker procedure is to use a set of commercially available lead shields of different wall thickness (and hence attenuation). The highly active sample is placed inside each shield and the apparent radioactivity is recorded. The observations can be plotted against the known attenuation factor of the shields and the linearity and slope of the line compared with standard readings.

It is standard practice to check the radioactivity of all preparations leaving the radiopharmacy for the nuclear medicine clinic or satellite departments, and for the radioactivity to be re-checked on receipt and before administration to the patient. Separate measuring instruments will be used in these locations and it is a wise precaution to check that all instruments remain in calibration by measuring the same standardised sample on each of them, correcting for decay if necessary.

Radionuclide identity

The British and European Pharmacopoeias describe tests for establishing the identity of the radionuclide. These may be a determination of the half-life, measurement of the energy of the radiations emitted, or a combination of both. Determination of the half-life of most medical radionuclides can be done in the radiopharmacy, by a modification of the method suggested for checking the linearity of the ionisation chambers described above. The BP gives some general guidance on the preparation of sources and the frequency and number of activity determinations needed to ensure a reliable result. Measurements at intervals of about half the expected half-life which extend over a period of three half-lives (i.e. six measurements) are considered satisfactory. The readings are converted to their logarithms and plotted against the time of measurement. The slope of the plot gives the decay constant, λ, defined by the relation:

$$\ln(A_t) = \ln(A_0) - \lambda t$$

where A_0 is the initial radioactivity and A_t is the radioactivity at time t, from which the half-life is calculated from the expression:

$$t_{1/2} = \ln(2)/\lambda$$

Determination of the energy spectrum of the radionuclide requires equipment not normally available in the radiopharmacy. In most cases the gamma spectrum is required. The gamma spectrum of a radionuclide that emits gamma rays and/or X rays is unique and characteristic and can be used as an identity test. The spectrum is best obtained with a Ge(Li) semiconductor detector, which gives a narrow photopeak (~2 keV), coupled to a multichannel analyser. The NaI(Tl) scintillation detector can be used for gamma spectroscopy, but suffers from a much lower intrinsic resolution (~50 keV), which may obscure the photopeak of any impurities. Both spectrometer systems need to be calibrated by determining the relationship between the photopeak channel number and standard sources of known gamma energy for identification of radionuclides.

The spectrometer system must also be calibrated for detection efficiency when used to determine radioactivities and levels of radionuclidic impurities. Standard sources of known radioactivity and gamma energy are required. These measurements are normally considered to be outside the activities of the radiopharmaceutical control laboratory. However, assessment of ^{99}Mo breakthrough from the ^{99}Mo/^{99}Tc^{m} generator is possible using an attenuation method involving a calibrated lead pot. Should the pharmacopoeial limit of 0.1% be exceeded, no further preparation of products from that generator may take place, and a replacement must be sought from the manufacturer.

Identification of pure beta emitters is sometimes performed in the radiopharmacy. The BP and EP method consists of determining the count rate of a sample and standard source when attenuated by a series of aluminium screens of increasing thickness and comparing their beta absorption curves. SOP 2 (Determination of Beta Absorption Curves) illustrates a typical procedure for this test.

Radionuclidic purity

The term 'radionuclidic purity' is defined in the BP as 'The ratio, expressed as a percentage, of the radioactivity of the radionuclide concerned to the total radioactivity of the source'. Standards for radionuclide impurities are given in the BP and EP monographs on all radiopharmaceuticals. Table 23.1 shows the impurity limits specified by the BP.

The principle underlying the control of radionuclidic impurities is protection of the patient from unnecessary radiation. Tight limits must be placed on all alpha emitters and long-lived radionuclides which may also have a long biological half-life.

No radionuclide sample is completely free of other radioactive species. The nature of the contaminants will depend on the method of radionuclide production, the impurity profile of the target or other starting material, and the production process employed. Sometimes the contaminants are radioisotopes of the desired radionuclide and these cannot, of course, be removed by chemical treatment. In these situations the only means of quality control lies in the method of production of the radionuclide, which is outside the province and control of the radiopharmacist.

The specified radionuclidic impurity limits reflect the radiological hazard associated with the impurity, the clinical use of the radiopharmaceutical, and the practicality of achieving tighter standards. For example, the BP specifies a limit of 1% for ^{60}Co and less than 2% total radionuclidic impurities in [^{58}Co] cyanocobalamin. The radionuclidic impurities have longer half-lives than the principal radionuclide so that the proportion of the radionuclidic impurity increases with time owing to the differential decay rates of principal and impurity radionuclides. Another important consequence is that the BP radionuclidic impurity limit also effectively defines a shelf-life for these materials.

A more complex set of radionuclidic impurity specifications is given for the most popular diagnostic radionuclide ^{99m}Tc. The radionuclidic purity specification of Sodium Pertechnetate [^{99m}Tc] Injection depends on the source of the parent ^{99}Mo. In the case of Non-Fission Pertechnetate (^{99}Mo produced by neutron bombardment of ^{98}Mo) not more than 0.1% of the total radioactivity is due to the parent ^{99}Mo, and not more than 0.01% of all other radionuclidic impurities. With Fission Sodium Pertechnetate (where the ^{99}Mo is extracted from uranium fission products) the radionuclidic purity specification is much more stringent. Six different impurities are controlled: ^{99}Mo (0.1%), ^{131}I (5×10^{-3}%), ^{103}Ru (5×10^{-3}%), ^{89}Sr (6×10^{-5}%), ^{90}Sr (6×10^{-6}%), and alpha-emitting impurities (1×10^{-7}); also other gamma-emitting impurities are limited to 1×10^{-2}%. In both sources of ^{99m}Tc an unspecified quantity of the long-lived isotope ^{99}Tc resulting from decay of the ^{99m}Tc is permitted.

However, it should be noted that high levels of the beta emitter ^{99}Tc can interfere with the labelling efficiency of a number of ^{99m}Tc radiopharmaceuticals through isotopic dilution and competition for binding sites on the ligands and the Sn(II) reductant, which is present in very slight excess. Manufacturers may specify a maximum regrowth time for ^{99m}Tc in a generator (i.e. maximum time between elutions) to limit the build-up and subsequent eluent content of this isotope and thus maintain the apparent efficiency of radiolabelling. A study of the effect of generator eluate on the quality of MAG3 labelling has been reported by Schomaker (1994).

Table 23.1 BP Standards for conventional radiopharmaceuticals

Preparation	Radionuclidic purity	Radiochemical purity	Details of method	pH	Chemical purity
Chromium [^{51}Cr] Edetate Injection	Gamma spectrum same as standard ^{51}Cr	$\geq$ 95% Cr edetate	Paper electrophoresis using barbitone + nitrate buffer	3.5–6.5	$\leq$ 1 mg/mL Cr
Cyanocobalamin [^{57}Co] Capsules	Gamma spectrum same as standard ^{57}Co $\leq$ 0.1% radionuclidic impurities	$\geq$ 90% in the form of cyanocobalamin	HPLC on C_8 silica with phosphate methanol pH 3.5 at a flow rate of 1 mL/min, UV detection at 361 nm and radiation detection of ^{57}Co	4.0–6.0	
Cyanocobalamin [^{57}Co] Solution	Gamma spectrum same as standard ^{57}Co $\leq$ 0.1% radionuclidic impurities	$\geq$ 90% in the form of cyanocobalamin	HPLC on C_8 silica with phosphate methanol pH 3.5 at a flow rate of 1 mL/min, UV detection at 361 nm and radiation detection of ^{57}Co	4.0–6.0	
Cyanocobalamin [^{58}Co] Capsules	$\leq$ 1% ^{60}Co and $\leq$ 2% total radionuclide imp. due to ^{60}Co + ^{57}Co + others	$\geq$ 84% in the form of cyanocobalamin	HPLC on C_8 silica with phosphate methanol pH 3.5 at a flow rate of 1 mL/min, UV detection at 361 nm and radiation detection of ^{58}Co	4.0–6.0	
Cyanocobalamin [^{58}Co] Solution	$\leq$ 1% ^{60}Co and $\leq$ 2% total radionuclide imp. due to ^{60}Co + ^{57}Co + others	$\geq$ 90% in the form of cyanocobalamin	HPLC on C_8 silica with phosphate methanol pH 3.5 at a flow rate of 1 mL/min, UV detection at 361 nm and radiation detection of ^{58}Co	4.0–6.0	
Gallium [^{67}Ga] Citrate Injection	Gamma spectrum similar to standard $\leq$ 0.2% ^{66}Ga	No test specified			Limit test for zinc (5 ppm)
Indium [^{111}In] Chloride Solution	$\geq$ 99.75% $\leq$ 0.25% ^{114m}In Specific activity $\geq$ 1.85 Bq/μg In	$\geq$ 95% as ionic In(III)	Activated ITLC-SG using 0.9%NaCl at pH 2.3; $InCl_3$ migrates with R_f 0.5–0.8	1.0–2.0	$\leq$ 0.4 μg/mL Cd 0.15 μg/mL Cu 0.60 μg/mL Fe; all by AA
Indium [^{111}In] Oxine Solution	$\geq$ 99.75% $\leq$ 0.25% ^{114m}In specific activity $\geq$ 1.85 GBq/μg	$\geq$ 90% as complex	Phase extraction from saline to octanol; measure activity in each washed layer	6.0 –7.5	
Indium [^{111}In] Pentetate Injection	Gamma and X-ray spectra similar to standard $\leq$ 0.2% ^{114m}In	$\geq$ 95% as pentetate	Activated ITLC-SG using 0.9% saline over 10–15 cm in 10 min. R_f = 1.0	7.0–8.0	$\leq$ 5 μg/mL Cd $\leq$ 0.4 mg/mL pentetic acid

(continued)

Table 23.1 *(continued)*

Preparation	Radionuclidic purity	Radiochemical purity	Details of method	pH	Chemical purity
Iobenguane [^{123}I] Injection	≥ 99.65% Specific activity ≥ 10 GBq/g base ≤ 0.35% other radionuclides	≥ 95% iobenguane ≤ 4% iodide ≤ 1% other radioactivity	HPLC on silica gel using NH_4NO_3:NH_4OH (1 : 27) at 1 mL/min, UV detection at 254 nm and radiation detection of ^{123}I	3.5–8.0	
Iobenguane [^{131}I] Injection for Diagnostic Use	≥ 99.9% Specific activity ≥ 206 GBq/g base	≥ 95% iobenguane ≤ 4% iodide ≤ 1% other radioactivity	HPLC as above	3.5–8.0	
Iobenguane [^{131}I] Injection for Therapeutic Use	≥ 99.9% Specific activity ≥ 400 GBq/g base	≥ 92% iobenguane ≤ 7% iodide ≤ 1% other radioactivity	HPLC as above		
Iodinated [^{125}I] Albumin Injection	≥ 99.9%	≥ 80% in albumin fractions II to V; ≤ 5% iodide	Size-exclusion chromatography on porous silica gel using phosphate-buffered saline as mobile phase	6.5–8.5	Albumin content to be declared, about 5 mg/mL
Iodinated [^{131}I] Norcholesterol Injection	Gamma spectrum same as standard 99.9% ^{131}I Specific activity 3.7–37 GBq/g	≥ 85% in the principal spot; ≤ 5% iodide	2 × TLC on silica gel using (a) chloroform and (b) chloroform–ethanol (1 : 1). In (a) the agent migrates with $R_f = 0.5$, iodide remaining at origin. In (b) the agent migrates near the solvent front and the iodide migrates with $R_f = 0.5$	3.5–8.5	
Krypton [^{81m}Kr] Inhalation Gas	≥ 99.9% ≤ 0.1% residual activity	–	–	–	
Sodium Iodide [^{123}I] Injection	≥ 99.65% ^{123}I No longer-lived radionuclides present	≥ 95% ^{123}I	HPLC on C_{18} silica using NaCl–octylamine in water–AcCN (100 : 5). Systems suitability test specified	7.0–10.0	
Sodium Iodide [^{123}I] Solution for Radiolabelling	≥ 99.7% ^{123}I	≥ 95% ^{123}iodide	HPLC on C_{18} silica using NaCl–octlylamine in water–AcCN (100 : 5). Systems suitability test specified	Strongly alkaline	

(continued overleaf)

Table 23.1 *(continued)*

Preparation	Radionuclidic purity	Radiochemical purity	Details of method	pH	Chemical purity
Sodium Iodide [^{131}I] Capsules for Diagnostic Use	Gamma spectrum same as standard. $\geq$ 99.9% radioactivity as ^{131}I no specific activity requirement	$\geq$ 95% as iodide	HPLC on C_{18} silica using NaCl–octlylamine in water–AcCN (100 : 5). Systems suitability test specified	–	$\leq$ 20 µg iodine per capsule
Sodium Iodide [^{131}I] Capsules for Therapeutic Use	Gamma spectrum same as standard. $\geq$ 99.9% radioactivity as ^{131}I no specific activity requirement	$\geq$ 95% as iodide	HPLC on C_{18} silica using NaCl–octlylamine in water–AcCN (100 : 5). Systems suitability test specified	–	$\leq$ 20 µg iodine per capsule
Sodium Iodide [^{131}I] Solution	Gamma spectrum same as standard. $\geq$ 99.9% radioactivity as ^{131}I No specific activity requirement	$\geq$ 95% as iodide	HPLC on C_{18} silica using NaCl–octlylamine in water–AcCN (100 : 5). Systems suitability test specified	7.0–10.0	$\leq$ 20 µg iodine per capsule
Sodium Iodide [^{131}I] Solution for Radiolabelling	Gamma spectrum same as standard. $\geq$ 99.9% radioactivity as ^{131}I No specific activity requirement	$\geq$ 95% as iodide	HPLC on C_{18} silica using NaCl–octlylamine in water–AcCN (100 : 5). Systems suitability test specified		Strongly alkaline
Sodium Iodohippurate [^{123}I] Injection	Gamma spectrum same as standard $\geq$ 99.65% radioactivity as ^{123}I $\leq$ 0.35% total impurities Specific activity 0.74–10 GBq/g	$\geq$ 96% as iodide 2-iodohippuric acid $\leq$ 2% each as 2-iodobenzoic acid or iodide	TLC on silica gel GF254 using toluene–butanol–glacial acetic acid–water (80 : 20 : 4:1) for 75 min or 12 cm and standards of 2-iodohippuric acid and 2-iodobenzoic acid	3.5–8.5	
Sodium Iodohippurate [^{131}I] Injection	Gamma spectrum same as standard $\geq$ 99.9% radioactivity as ^{131}I	$\geq$ 96% as 2-iodohippuric acid $\leq$ 2% as 2-iodobenzoic acid and/or iodide	TLC on silica gel GF254 using toluene–butanol–glacial acetic acid–water (80 : 20 : 4:1) for 75 min or 12 cm and standards of 2-iodohippuric and 2-iodobenzoic acids	6.0–8.5	
Sodium Molybdate[^{99}Mo] Solution (Fission)	^{131}I $\leq 5 \times 10^{-3}$% ^{103}Ru $\leq 5 \times 10^{-3}$% ^{132}Te $\leq 5 \times 10^{-3}$% ^{89}Sr, ^{90}Sr combined $\leq 6 \times 10^{-5}$% alpha emitters $\leq$ 1×10^{-7}% Other radionuclides $\leq$ 1×10^{-2}%	$\geq$ 95% [^{99}Mo] molybdate	TLC on silica gel using Na_2CO_3 solution; R_f about 0.9 for molybdate + pertechnetate		

(continued)

Table 23.1 *(continued)*

Preparation	Radionuclidic purity	Radiochemical purity	Details of method	pH	Chemical purity
Sodium Pertechnetate [^{99m}Tc] Injection (Fission)	^{99}Mo ≤ 1 × 10^{-1}% ^{131}I ≤ 5 × 10^{-3}% ^{103}Ru ≤ 5 × 10^{-3}% ^{89}Sr ≤ 6 × 10^{-5}% ^{90}Sr ≤ 6 × 10^{-6}% Other gamma emitters ≤ 1 × 10^{-2}% Alpha emitters ≤ 1 × 10^{-7}%	≥ 95%	Descending PC using methanol: water (80 : 20) for 2 h. TcO_4^- has R_f about 0.6		≤ 5 ppm Al
Sodium Pertechnetate [^{99m}Tc] Injection (Non-Fission)	^{99}Mo ≤ 0.1% ≤ 0.01% other radionuclides	≥ 95%	Descending PC as above		≤ 5 ppm Al
Sodium Phosphate [^{32}P]	Beta spectrum same as standard ^{32}P solution Specific activity ≥ 11.1 MBq ^{32}P/mg orthophosphate	≥ 95% phosphates: ≤ 0.0033% PO_4^- per 37 MBq	Ascending PC using propanol–water (75 : 25) with trichloroacetic acid and ammonia for 16 h with orthophosphoric acid as carrier; visualise carrier with perchloric acid followed by ammonium molybdate and exposure to H_2S to give a blue spot	6.0–8.0	
Strontium [^{89}Sr] Chloride Injection	≥ 99.6% ≤ 0.4% impurities ≤ 0.4% gammas other than ^{89m}Y Specific activity ≥ 1.8 MBq/ mg Sr	No RCP test	No test for RCP	4.0–7.0	Sr = 6–12.5 mg/mL ≤ 2 μg/mL Al ≤ 5 μg/mL Fe ≤ 5 μg/mL Pb All elements by emission spectroscopy
Thallous [^{201}] Chloride Injection	≥ 97% ^{201}Tl ≤ 2% ^{202}Tl Specific activity ≥ 3.7 GBq/ mg Tl	≥ 95% as thallium(I)	Cellulose acetate electrophoresis with 1.86% disodium edetate at 17 V/cm for 30 min. NLT: 95% activity migrates towards the cathode Limit test for Tl (10 ppm)	4.0–7.0	≤ 10 ppm Tl
Tritiated [^{3}H] Water Injection	No specification: compare LSC spectrum with standardised tritiated water	≥ 95%	Distillation and LSDC; radioactive concentrations before and after distillation within 5%	4.5–7.0	
Xenon [^{133}Xe] Injection	Gamma spectrum similar to standard; except for ^{131m}Xe and ^{133m}Xe; no residual activity after bubbling air for 30 min. 80–130% of stated activity	Not applicable			

Radionuclidic impurity is usually determined by gamma spectroscopy described above. In many cases the pharmacopoeias control radionuclidic impurities by specifying that the sample gamma spectrum does not differ significantly from that of a standardised solution, so that the limit for impurities is effectively that of the standard solution for which no details are provided. In other cases the characteristics of the impurities are listed so that they may be identified in the spectrum.

Sometimes a detailed method is provided in the BP. For example, the monograph on Sodium Molybdate (^{99}Mo) Solution (Fission) has a very detailed description of radiochemical separation of impurities and their determination, the strontium isotopes being determined by liquid scintillation spectrometry.

For Sodium Pertechnetate [^{99m}Tc] Injection several radionuclidic impurity tests are described. As discussed above, the standards are different for the injection derived from fission-produced ^{99}Mo parent and reactor (non-fission)-produced ^{99}Mo, the standard being more stringent in the first case as the fission product is a complex mixture of many radionuclides. An approximate method of parent ^{99}Mo estimation is described (preliminary test) that can be performed before clinical use of the material. The gamma spectrum of a 37 MBq sample is obtained through a 6-mm-thick lead shield which acts as a selective filter by absorbing virtually all the 0.140 MeV photons from ^{99m}Tc, but only 50% of the higher-energy 0.740 MeV photons from the parent ^{99}Mo. The resulting spectrum is that of the attenuated ^{99}Mo, and comparison with a standard allows a rapid estimation of the parent radionuclide contamination level. The definitive test is much more detailed and laborious and is intended for the manufacturer of the material.

Even this preliminary test is time-consuming, and most radiopharmacies perform a 'molybdenum breakthrough test' by placing the freshly eluted sample of Sodium Pertechnetate Injection in a 6-mm wall lead container, measuring the radioactivity and comparing this value with the radioactivity expected from the maximum permitted level of ^{99}Mo in the sample. Some commercial chambers give a direct readout of the ^{99}Mo content, thus further simplifying a measurement that must be done at the busiest period of the radiopharmacist's working day. An example of this test is shown in SOP3 (Molybdenum-99 Breakthrough Test for ^{99m}Tc eluates).

Chemical purity

The chemical identification and determination of purity of radiopharmaceuticals, precursors and kit additives is an essential part of the quality assurance of radiopharmaceuticals and specifications for these materials are gradually being introduced into the pharmacopoeias.

Radiopharmaceutical precursors

Standards for precursors such as iobenguane sulfate, medronic acid and sodium iodohippurate are official in the European Pharmacopoeia, but only the iobenguane and medronic acid monographs have been published in the BP 2010.

Chemical impurities

A related and important aspect is the control of chemical impurities, such as carrier and non-radioactive elements, metal ions, uncomplexed or unreacted precursors, and side-products of the labelling reaction which themselves are not radioactive. Standards for these impurities are fairly common. The (early) monographs on Chromium Edetate and Sodium Chromate Sterile Solution both have limits on chromium content (1 and 2.7 mg/mL respectively). The monograph for Ammonia [^{13}N] Injection has a limit of 2 ppm Al and that for Indium [^{111}In] Chloride Solution, used for protein and peptide labelling, has limits for a number of metal ions (Cd, Cu, Fe), which would compete with the radionuclide for binding or chelating sites on the biomolecule.

The monographs for the PET radiopharmaceuticals Flumazenil (N-[^{11}C]methyl) Injection, L-Methionine[^{11}C]-Methyl Injection, and Raclopride ([^{11}C]Methoxy) Injection have limits on intermediates, reagents and side products of labelling. Production of these radiopharmaceuticals is somewhat specialised and the agents must comply with the standard before administration, often through process control, etc., rather than after process testing.

Absolute determination of the chemical purity of any radiopharmaceutical is not possible in the radiopharmacy department and is the responsibility of the manufacturer of licensed radiopharmaceuticals. In the hospital radiopharmacy, however, chemical impurity tests such as the qualitative assessment of aluminium Al^{3+} ions are made on the first and last elution of each technetium generator and on days when products sensitive to this ion are being prepared. This is usually performed with a commercial test kit that depends upon a visual comparison of colour intensity between a sample of eluate and an Al^{3+} standard. Filter paper is impregnated with a colour complexing agent. A standard solution of aluminium Al^{3+} (10 µg/mL) is supplied. A spot of the standard solution causes a colour change in the paper. A spot of generator eluate is compared with the standard spot. If the colour is more intense in the eluate spot then the eluate contains more than 10 µg/mL aluminium Al^{3+} (the BP limit is 5 ppm = 5 µg/mL) and implies a lack of stability in the column; consequently the eluate should be discarded.

Radiochemical purity determinations

Introduction

Radiochemical purity is defined in the BP as 'The ratio, expressed as a percentage, of the radioactivity of the radionuclide concerned that is present in the source in the chemical form declared to the total radioactivity of that radionuclide present in the source'. Alternatively, radiochemical purity may be defined as the proportion of the total radioactivity in the sample associated with the desired radiolabelled species.

For most diagnostic radiopharmaceuticals a purity of above 95% is desirable (although not always achievable!) since the radiochemical impurities will almost certainly have a different biodistribution, which may distort the scintigraphic image and so invalidate a clinical diagnosis based on the scintigram. Radiochemical purities of radiopharmaceuticals described in the BP vary from 85% (Iodinated [^{131}I] Norcholesterol), 90% (e.g. Cyanocobalamin [^{57}Co] Solution) but most are specified to have a minimum radiochemical purity of 95%; in the latest monographs the purity requirement is considerably tightened to 97–99% for the newer introduced agents, reflecting the development of better analytical methods.

Radiochemical purity (or labelling yield) determinations are carried out in all radiopharmacies, either to check the quality of a standard formulation or kit, or to establish standards for an in-house preparation. Some form of physicochemical separation technique must be used in order to separate the various radioactive species in the sample prior to measurement of their radioactivity and subsequent calculation of their proportion in the sample.

Although extraction and phase separation methods are used, separation methods are universally employed in radiochemical purity determinations, planar, column chromatographic and electrophoresis being the most popular. The main advantage of planar over column and other elution methods is that all the applied radioactivity remains on the developed chromatoplate or electrophoretogram which can then be examined and quantitated by a number of techniques (e.g. scanned, autoradiographed, cut into regions or strips and the radioactivity associated with each area measured under identical conditions).

The BP specifies planar separation methods in many of the radiochemical purity tests described. These range from descending paper chromatography through thin-layer chromatography to paper electrophoresis. Whatever separation technique is used, the method of calculation of radiochemical purity is identical. The radioactivity in each spot, sample, or other sector is measured, corrected for background, and the percentage activity in each piece is expressed as a percentage of the total – a method known as 'normalisation', and is calculated from the formula:

$$\text{Per cent component} = 100 \times \frac{\text{radioactivity for component}}{\text{total radioactivity}}$$

The methods are illustrated in SOP11 (Radiochromatogram Quantitation). Chromatographic and other separation techniques for radiochemical purity determinations are extensively reviewed in Wieland *et al.* (1986). Methods for all currently used ^{99m}Tc radiopharmaceuticals are described in the recent book edited by Zolle (2007).

Insoluble radioactive species (colloids or highly lipophilic materials) are measured along with all other radioactive species in planar separations. Column chromatography methods invariably retain these species on the column, making their quantitation or estimation more difficult. Even so, the radioactivity associated with insoluble species must be distinguished from that due to lipophilic or slowly moving species by using a combination of separative methods. This problem has been known for many years, being addressed by Eckelman in an editorial for the *Journal of Nuclear Medicine* in 1976 (Eckelman 1976).

Many conventional radiochromatographic systems are unsatisfactory because only the impurity migrates and the principal component remains at the point of application. Systems must be developed that ensure that all potentially soluble components migrate. It is good analytical practice to employ several different stationary/mobile phase combinations to demonstrate the homogeneity of the spots or peaks for the components being measured. The BP gives extensive advice and descriptions on separation methods and specifications for the systems used, and many radiopharmaceutical monographs now specify two systems for complete separation of all species.

Calibration and validation

It is essential to calibrate the measuring or counting equipment and to validate the proposed counting or assay procedure. In most cases this will take the form of an assessment of the sensitivity and linearity of the counting or measuring system; the BP now gives detail for systems suitability testing on all separations methods. The thallium-activated sodium iodide scintillation detector is preferred for radiopharmaceutical gamma counting because of its sensitivity and ease of operation. All counting systems can show deviation from linearity at high count rates due to paralysis, coincidence, or pulse pile-up. The correct working conditions (detector voltage and threshold settings) and the range over which linearity is maintained must be determined by experiment. Measuring conditions must then be adjusted to maintain count rates within the linear region.

It is easy to paralyse the detector by applying too large a quantity of radioactivity in the sample. For example, a single drop of a 100 MBq/mL ^{99m}Tc radiopharmaceutical will contain about 2 MBq, an amount more than sufficient to cause paralysis of most detectors. In these situations the inverse square law can be used to advantage by placing samples for counting on a rigid jig held a suitable distance from the detector (after performing systems suitability tests).

Typical SOPs for optimising operating conditions and detector linearity checks are illustrated in SOP 4 (Scintillation Detector Performance Optimisation) and SOP 5 (Scintillation Detector Linearity Checking).

Planar chromatography

Planar chromatography includes paper, thin-layer, and high performance thin-layer chromatography. The techniques are similar in that a sample is applied to the stationary medium and, after equilibration in a closed vessel with the mobile phase, is then developed for an appropriate distance or time.

The developing tank or vessel should be transparent and fitted with an airtight lid or seal to ensure constant composition of the vapour phase throughout the chromatographic run.

The choice of mobile phase for a particular product is made primarily by referring to the Product Data Sheet supplied by the manufacturer, or as a result of data published in the nuclear medicine literature. Each mobile phase must be validated using systems to ensure that separation of product from impurities can clearly be seen. Mobile phases should be changed daily and again if a repeat chromatogram has to be run. Sufficient volume is added to just cover the base of the tank and the lower few millimetres of the chromatoplate.

Paper chromatography

Paper chromatography has been largely replaced by thin-layer chromatography (TLC) methods but is still applied to a number of BP radiopharmaceuticals. The disadvantages of this medium are the poor resolution compared with other planar thin-layer support media and the long development times required for both ascending and descending techniques. In radiopharmacy these are often outweighed by the ease of cutting a developed paper chromatogram into strips or segments for counting or scanning of the radioactivity profile.

It is good practice to mark the (starting) line of application and the expected solvent front (finishing line) with a sharp, soft pencil before applying the sample. Paper is manufactured with a 'grain' lying in one direction (the machine direction) and it is recommended that the machine direction be marked on the paper and the chromatogram run in the same direction to ensure reproducibility between runs.

On a multiple sample paper chromatogram the width of the chromatographic lanes should be wider than customary on TLC plates to accommodate the greater lateral diffusion of bands encountered in this technique. Edge effects are also common; band development and band shape are affected by the solvent flow characteristics induced by evaporation at the paper edges. It is prudent to ensure that samples are not applied too close to the edges – a margin of 10 mm is satisfactory – and to spot at intervals of not less than 25 mm across the width of the paper.

Single-sample paper chromatograms are perhaps more common in the radiopharmacy, using strips of dimensions about 20 × 200 mm. These have the advantage of simple development in a tall jar such as a measuring cylinder with minimum mobile phase volumes. A typical procedure is illustrated in SOP 6 (Paper Chromatography of Radiopharmaceuticals). As with all planar chromatography methods, the paper should be equilibrated with the mobile phase vapour in the developing tank before running the chromatogram.

Chromatography papers

Whatman No. 1 paper is a good, general-purpose medium for paper chromatography but tears easily when wetted with aqueous solvents. It is unsuitable for ascending chromatographic techniques (unless supported in some kind of frame, or wrapped and clipped into a cylinder) because of this property. Whatman 3MM paper is a thicker paper having similar chromatographic characteristics to No. 1. Its advantage lies in the increased mechanical strength and the ability to absorb a sample spot with less spreading. The paper is used quite successfully in miniature chromatography systems. Whatman 31ET is a more open-textured paper that runs faster than No. 1 or 3MM but has a lower intrinsic resolution.

A number of ion-exchange papers are also available: DE81, a weak basic anion exchanger, and P81, a strong cation exchanger. They can be used to advantage in the separation of differently charged species. Control of mobile phase pH is essential with these materials to ensure the correct degree of ionisation of both the paper-bound exchanger groups and the migrating solute.

Strips of chromatography paper are cut from bulk rolls of the relevant support media and are normally 2.5 × 12 cm in dimensions unless otherwise stated in the product specification.

Thin-layer chromatography

Thin layer chromatography (TLC) is the most popular planar chromatographic method. The technique is simple and acceptable results are easily obtained. TLC is probably the most useful method for radiopharmaceutical work, although development times of several hours can be a disadvantage with radiopharmaceuticals containing short-lived radionuclides. High performance thin-layer plates are made from finer silica gel particles, and modified silica types are available, similar to those used in HPLC.

Thin-layer chromatoplates may be prepared 'in-house' but commercial TLC materials are preferable for radiopharmaceutical quality control applications. The normal thickness of the layer is 0.25 mm (250 μm). Glass-backed plates are traditional, but are not easily cut or segmented. Plastic-backed and metal-foil-backed plates are more versatile; they can be cut with scissors or a sharp scalpel to any required size. Similarly, after development these chromatoplates can be cut into suitable segments for counting and quantitation. Some plates have a tendency to flake or crumble when being cut, leading to loss of radioactive material. This can be overcome by covering the layer with adhesive tape before cutting.

Many different stationary phases are available for TLC work, but for radiopharmaceutical purposes silica gel is to be preferred in view of the large number of chromatograms reported. Plates incorporating a fluorescent indicator, although useful for locating the solvent front (by virtue of the concentration of UV-absorbing impurities at the solvent front) and location of UV-absorbing species, are not normally required in radiopharmacy since the quantitation is made through the radioactivity distribution on the plate. The pharmacopoeias advise preconditioning of plates, sometimes washing by preliminary development or, more usually, by activating at 110–120 °C for 20 minutes.

ITLC materials

Instant thin-layer chromatography (ITLC) materials are specified in many BP monographs. Produced by the Pall Company,* they consist of a glass fibre web impregnated with the modified silica stationary phases, silica gel (ITLC-SG) and silicic acid (ITLC-SA). The ITCL-SG material is very popular among radiopharmacists for routine radiochemical purity determinations. ITLC supports/stationary phases are fast-running variants of conventional TLC systems. The mobile phase migration speed is increased by the fine random mesh construction of the material, but the resolution is poorer than that of conventional TLC supports and is similar to that of paper. ITLC chromatographic systems for radiochemical purity determinations of radiopharmaceuticals are included in Tables 23.3–23.5. A typical method for ITLC chromatography is illustrated in SOP 7 (ITLC of Radiopharmaceuticals).

Sample application techniques

Chromatographic separation and quantitation depend in part on the technique, accuracy and reproducibility of the sample application. For optimal resolution the sample spot must be kept small, about 3 mm for standard 200 mm length plates, and proportionally smaller for shorter length plates. If the sample is applied as a band, then it too must be kept narrow – about 1–2 mm in width. The volume applied will depend on the radioactivity of the sample and the purpose of the chromatogram. Detection of small amounts of impurities will require higher applied radioactivity than studies aimed at determining the major radiolabelled components. The BP suggests that volumes equal to or less than 10 μL should be applied to the line of application, or origin. Volumes between 2 and 5 μL are generally applied in practice, either from a microsyringe or, more conveniently with radiopharmaceuticals, from disposable capillary micropipettes. These are available in several volumes with an accuracy of about ±2% of the stated volume. This is sufficient since the main purpose of controlling the sample volume is to control the chromatographic conditions not the amount of sample, because percentage purities are computed from the distribution of radioactivity along the chromatogram.

Many radiopharmacists prefer to apply samples by expelling a single hanging drop from a narrow-bore needle attached to a 1 mL syringe and touching the drop onto the application line of the chromatoplate. There are many advantages to this technique; with practice a single drop of reproducible size can be formed and transferred to the chromatoplate. The size of the drop does not depend too much on the needle size and a 25G (orange) needle is very satisfactory.

Multiple sample applications may be necessary to load the chromatoplate with sufficient radioactivity, but care should be taken in drying the spots between applications. Heating the plate between applications is not advised with ^{99m}Tc radiopharmaceuticals since sample decomposition or oxidation may occur during the drying, leading to overestimation of impurities. If spots have to be dried between applications then the use of a gentle current of nitrogen directed at the spot through a Pasteur pipette is a better option than a heat lamp or hot air blower.

Radiopharmaceutical applications

Standard chromatography

Most scientists will have used conventional TLC methods in their training and few words are needed here to describe the technique. In radiopharmaceutical quality control, samples are applied and the chromatoplate is developed in a closed tank, after an equilibration period with the plate suspended in the mobile phase vapour before developing. The BP specifies standard TLC methods for a number of the radiopharmaceuticals listed in Table 23.2.

---

* This company has stopped manufacture of ITLC materials. An essentially equivalent material is now available from Varian. All ITLC methods should be re-validated when using this new source.

Table 23.2 BP standards for technetium-99m radiopharmaceuticals

Preparation	Radiochemical purity method	Other tests	pH
Sodium Pertechnetate [^{99m}Tc] Injection (Fission and Non-Fission)	Descending PC using methanol–water (80 : 20) as mobile phase for 2 h. Pertechnetate migrates with $R_f = 0.6$. ≥ 95% radioactivity as pertechnetate	≤ *5ppm Aluminium:* colorimetric limit test by comparison against standard using chromazurol S	4.0–8.0
Technetium [^{99m}Tc] Human Albumin Injection	Activated ITLC-SG using butan-2-one for 10–15 cm in 10 min; labelled albumin remains at origin. TcO_4^- migrates behind solvent front. ≤ 5% pertechnetate HPLC-SEC on silica gel FC with phosphate azide buffer at 0.6 mL/min. Multiple peaks eluted but ≥ 80% of radioactivity associated with albumin fractions II, III, IV and V	*Albumin* by colorimetry; *Tin* by colorimetry; ≤ 1 mg/mL *Physiological distribution*–≤ 15% in liver, ≥ 3.5% in blood of 2/3 rats	2.0–6.5
Technetium [^{99m}Tc] Bicisate Injection	TLC on silica gel using ethyl acetate as mobile phase, allowing spots to dry before development. Bicisate complex $R_f \geq 0.4$, impurities $R_f \leq 0.2$. ≥ 94% bicisate complex, ≤ 4% of 6 named impurities		
Technetium [^{99m}Tc] Colloidal Rhenium Sulfide	Ascending PC using 0.9% NaCl; over 10–15 cm. Colloid remains at origin, pertechnetate migrates with R_f about 0.6. ≥ 92% colloidal activity	*Re by colorimetry:* ≤ 0.22 mg Re/mL *Physiological distribution:* ≥ 80% in liver and spleen, ≤ 5% in lungs in 3/3 mice else repeat the test	4.0–7.0
Technetium [^{99m}Tc] Colloidal Sulphur Injection	Ascending PC using 0.9% NaCl over 10–15 cm. Pertechnetate migrates with $R_f = 0.6$. Other ^{99m}Tc impurities with $R_f = 0.8$–0.9, ≥ 92% radioactivity as colloid	*Physiological distribution*: ≥ 80% in liver and spleen, ≤ 5% in lungs of 3/3 mice, else repeat test	4.0–7.0
Technetium [^{99m}Tc] Colloidal Tin Injection	Activated ITLC-SG using N_2-purged 0.9% saline for 10–15 cm over 10 min. Colloid remains at origin, pertechnetate at solvent front; ≥ 95% radioactivity as colloid	*Tin:* ≤ 1 mg/mL by colorimetry *Physiological distribution:* ≥ 80% in liver and spleen, ≤ 5% in lungs of 3/3 mice, else repeat test	4.0–7.0
Technetium [^{99m}Tc] Etifen Injection	Activated ITLC-SA using 0.9% saline for 10–15 cm in 10 min. Colloid remains at origin, complex at $R_f = 0.5$ and pertechnetate at solvent front. ≥ 95% as complex	*Identification:* HPLC on C_{18}-silica using pH 2.5 phosphate buffer–methanol (80 : 20)as mobile phase; Etifen EPCRS used as reference *Physiological distribution*- ≥ 80% in gallbladder + intestines; ≤ 3% in liver, ≤ 2% in kidney of 2/3 mice	4.0–6.0
Technetium [^{99m}Tc] Exametazime Injection	Complex + *meso* isomer: ≥ 80% by ITCL-SG using butan-2-one; complex + *meso* + TcO_4^- $R_f = 0.8$–1.0, colloid and non-lipophilic complexes at origin. *Meso*-complex: ≤ 5% by HPLC on spherical base-deactivated end-capped C_{18} silica of pore size 13 nm and C-loading of 11% Pertechnetate: ≤ 10% by ITLC-SG using 0.9% saline for 2/3 of the plate	No physiological distribution test	5.0–10.0

(continued overleaf)

Table 23.2 *(continued)*

Preparation	Radiochemical purity method	Other tests	pH
Technetium [^{99m}Tc] Gluconate Injection	Activated ITLC-SA using (a) 0.9% saline for 10–15 cm in 10 min; complex + pertechnetate near solvent front; (b) butan-2-one; pertechnetate near solvent front	*Physiological distribution:* $\geq$ 15% in kidney, $\geq$ 20% in bladder + urine, $\leq$ 5% in liver in 2/3 rats	6.0–8.5
Technetium [^{99m}Tc] Macrosalb Injection	Non-filterable radioactivity: by 3 μm polycarbonate filter retention; $\geq$ 90%	*Particle size:* $\leq$ 10/5000 > 100 μm; none > 150 μm *Aggregated albumin:* by UV $\geq$ 37 MBq ^{99m}Tc per mg albumin *Physiological distribution:* $\geq$ 80% in lungs, $\leq$ 5% in liver + spleen in 2/3 rats	3.8–7.5
Technetium [^{99m}Tc] Medronate Injection	Activated ITLC-SG using 13.6% sodium acetate; colloids remain at origin, complex and pertechnetate at solvent front. Repeat chromatography on activated ITLC-SG using butan-2-one for 10–15 cm in 10 min; medronate and colloid both remain at origin, $\leq$ 2% pertechnetate at solvent front. From both chromatograms $\leq$ 5% total impurities	*Tin:* $\leq$ 3 mg/mL by colorimetry *Physiological distribution-* $\geq$ 1.5% in femurs, $\leq$ 1% in liver; $\leq$ 0.05% in blood	4.0–9.0
Technetium [^{99m}Tc] Mertiatide Injection	$\geq$ 94% $\leq$ 3% hydrophilic impurity $\leq$ 4% lipophilic impurity	Ascending PC over 15 cm using water–acetonitrile (40 : 60); $\leq$ 2% at origin. HPLC on C_{18} silica with gradient elution from A – ethanol–phosphate pH 6 (9 : 93) and B – water–methanol (10 : 90)	5.0–7.5
Technetium [^{99m}Tc] Microspheres Injection	Non-filterable radioactivity: by 3 μm polycarbonate. Filter retention: $\geq$ 95%	*Particle size*: $\leq$ 10/5000 > 75 μm and none > 100 μm *Number of particles*: by counting in haemocytometer $\geq$ 185 MBq ^{99m}Tc per 10^6 particles *Tin:* $\leq$ 3 mg/mL by colorimetry *Physiological distribution-* $\leq$ 5% in liver and spleen, $\geq$ 80% in lungs of 2/3 rats	4.0–9.0
Technetium [^{99m}Tc] Pentetate Injection	Activated ITLC-SG using butan-2-one for 10–15 cm in 10 min. Complex and colloid at origin, pertechnetate behind solvent front. Repeat chromatography using 0.9% NaCl; colloid at origin, complex and pertechnetate at solvent front. From both chromatograms $\leq$ 5% total impurities	*Tin:* $\leq$ 1 mg/mL by colorimetry	4.0–7.5
Technetium [^{99m}Tc] Tin Pyrophosphate Injection	Activated ITLC-SG using butan-2-one degassed with N_2 for 10–15 cm in 10 min. Dry spots under N_2. Complex remains at origin, pertechnetate migrates with R_f = 0.95–1.0. Repeat chromatography with 1 mol/L sodium acetate; develop immediately; both complex and pertechnetate migrate with R_f = 0.9–1.0; colloid remains at origin. $\leq$ 10% total impurity	*Tin:* $\leq$ 3 mg/mL by colorimetry	6.0–7.5

(continued)

Table 23.2 *(continued)*

Preparation	Radiochemical purity method	Other tests	pH
Technetium [^{99m}Tc] Sestamibi Injection	TcO_4^- and other polar impurities: HPTLC on C_{18} silica gel using tetrahydrofuran, ammonium acetate, methanol, acetonitrile (10 : 20 : 30 : 40). Develop over 6 cm. Colloidal Tc at origin; complex R_f 0.3–0.6; pertechnetate and other polar impurities at solvent front Unsaturated sestamibi impurity: HPLC on spherical base-deactivated end-capped C_{18} silica gel using acetonitrile, 0.66% ammonium sulfate, methanol (20 : 35 : 45). Main complex $\geq$ 94%, $\leq$ 3% unsaturated impurity	No test for tin; no physiological distribution test	5.0–6.0
Technetium [^{99m}Tc] Succimer Injection	Activated ITLC-SG using butan-2-one for 10–15 cm in 10 min. Complex at origin, pertechnetate at solvent front. $\leq$ 2% pertechnetate, $\geq$ 95% complex	*Tin:* $\leq$ 1 mg/mL by colorimetry *Physiological distribution-* $\geq$ 40% in kidneys, $\leq$ 10% in liver, $\leq$ 2% in stomach, $\leq$ 5% in lungs of 2/3 rats	2.3–3.5

Size of chromatogram

Radiopharmacists have developed a number of miniature and micro-chromatographic methods for speed and ease of handling in the radiopharmaceutical quality control laboratory. Mini-chromatography: was introduced by Zimmer and Pavel (1977) and described in the UK by Frier and Hesslewood (1980). A practical guide and methods manual based on this technique was produced for the USA Society of Nuclear Medicine by Robbins (1984) Mini-chromatography employs single strips, about 10 × 50 mm, for each chromatogram. The support is usually ITLC-SG, although some workers have used paper. The strips are marked in pencil 8 mm (origin) and 46 mm (solvent front) from the base and the sample is applied as a single spot on the 8 mm line. Without drying the spot, the strip is placed in a suitable vial (a liquid scintillation vial, or Universal container is suitable) containing a layer of mobile phase some 1–2 mm deep and allowed to develop to the marked solvent front. A typical SOP is shown in SOP 8 (Minichromatography of ^{99m}Tc radiopharmaceuticals) and Table 23.3 shows some applications of the method. Table 23.4 lists some published applications of TLC to radiopharmaceuticals.

It can be difficult to observe the progress of the mobile phase on these small chromatograms. Back illumination from a diffused source (e.g. an X-ray viewer) is helpful since the wetted strip is translucent

Table 23.3 Minichromatography applications for ^{99m}Tc radiopharmaceuticals

No.	Support	Mobile phase	Useful for[a]
A. Free pertechnetate determinations only			
1	Whatman 3MM	95% acetone	MDP, GH, DTPA, DMSA, HAS, MAA, μS
2	Whatman 3MM	0.9% saline	SC, MAA, SbC, PyP
3	ITLC-SG	85% methanol	SC, MAA
B. Free pertechnetate and hydrolysed Tc (remains at origin)			
4	Whatman 3MM	95% acetone 0.9% saline[b]	DTPA, HIDA
5	ITLC-SG	(a) 95% acetone[c] (b) 0.9% saline[b]	MDP, PyP, EHDP

[a] Abbreviations: DMSA, succimer (dimercaptoacetic acid). DTPA, pentetate (diethylenetriamine pentaacetate). EHDP, editronate (hydroxyethyl diphosphonate). GH, glucoheptonate. HAS, human serum albumin. HIDA, lidofen (2, 6-dimethylacetanilidoiminodiacetate). MAA, Macrosalb (macroaggregated albumin). MDP, medronate (methylene diphosphonate). PyP, pyrophosphate. SbC, antimony sulfide colloid. SC, sulfur colloid. μS, HAS microspheres.

[b] Secondary solvent runs to 20 mm above origin.

[c] Wet spot – do not dry before development.

Table 23.4 Thin-layer chromatography of selected radiopharmaceuticals

Radiopharmaceutical			Support	Mobile phase	R_f values			Reference
					Complex	TcO_4^-	Colloid	
Pertechnetate	a		ITLC-SG	Acetone		1		Robbins (1984)
	b		ITLC-SG	0.9% NaCl		1		
	c		Wh 1	Acetone		1		
	d		Silica gel	0.9% NaCl		1		
Colloids								
Tc-S (sulfur colloid)	a		Wh31ET	Acetone		1	0	Robbins (1984)
Tc-SbS (antimony sulfide)	b		ITLC-SG	0.9% NaCl		1	0	Robbins (1984)
Tc-ReS (rhenium sulfide)	c		Wh1	0.9% NaCl		0.6–0.7	0	Ph Eur
Tc-Sn colloid	d		ITLC-SG	0.9% NaCl		1	0	Zolle (2007)
Tc-Albumin microcolloid	e		ITLC-SG	85% MeOH		0.6–0.7	0	Zolle (2007)
Tc-Albumin millimicrospheres	f		ITLC-SG	85% MeOH		0.6–0.7	0	Zolle (2007)
Tc-ReS nanocolloid	g		Wh1	MEK		1	0	Zolle (2007)
Tc-Albumin microcolloid	h		Wh1	0.9% NaCl		0.75	0	Manufacturer
	j		ITLC-SG	Acetone		1	0	Zolle (2007)
Lung imaging agents								
Tc-MAA (Macrisalb)	a		Wh 31ET	Acetone	0	1		Robbins (1984)
	b		Wh1	70% MeOH	0	0.6	0	USP
	c		ITCL-SG	Acetone	0	1	0	
Tc-HAM (microspheres)	a		Wh31ET	Acetone	0	1		Robbins (1984)
	b		ITLC-SG	Acetone	0	1	0	Zolle (2007)
	c		Wh 1	80% MeOH	0	0.6–0.7	0	Zolle (2007)
Renal agents								
Tc-Pentetate (DTPA)	a		Wh 31Et	Acetone	0	1	0	Robbins (1984)
	b		ITLC-SG	Water	1	1	0	
	c	I	ITLC-SG	Butanone	0	1	0	PhEur
		II	ITLC-SG	0.9% NaCl	1	1	0	
Tc-Ferpentate	a		Wh31ET	Acetone	1	1	0	Robbins (1984)
	b		ITLC-SG	Water	1	1	0	
Tc-Gluceptate	a		Wh31ET	Acetone	1	1	0	Robbins (1984)
	b		ITLC-SG	Water	1	1	0	

(continued)

Table 23.4 *(continued)*

Radiopharmaceutical			Support	Mobile phase	R_f values			Reference
					Complex	TcO_4^-	Colloid	
Tc-Succimer (DMSA)	a		ITLC-SA	*n*-BuOH + 0.3 mol/L HCl	0.5	1	0	Robbins (1984)
	b	I	ITLC-SG	Butanone	0	1	0	PhEur
		II	ITLC-SG	0.9% NaCl	1	1	0	
	c		ITLC-SG	0.5M AcOH	1	1	0	
	d		ITLC-SG	96% EtOH	0.5	1	0	Ph Eur
Tc-MAG3	a		ITLC-SG	NaCl	1	1	0	Chen, 1993
	b		ITLC-SG	Acetone	0	1	0	
	c		Wh1	MeCN–H_2O (60 : 40)	Nd	Nd	0	Ph Eur
Albumin								
Tc-I (human albumin)	a		Wh31ET	Acetone	0	1	0	Robbins (1984)
	b		ITLC-SG	Mek	0	1	0	BP 2008
	c		ITLC-SG	EtOH + NH_3 + H_2O	1	1	0	
Bone agents								
Tc-Editronate (EHDP)	a		Wh31ET	Acetone	1	1	0	Robbins (1984)
	b		ITLC-SG	Water	1	1	0	
Tc-Medronate (MDP)	a		Wh31ET	Acetone	1	1	0	Robbins (1984)
	b		ITLC-SG	Water	1	1	0	
Tc-Oxidronate	a		Wh31ET	Acetone	1	1	0	Robbins (1984)
	b		ITLC-SG	Water	1	1	0	
Tc-Pyrophosphate (PyP)	a		Wh31ET	Acetone	1	1	0	Robbins (1984)
Tc-Pyrophosphate	b	I	ITLC-SG	Butan-2-one	0	1	0	BP
		II	ITLC-SG	13.6% Sodium acetate	1	1		
Tc-Diphosphonates		I	ITLC-SG	Butan-2-one	0	1	0	BP
		II	ITLC-SG	13.6% Sodium acetate	1	1		
Tc-Tetrafosmin	a		ITLC-SG	Acetone: CH_2Cl_2 (35 : 65 v/v)	0.4–0.7	1	0	Zolle (2007)
Hepatobiliary agents								
Tc-Lidofen (HIDA)	a		ITCL-SA	20% NaCl	0	1	0	Robbins (1984)
	b		ITLC-SG	Water	1	1	0	

(continued overleaf)

Table 23.4 *(continued)*

Radiopharmaceutical			Support	Mobile phase	R_f values			Reference
					Complex	TcO_4^-	Colloid	
Tc-Iprofen (PIPIDA)	a		ITCL-SA	20% NaCl	0	1	0	Robbins (1984)
	b		ITLC-SG	Water	1	1	0	
Tc-Diosfenin	a		ITCL-SA	20% NaCl	0	1	0	Robbins (1984)
	b		ITLC-SG	Water	1	1	0	
Tc-Etifenin (EHIDA)	a		ITLC-SG	0.9% NaCl	0.4-0.5	1	0	Ph Eur
Brain imaging agents								
Tc-Exametazime 3-system method (See text for details)	a	I	ITLC-SG	Butan-2-one	1	1	0	
		II	ITLC-SG	0.9% NaCl	0	1	0	Manufacturer
		III	Wh 1	MeCH–H_2O (1 : 1)		1	0	
Tc-Exametazine (HMPAO) 2-system method	b	I II	ITLC-SG ITLC-SG	butan-2-one 0.9% NaCl	0	1 1	0 0	Neirinckx *et al.* (1987), Ph Eur
	c		ITLC-SG	0.9% NaCl	0.1	1	0	
	d		Wh1	MeCN:H_2O	1	1	0	
	e		WhDE81	Butan-2-one	1	0	0	Solanki *et al.* (1988)
	f		Wh1	Et_2O	1	0	0	Hung *et al.* (1988)
Tc-Bicisate (ECD)	a		ITLC-SG	Acetone	0	1	0	Verbruggen *et al.* 1992
Tc-ECD	b		WhMKC18	Acetone + 0.5 mol/L NH_4Ac				Leveille *et al.* (1992)
	c		Baker-flex SG 18-F	Ethyl acetate	1	1	0	Manufacturer, Zolle (2007)
	d		Wh3MM	Ethyl acetate	1			Amin (1997)
Heart imaging agents								
Tc-Tetrafosmin			ITLC	CH_2Cl_2/Me_2CO	0.5	1	0	Geyer *et al.* (1995)
Tc-Tetrafosmin			ITLC-SG	Butan-2-one	0.5	1	0	Metaye *et al.* (1991)
Tc-MIBI	a		Alumina	EtOH	0.5–1	0–0.5	0	Proulx *et al.* (1989)
	b		ITLC-SG	Acetone	0.5–1	0–0.5	0	
	c		ITLC-SG	0.9% NaCl	0–0.25	0.75–1	0	
	d		ITLC-SG	$CHCl_3$:MeOH (9 : 1)	0.5–1	0–0.5	0	
	e		Wh1	Acetone	0.75–1	0.75–1	0	
	f		Wh1	0.9% NaCl	0–0.5	0.5–1	0	

(continued)

Table 23.4 *(continued)*

Radiopharmaceutical			Support	Mobile phase	R_f values			Reference
					Complex	TcO_4^-	Colloid	
	g		Wh1	$CHCl_3$:MeOH (9 : 1)	0.5–1	0–0.25	0	
	h		ITCL-SG	Butan-2-one	0.5	1	0	Van Wyk *et al.* (1991)
	i		Wh3MM	Et acetate	0.5–0.7	1	0	Patel (1995)
Tumour imaging agents								
Tc(V)-DMSA	a		Silica gel	BuOH–AcOH–H_2O (3 : 2:3)	0.5	0.7	0	Westera *et al.* (1985)
	b		Silica gel	Butan-2-one	0.0	1.0	0	
Tc-Depreotide	a	I	ITLC-SG	Methanol–1 mol/L ammonium acetate (1 : 1)	1.0	1.0	0	Manufacturer, Zolle (2007)
		II	ITLC-SG	Saturated NaCl	0	1.0	0	
Tc-Arcitumomab	a		ITLC-SG	Acetone	0	1.0	0	Manufacturer
Tc-Sulesomab	a		ITLC-SG	Acetone	0	1.0	0	Manufacturer

and the solvent front can be seen. Some authorities recommend marking the support with a dye marker pen just below the expected final solvent front. The dye moves with the mobile phase, enabling the progress to be monitored visually near the end of the development.

The main difficulties with the method are its reproducibility and poor resolution of migratory species. It is most useful when the radiolabelled species either remain at the origin or migrate with the solvent front. Chromatogram scanning is not easy, but cutting and counting is rapid and simple. Millar has reported the results of a survey into the use of this method by a panel of UK radiopharmacists and concluded that the results from this method improve with experience (Millar, 1989). A summary of the quality specifications for BP radiopharmaceuticals is given in Table 23.5

Examination and quantitation of chromatoplates

In conventional chromatography, separated bands or spots on the developed chromatoplate are visualised by spraying with a chromogenic reagent or by some other treatment and the band positions and intensities are assessed in a semiquantitative manner. Radiochromatograms can be evaluated in a quantitative manner provided that the detection and measuring systems are properly calibrated.

Autoradiography

Radiochromatograms can be visualised by autoradiography, in which a sheet of photographic film is placed on the radiochromatogram, exposed for a suitable period of time, and then developed. The method is very good for ^{14}C- and ^{3}H-labelled radiochemicals and special film can be obtained for the purpose. Very low radioactivities of these isotopes can be detected with long exposures since the film responds to all the β-particles detected over the exposure and the density of blackening is proportional to the number of particles captured.

Conventional double-sided X-ray film can be used for autoradiography of ^{99m}Tc radiopharmaceuticals. A piece of the film is clipped to the chromatogram and left to expose for 30–60 minutes in the dark. Over-development in X-ray developer usually heightens the contrast of the spots. Although autoradiograms from ^{14}C and ^{3}H sources can be quantitated, this is less

Table 23.5 BP Standards for PET radiopharmaceuticals

Preparation	Precursor purity	Precursor methods	Radiochemical purity	Details of method	pH	Chemical purity	Details of method
Ammonia [^{13}N] Injection	–	–	≥ 99%	LC on cation-exchange resin with 0.002 mol/L nitric acid	5.5–8.5	≤ 2 ppm Al	
Carbon Monoxide [^{15}O]	–	–	≥ 97%	GC using concentric columns flushed with helium and thermal conductivity detection	–	–	
Fludeoxyglucose [^{18}F] Injection	1,3,4,6-Tetra-*O*-acetyl-2-*O*-trifluoro-methane-sulfonyl-β-D-mannopyranose: IR, MPt 119–122°C. 3,4,6-Tri-*O*-acetyl-D-glucal: IR, MPt 53–55°C	Comparison of IR spectrum with PhEur reference spectrum; melting point	≥ 95% of FDG and FDM ≤ 10% FDM ≥ 95% FDG	LC using strongly basic anion-exchange resin with 0.1 mol/L NaOH mobile phase at 1 mL/min TLC on silica gel using water–MeCN		2-Fluoro-2-deoxy-D-glucose: ≤ 10 mg/V 2-Chloro-2-deoxy-D-glucose/;≤ 0.5mg/V Aminopolyether: ≤ 2.2 mg/V Tetra-alkylammonium salts: ≤ 2.75mg/V	LC using strongly basic anion-exchange resin with 0.1M NaOH mobile phase at 1 mL/min TLC on silica gel with ammonia–methanol LC on C_{18} silica with tosyl acid: MeCN mobile phase
Flumazenil (*N*-[^{11}C]methyl)} Injection	Demethylflumazenil	IR spectrum, MPt 286–289°C	≥ 95%	LC on spherical C_{18} silica of specific surface area 400 m^2/g and C loading of 19% Methanol–water mobile phase	6.0–8.0	Flumazenil: ≤ 50 µg/V Impurity A: ≤ 5 µg/V Other: 1 µg/V	LC on spherical C_{18} silica of specific surface area 400 m^2/g and C loading of 19% Methanol–water mobile phase
L-Methionine ([^{11}C]-Methyl) Injection	L-Homocysteine thiolactone HCl	Specific optical rotation, IR spectrum	≥ 95% Enantiomeric purity: ≤ 10%	LC on spherical C_{18} silica of specific surface area 220 m^2/g and C loading of 6.2%; KH_2PO_4 solution as mobile phase	4.5–8.0	Impurity A: ≤ 0.6 mg/V Impurity B: ≤ 2 mg/V Methionine: ≤ 2 mg/V	LC on spherical C_{18} silica of specific surface area 220 m^2/g and C loading of 6.2%; KH_2PO_4 solution as mobile phase
Oxygen [^{15}O]	–	–	≥ 97%	GC using concentric columns flushed with helium and thermal conductivity detection	–		
Raclopride ([^{11C}] Methoxy) Injection	(*S*)-3,5-Dichloro-2,6-dihydroxy-*N*-[(1-ethylpyrrolidin-2-yl) methyl]benzamide	Melting point, specific optical rotation	≥ 95%	LC on spherical end-capped silica gel of specific surface area 175 m^2/g, pore volume 0.7 cm^2/g and C loading 15%	4.5–8.5	Raclopride: ≤ 10 µg/V Impurity A: ≤ 1 µg/V	LC on spherical end-capped silica gel of specific surface area 175 m^2/g, pore volume 0.7 cm^2/g and C loading 15%
Sodium Acetate (1-[^{11}C]) Injection	–	–	≥ 95%	LC on strongly basic ion-exchange resin with 0.1 mol/L NaOH mobile phase		Residual solvents Acetate: ≤ 20 mg/V	LC on strongly basic ion-exchange resin with 0.1 mol/L NaOH mobile phase
Sodium Fluoride [^{18}F] Injection			≥ 98.5%	LC on strongly basic ion-exchange resin with 0.1 mol/L NaOH mobile phase		Fluoride: ≤ 4.52 mg/V	LC on strongly basic ion-exchange resin with 0.1 mol/L NaOH mobile phase
Water [^{15}O] Injection			≥ 99%	LC on aminopropylsilyl silica gel, phosphate buffer pH 3 as mobile phase	5.5–8.5	Ammonium: ≤ 10ppm	Limit test
						Nitrates: ≤ 10ppm	Colour test

convenient with the gamma-emitting radionuclides employed in radiopharmaceuticals and the method is used primarily to provide a permanent record of the radiochromatogram. A typical method is shown in SOP 9 (Autoradiography of Chromatograms). However, recent advances in radiochromatogram scanners and phosphor imagers have largely removed the need for autoradiography.

Chromatogram scanning

A simple scanner may be constructed from a slit-collimated NaI(Tl) detector coupled to a scaler-ratemeter with the ratemeter output signal passed to a chart recorder. If the radiochromatogram is attached to the chart recorder then a full-size tracing of the radioactivity profile may be obtained. A useful addition is a chromatography integrator to measure the areas of radioactive peaks and generation of percentage purity reports. The exact details of the system will depend on availability of equipment.

Commercial radiochromatogram scanners are available that work along the lines described above, and others (known as linear analysers) that simultaneously count the activity detected in a fixed number of channels along the length of the chromatogram and present the result as a histogram. A typical SOP is shown in SOP 12 (Performance Checks on Berthold Scanner) Some departments of nuclear medicine use their gamma cameras as chromatogram scanners by displaying an image of the chromatoplate and generating an activity profile along the image.

After developing and drying, the strip is placed on a suitable scanner (e.g. Veenstra, Lab Logic, Berthold or Gita) and a trace of the radioactivity profile is obtained. Visual assessment of the trace is made to ensure that the R_f of the peak(s) obtained corresponds to the values expected for the radiopharmaceutical under test. If other peaks are seen, and then measured (area under the curve; the software provided with these scanners will automatically calculate this and also perform background subtraction), a decision can be made whether the product has met the Product Specification.

Calibration and validation

Whichever system is used, it is important to confirm that it is capable of producing reproducible radioactivity profiles from the chromatogram. It is also important to check the detection system for resolution and linearity using the tests described below.

Scanner resolution is difficult to evaluate quantitatively, but a working estimate can be obtained by scanning a dummy chromatogram prepared with spots about 2 mm in diameter placed at decreasing intervals along the line of the scan (say 32, 16, 8, 4, and 2 mm). The 'chromatogram' is scanned under a variety of conditions, and inspection of the radioactivity profile will determine which pair of spots is incompletely resolved. A more elegant solution is to construct a test plate having narrow strips of a long-lived radionuclide (e.g. ^{57}Co) permanently embedded at decreasing intervals and to periodically scan this plate and check that the resolution is satisfactory.

The resolution of the scanner will depend on the design of the collimator, the detector–chromatoplate distance, and the window settings on the scaler. The optimum conditions for any system must be found by experiment. A typical procedure is shown in SOP 10 (Radiochromatogram Scanner: Operation and Performance Checks).

Scanner response linearity must be checked and verified if quantitation is wanted. The band or peak area is the quantity sought, not simply the count rate, so that the linearity must be checked under normal scanning conditions. A suitable method is described in SOP 10.

Stability of band area must be evaluated under the normal operating conditions. The radioactivity peak profile of bands on the chromatogram will depend on their activity and resolution, but the area of the band should remain constant and proportional to the radioactivity. The condition can be tested by applying the same radioactivity as differently sized spots onto the chromatoplate and scanning under normal operating conditions.

Measurement of band area

Measurement of band area from the radioactivity profile is an important stage in quantitating the radiochromatogram. The precision of the final radiochemical purity value will depend on the reliability of these band area measurements.

Chromatographic band areas can be determined by a number of methods. The simplest is triangulation: the area is calculated as $0.5(h \times w)$, where h is the band height and w is the full width at half the maximum height (also known as FWHM), both expressed in the same arbitrary units (e.g. mm on the chart). The method is acceptable only where the bands are perfectly symmetric, and the BP systems suitability test requires the peak symmetry, or ratio of widths of the leading and trailing sides at FWHM, to be 0.8–1.5. In most radiochromatograms the bands are far from symmetric; tailing and distortion are commonly seen. A chart recorder fitted with an integrator is much more useful in determining the areas of these bands. A dedicated chromatography integrator is the best option. These instruments, although designed for HPLC and other column chromatographic methods, are easily connected to a ratemeter and act just like a chart recorder with the advantage of producing a report on the percentage radioactivity in each detected band. Peak positions are expressed in time units, but these are easily converted to distances along the chromatogram if the scan speed is accurately known. Their one disadvantage is the tendency to assign peaks to a noisy background; this can be overcome by (a) increasing the time constant of the ratemeter and accepting some distortion in the band shape, or (b) resetting the signal threshold for initiation of peak integration.

An alternative to band area determination is to cut the radiochromatoplate into segments corresponding to the peaks identified from the radioactivity profile and to count the radioactivity in each one as described in the next section.

Chromatogram counting

If chromatogram scanning is not possible, then cutting and counting is the only practical alternative. The chromatoplate can be cut into sections, each corresponding to a component, main or impurity, and the segments counted in suitable counting equipment. If the radioactivity distribution is unknown, the chromatoplate can be cut into equal-width segments, the radioactivity counted, and the radioactivity profile constructed as a histogram. This method will have to be used where the applied radioactivity is too low for reliable peak discrimination by scanning but has the definite advantage of allowing extended counting times for each segment and improvement of counting statistics. A suitable method is shown in SOP 11 (Radiochromatogram Quantitation).

The counting efficiency will depend on the design and operating characteristics of the detector, but for most NaI(Tl) well detectors an efficiency approaching or exceeding 10% can be expected with ^{99m}Tc and radionuclides of similar gamma energy. When counting in a well detector it is important to maintain the same counting geometry for all segments of the chromatogram, large or small pieces. This is achieved by rolling or compressing the material into the bottom of a counting vial before placing it in the detector.

The linearity of detection should be verified by counting a series of dilutions (or simulated spots on the chromatogram) covering the range 1–200% of the expected radioactivity and plotting the count rate against applied radioactivity (in kBq) as described under chromatogram scanners. A suitable procedure for linearity checking and use of a well crystal counter is shown in SOP 5 (Scintillation Detector Linearity Checking).

Interpreting the results from chromatography

Visual assessment of the trace (or histogram) is made to ensure that the R_f of the peak(s) obtained corresponds to those expected for the radiopharmaceutical under test. If other peaks are seen, then they are measured (area under the curve) (the software provided with these scanners will automatically calculate this and also perform background subtraction), and a decision is made whether the product has met the Product Specification.

If the RCP shows that the product is outside the specification then replicate analyses are performed using fresh mobile phase and cleaned containers. An alternative method of determining RCP may be used if appropriate. Should this duplicate sample also show a substandard product, the batch must be withdrawn. An established recall procedure should be put into effect if necessary.

Artefacts in planar chromatography

Artefacts and non-reproducible results can arise from a number of sources in radiochromatography. The following checklist is based on Levit (1980) but is still relevant.

1. Reaction with the support, especially by drying the spots
2. Splashing when spotting
3. Interaction with dyes used to visualise the solvent front

4 Grease from fingers
5 Strips touching wet walls of the developing chamber
6 Contamination with other radiopharmaceuticals when spotting
7 Incorrect mobile phase
8 Correct, but contaminated mobile phase
9 Insufficient mobile phase to allow full development to the required solvent front
10 Contaminated forceps and scissors
11 Poor mixing of mobile phase components
12 Uneven sample spotting
13 Sample washed off by using too much mobile phase in the chamber
14 Selective evaporation of mobile phase component on storage.

Column chromatography

A number of column methods are used in radiopharmaceutical quality control and their use is increasing each year with the introduction of new pharmacopoeial monographs and the development of novel molecular imaging agents. Liquid column chromatography has become the most useful method for assay, impurity determination and stability studies of all pharmaceuticals, including radiopharmaceuticals. The most popular are HPLC and gel filtration (size-exclusion) techniques, although gas chromatographic (GC) methods are employed for the newer PET gases (carbon monoxide, oxygen, ammonia).

Size-exclusion chromatography(SEC) of radiopharmaceuticals

Gel filtration, or size-exclusion chromatography, is a technique in which a sample is applied to a vertical column and eluted under gravity or low pressure with a solvent. Small solute molecules can penetrate the interstices of the three-dimensional mesh in porous beads of the gel, while larger molecules are excluded. Consequently, unlike other forms of chromatography, the smaller solutes are retained longer than larger molecules, which elute first from the column. The eluate can be collected as fractions for radioassay, or an on-line detector can be constructed as described in the section on HPLC to give the eluted radioactivity profile.

The gel filtration method is applied mainly to macromolecules but has several interesting uses in radiopharmacy. The obvious application is in the assessment of radiolabelling of proteins, iodinated or ^{111}In-labelled through a bifunctional chelate. The radiolabelled protein is eluted first, followed by the radiolabelled unbound bifunctional chelate and other small radiolabelled species. The technique is easily adapted as a purification method for radiolabelled macromolecules by using short bed columns in 10 mL polypropylene syringe barrels and collecting the first few fractions eluted. The BP now specifies a size-exclusion method for Technetium [^{99m}Tc] Albumin Injection that uses a porous silica gel stationary phase in a standard HPLC system.

High performance liquid chromatography

One of the biggest drawbacks to paper and thin-layer chromatography methods of determining RCP is the resolving power of the methods. Most methods commonly used will only resolve one component and so two or three methods may be needed to identify all the major contaminants in a product. Time can also be a limiting factor, with some methods taking 20–30 minutes to develop, or even longer. Indeed some TLC RCP methods may not be sufficient to identify all the compounds that are present in a product. High performance liquid chromatography (HPLC) has a higher sensitivity and resolving power than simple TLC methods. HPLC separation operates on the hydrophilic/lipophilic properties of the components of a sample applied. Gamma emitters are detected using a well scintillation counter connected to a ratemeter and recording device – chart or screen. Other detectors (UV or refractive index) can be connected in series, allowing simultaneous identification of compounds.

It should not be necessary to perform HPLC on radiopharmaceuticals reconstituted from licensed cold kits. It is useful to have techniques available for the purpose of eliminating a cause of any abnormal patient scan. For radiopharmaceuticals prepared ‘in-house’ or novel compounds for research purposes, an HPLC method for estimating radiochemical purity is essential. It should be noted that HPLC does not detect colloidal contaminants and that this component should be estimated using TLC methods.

HPLC uses very small particles of absorbent coated with stationary phase (5–10 μm) tightly packed in small-diameter columns (4 mm × 100–200 mm). The large surface area available for exchange and partitioning within the compact column gives excellent resolution of many substances including radiopharmaceuticals. The pressure drop across the length of an HPLC column can be considerable, and driving pressures of 7 MPa (1000 psi) are not unusual, necessitating the use of specially designed pumps and sample injector systems.

HPLC is a highly popular technique in pharmaceutical analysis and development since it allows separation of most, if not all, impurities and degradation products, and permits the development of stability-indicating assays. The method has a place in radiopharmaceutical quality control but is more expensive in first cost and running costs for consumables.

Equipment

The basic equipment for HPLC consists of a reservoir of mobile phase that is pumped through a sample injector device and chromatographic column to a detector and a collection vessel. A wide range of commercial equipment is available and the overriding consideration with radioactive materials is reliability and ease of decontamination. Chromatography pumps for HPLC are mainly piston-actuated pumps and come in a variety of pump actions, some with damping cylinders to smooth the pulses from the piston stroke (essential with high-sensitivity UV detectors).

Samples are applied with an injector valve in which a sample loop is pre-loaded and the mobile phase flow is switched through the loop during injection. This enables safe filling of the constant-volume loop. The normal technique is to inject excess sample through the sample loop into a plastic tube fitted with a needle inserted in a shielded vial. Preliminary injection of an air bubble helps in visualising the progress of the loop filling.

Radiopharmaceutical applications

Radiopharmaceutical applications of HPLC have been reviewed by several authors (de Groot *et al.* 1985; Wieland *et al.* 1986) and should be consulted for practical and specific details of a particular application. HPLC methods are now available for a range of routine diagnostic radiopharmaceuticals and some typical analytical systems are shown in Table 23.6. The method is specified for nearly all new BP radiopharmaceuticals including cyanocobalamin solutions and ^{99m}Tc-labelled radiopharmaceuticals.

A number of problems have been reported with HPLC of technetium radiopharmaceuticals. The analytical method relies on the complete elution of all radioactive species injected or applied to the column. This is not possible when the sample contains colloidal or reduced Tc_2O since this component will become trapped on the column and purity determinations based on the areas of eluted components will overestimate the purity of the sample. Some kind of radioactivity-balance must be sought, and a method employing calibrated pre-column and post-column detection loops is recommended.

A second problem arises with the use of excess Sn(II) salts as reducing agents in technetium kits. Chromatography usually causes some of the Sn(II) to be retained or trapped at the top of the column; this will reduce any TcO_4^- present in succeeding samples. A second and subsequent sample will appear to be free of TcO_4^- impurity owing to on-column reduction, again giving falsely high radiochemical purity values. The effect can be detected with the dual detector loop system but the loss may be due to colloid, reduction of free pertechnetate, or both. Under these circumstances planar chromatographic methods have the advantage since all radiolabelled species will be separated or detected under proper conditions. Consequently, HPLC is not specified for most BP ^{99m}Tc-labelled radiopharmaceuticals.

Radiolabelled proteins

Radiolabelled protein radiopharmaceuticals require different HPLC conditions from small-molecule radiotracers. Radio-HPLC can be used to purify labelled proteins from precursor reagents and unbound radiolabel, and similar systems are applied to the radiochemical analysis of these materials.

Several different physicochemical processes can be used in the separation and purification of proteins. Separation according to molecular size can be achieved through size-exclusion chromatography, with Sephadex and porous-silica stationary phase materials. Macromolecules are separated by a 'sieving' process according to their size, the smaller molecules being eluted last. A typical example is the chromatography of ^{99m}Tc-labelled human serum albumin by Hosain and Hosain (1982).The revised monograph

Table 23.6 Some HPLC methods for radiopharmaceuticals

Radiopharmaceutical	Column	Isocratic or gradient	Mobile phase(s)	Reference
^{99m}Tc-Pertechnetate	Spherisorb amino bonded	Isocratic	Sodium acetate pH 4.5	Deutsch *et al.* (1982)
^{99m}Tc-Pertechnetate	Waters Sepralyte C_{18}	Isocratic	BuN^+OH in 40% MeOH	Bonnyman (1983)
^{99m}Tc-HSA	Spherogel TSK 3000	Isocratic	0.1 mol/L phosphate	Vallabhajosula *et al.* (1982)
^{99m}Tc-EHDP	TSK G2000PW	Isocratic	0.9% NaCl, 10 mmol/L EHDP, 1 mmol/L Sn(II)	Huigen *et al.* (1988)
^{99m}Tc-EHDP	Aminex A28	Isocratic	0.85 mol/L sodium acetate	Huigen *et al.* (1988)
^{99m}Tc-EHDP	C_{18}	Isocratic	50 mmol/L EHDP + 10 mmol/L NaAc + 3 mmol/L Bu_4NOH	Niewland (1989)
^{99m}Tc-Exametazime	PRP-1	Gradient	A: 20 mmol/L phosphate buffer pH 7.4 B: tetrahydrofuran 0% B to 25% B over 6 min	Neirinckx *et al.* (1987)
^{99m}Tc-Exametazime	Chiracel OD	Isocratic	Hexane: isopropanol: analysis of labelled stereoisomers	Nowotnik *et al.* (1995)
^{99m}Tc-Exametazime	PRP-1	Gradient	A: 10 mmol/L potassium phosphate pH 7 or water containing 1% methanol B: acetonitrile 0% B to 50% B over 5 min	Hunt (1988)
^{99m}Tc-Exametazime	PRP-1	Gradient	A: 50 mmol/L sodium acetate pH 5.6 B: tetrahydrofuran 0% B to 100% B over 17 min	Weisner *et al.* (1993)
^{99m}Tc-MDP	Aminex	Isocratic	0.85 mmol/L Na acetate	Tanabe *et al.* (1983)
^{99m}Tc-HIDAs	μBondapak C18	Isocratic	0.025 mmol/L phosphate, pH 6.0	Nunn (1983)
^{99m}Tc-HIDAs	Ultrasphere ODS 5 μm	Isocratic	0.01 mmol/L phosphate pH 6.8 + MeOH (1 : 1)	Fritzberg and Lewis (1980)
^{99m}Tc-DADS derivatives	Ultrasphere ODS 5 μm	Gradient	0.01 mmol/L phosphate + MeCN 1 : 9 to 4 : 6 in 10 min.	Fritzberg *et al.* (1981)
^{99m}Tc-Bisaminophenols	PRP-1 RP	Isocratic	MeCN–water (85 : 15)	Kung *et al.* (1984)
^{99m}Tc-$DMPE_2Cl_2$	C_8	Isocratic	MeOH + water (7 : 3) + 0.02 mmol/L hexanesulfonic acid + 0.003 mmol/L phosphate	Vandenheyden *et al.* (1983)
^{99m}Tc-MAG3	C_{18}	Isocratic	EtOH–0.1 mmol/L phosphate pH 6.5 (5 : 95)	Fritzberg *et al.* (1986), Taylor and Eshina (1988)

(continued overleaf)

Table 23.6 *(continued)*

Radiopharmaceutical	Column	Isocratic or gradient	Mobile phase(s)	Reference
^{99m}Tc-MAG3	C_{18}	Isocratic	10% MeOH in 0.05 mmol/L phosphate pH 7.0	Brandau *et al.* (1988)
^{99m}Tc-MAG3	C_{18}	Isocratic with wash	A: Ethanol B: 10 mmol/L phosphate buffer pH 6 A:B 5 : 95 After peak, wash with methanol–water 90 : 10	Millar *et al.* (1990)
^{99m}Tc-MAG3	C_{18}	Gradient	A: 10 mmol/L potassium phosphate with 1% triethylamine pH 5 B: Tetrahydrofuran 0% B to 8% B over 30 min	Shattuck *et al.* (1994)
^{99m}Tc-Sestamibi	C_8	Gradient	A: 50 mmol/L ammonium sulfate B: Methanol 0% B to 95% B over 5 min	Carvalho *et al.* (1992)
^{99m}Tc-Sestamibi	C_{18}	Isocratic	A: Methanol B: 50 mmol/L ammonium sulfate C: Acetonitrile A:B:C 45 : 35 : 20	Hung *et al.* (1991)
^{99m}Tc-Tetrofosmin	PRP-1	Gradient	A: 10 mmol/L phosphate buffer pH 7.5 B: Tetrahydrofuran 0% B to 100% B over 17 min	Kelly *et al.* (1993)
^{99m}Tc-Tetrofosmin	PRP-1	Isocratic	A: Acetonitrile B: 10 mmol/L ammonium carbonate A:B 70 : 30	Graham and MIllar (1999)
^{99m}Tc-Tetrofosmin	PRP-1	Isocratic	A: 5 mmol/L monopotassium phosphate B: Acetonitrile A:B 50 : 50	Cagnolini *et al.* (1998)
^{99m}Tc-Depreotide	C_{18}	Gradient	A: 0.1% TFA in water B: 0.1% TFA in acetonitrile 20% B to 27% B over 30 min	Zinn *et al.* (2000)
[$^{123/131}$I]MIBG	C_{18}	Isocratic	A: 100 mmol/L sodium phosphate B: Tetrahydrofuran A:B 88 : 12	Wieland *et al.* (1980)
[^{131}I]MIBG	µBondapak, C_{18}	Isocratic	0.2 mmol/L ammonium phosphate pH 7.0: THF (80 : 20)	Mangner (1986)
[^{123}I]Iodohippurate	Hypersil SAS	Isocratic	MeOH: 0.1 mmol/L AcOH (30 : 70) pH 4.0	Millar (1982)

(continued)

Table 23.6 *(continued)*

Radiopharmaceutical	Column	Isocratic or gradient	Mobile phase(s)	Reference
p-[^{123}I] Iodophenylsulfonamide	PRP-1	Isocratic	60% MeOH–sodium citrate pH 8.0 (60 : 40)	Hunt (1988)
[^{123}I]HIPDM	μBondapak, phenyl	Isocratic	1% ammonium acetate pH 5.5–MeOH (30 : 70)	Mangner (1986)
[^{123}I]Iodo-α-methyltyrosine	RP-18	Gradient	MeOH–water–AcOH (40 : 60 : 1)	Biersack *et al.* (1989)
[^{123}I]Ioflupane	C_{18}	Isocratic	A: Methanol B: Water C: Triethylamine A:B:C 85 : 15 : 0.2	Baldwin *et al.* (1995)
[^{123}I]Iomazenil	C_{18}	Isocratic	A: Methanol B: Water A:B 55 : 45	Zoghbi *et al.* (1992)
^{125}I-Albumin	C_4	Gradient	A: 0.1% TFA in water B: 0.1% TFA in acetonitrile 35% B to 90% B in 10 min	Maltby, unpublished method
^{111}In-DTPA	Alltech C_{18}	Isocratic	5 mmol/L phosphate–2.5 mmol/L octylamine in MeCN	Vora (1991)
^{111}In-Octreotide	C_{18}	Gradient	A: Saline B: Methanol 40% B to 80% B in 20 min	Krenning *et al.* (1992)
[^{18}F]FDG	Amino	Isocratic	A: Acetonitrile B: Water A:B 95 : 5	Hamacher *et al.* (1986)
^{68}Ga- and ^{111}In-LDL	TSKGel G500PW	Isocratic	0.15 mmol/L NaCl	Moerlein *et al.* (1991)

for Iodinated [^{125}I] Albumin Injection specifies a silica gel size-exclusion chromatographic method, eluting the sample with phosphate-buffered saline and requiring a minimum of 80% of the radioactivity to be eluted in fractions II to V (polymeric and monomeric HAS) and a maximum of 5% in fraction VI (iodide).

Separation according to overall charge is performed with ion-exchange columns and carefully buffered mobile phases, often by gradient elution to modify the pH (and thus retention) during the chromatographic run. Ionic strength is as important as pH in this separation mode, and gradient elution (either by pH or ionic strength) can be employed to hasten elution. The BP specifies ion-exchange stationary phases for a number of PET radiopharmaceuticals with strong acid or alkaline mobile phases.

Separation according to the degree of hydrophobic interaction is achieved with a number of reversed-phase (rp) columns. Silica C_{18} rp can be used at acidic pH values, although polymer-based columns (prp-18, etc.) are to be preferred because of their wider operating pH range (1 to 13). Newer column materials such as TSK 5PW-phenyl and graphitised carbon (Hypercarb) are reported to be useful. Proteins are strongly retained on these column materials and gradient elution methods are frequently necessary, decreasing the proportion of organic modifier and neutral salt concentrations to hasten elution.

An ultraviolet absorbance detector in tandem with the radiation detector is essential to ensure that the radioactivity and protein are co-eluted. Aromatic amino acids absorb strongly at 280 nm, the monitoring wavelength usually chosen.

Detector linearity

The problem of assuring detector linearity has been discussed earlier under planar chromatography. Similar considerations apply here; the detection system must be shown to have a linear response to peak area over the range of radioactivities expected. The normal radioactivity injected in the sample will depend on local conditions and customs. In general, a sample volume of 10–50 μL is appropriate and the sample is injected through the loop of the injector set in the fill position, which is then switched to sweep the slug of sample through to the column. A test of the linearity and dynamic range of the detector system requires a series of dilutions of a non-retained radiopharmaceutical covering the range 1–200% of the expected radioactivities. Equal volumes of these solutions are chromatographed by injection through the sample loop, even though the exact volume of the loop is unknown. The practice of partly filling the injector sample loop with smaller volumes delivered from a microsyringe cannot be relied upon to give reproducible sample volumes.

The plot of peak area against injected radioactivity will soon reveal any paralysis of the detection system by curvature. If the curvature is unacceptable then one solution is to employ a smaller-volume detector loop or coil, and some authorities recommend a set of interchangeable detector loops for specific purposes. A suitable systems performance test is described in SOP 13 (HPLC of Radiopharmaceuticals: Performance Checks).

Incomplete sample recovery

As mentioned under the discussion of technetium radiopharmaceuticals, some of the radioactivity may not be eluted from the column for various causes and it becomes necessary to check for incomplete elution. One method is to use two detector loops or coils, one connected to the column outlet as normal and another identical loop connected between the injector system and the column. All the injected radioactivity then passes through the pre-column detector and is recorded as a single, large peak which can be used as a standard (area) for the peaks eluted from the column. Eluted component radioactivities can then be reported as percentages of the pre-column standard peak and the recovery easily computed.

The practical application of this idea requires some thought and any system needs to be rigorously tested before use. The pre-chromatography peak will be sharp and intense compared with the eluate peaks and the detector and recorder settings may not be appropriate for both. A smaller pre-column loop can be used and calibrated against the post-column loop by chromatography of a series of dilutions of a non-retained species such as pertechnetate. Accurate calibration and validation of the assay method must be assured when using these techniques.

If the eluted components are trapped or adsorbed in the detector loop then the recovered radioactivity may be greater than 100%. This is usually indicated as a higher than normal baseline. The only solution is to replace the detector loop with one made from material less prone to adsorbing the component in question. Teflon loops are satisfactory for most post-column purposes even though they cannot be permanently bent or shaped into a neat loop. They cannot be used before the column under the high pressures encountered at this end of the system.

Solid-phase extraction (SPE) methods

Solid-phase extraction utilises the same analyte/sorbent interactions that are exploited in HPLC. A variety of bonded sorbents are available packed into disposable cartridges or columns. The sorbent will selectively retain specific types of chemical compounds from the sample loaded on the column. There are many different sorbents available and many suppliers and manufacturers of SPE columns and cartridges. Components can be selectively eluted by careful choice of solvents. Eluates are collected and have sufficient activity that they can be counted in a radionuclide calibrator. Thus, in contrast to paper chromatography, the radiation dose to operators can be significant, and steps to reduce this should be taken. However, the procedure takes about 5 minutes, ensuring that RCP determination can be carried out before administration of the patient dose. A number of SPE methods have been collected by the UK Radiopharmacy Groups and are reproduced here in Table 23.7.

Electrophoretic methods

Electrophoresis is a separation technique that relies on the different migration velocities of charged solute species dissolved in an electrolyte solution under the influence of an electric field gradient. Solute migration will depend on a number of factors including the sign and multiplicity of the charge, and the effective hydrodynamic volume.

The direction of migration will depend on the sign of the charge: cationic species C^+ will travel towards the cathode (negative electrode) while anionic species A^- travel towards the anode (positive electrode). Neutral molecules and insoluble species will not migrate but may be carried a small distance by the flow of electrolyte generated by electroendosmosis.

The degree of separation can be changed to a small extent by altering the electrolyte environment and thus the hydrodynamic radius. The migration of weak acids and bases can be modified by pH changes, which alter the degree of ionisation of these species.

Electrolyte solutions

Conductive electrolyte solutions are essential for electrophoresis to ensure a uniform electric field gradient and an acceptable current flow. In most radiopharmaceutical applications, buffered aqueous electrolyte solutions are used.

When dealing with low-solubility lipophilic radiopharmaceuticals, a mixed hydro-organic electrolyte solution may be employed such as *n*-propanol containing cetyltrimethylammonium bromide (Cetrimide) or another long-chain alkylammonium halide as conductive electrolyte.

Support media

Although electrophoresis is possible in tubes of aqueous electrolyte, diffusion and convection currents distort any separation that might be achieved and it is customary to use a fairly rigid support medium to reduce these effects. Paper and cellulose acetate strips soaked in the electrolyte solution are commonly used in radiopharmacy and can be scanned or evaluated in the same way as radiochromatograms described in another section. Starch and polyacrylamide gels are used as supports for protein and macromolecular electrophoresis including radiolabelled antibodies and other proteins.

Of the paper supports, Whatman No. 1 is satisfactory for electrophoresis. It needs careful handling when wetted by electrolyte but has sufficient mechanical strength when dried. Cellulose acetate strips are quite strong when wet but need careful handling when dry, being brittle and prone to cockling. Some mechanical strength can be retained in the dry state by using 10% v/v glycerol in the electrolyte solution. The dried strip retains its flexibility and the added glycerol can sometimes improve the resolution by suppressing band spreading by diffusion.

Electrophoresis equipment

The horizontal technique is satisfactory for most radiopharmaceutical applications and good commercial equipment is available at a reasonable cost. Home-made equipment is unsuitable for this technique in view of the hazards associated with the high voltages necessary for the separation.

The basic equipment consists of a tank having two electrode compartments and a frame or cooled platen for supporting the strips. The strips are placed on the horizontal supports and connected to the electrode compartments by paper wicks pre-soaked in the electrolyte and placed over the ends of the strip and dipping into the electrode compartments. A transparent cover fitted with a safety cut-out is placed over the tank before electrical connection is made to the power supply.

Power supplies come in many shapes and specifications depending on the nature of the electrophoresis experiment. Constant-voltage (V), constant-current (i), or constant-power ($V{\cdot}i$) operation modes are available. Each has its advantages and disadvantages. Constant voltage operation (about 10–30 V/cm of strip = about 300 V) is traditional, but overheating of the strip can occur and, in extreme cases, charring with citrate buffers! A typical set of instructions is shown in SOP 14 (Electrophoresis of Radiopharmaceuticals).

Table 23.7 Solid-phase extraction methods

General procedure:

1. Pre-wet ('activate') the cartridge with 2-5 mL ethanol or methanol.
2. Prepare the cartridge with 2–10 mL of preparation solvent.
3. Place a drop of the radiopharmaceutical in the inlet of the cartridge.
4. Elute sequentially with 2–10 mL quantities of eluates A, B, C and collect each in a separate tube; after the last eluate, force air through the cartridge to dry it.
5. Place the cartridge in another tube for measurement of residual activity.
6. Measure the activity in each tube in an ionisation chamber.
7. Calculate radiochemical purity according to the table.

Radiopharmaceutical	Type of cartridge	Preparation solvent	Eluates				Purity
			A	B	C	D	
^{99m}Tc-Sestamibi	Alumina N	0.5 mL ethanol	10 mL ethanol	cartridge residue			A/total
^{99m}Tc-Sestamibi	C_{18}	2 mL saline	2 mL saline	5 mL ethanol	Cartridge residue		B/total
^{99m}Tc-Tetrofosmin	C_{18}	2 mL saline	2 mL saline	5 mL ethanol	Cartridge residue		B/total
^{99m}Tc-Tetrofosmin	Silica	5 mL saline then 1 mL air	10 mL methanol–water (70 : 30) over 2 min	Cartridge residue			B/total
^{99m}Tc-Tetrofosmin	Silica	5 mL saline then 1 mL air	10 mL methanol–water (70 : 30) over 2 min	10 mL methanol–saline (80 : 20)	Cartridge residue		B/total
^{99m}Tc-MAG3	C_{18}	10 mL 1 mmol/L HCl	10 mL 1 mmol/L HCl	10 mL 50% ethanol	Cartridge residue		B/total
^{99m}Tc-MAG3	C_{18}	10 mL 1 mmol/L HCl	5 mL 1 mmol/LHCl	5 mL 0.5% ethanol in 10 mM sodium phosphate buffer, pH6	10 mL 7% ethanol in PB	Cartridge residue	C/total
^{99m}Tc-Exametazime	C_{18}	5 mL saline	5 mL saline	Cartridge residue			B/total
^{99m}Tc-Exametazime	C_{18}	5 mL saline	5 mL saline	5 mL ethanol	Cartridge residue		B/total
^{111}In-Octreotide	C_{18}	10 mL water	5 mL water	5 mL methanol	Cartridge residue		B/total
[^{123}I]Ioflupane	C_{18}	5 mL water	5 mL water	5 mL ethanol	Cartridge residue		B/total
[$^{123/131}$I]MIBG	C_{18}	5 mL water	5 mL water	10 mL 100 mM monosodium phosphate buffer–THF (3 : 1)	Cartridge residue		B/total
[$^{123/131}$I]MIBG	C_{18}	5 mL water	5 mL10 mmol/L NaOH	Cartridge residue			B/total

Radiopharmaceutical applications

The main application is in the radiochemical purity determination of labelled proteins where separation cannot easily be achieved with chromatographic techniques. The BP 1988 specified paper electrophoresis for the radiochemical purity of Iodinated [^{125}I] Albumin Injection, now replaced by a size-exclusion chromatography method in the current pharmacopoeia.

The radiochemical purity of Chromium [^{51}Cr] Edetate Injection is determined by paper electrophoresis using a barbitone-buffered electrolyte. A 10 µL sample is applied as a 3-mm band at a point 10 cm from the cathode on 120 g/m^2 paper. Electrophoresis is performed at 30 V/cm for 30 minutes when the desired anionic edetate complex migrates some 5 cm towards the anode. The expected radiochemical impurities are [^{51}Cr]CrO_4^-, which migrates faster towards the anode (about 10 cm), and the cationic $^{51}Cr^{3+}$ ion, which migrates in the opposite direction, some 7 cm towards the cathode. Thallous [^{201}Tl] Chloride Injection is tested for radiochemical purity by electrophoresis on cellulose acetate strips using an edetate buffer as supporting electrolyte. The separation of principal component from two differently charged impurities is clearly demonstrated by electrophoresis; chromatographic methods are less successful at this separation.

High-voltage capillary zone electrophoresis

High-voltage capillary zone electrophoresis (HVCZE) has been hailed as an answer to many difficult analytical separations by virtue of its non-chromatographic electrophoretic mobility mode of separating components. The technique employs fine glass capillaries of about 50 µm internal diameter, which allow fast and efficient heat dissipation and permit the use of high voltages in the 15–30 kV range for fast and efficient separation of a variety of analytes including peptides and proteins. Commercial equipment uses on-line UV detection and produces separations seemingly indistinguishable from HPLC traces in terms of speed and resolution. Radiopharmaceutical applications are few, but are expected to increase once the problem of on-line radioactivity detection is solved.

Capillary electrophoresis techniques available

Capillary zone electrophoresis (CZE), also known as free-solution CE (FSCE), is the simplest form of capillary electrophoresis. The separation mechanism is based on differences in the charge-to-mass ratio of the analytes. Fundamental to CZE are homogeneity of the buffer solution and constant field strength throughout the length of the capillary. The separation relies principally on the pH-controlled dissociation of acidic groups on the solute or the protonation of basic functions on the solute.

Capillary gel electrophoresis (CGE) is the adaptation of traditional gel electrophoresis into the capillary using polymers in solution to create a molecular sieve, also known as replaceable physical gel. This allows analytes having similar charge-to-mass ratios to be resolved by size. This technique is commonly employed in SDS–gel molecular weight analysis of proteins and the sizing of applications of DNA sequencing and genotyping. SDS-PAGE is described in detail elsewhere in this book.

Capillary isoelectric focusing (CIEF) allows amphoteric molecules, such as proteins, to be separated by electrophoresis in a pH gradient generated between the cathode and anode. A solute will migrate to a point where its net charge is zero. At the solute's isoelectric point (pI), migration stops and the sample is focused into a tight zone. In CIEF, once a solute has focused at its pI, the zone is mobilised past the detector by either pressure or chemical means. This technique is commonly employed in protein characterisation as a mechanism to determine a protein's isoelectric point.

Radiopharmaceutical applications are limited but are expected to increase once the problem of on-line radioactivity detection is solved.

Partition methods

Recently a number of workers have used a modified form of the classical shake flask solvent partition technique used for determination of log *P* values. The method has the advantage that equilibrium is established between the phases within a few minutes and samples can be withdrawn and the phases assayed for radioactivity.

In a typical experiment a small sample of the radiopharmaceutical is diluted with aqueous buffer and the same volume of immiscible organic solvent is added (octanol, chloroform, and diethyl ether are all popular). The tube is capped and the phases are mixed (often with a whirlmixer) and then allowed to separate; then samples are counted. The results are expressed as percentage of the 'lipophilic' radioactivity in the organic phase calculated from the expression:

$$\text{Per cent lipophilic} = 100 \times \frac{C\ (\text{organic at equilibrium})}{C\ (\text{organic at start})}$$

The method has been used by Tubergen *et al.* (1991) for extraction of lipophilic ^{99m}Tc-d,l-HMPAO with diethyl ether. Bossuyt *et al.* (1991) used extraction into water-saturated octanol for rapid radiochemical purity determinations of MRP20.

The method is specified in the BP for the radiochemical purity of Indium [^{111}In] Oxine Solution.

Particle sizing

Two major types of diagnostic radiopharmaceuticals consist of particulate suspensions. One group is used for the investigation of perfusion defects and includes preparations such as macroaggregated human serum albumin and microspheres. The other group is used for investigation of the reticuloendothelial system and includes colloidal preparations.

Particulate preparations

Safe and reproducible use of these preparations requires control over the number and size of the particles in the product. The preferred range of particle size is 20–80 μm with no particles larger than 100 μm and the minimum of particles below 20 μm.

Light microscopy is the best method for determination of particle number and size in these preparations. A sample is placed in a standard haemocytometer chamber and the number of particles is estimated by counting particles in the centre and four corner squares: multiplication by the appropriate factor will give the number of particles per cubic centimetre.

Particle sizing is best done from a photograph of the haemocytometer chamber. At least 600 particles should be examined and their sizes estimated from the known magnification of the photograph. Alternatively, a Zahlstreifen eyepiece can be used. This has adjustable parallel counting lines and is used by counting about 200 particles along a section of known length (1–2 mm). From this number the length containing 5000 particles is estimated. This length is then scanned, counting only those particles that are over size. The maximum percentage of oversize particles can then be calculated from confidence limits based on the Poisson distribution.

Colloidal preparations

Not all radiopharmaceutical colloids are true colloids, and the mean particle size of colloidal preparations varies widely between different formulations of the same agent, and between different agents. Some sulfur colloids have mean particle sizes of around 0.4–0.6 μm, while antimony trisulfide colloids have mean sizes below 0.1 μm. No single technique is suitable for sizing over such a large range.

Filtration through Nuclepore membranes (polycarbonate membranes having closely controlled etched pores) gives useful data for routine quality control. Samples of the preparation are filtered through a number of separate filters of known, different pore sizes and the percentage of radioactivity retained by each filter is calculated. The percentage retention may be plotted against filter pore size to give an 'activity–size' distribution, approximating to a number distribution. The method is not suitable for particles smaller than 0.05 μm. A typical method is shown in SOP 15 (Particle Sizing of ^{99m}Tc Colloids by Filtration).

Electron microscopy of samples evaporated on carbon grids has been used for accurate sizing of some colloids but cannot be recommended for routine examination. Some colloidal particles (especially of sulfur) will evaporate under the conditions of high vacuum and electron bombardment and results are not easily comparable with those from filtration studies.

Light scattering and photon correlation techniques are now used for estimation of colloidal particle size distributions. These methods are quick and return a weight distribution that may not reflect the radioactivity associated with the individual size fractions.

Particulate contamination

All products for administration by injection should be free from gross particulate contamination. Control is exercised by using glassware, vials and reagents that are themselves free from particulate matter. Visual examination of the product either directly through a lead-glass screen or between illuminated cross-Polaroid screens provides adequate control of most small volume radiopharmaceuticals. Those that cannot be examined visually (e.g. colloids, macroaggregates, microspheres) must be controlled through strict control of glassware, reagents and containers.

Control of pH

Measurement of pH presents problems both from the low volume of sample that is available and from the inherent radioactivity. Glass electrodes and pH meters are universally employed for measurement and checking of solution pH of pharmaceuticals. They are not always suitable for radiopharmaceutical quality control in view of the health and contamination hazards associated with handling unsealed sources.

Narrow-range indicator papers are suitable if standard pH buffers are used in conjunction with the sample to give reference colours corresponding to upper and lower pH limits. A drop of each pH standard should be placed on the paper along with a drop of the sample, so providing a permanent visual record of the pH test. Alternatively, a (low-cost) small-volume pH meter can be purchased specifically for the purpose (e.g. ISFET pH Meter Pocket Size IQ125 from Camlab). This employs a robust ion-selective field-effect transistor (ISFET) silicon sensor and can measure the pH of single-drop samples. Calibration is required, usually with two standard buffer solutions spanning the expected range of pH to be measured.

Biological distribution tests

Biological distribution tests are performed in the development of new radiopharmaceuticals and are specified for some radiopharmaceuticals in the BP. In most cases the test is performed on 3 mice or rats and the test is valid if results in 2 of 3 animals are acceptable. A number of particulate radiopharmaceuticals are controlled in respect of abnormal lung (colloid) or liver (lung perfusion agents) uptake in the subjects. Biological distribution tests are not normally performed in the hospital radiopharmacy; their proper place is in the radiopharmacy research laboratory or in the radiopharmaceutical manufacturer's quality control laboratories.

Sterility testing

The sterility testing of short-lived and PET radiopharmaceuticals is an issue that can reveal differences in opinion, especially if doubt can be cast upon results obtained when testing is not commenced immediately. Sterility testing of radiopharmaceuticals following patient dose preparation may not confirm the sterility of the manufacturers' products but merely ensure that the procedures used in the radiopharmacy result in sterile products. Radiopharmaceuticals are made in very small batches. Thus, to provide a control of the quality of production the frequency of testing should allow the detection of non-sterile preparations, and must allow a history of the performance of the unit to be reviewed. The frequency of testing should be reviewed in the light of the proven performance of the unit. It is preferable that testing be initiated within the Radiopharmacy Unit as soon as possible. Owing to the possibility of ingredients interfering with the sterility test, samples chosen for testing (e.g. kit residues) should initially have been validated by the use of positive controls. If samples are to be transferred to a separate Pharmacy Quality Control Laboratory for testing, they should first be stored in the Radiopharmacy Unit and time allowed for the radioactivity to decay for an appropriate period. It should be noted, however, that while contaminated radiopharmaceuticals have been detected in some instances by sterility testing in this manner, there is clear evidence that in certain cases the number of viable organisms in some radiopharmaceuticals decreases during the storage time required for radioactive decay. It is preferable, therefore, that testing be initiated within the Radiopharmacy Unit as soon as possible.

Sterility testing of short-lived radiopharmaceuticals should therefore be carried out by inoculating broth culture media with a small volume of the preparation (0.3 mL) under aseptic conditions. The broth can then be incubated, for about 2 weeks, and examined for growth. If the facilities are available this can be performed in the laboratory, but this is not possible for most hospital radiopharmacies. In this case the inoculated broths are stored at room temperature behind suitable shielding until the radioactivity has decreased enough for the samples to be transported to a quality control testing laboratory. An alternative to this method is filtration of the sample under aseptic conditions using a 0.2 μm filter. The filter is then cultured in a mixture of broths.

The results of sterility testing for short lived radiopharmaceuticals are retrospective and are chiefly a control of quality of production. Retrospective sterility testing of products may be undertaken three times a week. Ideally, a sample (0.3–0.5 mL) of the first elution (used) of each new generator is aseptically transferred to two different sterile culture media contained in 100-mL vials. These are then incubated (shielded) within the radiopharmacy department at room temperature and kept for at least one week to ensure total radioactive decay. They are then transported to a Pharmacy Microbiological Testing Laboratory for further culturing as necessary. In a similar fashion, the last elution from each generator (unused) is tested, as is a sample taken from the remnants of a product that has been prepared during the week and from which patient doses have been dispensed. If a positive growth is found, an investigation must be held to determine possible cause(s). Corrective action, e.g. a total cleandown, may be undertaken if deemed appropriate. Results of all microbiological testing are held in the radiopharmacy and logged accordingly. Where it is not practicable to test the residues of kits, for example because doses are drawn up outside the radiopharmacy, the remnants of a further vial of eluate from the generator should be tested instead. As an alternative to sampling from the vial into broth, it may also be worth considering the possibility of adding broth (or double-strength broth) to the vial.

Long-lived radiopharmaceuticals manufactured on a commercial scale, e.g. ^{125}I-iodinated albumin and ^{51}Cr-EDTA, are prospectively sterility tested before release due to the longer shelf-life of these products.

Pyrogenicity testing

Bacterial endotoxins (pyrogens) are polysaccharides from bacterial membranes. They are water soluble, heat stable, and filterable. If they are present in a preparation and administered to a patient, they can cause fever and also leukopenia in immunosuppressed patients. To minimise the chances that pyrogens are present it is important that preparations are manufactured and dispensed under aseptic conditions and that all consumables and equipment used have been heat treated and are known to be pyrogen free. Most licensed products are guaranteed pyrogen free. The EP sets a limit of (175/V) EU (Endotoxin Units)/mL where V is the maximum recommended dose in millilitres.

However for PET radiopharmaceutical producers, pyrogen testing and proof of absence of pyrogens prior to injection into patients is becoming the industry standard. A fast, reliable method thus is necessary. Limulus amoebocyte lysate (LAL) testing was introduced some years ago, but reliable results were not always produced because of many artefacts, including false positives. More recently the FDA have approved the use of specific kits performing a kinetic chromogenic method, using improved LAL reagents coupled with endotoxin-specific software validated to 21 CFR Part 11 requirements, which use only a small amount of product at non-interfering dilution and require no preparation of endotoxin standards. This hand-held reader plus disposable test cartridge gives quantitative results in 15 minutes and can detect endotoxin levels from as low as 0.01 EU/mL to as high as 10 EU/mL. This has been licensed by the FDA for both in-process and final product testing and means that all 'longer-lived' PET radiopharmaceuticals, e.g. ^{18}F-fluorinated compounds, can be prospectively tested.

Quality control of PET radiopharmaceuticals

PET radiopharmaceuticals, by virtue of their very short half-life, cannot be quality assured in a separate and independent operation before administration, and their production and quality control are part and parcel of the same manufacturing process, which is similar to that of conventional pharmaceuticals but very much faster. Much of the testing takes place before production commences: identity and purity of precursors, ligands and reagents; systems suitability tests on maintenance, operation of chemical reactors and purification processes for the product will have been undertaken and the process validated. Some retrospective testing will have been done on pilot batches to demonstrate suitability, etc.

The pharmacopoeias recognise the problems with PET production and allow a range of processes, synthetic routes, etc., to be adopted provided the final material complies with the standard. The monograph for Fludeoxyglucose [^{18}F] Injection recognises several production routes: phase transfer catalysed nucleophilic substitution of 1,2,4,5-tetra-*O*-acetyl-2-*O*-trifluoromethanesulfonyl-β-D-mannopyranose with [^{18}F]fluoride, and electrophilic substitution of 3,4,6-tri-*O*-acetyl-D-glucal with molecular [^{18}F]fluorine or [^{18}F]acetylhypofluorite. Specifications are provided for both starting materials including chemical purity by HPLC, the phase transfer catalyst, solid-phase derivatisation agent, residual solvents, etc. Radiochemical purity is determined by HPLC and TLC.

Summary and conclusions

Quality control of radiopharmaceuticals is a complex and time-consuming activity in the hospital radiopharmacy. It should be envisaged as part of an ongoing scheme of quality assurance which embraces all aspects of the work done in the radiopharmacy. Not all the tests described can, or should, be performed on each diagnostic agent every time it is dispensed or manufactured. A proper scheme is necessary to ensure that all radiopharmaceuticals are regularly checked, and a combination of radiochemical analysis, environmental control and monitoring, and adequate training of personnel will go a long way towards achieving satisfactory quality assurance.

Appendix: Standard Operating Procedures

SOP 1: Calibration of ionisation chamber

Ionisation chambers used for routine measurement of radioactivities of received and dispensed radiopharmaceuticals need to be checked for calibration accuracy and linearity of response every 3 months.

1 *Calibration accuracy*
For this test a standard radioactive source is required. A suitable source is ^{226}Ra having an activity of about 3.7 MBq (100 μCi) obtainable from Amersham International and provided with a calibration certificate traceable to NPL.
- a Set the ionisation chamber controls to read ^{226}Ra.
- b Place the standard source in the measuring volume of the ionisation chamber. Allow the instrument to settle for several minutes before taking a reading. It may be necessary to switch to a 'slow' setting of the readout device to reduce the random fluctuations.
- c Take at least three readings of the source activity at about 5-minute intervals and record their average and standard deviation.
- d If necessary with an indirect reading instrument, calculate the radioactivity of the standard source.
- e Compare the measurements with the stated radioactivity of the standard source.
- f Confirm that the measured radioactivity lies within 5% of stated radioactivity. If the measurement lies outside this tolerance the instrument must be taken out of use and services or recalibrated by the manufacturer.

2 *Linearity checks*
The linearity of response over the dynamic range of the instrument should be confirmed as follows.
- a Obtain a sample of the highest ^{99m}Tc activity expected in the radiopharmacy, usually in the GBq range.
- b Taking all radiation safety precautions, measure the radioactivity of this sample. Note the activity and time of measurement.
- c Repeat the measurement at intervals of 6–12 hours, noting the time and activity at each measurement, until the radioactivity has fallen to a level indistinguishable from background.

d Convert the recorded radioactivities to their logarithms and plot as ordinate against elapsed time since the initial observations.

e Examine the plot visually for linearity. If programs are available, then perform a linear regression on the data and examine the residuals for evidence of non-linearity.

f Carefully note the radioactivity regions which appear non-linear (usually the high and low ends of the overall range) and record the usable range on the instruction sheet for the instrument.

SOP 2: Determination of beta absorption curves

Beta absorption curves are specified in the BP as a means of identification of beta-emitting radionuclides. The equipment consists of a lead castle fitted with shelves for the source and interposed screens all below a GM detector. Aluminium screens or filters are placed between the source and the GM detector and the decrease in count rate with increasing aluminium thickness is followed until all the particles are absorbed as shown by a fairly constant background count rate. The absorption curve is compared with that of a standard sample measured under identical conditions.

Preparation of the radioactive source is critical; the BP directions for source preparation must be followed.

Method

1. Check the controls and operation of the scaler. Set the high voltage to its specified level.
2. With no source present in the assembly, count the background for 5 minutes.
3. Place the metal shield on SHELF 1 of the castle and leave it in position at all times *except when taking a count*.
4. Place the unknown source in a plastics holder and insert in SHELF 4 of the castle. Place an absorber holder on SHELF 3.
5. Take 1-minute counts (or longer as appropriate) with increasing thickness of aluminium absorbers placed in SHELF 3. At least six screens should be used, of increasing mass per unit area (mg/cm^2), with the thickest screen absorbing all the particles and thus giving a background count.
6. Correct all counts for background and paralysis using the formula:

$$C_{\text{true}} = \frac{C_{\text{obs}}}{1 - C_{\text{obs}}\tau}$$

   where C_{obs} is the observed count rate (in cpm) after background subtraction and τ is the paralysis time of the equipment expressed in seconds.
7. Repeat steps 4 to 6 with the standard source of the radionuclide being identified.
8. Plot the logarithm of the true count rate (ordinate) against the superficial density (mg/cm^2) for both sample and standard.
9. Calculate the coefficient of mass attenuation by the following method:

   a Inspect the plots and identify the portion of the curve that is the most linear.

   b Identify the lightest screen, m_l, and the heaviest screen, m_z, lying within the linear region of the plots.

   c Calculate the coefficient from the formula:

$$\mu_m = \frac{2.303}{m_z - m_l}(\log A_l - \log A_z)$$

   where A_l, A_z are the corrected count rates obtained with the lightest and heaviest screens within the linear part of the curve.
10. Compare the mass absorption coefficients of the sample and standard.
11. Accept the sample identity if the difference between the coefficients is less than 10%.

SOP 3: Molybdenum-99 breakthrough test for ^{99m}Tc eluates

Every eluate obtained from a ^{99}Mo/^{99m}Tc generator system should be examined for ^{99}Mo breakthrough. The rapid method described below depends on the selective transmission of high-energy gamma photons from ^{99}Mo impurity through a 7-mm-thick lead shield.

The maximum permissible radioactivity due to the parent ^{99}Mo is 0.1% of the measured ^{99m}Tc radioactivity (or 1 kBq of ^{99}Mo activity for every 1 MBq of ^{99m}Tc activity).

Method

1 Measure the ^{99m}Tc radioactivity of the generator eluate as described in the SOP for the ionisation chamber.
2 Reset the ionisation chamber to measure ^{99}Mo radioactivity by changing the attenuator settings to those appropriate to ^{99}Mo.
3 Transfer the eluate vial to the 7-mm-wall lead shield and replace in the ionisation chamber.
4 Note the reading corresponding to ^{99}Mo activity and calculate the percentage present.

SOP 4: Scintillation detector performance optimisation

Scintillation detectors must be set to maximum counting efficiency by adjustment of the photomultiplier high voltage and the pulse threshold or window settings. This SOP describes a generic procedure for optimising scintillation counters, either plastics or thallium-activated sodium iodide.

Method

1 Set the threshold to about 20% of its maximum value. If an energy window is available, then set this to 'integral' or a wide value to ensure collection of high numbers of pulses.
2 Place a gamma-emitting sample of activity 1–5 kBq near the detector (or in the well of well detector).
3 Slowly increase the high-voltage (HV) setting until the scaler begins to count.
4 Set the equipment to record 10-second counts.
5 Starting at a rational value just below the HV determined above, increase the HV in steps of 10 volts and record the 10-second count. Continue as the count rises with voltage and stop when it is obvious that the counter is 'racing'.
6 Remove the radioactive source and repeat the previous step to obtain a series of background counts at the same voltages.
7 Plot the sample (S) and background (B) count rates against HV to determine the length of the counting plateau and to select an operating voltage within that range.
8 Alternatively, calculate the function S^2/B and plot at each HV setting. The optimum HV corresponds to the peak on this plot.
9 As a further check, the detector linearity should be determined with standards of known radioactivity.

SOP 5: Scintillation detector linearity checking

The working voltage and energy window of a NaI(Tl) scintillation detector must be adjusted to detect the photopeak of the specified radionuclide (^{99m}Tc in this case) to ensure maximum counting efficiency. The instrument settings should have already been adjusted for optimum counting efficiency according to SOP 4: Scintillation Detector Performance Optimisation and should not be changed.

Method

1 Prepare a stock solution containing about 1 MBq/mL of ^{99m}Tc radioactivity by dilution from a generator eluate. Note the eluate label details (radioactivity, volume, time of measurement) for use in calculations later.
2 Prepare a series of calibration standards by diluting 0.2, 0.4, 0.6, 0.8 and 1.0 mL of the stock solution to 100 mL with water. Label the calibration standards.
3 Dispense 1 mL aliquots of each standard into 5 mL plastic counting vials by using a *fresh* 1 mL disposable syringe for each. Ensure the tubes are securely capped and label them.
4 Take a 10-second background count and then count each calibration standard for 10 seconds. Correct the counts by subtracting the background. Note the time of measurement.

5 Calculate the radioactivity of the standards counted from the expression:

$$A(\text{dps}) = \frac{S(\text{MBq/mL}) \times V(\text{mL}) \times 10^6 \times f}{100}$$

where S (MBq/mL) is the radioactive concentration of the stock solution (from label details), V(mL) is the volume of eluate taken for dilution, and f is the *decay factor* for ^{99m}Tc obtained from tables for the *elapsed time* $(t - t_{ref})$ between the reference time and completion of the counting in step 4. The factor 10^6 converts radioactivity in MBq to disintegrations per second.

6 Convert the observed 10-second counts to count rate (in cps) and plot observed count (cps) against the true radioactivity (in dps, step 5). Examine the plot and check that points at the higher radioactivities are linear and do not show a drop in count rate.

7 By drawing the best line through the points or using a graphics/statistics program to generate the best line, calculate the counting efficiency from the slope of the graph. (A slope of 1 indicates 100% efficiency, 0.2 is 20%.)

SOP 6: Paper chromatography of radiopharmaceuticals

Whatman 3MM paper is recommended for radiochromatography as it is fast running and mechanically strong in the wet condition.

Method

1 Cut a piece of Whatman 3MM paper and mark in sharp, soft pencil as in the diagram:

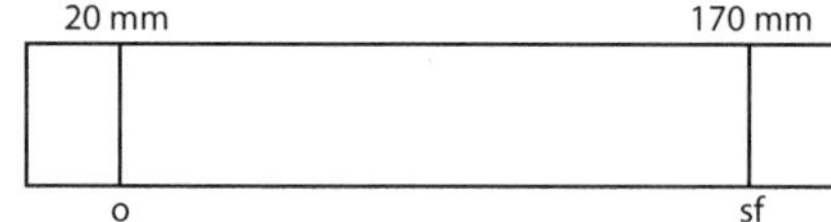

2 Take a tall cylinder (250 × 40 mm diam.) and place enough mobile phase to give a 10 mm deep pool at the bottom. Moisten a solvent saturation pad with the mobile phase and slide it down the inside wall of the cylinder until it touches the pool of mobile phase.

3 As an aid to visualising the solvent migration make a mark about 3 mm below the solvent front line with a suitable felt-tip marker.

4 Using either a 5 μL capillary pipette or a drop hanging from the end of a 25G (orange) needle, place a single spot of the radiopharmaceutical at the origin of the paper strip.

5 Immediately clip the strip to the hanger and lower gently into the cylinder until the bottom edge is immersed some 2–3 mm in the pool.

6 Place the assembly in front of the cold light and allow development to proceed until the mobile phase reaches the solvent front line.

7 Immediately remove the strip from the cylinder and dry under the infrared lamp or in a stream of warm air.

8 Examine and quantitate the strip by any of the approved methods for the particular radiopharmaceutical.

SOP 7: ITLC chromatography of radiopharmaceuticals

The ITLC system consists of a glass microfibre mat impregnated with silica gel or silicic acid. The material is extremely fragile and should be handled with great care. In particular the surfaces should not be touched with the bare fingers as fingerprints are known to cause artefacts in the chromatograms.

Method

1 Cut a piece of ITLC material and mark in sharp, soft pencil as in the diagram. Activate the silica by heating in an oven at 110°C for 10 minutes, then allowing the strip to cool before use.

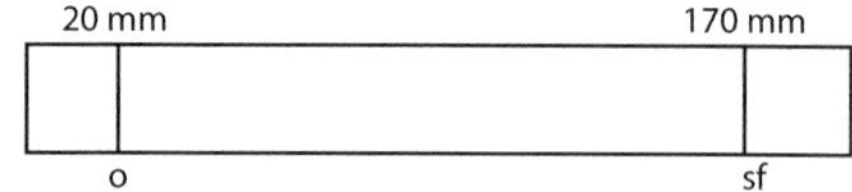

2 Take a tall cylinder (250 × 40 mm diameter) and place enough mobile phase to give a 10 mm deep pool at the bottom. Moisten a solvent saturation pad with the mobile phase and slide it down the inside wall of the cylinder until it touches the pool of mobile phase.

3 As an aid to visualising the solvent migration, make a mark about 3 mm below the solvent front line with a suitable felt-tip marker.
4 Using either a 5 µL capillary pipette or a drop hanging from the end of a 25G (orange) needle, place a single spot of the radiopharmaceutical at the origin of the ITCL strip.
5 Immediately clip the strip to the hanger and lower gently into the cylinder until the bottom edge is immersed some 2–3 mm in the pool.
6 Place the assembly in front of the cold light and allow development to proceed until the mobile phase reaches the solvent front line.
7 Immediately remove the strip from the cylinder and dry under the infrared lamp or in a stream of warm air.
8 When dry, protect the ITLC strip by sandwiching between two layers of adhesive tape.
9 Examine and quantitate the strip by any of the approved methods for the particular radiopharmaceutical.

SOP 8: Minichromatography for ^{99m}Tc radiopharmaceuticals

Method

1 Prepare strips of Gelman ITLC-SG material or Whatman 3MM paper according to the diagram:

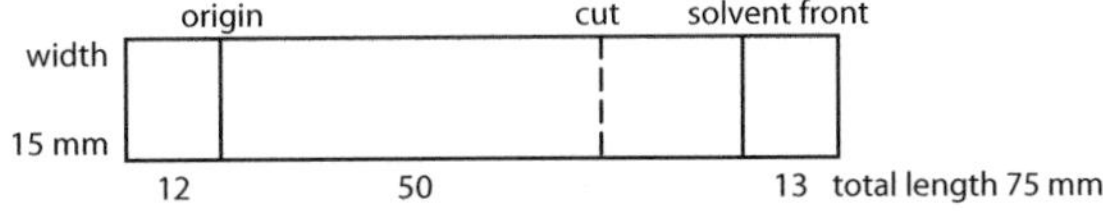

2 Prepare developing tanks by placing about 1 mL of the mobile phase into glass Universal tubes or scintillation vials.
3 Apply 5 µL spots of samples to separate strips using calibrated capillary pipettes.
4 Immediately develop the chromatograms until the mobile phase reaches the solvent front line.
5 Remove the strips from the developing tube and dry them under the IR lamp.
6 Divide each strip into upper and lower sections by cutting across the pre-marked line.
7 Roll each section and place in a counting tube.
8 Determine which is the most radioactive section and count this for 50 or 60 seconds, or until at least 10 000 counts have been accumulated, whichever is the longer, C_h.
9 Count the less active section for the same time period, C_l.
10 Count the background for the same period of time, B.
11 Calculate the percentage of radioactivity in each section of the strip from the formula:

$$\text{Per cent radioactivity} = 100 \times \frac{C_{h \text{ or } l} - B}{C_h + C_l - 2 \times B}$$

SOP 9: Autoradiography of chromatograms

Autoradiography of radiochromatograms provides a permanent record of the distribution of radioactivity on the chromatoplate but cannot give reliable information on the distribution of radioactivity between peaks, spots or regions.

Method

1 Develop and dry the chromatogram as usual.
2 Take the chromatoplate and light-proof cassette or envelope into the darkroom.
3 Once in the darkroom switch on the safelight and switch off the normal lighting. Wait a few minutes for the eyes to adjust to the new lighting level.
4 Unwrap a sheet of X-ray film and cut a piece the same size as the chromatoplate. Replace unused film in its envelope. Fix the plate and film together using clips and mark the orientation and identity of both by clipping a distinctive pattern on one edge of the plate–film pair. Place the assembly in the light proof cassette and leave for at least 30 minutes or preferably overnight.
5 After exposure of the film re-enter the darkroom and assemble the developing tanks and dishes. Half fill the developing tank with developer, and similarly half fill the stop tank with stop solution and fixer tank with fixer solution.

6 Switch on the safelight and switch off the normal lighting. Wait a few minutes for the eyes to adjust to the new lighting level. Remove the plate–film pair from the lightproof cassette. Separate the two components and gently place the film in the developer.
7 Develop the film for about 5 minutes until the radioactive areas are clearly shown as dark spots. gently rock the tank during development to ensure even mixing and exposure to the developing solution.
8 Stop development by transferring the film to the stop bath and immersing in the stop solution for about 1 minute.
9 Transfer the film from the stop bath to the fixer bath and gently rock the bath until the unexposed areas of the film are dissolved and appear uniformly clear when viewed against the safelight.
10 Transfer the film to the wash tank and wash in running water for at least 10 minutes. Remove the finished film, squeeze off excess water and hang on clips to dry.

SOP 10: Radiochromatogram scanner: operation and performance checks

The radiochromatogram scanner consists of a motor- and gearbox-driven scanner base-plate which carries the chromatoplate beneath a slit-collimated 12.5 mm (0.5 inch) diameter NaI(Tl) detector. This is connected to a NE 5 scaler ratemeter from which a 100 mV full scale deflection (fsd). output is fed to a Spectra-Physics integrator.

Operating instructions

1 Switch ON all units and allow to stabilise for a few minutes.
2 For normal work set the integrator settings as follows:
   - chart speed 4 cm/min
   - attenuation 128
3 Place the chromatogram on the bedplate underneath the acetate cover sheet and adjust the detector head to scan the required channel on the chromatogram.
4 Set the ratemeter to a sensitive range, set the bedplate gearbox in neutral, and manually scan the chromatogram to locate the main peak. Adjust the sensitivity of the scaler to give a reading greater then 0.5 fsd. Also adjust the response time (time constant) of the scaler to remove most, but not all, of the ratemeter fluctuations.
5 Move the chromatoplate so that a low activity (background) region is under the detector. Set the integrator to evaluate the background by pressing PTEVAL on the control panel and wait until the instrument completes its evaluation.
6 Move the chromatoplate so that the lower edge lies under the detector slit. Change the gearbox setting to a speed of 4.41 cm/min (marked on the case).
7 To scan the chromatogram, simultaneously press the SCAN button on the bedplate and the INJ A pad on the integrator. The chromatoplate will move under the detector at a speed of 4.41 cm/min and the integrator will plot the radioactivity profile at a chart speed of 4 cm/min.
8 Significant peaks on the chromatogram will be marked with their ‘retention time’ during the scan.
9 To stop the scan press the INJ A pad on the integrator and then the STOP button on the scanner. The integrator then prints out a report listing the retention times and peak areas of all detected peaks.

Linearity and resolution checks

The radiochromatogram scanning system must be periodically checked for linearity of response and resolving power.

Method

1 Prepare a solution of sodium pertechnetate containing between 8 and 12 MBq/mL of ^{99m}Tc radioactivity.
2 Take a piece of Whatman No. 1 chromatography paper of size 2 × 20 cm. Draw a central pencil line down the length of the strip and mark off six sets of cross lines 2 cm apart.

3 Using a 20 μL syringe, carefully dispense 1, 2, 5, 10, 15 and 20 μL volumes at successive cross lines to simulate spots on a chromatogram. Dry the spots under an infrared lamp.
4 Place the prepared strip on the scanner bedplate and scan the 'chromatogram' under the standard conditions to be used for the ^{99m}Tc chromatograms.
5 Examine the radioactivity profile and the peak report. Calculate the amount of radioactivity in each of the spots and plot this against the measured/reported peak areas (expressed as counts) for each simulated peak.
6 Examine the plot and confirm that it is linear over the range of radioactivity examined. In particular, ensure that the difference between the measured count for the 20-μL peak and the best-fitting line is not more than more than 3% for that sample.

Resolution checks

The peak resolving power of the scanning system must be checked periodically to ensure that recorded radioactivity profiles are acceptable and are undistorted. Peak profiles may appear distorted through the selection of long time constants (response times) which produce a trailing distortion to the profile.

Method

1 Prepare a solution of sodium pertechnetate containing between 8 and 12 MBq/mL of ^{99m}Tc radioactivity.
2 Take a piece of Whatman No. 1 chromatography paper 20 × 2 cm and draw a central line down the length of the paper strip. Mark off six sets of cross lines at spacings of 4, 6, 8, 10, 12, 16, 18, and 20 mm.
3 Using a glass microsyringe dispense 5 μL volumes of the pertechnetate solution at each cross line. Ensure that the spot diameter is less than 3 mm by making multiple applications if necessary, then dry the spots under an infrared lamp.
4 Place the prepared strip on the scanner bedplate and accumulate the 'chromatogram' under the standard conditions to be used for the ^{99m}Tc chromatograms.
5 Examine the radioactivity profile for the strip and locate the pair of spots where the baseline is not cleanly separated but the height of the trough above the baseline is about one-tenth of the average adjacent peak heights. The distance between the spots is the approximate resolution of the detection system.

SOP 11: Radiochromatogram quantitation

Methods for determining the radioactivities of multiple peaks on chromatograms or electrophoretograms are described in this SOP. General principles only are discussed. The user should obtain exact details from the SOP for a particular radiopharmaceutical

If chromatogram scanning is not possible, then cutting and counting is the only practical alternative. The chromatoplate can be cut into sections each corresponding to a component, main or impurity, and the segments counted in suitable counting equipment. If the radioactivity distribution is unknown the chromatoplate can be cut into equal width segments, the radioactivity counted, and the radioactivity profile constructed as a histogram. This method will have to be used where the applied radioactivity is too low for reliable peak discrimination by scanning.

The counting efficiency will depend on the design and operating characteristics of the detector, but for most NaI(Tl) well detectors an efficiency approaching or exceeding 50% can be expected with ^{99m}Tc and radionuclides of similar gamma energy.

When counting in a well detector it is important to maintain the same counting geometry for all segments of the chromatogram, large or small pieces. This may be achieved by rolling or compressing the material into the bottom of a counting vial before placing in the detector.

The linearity of detection should be verified by counting a series of dilutions (or simulated spots on the chromatogram) covering the range 1 to 200% of the expected radioactivity and plotting the count rate against applied radioactivity (in kBq).

Detector linearity

1. Prepare a solution of pertechnetate at approximately the same radioactive concentration as the radiopharmaceutical being examined. Alternatively, the radiopharmaceutical itself may be used as the radioactivity standard in this test.
2. Prepare a series of at least five radioactivity standards by dispensing from a microsyringe 1, 3, 5, 7 and 10 μL volumes of the radioactive solution onto small strips of the chromatographic medium to be used in the main radiochemical purity test.
3. Dry the strips and 'Swiss roll' them into counting tubes ensuring that the final size of the rolled strips is similar in all tubes.
4. Count the strips under the standard conditions specified for counting on the equipment used.
5. Plot the count rate (cps) against the decay-corrected radioactivity of the samples applied in step 2.
6. Examine the plot for linearity and ensure that the plotted point for the highest radioactivity does not differ by more than 3% from the value predicted from the best-fitting line.

Cut and count

This method can be used when the migration distances of the various radioactive species are known. The developed strip is cut into two or three pieces corresponding to the regions where the radioactive components are expected to lie.

1. Before running the chromatogram, mark off in soft pencil the cutting lines (as well as the conventional origin and solvent front lines).
2. Dry the developed chromatogram as usual. Cut the chromatogram into two or three sections according to the method directions. Roll each section and place in a counting tube. mark the tube with a code indicating its contents.
3. Ensure that the detector–scaler is set to the specified operating conditions for that particular radionuclide and that all pre-counting checks have been performed.
4. Count the background radiation for 50 or 60 seconds and calculate the background rate (cps).
5. Count the rolled sections in their counting tubes for 50 or 60 seconds. Calculate the raw rate (cps) for each section.
6. Subtract the background count rate from each section count rate.
7. Calculate the percentage of the total radioactivity in each section from the formula:

$$\text{Per cent in section} = 100 \times \frac{\text{corrected cps}}{\text{sum of corrected cps for all sections}}$$

Histogram method

1. Dry the developed chromatogram as usual. In the case of ITLC chromatograms seal the surface by applying a strip of adhesive tape to each side.
2. Starting from the bottom of the chromatogram, mark off 5-mm segments with a soft pencil or ball point pen. *Number each segment before proceeding.*
3. Cut the segments with scissors or a sharp knife and place each one in a coded sample tube.
4. Ensure that the detector–scaler is set to the specified operating conditions for that particular radionuclide and that all pre-counting checks have been performed.
5. Count the background radiation for 50 or 60 seconds and calculate the background rate (cps).
6. Count the rolled sections in their counting tubes for 50 or 60 seconds. Calculate the raw rate (cps) for each section.
7. Subtract the background count rate from each section count rate.
8. Plot a histogram of the corrected cps against strip number and use this to identify the main and impurity peaks in the chromatogram. *It is often helpful to plot a second histogram showing the corrected cps on a log scale as an aid in locating small impurity peaks.*
9. Add together the counts for all segments contributing to the particular peak and calculate

the percentage of total radioactivity under each peak from the formula:

$$\text{Per cent peak} = 100 \times \frac{\text{sum of segment counts for the peak}}{\text{sum of all segment counts}}$$

SOP 12: Performance checks on Berthold system

The Berthold chromatogram linear analyser system must be periodically checked for linearity of response over the length of the plate and for linearity of radioactivity response. The following SOP describes methods for both these tests.

Linearity of response

1. Obtain a 25–30-cm long intravenous cannula and adhesive tape it across a standard 20 × 20 cm TLC glass plate so that tube is straight and taut and the ends project over the edge of the plate.
2. Fill a 2-mL disposable syringe with a solution of sodium pertechnetate of radioactivity 1–5 MBq/mL. Attach to the cannula plate assembly and carefully fill the cannula tubing with the solution, ensuring no trapped air bubbles or voids in the line.
3. Remove the syringe and plug the ends of the cannula with Parafilm or similar. Insert the cannula-plate assembly into the stainless steel bedplate system of the Berthold scanner. Cover the projecting ends with thin lead sheeting to shield them. Ensure the ends of the cannula are away from the detection zone of the head.
4. Set up the Berthold linear analyser for standard ^{99m}Tc scanning of the TLC plate and accumulate data under the standard conditions to be used in the routine analysis.
5. Examine the computer plot for linearity of response across the length of the detection zone. Faults likely to occur are:
   a. loss of sensitivity at either end of the zone
   b. loss of sensitivity in middle region of the zone
   c. localised loss of sensitivity.
6. Faults (a) and (b) are likely to be caused by incorrect setting of the HV to the proportional counter head. Fault (c) is often due to dirt or particles on the anode wire.
7. Report all faults to the technician who will take remedial action.

Detector linearity

The Berthold linear analyser system must be periodically checked for linearity of radioactive response over the expected range of ^{99m}Tc activities.

1. Prepare a solution of sodium pertechnetate containing between 8 and 12 MBq/mL of ^{99m}Tc radioactivity.
2. Take a piece of Whatman No. 1 chromatography paper of size 2 × 20 cm. Draw a central pencil line down the length of the strip and mark off six sets of cross lines 2 cm apart.
3. Using a 20 μL syringe, carefully dispense 1, 2, 5, 10, 15 and 20 μL volumes at successive cross lines to simulate spots on a chromatogram. Dry the spots under an infrared lamp.
4. Place the prepared strip on the Berthold linear analyser bedplate assembly and accumulate the 'chromatogram' under the standard conditions to be used for the ^{99m}Tc chromatograms.
5. Examine the radioactivity profile and the peak report. Calculate the amount of radioactivity in each of the spots and plot this against the measured/reported peak areas (expressed as counts) for each simulated peak.
6. Examine the plot and confirm that it is linear over the range of radioactivity examined. In particular, ensure that the difference between the measured count for the 20-μL peak and the best-fitting line is not more than 3% for that sample.

Resolution test

The Berthold linear analyser system must be periodically checked for detector resolution when used with ^{99m}Tc radiopharmaceuticals.

1. Prepare a solution of sodium pertechnetate containing between 8 and 12 MBq/mL of ^{99m}Tc radioactivity.
2. Take a piece of Whatman No. 1 chromatography paper 20 × 2 cm and draw a central line down the

length of the paper strip. Mark off six sets of cross lines at spacings of 4, 6, 8, 10, 12, 16, 18, and 20 mm.

3 Using a glass microsyringe dispense 5 µL volumes of the pertechnetate solution at each cross line. Ensure that the spot diameter is less than 3 mm by making multiple applications if necessary, then dry the spots under an infrared lamp.

4 Place the prepared strip on the Berthold linear analyser bedplate assembly and accumulate the 'chromatogram' under the standard conditions to be used for the ^{99m}Tc chromatograms.

5 Examine the radioactivity profile for the strip and locate the pair of spots where the baseline is not cleanly separated but the height of the trough above the baseline is about one-tenth of the average adjacent peak heights. The distance between the spots is the approximate resolution of the detection system.

SOP 13: HPLC of radiopharmaceuticals: performance checks

HPLC systems must be checked for compliance with performance specifications before use in radiopharmaceutical quality control. The main specification and tests are column resolution and detector linearity performance.

Column resolution

1 Set up the HPLC system to the operating conditions specified for the particular radiopharmaceutical. Note especially:
  a mobile phase flow rate
  b detector sensitivity setting and electronic damping
  c integrator attenuation
  d peak threshold detection setting
  e integrator chart speed.

2 Prepare a solution of sodium pertechnetate at the same radioactive concentration as recommended for the radiopharmaceutical. *The use of the radiopharmaceutical itself is not recommended for this test.*

3 Set the HPLC system to its operating conditions and allow the column to equilibrate for about 15 minutes before proceeding.

4 Inject a 20 µL sample of the pertechnetate solution onto the column through the injector device and record the chromatogram.

5 Examine the chromatogram and ensure that:
  a The peak is symmetric with little evidence of tailing.
  b The apex of the peak lies within the upper half of the chart record and does not go off scale.

6 Determine the column efficiency from the expression:

$$N = \frac{5.54}{L}\left(\frac{V_r}{W_h}\right)^2$$

where V_r is the distance along the baseline between the point of injection and a perpendicular dropped from the maximum of the peak of interest, L is the length of the column in metres, and w_h is the width of the peak of interest at half-height, measured in the same units as V_r.

7 When examining radiopharmaceuticals containing several components, ensure that the resolution of the column is at least 1.0 as defined by the formula:

$$R = 2(V_{ra} - V_{rb})/(y_a + y_b)$$

where V_{ra} and V_{rb} are the distances along the baseline between the point of injection and perpendiculars dropped from the maxima of two adjacent peaks, and y_a and y_b are the respective baseline peak widths.

Detector linearity

1 Prepare a series of five dilutions of sodium pertechnetate solution which contain 20, 50 100, 150 and 200% of the expected activity of the radiopharmaceutical to be chromatographed.

2 *In random order*, inject 20 µL samples of each dilution and record the chromatograms and peak areas.

3 If time permits, repeat the injections in a different random order, recording the chromatograms and peak areas as before.

4 Plot the recorded peak areas against the concentrations (expressed preferably in MBq/mL, although % dilutions are acceptable in some situations).

5 Examine the plot and confirm that it is linear over the range of radioactivity examined. In particular ensure that the difference between the recorded peak area for the highest activity (200%) peak and the best-fitting line is not more than 3%.

SOP 14: Electrophoresis of radiopharmaceuticals

Introduction

Although planar chromatography (paper, TLC, ITLC) is the most popular technique, electrophoretic separations add an extra dimension to the purity/impurity profile of radiopharmaceuticals. Unlike chromatography there is no solvent front for determining R_f values. A suitable alternative is to run a spot of pertechnetate [$^{99m}TcO_4^-$] under the same conditions as the sample and report sample migrations as the ratio

$$R_S = \frac{\text{migration (mm) of sample}}{\text{migration (mm) of } TcO_{4^-}}$$

Since TcO_4^- is anionic, any cationic ^{99m}Tc species will have negative R_S values under this convention.

Method

1 Set up the Shandon electrophoresis tank and fill both compartments with the chosen electrolyte solution (usually a pH 6.8 phosphate, or 9.2 carbonate–bicarbonate buffer) ensuring that the two chambers are equally filled.

2 For *paper electrophoresis*, take a piece of Whatman No. 1 paper (10 × 30 cm) and mark an application line at the mid-point with a soft pencil, marking off application points along the line at 2-cm intervals.

3 Dip the paper in the electrolyte solution. Gently blot between paper towels, and place in position in the electrophoresis tank. Close the lid and pass current for about 5 minutes at a voltage of 10 V/cm to equilibrate the paper.

4 Remove the lid (the current cuts off automatically) and spot the radiopharmaceutical on the pre-marked spots from a 1-mL syringe fitted with an orange needle. Replace the lid and run the electrophoretogram for 30–40 minutes.

5 For *cellulose acetate (Celagram) electrophoresis*, carefully remove the strip from its packing and with a soft pencil gently mark the point for application. Place the marked strip shiny side up on the surface of the buffer electrolyte contained in a shallow dish and allow to float for 2–3 minutes (until the pores are filled with the liquid).

6 Remove the strip with forceps and very gently blot semi-dry between paper towels. Transfer the strip to the electrophoresis tank and place paper wicks over each end dipping into the buffer. Replace the lid and pass current for 5 minutes at about 10 V/cm to equilibrate the cellulose.

7 Remove the lid (the current cuts off automatically), spot the radiopharmaceutical and proceed as in step 4.

8 When electrophoresis is finished, remove the paper or cellulose strips (*care:* soggy paper tears easily) and hang to dry in front of the heat lamp. The cellulose acetate strips tend to curl at this stage and become very friable. One solution is to coat them with a strip of adhesive tape before they are completely dry. Another solution is to add about 10% glycerol to the electrolyte buffer used to pre-soak the strips to prevent complete dehydration under the heat lamp.

9 The dried electrophoretograms can be examined and quantitated by any of the methods described under chromatography.

SOP 15: Particle sizing of ^{99m}Tc colloids by filtration

The biodistribution of any colloid preparation will depend largely on its particle size distribution. Small particles (about 10–100 nm) are taken up by circulating RES cells and lymph nodes, while larger particles (about 200–800 nm) are extracted by the liver and spleen.

Nuclepore filtration

Nucleopore filters are polycarbonate membranes that have been treated to produce submicroscopic pores of accurately known diameter; they may be regarded as 'sieves' for submicrometre particles. Unlike with sieves, however, the mass of material retained by a particular mesh cannot be measured. With radiolabelled colloids, the radioactivity retained by a filter can be compared with the activity that passes through, and the percentage activity retained can be calculated. The test can be carried out with a range of nucleopore filters and a cumulative particle size distribution curve constructed.

Small samples of the radiolabelled colloid are filtered through a range of filters (0.03–8.0 μm) and the percentage activity retained is calculated. The results are plotted as a cumulative frequency (percentage oversize) curve and as a normal distribution.

Method

1. Prepare a series of nucleopore filters by fitting membranes to filter holders. Mark each one with its pore size.
2. Dilute the colloid preparation with isotonic saline to a radioactive concentration of about 500 kBq/mL.
3. Using a 1-mL disposable syringe, carefully inject about 0.1 mL of the sample into one of the prepared filter holders.
4. Attach a 2 mL Luer-lock syringe (preloaded with 2 mL of saline) to the filter holder and wash the colloid through the filter into a small plastic vial.
5. Remove the syringe, refill it with air, and force the solution remaining inside the holder through the filter by air pressure.
6. Securely cap both vial and filter and count the activity on a calibrated scintillation detector. Correct all counts for background.
7. If necessary, correct the filtrate counts for any free pertechnetate activity found by chromatography of the colloid sample.
8. Calculate the percentage activity retained by the filter using the formula:

$$\text{Per cent retained} = 100 \times \frac{F - B}{S + F - 2B}$$

   where F and S are count rate of filter and solution, respectively, and B is the background.
9. Plot the percentage retained against log (pore size) to obtain a sigmoid curve. Locate the 50% retention point and read off the average particle size of the preparation.
10. Re-plot the data using log probability paper. Determine the mean particle size and the log standard deviation from the plot.

References

Amin KC, Saha GB, Go RT (1997). A rapid chromatographic method for quality control of technetium-99m-bicisate. *Nucl Med Technol* 25: 49–51.

Baldwin RM *et al.* (1995). Regional brain uptake and pharmacokinetics of [^{123}I]fluoroalkyl-2-carboxy-3-(4-iodophenyl)nortropane esters in baboons. *Nucl Med Biol* 22: 211–219.

Biersack HJG *et al.* (1989). Imaging of brain tumours with L-3 [^{123}I]iodo-α-methyltyrosine and SPECT. *J Nucl Med* 30: 110–112.

Bonnyman J (1983). Effect of milking efficiency on ^{99}Tc content of ^{99m}Tc derived from ^{99m}Tc generators. *Int J Appl Radiat Isot* 34: 901–906.

Bossuyt SM *et al.* (1991). Tc-99m-MRP20; a potential brain perfusion agent; in vivo distributions and SPECT studies in normal volunteers. *J Nucl Med* 32: 399–403.

Brandau W *et al.* (1988). Technetium-99m labelled renal function and imaging agents. III Synthesis of ^{99m}Tc-MAG3 and biodistribution of by-products. *Appl Radiat Isot* 39: 121–129.

British Institute of Radiology (1979). *Guidelines for the Preparation of Radiopharmaceuticals in Hospitals*. London: British Institute for Radiology.

Cagnolini A *et al.* (1998). Comparison of the kit performance of three ^{99m}Tc myocardial perfusion agents. *Nucl Med Biol* 25: 435–439.

Carvalho PA *et al.* (1992). Subcellular distribution and analysis of technetium-99m-MIBI in isolated perfused rat hearts. *J Nucl Med* 33: 1516–1522.

de Groot GJ *et al.* (1985). A system for high performance liquid chromatography of ^{99m}Tc complexes with on-line radiometric detection and data processing. *Int J Appl Radiat Isot* 36: 349–355.

Deutsch E *et al.* (1982). Preparation of no carrier added technetium-99m complexes: determination of total technetium content of generator eluates. *Int J Appl Radiat Isot* 33: 843–848.

Eckelman WC (1976). Radiochemical purity of new radiopharmaceuticals. *J Nucl Med* 17: 865.

Frier M, Hesslewood S, eds. (1980). *Quality Assurance of Radiopharmaceuticals – A Guide to Hospital Practice*. Special issue of Nuclear Medicine Communications. London: Chapman and Hall.

Fritzberg AR, Lewis D (1980). HPLC analysis of Tc-99m iminodiacetate hepatobiliary agents and a question of multiple peaks. *J Nucl Med* 21: 1180–1184.

Fritzberg AR *et al.* (1981). Chemical and biological studies of Tc-99m *N,N′* bis(mercaptoacetamido)-ethylenediamine; a potential replacement for I-131 hippurate. *J Nucl Med* 22: 258–263.

Fritzberg AR *et al.* (1986). Synthesis and biological evaluation of technetium-99m MAG3 as a hippuran replacement. *J Nucl Med* 27: 111–116.

Geyer MC *et al.* (1995). Rapid quality control of technetium-99m-tetrofosmin: comparison of miniaturized and standard chromatography systems. *J Nucl Med Technol* 23: 186–189.

Graham D, Millar AM (1999). Artefacts in the thin-layer chromatographic analysis of ^{99m}Tc-tetrofosmin injections. *Nucl Med Commun* 20: 439–444.

Hamacher K *et al.* (1986). Efficient stereospecific synthesis of no-carrier-added 2-[18F]-fluoro-2-deoxy-D-glucose using aminopolyether supported nucleophilic substitution. *J Nucl Med* 27: 235–238.

Hauser W, Cavallo L (1977). Measurement and quality assurance of the amount of administered tracer. In: Rhodes BA, ed. *Quality Control in Nuclear Medicine*. St Louis, MO: Mosby, 154–163.

Hosain P, Hosain F (1982). High performance size exclusion chromatography of human serum albumin labelled with technetium-99m. In: Raynaud C, ed. *Nuclear Medicine and Biology Advances. Proceedings of the 3rd World Congress in Nuclear Medicine and Biology*, Vol 1. Oxford: Pergamon Press, 238–241.

Huigen YM *et al.* (1988). Effect of the composition of the eluent in the chromatography of ^{99m}Tc-diphosphonate complexes. *Appl Radiat Isot* 39: 381–384.

Hung JC *et al.* (1991). Rapid preparation and quality contol method for technetium-99m-2-methoxy isobutyl isonitrile (technetium-99m sestamibi). *J Nucl Med* 32: 2162–2168.

Hung CY *et al.* (1988). A kinetic analysis of Tc-99m d,l-HMPAO decomposition in aqueous media. *J Nucl Med* 29: 1568–1576.

Hunt FC (1988). Reversed phase high performance liquid chromatography of gallium-67 and indium-111 chelates of EHPG, HBED and their derivatives. *Appl Radiat Isot* 39: 349–352.

Kelly JD *et al.* (1993). Technetium-99m-tetrofosmin as a new radiopharmaceutical for myocardial perfusion imaging. *J Nucl Med* 34: 222–227.

Kloster G, Laufer P (1984). Identification of radiopharmaceuticals by their retention on HPLC; a caveat. *Int J Appl Radiat Isot* 35: 545.

Krenning EP *et al.* (1992). Somatostatin receptor scintigraphy with indium-111-DTPA-D-Phe-1-octreotide in man: metabolism, dosimetry and comparison with iodine-123-Tyr-3-octreotide. *J Nucl Med* 33: 652–658.

Kung HF *et al.* (1984). Synthesis and biodistribution of neutral lipid-soluble tc-99m complexes that cross the blood–brain barrier. *J Nucl Med* 25: 326–332.

Leveille J *et al.* (1992). Intrasubject comparison between technetium-99m ECD and technetium-99m HMPAO in healthy human subjects. *J Nucl Med* 33: 480–484.

Levit N, ed. (1980). *Radiopharmacy Laboratory Manual for Nuclear Medicine Technologists*. Albuquerque, NM: University of New Mexico College of Pharmacy, 69–80.

Mangner TJ (1986). Potential artefacts in the chromatography of radiopharmaceuticals In: Wieland DM *et al.*, eds. *Analytical and Chromatographic techniques in Radiopharmaceutical Chemistry*. New York: Springer-Verlag, 261–278.

Metaye T *et al.* (2001). Rapid quality control for testing the radiochemical purity of 99Tc(m) tetrofosmin. *Nucl Med Commun* 22(10): 1139–1144.

Millar AM (1982). HPLC of Iodohippuric acid [^{123}I] Injection. *J Pharm Pharmacol* 34: 14–17.

Millar AM (1989). Quality assurance of radiopharmaceuticals In: Theobald AE, ed. *Radiopharmaceuticals and Radiotracers in Pharmacy*. Chichester: Ellis Horwood, 83–102.

Millar AM *et al.* (1990). ^{99}Tc^{m}-MAG3: *in vitro* stability and *in vivo* behaviour at different times after preparation. *Nucl Med Commun* 11: 405–412.

Moerlein SM *et al.* (1991). Metabolic imaging with gallium-68- and indium-111-labelled low-density lipoprotein. *J Nucl Med* 32: 300–307.

Neirinckx RD *et al.* (1987). Technetium-99m d,l-HM-PAO: a new radiopharmaceutical for SPECT imaging of regional cerebral blood flow. *J Nucl Med* 28: 191–202.

Niewland RJA (1989). Improvement of the reproducibility of ion-pair HPLC of ^{99m}Tc(Sn)EHDP complexes and the influence of the Sn(II) concentration on the composition of the reaction mixture. *Appl Radiat Isot* 40: 153–157.

Nowotnik DP *et al.* (1995). Separation of the stereoisomers of hexamethyl-propyleneamine oxime (HMPAO) by high performance liquid chromatography. *J Liq Chromatogr* 18: 673–687.

Nunn AD (1983). Structure–distribution relationships of radiopharmaceuticals: correlation between the reversed-phase capacity factors for Tc-99m phenylcarbamoylmethyl iminodiacetic acids and their renal elimination. *J Chromatogr* 255: 91–100.

Patel M (1995). A minaturised rapid paper chromatographic procedure for quality control of technetium-99m sestamibi. *Eur J Nucl Med* 22: 1416–1419.

Proulx A *et al.* (1989). Routine determination of ^{99m}Tc-MIBI. *Appl Radiat Isot* 40: 95–97.

Rhodes BA, ed. (1978). *Quality Control in Nuclear Medicine*. St Louis, MO: Mosby.

Robbins PJ (1984). *Chromatography of Technetium-99m Radiopharmaceuticals – A Practical Guide*. New York: The Society of Nuclear Medicine, Inc.

Schomaker K *et al.* (1994). [^{99m}Tc-generator eluates: effects on the radiochemical purity of the labelling products]. *Nuklearmedizin* 33: 33–39.

Shattuck LA *et al.* (1994). Evaluation of the hepatobiliary excretion of technetium-99m-MAG3 and reconstitution factors affecting radiochemical purity. *J Nucl Med* 35: 349–355.

Solanki KK *et al.* (1988). A rapid method for the preparation of ^{99m}Tc hexametazime-labelled leucocytes. *Nucl Med Commun* 9: 753–761.

Tanabe S *et al.* (1983). Effect of pH on the formation of Tc ($NaBH_4$)-MDP radiopharmaceutical analogues. *Int J Appl Radiat Isot* 34: 1577–1584.

Taylor AT, Eshina D (1988). Effects of altered physiologic states on clearance and biodistribution of technetium-99m MAG3, iodine-131 OIH, and iodine-125 iothalamate. *J Nucl Med* 29: 616–622.

Tubergen K *et al.* (1991). Sensitivity of technetium-99m-d,l-HMPAO to radiolysis in aqueous solution. *J Nucl Med* 32: 111–115.

Vallabhajosula S *et al.* (1982). Radiochemical analysis of Tc-99m human serum albumin with high-pressure liquid chromatography. *J Nucl Med* 23: 326–329.

Vandenheyden JL *et al.* (1983). Preparation and characterisation of [$^{99m}Tc(DMPE)_2X_2$], X = Cl, Br; DMPE = 1,2 bis (dimethylphosphinoethanol. *Int J Appl Radiat Isot* 34: 1611–1615.

Van Wyk *et al.* (1991). Synthesis and ^{99m}Tc labelling of MMI (MIBI) and its ethyl analogue. EMI. *Appl Radiat Isot* 42: 687–689.

Verebruggen AM *et al.* (1992). Technetium-99m-L,L-ethylenedicysteine: a renal imaging agent. I. Labeling and evaluation in animals. *J Nucl Med* 33: 551–557.

Vora MM (1991). HPLC analysis of indoium-111 diethylenetriaminepentaacetic acid (In-111 DTPA) radiopharmaceutical. *Int J Appl Radiat Isot* 42: 19–24.

Weisner PS *et al.* (1993). A method for stabilising technetium-99m exametazime prepared from a commercial kit. *Eur J Nucl Med* 20: 661–666.

Westera G *et al.* (1985). A convenient method for the preparation of ^{99m}Tc(V) dimercaptosuccinic acid (^{99m}Tc(V)-DMSA). *Int J Appl Radiat Isot* 36: 349–355.

Wieland DM *et al.* (1980). Radiolabeled adrenergic neuron-blocking agents: adrenomedullary imaging with [^{131}I]iodobenzylguanidine. *J Nucl Med* 21: 349–353.

Wieland *et al.*, eds. (1986). *Analytical and Chromatographic Techniques in Radiopharmaceutical Chemistry*. New York: Springer-Verlag.

Zimmer AM, Pavel DG (1977). Rapid miniaturised chromatographic quality-control procedures for Tc-99m radiopharmaceuticals. *J Nucl Med* 18: 1230–1233.

Zinn KR *et al.* (2000). Noninvasive monitoring of gene transfer using a reporter receptor imaged with a high-affinity peptide radiolabeled with ^{99m}Tc or ^{188}Re. *J Nucl Med* 41: 887–895.

Zoghbi SS *et al.* (1992). Pharmacokinetics of the SPECT benzodiazepine receptor radioligand [^{123}I]iomazenil in human and non-human primates. *Nucl Med Biol* 19: 881–888.

Zolle I, ed. (2007). *Technetium-99m Radiopharmaceuticals: Preparation and Quality Control in Nuclear Medicine*. Berlin: Springer.

24

Radiolabelling of blood cells: theory and practice

Beverley Ellis

Introduction

Blood cellular elements can be radiolabelled with radionuclides such as indium-111, technetium-99m and chromium-51 for a variety of clinical procedures. Radiolabelling may be carried out by *in-vitro* techniques, e.g. radiolabelled leukocytes, or by *in-vivo* methods, e.g. radiolabelled red cells. *In-vitro* methods involve the initial isolation of blood cells, radiolabelling with a cell labelling agent and subsequent re-injection of the cells into the patient. The clinical applications of radiolabelled blood cells are many and diverse. A summary of these applications appears in Table 24.1.

Table 24.1 Clinical applications of radiolabelled cells

Clinical application	Radiolabelled blood cellular element
Non-quantitative imaging of infection and inflammation	^{111}In-labelled mixed leukocytes or ^{99m}Tc-labelled mixed leukocytes
Quantitative imaging of infection and inflammation	^{111}In-labelled granulocytes or neutrophils
Cell kinetic studies of granulocytes or neutrophils	^{111}In-labelled granulocytes or neutrophils
Lymphocyte migratory patterns and kinetic studies	^{111}In-labelled lymphocytes
Abnormal platelet deposition	^{111}In-labelled platelets
Platelet kinetic and survival studies	^{111}In-labelled platelets
GI bleeding	^{99m}Tc-labelled red cells
Spleen imaging	^{99m}Tc-labelled red cells (heat-damaged)
Red cell survival studies	^{51}Cr-labelled red cells
Blood volume and red cell volume	^{51}Cr-labelled red cells
Cardiac and vascular imaging	^{99m}Tc-labelled red cells

Types of blood cell

The different types of blood cells are shown in Figure 24.1. Red blood cells (erythrocytes) are biconcave discs and do not contain a nucleus. They are the most abundant of all the blood cellular elements (5×10^9/mL of blood). Each erythrocyte is approximately 8 μm in diameter and approximately 2 μm thick in the widest part. Red blood cells are produced in the bone marrow and have a lifespan of approximately 120 days before being destroyed in the spleen. The large surface area and elastic properties of the erythrocyte allow the cells to pass through the capillaries enabling their main function of oxygen transport to be carried out. The most important component of the red blood cell is haemoglobin which contains two α polypeptide chains (141 amino acid residues each) and two β polypeptide chains (146 amino acid residues each). Each chain contains a haem group, which consists of a tetrapyrrole porphyrin ring containing ferrous iron. Each haem group can carry one O_2 molecule bound reversibly to the Fe^{2+}. A histidine residue of the globin chain is attached to the haem group. Haemoglobin and other cellular proteins (intracellular and membrane) may contribute to the binding of radiolabels to the erythrocyte.

Leukocytes include granulocytes, monocytes and lymphocytes. Granulocytes (polymorphonuclear cells) have multilobed nuclei and consist of neutrophils, eosinophils and basophils according to the staining properties of the granules in their cytoplasm. Neutrophils are the most abundant type of leukocyte and in normal individuals account for about 70% of the total leukocyte population. Neutrophils are 12–15 μm in diameter and constitute over 90% of circulating polymorphonuclear cells. Granulocytes are produced in the bone marrow and have a half-time in the circulation of 6–7 hours. The total granulocyte pool consists of a marginating granulocyte pool and a circulating granulocyte pool. Granulocytes released from the bone marrow distribute between the two pools, which are in dynamic equilibrium. The granulocytes in the marginating pool are found in the spleen, liver, lung and possibly bone marrow. Granulocytes migrate to sites of infection and inflammation. The primary function of polymorphonuclear cells is to phagocytose and destroy bacteria. It is this function which is exploited in detecting sites of infection and inflammation. Granulocytes are destroyed predominately in the liver, spleen and bone marrow.

Lymphocytes constitute about 20–30% of the leukocyte population. They are variable in size; small lymphocytes are about 7–8 μm in diameter and medium and large lymphocytes range from 9 to 15 μm

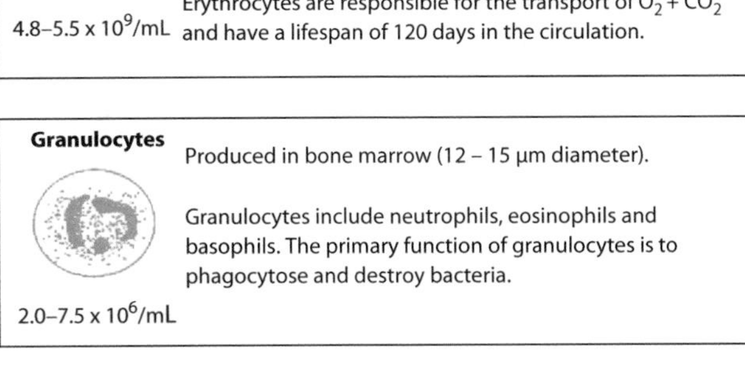

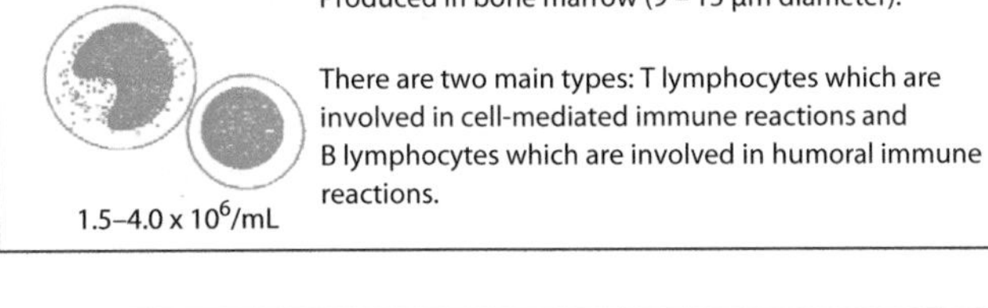

Lymphocytes
Produced in bone marrow (9 – 15 μm diameter).
There are two main types: T lymphocytes which are involved in cell-mediated immune reactions and B lymphocytes which are involved in humoral immune reactions.
1.5–4.0 x 10^6/mL

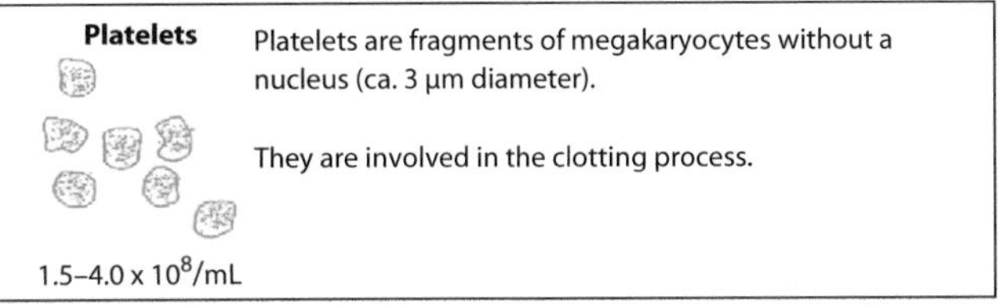

Platelets
Platelets are fragments of megakaryocytes without a nucleus (ca. 3 μm diameter).
They are involved in the clotting process.
1.5–4.0 x 10^8/mL

Figure 24.1 Types of blood cells.

in diameter. Lymphocytes migrate from the blood to the spleen, lymph nodes and other lymphatic tissues. Lymphocytes are of two types; T lymphocytes originate in the bone marrow and migrate to the thymus where they mature. These lymphocytes are primarily responsible for cell-mediated immune reactions. B lymphocytes are produced in the bone marrow and are involved in humoral immune reactions. 'Pure' granulocyte or neutrophil populations may be used in the imaging of infection and inflammation. Generally, for non-quantitative studies 'mixed' leukocytes are used because of the ease of preparation. However, for granulocyte kinetics and quantitative imaging, preparations of granulocytes or neutrophils are required.

Platelets are derived from megakaryocytes in the bone marrow and are non-nucleated discs. They are about 3 μm in diameter and 0.8 μm in thickness and are present at a concentration of approximately $1.5–4.0 \times 10^8$ per millilitre of blood. Platelets circulate in the bloodstream for 7.3–9.5 days (ICSH 1988), after which they are destroyed by the reticuloendothelial system. However on contact, with damaged vascular surfaces, they form a plug and stick to damaged vessels to prevent bleeding. This property has been utilised in the imaging of thrombus.

Characteristics required of cell-labelling agents

It is an important requirement in the radiolabelling of leukocytes and platelets for the investigation of normal and pathological conditions that the cells follow their natural behaviour when returned to the patient. Therefore, it is essential that the radiolabelled cells behave in exactly the same manner as their unlabelled counterparts. If the leukocytes are damaged by the cell-labelling agent, the chemotactic response may be altered, and this could affect the migration to sites of infection and inflammation. Cellular damage may arise from the labelling process itself, particularly from centrifugation and pipetting; hence centrifugation speed and time, and contact with the cells should be kept to a minimum. In addition, chemical or radiation exposure from the radionuclide or ligand should be kept to a minimum to avoid damage to the cells.

Generally, in leukocyte labelling, the labelling agent penetrates the cell membrane by passive diffusion, followed by retention of the radionuclide within the cell. Thus the agent must be neutral and sufficiently lipophilic to cross cell membranes. Retention of the radionuclide in the cell for the length of the clinical investigation is an essential requirement. Even though an agent penetrates the cell membrane it does not necessarily mean that it will be retained inside the cell. Elution of radioactivity from the cell during the course of an investigation could result in localisation in other organs or tissues, giving false information and unnecessary irradiation of these areas (Thakur 1981).

There is a need for a radioactive agent that, ideally, will specifically label one type of blood cell in whole blood or *in vivo*, thereby eliminating the requirement for cell separation. Such an agent would reduce the preparation time of the cell labelling process. However, at present no agent is available that fits all the criteria as a specific cell-labelling agent, although anti-granulocyte antibodies have been used with some success in Europe. The ability to radiolabel cells in the presence of plasma is also an important aspect; cells that are deprived of plasma may become metabolically activated and are retained in the lungs (Peters, Saverymuttu 1987).

The radionuclide should emit gamma radiation suitable for external detection (if imaging is required) and have a half-life long enough for the clinical investigation but short enough to minimise unnecessary radiation to the patient.

Agents used for cell labelling

The principal radionuclides used in cell labelling are shown in Table 24.2. The choice of radionuclide is dependent upon its physical properties and the length of the clinical study.

Table 24.2 Radionuclides used for cell labelling

Radionuclide	Half-life	Principal emissions (keV)
^{99m}Tc	6 hours	140
^{111}In	67.9 hours	171, 245
^{51}Cr	27.7 days	320

Currently, all ligands used in cell labelling with indium or technetium form lipophilic complexes that are non-selective, i.e. they label all cells indiscriminately. For example, if an indium or technetium complex is added to a sample of whole blood all the cells become labelled, but as the red cells are more numerous, most of the activity is associated with these cell types (Osman, Danpure 1987). Therefore, it is necessary to isolate the cells required prior to labelling. It is this separation of cells that is time-consuming and requires skilled staff.

Indium ligands

Indium-111 is supplied in high specific activity, with no carrier added, as the chloride in 0.04 mol/L HCl. Hydrolysis of $InCl_3$ occurs above pH 3.5 to the insoluble indium trihydroxide; thus when diluting solutions of indium chloride, it is important to use 0.04 mol/L HCl instead of water or saline. Intravenous administration of [^{111}In]indium chloride to a patient will result in the indium becoming bound to plasma proteins, predominantly transferrin (Hosain *et al.* 1969). Ionic indium as [^{111}In]$InCl_3$ will not penetrate cell membranes and thus is not suitable in this form as a cell labelling agent. The presence of a complexing ligand is required to label cells at physiological pH and also to avoid precipitation (Moerlein, Welch, 1981).

Oxine (8-hydroxyquinoline) was the first ligand to be used for the ^{111}In-labelling of leukocytes (McAfee, Thakur 1976). Oxine forms a 3 : 1 complex with indium that is neutral and highly lipophilic. This property allows rapid diffusion of the complex across cell membranes. It has been proposed that, once inside the cell, the indium complex completely (Thakur *et al.* 1977b) or partially dissociates (H. Jackson, unpublished work), allowing the indium to bind to intracellular proteins. One of the drawbacks of oxine is that it will also label the transferrin present in the plasma. Therefore, the cells have to be washed thoroughly to remove plasma. However ^{111}In-oxine is still widely used clinically and has a UK Product Licence. In 1981 tropolone (2-hydroxy-2,4,6-cycloheptatrienone) was introduced as an alternative to oxine (Dewanjee *et al.* 1981). This agent also forms a neutral lipophilic 3 : 1 complex with indium. The advantage of tropolone over oxine is that cells can be labelled in the presence of small amounts of plasma (Danpure *et al.* 1982a). Tropolone has also been widely used clinically in the UK.

Technetium ligands

Technetium-99m (see Chapter 8) has been widely used for radiolabelling cells. In 1985 ^{99m}Tc-HMPAO (hexamethylpropyleneamineoxime, Ceretec) was introduced as a regional cerebral perfusion agent (Nowotnik *et al.* 1985) and later developed as a cell-labelling agent (Peters *et al.* 1986). HMPAO, or exametazime, is commercially available (Ceretec) and will form a neutral complex with technetium, provided the technetium is reduced to +5 oxidation state using stannous ion. The complex (Figure 24.2) contains technetium in the +5 oxidation state, with a single oxygen atom attached directly to the metal.

The metal is coordinated to the four nitrogen atoms. It has a zero net charge and is highly lipophilic. HMPAO exists in two diastereomeric forms: *meso*- and *d,l*-. The *d,l*-HMPAO has superior brain uptake and retention compared with the mixture containing the two forms and consequently was developed as a cell-labelling agent (Neirinckx *et al.* 1987). An advantage of this agent is that cells may be radiolabelled in the presence of plasma. The mechanism of cell labelling with this agent is not fully understood, but it is thought that the agent passes into the cell by passive diffusion. In the cell, the complex breaks down into a hydrophilic form that is unable to cross the cell membrane, thus allowing the technetium to be retained within the cell (Neirinckx *et al.* 1987). It has been suggested that intracellular glutathione may be involved in the *in-vivo* conversion of the primary to secondary complex (Neirinckx *et al.* 1988), though this mechanism has been debated (Babich 1991). The instability of the agent is also a drawback; the radiopharmaceutical must be used within 30 minutes after reconstitution because of this conversion from the primary complex to the secondary complex. The amount of stannous chloride in the kit is very low (7.6 μg). The reason for this is that the concentration of stannous ion is directly related to the degradation of the primary to the secondary complex (Hung *et al.* 1988). The age and radioactive concentration of the technetium eluate is another factor that can affect the

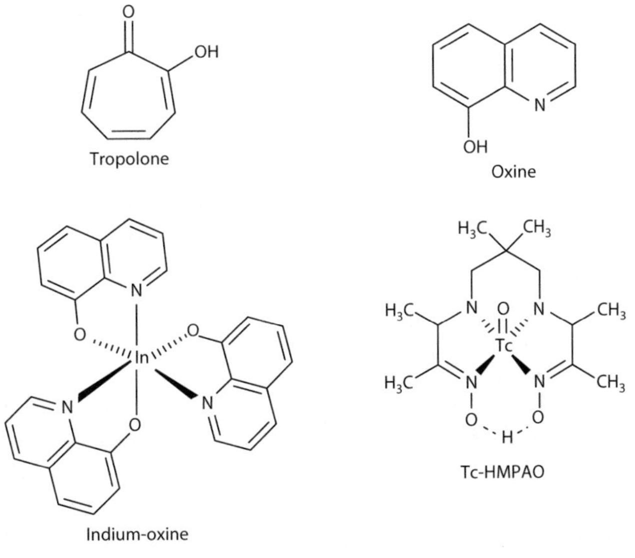

Tropolone

Oxine

Indium-oxine

Tc-HMPAO

Figure 24.2 Structures of tropolone, oxine, indium-oxine and technetium-HMPAO.

formation of the primary complex. The extent of degradation increases with generator eluates older than 2 hours and with eluates from generators not previously eluted within the last 24 hours, as a result of radiolytic oxidation and a low stannous ion content. This limitation has led to the development of methods to enhance the stability and cost-effectiveness of ^{99m}Tc-HMPAO. Reconstitution of the unlabelled HMPAO kit with saline and subsequent subfractionation followed by storage at – 70°C (Morrissey, Powe 1993), –66°C (Hawkins *et al.* 1991) or –10°C (Sampson *et al.* 1991) has been used as a cost-effective method. An approach to improving cost-effectiveness and stabilisation of the ^{99m}Tc-HMPAO using a tin enhancement method has been reported by Solanki *et al.* (1993). Exametazime solution, 0.3 mL (25 μg exametazime) and 0.1 mL stannous fluoride (0.66 μg Sn^{2+}) solution are mixed, followed by the addition of 400–500 MBq of [^{99m}Tc]pertechnetate. The ^{99m}Tc-HMPAO is reported to be stable up to 1.5 hours after preparation and up to 15 doses may be obtained from one vial of exametazime up to a period of 150 days, provided that the sub-fractionated vial has been kept at –10°C.

Ceretec is licensed as a single-dose product. Any method of preparation other than that recommended by the manufacturer absolutely transfers the onus of liability from the manufacturer to user. Any deviation by the user from the manufacturer's instructions should be carefully validated and rigid quality assurance procedures performed.

Isolation of leukocytes and platelets from whole blood

Collection of blood for leukocyte labelling

Whole blood is usually taken from the antecubital fossa into a 60-mL syringe (containing an anticoagulant) and fitted with a 19G needle or butterfly (to minimise damage to the cells). The anticoagulant of choice is acid-citrate–dextrose (ACD, NIH, Formula A). The typical concentration of ACD is 1.5 parts to 8.5 parts of whole blood (Saverymuttu *et al.* 1983). The amount of blood taken varies from centre to centre, but typically 51 mL of blood is taken into a syringe containing 9 mL ACD. The blood should be taken slowly, avoiding froth and bubble formation, and ensuring that the blood is mixed with the anticoagulant. Heparin is not recommended as it has been reported to cause microaggregation of cells and has a tendency to adhere to plastic centrifuge tubes (Peters *et al.* 1983; McAfee *et al.* 1984).

Separation of leukocytes

The separation of mixed leukocytes is most commonly achieved by erythrocyte sedimentation of anticoagulated blood. Simple centrifugation of anticoagulated whole blood forming a buffy coat is not an efficient method for obtaining leukocytes (McAfee *et al.* 1984). Erythrocyte sedimentation may be accelerated by the use of sedimentation agents such as methylcellulose (2% in saline), 6% dextran and 6% hydroxyethyl starch (hetastarch, Hespan; molecular weight 450 000 daltons; molar substitution 0.7 (450/0.7)). These agents accelerate erythrocyte sedimentation by affecting the charge of the sialic acid groups on the outer membrane of the red cell; this is thought to result in some erythrocytes becoming less charged than their neighbours and aggregating to form rouleaux, which then sediment (Sewchand, Canham 1979). Methylcellulose and dextran have been found to cause allergic reactions in some patients (Peters *et al.* 1982). Hydroxyethyl starch (450/0.7) is generally the preferred sedimentation agent as it has been reported to induce a more rapid red cell sedimentation and greater leukocyte recovery and its use has not been associated with allergic reactions (McAfee *et al.* 1984). Normally, 3 mL of hetastarch per 30 mL of blood is employed (Danpure *et al.* 1982a). The sedimentation time varies from patient to patient, but is generally 45–60 minutes.

Sedimentation may be affected by a variety of factors such as the volume of blood, number of cells and certain disease states, e.g. sickle cell anaemia. After sedimentation, two distinct layers of approximately equal volume are formed. The lower layer contains erythrocytes and the upper layer contains leukocytes and platelets (leukocyte-rich platelet-rich plasma). The leukocyte-rich platelet-rich plasma is carefully removed and centrifuged at low centrifugation speeds, e.g. 150g for 5 minutes to pellet the leukocytes, leaving the platelets in the supernatant (platelet-rich plasma). The leukocyte pellet will

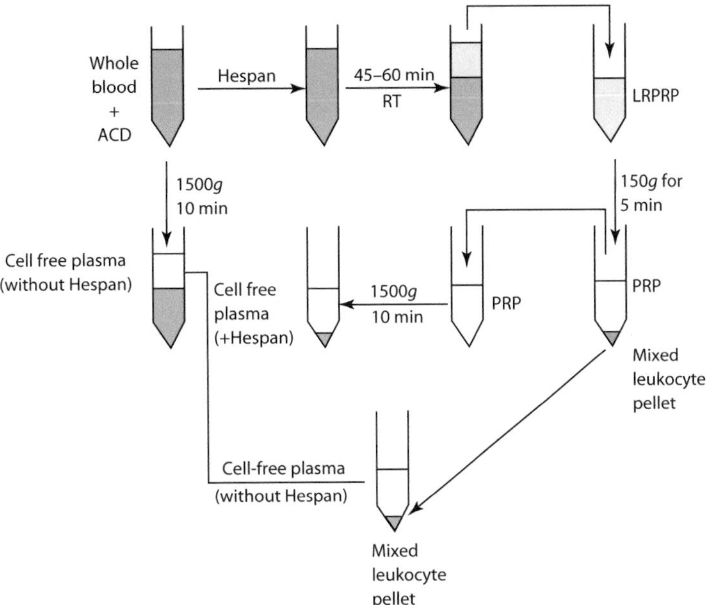

Figure 24.3 Separation of mixed leukocytes. LRPRP = leukocyte-rich platelet-rich plasma; PRP = platelet-rich plasma.

generally contain granulocytes, lymphocytes, monocytes and also small amounts of contaminating red cells and platelets. The platelet-rich plasma is removed and centrifuged at 1500g for 10 minutes, causing the platelets to pellet and leaving cell-free plasma as the supernatant. The cell-free plasma is used for washing the cells after labelling. Cell-free plasma may also be obtained from the centrifugation of whole blood at 1500g for 10 minutes. Cell-free plasma is used for resuspending the cells after labelling for re-injection (Figure 24.3). It is also used as a diluent for cells to be labelled with ^{111}In-tropolonate or ^{99m}Tc-HMPAO and saline should be used as a diluent for ^{111}In-oxine. Methods for the separation of leukocytes from whole blood and radiolabelling with ^{111}In-tropolonate and ^{99m}Tc-HMPAO are given in Appendices 1 and 2.

Separation of neutrophils or granulocytes

Some clinical studies may require the use of granulocytes or neutrophils. These cells cannot be separated from monocytes and lymphocytes by differential centrifugation because they only have slight differences in density. Thus the separation of these cells requires the use of isopycnic density gradients. This method of separation is based on Stokes' law; the rate of centrifugation in a centrifugal field is zero when the cell encounters a medium of identical density (McAfee *et al.* 1984). Therefore, centrifuging the cells in media with discontinuous density gradients will cause the cells to migrate until they reach the interface with a solution of density equal to or greater than their own. Hence, cells of different densities reside at different depths. Ficoll-Hypaque gradients have been used for the separation of granulocytes from whole blood (Weiblen *et al.* 1979), but it has been reported that this medium may have an adverse metabolic effect on leukocytes (Dooley *et al.* 1982). Percoll–plasma density gradients have been used for the separation of granulocytes for radiolabelling with ^{111}In-tropolonate (Danpure 1985). Percoll consists of polyvinylpyrrolidone-coated silica particles 15–30 nm in diameter. Discontinuous Percoll–plasma gradients may be prepared by mixing 9 volumes of Percoll (specific gravity 1.13 g/mL) with 1 volume of 1.5 mol/L sodium chloride to give iso-osmotic Percoll (100%). The Percoll is then diluted with the patient's cell-free plasma to obtain 65%, 60% and 50% v/v solutions of Percoll in plasma. The solutions are then carefully layered in order of decreasing density in a 10-mL

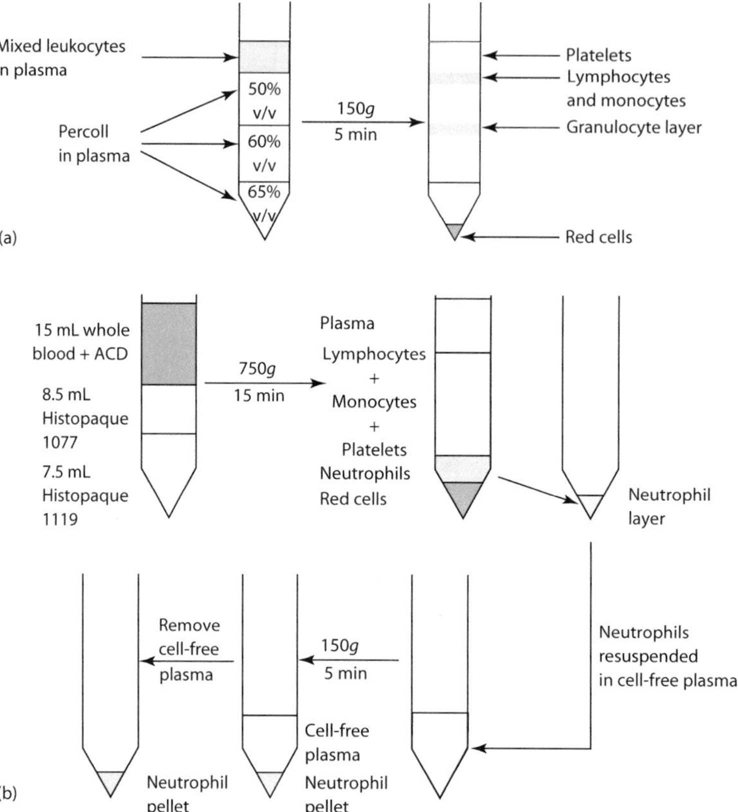

Figure 24.4 Separation of pure granulocytes (a) and pure neutrophils (b) from whole blood.

centrifuge tube. The suspension of leukocytes is then layered on top and the tube is centrifuged at 150*g* for 5 minutes. This results in the formation of a series of bands containing different types of blood cells (Figure 24.4). The granulocyte layer is carefully removed by pipetting, washed, and resuspended in cell-free plasma. A method of preparation is given in Appendix 4.

A simple method for the separation of neutrophils, without the necessity of obtaining a leukocyte suspension has been developed by Sampson, Solanki (1992) (Appendix 3). The method uses density gradients of Histopaque (1119 and 1077) that contain Ficoll 400 (a synthetic high-molecular-weight polymer of sucrose and epichlorohydrin) and sodium diatrizoate (sodium salt of 3,5-diacetamido-2,4,6-triiodobenzoic acid), which are used in conjunction to form solutions with the required physical properties. A double gradient is formed by carefully pouring 7.5 mL of Histopaque 1119 (density 1.119 g/mL) into a Universal tube and 8.5 mL of Histopaque 1077 (density 1.077 g/mL) is layered onto the latter, without allowing mixing of the two layers. 15 mL of whole blood is layered onto the top of the double gradients layer (see Figure 24.4). The tube is then centrifuged at 750*g* for 15 minutes. This results in a neutrophil layer above the sedimented red cells. The neutrophil layer is carefully removed, washed with cell-free plasma and resuspended in cell-free plasma for radiolabelling. The purity of the neutrophils is reported to be 96% ± 3 SD.

Separation of lymphocytes

The use of lymphocytes in clinical studies has been limited owing to reports of radiation damage caused by the low-energy Auger electrons and the chemical toxicity of the ligand (Segal *et al.* 1978; Chisholm *et al.* 1979; ten Berge *et al.* 1983; Balaban *et al.* 1986). Several workers have reported that radiation damage from intracellular ^{111}In may induce a mutagenic change that can result in the formation of malignant tumour (Frost, Frost 1978; ten Berge *et al.* 1983).

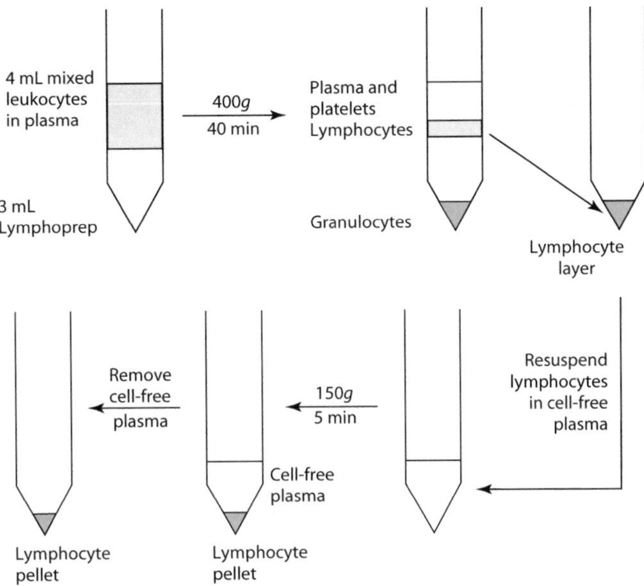

Figure 24.5 Separation of lymphocytes.

However, such carcinogenesis has never been proven (Alavi, Hansell 1984). As a consequence, lymphocytes radiolabelled with ^{111}In have not yet found favour with clinicians. Lymphocytes have been radiolabelled using ^{99m}Tc-HMPAO and, even though cellular damage has been reported with technetium (Schmidt *et al.* 1990), it is considerably less than that caused by ^{111}In and this may be a more favourable label for clinical use in the future.

A difficulty associated with lymphocytes is that of obtaining a sufficient number of cells to radiolabel. Lymphocytes normally comprise only 20–30% of the total leukocyte count; therefore, large volumes of blood are required for labelling. Lymphocytes have been harvested from whole blood using density gradients. Ficoll–Hypaque has been used (Wagstaff *et al.* 1981), although the lymphocytic response to stimulation with a mitogen or antigen may be reduced using this method (Berger, Edelson 1979). A procedure for the isolation of lymphocytes from whole blood has been described by Sampson and Goffin (1991). The method involves the isolation of leukocytes by mixing two 50-mL portions of ACD anticoagulated blood with hetastarch in two 50-mL Falcon tubes. After sedimentation, the supernatants are removed and centrifuged at 100*g* for 7 minutes to pellet the leukocytes, which are combined and resuspended in 4 mL of cell-free plasma. The cell suspension is layered onto 3 mL of 'Lymphoprep' (Axis-Shield) and centrifuged at 400*g* for 40 minutes (Figure 24.5). This results in several bands of cells, of which the lymphocyte and monocyte layer is carefully removed, washed with cell-free plasma and resuspended in cell-free plasma for radiolabelling. The percentage purity of the lymphocytes in the cell-suspension was found to be 81% ± 8 SD (Sampson, Goffin 1991). Details of this method are given in Appendix 5.

Separation of platelets from whole blood

Many different methods have been published for the radiolabelling of platelets. The volume of blood needed is variable, but usually small quantities (17–60 mL) are employed. Blood is withdrawn using a large-diameter needle (minimum 19G) into a syringe containing acid-citrate solution (Hawker *et al.* 1980). The preferred amount of acid-citrate solution is 1 mL per 6 mL blood (Thakur, McKenny 1985). This results in the lowering of the blood pH to 6.5 (if, for example, 3 mL of acid-citrate solution is mixed with 17 mL of blood), which prevents gross platelet aggregation during centrifugation. Other workers have withdrawn the blood into a syringe containing ACD (NIH, Formula A) using 1.5 volumes of ACD to 8.5 volumes of blood (Danpure, Osman 1988a).

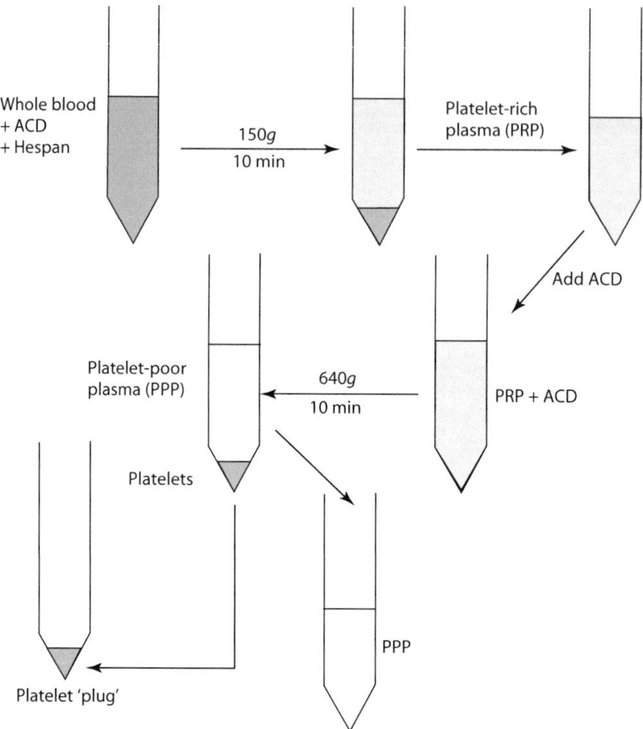

Figure 24.6 Separation of platelets.

The anticoagulated blood is carefully transferred to a sterile polypropylene tube and centrifuged at 200*g* for 10 minutes to obtain a pellet of erythrocytes and leukocytes and a supernatant containing platelet-rich plasma (PRP). Hetastarch may also be mixed with the anticoagulated blood prior to centrifugation (Danpure, Osman 1994). High centrifuge speeds and long centrifuge times should be avoided as these may affect platelet function. The platelet-rich plasma is removed and at this stage ACD is added to acidify the plasma. One volume of ACD to 10 volumes of PRP may be used (Danpure, Osman 1994). Alternatively, antiaggregating agents such as prostaglandin E_1 in calcium-free Tyrode's buffer may be added (Hawker *et al.* 1980). The reason for the addition of ACD or antiaggregating agents to the PRP is to prevent aggregation of the platelets on centrifugation. The PRP is centrifuged at 640*g* for 10 minutes to obtain a pellet of platelets and platelet-poor plasma (PPP). The medium in which the platelet pellet is resuspended for radiolabelling depends upon which ^{111}In-complex or ^{99m}Tc-complex is employed. If the platelets are labelled with ^{111}In-tropolonate or ^{99m}Tc-HMPAO then the pellet may be resuspended in PPP. However if ^{111}In-oxine is used, the pellet may be resuspended in plasma-free media such as Modified Tyrode's Solution (Thakur *et al.* 1981), ACD-saline (ICSH 1988) and Calcium Free Tyrode's Solution containing prostaglandin E_1 (Hawker *et al.* 1980) after the pellet is washed to remove traces of plasma. The radiolabelling of platelets with ^{111}In-tropolonate or ^{99m}Tc-HMPAO provides a relatively simpler method as the platelets do not need to be completely deprived of plasma. A method for the separation of platelets from whole blood is given in Appendix 6 and shown diagrammatically in Figure 24.6.

Radiolabelling of cells and labelling efficiency

Leukocytes

Once the cells required for radiolabelling have been isolated, they are resuspended in saline (if labelling with ^{111}In-oxine) or plasma (if labelling with ^{111}In-tropolonate or ^{99m}Tc-HMPAO). The ^{111}In complex or ^{99m}Tc-HMPAO is added to the cell suspension and incubated for 5–10 minutes. Cell-free plasma is then added to the suspension to remove any unbound radionuclide and after centrifugation to obtain the plug of cells, the supernatant is removed, and the cells are resuspended in cell-free plasma for re-injection. Some workers withdraw larger volumes of blood from the patient, of which an aliquot is transferred to a sterile tube not containing hetastarch or other sedimentation agent and centrifuged at 2000*g* for 10 minutes to obtain cell-free plasma that is used for resuspending the cells for injection and as the cell labelling medium.

Platelets

Platelets are incubated with ^{111}In complexes or ^{99m}Tc-HMPAO in plasma or a plasma-free medium. The times of incubation vary from 60 seconds to 30 minutes. Generally for ^{111}In-oxine the incubation time is 60 seconds to 2 minutes. For ^{111}In-tropolonate or ^{99m}Tc-HMPAO in plasma, incubation times of 5 minutes and 30 minutes, respectively, are recommended (Danpure, Osman 1988a, 1994). As with leukocyte labelling, unbound radionuclide is removed by the addition of platelet-poor plasma (cell-free plasma), followed by centrifugation to obtain a platelet pellet. The platelet pellet is resuspended in platelet-poor plasma for re-injection.

Labelling efficiency

The labelling efficiency is usually described as the percentage radioactivity incorporated into the cells: the radiolabelled cells are separated from the labelling medium by centrifugation and the radioactivity on the labelled cells and radioactivity remaining in the labelling medium are measured and the percentage labelling efficiency is calculated as shown below:

$$\%\ \text{Labelling efficiency} = \frac{\text{Radioactivity on cells}}{\text{Radioactivity on cells} + \text{Radioactivity remaining in supernatant}} \times 100$$

Ideally, a high labelling efficiency is desirable, incorporating as much activity as possible on a first attempt, as re-labelling may result in damaged cells. It must be stressed that achieving a high labelling efficiency is not necessarily indicative of a good labelling procedure or viable cells. It is important to obtain a viable population of cells for re-injection; thus a labelling efficiency of 50% with viable cells is better than a 90% labelling efficiency with non-viable cells. However there must be enough activity on the cells to obtain reliable results.

Factors affecting the labelling efficiency

Many factors affect the labelling efficiency and these are summarised in Table 24.3.

Table 24.3 Factors that may affect the labelling efficiency

- Plasma concentration
- Types of cell collected
- Method of radiolabelling
- Choice of sedimentation agent
- Choice of anticoagulant
- Presence of disease in patient
- Stability of cell chelator
- Concentration of ligand and radionuclide
- Concentration and number of cells and volume of ingredients
- pH
- Temperature
- Cell damage
- Drugs
- Operator inter-variability

Plasma concentration of the labelling medium

The amount of plasma in the labelling medium will affect the labelling efficiency. If cells are labelled in a medium containing 90% plasma using ^{111}In-oxine, the ^{111}In preferentially binds to plasma proteins resulting in a labelling efficiency of only 5%. On the other hand, if the cells are washed free of plasma and labelled in buffered saline, the labelling efficiency may be as high as 95% (Danpure *et al.* 1982b). Cells deprived of plasma may become metabolically activated (Saverymuttu *et al.* 1983), but small amounts of plasma (10%) can have a protective effect on the cells (Roddie *et al.* 1988). Labelling cells with ^{111}In-tropolonate or ^{99m}Tc-HMPAO in the presence of plasma will achieve labelling efficiencies that are satisfactory but lower than those achieved by labelling in saline. This is because the plasma proteins and cells will compete for uptake of the ^{111}In or ^{99m}Tc (Danpure, Osman 1988b).

pH of the labelling medium

The pH of the labelling medium affects the labelling efficiency. Optimal labelling efficiencies for labelling platelets with ^{111}In-tropolonate in saline are obtained at pH 9 (Dewanjee *et al.* 1981) and an increase in labelling efficiency is observed with ^{111}In-mercapto-pyridin-*N*-oxide (Merc) when the pH is increased from 4.5 to 7 (Thakur, Barry 1982). Solanki *et al.* (1988) report that optimal labelling efficiencies with ^{99m}Tc-HMPAO labelled leukocytes are achieved at a pH of approximately 7.5. However the optimal pH for cell labelling may not be the pH required to maintain the viability and function of cells. Thus cells are usually labelled at pH 6.5–7.4. With the addition of ACD to whole blood, the pH of the plasma is reduced from 7.4 to 7.2; however, this does not appear to compromise the labelling efficiency or viability of the leukocytes. Radiolabelling of platelets may require the further addition of ACD, to reduce the pH of the medium to 6.5. Lowering of pH minimises the spontaneous aggregation of the platelets that may occur at higher pH.

Cell concentration, number and volume of ingredient

An increase in labelling efficiency is observed with an increase in the number of cells if cells are labelled in saline (Thakur *et al.* 1977a). If the cells are labelled in plasma with ^{111}In-tropolonate, the labelling efficiency increases with cell concentration because of the competition between the cells and plasma for the uptake of the radionuclide. Therefore, if cells are labelled in 1 mL of 90% plasma containing 10^8 granulocytes, labelling efficiencies of approximately 90% are achieved, but if the volume of plasma is 10 mL containing the same number of cells, the labelling efficiency is reduced to 30% (Danpure, Osman 1988b).

The concentration of cells will also be affected by the volume of ingredients such as the volumes of ligand and radionuclide. Sampson *et al.* (1991) reported that when leukocytes ($2–5 \times 10^7$) were incubated with aliquots of exametazime solution ranging from 0.25 to 2 mL (from a vial of Ceretec reconstituted with 4 mL saline), the labelling efficiency decreases from $65\% \pm 10$ SD to $45\% \pm 8$ SD.

Concentration of ligand and radionuclide

Bidentate ligands such as oxine and tropolone bind to indium to form a 3 : 1 complex; thus three ligand molecules bind to one indium atom. Therefore, an excess of ligand is required to ensure that the indium is completely complexed. Preparations of ^{111}In complexes for cell labelling may contain 10^2 to 10^6 times more ligand than indium, even though picomole amounts of radioactive complex are formed (Danpure 1985). Technetium complexes used in cell labelling such as ^{99m}Tc-HMPAO also contain excess ligand; for example, commercial preparations contain 0.5 mg of HMPAO (1.8×10^{-6} moles), which is reconstituted with 5 mL of [^{99m}Tc]pertechnetate (500 MBq) (2.6×10^{-11} moles of technetium), and 4 mL of this preparation is used for leukocyte labelling (Ceretec Package Insert, GE Healthcare, 2006). However, it has been reported that the primary lipophilic complex is still obtained using smaller amounts of HMPAO.

The effect of temperature

Cells are usually radiolabelled at room temperature. They may also be radiolabelled at 37°C. This temperature does not necessarily result in higher rates of labelling or labelling efficiencies. However, if cells are radiolabelled at 4°C, a decrease in the rate of labelling is observed (Danpure 1985).

Cell viability of leukocytes and platelets

It is essential that cells are viable when returned to the body. Labelled cells may be damaged from the harvesting and labelling procedures. Methods of assessing leukocyte function such as chemotaxis, phagocytosis, adherence to nylon columns and superoxide anion production have been reported (Colas-Linhart *et al.* 1983; Thakur *et al.* 1984; Mortelmans *et al.* 1989; Lang *et al.* 1993). The proliferative capacity of labelled lymphocytes to a mitogenic response such as concanavalin A or phytohaemagglutinin has been used to assess their function (Segal *et al.* 1978; Balaban *et al.* 1986). Leukocyte viability has been assessed with trypan blue solution (0.5%), which is incorporated into dead cells; with propidium iodide, which is taken up by dead or decaying cells; with nitroblue tetrazolium, which labels activated cells; and with monoclonal antibody CD-45 which is taken up by intact cells (Sampson 1998). Many reports have been published of platelet function tests such as aggregation (Mathias, Welch 1984). Many of these tests are time-consuming and unsuitable for routine *in-vitro* testing prior to re-injection, but are useful in the development of new labelling methods. A simple test for leukocytes is to observe the final preparation of labelled cells for clumps or aggregates (Sampson 1998). Similarly for platelets, the final preparation may be observed for the 'swirling' motion of viable platelets.

An *in-vivo* test of leukocyte integrity is usually carried out by investigating the biodistribution of labelled cells over a period of 15–30 minutes after re-injection. Viable cells pass rapidly through the lungs, followed by uptake in the spleen and liver (Danpure *et al.* 1982b). Damaged cells are retained in the lungs and have a high uptake in the liver and a slower uptake into inflammatory lesions (Saverymuttu *et al.* 1983). However, retention in the lungs and high liver uptake may not necessarily indicate damaged cells as it may occur in certain lung and liver pathology.

Problems encountered with leukocyte or platelet radiolabelling

The radiolabelling of blood components is uniquely different from the radiolabelling of a stable chemical moiety. Each blood sample is different from its predecessor and labelling is dependent on many patient related factors. These include the number of cells, the ratio of different cell types, volume of plasma and amount of protein, to name but a few. It is not surprising that difficulties sometimes arise during labelling and this section will deal with some of the most commonly reported problems.

Difficulties with white cell labelling occur during the initial sedimentation step to reduce the red cells. Red cells may remain floating in the supernatant (leukocytes and platelets). If an excessive number of red cells are present in the leukocyte suspension, they will also take up the radiolabel, which may consequently result in a high blood background when re-injected. Haemolysing agents such as ammonium chloride have been used, but these agents may also damage the cells to be labelled.

The sedimentation process usually takes 45–60 minutes, but occasionally red cells may fail to sediment. The usual cause is the presence of fine threads of fibrin owing to insufficient anticoagulation. Although the correct amount of acid-citrate–dextrose may have been drawn into the syringe, inadequate mixing with the blood results in only partial anticoagulation. It has been suggested that certain drugs such as azathioprine and digoxin which affect cell membranes may also cause problems during sedimentation. Difficulties have also been reported in patients with sickle-cell anaemia, because of the slow erythrocyte sedimentation rate of sickled blood. Red cell sedimentation in these patients has been successfully improved by using an increased proportion of hetastarch (Webber *et al.* 1994).

A pressing problem for operators is what to do if blood fails to sediment. Blood should normally sediment within 20–60 minutes of adding the sedimentation agent. If at the end of that period the blood has just started to sediment, it should be left for another 30 minutes. However, if no sedimentation occurs after this time, the blood should be centrifuged at 14*g* for 15 minutes; if this does not improve sedimentation, the centrifugation speed may be increased in 2–3*g* increments for 15 minutes at each increment. As soon as the red cells begin to sediment, the same speed should be continued until sedimentation is complete. If difficulties occur it is good practice to confirm the composition of the leukocyte-rich platelet-rich plasma (Sampson 1996).

An unusual appearance of the leukocyte-rich platelet-rich plasma may not necessarily indicate problems with radiolabelling. For instance, in milky yellow blood samples from patients with hypercholesterolaemia, sedimentation and radiolabelling are not affected (Sampson, Solanki 1989).

Many factors affect the labelling efficiency as described earlier. If there are too few cells to label adequately, e.g. leukopenic patients, the labelling efficiency will be low. Difficulties may also arise in the radiolabelling of lymphocytes, where there may be insufficient activity on the cells for imaging because of the small number of cells. As a consequence, larger volumes of blood may be required.

Damage may be caused to the cells during the separation and radiolabelling procedure. It is therefore essential to obtain a viable cell population for re-injection. All handling of the cells such as pipetting and centrifugation should be kept to a minimum and the cells treated as gently as possible. Centrifugation times and speeds should also be kept to a minimum. Platelets are sensitive to manipulations and can easily aggregate and become irreversibly damaged.

Radiolabelled red blood cells

Red blood cells may be radiolabelled by several techniques: *in-vivo*, *in-vitro* and a combination of the two methods. The radionuclides that are commonly used for red cell labelling are ^{51}Cr and ^{99m}Tc (see Table 24.2). The choice of radionuclide and radiolabelling technique is dependent on the type of clinical investigation, a summary of which is shown in Table 24.1. For diagnostic imaging, several properties of the cell labelling agent are required. The radionuclide should emit a gamma-ray suitable for imaging and have a half-life suitable for the duration of the clinical study. The *in-vivo* function and biochemical properties of the cells should not be altered and the radionuclide should remain firmly bound to the cell for the length of the study and not be re-utilised after the destruction of the cell (Srivastava, Chervu 1984).

In-vitro labelling with technetium-99m

In-vitro labelling of red blood cells has been used for the determination of red cell and blood volume. The *in-vitro* method may also be employed in patients who are taking certain drugs such as heparin or hydralazine or who have previously been given iodinated contrast media. These substances may interfere with or inhibit Sn^{2+} transport through the red cell membrane, resulting in lower labelling efficiencies with technetium (Saha 2004). Several methods have been described in the literature for *in-vitro* labelling with technetium. As before, the labelling efficiency is usually expressed as a percentage of ^{99m}Tc incorporated into the cells. An early method was that of the Brookhaven National Laboratory using a kit (Srivastava, Chervu 1984). The method has since been modified (Srivastava, Straub 1990) and is commercially available as Ultratag RBC. The kit contains stannous citrate and acid-citrate–dextrose in a freeze-dried mixture, with which 1 mL of heparinised blood is incubated for 5 minutes. This is followed by the addition of 0.1% sodium hypochlorite and ACD solution. This results in any excess tin(II) being oxidised to tin(IV) and plasma-bound tin may be removed as a tin–citrate complex. Subsequent addition of [^{99m}Tc]pertechnetate, followed by incubation for 20 minutes, results in ^{99m}Tc-labelled red blood cells. The labelling efficiency is reported to be greater than 97%. Another method of *in-vitro* labelling involves the reconstitution of a lyophilised kit containing a stannous agent, e.g. stannous pyrophosphate or sodium medronate with sterile saline. An aliquot of this stannous ion solution is diluted with sterile saline and incubated with anticoagulated blood for 5–10 minutes. After centrifugation, the plasma is removed and the red cells are mixed and incubated with [^{99m}Tc]pertechnetate. The labelled cells are then re-injected into the patient (Owunwanne *et al.* 1995).

In-vivo labelling with technetium-99m

The method of labelling cells *in vitro* produces good results but it is time consuming. Pavel *et al* introduced the *in-vivo* method of radiolabelling red cells with technetium (Pavel *et al.* 1977). This technique was discovered following the observation that there were high levels of blood background activity when [^{99m}Tc] pertechnetate brain scans were performed several days after ^{99m}Tc-pyrophosphate bone scans. This was likely to be the result of unreacted stannous ions in the bone-scanning agent attaching to the red blood cells.

The *in-vivo* method involves 'pre-tinning' of the red cells by injection of stannous compounds such as stannous pyrophosphate, followed after a time interval by the injection of [^{99m}Tc]pertechnetate. Injection of pertechnetate alone will not result in the ^{99m}Tc binding strongly to cells, as it freely diffuses in and out of cells. The exact mechanism of labelling is not entirely understood, but it is thought that the stannous agent diffuses into the cell and becomes firmly bound to cellular components. The stannous agent is usually a complex, e.g. stannous pyrophosphate. Stannous ions are susceptible to hydrolysis at physiological pH and will precipitate, resulting in their rapid clearance from the blood by the reticuloendothelial system. However, when complexed with soluble chelates, hydrolysis will be resisted but the stannous ions are not so tightly bound to the chelate that they will be unable to dissociate and become attached to the red blood cell. The pertechnetate diffuses freely in and out of the cells but in the presence of Sn(II) in the cell it becomes reduced and subsequently binds to the beta chain of haemoglobin (Srivastava, Chervu 1984). The amount of stannous ion required for optimal labelling is 10–20 μg per kilogram of body weight.

Combined *in-vivo/in-vitro* labelling methods with technetium-99m

A disadvantage of the *in-vivo* technique is a variable labelling efficiency. Low labelling yields may be owing to the excess tin(II) not being incorporated into the cell, thus reducing the pertechnetate outside the red blood cells. Reduced technetium is not able to diffuse across the red cell membrane. To overcome the problem of variability in labelling efficiency, combinations of both the *in-vivo* and *in-vitro* techniques have been used. The modified *in-vivo/in-vitro* technique involves the intravenous administration of a stannous agent, followed 20–30 minutes later by withdrawing an aliquot of 'tinned' blood into a heparinised syringe. The blood is diluted with saline and centrifuged to obtain red cells. The washing step is repeated to remove any excess tin(II) not incorporated into cells. The red cells are then incubated with [^{99m}Tc]pertechnetate, followed by washing and centrifugation to remove unincorporated ^{99m}Tc. The cells are re-injected after resuspension in saline (Bauer *et al.* 1983) (Appendix 7). Another method involving a combination of the *in-vitro* and *in-vivo* techniques has been described as the modified *in-vivo* method (Callahan *et al.* 1982). This method involves the *in-vivo* 'tinning' of cells, followed after 10–20 minutes by the withdrawal of blood into a heparinised syringe containing [^{99m}Tc]pertechnetate. The contents of the syringe are mixed at room temperature and the blood is re-injected into the patient (Appendix 8).

Heat-damaged red blood cells

Heat-damaged red cells have been used for spleen imaging studies. Inadequately damaged cells will result in activity in the blood pool and well-perfused organs such the liver and kidney. Various methods are available for preparing heat-damaged red cells. Generally the blood is initially mixed with stannous ion by *in-vivo* or *in-vitro* methods previously described. The 'tinned' cells are separated from plasma. Red cells do not sufficiently denature in plasma (Vaik, Guille 1984). The red cells are incubated with [^{99m}Tc]pertechnetate and then heated in a water-bath at 49.5°C for 15 minutes as described in Appendix 9. The temperature of 49.5°C is critical. Too hot a temperature will burst the red cells and too low a temperature will not denature the cells sufficiently. It is also essential to maintain the whole of the cell suspension for 15 minutes. It should therefore be shaken gently throughout the procedure. A number of workers recommend centrifugation of the damaged cells, as the burst fragments will be visible in the supernatant layer. Injection of cell fragments may localise in the liver and produce a poor-quality image.

In-vitro labelling with chromium-51

Chromium-51 in the form of sodium chromate has been used for the *in-vitro* labelling of red cells. Chromium-51 is not suitable for imaging using a gamma camera because of the low photon yield (less than 10% abundance) of the 320 keV gamma-ray and long half-life of 27.7 days. Sodium [^{51}Cr]chromate in the hexavalent state diffuses through the red cell membrane and is enzymatically reduced to the trivalent state, which binds firmly to the beta globin chain of the haemoglobin molecule. In the trivalent state, chromium will not pass through the cell membrane but will bind to plasma proteins. ^{51}Cr elutes from labelled red cells at the rate of approximately 1% per day (Swanson 1990). In order to avoid toxicity to cells and to achieve high labelling efficiencies, sodium [^{51}Cr]chromate should be used in a high specific activity (less than 2 µg of chromium per mL of packed red cells). A method for red cell labelling with ^{51}Cr is given in Appendix 10.

Direct blood labelling agents

The main advantages in using direct blood labelling agents that are cell-selective is that lengthy procedures and skilled personnel are not needed to isolate specific cell types. This avoids the possibility of cell damage. High-grade laboratories are unnecessary for these procedures. Cell-selective agents would reduce the risk to operators of working with blood which may be contaminated with HIV and hepatitis B.

Whole monoclonal antibodies

Monoclonal antibodies (MABs) have been in use for several years and are directed against antigenic receptors on the surface of blood cells thus avoiding the need to separate the cells. The ideal properties of a cell labelling antibody have been described by Danpure and Osman (1986). As with ^{99m}Tc and ^{111}In complexes the *in-vivo* behaviour of the labelled cells should not be affected and the MAB should remain attached to the cells during the course of the clinical study. The MAB must be specific for the blood cell type and not cross-react with other blood cells or endothelial cells. The antibody should be specific for the antigens on the surfaces of the cells. The major drawbacks that have been found with these agents for imaging infection and inflammation include (a) a low cell-bound activity, (b) a long plasma half-life requiring a long interval between injection and imaging to achieve a good target-to-background ratio, and (c) a higher incidence of a HAMA response with mouse-derived antibodies (Signore *et al.* 2006). As a consequence, whole MABs such as BW250/183 (Becker *et al.* 1992) (an IgG1 labelled with ^{99m}Tc directed against cross-reacting antigen 95 (NCA-95) expressed on granulocytes) and ^{99m}Tc-fanolesomab (Love *et al.* 2006) (an IgM that binds to CD15 antigen expressed on neutrophils) have been used with limited success for infection/inflammation imaging but have not become widely used in clinical practice.

Monoclonal antibody fragment

Sulesomab (Leukoscan) is a small murine monoclonal antibody Fab′ fragment (IMMU-MN3) that can be radiolabelled with ^{99m}Tc. The antibody reacts with the glycoprotein, non-specific cross-reactive antigen (NCA-90) on the surface of granulocytes. It also cross-reacts with the carcinoembryonic antigen (CEA). The kit formulation for the preparation of ^{99m}Tc-sulesomab consists of 0.31 mg sulesomab, 0.22 mg stannous chloride, sodium chloride, potassium sodium tartrate, sodium acetate, sucrose and is buffered to pH 5–7. The kit is reconstituted to 0.5 mL with isotonic sodium chloride injection and 1 mL [^{99m}Tc]pertechnetate (750–1110 MBq) and the recommended adult dose is 0.25 mg of Fab′ fragment labelled with 900 ± 200 MBq of ^{99m}Tc. The indications for ^{99m}Tc-sulesomab are infection/inflammation imaging in bone in patients with suspected osteomyelitis, including patients with diabetic foot ulcers (Becker *et al.* 1994). Leukoscan has not been associated with HAMA reactions following a single administration and has been accepted into clinical practice.

Practical aspects of cell labelling

Health and safety

Personnel should be fully aware of the dangers of working with blood samples, especially with the risks of HIV and hepatitis. Some authorities recommend that operators who work with blood should be vaccinated against hepatitis B. Instruction in the safe handling and disposal of radioactive blood waste is important and there should be written protocols for these procedures. The use of needles should be minimised or eliminated from blood radiolabelling procedures to avoid the possibility of needle-stick injuries. Cell labelling techniques should be carried out by personnel who have been carefully trained in aseptic manipulations and in the preparation of radiolabelled cells. It is generally accepted that no change in procedure needs to be employed in handling blood known to be infected with hepatitis C or HIV.

Facilities for cell labelling

Pharmaceutical isolators are increasingly used for these procedures. A Type 2 (negative pressure) isolator provides filtered air to Grade A/B (Orange Guide: MHRA 2007) is recommended and this type of unit offers protection to the product, operator and environment. For the manufacturing of radiopharmaceuticals, the isolator is required to be sited in a Grade D environment (Orange Guide; MHRA 2007). It is recommended that the radiolabelling of autologous blood products, an open procedure, should be undertaken in a separate room, ideally designated for such manipulations, with separate changing facilities to ensure that there is no possibility of cross-contamination of other products. A more detailed discussion on facilities is given in Chapter 27.

All materials introduced into the isolator should be sprayed with a sanitising agent, e.g. sterile 70% w/v isopropyl alcohol (spore free), although 70% IPA will not kill blood spores. The workstation should be thoroughly disinfected before commencing any preparation of radiolabelled cells. It is good practice that all blood work should be undertaken on a tray to contain spillages. After each patient blood labelling, all non-disposable materials including the centrifuge buckets and workstation, should be thoroughly disinfected with an agent that is active against blood organisms and spores. Disposable items such as universal tubes, pipettes, kwills and syringes, should be discarded according to written local procedures. Wrist-change gloves should be discarded and gauntlets disinfected after each blood labelling session to prevent any cross-contamination.

Documentation

All the details of the blood labelling procedure should be recorded such that a history of all the ingredients may be easily traced. Details that are required to be recorded for radiolabelled leukocytes include:

- Date of procedure
- Patient's name, radiopharmaceutical and dose
- Name of radionuclide/radiopharmaceutical, batch number, expiry, activity and volume
- Saline batch number and expiry
- ACD batch number, expiry
- Sedimentation agent, e.g. Hetastarch batch number, expiry
- Name of ligand, batch number and expiry
- Activity in supernatant
- Activity at a specified time and volume of final injection
- Labelling efficiency
- Signature of dispenser and checker.

Patient

Patient identification is a very important aspect and stringent procedures should be in force to ensure that the radiolabelled cells are re-injected into the person from whom the blood was taken. In laboratories where blood cells from more than one patient are radiolabelled simultaneously, it is important to identify the blood taken from each patient and the corresponding blood manipulation tubes. A simple system using a three-part Yellow Label has been developed by Sampson (1993). The label consists of three parts each having the same sequential number, the name of the patient, radiopharmaceutical and the dose required. On completion of the radiolabelling procedures the dose and volume at a specified time are recorded. The three-part label is initially attached to the syringe of blood and the second portion of the label is removed and affixed to the procedure book. The third section of the label is attached to the blood manipulation tube. After radiolabelling, the third portion of the label is removed from the blood manipulation tube and attached to the final syringe of labelled cells. At the end of the procedure, all the three labels are matched and the patient is identified by several parameters, e.g. hospital number, patient's name and date of birth. The details are then matched with those on the syringe. A schematic diagram of the three-part Yellow Label is given in Figure 24.7.

Working with animal blood

Nuclear medicine is becoming recognised as an important diagnostic modality in the veterinary world. One of the tests that may be requested is labelled white cells. The indications for leukocyte scintigraphy are as follows:

1. Identification or location of sepsis in animals with known or suspected inflammatory disease in:
   a. multisystemic infections or generalised septicaemia

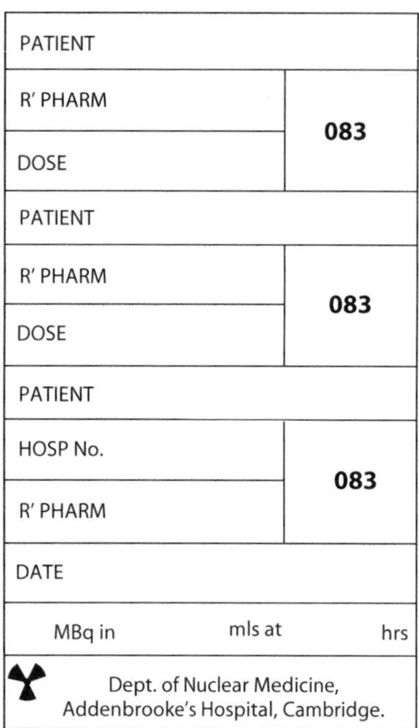

PATIENT	
R' PHARM	083
DOSE	
PATIENT	
R' PHARM	083
DOSE	
PATIENT	
HOSP No.	083
R' PHARM	
DATE	
MBq in mls at hrs	
Dept. of Nuclear Medicine, Addenbrooke's Hospital, Cambridge.	

Figure 24.7 Patient identification using a three-part yellow label system.

   b septic arthritis, discospondylitis, osteomyelitis
   c rheumatoid arthritis
   d inflammatory bowel disease.
2 Identification of fever of unknown origin.
3 Evaluation of surgical sites or implants as in:
   a drainage
   b delayed unions
   c excessive pain or swelling
   d postoperative fever
   e loosening or infection of orthopaedic prostheses.
4 Evaluation of disease progression and response to treatment.
5 Evaluation of lesions identified radiographically, e.g. lytic regions in bone and soft tissue masses.

Radiolabelling techniques and facilities for animal work

Blood labelling techniques used in animal work are similar to those used with humans. Briefly, for dogs and cats, 50 mL of blood should be taken and sedimented onto 10 mL hetastarch. It is essential to sediment the blood using sedimentation agents rather than slow centrifugation. The leukocyte-rich platelet-rich plasma is obtained as described earlier (Separation of leukocytes) and a leukocyte plug is obtained by centrifugation. Radiolabelling can be undertaken using ^{111}In-tropolonate or ^{99m}Tc-HMPAO.

For work on horses, 100 mL of blood is usually taken and sedimented using sedimentation agents. The time taken for sedimentation of horse blood is greatly reduced and may only take 5–10 minutes.

Animal work should be undertaken in facilities dedicated for that particular use. The blood should be processed in a total-containment workstation sited in a separate laboratory from that used for humans. Rigid disinfection and sanitisation procedures should be carried out before and after working with animal blood. The procedures should be documented. The final syringe of blood should be checked by an independent operator before issue.

Acknowledgments

The author would like to thank Harry Heyes for assistance with the diagrams.

Appendices

1. Labelling of leukocytes with ^{111}In-tropolonate

1 Dispense 9 mL of ACD (NIH, Formula A) into each of two 60-mL syringes.
2 Withdraw 51 mL of the patient's blood into each syringe using a 19G butterfly.
3 Dispense 2 mL of 6% w/v hydroxyethyl starch (molecular weight 450 000 daltons; molar substitution 0.7) into 5 Universal tubes.
4 Dispense 20 mL of anticoagulated blood into each of the Universal tubes containing the sedimentation agent, mix by one gentle inversion and leave for 45–60 minutes to sediment the red cells.
5 Dispense the remaining 20 mL of blood into a Universal tube not containing a sedimentation agent and centrifuge at 1500*g* for 10 minutes. The supernatant contains cell-free plasma and

ACD which is used as the cell-labelling medium and for suspending the radiolabelled cells for reinjection.

6 After the red cells have sedimented (step 4), remove 15-mL aliquots of the leukocyte-rich platelet-rich plasma (LRPRP) into sterile Universal tubes.

7 Centrifuge the LRPRP at 150*g* for 5 minutes to give a pellet of leukocytes and a supernatant containing platelet-rich plasma (PRP).

8 Transfer the PRP to a Universal tube and centrifuge at 1500*g* for 10 minutes to obtain cell-free plasma. This is used for washing the cells after labelling.

9 Resuspend the leukocytes in 1 mL of cell-free plasma from step 5.

10 Add 0.1 mL of tropolone solution (0.054% w/v in Hepes–saline buffer, pH 7.6), followed by 30 MBq of $^{111}InCl_3$ to the cells.

11 Incubate the cells for 5–10 minutes at room temperature.

12 Add 5–10 mL of cell-free plasma from step 8 and centrifuge at 150*g* for 5 minutes.

13 Remove the supernatant and retain for determining the labelling efficiency.

14 Resuspend cells in 3–4 mL of cell-free plasma from step 5. Check the activity (20 MBq is the diagnostic reference level) and calculate the labelling efficiency.

Alternatively 50 mL of blood may be taken into 60-mL syringes containing 6 mL ACD (NIH, Formula A), and similar steps taken as described above except the cell-free plasma is obtained from the PRP containing 6% w/v hydroxyethyl starch (450/0.7) and the leukocytes to be labelled are resuspended in 0.25 mL of cell-free plasma.

The method for labelling leukocytes with ^{111}In-oxine is described in the [^{111}In]-oxine package insert (GE Healthcare).

2. Labelling of leukocytes with ^{99m}T-HMPAO

The official method for labelling leukocytes with ^{99m}Tc-HMPAO is described in the Ceretec package insert (GE Healthcare). An alternative method by Solanki *et al.* (1993) is described below.

1 Dispense 6 mL of ACD (NIH, Formula A) into a 60-mL syringe.

2 Withdraw 50 mL of blood into the syringe using a 19G butterfly.

3 Transfer to a 50-mL Falcon tube containing 10 mL of 6% w/v hydroxyethyl starch (450/0.7) and leave for 45–60 minutes to allow the red cells to sediment.

4 After sedimentation, remove the LRPRP to another Falcon tube and centrifuge at 150*g* for 5 minutes.

5 Remove the PRP and centrifuge at 1500*g* for 10 minutes to obtain cell-free plasma.

6 Resuspend the leukocyte pellet in 0.25 mL of cell-free plasma.

7 Reconstitute a vial of HMPAO (Ceretec) with 6 mL of sterile nitrogen-flushed saline. Store in a freezer when not in use (expiry 6–9 months).

8 Add 6 mL of sterile saline to a vial of stannous medronate. Withdraw a volume of 0.1 mL of this solution and dilute to 10 mL with sterile saline. The stannous solution must be freshly prepared.

9 Withdraw 0.3 mL of the reconstituted HMPAO solution from step 7 and withdraw 0.1 mL of the stannous solution prepared in step 8 into the syringe. Add 500 MBq of [^{99m}Tc]pertechnetate to the contents of the syringe. To ensure a good label it is essential to keep the volume of pertechnetate small, i.e. 0.2–0.3 mL.

10 Add the ^{99m}Tc-HMPAO solution to the resuspended cells from step 6 and incubate at room temperature for 10 minutes.

11 Add 3 mL of cell-free plasma to the labelling medium and centrifuge at 150*g* for 5 minutes.

12 Remove the supernatant and retain for determining the labelling efficiency.

13 Resuspend the radiolabelled cells in 3–4 mL of cell-free plasma. Check the activity (200 MBq is the diagnostic reference level) and calculate the labelling efficiency.

3. Separation of neutrophils

This method has been described by Sampson and Solanki (1992) for radiolabelling neutrophils with ^{99m}Tc-HMPAO and the purity of the separated neutrophils is reported to be 96%.

1 Dispense 6 mL of ACD (NIH, Formula A) into a 60-mL syringe.
2 Withdraw 50 mL of blood into the syringe using a 19G butterfly.
3 Dispense 7.5 mL of density gradient 1.119 g/mL (Histopaque 1119, Sigma-Aldrich) into a Universal tube.
4 Carefully layer 8.5 mL of density gradient 1.077 g/mL (Histopaque 1077, Sigma-Aldrich) onto the first gradient, but do not allow the two layers to mix.
5 Carefully layer 15 mL of anticoagulated blood onto the double density gradient, ensuring the layers are not mixed.
6 Centrifuge the tube at 750*g* for 15 minutes. This will result in the formation of two layers.
7 Remove the second layer containing the neutrophils and resuspend in 2 mL cell-free plasma. (Cell-free plasma may be obtained by the centrifugation of 15 mL of anticoagulated whole blood at 1500*g* for 10 minutes).
8 Centrifuge the resuspended neutrophils at 150*g* for 5 minutes and remove the supernatant.

This procedure may require two or three samples of 15 mL of anticoagulated blood for collection of sufficient cells for clinical studies. The separated cells may be collected and resuspended in cell-free plasma for radiolabelling.

4. Separation of granulocytes

This method has been described by Danpure and Osman (1994) for the radiolabelling of granulocytes with ^{111}In-tropolonate or ^{99m}Tc-HMPAO.

1 Dispense 9 mL of ACD (NIH, Formula A) into each of two 60-mL syringes.
2 Withdraw 51 mL of the patient's blood into each syringe using a 19G butterfly.
3 Dispense 2 mL of 6% w/v hydroxyethyl starch (450/0.7) into 5 Universal tubes.
4 Dispense 20 mL of blood into each of the Universal tubes containing the sedimentation agent, mix by one gentle inversion and leave for 45–60 minutes to sediment the red cells.
5 Dispense the 40 mL of blood into a Universal tube not containing a sedimentation agent and centrifuge at 1500*g* for 10 minutes. The supernatant contains cell-free plasma and ACD which is used as the cell-labelling medium, preparing Percoll/plasma gradients and for suspending the radiolabelled cells for reinjection.
6 After the red cells have sedimented (step 4), remove 15-mL aliquots of the leukocyte-rich platelet-rich plasma (LRPRP) into sterile Universal tubes.
7 Centrifuge the LRPRP at 150*g* for 5 minutes to give a pellet of leukocytes and a supernatant containing platelet-rich plasma (PRP).
8 Transfer PRP to a Universal tube.
9 Resuspend the leukocytes in 4 mL of PRP from step 8.
10 Centrifuge the remaining PRP at 1500*g* for 10 minutes to obtain cell-free plasma, which is used for washing the cells after labelling.
11 Prepare iso-osmotic Percoll (IOP = 100%) by mixing 9 volumes of Percoll (specific activity 1.13 g/mL) with 1 volume of 1.5 mol/L sodium chloride (90 g/L).
12 Dilute the IOP with the patient's cell-free ACD-plasma prepared in step 5, to obtain 65%, 60% and 50% v/v solutions of Percoll in plasma.
13 Prepare two 3-step discontinuous density-gradients by carefully layering 2 mL of each solution in order of decreasing density into a sterile 10 mL centrifuge tube. One gradient is needed for the leukocytes from 50 mL of blood.
14 Gently overlay 2 mL of the leukocytes in plasma onto each gradient.
15 Centrifuge the gradients at 150*g* for 5 minutes.
16 Discard the plasma and the cells (platelets and mononuclear cells) at the plasma/50% interface and sample the granulocytes from the 50/60% interface.
17 Wash the granulocytes free of Percoll by adding 10 mL of cell-free plasma containing 6% w/v hydroxyethyl starch from step 10 and centrifuge

the cells at 150*g* for 5 minutes. Discard the supernatant.

18 Resuspend the cells in 1 mL of cell-free plasma obtained from step 5 for radiolabelling.

5. Separation of lymphocytes

This method has been described by Sampson and Goffin (1991) for the labelling of lymphocytes using ^{99m}Tc-HMPAO.

1. Dispense 6 mL of ACD (NIH, Formula A) into two 60-mL syringes.
2. Withdraw 50 mL of venous blood into each syringe.
3. Transfer the anticoagulated blood into two 50-mL Falcon tubes each containing 10 mL of 6% w/v hydroxyethyl starch (450/0.7) and leave for 45-60 minutes for the red cells to sediment.
4. Remove the LRPRP from each tube and centrifuge at 100*g* for 7 minutes.
5. Remove the supernatant (PRP) and centrifuge at 1500*g* for 10 minutes to obtain cell-free plasma.
6. Resuspend the leukocyte pellets in 4 mL of cell-free plasma.
7. Carefully layer the cell suspension onto 3 mL of 'Lymphoprep' (Axis-Shield) in a 10 mL Falcon tube.
8. Centrifuge the tube at 400*g* for 40 minutes.
9. Remove the top layer containing plasma.
10. Remove the first band containing mainly lymphocytes and resuspend with 1 mL of cell-free plasma in a 10-mL Falcon tube.
11. Centrifuge the tube at 150*g* for 5 minutes and discard the supernatant.
12. Resuspend the cells in cell-free plasma for radiolabelling.

6. The labelling of platelets with ^{111}In-tropolonate or ^{99m}Tc-HMPAO

This method has been described by Danpure and Osman (1994). An alternative method for labelling platelets with ^{111}In-oxine is described in the ^{111}In-Oxine Solution package insert (GE Healthcare, 2010 http://md.gehealthcare.com/shared/pdfs/pi/Indoxy.pdf).

1. Dispense 9 mL ACD (NIH, Formula A) into a 60-mL syringe.
2. Withdraw 51 mL of venous blood using a 19G butterfly needle.
3. Dispense the anticoagulated blood into 3 Universal tubes each containing 2 mL of 6% w/v hydroxyethyl starch. Mix the contents of each tube and centrifuge at 150*g* for 10 minutes to obtain a pellet of leukocytes and red cells and supernatant containing platelets in plasma (PRP).
4. Carefully remove the PRP (without using a needle). Acidify the PRP by adding 1 volume ACD to 10 volumes of PRP.
5. Centrifuge the acidified PRP at 640*g* for 10 minutes to obtain a pellet of platelets.
6. Remove the supernatant (cell-free plasma, pH 6.5) and retain. This plasma may be used for the platelet labelling medium, washing the platelets after labelling and resuspending the platelets for re-injection.
7. Resuspend the platelets in 1 mL of acidified cell-free plasma for radiolabelling.

For labelling with ^{111}In-tropolonate:

a. ^{111}In-Tropolonate is prepared by the addition of the required amount of $^{111}InCl_3$ to 0.1 mL of tropolone solution (0.054% w/v in Hepes-saline buffer pH 7.6) just before addition to the platelet suspension.
b. Add the ^{111}In-tropolonate to the platelets in 1 mL cell-free plasma.
c. Incubate the platelets at room temperature for 5 minutes.
d. Add 5 mL of acidified cell-free plasma (pH 6.5) and centrifuge the platelet suspension at 640*g* for 10 minutes.
e. Remove the supernatant and retain for determining the labelling efficiency.
f. Resuspend the radiolabelled platelets in 5 mL of acidified cell-free plasma (pH 6.5) and measure the activity. Calculate the labelling efficiency.

For labelling with ^{99m}T-HMPAO:

a Prepare the ^{99m}Tc-HMPAO as recommended by the manufacturer's instructions.

b Add 4 mL of ^{99m}Tc-HMPAO to the platelets resuspended in 1 mL cell-free plasma (pH 6.5). Incubate for 30 minutes at room temperature.

c Add 10 mL of cell-free plasma (pH 6.5) and centrifuge at 640*g* for 10 minutes.

d Remove the supernatant and retain for determining the labelling efficiency.

e Resuspend the radiolabelled platelets in 5 mL of acidified cell-free plasma (pH 6.5) and measure the activity. Calculate the labelling efficiency.

7. Modified *in-vivo/in-vitro* labelling of red cells with technetium-99m

1 Pre-tin the red cells *in vivo* as follows:
   a Reconstitute the Amerscan Stannous Agent vial (GE Healthcare, containing 4 mg of stannous fluoride and 6.8 mg of sodium medronate) with 6 mL of sterile saline.
   b Inject 0.03 mL per kg body weight.

2 Between 15 and 30 minutes after injection, withdraw 3–5 mL of pre-tinned blood into a syringe rinsed with heparin.

3 Incubate 3 mL of the blood with the required amount of [^{99m}Tc]pertechnetate for 20 minutes at room temperature.

4 After incubation, add 5 mL of sterile saline and centrifuge at 500*g* for 10 minutes.

5 Remove the supernatant and measure the activity in the red cell pellet and supernatant and determine the labelling efficiency.

6 Resuspend the red cells in sterile saline and re-inject the patient with 1-1.5 mL of blood containing the required amount of ^{99m}Tc (for cardiovascular and vascular imaging, 800 MBq is the diagnostic reference level; for GI bleed, 400 MBq is the diagnostic reference level).

8. Modified *in-vivo* labelling of red cells with technetium-99m

This method has been described by Callahan *et al.* (1982).

1 Pre-tin the red cells *in-vivo* as described above.

2 20 minutes after injection, withdraw 4 mL of pre-tinned blood into a shielded syringe containing the required amount of [^{99m}Tc]pertechnetate using a 19G butterfly needle.

3 Remove the shielded syringe from the butterfly and cap the syringe.

4 Invert the syringe for 5–10 minutes.

5 Re-inject the labelled cells. (For diagnostic reference levels see Appendix 7.)

9. Red cell labelling with technetium-99m: heat-damaged erythrocytes (Merseyside and Cheshire Radiopharmacy Services)

1 Pre-tin the red cells *in vivo* as described above.

2 20 minutes after injection, withdraw 16 mL of pre-tinned blood into a vial containing 4 mL ACD solution.

3 Centrifuge at 1000*g* for 10 minutes and remove the supernatant.

4 Add the required amount of [^{99m}Tc]pertechnetate and agitate the cells gently.

5 Incubate in a water-bath at 49.5°C for 15 minutes. The temperature is critical and must be carefully controlled.

6 Add 10 mL sterile 0.9% sodium chloride solution and centrifuge at 1000*g* for 10 minutes and remove the supernatant.

7 Add another 10 mL of sterile saline solution and centrifuge at 1000*g* for 10 minutes and remove the supernatant.

8 Resuspend the cells in sterile saline to a total volume of 15 mL.

9 After measuring the activity, re-inject the required amount (100 MBq is the diagnostic reference level).

10. Red cell labelling with chromium-51

This method has been described by Danpure and Osman (1994).

1 Withdraw 8.5 mL of blood into a syringe containing 1.5 mL ACD (NIH, Formula A).
2 Transfer the anticoagulated blood to a 10-mL sterile polypropylene tube and centrifuge at 1200–1500*g* for 5 minutes.
3 Remove the supernatant (plasma) and the white buffy coat on top of the red cells which contains the leukocytes and platelets.
4 Add the required amount of sodium [^{51}Cr] chromate in at least 0.2 mL of saline. The addition should be slow with continuous mixing.
5 Incubate for 15 minutes at room temperature.
6 Wash the cells with 4–5 volumes of saline.
7 Resuspend the cells in 11–12 mL of saline. Withdraw 10 mL into a pre-weighed syringe for re-injection. (0.8 MBq is the diagnostic reference level for red cell volume; 2 MBq is the diagnostic reference level for red cell survival studies.) Weigh the syringe after injection.

References

Alavi JB, Hansell J (1984). Labeled cells in the investigation of hematologic disorders. *Semin Nucl Med* 14: 208–225.

Babich JW (1991). Technetium-99m-HM-PAO retention and the role of glutathione: the debate continues. *J Nucl Med* 32: 1681–1683.

Balaban EP *et al.* (1986). Effect of the radiolabel mediator tropolone on lymphocyte structure and function. *J Lab Clin Med* 107: 306–314.

Bauer R *et al.* (1983). In vivo/in vitro labelling of red blood cells with ^{99m}Tc. *Eur J Nucl Med* 8: 218–222.

Becker W *et al.* (1992). The single late Tc-99m granulocyte antibody scan in inflammatory diseases. *Nucl Med Commun* 13: 186–192.

Becker W *et al.* (1994). Detection of soft-tissue infections and osteomyelitis using a technetium-99m-labeled anti-granulocyte monoclonal antibody fragment. *J Nucl Med* 35: 1436–1443.

Berger CL, Edelson RL (1979). Comparison of lymphocyte function after isolation by Ficoll-Hypaque flotation or elutriation. *J Invest Dermatol* 73: 231–235.

Callahan RJ *et al.* (1982). A modified method for the in vivo labelling of red blood cells with Tc-99m: concise communication. *J Nucl Med* 23: 315–318.

Chisholm PM *et al.* (1979). Cell damage resulting from the labelling of rat lymphocytes and HeLa S3 cells with In-111 oxine. *J Nucl Med* 20: 1308–1311.

Colas-Linhart N *et al.* (1983). Five leucocyte labelling techniques: a comparative in-vitro study. *Br J Haematol* 53: 31–41.

Danpure HJ (1985). Cell-labelling with ^{111}In-complexes. In: Theobald AE, ed. *Radiopharmacy and Radiopharmaceuticals*. London: Taylor and Francis, 51–185.

Danpure HJ, Osman S (1986). Iodine-labelled monoclonal antibodies for cell-labelling. Principles and prospects. *Int J Rad Appl Instrum A* 37: 735–739.

Danpure HJ, Osman S (1988a). Investigations to determine the optimum conditions for radiolabelling human platelets with 99Tcm-hexamethyl propylene amine oxime (99Tcm-HM-PAO). *Nucl Med Commun* 9: 267–272.

Danpure HJ, Osman S (1988b). Optimum conditions for radiolabelling human granulocytes and mixed leucocytes with ^{111}In-tropolonate. *Eur J Nucl Med* 13: 537–542.

Danpure HJ, Osman S (1994). Radiolabelling of blood cells – methodology. In: Sampson CB, ed. *Textbook of Radiopharmacy*. London: Gordon and Breach, 75–86.

Danpure HJ *et al.* (1982a). The labelling of blood cells in plasma with ^{111}In-tropolonate. *Br J Radiol* 55: 247–249.

Danpure HJ *et al.* (1982b). The advantages of labelling granulocytes in plasma with In-111 tropolonate. In: Raynaud C, ed. *Proceedings of the Third World Congress of Nuclear Medicine and Biology*. Oxford: Pergamon Press, 2395–2398.

Dewanjee MK *et al.* (1981). Indium-111 tropolone, a new high-affinity platelet label: preparation and evaluation of labelling parameters. *J Nucl Med* 22: 981–987.

Dooley DC *et al.* (1982). Isolation of large numbers of fully viable human neutrophils: a preparative technique using Percoll density gradient centrifugation. *Exp Haematol* 10: 591–599.

Frost P, Frost H (1978). Recirculation of lymphocytes and the use of indium-111. *J Nucl Med* 20: 169.

Hawker RJ *et al.* (1980). Indium (^{111}In)-labelled human platelets: optimal method. *Clin Sci* 58: 243–248.

Hawkins T *et al.* (1991). The long-term stability of reconstituted exametazime; a clinical and laboratory evaluation. *Nucl Med Commun* 12: 1045–1055.

Hosain F *et al.* (1969). Binding of trace amounts of ionic indium-113m to plasma transferrin. *Clin Chim Acta* 24: 69–75.

Hung JC *et al.* (1988). Kinetic analysis of technetium-99m d, l-HM-PAO decomposition in aqueous media. *J Nucl Med* 29: 1568–1576.

ICSH (International Committee for Standardization in Haematology) (1988). Recommended method for indium-111 platelet survival studies. *J Nucl Med* 29: 564–566.

Lang EL *et al.* (1993). Quality assurance of white blood cell labelling with a test based adherence. *J Nucl Med* 34: 345–348.

Love C *et al.* (2006). Imaging of infection and inflammation with ^{99m}Tc-Fanolesomab. *Q J Nucl Med Mol Imaging* 50: 113–120.

Mathias CJ, Welch MJ (1984). Radiolabelling of platelets. *Semin Nucl Med* 14: 118–127.

McAfee JG, Thakur ML (1976). Survey of radioactive agents for in-vitro labelling of phagocytic leucocytes. I. Soluble agents. *J Nucl Med* 17: 480–487.

McAfee JG *et al.* (1984). Technique of leucocyte harvesting and labelling: problems and perspectives. *Semin Nucl Med* 14: 83–107.

MHRA (Medicines and Healthcare products Regulatory Agency) (2007). *Rules and Guidance for Pharmaceutical Manufacturers and Distributors* (Orange Guide). London: Pharmaceutical Press.

Moerlein BSM, Welch MJ (1981). The chemistry of gallium and indium as related to radiopharmaceutical production. *Int J Nucl Med Biol* 8: 277–287.

Morrissey GJ, Powe JE (1993). Routine application of fractionated HM-PAO stored at −70°C for WBC scintigraphy. *J Nucl Med* 34: 151–155.

Mortelmans L *et al.* (1989). In-vitro and in-vivo evaluation of granulocyte labelling with [^{99m}Tc] d,l-HM-PAO. *J Nucl Med* 30: 2022–2028.

Neirinckx RD *et al.* (1987). Technetium-99m d,l-HM-PAO: A new radiopharmaceutical for SPECT imaging of regional cerebral blood perfusion. *J Nucl Med* 28: 191–202.

Neirinckx RD *et al.* (1988). The retention mechanism of technetium-99m-HM-PAO intracellular reaction with glutathione. *J Cereb Blood Flow Metab*, S4–S12.

Nowotnik DP *et al.* (1985). Development of a 99Tcm-labelled radiopharmaceutical for cerebral blood flow imaging. *Nucl Med Commun* 6: 499–506.

Osman S, Danpure HJ (1987). A simple in-vitro method of labelling human erythrocytes in whole blood with ^{113m}In-tropolonate. *Eur J Haematol* 39: 125–127.

Owunwanne A *et al.*, eds (1995). *The Handbook of Radiopharmaceuticals*. London: Chapman and Hall Medical, 70–74.

Pavel DG *et al.* (1977). In vivo labelling of red blood cells with ^{99m}Tc: a new approach to blood pool visualization. *J Nucl Med* 18: 305–308.

Peters AM, Saverymuttu SH (1987). The value of indium-labelled leucocytes in clinical practice. *Blood Rev* 1: 65–76.

Peters AM *et al.* (1982). A comparison of indium-111-oxine and indium-111-acetylacetone labelled leucocytes in the diagnosis of inflammatory disease. *Br J Radiol* 55: 827–832.

Peters AM *et al.* (1983). Imaging of inflammation with indium-111 tropolonate labeled leucocytes. *J Nucl Med* 24: 39–44.

Peters AM *et al.* (1986). Clinical experience with ^{99m}Tc-hexamethylpropylene-amineoxime for labelling leucocytes and imaging inflammation. *Lancet* ii: 945–949.

Roddie ME *et al.* (1988). Inflammation: imaging with Tc-99m HMPAO-labeled leucocytes. *Radiology* 166: 767–772.

Saha GB, ed. (2004). *Fundamentals of Nuclear Pharmacy*, 5th edn. New York: Springer-Verlag, 116–118.

Sampson CB (1993). Radiolabelling and reinfusion of blood cells. *Nucl Med Commun* 14: 1041.

Sampson CB (1996). Complications and difficulties in radiolabelling blood cells: a review. *Nucl Med Commun* 17: 648–658.

Sampson CB (1998). Labelled cells for imaging infection. In: Cox PH, Buscombe J, eds. *The Imaging of Infection and Inflammation*. Dordrecht: Kluwer Academic Publishers, 31–60.

Sampson CB, Goffin E (1991). Technetium-labelled autologous lymphocytes: clinical protocol for radiolabelling using a high concentration and low volume of 99Tcm-exametazime. *Nucl Med Commun* 12: 875–878.

Sampson CB, Solanki C (1989). Does plasma fat, viscosity, or erythrocyte sedimentation rate affect the radiolabelling of leucocytes? *Nucl Med Commun* 10: 224.

Sampson CB, Solanki C (1992). Separation and technetium labelling of pure neutrophils: development of a simple and rapid clinical protocol. *Nucl Med Commun* 13: 210.

Sampson CB *et al.* (1991). ^{99}Tc^{m}-exametazime-labelled leucocytes: effect of volume and concentration of exametazime on labelling efficiency, and clinical protocol for high efficiency multi-dose radiolabelling. *Nucl Med Commun* 12: 719–723.

Saverymuttu SH *et al.* (1983). Lung transit of ^{111}indium-labelled granulocytes. Relationship to labelling techniques. *Scand J Haematol* 30: 151–160.

Schmidt KG *et al.* (1990). Tc-99m-HMPAO as a lymphocyte label. In: Thakur ML, ed. *Radiolabeled Cellular Blood Elements*. New York: Wiley-Liss, Inc., 209–218.

Segal AW *et al.* (1978). Indium-111 labelling of leucocytes: a detrimental effect on neutrophil and lymphocyte function and an improved method of cell labelling. *J Nucl Med* 19: 1238–1244.

Sewchand LS, Canham PB (1979). Modes of rouleaux formation of human red blood cells in polyvinylpyrrolidone and dextran solutions. *Can J Physiol Pharmacol* 57: 1213–1222.

Signore A *et al.* (2006). Receptor targeting agents for imaging inflammation/infection: where are we now? *Q J Nucl Med Mol Imaging* 50: 236–242.

Solanki C *et al.* (1993). Multidose use of exametazime for leucocyte labelling: a new approach using tin enhancement. *Nucl Med Commun* 14: 1035–1040.

Solanki KK *et al.* (1988). A rapid method for the preparation of 99Tcm hexametazime-labelled leucocytes. *Nucl Med Commun* 9: 753–761.

Srivastava SC, Chervu LR (1984). Radionuclide-labeled red blood cells: current status and future prospects. *Semin Nucl Med* 14: 68–82.

Srivastava SC, Straub RF (1990). Blood cell labelling with ^{99m}Tc: progress and perspectives. *Semin Nucl Med* 20: 41–51.

Swanson D. (1990) Radiopharmaceuticals for hematological applications, 1. Blood volume measurements. In: Swanson DP *et al.*, eds. *Pharmaceuticals in Medical Imaging*. New York: Macmillan, 616–621.

ten Berge RJM *et al.* (1983). Labelling with indium-111 has detrimental effects on human lymphocytes: concise communication. *J Nucl Med* 24: 615–620.

Thakur ML (1981). Editorial. Cell labelling: achievements, challenges, and prospects. *J Nucl Med* 22: 1011–1014.

Thakur ML, Barry MJ (1982). Preparation and evaluation of a new indium-111 agent for efficient labelling of human platelets in plasma. *J Labelled Comp Radiopharm* 19: 1410–1412.

Thakur ML, McKenny S (1985). Techniques of cell labelling: an overview. In: Ezikowitz MD, Hardeman MR, eds. *Radiolabeled Cellular Blood Elements, Pathology, Techniques and Scintigraphic Applications*. New York: Plenum Press, 67–87.

Thakur ML *et al.* (1977a). Indium-111-labeled leucocytes for the localization of abscesses: preparation, analysis, tissue distribution, and comparison with gallium-67 citrate in dogs. *J Lab Clin Med* 89: 217–228.

Thakur ML *et al.* (1977b). Indium-111-labeled cellular blood components: mechanism of labelling and intracellular location in human neutrophils. *J Nucl Med* 18: 1020–1024.

Thakur ML *et al.* (1981). Indium-111-labeled human platelets: improved method, efficacy, and evaluation. *J Nucl Med* 22: 381–385.

Thakur ML *et al.* (1984). Neutrophil labelling. Problems and pitfalls. *Semin Nucl Med* 14: 107–117.

Vaik PE, Guille J (1984). Measurement of splenic function with heat-damaged RBCs: effect of heating conditions: concise communication. *J Nucl Med* 25: 965–968.

Wagstaff J *et al.* (1981). A method for following human lymphocyte traffic using indium-111 oxine labelling. *Clin Exp Immunol* 43: 435–442.

Webber D *et al.* (1994). The effect of varying type and volume of sedimenting agents on leucocyte harvesting and labelling in sickle cell patients. *Nucl Med Commun* 15: 735–741.

Weiblen BJ *et al.* (1979). Studies of the kinetics of indium-111-labeled granulocytes. *J Lab Clin Med* 94: 246–255.

25

Particulate radiopharmaceuticals

Peter Williamson, Pei-San Chan and Richard Southworth

Introduction

Therapeutic and diagnostic radiopharmaceuticals can be divided into three main groups; molecular ([^{18}F]FDG, [^{67}Ga]gallium citrate), macromolecular ([^{125}I]-HSA, ^{125}I-monoclonal antibodies), and particulate. Radiopharmaceutical particulates (also known as microparticulates, radiocolloids or radiofluids) vary in size from just a few nanometres to hundreds of micrometres in diameter, and have a variety of formulations, including colloids, liposomes, suspensions, aerosols, nanocapsules, and microcapsules, summarised in Table 25.1.

Many microparticulates are labelled with technetium-99m (^{99m}Tc), exploiting its excellent imaging characteristics for diagnostic purposes. However, microparticulates have been variously labelled with a variety of radionuclides for both imaging and therapeutic purposes, including rhenium-186 (^{186}Re), rhenium-188 (^{188}Re), indium-111 (^{111}In), gallium-67 (^{67}Ga), ytrrium-90 (^{90}Y), and phosphorus-32 (^{32}P). Some of these agents (and their clinical applications) are discussed below.

Nanoscale devices in nanomedicine and biotechnology offer an attractive platform for the combination of biomedical imaging and nuclear therapeutic devices. Multifunctional nanocarriers capable of selectively targeting disease sites by virtue of targeting moieties on their surface could potentially be used for both diagnostic imaging and carrying large payloads of therapeutic drugs or therapeutic radionuclides. These same agents could then be used in follow-up imaging to evaluate the effectiveness of their therapy. An increasingly common approach in diagnostic imaging is the use of multimodal imaging techniques, utilising the respective advantages of different modalities to provide more powerful and accurate information. The combination of positron emission tomography (PET) and magnetic resonance imaging (MRI) technologies into hybrid systems is still in its infancy, but the respective high sensitivities and high resolution of these two techniques are complementary; the development of dual

Table 25.1 Summary of the range of microparticulates currently available

Nanospheres or microspheres	Spherical objects ranging from tens to hundreds of nanometres in size, composed of synthetic or natural polymers. The drug/agent of interest can be dissolved, entrapped, attached or encapsulated into or with the polymer matrix.
Macroaggregates	Aggregates of particles are defined as microaggregates if below 10 μm in diameter, and macroaggregates if they are larger. Often consisting of a range of sizes owing to their preparation procedures, which include precipitation, coagulation or co-precipitation.
Microcapsules	Microcapsules can be spherical, non-spherical, or aggregates. A core is surrounded by a wall or coating. The capsule or coating can improve pharmaceutical properties in various ways.
Liposomes	Liposomes are closed vesicles that form on hydration of dry phospholipids above their transition temperature. They can be classified by their size and number of bilayers. Multilamellar liposomes consist of several bilayers, each separated by aqueous spaces. Sizes range from a few hundred to thousands of nanometres in diameter. Small unilamellar vesicles (SUVs) are <100 nm, while large unilamellar vesicles (LUVs) are >100 nm. Drugs/agents can be entrapped in the aqueous space or intercalated in the bilayer, i.e. the surface can be modified with targeting ligands or polymers.
Micelles	An aggregate of molecules in solution, composed of hydrophilic and hydrophobic components generally arranged in a spherical shape, with the hydrophobic core shielded from water by the hydrophilic groups.
Nanocrystals	Nanocrystals are aggregates made up of around 100 molecules in a single crystal surrounded by coating of surfactant. They can be produced via procedures such as nanoionisation, pearly milling and high-pressure homogenisation. Nanocrystals help to overcome problems such as bioavailability of poorly soluble drugs, e.g. by increasing the surface area and rate of dissolution, making them good candidates for orally absorbed drugs/agents.
Quantum dots	Nanoscale crystalline structures that can transform the colour of light utilising quantum effects. White light is absorbed, and re-emitted a couple of nanoseconds later at a different wavelength. Varying the size and composition of the quantum dot allows tuneable emission wavelength from blue to near infrared.
Dendrimers	Highly branched macromolecules with a number of chains radiating from a central atom or a cluster of atoms. They have controlled monodisperse 3D architecture, growing outwards from a central core in a series of polymerisation reactions, allowing precise control of their size. Folding and cavities in the core structure can create cages and channels. The surface groups of dendrimers can also be modified, allowing for a variety of applications.

PET/MRI microparticulate imaging agents to exploit this technology is a likely avenue of microparticulate research in the near future.

Microparticulate properties and biodistribution

When considering microparticulate biodistribution *in vivo*, surface chemistry, particle size, and morphology play important roles in interactions with cells and tissues of the body. Historically, non-uniformity in many of these parameters has been a significant problem in microparticulate manufacture, having implications for their labelling affinities and efficiencies. Ultimately, these non-uniformities result in variable biodistributions and rates of clearance from the body, which perhaps has limited the exploitation of microparticulate approaches to their full potential. The recent resurgence of interest in the nanomaterials field can be attributed to recent advances in techniques for microparticulate synthesis, allowing greater control over particulate size, shape, surface structure, charge and functionality than ever previously possible.

Microparticulate size

Microparticulate size influences many aspects of their behaviour; a topic widely reviewed (Illum *et al.* 1982; Dunne *et al.* 2000; Lamprecht *et al.* 2001; Shinde-Patil *et al.* 2001). The size of a particle determines its velocity in the bloodstream, and its capacity for diffusion across and adhesion to blood vessels and airways and the extracellular matrix. Following intravenous injection, microparticulates in the range of 300–1000 nm typically collect in the liver, where they are phagocytised by Kupffer cells (Illum *et al.* 1982; Storm *et al.*, 1995). Particles larger than 2000 nm have a greater tendency to be trapped in the spleen, whereas those smaller than 100 nm can potentially cross blood vessel membranes and accumulate in bone marrow. Particulates larger than 10 μm are also known to lodge in lung capillaries (Al-Janabi, Moussa 1989; CIS-US package insert, *Pulmolite*, CIS-US, Bedford MA, USA). After administration by inhalation (a common approach for radioaerosol visualisation of lung ventilation), particles smaller than 2 μm in diameter have been shown to collect in alveoli, while those greater than 5 μm in diameter remain in the upper airway regions, bronchial tubes and trachea (Edwards *et al.* 1997; Bennett *et al.* 2002; Kreyling *et al.* 2006).

Whatever the route of administration, macrophages phagocytose particulates above 500 nm in diameter, while smaller particles are commonly endocytosed by both phagocytic and non-phagocytic cell types (Peltier *et al.* 1992; Aderem, Underhill 1999; Kwiatkowska, Sobota 1999; May, Machesky 2001; Rejman *et al.* 2004).

Surface chemistry

The interaction between microparticulates and the cells and tissues of the body is also highly dependent on microparticulate surface chemistry. Opsonisation often takes place in the blood circulation, where blood serum components (commonly complement proteins C3, C4, C5 and immunoglobulins) bind to the particle surface, modifying them in such a way as to promote their recognition and phagocytic engulfment by macrophages of the RES (reticuloendothelial system), thereby preventing the particle from reaching its desired target (Frank, Fries 1991; Moghimi *et al.* 2001). Particulate surface characteristics such as charge are therefore important in determining particulate serum half-life; neutral particles will have a slower opsonisation rate in comparison with those that are highly charged (Roser *et al.* 1998). Microparticulate surfaces are therefore often decorated with groups that prevent or delay opsonisation to increase plasma half-life, such as hydrophilic polymers and non-ionic surfactants like PEG (poly (ethylene glycol)) (Torchilin 1994; Storm *et al.* 1995). Functionalisation of surfaces with targeting agents can also be used to specifically direct microparticles to biologically relevant sites to demarcate a disease process. Antibodies, small molecules, carbohydrates and peptides are increasingly being used as targeting ligands for tissue or disease-specific accumulation in the brain, liver, spleen and tumours (Kreuter 2001; Peer *et al.* 2007; Kairemo *et al.* 2008). These applications will be discussed in more detail later. The surface chemistry of microparticulates is also important when considering the interaction of particles with each other. Unchecked, many microparticulates in suspension tend to agglomerate, producing poor dispersity and inhomogeneous labelling. This issue is commonly combated by functionalisation with highly charged ligands to repel each other, or branched polymers to sterically stabilise the particles in solution; however, this must obviously be undertaken with care to prevent problems associated with *in-vivo* opsonisation.

Microparticulate morphology

Many recent reviews identify particulate shape as an important parameter controlling blood half-life, suggesting that phagocytic mechanisms depend on shape recognition; long rod-shaped microparticulates are taken up in cells four times faster than short cylinders, for example (Euliss *et al.* 2006; Champion *et al.* 2007; Geng *et al.* 2007; Gratton *et al.* 2008). It is possible that mimicking of the distinctive shapes of bacteria, fungi and blood cells, may therefore ensure rapid and cell-specific uptake of microparticulates. Utilising modern methods of particle synthesis including lithography and microfluidics, it is now possible to produce a myriad of shapes that are uniform in chemistry, including boomerangs, doughnuts, cylinders and cubes, for this purpose (Euliss *et al.* 2006; Champion *et al.* 2007). While particle shape seems to be one important determinant of uptake rate, it must be appreciated that it is only one of a range of particulate properties that determines uptake and biodistribution; highly negatively charged particles have a relatively low cellular uptake rate regardless of their shape, for example (Gratton *et al.* 2008). Thus it seems that a variety of particulate properties must be addressed to achieve the 'ideal' microparticulate agent for a particular purpose.

Synthesis of particulate structures

The synthesis of nanoparticles can be achieved by a variety of methods, adopting both 'top-down' and 'bottom-up' approaches (Euliss *et al.* 2006; Champion *et al.* 2007; Ozin *et al.* 2009). 'Top-down' approaches such as ball milling (or attrition) or lithography start with a material that is then sculpted down. Ball milling mechanically degrades a starting material to yield building blocks, which are subsequently converted into bulk materials. This approach has been employed to achieve magnetic samarium–cobalt particles as small as 25 nm (Kirkpatrick *et al.* 1996), which can then be coated with gold for biological application (Berning *et al.* 2007). While attrition methods such as this can produce nanoparticles in a range of sizes, the size distribution is often wide, with variable particle morphologies.

Photolithography uses light to etch a pattern or image onto a poly(ethylene glycol) diacrylate polymer film, giving the capacity to generate microparticulates in a variety of shapes, which to date have included cubes, crosses and cylinders in the micrometre range (Meiring *et al.* 2004). Photolithography is currently the most widely used technology in the photelectronics industry, but it faces challenges with respect to its high cost and ability to reach sub-100 nm particle sizes. A recent exciting prospect is the development of IMPRINT lithography, produced at lower costs and capable of such small sizes. Here, a mask mould is brought into contact with a liquid precursor or non-wettable substrate, which is cured by heat or UV light during the printing process. Gratton *et al.* have successfully used perfluoropolyether-based elastomers (PFPEs) as moulds, which are relatively easy to then remove from the substrate, thereby generating nanoparticle cubes and cylinders with controllable size, shape and charge (Gratton *et al.* 2008).

'Bottom-up' methods are currently more popular for nanoparticle synthesis owing to their greater versatility and control over the resultant nanoparticle properties. Most approaches involve either self-assembly (creating liposomes, micelles or polymeric particles) or chemical synthesis (creating dendrimers or miniemulsions). These methods first take a nanomaterial building block, and assemble it into the final material, using either thermodynamic equilibrium or kinetic approaches. Thermodynamic equilibrium synthesis involves generating supersaturation, nucleation and growth, while kinetic approach synthesis is achieved either by limiting the respective amounts of precursors available for growth or by confining the space available for growth, by utilising micelles, for example.

Self-assembly occurs as a result of the spontaneous organisation of nanometre-scale building blocks, which may be organic, inorganic or polymeric materials, and is a common approach for the synthesis of vesicles or liposomes (Bangham, Horne 1964; De Cuyper *et al.* 2007). Liposomes consist of a phospholipid bilayer surrounding an aqueous or hydrophilic core. Under certain conditions the amphiphilic phospholipid structures will spontaneously arrange (self-assemble) to form vesicles. Not only can these vesicles be loaded with drugs, they are biocompatible and easily surface functionalised. Doxil is a clinically available 'stealth' liposome used in the treatment of ovarian cancer. Doxorubicin, an anticancer drug, is encapsulated by phospholipid layer coated in polyethylene glycol (PEG) to help avoid the immune system (Ortho-Biotech 2001). Self-assembly processes are highly dependent on the interaction between particles, their size and their shape. The surface properties of a particular particle/building block (such as charge and functionality) will affect how they interact, and thus govern the geometry and distances at which they will achieve equilibrium.

The chemical synthesis of nanoparticulate materials is commonly achieved via precipitation reactions, while various other microparticulates have been obtained using suspension or emulsion polymerisation reactions and solvent evaporation. While both inorganic and organic methods have been employed in the past, the latter are most commonly used currently, owing to recent advances in synthetic organic polymer chemistry. More recently a kinetic approach utilising microemulsion systems has been adopted, producing narrow particulate size distributions (Rauscher *et al.* 2005; Voigt *et al.* 2005). Microemulsions consist of liquid mixtures of oil and water containing a surfactant. The surfactant forms a monolayer at the interface of the oil and water phases, with the hydrophobic tails facing the oil phase and polar heads facing the water phase. The resultant micelle 'nanodroplets' formed can be used as reactors for chemical synthesis. A fission–fusion mechanism between the droplets results in a controlled micromixing process and in turn a more monodisperse particle synthesis. In this way, Munshi *et al.* have produced highly monodisperse polyacrylamide particles smaller than 100 nm in diameter, using reverse micelles as reactors for polymerisation reactions (Munshi *et al.* 1997).

Practical use

Mean particle size often varies between different products and between formulations of the same agent by different manufacturers. The resultant biodistributions of theses formulations may therefore differ significantly, and careful consideration must be employed when introducing new products or replacing one agent with another.

Particulate radiopharmaceuticals are generally commercially available as pre-formed particles of a determined size and number in the product. They may be pre-labelled with the radioisotope, ready to use (e.g. therapy applications) or require in-house radiolabelling as for ^{99m}Tc kits (via the standard reduction of pertechnetate by stannous ions).

The visual appearance of particulate suspensions should be homogeneous and, owing to possible sedimentation of the particulates, the product should be shaken or mixed before each withdrawal from the vial and measuring the radioactivity in its container. The syringe should also be swirled immediately prior to injection to prevent particles lodging in the syringe or administration line.

In-house determination of ^{99m}Tc particulate radiopharmaceuticals for particle size and numbers of particles in a specific volume of fluid may be undertaken for quality control purposes, utilising either membrane filtration methods or light microscopy (Pederson *et al.* 1981).

Nanoparticulates and microparticulates in routine use

Lung imaging

The main function of the lung is to exchange inhaled oxygen with carbon dioxide from the blood. This gas exchange takes place in the alveoli, which are small densely capillaried sac-like structures which allow diffusion of gasses between blood and air. The flow of air into and out of the lungs is referred to as ventilation, and the flow of blood through the lungs as perfusion.

Nuclear imaging of the lung (or lung scintigraphy) is widely used to visualise and quantify lung ventilation, perfusion and mucociliary clearance to aid in the diagnosis of conditions such as pulmonary thromboemboli (Secker-Walker 1968; Peltier *et al.* 1992), chronic obstructive pulmonary disease (COPD), interstitial pulmonary disease (IPD), and asthma (Sasaki *et al.* 1998; Pellegrino *et al.* 2001; Magnant *et al.* 2006). While single-photon-emitting gases like ^{133}Xe and ^{81m}Kr may be used for measuring ventilation, radiolabelled aerosol suspensions including molecular ^{99m}Tc-DTPA and the particulate ^{99m}Tc-labelled Technegas do not result in significant diagnostic differences, and have several advantages (Tägil *et al.* 2000; Hartmann *et al.* 2001; Rizzo-Padoin *et al.* 2001; Magnant *et al.* 2006). First, microparticulate size can be tailored to target different regions of the lung (Bennett *et al.* 2002); second, the greater retention time of microparticulates allows longer scan times, or sequential imaging to be performed; and third, labelling with ^{99m}Tc offers favourable radiopharmaceutical properties, such as a highly abundant 140 keV gamma-ray, a short half-life (6.01 hours), and favourable dosimetry, as well as being readily available via ^{99}Mo/^{99m}Tc generator production.

^{99m}Tc-Macroaggregated albumin (MAA)

^{99m}Tc-macroaggregated albumin (MAA) is commonly used to measure lung perfusion (Secker-Walker 1968; Schuster 1998; Sasaki *et al.* 1998; Palmer *et al.* 2001), using a number of commercially available kits (Draximage, CIS-US). ^{131}I-MAA was the first radiolabelled MAA to be used in humans (Taplin *et al.* 1964), but ^{131}I was soon replaced by the more readily available ^{99m}Tc. MAA microparticles are formed by the thermal aggregation of human serum albumin; typically, a solution of human serum albumin (HAS) is mixed with solution of stannous chloride to form Sn-MAA in a 0.1 mol/L acetate solution buffered at pH 5.4. Sample solutions are then stirred before heating to 70–80°C to form MAA aggregates. The aggregates are washed via centrifugation before resuspension in buffer solutions for labelling with [^{99m}Tc]pertechnetate (Webber *et al.* 1973; Lyster *et al.* 1974; Al-Janabi, Moussa 1989). Hunt *et al.* have produced an alternative formulation of MAA aggregates using a recombinant human albumin amid fears of contaminated blood derived agents spreading infectious diseases (Hunt *et al.* 2006).

Reproducible generation of MAA microparticulates of a specific size is fundamental to the accuracy of this technique. MAA size and labelling properties are highly dependent on temperature, stir time, pH, and reactant concentrations during preparations (Secker-Walker 1968; Al-Janabi, Moussa 1989). Adjusting preparation conditions in the aggregation step is key to controlling the final particulate properties. The introduction of a dispersing agent such as Tween 80, for example, before heating can produce a narrower size distribution (Al-Janabi, Moussa 1989).

For perfusion studies, it is recommended that 90% of the particles are within the size range 10–90 μm (although typically most are in the size range 20–40 μm), and no particles should be larger than 150 μm (Draximage, CIS-US). The average diameter of lung capillaries is around 7 μm, while the average diameter of ^{99m}Tc-MAA is considerably larger. When injected intravenously, ^{99m}Tc-MAA temporarily lodges in lung capillaries, providing the capacity to image the lung vasculature, and generate an index of lung perfusion. If pulmonary flow is normal, ^{99m}Tc-MAA distributes to the entire pulmonary area. Defects in perfusion indicate a high probability of pulmonary embolism. ^{99m}Tc-MAA is typically retained in the lung with a half-life of 1–5 hours (with larger aggregates having a longer half-life), before being broken down mechanically by the pressure of the blood, metabolised by the reticuloendothelial system, and then excreted via the kidneys (Darte *et al.* 1976; Malone *et al.* 1983). The number of particles administered per dose should be in the range 60 000–700 000 with a usual average of 400 000 particles (Bajc *et al.* 2009). A typical injection would block approximately 1% of lung capillaries, and should not exceed 1.5×10^6 microparticles carrying 148 MBq of activity, resulting in an estimated whole body radiation dose of 0.60 mGy (Draximage, CIS-US). Contraindications may include hypersensitivity to HSA, and the technique may not be suitable for patients with pulmonary hypertension (CIS-US, Draximage; Whinnery, Young 1980).

Technegas and Pertechnegas

Radioaerosols are inhaled by the patient via a nebuliser or special ventilation equipment for visualisation of lung ventilation, their lung distribution being dependent on particulate size. Droplets must be smaller than 2 μm to reach the lower regions of the lungs, and for uniform distribution throughout the lower lungs, particle sizes smaller than 0.5 μm are recommended (Edwards *et al.* 1997; Bennett *et al.* 2002; Kreyling *et al.* 2006). When targeting the central airways, particles greater than 5 μm are employed; in this way mucociliary function can be studied in pathologies such as asthma and cystic fibrosis.

Radioaerosols that have been routinely used include ^{99m}Tc-DTPA (diethylenetriamine pentaacetic acid), ^{99m}Tc-Sn-phytate, ^{99m}Tc-sulfur colloid, Technegas and Pertechnegas (Peltier *et al.* 1992; Scalzetti, Gagne 1995; Lloyd *et al.* 1995; Rizzo-Padoin *et al.* 2001; Magnant *et al.* 2006). ^{99m}Tc-DTPA is hampered by the fact that it crosses lung membranes too quickly, meaning that successive scans will differ, with knock-on effects on image quality (Brådvik *et al.* 1994). The radioaerosols ^{99m}Tc-sulfur colloid and ^{99m}Tc-Sn-phytate have slower lung clearance and help to overcome the image stability issue (Isitman *et al.* 1974; Peltier, Chatal 1986). However, ^{99m}Tc-colloid and ^{99m}Tc-phytate are known to cause intense foci of parasitic bronchial activity, as a result of accumulation in bronchial trunks, which hinders image interpretation (Peltier *et al.* 1992). Technegas and Pertechnegas, now most commonly used for ventilation studies, consist of smaller carbon-based particles. They remain stable to transmembrane transfer and have lower proximal bronchial activity.

Technegas is a ^{99m}Tc-labelled aerosol produced by evaporating pertechnetate to dryness a graphite crucible. The pertechnetate-coated crucible is then rapidly heated to 2500°C in an inert atmosphere of argon to produce a fine dust of ^{99m}Tc-labelled carbon particles (Lemb *et al.* 1993; Senden *et al.* 1997; Howarth *et al.* 1999). Faulty equipment may lead to large particles being produced, which will impair the image quality. For a typical ventilation study, approximately 40 MBq of the radioaerosol is inhaled (Administration of Radioactive Substances Advisory Committee (ARSAC) guidelines) and up to 4–6 images of the lungs are taken with up to 200 000 counts per view (Peltier *et al.* 1992; Howarth *et al.* 1999).

Technegas distributes to alveoli and distal non-ciliated airways, avoiding accumulation in the central regions of the lung (Isawa *et al.* 1991), clearing very slowly, with a biological half-life of up to 135 hours in the lung (Burch *et al.* 1986; Strong, Agnew 1989; Sasaki *et al.* 1998).

The morphology of Technegas was originally thought to resemble that of buckminsterfullerene (Burch *et al.* 1986). However, since Technegas particle sizes larger than 1 nm have been reported, this is not necessarily the case. Lemb *et al.* described Technegas as agglomerated graphite 60–160 nm particles, consisting of hexagonal primary particles 7–23 nm in size (Lemb *et al.* 1993). More recently, Senden *et al.* reported Technegas microparticles to be hexagonal platelets of metallic technetium contained within a thin layer of graphitic carbon 30–60 nm in size (Senden *et al.* 1997).

Pertechnegas is produced in a similar fashion to Technegas, but in the presence of oxygen (Scalzetti, Gagne 1995). As little as 0.1% oxygen leads to its formation rather than Technegas (Scalzetti, Gagne 1995). The particulate size is comparable to that found in Technegas (30–100 nm), while mass spectrometry reveals the presence of a variety of gas-phase technetium oxides (Mackey *et al.* 1997). In terms of image quality, Pertechnegas is much the same as Technegas. However, its distinguishing property is its rapid rate of clearance from the lungs, 7–10 minutes, which means that its biological behaviour is similar to [^{99m}Tc]pertechnetate (Monaghan *et al.* 1991; Mackey *et al.* 1997). In this respect it could be seen as advantageous to avoid a large radiation dose to the lungs.

Both ^{99m}Tc-MAA and Technegas are routinely used in lung ventilation and perfusion and studies, often used sequentially, with the images being matched (Sasaki *et al.* 1998). However, there are many non-particulate agents used for lung ventilation imaging, such as xenon-133, xenon-127, and krypton-81m. The choice is highly dependent on cost, diagnostic quality, use and safety (Rizzo-Padoin *et al.* 2001).

Reticuloendothelial system (RES) imaging

The reticuloendothelial system (RES) consists of organs containing phagocytic cells (Kupffer cells in the liver, reticular cells in lymph nodes, spleen and bone marrow, tissue histiocytes and macrophages in the lung (Sacks 1926; Marshall 1965)), whose main function is to ingest and destroy pathogens such as bacteria, protozoa and damaged cells as part of the immune response (Aderem, Underhill 1999; Kwiatkowska, Sobota 1999; May, Machesky 2001). The liver, spleen and bone marrow make up 80–90%, 5%, and 5% of RES cells, respectively. Their generally phagocytic nature makes them very amenable to imaging approaches utilising radiocolloids. Microparticles smaller than 100 nm accumulate in bone marrow, while those in the size range 300–1000 nm tend to accumulate in liver, and particles greater than 1 μm in size tend to accumulate to a greater extent in the spleen (Davis *et al.* 1974). A number of radiocolloids have been used for imaging the RES, including ^{198}Au-colloid, ^{99m}Tc-macroaggregated albumin, ^{99m}Tc-albumin colloid, ^{99m}Tc-sulfur colloid, ^{99m}Tc-Sn-colloid, and ^{99m}Tc-calcium phytate (Mundschenk *et al.* 1971; Lin, Winchell 1972; Klingensmith *et al.* 1983; Groshar *et al.* 2002).

[^{98}Au]Gold colloid

Colloidal gold first appeared as a radiopharmaceutical in the 1940s and was identified as a clinical tool for liver, bone marrow, lymph imaging in the 1950s and 1960s (Sherman, Ter-Pogossian 1953; Carter, Ankeney 1964; Edwards *et al.* 1964; Sage *et al.* 1964). Colloidal gold has also been applied as a radiotherapeutic agent in the treatment of arthritis and certain cancers by intracavity injection (Swanson 1949; Fountain, Malkasian Jr 1981). Although still available commercially in some countries, it has largely been superseded by other radiocolloids for imaging purposes due to its undesirable beta- and high gamma-radiation doses. To this end, it is reviewed purely from a historical point of view as one of the first colloidal particulates.

Gold-198 decays with a half-life of 2.7 days, emitting a high-energy gamma-ray (412 keV) and beta-particle (0.96 MeV). While the beta-radiation has applications in radiation therapy, in terms of imaging, the high radiation dose may cause radiation necrosis and damage to organs such as the liver, kidney and spleen (Upton *et al.* 1956).

A comprehensive study and synthesis of colloidal gold particles from gold chloride and sodium citrate was first completed by Faraday in 1857 (Faraday 1857). Methods remain much the same today, reducing chlorauric acid (Au^{3+}, $HAuCl_4$) to Au(0) with sodium citrate (Turkevich *et al.* 1951; Turkevich *et al.* 1953), the resultant particles being in the size range 10–30 nm (Milligan, Morriss 1964), making them ideal for localisation in bone marrow and lymphoscintigraphy (discussed below). However, bone marrow imaging was largely redundant until the advent of preferable ^{99m}Tc colloids. Although originally attributed to pharmacological toxicity, the pathological effects of colloidal gold microparticles are actually mediated by the associated radiation exposure. Colloidal gold therefore still represents a versatile platform for biomedical applications (Glomm 2005; Sharma *et al.* 2006). In the early 1990s Giersig, Mulvaney prepared stabilised gold particles capped with thiol groups, making them soluble in non-polar solvents and amenable to diverse reactions (Giersig, Mulvaney 1993). The thiol groups can also be used as an anchor for surface functionalisation with other ligands and molecules, in preparation for biological applications (Brust, Kiely 2002).

^{99m}Tc-Sulphur colloid

^{99m}Tc-Sulphur colloid has a blood clearance half-life of 2–2.5 minutes by the RES (Frier *et al.* 1981; Kashiwaya *et al.* 1994; Manchester *et al.* 1994). Uptake depends on blood flow to the particular organ and content of phagocytic cells. For liver and spleen imaging, the recommended dose is between 37 and 296 MBq, and for bone marrow imaging a dose of 111–444 MBq is recommended (Malinkrodt-US 1985; CIS-US 2002). Around 90% accumulates in the liver, with 5–10% distributing to the spleen and bone marrow, dependent on kit formulation (Frier *et al.* 1981).

^{99m}Tc-Sulphur colloid was first developed by Harper *et al.* in 1964. Preparation involved bubbling hydrogen sulfide gas through an acidified solution of sodium pertechnetate, using gelatin as a stabilising agent (Harper *et al.* 1964). However, the requirement for purification made for an impracticably long synthesis. Today, commercial kits are based on methods developed by Stern and Larson and colleagues (Larson, Nelp 1966; Stern *et al.* 1966). Pertechnetate is reacted with sodium thiosulfate and acid in the presence of carboxymethylcellulose as a stabilising agent. Sulfur colloid kits are commercially available with different formulations (Krogsgaard 1976; Kashiwaya *et al.* 1994; Manchester *et al.* 1994), used for liver, spleen, marrow and lymphoscintigraphy (Petasnick, Gottschalk 1966; Mundschenk *et al.* 1971; Klingensmith *et al.* 1983; Hung *et al.* 1995; Eshima *et al.* 1996).

Typically for thiosulfate kit procedures, 15% of particles generated are less than 0.1 µm, 80% in the range 0.1–1.0 µm, and 5% greater than 1 µm (Davis *et al.* 1974). For lymphoscintigraphy, particle size is particularly important, requiring particles smaller than 0.1 µm to ensure uptake in the lymph nodes (Strand, Persson 1978; Bergqvist *et al.* 1983; Eshima *et al.* 1996). In an attempt to produce narrower size ranges and smaller particle sizes, colloidal preparations have been filtered to achieve average sizes of 10 nm and 38 nm (Hung *et al.* 1995; Eshima *et al.* 1996). Traditional labelling procedures currently involve heating to increase the rate of ^{99m}Tc incorporation (Larson, Nelp 1966; Stern *et al.* 1966). However, such heating encourages agglomeration, and is therefore a confounding factor when attempting to obtain appropriately small particle sizes. As such, there is commonly a trade-off between particle size and rate of production.

More recently, alternatives for imaging the RES have become favourable. The labelling procedures and formulation of sulphur colloid kits are commercially undesirable, involving multiple steps. ^{99m}Tc-albumin colloid (nanocolloid), antimony sulfide and ^{99m}Tc-phytate (Hamilton *et al.* 1977; Martindale *et al.* 1980) are some alternative examples used for bone marrow imaging.

Lymphoscintigraphy

Lymph node imaging is used for imaging lymphatic obstruction, for example in cases of lymphoedema, but sentinel node imaging has driven the most recent interest in colloidal nanoparticulates. Sentinel lymph nodes (SLNs) are the first lymph nodes receiving lymph draining directly from a tumour site, and are therefore the most likely to be in involved in metastatic disease (Kapteijn *et al.* 1997; Krag *et al.* 1998). Many solid tumours, including breast cancer, prostate cancer, malignant melanoma, head and neck cancers and penile and gynaecological (cervical, vulval) cancers spread via lymphatic drainage, and the presence of lymph node metastases is an important prognostic biomarker.

The aim of SLN imaging is to find the precise location of the node for biopsy and to detect microscopic nodal disease by identifying all potentially involved nodes. This approach offers significantly higher sensitivity than traditional blue dye methods (De Cicco *et al.* 1998). Selective biopsy of the sentinel node offers an alternative diagnostic procedure for tumour staging rather than removing all regional lymph nodes, which often leads to lymphoedema (Cabanas 1977; Wilhelm *et al.* 1999). A wide variety of radiopharmaceuticals have been used for SLN lymphoscintigraphy including ^{99m}Tc-labelled dextran (Henze *et al.* 1982), ^{99m}Tc- HSA (Bedrosian *et al.* 1999), [^{198}Au]gold colloid (Sage *et al.* 1964), ^{99m}Tc-stannous phytate (Alavi *et al.* 1978), ^{99m}Tc-sulfur colloid (^{99m}Tc-SC) (Hung *et al.* 1995; Eshima *et al.* 1996), ^{99m}Tc-antimony trisulfide colloid (^{99m}Tc-ATC) (Alazraki *et al.* 1997; Wilhelm *et al.* 1999) and ^{99m}Tc-colloidal albumin (^{99m}Tc-CA (nanocolloid)) (Rink *et al.* 2001) and ^{99m}Tc-colloidal rhenium sulfide (Watanabe et al. 2001).

After interstitial injection, particulates are transported by the lymphatic system, localising via drainage into the lymph nodes. For melanoma, colloids are administered intradermally or subcutaneously; for breast cancer, intratumoral or peritumoral administration have also been successfully used (Wilhelm *et al.* 1999). Both stability and particle size are again important factors here. Particles must be absorbed by peripheral lymph receptors before entering the lymph system and must be smaller than 100 nm to reach the lymph nodes (Strand, Persson 1978; Bergqvist *et al.* 1983; Ikomi *et al.* 1995), but larger than 5 nm to avoid penetration into capillary membranes and subsequent filtration and excretion (Henze *et al.* 1982). Optimal uptake has been observed for particulates in the size range 5–15 nm (Strand, Persson 1978).

Inflammation and infection imaging

Inflammation scintigraphy is frequently used to identify and localise pulmonary and abdominal infections and fevers of unknown origin, and to distinguish tumours from inflammation (McAfee, Thakur 1976; Pike 1991; Hughes 2003). Early approaches attempted to use leukocyte phagocytosis of sulfur, gold and albumin colloids, but poor labelling efficiency and label stability have generally proved to be significant limiting factors (Hanna, Lomas 1986). Non-phagocytic approaches utilising white blood cells labelled with ^{111}In-oxine and ^{99m}Tc-HMPAO have therefore largely replaced these early colloidal approaches. ^{111}In-oxine and ^{111}In-tropololnate (McAfee, Thakur 1976) have both demonstrated accuracy and sensitivity in the detection of bowel disease (Saverymuttu *et al.* 1981); however, ^{111}In radiopharmaceuticals are expensive compared with ^{99m}Tc. While radiolabelling yields are high, cell labelling in general involves lengthy procedures owing to the non-specificity of the labelling procedures, requiring leukocyte separation from whole blood before labelling. Therefore, interest is returning to colloidal radiopharmaceuticals for leukocyte labelling using colloidal stannous fluoride (SnF_2). ^{99m}Tc-SnF_2 is widely available in Europe and Australia, cheap to produce, and capable of directly and specifically labelling leukocytes in whole blood without the need for time consuming or complicated separation methods (Schroth *et al.* 1981).

Stannous fluoride colloid

Stannous fluoride colloid, ^{99m}Tc-SnF_2, is a commercially available radiopharmaceutical, primarily used to radiolabel leukocytes for imaging inflammation and infection; the mode of this labelling is currently unclear, but may involve phagocytosis, specific cell surface adherence, or even both (Hanna *et al.* 1984; Hanna, Lomas 1986; Mock, English 1987; Boyd *et al.* 1993; Tsopelas *et al.* 2003; Tsopelas 2006). The biological clearance of labelled leukocytes in the blood and lung is rapid, with biological half-lives of 1.2 and 2.7 hours, respectively. Clearance is slow in the liver, spleen and bone marrow, remaining constant over 15 hours.

^{99m}Tc-SnF_2 colloids comprise aggregates of coiled and branched chains ranging from 0.1 to 3 µm in diameter, which can be narrowed to 0.33 to 1.12 µm using a 0.1 µm filter (McClelland *et al.* 2003). Particle size has previously been shown to be the single most important factor affecting phagocytic engulfment of

^{99m}Tc stannous colloid, with the optimal mean particle size being 2.1 μm (Hanna, Lomas 1986). Various labelling procedures have been described (Schroth *et al.* 1981; Hanna, Lomas 1986; Mock, English 1987; Hirsch *et al.* 1989), but the work of Hanna *et al.* in 1984, demonstrating that using fresh stannous fluoride improved labelling efficiency and cell viability and reduced spleen and liver uptake (Hanna *et al.* 1984), has endured as the core of most commercially available kits, such as the Radpharm Scientific Leukocyte Labelling Kit (RadPharm-Scientific 2008). The colloid is first prepared by mixing the aqueous sodium fluoride with stannous fluoride; then it is filtered and [^{99m}Tc]pertechnetate is added. The mixture is incubated for 1 hour, producing radiolabelled stannous fluoride colloid in high radiochemical yield (99%) (RadPharm-Scientific 2008). This colloid is then incubated in whole blood for 1 hour to specifically label leukocytes.

Other diagnostic uses of radiopharmaceutical particulates

Blood pool imaging and shunts

Intravenous administration of ^{99m}Tc-colloids (which do not bind to red blood cells) has been used in the detection of gastrointestinal bleeds, but this has been superseded by techniques that label red blood cells with ^{99m}Tc directly. ^{99m}Tc-MAA is also used to assess arteriovenous anastomoses, or shunts, where there is a breakthrough from arterioles to venules, characteristic of tumour vasculature, and particularly common in primary and metastatic liver cancers. Such shunts are problematic in that therapeutic microspheres could potentially bypass their tumour target and lodge in radiosensitive non-tumour tissues such as the lung. Assessing the extent of shunting utilising ^{99m}Tc-MAA is therefore useful in determining suitability of treatment and appropriate dosing regimes for selective internal radiation therapy using therapeutic radiopharmaceuticals.

Gastrointestinal Imaging

Radionuclide imaging of the gastrointestinal tract with microparticulates allows functional evaluation of oesophageal transit, gastro-oesophageal reflux and gastric emptying. Various particulates have been used for these purposes, including sulfur colloids, rhenium and antimony sulfide, and MAA (Taillefer *et al.* 1987; Nightingale *et al.* 1993; Bestetti *et al.* 2000). The radiolabelled colloid is incorporated into specific liquid or solid foods (e.g. mashed potato, porridge, scrambled egg) and is ingested by the patient.

Radionuclide therapy

Microparticulates have been employed to deliver a localised dose of beta-emitting radionuclides for the therapy of rheumatoid arthritis and some cancers. Microparticulates can be injected such that they become trapped within a desired target, such as inside a joint, localised within a body cavity, or directly injected inside a tumour. While many of these approaches are non-specific, there is increasing research into site-specific targeting of particulates to cellular or vascular receptors by conjugating particulates with peptides or antibodies.

Synovectomy

Inflammatory joint disease affects at least 1% of the world's population (Jacobson *et al.* 1997). Synovial joints consist of a fibrous capsule, ligaments and articular discs. Inside the capsule is a synovial lining, composed of two cells types, phagocytic (type A) and fibroblast-like (type B) synoviocytes. In inflammatory conditions, the type A synoviocyte predominates, resulting in swelling and enlargement of the synovial membrane and increased synovial fluid secretion (Firestein 1996; Iwanaga *et al.* 2000).

Rheumatoid arthritis and synovial disease are typically treated by systemic antirheumatic therapies such as non-steroidal anti-inflammatory drugs (NSAIDs), glucocorticoids and disease-modifying antirheumatic drugs (DMARDs) (Smith 2005). When these traditional therapies fail, local articular radiotherapeutic treatments such as synovectomy can be applied. Radioparticulates can be used for ablation of the synovial lining, thereby decreasing fluid secretion, and reducing intra-articular pressure. Since synoviocytes phagocytose particulates, they are also a useful target for microparticulate-mediated irradiation.

The importance of particulate size is not completely understood, but generally, smaller particles tend to leak from the joint space; resulting in their undesirable accumulation in the reticuloendothelial system (Gedik *et al.* 2006). Colloidal gold particles in the size range 20–30 nm result in a leakage of 3–18% (Virkkunen *et al.* 1967), while a particulate size of 300 nm results in a more acceptable leakage of 1% (Correns *et al.* 1969). Preparations with a mean particle size between 2 and 5 μm have favourable cellular uptake, with minimal extra-articular leakage by lymphatic or venous drainage.

Early examples of radiocolloids used for synovectomy include chromic [^{32}P]phosphate (Winston *et al.* 1973) and [^{198}Au]gold colloids (Ansell *et al.* 1963), which have been superseded by ^{90}Y-colloids (e.g. silicate, resin, citrate), and ^{186}Re-sulfide (Klett *et al.* 2007), ^{169}Er-citrate (Manil *et al.* 2001), ^{188}Re-tin colloid (Shukla *et al.* 2007), ^{177}Lu-hydroxyapatite (Chakraborty *et al.* 2006) and ^{166}Ho-macroaggregates (Kraft *et al.* 2007), and ^{165}Dy-ferric hydroxide macroaggregates (FHMA) (Barnes *et al.* 1994). The choice of radionuclide depends largely on its ability to penetrate tissues, and on its half-life, which must be sufficient to impart the prerequisite dose but not so long as to cause damage to bone, cartilage or skin. Table 25.2 lists some properties of radionuclides used (Klett *et al.* 2007).

Yttrium-90 citrate colloid (^{90}YCC)

Yttrium-90 colloids are widely used for synovectomy, predominantly in knee joints (Gumpel *et al.* 1974; Gumpel 1978; Kampen *et al.* 2006; Chrapko *et al.* 2007) and are commercially available throughout Europe in two different forms, resin and citrate, and previously as silicate (now discontinued in Europe).

A typical routine kit preparation, such as YMM-1, ^{90}Y-citrate, (CISBio-International 2008) has the following composition: a colloidal suspension with a pH between 5.5 and 7.5, radiochemical purity no less then 95%. The colloidal suspension of ^{90}YCC is administered via intra-articular injection and a recommended activity of 111–222 MBq per joint. Fifty per cent of the particles have an average diameter between 3 and 6 μm (CISBio-International 2008).

Table 25.2 Properties of radionuclides used for synovectomy[a]

Isotope	$t_{1/2}$	Penetration depth	Joint suitability
^{90}Y	2.7 days	2.8 mm	Large joints – knee
^{186}Re	9.4 days	1.0 mm	Medium joints – hip, shoulder, wrists
^{169}Er	3.7 days	0.3 mm	Small joints – fingers, toes

[a] Adapted from Klett *et al.* (2007).

Malignant pleural effusions and peritoneal ascites

Recurrent malignant pleural effusions in the chest or peritoneum in abdominal cavities, as a result of ovarian or renal cell cancers, for example, have been treated with [^{198}Au]gold-colloid (Mohlen and Beller 1979), colloidal chromic [^{32}P]phosphate (Young *et al.* 2003) and ^{90}Y-silicate. These approaches are generally used when conventional chemotherapy or radiotherapy has failed. The radioparticulates are instilled directly into a body cavity for local therapy. The localisation is non-selective, depositing randomly on the cavity surfaces, requiring the patient to be rotated and change position to mix the colloid suspension within the intracavity fluid. A more targeted approach is being sought with radioimmunotherapy.

Treatment of hepatocellular cancer

If a primary liver tumour or its metastases are in an inoperable position, radioparticulates may be used to reduce symptoms and improve quality of life, or to shrink large tumours to enable surgical resection. The dominance of hepatic arterial blood flow to tumour tissue is exploited as normal hepatic tissue receives the majority of blood flow from the portal vein. With intra-arterial administration, the particulate radiopharmaceutical is implanted directly into a tumour, lodging preferentially in the capillaries feeding the tumour to deliver a radiation dose to the surrounding tissue.

^{90}Y-Microspheres

Radioparticulates used in the treatment of hepatocellular cancer include SIR-Spheres (Sirtex Medical) and Theraspheres (MDS Nordion). SIR-Spheres are a suspension of biocompatible resin microspheres, between 20 and 60 μm in diameter, containing ^{90}Y. The dose administered may range between 1.5 and 3 GBq with a typical 3–8 million microspheres delivered per dose, based on the estimated degree of tumour involvement in the liver or patient body surface area. TheraSpheres are ^{90}Y glass microspheres with a mean particle size of 20–30 μm with 30–60 million microspheres delivered per dose. The lower particle size prevents the microspheres passing from the tumour vasculature and into the venous circulation. The microspheres do not degrade and remain permanently trapped within the tumour vasculature. TheraSpheres have been studied more in HCC and SIR-Spheres more in liver metastases. There are no direct comparative studies between the two products, but a review found that 3-month response rates and toxicity profiles were comparable between TheraSpheres and SIR-Spheres (Kennedy *et al.* 2005).

Other agents under development for hepatic tumours include ^{177}Lu-hydroxypatite with particle diameters of 20–60 μm (Chakraborty *et al.* 2008), ^{166}Ho-loaded poly(L-lactic acid) microspheres (^{166}Ho-PLLA-MS) with 92–96% of particles between 20–50 μm (Zielhuis *et al.* 2006), and ^{16}Ho-alginate microspheres with a mean size of 159 μm (Zielhuis *et al.* 2007). Whereas ^{90}Y is a pure beta emitter, ^{166}Ho is a combined beta–gamma emitter and highly paramagnetic. It therefore offers imaging possibilities, through both single-photon emission computed tomography (SPECT) and magnetic resonance imaging (MRI).

Particulates in cancer imaging and therapy

The current use of particulates in tumour and cancer therapy is mainly limited to intracavity or intratumoral injection. This approach is significantly hampered, however, by radionuclide leakage from the site of injection. As previously mentioned, the functionalisation of nanoparticles is a highly active field of research, with biological targeting of molecules such as peptides, proteins and nucleic acids imparting specificity for a particular target. The large surface area of microparticulates has the potential to allow multiple imaging radionuclides or a high therapeutic payload to be conjugated to the particle surface. The surface can be functionalised by a variety of groups, offering the opportunity to introduce different agents simultaneously for multimodality imaging, for example, or for simultaneously delivering a drug or radionuclide payload, as well as providing biodistribution information by imaging.

Targeting strategies for cancer therapy and imaging

Passive targeting

Nanoparticles passively accumulate in tumours through an effect called enhanced permeability and retention (EPR). The rapid and poorly controlled growth of tumour blood vessels results in large gaps (up to 800 nm across) between tumour endothelial cells (Hobbs *et al.* 1998). Tumours also lack an effective lymph drainage system. These effects combine to produce a leaky, tortuous vasculature that is predisposed to retaining nanoparticles in the range 10–100 nm (Sunderland *et al.* 2006; Kairemo *et al.* 2008). Utilising nanoparticles in this size range, and making them hydrophilic (to avoid plasma protein adsorption), optimises their capacity for passive uptake in small tumours of this type. Further modification in terms of size and surface properties to avoid uptake by macrophages in the RES can also be used to optimise them for passive targeting approaches.

Active targeting

In larger tumours with larger and more patent blood vessels, passive uptake is less prevalent. Nanoparticle accumulation is therefore augmented by conjugation of biological molecules that bind preferentially to specific tumour cell antigens or receptors. The folic acid receptor, angiogenic markers such as the αvβ3 integrins, and specific antigens for monoclonal antibodies expressed by tumour cells have all been used for this purpose (Schiffelers *et al.* 2003; Itoa *et al.* 2004; Park *et al.* 2004; Sun *et al.* 2006). The cell surface expression of receptors and antigens offers a pathway for nanoparticle/drug uptake via receptor-mediated endocytosis. Glycoproteins cannot remove polymer-conjugated drugs from cells that have entered via endocytosis, and therefore also hold some promise in overcoming multidrug resistance (MDR).

To date, the use of nanoparticulates in nuclear medicine involving these targeted approaches is limited to research rather than clinical exploitation, but examples are becoming ever more frequent. Some more recent examples involving bioconjugates for both active and passive targeted delivery include the use of ^{211}At (Kučkaa *et al.* 2006), ^{188}Re (Bao *et al.* 2003), ^{64}Cu (Rossin *et al.* 2005), ^{18}F (Devaraj *et al.* 2009), ^{153}Sm (Ascencio *et al.* 2005), and ^{111}In (DeNardo *et al.* 2005). Rossin *et al.* (2005) developed ^{64}Cu-radiolabelled folate conjugated to shell cross-linked nanoparticles (SCKs) to target tumours expressing the folate receptor. The SCKs were functionalised with folate, fluorescein thiosemicarbazide, and 1,4,8,11-tetraazacyclotetradecane-*N*,*N*′,*N*″,*N*‴-tetra-acetic acid (TETA) (Rossin *et al.* 2005).

DeNardo *et al.* have prepared ^{111}In-Chimeric (ChL6) monoclonal antibody (mAb) bioprobes for thermal ablation of cancer cells. ^{111}In-DOTA-(ChL6)-mAb was conjugated to poly(ethylene glycol) (PEG) on an iron oxide core. Anti-tumour monoclonal antibody (mAb) targets the particles to specific cancer cells where an alternating magnetic field can induce thermal therapy (DeNardo *et al.* 2005).

Kučkaa *et al.* have designed astatine-labelled nanoparticles for accumulation in smaller tumours by virtue of the EPR effect. The affinity of astatine for silver was exploited via the use of silver nanoparticles. The silver core was covalently coated with a poly(ethylene oxide) (PEO) shell to help avoid opsonisation (Kučkaa *et al.* 2006).

Liposomes in cancer therapy and imaging

Liposomes can be used as nanocarriers for the delivery of drugs or imaging agents (Torchilin 1994; Torchilin, Trubetskoy 1995; Bao *et al.* 2003; Bao *et al.* 2004). Drugs/agents can be entrapped in the aqueous space or intercalated into the bilayer itself. It is also possible to modify the surface of the particles to alter their pharmacological profile or introduce a targeting functionality. Attachment of the hydrophilic polymer poly (ethylene glycol) (PEG) is a common modification to avoid degradation and minimise toxicity. Liposomes are typically in the diameter range 80–300 nm, and in this respect their passive uptake and accumulation in tumours may be limited by their large size. They are therefore better suited to active targeting approaches in larger tumours. Larger liposomes will accumulate in the RES system, potentially giving a high radiation dose to bone marrow, spleen and liver. A direction for future research is the generation and labelling of smaller unilaminar liposomes, which may overcome this problem.

Two approaches can be taken for incorporation of the radionuclide. First, the radionuclide can be entrapped within the liposome aqueous space, either during liposome formulation or through the use of a suitable chelating agent that will pass through the lipid layer. Examples of lipophilic chelators used include hexamethylpropyleneamine oxime (HMPAO) and diethylenetriaminepentaacetic acid (DTPA) (Espinola *et al.* 1979; Goins *et al.* 1994). Second, the chelating agent can be derivatised with a hydrophobic anchor that will embed itself in the lipid bilayers, such that chelating agent is studded on the liposome, surface ready for chelation. DTPA has been bound to long-chain hydrocarbons (stearylamine-DTPA) and used to chelate ^{67}Ga and ^{99m}Tc to the surface of liposomes in this manner (Hnatowich *et al.* 1981). A great number of studies involving the development of liposomes for nuclear imaging have been undertaken in recent years, most commonly including radiolabelling with ^{99m}Tc (Bao *et al.* 2004), ^{111}In (Syrigos *et al.* 2003), ^{186}Re (Bao *et al.* 2003) and ^{67}Ga (Ogihara *et al.* 1986). Many of them demonstrate good accumulation in tumours and sites of inflammation (Phillips *et al.* 2009) and are likely to become increasingly prevalent in clinical practice in the future.

Towards dual modality

Dual modality is an increasingly desirable approach for medical and experimental imaging. Combining imaging modalities potentially provides complementary information, and allows the advantages of one technique to compensate for the shortcomings of another. PET/CT and SPECT/CT machines are now the clinical norm, allowing the superimposition of high-sensitivity biological information on high-resolution structural images. The next generation of these hybrid imaging machines is likely to combine PET and MRI. MRI has significant advantages over CT as a complementary technique, in that not only does it provide high resolution structural detail but it provides a host of other biophysical datasets, such as blood oxygenation and spectroscopic information, and itself has a host of contrast agents for providing more than just anatomical information. The fact that it is a non-ionising technique (unlike CT) is also an advantage in limiting the radiation dose that a patient is exposed to. The design of 'smart' multimodality nanoparticles to exploit emerging PET/MR technology is therefore an attractive proposal. Nanoparticles are widely used in MRI to deliver a large local concentration of contrast agent, thereby overcoming MRI's low inherent sensitivity (in the millimolar range). Most MRI contrast agents utilise either iron or gadolinium to modify the relaxation characteristics of protons in surrounding water molecules to provide contrast, although other approaches such as [^{19}F]perfluorocarbon-filled liposomes are also being explored (Winter *et al.* 2007). It would therefore seem likely that these agents would constitute any multimodal contrast agent, while the PET component is potentially more flexible. Although the MRI and PET component of these agents need not necessarily be isotopes of the same element, it may be an advantage in terms of their chemistry and synthesis. Likely PET/MR pairings for such approaches would therefore potentially be ^{52}Fe/^{56}Fe, or ^{18}F/^{19}F.

References

Aderem A, Underhill DM (1999). Mechanisms of phagocytosis in macrophages. *Ann Rev Immunol* 17: 593–623.

Alavi A *et al.* (1978). Technetium 99m stannous phytate as an imaging agent for lymph nodes. *J Nucl Med* 19: 422–426.

Alazraki NP *et al.* (1997). Lymphoscintigraphy, the sentinel node concept, and the intraoperative gamma probe in melanoma, breast cancer, and other potential cancers. *Semin Nucl Med* 27: 55–67.

Al-Janabi MA, Moussa SO (1989). A modified procedure for the preparation of macroaggregated albumin (MAA) kits to be labelled with ^{99m}Tc for lung scanning. *J Labelled Compd Radiopharm* 28: 519–523.

Ansell BM *et al.* (1963). Evaluation of intra-articular colloidal gold Au-198 in the treatment of persistant knee infusions. *Ann Rheum Dis* 22: 435–439.

Ascencio JA *et al.* (2005). Synthesis and theoretical analysis of samarium nanoparticles: perspectives in nuclear medicine. *J Phys Chem B* 109: 8806–8812.

Bajc M *et al.* (2009). EANM guidelines for ventilation/perfusion scintigraphy. Part 1. Pulmonary imaging with ventilation/perfusion single photon emission tomography. *Eur J Nucl Med Mol Imaging* 36: 1356–1370.

Bangham AD, Horne RW (1964). Negative staining of phospholipids and their structural modification by surface-active agents as observed in the electron microscope. *J Mol Biol* 8: 660–668.

Bao A *et al.* (2003). ^{186}Re-liposome labeling using ^{186}Re-SNS/S complexes: in vitro stability, imaging, and biodistribution in rats. *J Nucl Med* 44: 1992–1999.

Bao A *et al.* (2004). Direct ^{99m}Tc labeling of pegylated liposomal doxorubicin (Doxil) for pharmacokinetic and non-invasive imaging studies. *J Pharmacol Exp Ther* 308: 419–425.

Barnes CL *et al.* (1994). Intra-articular radiation treatment of rheumatoid synovitis of the ankle with dysprosium-165 ferric hydroxide macroaggregates. *Foot Ankle Int* 15(6): 306–310.

Bedrosian I *et al.* (1999). ^{99m}Tc-Human serum albumin: an effective radiotracer for identifying sentinel lymph nodes in melanoma. *J Nucl Med* 40: 1143–1148.

Bennett WD *et al.* (2002). Targeting delivery of aerosols to different lung regions. *J Aerosol Med* 15: 179–188.

Bergqvist L *et al.* (1983). Particle sizing and biokinetics of interstitial lymphoscintigraphic agents. *Sem Nucl Med* 13: 9–19.

Berning, D E. *et al.* (2007). Gold-coated nanoparticles for use in biotechnology applications. Los Alamos, NM: United States Los Alamos National Security, LLC. http://www.freepatentsonline.com/7226636.html (accessed 2 July 2010).

Bestetti A *et al.* (2000). ^{99m}Tc-sulfur colloid gastroesophageal scintigraphy with late lung imaging to evaluate patients with posterior laryngitis. *J Nucl Med* 10: 1597–1602.

Boyd SJ *et al.* (1993). Evaluation of white cell scintigraphy using indium-Ill and technetium-99m labelled leucocytes. *Eur J Nucl Med* 20: 201–206.

Brådvik I *et al.* (1994). Different kinetics of lung clearance of technetium-99m labelled diethylene triamine penta-acetic acid in patients with sarcoidosis and smokers. *Eur J Nucl Med* 21: 1218–1222.

Brust M, Kiely CJ (2002). Some recent advances in nanostructure preparation from gold and silver particles: a short topical review. *Surf A Physicochem Eng Aspects* 202: 175–186.

Burch WM *et al.* (1986). Technegas – a new ventilation agent for lung scanning. *Nucl Med Commun* 7: 865–871.

Cabanas RM (1977). An approach for the treatment of penile carcinoma. *Cancer* 39: 456–466.

Carter TL, Ankeney JL (1964). Hepatic blood flow determined by colloidal gold clearance compared with direct flow measurements. *J Nucl Med* 5: 901–912.

Chakraborty S *et al.* (2006). Preparation and preliminary biological evaluation of ^{177}Lu-labelled hydroxyapatite as a promising agent for radiation synovectomy of small joints. *Nucl Med Commun* 27(8): 661–668.

Chakraborty S *et al.* (2008). Preparation and preliminary studies on ^{177}Lu-labeled hydroxyapatite particles for possible use in the therapy of liver cancer. *Nucl Med Bio* 35(5): 589–597.

Champion JA *et al.* (2007). Particle shape: a new design parameter for micro- and nanoscale drug delivery carriers. *J Control Release* 121: 3–9.

Chrapko B *et al.* (2007). Radiation synovectomy with ^{90}Y colloid in the therapy of recurrent knee joint effusions in patients with inflammatory joint diseases. *Rheumatol Int* 27: 729–734.

CISBIO-International (2008). Package insert, YMM-1: Yttrium [90Y] citrate colloid. Cèze: CisBio International.

CIS-US (2002). Package insert, *CIS-Sulfur Colloid.* Bedford MA: CIS-US.

CIS-US Package insert, *Pulmolite.* Bedford MA: CIS-US.

Correns H *et al.* (1969). Intraartikuläre Behandlung der chronischen Polyarthritis mit grob-kolloidalem Au-198. *Radiobiol Radiother* 10: 505–509.

Darte L *et al.* (1976). Quality control and testing of ^{99m}Tc-macroaggregated albumin. *Nuklearmedizin* 15: 80–85.

Davis MA *et al.* (1974). A rapid and accurate method for sizing radiocolloids. *J Nucl Med* 15: 623–628.

De Cicco C *et al.* (1998). Intraoperative localization of the sentinel node in breast cancer: technical aspects of lymphoscintigraphic methods. *Semin Surg Oncol* 15: 268–271.

De Cuyper M *et al.* (2007). Surface functionalization of magnetoliposomes in view of improving iron oxide-based magnetic resonance imaging contrast agents: anchoring of gadolinium ions to a lipophilic chelate. *Anal Biochem* 367: 266–273.

DeNardo SJ *et al.* (2005). Development of tumor targeting bioprobes ^{111}In-chimeric L6 monoclonal antibody nanoparticles) for alternating magnetic field cancer therapy. *Clin Cancer Res* 11: 7087–7092.

Devaraj NK *et al.* (2009). ^{18}F labeled nanoparticles for in vivo PET-CT imaging. *Bioconjug Chem* 20: 397–401.

Dunne M *et al.* (2000). Influence of particle size and dissolution conditions on the degradation properties of polylactide-coglycolide particles. *Biomaterials* 21: 1659–1668.

Edwards CL *et al.* (1964). Clinical bone marrow scanning with radioisotopes. *Blood* 23: 741–756.

Edwards DA *et al.* (1997). Large porous particles for pulmonary drug delivery. *Science* 276: 1868–1871.

Eshima D *et al.* (1996). Technetium-99m-sulfur colloid for lymphoscintigraphy: effects of preparation parameters. *J Nucl Med* 37: 1575–1578.

Espinola LG *et al.* (1979). Radiolabeled liposomes as metabolic and scanning tracers in mice. II. In-111 oxine compared with Tc-99m DTPA, entrapped in multilamellar lipid vesicles. *J Nucl Med* 20: 434–440.

Euliss LE *et al.* (2006). Imparting size, shape, and composition control of materials for nanomedicine. *Chem Soc Rev*, 1095–1104.

Faraday M (1857). Experimental relations of gold (and other metals) to light. *Phil Trans R Soc Lond* 147: 145–181.

Firestein GS (1996). Invasive fibroblast-like synoviocytes in rheumatoid arthritis. Passive responders or transformed aggressors? *Arthritis Rheum* 39: 1781–1790.

Fountain KS, Malkasian GD Jr (1981). Radioactive colloidal gold in the treatment of endometrial cancer: Mayo Clinic experience, 1952–1976. *Cancer* 47: 2430–2432.

Frank MM, Fries LF (1991). The role of complement in inflammation and phagocytosis. *Immunol Today* 12: 322–326.

Frier M *et al.* (1981). The biological fate of sulphur colloid. *Eur J Nucl Med* 6: 371–374.

Gedik GK *et al.* (2006). Comparison of extraarticular leakage values of radiopharmaceuticals used for radionuclide synovectomy. *Ann Nucl Med* 20: 183–188.

Geng Y *et al.* (2007). Shape effects of filaments versus spherical particles in flow and drug delivery. *Nat Nanotechnol* 2: 249–255.

Giersig M, Mulvaney P (1993). Preparation of ordered colloid monolayers by electrophoretic deposition. *Langmuir* 9: 3408–3413.

Glomm WR (2005). Functionalized gold nanoparticles for applications in bionanotechnology. *J Dispers Sci Technol* 26: 389–414.

Goins B *et al.* (1994). Use of technetium-99m-liposomes in tumor imaging. *J Nucl Med* 35: 1491–1498.

Gratton SEA *et al.* (2008). The effect of particle design on cellular internalization pathways. *Proct Natl Acad Sci U S A* 105: 11613–11618.

Groshar D *et al.* (2002). Quantitation of liver and spleen uptake of ^{99m}Tc-Phytate colloid using SPECT: detection of liver cirrhosis. *J Nucl Med* 43: 312–317.

Gumpel JM (1978). Intra articular yttrium 90 in rabbits. Comparison of behaviour of various radiocolloids in rabbits and in man. *Ann Rheum Dis* 37: 195–197.

Gumpel JM *et al.* (1974). Use of yttrium 90 in persistent synovitis of the knee. II. Direct comparison of yttrium colloid resin and yttrium citrate. *Ann Rheum Dis* 33: 126–128.

Hamilton RG *et al.* (1977). Technetium 99m phytate as a bone marrow imaging agent: biodistribution studies in animals. *J Nucl Med* 18: 563–565.

Hanna RW, Lomas FE (1986). Identification of factors affecting technetium 99m leucocyte labelling by phagocytic engulfment and development of an optimal technique. *Eur J Nucl Med* 12: 159–162.

Hanna R *et al.* (1984). Radiochemistry and biostability of autologous leucocytes labelled with ^{99m}Tc-stannous colloid in whole blood. *Eur J Nucl Med* 9: 216–219.

Harper PV *et al.* (1964). ^{99m}Tc as a radiocolloid. *J Nucl Med* 5: 382.

Hartmann IJC *et al.* (2001). Technegas versus ^{81m}Kr ventilation–perfusion scintigraphy: a comparative study in patients with suspected acute pulmonary embolism. *J Nucl Med* 42: 393–400.

Henze E *et al.* (1982). Lymphoscintigraphy with Tc-99m-labeled dextran. *J Nucl Med* 23: 923–929.

Hirsch JI *et al.* (1989). Preparation and evaluation of a ^{99m}Tc-SnF_2 colloid kit for leukocyte labeling. *J Nucl Med Technol* 30: 1257–1263.

Hnatowich DJ *et al.* (1981). Labeling of preformed liposomes with Ga-67 and Tc-99m by chelation. *J Nucl Med* 22: 810–814.

Hobbs SK *et al.* (1998). Regulation of transport pathways in tumor vessels: role of tumor type and microenvironment. *Proc Natl Acad Sci U S A* 95: 4607–4612.

Howarth DM *et al.* (1999). ^{99m}Tc Technegas ventilation and perfusion lung scintigraphy for the diagnosis of pulmonary embolus. *J Nucl Med* 40: 579–584.

Hughes DK (2003). Nuclear medicine and infection detection: the relative effectiveness of imaging with ^{111}In-oxine–, ^{99m}Tc-HMPAO–, and ^{99m}Tc-stannous fluoride colloid–labeled leukocytes and with ^{67}Ga-citrate. *J Nucl Med Technol* 31: 196–201.

Hung JC *et al.* (1995). Filtered technetium-99m-sulfur colloid evaluated for lymphoscintigraphy. *J Nucl Med* 36: 1895–1901.

Hunt AP *et al.* (2006). Preparation of Tc-99m-macroaggregated albumin from recombinant human albumin for lung perfusion imaging. *Eur J Pharm Biopharm* 62: 26–31.

Ikomi F *et al.* (1995). Mechanism of colloidal particle uptake into the lymphatic system: basic study with percutaneous lymphography. *Radiology* 196: 107–113.

Illum L *et al.* (1982). Blood clearance and organ deposition of intravenously administered colloidal particles—the effects of particle-size, nature and shape. *Int J Pharm* 12: 135–146.

Isawa T *et al.* (1991). Technegas for inhalation lung imaging. *Nucl Med Commun* 12: 47–55.

Isitman AT *et al.* (1974). An assessment of alveolar deposition and pulmonary clearance of radiopharmaceuticals after nebulization. *Am J Roentgenol Radium Ther Nucl Med* 120: 776–781.

Itoa A *et al.* (2004). Magnetite nanoparticle-loaded anti-HER2 immunoliposomes for combination of antibody therapy with hyperthermia. *Cancer Lett* 212: 167–175.

Iwanaga T *et al.* (2000). Morphology and functional roles of synoviocytes in the joint. *Arch Histol Cytol* 63: 17–31.

Jacobson DL *et al.* (1997). Epidemiology and estimated population burden of selected autoimmune diseases in the United States. *Clin Immunol Immunopathol* 84: 223–243.

Kairemo K *et al.* (2008). Nanoparticles in cancer. *Curr Radiopharm* 1: 30–36.

Kampen WU *et al.* (2006). Therapeutic status of radiosynoviorthesis of the knee with yttrium [^{90}Y] colloid in rheumatoid arthritis and related indications. *Rheumatology* 46: 16–24.

Kapteijn BAE *et al.* (1997). Validation of gamma probe detection of the sentinel node in melanoma. *J Nucl Med* 38: 362–366.

Kashiwaya Y *et al.* (1994). Control of glucose utilization in working perfused rat heart. *J Biol Chem* 269: 25502–25514.

Kennedy A *et al.* (2005). Liver brachytherapy for unresectable colorectal metastases. *GI Cancer Symposium.* Alexandria, VA: American Society of Clinical Oncology, 145.

Kirkpatrick EM *et al.* (1996). Magnetic properties of single domain samarium cobalt nanoparticles. *IEEE Trans Magn* 32: 4502–4504.

Klett R *et al.* (2007). Radiosynoviorthesis of medium-sized joints with rhenium-186-sulphide colloid: a review of the literature. *Rheumatology* 46: 1531–1537.

Klingensmith WC *et al.* (1983). Normal appearance and reproducibility of liver-spleen studies with Tc-99m Sulfur colloid and Tc-99m Microalbumin colloid. *J Nucl Med* 24: 8–13.

Kraft O *et al.* (2007). Radiosynoviorthesis of knees by means of ^{166}Ho-holmium-boro-macroaggregates. *Cancer Biother Radiopharm* 22(2): 296–302.

Krag D *et al.* (1998). The sentinel node in breast cancer a multicenter validation study. *N Engl J Med* 339: 941–946.

Kreuter J (2001). Nanoparticle systems for brain delivery of drugs. *Adv Drug Deliv Rev* 47: 65–81.

Kreyling WG *et al.* (2006). Ultrafine particle–lung interactions: does size matter? *J Aerosol Med* 19: 74–83.

Krogsgaard OW (1976). Technetium-99m-sulfur colloid in vitro studies of various commercial kits. *Eur J Nucl Med* 1: 31–35.

Kučkaa J *et al.* (2006). Astatination of nanoparticles containing silver as possible carriers of ^{211}At. *Appl Radiat Isotopes* 64: 201–206.

Kwiatkowska K, Sobota A (1999). Signaling pathways in phagocytosis. *Bioessays* 21: 422–431.

Lamprecht A *et al.* (2001). Size-dependent bioadhesion of micro- and nanoparticulate carriers to the inflamed colonic mucosa. *Pharm Rev* 18: 788–793.

Larson SM, Nelp WB (1966). Radiopharmacology of a simplified technetium-99m-colloid preparation for photoscanning. *J Nucl Med* 7: 817–826.

Lemb M *et al.* (1993). Technegas: a study of particle structure, size and distribution. *Eur J Nucl Med* 20: 576–579.

Lin MS, Winchell HS (1972). A "kit" method for the preparation of a technetium-tin(II) colloid and a study of its properties. *J Nucl Med* 13: 58.

Lipskaya T *et al.* (1995). Compartmentation and metabolic parameters of mitochondrial hexokinase and creatine kinase depend on the rate of oxidative phosphorylation. *Biochem Mol Med* 55: 81–89.

Lloyd JJ *et al.* (1995). Technegas and pertechnegas particle size distribution. *Eur J Nucl Med* 22: 473–476.

Lyster DM *et al.* (1974). Preparation of a ^{99m}Tc-Sn-MAA kit for use in nuclear medicine. *J Nucl Med* 15: 198–199.

Mackey DW *et al.* (1997). Physical properties and use of pertechnegas as a ventilation agent. *Eur J Nucl Med* 35: 163–167.

Magnant J *et al.* (2006). Comparative analysis of different scintigraphic approaches to assess pulmonary ventilation. *J Aerosol Med* 19: 148–159.

Malinkrodt-US (1985). Package insert, *TechneColl.* Hazellwood, MO: Malinkrodt-US, Rev 3/85.

Malone LA *et al.* (1983). Kinetics of technetium 99m labelled macroaggregated albumin in humans. *Br J Radiol* 56: 109–112.

Manchester J *et al.* (1994). Glucose transport and phosphorylation in single cardiac myocytes: rate-limiting steps in glucose metabolism. *Am J Physiol* 266: E326–333.

Manil L *et al.* (2001). Physical and biological dosimetry in patients undergoing radiosynoviorthesis with erbium-169 and rhenium-186. *Nucl Med Commun* 22: 405–416.

Marshall AHE (1965). The reticular tissue and the reticuloendothelial system. *J Pathol Bacteriol* 65: 29–48.

Martindale AA *et al.* (1980). Technetium-99m antimony colloid for bone-marrow imaging. *J Nucl Med* 21: 1035–1041.

May RC, Machesky LM (2001). Phagocytosis and the actin cytoskeleton. *J Cell Sci* 114: 1061–1077.

McAfee JG, Thakur ML (1976). Survey of radioactive agents for In vitro labeling of phagocytic leukocytes. ii. Particles. *J Nucl Med* 17: 488–492.

McClelland CC *et al.* (2003). ^{99m}Tc-SnF$_2$ colloid LLK: particle size, morphology, leucocyte labelling behaviour. *Nucl Med Commun* 24: 191–202.

Meiring JE *et al.* (2004). Hydrogel biosensor array platform indexed by shape. *Chem Mater* 16: 5574–5580.

Milligan WO, Morriss RH (1964). Morphology of colloidal gold – comparative study. *J Am Chem Soc* 86: 3461.

Mock BH, English D (1987). Leukocyte labeling with technetium-99m tin colloids. *J Nucl Med* 28: 1471–1477.

Moghimi SM *et al.* (2001). Long-circulating and targetspecific nanoparticles: theory to practice. *Pharm Rev* 53: 283–318.

Möhlen KH, Beller FK (1979). Use of radioactive gold in the treatment of pleural effusions caused by metastatic cancer. *J Cancer Res Clin Oncol* 94(1): 81–85.

Monaghan P *et al.* (1991). An improved radionuclide technique for the detection of altered pulmonary permeability. *J Nucl Med* 32: 1945–1949.

Mundschenk H *et al.* (1971). Phagocytic activity of the liver as a measure of hepatic circulation – a comparative study using ^{198}Au and ^{99m}Tc-sulfur colloid. *J Nucl Med* 12: 711.

Munshi N *et al.* (1997). Size modulation of polymeric nanoparticles under controlled dynamics of microemulsion droplets. *J Colloid Interface Sci* 190: 387–391.

Ng CK *et al.* (1991). Sensitivity of myocardial fluorodeoxyglucose lumped constant to glucose and insulin. *Am J Physiol* 260: H593–603.

Nightingale JM *et al.* (1993). Disturbed gastric emptying in the short bowel syndrome. Evidence for a 'colonic brake'. *Gut* 34: 1171–1176.

Ogihara I *et al.* (1986). Tumor uptake of ^{67}Ga-carrying liposomes. *Eur J Nucl Med* 11: 405–411.

Ortho-Biotech (2001). Package insert, *Doxil*. Horsham, PA: Ortho-Biotech.

Ozin GA *et al.* (2009). *Nanochemistry: A Chemical Approach to Nanomaterials*. Cambridge: Royal Society of Chemistry.

Palmer J *et al.* (2001). Comprehensive ventilation/perfusion SPECT. *J Nucl Med* 42: 1288–1294.

Park J *et al.* (2004). Evaluation of 2-methacryloyloxyethyl phosphorylcholine polymeric nanoparticle for immunoassay of C-reactive protein detection. *Anal Chem* 76: 2649–2655.

Peer D *et al.* (2007). Nanocarriers as an emerging platform for cancer therapy. *Nat Nanotechnol* 2: 751–760.

Pellegrino R *et al.* (2001). Regional expiratory flow limitation studied with Technegas in asthma. *J Appl Physiol* 91: 2190–2198.

Peltier P, Chatal JF (1986). 99mTc-DTPA and 99mTc-rhenium sulfur aerosol compared as adjuncts to perfusion scintigraphy in patients with suspected pulmonary embolism. *Eur J Nucl Med* 12: 254–257.

Peltier P *et al.* (1992). Comparison of technetium-99mC and phytate aerosol in ventilation studies. *Eur J Nucl Med* 19: 349–354.

Pendersen B, Kristensen K (1981). Evaluation of methods for sizing of colloidal radio pharmaceuticals. *Eur J Nucl Med* 6: 521-526.

Petasnick JP, Gottschalk A (1966). Spleen scintiphotography with technetium-99m sulfur colloid and the gamma ray scintillation camera. *J Nucl Med* 7: 733–739.

Phillips WT *et al.* (2009). Radioactive liposomes. *Nanomed Nanobiotechnol* 1: 69–83.

Pike MC (1991). Imaging of inflammatory sites in the 1990s: new horizons. *J Nucl Med* 32: 2034–2036.

Radpharm-Scientific (2008). Package insert, *Leucocyte labelling kit*. Canberra, ACT: RadPharm Scientific.

Rauscher F *et al.* (2005). Analysis of a technical-grade w/o-microemulsion and its application for the precipitation of calcium carbonate nanoparticles. *Colloids Surf A Physicochem Eng Asp* 254: 183–191.

Rejman J *et al.* (2004). Size-dependent internalization of particles via the pathways of clathrin and caveolae-mediated endocytosis. *Biochem J* 377: 159–169.

Rink T *et al.* (2001). Lymphoscintigraphic sentinel node imaging and gamma probe detection in breast cancer with Tc-99m nanocolloidal albumin results of an optimized protocol. *Clin Nucl Med* 26: 293–298.

Rizzo-Padoin N *et al.* (2001). A comparison of radiopharmaceutical agents used for the diagnosis of pulmonary embolism. *Nucl Med Commun* 22: 375–381.

Roser M *et al.* (1998). Surface-modified biodegradable albumin nano- and microspheres. II: effect of surface charges on in vitro phagocytosis and biodistribution in rats. *Eur J Pharm Biopharm* 46: 255–263.

Rossin R *et al.* (2005). ^{64}Cu-Labeled folate-conjugated shell cross-linked nanoparticles for tumor imaging and radiotherapy: synthesis, radiolabeling, and biologic evaluation. *J Nucl Med* 46: 1210–1218.

Sacks B (1926). Reticulo-endothelial system. *Physiol Rev* 6: 504–545.

Sage HH *et al.* (1964). Radioactive colloidal gold measurements of lymph flow and functional patterns of lymphatics and lymph nodes in the extremities. *J Nucl Med* 5: 626–642.

Sasaki Y *et al.* (1998). Estimation of regional lung function in interstitial pulmonary disease using ^{99m}Tc-Technegas and ^{99m}Tc-macroaggregated albumin single-photon emission tomography. *Eur J Nucl Med* 25: 1623–1629.

Saverymuttu SH *et al.* (1981). Indium-111 labelled autologous leucocytes in inflamotory bowel disease. *Gastroenterology* 80: 1273.

Scalzetti EM, Gagne GM (1995). The transition from Technegas to Pertechnegas. *J Nucl Med* 36: 267–269.

Schiffelers RM *et al.* (2003). Antitumor efficacy of tumor vasculature-targeted liposomal doxorubicin. *J Control Release* 91: 115–122.

Schroth HJ *et al.* (1981). Cell labelling with colloidal substances in whole blood. *Eur J Nucl Med*, 469–472.

Schuster DP (1998). The evaluation of lung function with PET. *Semin Nucl Med* 28: 341–351.

Secker-Walker RH (1968). Scintillation scanning of lungs in diagnosis of pulmonary embolism. *Br Med J* 2: 206–208.

Senden TJ *et al.* (1997). The physical and chemical nature of Technegas. *J Nucl Med* 38: 1327–1333.

Sharma P *et al.* (2006). Nanoparticles for bioimaging. *Adv Colloid Interface Sci* 123–126: 471–485.

Sherman A, Ter-Pogossian M (1953). Lymph-node concentration of radioactive colloidal gold following interstitial injection. *Cancer* 6: 1238–1240.

Shinde-Patil VR *et al.* (2001). Particle diameter influences adhesion under flow. *Biophys J* 80: 1733–1743.

Shukla J *et al.* (2007). Characterization of Re-188-Sn microparticles used for synovitis treatment. *Int J Pharm* 338 (1-2): 43–47.

Smith RJ (2005). Therapies for rheumatoid arthritis: hope springs eternal. *Drug Discov Today* 10: 1598–1606.

Southworth R *et al.* (2005). The low oxygen-carrying capacity of Krebs buffer causes a doubling in ventricular wall thickness in the isolated heart. *Can J Physiol Pharmacol* 83: 174–182.

Stern HS *et al.* (1966). Preparation, distribution and utilization of technetium-99m-sulfur colloid. *J Nucl med* 7: 665–675.

Storm G *et al.* (1995). Surface modification of nanoparticles to oppose uptake by the mononuclear phagocyte system. *Adv Drug Deliv Rev* 17: 31–48.

Strand SE, Persson BAA (1978). Quantitative lymphoscintigraphy I: basic concepts for optimal uptake of radiocolloids in the parasternal lymph nodes of rabbits. *J Nucl Med* 20: 1038–1046.

Strong JC, Agnew JE (1989). The particle size distribution of Technegas and its influence on regional lung deposition. *Nucl Med Commun* 10: 425–430.

Sun C *et al.* (2006). Folic acid-PEG conjugated superparamagnetic nanoparticles for targeted cellular uptake and detection by MRI. *J Biomed Mater Res A* 78: 550–557.

Sunderland CJ *et al.* (2006). Targeted nanoparticles for detecting and treating cancer. *Drug Dev Res* 67: 70–93.

Swanson JN (1949). Repeated colloidal gold tests in rheumatoid arthritis. *Ann Rheum Dis* 8: 232–237.

Syrigos KN *et al.* (2003). Biodistribution and pharmacokinetics of ^{111}In-dTPA-labelled pegylated liposomes after intraperitoneal injection. *Acta Oncol* 42: 147–153.

Tägil K *et al.* (2000). Efficient lung scintigraphy. *Clin Physiol* 20: 95–100.

Taillefer R *et al.* (1987). Comparison of technetium-99m sulfur colloid and technetium-99m albumin colloid labeled solid meals for gastric emptying studies. *Clin Nucl Med* 12: 597–600.

Taplin GV *et al.* (1964). Suspensions of radioalbumin aggregates for photoscanning the liver, spleen, lung and other organs. *J Nucl Med* 5: 259–275.

Torchilin VP (1994). Immunoliposomes and PEGylated immunoliposomes: possible use for targeted delivery of imaging agents. *Immunomethods* 4: 244–258.

Torchilin VP, Trubetskoy VS (1995). In vivo visualizing of organs and tissues with liposomes. *J Liposome Res* 5: 795–812.

Tsopelas C (2006). Physico-chemical characterisation of ^{99m}Tc–tin fluoride colloid agent used for labelling white cells. *J Labelled Comp Radiopharm* 49: 505–516.

Tsopelas C *et al.* (2003). Preparation and biological evaluation of ^{99m}Tc-stannous fluoride colloid-labelled leucocytes in rats. *J Labelled Comp Radiopharm* 46: 751–763.

Turkevich J *et al.* (1951). A study of the nucleation and growth processes in the synthesis of colloidal gold. *Discuss Faraday Soc* 11: 55–75.

Turkevich J *et al.* (1953). The formation of colloidal gold. *J Phys Chem* 57: 670–673.

Upton AC *et al.* (1956). Liver damage and hepatomas in mice produced by radioactive colloidal gold. *Cancer Res* 16: 211–215.

Virkkunen M *et al.* (1967). Experiences of intra-articular administration of radioactive gold. *Acta Rheumatol Scand* 13: 81–91.

Voigt A *et al.* (2005). Size and distribution prediction for nanoparticles produced by microemulsion precipitation: a Monte Carlo simulation study. *Nanotechnology* 16: S429–S434.

Watanabe T *et al.* (2001). Sentinel node biopsy with technetium-99m colloidal rhenium sulphide in patients with breast cancer. *Br J Surg* 88: 704–707.

Webber MM *et al.* (1973). Rapid preparation of ^{99m}Tc-labeled albumin macroaggregates. *Radiology* 108: 435–436.

Whinnery JE, Young JT (1980). Granulomatous interstitial pneumoniain a miniature swine associated with repeated intravenous injections of Tc-99m human serum albumin. *J Nucl Med* 21: 207–210.

Wilhelm AJ *et al.* (1999). Radiopharmaceuticals in sentinel lymph-node detection – an overview. *Eur J Nucl Med* 26: s36–s42.

Winston MA *et al.* (1973). Radioisotope synovectomy with ^{32}P-chromic phosphate – kinetic studies. *J Nucl Med* 14: 886–889.

Winter PM *et al.* (2007). Emerging nanomedicine opportunities with perfluorocarbon nanoparticles. *Expert Rev Med Devices* 4: 137–145.

Young RC *et al.* (2003). Adjuvant treatment for early ovarian cancer: a randomized phase III trial of intraperitoneal ^{32}P or intravenous cyclophosphamide and cisplatin – a gynecologic oncology group study. *J Clin Oncol* 21(23): 4350–4355.

Zielhuis SW *et al.* (2006). Production of GMP-grade radioactive holmium loaded poly(L-lactic acid) microspheres for clinical application. *Int J Pharm* 311: 69–74.

Zielhuis SW *et al.* (2007). Characterization of holmium loaded alginate microspheres for multimodality imaging and therapeutic applications. *J Biomed Mater Res A* 82(4): 892–898.

SECTION E

Radiopharmacy practice

26

Design and operation of radiopharmacy facilities

Tom Murray and David Graham

Introduction

Radiopharmacy or PET production facilities are primarily designed and operated to safely prepare radioactive medicinal products, otherwise known as radiopharmaceuticals. Radiopharmaceuticals that contain radionuclides with long half-lives are normally obtained as market-authorised finished products from commercial suppliers. However, the vast majority of radiopharmaceuticals contain radionuclides with short half-lives for which commercial supply is impractical, and such products tend to be prepared locally in radiopharmacies. The majority of radiopharmaceuticals are produced as sterile preparations intended for parenteral administration. It is therefore necessary in the design and operation of a radiopharmacy to maintain the sterility of the product throughout the dispensing process.

As a result, radiopharmacy practice has become firmly established as an integral part of the multidisciplinary team providing services to nuclear medicine departments in the UK, Europe and the USA. Traditionally these have been designed with the intention of preparing in a 'ready to administer' form SPECT radiopharmaceuticals, particularly but not exclusively involving ^{99m}Tc. More recently with the development of PET as a routine service, the PET production facility must be designed differently to meet the challenges of preparing and handling positron-emitting radiopharmaceuticals. Facilities for the preparation of these two types of radiopharmaceuticals have tended to develop in two patterns – one in which each nuclear medicine facility has its own department, the other in which a number of nuclear medicine facilities are supplied by a centralised department. The specialised requirements for PET production are detailed later as a separate issue in this chapter, but the principles of facility design together with aspects of good operational practice will be common to both.

Radiopharmacy design

Various factors need to be taken into consideration in the planning of a radiopharmacy. While the present and future needs of the local department will always be the main driving force in shaping the final plan, compliance with regulatory requirements must also be taken into account. With these factors in mind, it is important that the design be primarily concerned with the safe production of radiopharmaceuticals in terms of good manufacturing, and radiation protection practices. It is important that the aim of the radiopharmacy design is based on the following principles.

- *Product protection*: The product must be protected from contaminants (viable and non-viable particulates) both from the environment and from operators. Care must also be taken to avoid cross contamination from other products.
- *Operator protection*: The operator must be protected from the radiation hazards that are a consequence of preparing radioactive medicines and, if relevant, the additional biohazard that may be present when radiolabelling blood components, as routinely performed in modern radiopharmacy units.
- *Protection of the environment:* Radioactive and microbial contamination must be prevented from escaping or being accidentally spread to other equipment, other personnel and the general environment.

It must be stressed that all of these cannot be achieved by facility design alone, which must be combined with good understanding and design of the processes that will be carried out within the facility. It is important when undertaking facility design to consider process flow and how materials and personnel are brought together in the unit to achieve the finished product.

At an early stage in the planning process it is important to consider how any new facility will be brought into operation. The process known as commissioning consists of validation, firstly of the design and ultimately of the new facility. Validation is a documented process whereby the facility is tested to show that it performs to the requirements of the design specification and will be discussed more fully later in the chapter.

Factors affecting design

The two basic functions of a radiopharmacy or PET facility are the manipulation of unsealed radioactive materials and the preparation of these in a pharmaceutical form suitable for intravenous administration. Therefore, the regulations and guidelines that govern these functions will have an influence on the design as well as the way in which the processes are carried out. Different countries will have their own national regulation and guidelines although the Pharmaceutical Inspection Convention and Pharmaceutical Inspection Co-operation Scheme (PIC/S) is developing harmonised guidance.

Pharmaceutical aspects

In the UK the preparation of diagnostic and therapeutic radiopharmaceuticals falls under the legislative control of the Medicines Act 1968. Commercial organisations will require a full manufacturing licence with the Medicines and Healthcare products Regulatory Authority (MHRA) or the European Medicines Evaluation Agency (EMEA), whereas organisations working within NHS have two options open to them:

1. Licensing by the MHRA with a Manufacturer's 'Specials' Licence.
2. Working under a Section 10 exemption of the Medicines Act 1968, where medicinal products are dispensed under the direct supervision of a pharmacist.

When manufacturing, the guidelines given in *Rules and Guidance for Pharmaceutical Manufacturers and Distributors* (GMP) (MHRA 2007) must be followed.

Radiation protection aspects

The handling, storage and disposal of radioactive substances are governed by both the Ionising Radiation Regulations 1999 and the Radioactive Substances Act 1993. Practical guidelines can also be found in *Medical and Dental Guidance: A good practice guide on all aspects of ionising radiation protection in the clinical environment* (IPEM 2002). Further attention must also be paid to the Work with Ionising Radiation Approved Code of Practice and practical guidance on the Ionising Radiation Regulations 1999. For more detailed information see Chapter 3.

Local considerations

In the drawing up of plans at a local level, many factors have to be taken into consideration, and perhaps the most important of these are discussed below:

Budget

The budget requirements may be considered in the context of premises, equipment and staffing. The cost of building a new department on a 'greenfield' site will be considerably larger compared with converting or upgrading an existing area. There are pros and cons with both approaches and much will depend on the local situation. Budget estimates will be more easily achieved by preparing a detailed project specification written by a multidisciplinary team that will have to include electrical and mechanical engineers as well as architects. This specification can then be used in a tendering exercise to price the construction work. With any design it is important to identify any new equipment that will be required so that costs can be identified, not just the capital costs but also the cost of maintenance as well as the price of service contracts. Finally, once a budget cost has been calculated, some contingency should be added into the budget for the project to cover any unforeseen problems or oversights. Staffing of the facility is a major budgetary item.

Nature and volume of work

The design of any radiopharmacy or PET facility will depend on what services are to be provided from the facility. Both of these specialities are most likely to be preparing radiopharmaceuticals for intravenous use and this will need cleanroom facilities within which will be housed workstations for carrying out any aseptic manipulations. A cleanroom will require a support room and a change facility. The size of these will largely depend on the volume of work and the number of personnel needed in the department. If cell labelling procedures are to be undertaken, then a separate facility of cleanroom, support room and change room will also be required. A separate area should be provided for performing quality control tests and the housing of equipment such as radio chromatogram scanners, HPLC equipment, etc. Consideration should also be given to where microbiological samples will be handled since this will need separate facilities from production areas. The research and development commitments of a department will also have to be taken into account since, depending on the techniques and procedures, a more sophisticated laboratory would be required if, for example, synthetic chemistry were being undertaken rather than just in-house quality testing. The housing and use of animals must be in a completely separate facility from those used as production areas and separated from any hospital patient areas (MHRA 2007).

Location and site selection

When considering the location of a new radiopharmacy there are a number of criteria that should be considered. Location may contribute to the quality of the products. If the radiopharmacy is situated next to areas that may discharge large amounts of dust, for example, this might lead to increased risk of contamination or increased maintenance of the cleanroom plant (i.e. more frequent change of pre-filters, bag filters or even HEPA filters).

Ideally the radiopharmacy or PET facility should be in close proximity to the scanning department, but at the same time should not create a radiation hazard to either other areas or personnel. If a central radiopharmacy supplying a number of sites is being designed then its location with respect to transport links is of paramount importance. This is particularly crucial if the supply of PET radiopharmaceuticals is being considered because of the short half-lives of these radionuclides.

The location should allow for easy access for deliveries (and where relevant dispatch of materials) in order to receive radioactive goods and create no radiation risk to adjacent areas. Consideration must also be given to how and when deliveries are made so their security can be confirmed.

Any facility design must provide rooms of sufficient size to allow for efficient workflow and for the staff to work comfortably. Rooms that are too small may when occupied prove difficult to control to the required specifications of temperature, humidity and even cleanliness.

Structure and finishes of the cleanroom

The requirements for pharmaceutical cleanrooms and those used for handling 'open' radioactive sources are broadly similar. The GMP guidelines recommend that walls, floors and ceilings should have a smooth, impervious, and non-shedding surface that should allow sanitation and disinfection. Bare wood and other unsealed surfaces must be avoided and sinks must be carefully positioned in the facility (see later). The junction between walls, floors and ceilings should be coved to facilitate cleaning, and to reduce dust accumulation there should be a minimum of shelves and other projected fittings. Cleanrooms should be built as airtight structures, since they should be operated at a positive pressure. The construction has to be of high quality with well-sealed joints since openings may harbour dirt. Materials need to be tough enough to resist scratching or chipping since if present these might also be places where dirt could accumulate. Windows must not open to the outside and if present internal glazing must be flush with the walls and without ledges. Light fixtures should fit flush with the ceiling and give good-quality lighting (500 lux at bench level). Their design should allow for easy change of the light elements without compromise of the cleanroom integrity. Within the unit internal windows or vision panels should be considered since it allows management and visitors to observe the cleanroom without entering it. Additionally, for health and safety reasons, it would be better to have operators visible within the cleanroom area. Shielding may have to be incorporated into the wall construction for radiation protection of operators as well as adjacent areas. Cleanroom doors are laminates of glass-reinforced plastic (GRP) and are usually supplied without handles. They normally have a self-closing mechanism to minimise loss of pressure in the cleanroom. For the same reason, doors should also be interlocking within a cleanroom suite. Ceilings should be suspended or self-supporting since access to carry out maintenance on the cleanroom services might be required and access panels should be fitted to allow this in a way that would minimise disruption of the cleanroom. Filter modules also require to be fitted and designed to allow ease of filter change as well as integrity testing.

Design and layout overview

The radiopharmacy should be designed not only to take the existing service into account but also to allow for future developments. In the design of any new radiopharmacy consideration ought to be given for the inclusion of the following areas in the plan:

1. Cleanroom suite or facility
2. Laboratory
3. Radionuclide store
4. Office
5. Staff welfare facilities
6. Storeroom
7. Radioactive materials reception area.

A section of the radiopharmacy premises may have to be defined as a controlled or supervised area under the Ionising Radiation Regulations 1999 (Stationery Office 1999), depending on the type and quantity of the radionuclides being handled. A controlled area is defined as any area where the instantaneous dose rate exceeds 7.5 μSv/h or is likely to exceed this level. A radiopharmacy which handles more than 30 GBq of ^{99m}Tc or 10 MBq of ^{131}I, for example, will need to be classed as a controlled area (see Chapter 3).

Cleanroom suite or facility

It is generally accepted that the aseptic preparation of sterile radiopharmaceuticals for intravenous administration must be carried out in some type of a cleanroom. However, the cleanroom cannot function in isolation and requires a number of support rooms. It is these together that form the cleanroom suite. Consideration of the grade of these rooms will be discussed in detail later, but a layout is described in Figure 26.1, which illustrates what might be required.

Personnel will have to enter into and leave the cleanroom through a changing room. Depending on the grade of room being entered, changing may have to be considered within two distinct zones: first a pre-change zone where personnel change out of outdoor clothing and don cleanroom undergarments; they then progress into another changing room where sterile cleanroom clothing is donned. This two-stage changing method minimises the microbial and particulate contamination entering the room.

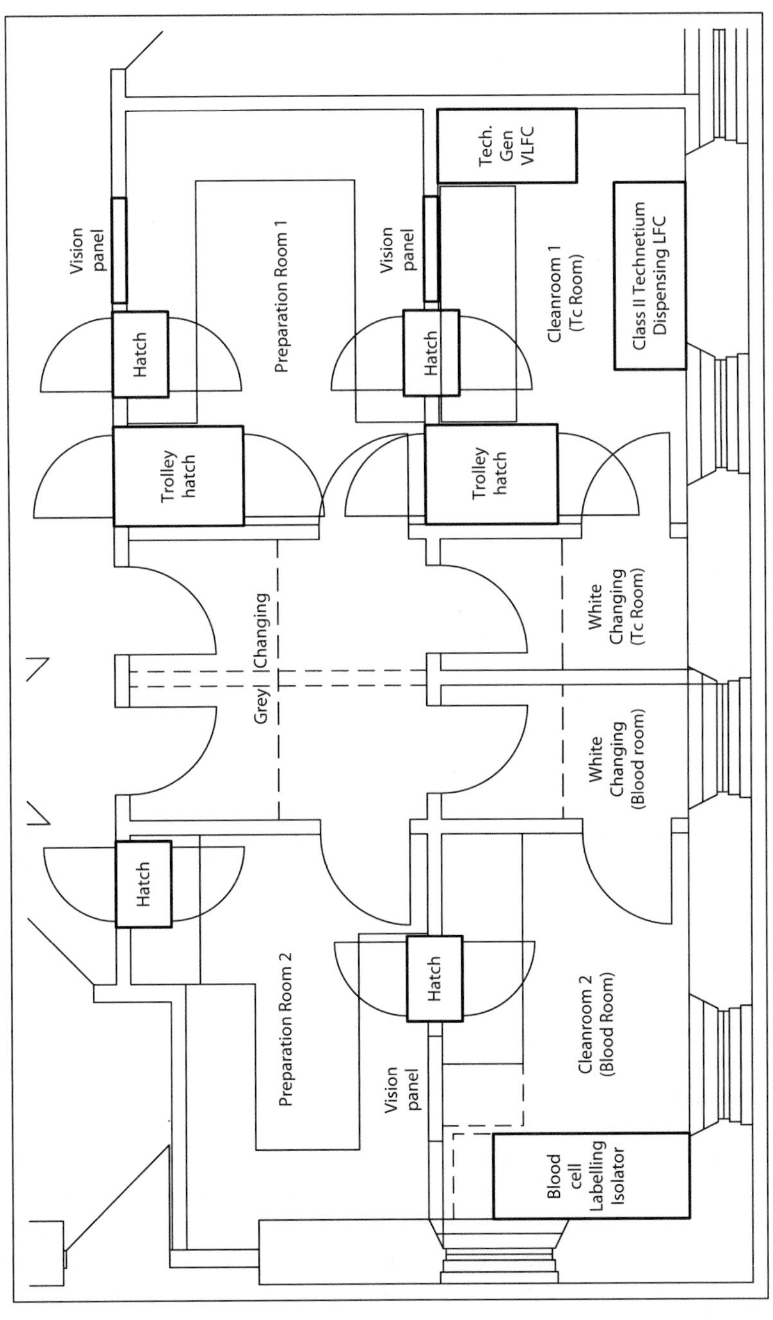

Figure 26.1 Plan of proposed cleanroom suite, Aberdeen Radiopharmacy. In relation to the text: support rooms are labelled 'Preparation Room'. Reproduced with kind permission of CCDP, © Springer-Verlag London Ltd.

A support room lying adjacent to the cleanroom allows servicing of the cleanroom where materials are passed into and out of the cleanroom. This should be achieved via hatch(es) systems where the doors are interlocked to prevent both sides being opened at the same time. The function of this support room would also include the checking, labelling and packaging of finished products.

Quality control laboratory

A laboratory area allows for the performance of routine quality control procedures as well as research and development work. The laboratory should be suitably equipped to perform these functions and would normally be supplied with such services as chemical safety cabinets, vacuum, and compressed air.

Radionuclide store

A room that can be securely locked should be part of the design to ensure the safe storage of radioactive stock materials. This room can also act as a decay store, facilitating the safe storage of radioactive residues and other contaminated waste materials.

A feature of such a store may include a shielded facility (i.e. bunker) for the storage of high-activity as well as long-lived radionuclides including ^{99m}Tc-generators. A refrigerator and freezer may be located here for the storage of products that require these conditions, and this in turn may need to have some shielding.

Office

Space permitting, it is beneficial to include an office in the design of any radiopharmacy. This provides an area for the storage of documents required for radiopharmaceutical production. These are best kept in a location distinct from and preferably at a distance from those areas where radioactive materials are stored or dispensed.

Staff welfare facilities

It is a requirement to provide toilet and cloakroom facilities for staff working in the radiopharmacy and PET facility. One consequence of the removal of sinks from the cleanroom suite, as required to comply with GMP, is that hand wash facilities will have to be provided in a suitable location to allow hand washing prior to entry into the cleanroom and support areas. Sinks will also be needed to allow hand washing prior to exit from a controlled or supervised area. To comply with GMP and HOS, sink and hand wash location must be outside changing rooms that give direct entry into a cleanroom, but within the controlled or supervised area, to allow monitoring and washing prior to exit. Shower facilities can be provided for decontamination of radiopharmacy personnel in case of accidental spillage.

Storeroom

Sundry items (non-radioactive kits, syringes, etc.) used in the production process will have to be stored outside the cleanroom suite. Here, orders may be received, unpacked and stored before being transferred as required to the clean support rooms via a suitable hatch or designated route.

Radioactive materials reception area

The security of radioactive and other dangerous substances has recently become an issue. Burglar alarms that communicate to the police should be considered for these areas where radioactive substances are stored. Also, consideration should be given to how and when deliveries of radioactive goods are made so that these materials are stored securely and their whereabouts confirmed.

Cleanroom design

General principles

A cleanroom is defined as a room where the concentration of particles is controlled and which is constructed and operated in a manner that minimises the introduction, generation and retention of particles inside the room. Other parameters such as temperature, humidity and air pressure are also controlled as necessary. There are a number of systems used to classify cleanrooms (US Federal Standard 20, International Standard Organisation (ISO) Standard 14644-1), but the GMP definition will be used here (Tables 26.1 and 26.2) and will be used later in this

Table 26.1 EU GMP Guide 2007, cleanroom air particle classification system for the manufacture of sterile products

GMP grade	Maximum permitted number of particles/m^3 equal to or above				Transfer of classes (all operational)		
	At rest[a]		Operational		US Fed 209D	US Fed 209E	ISO
	0.5 μm	5 μm	0.5 μm	5 μm			
A	3 500	1[b]	3 500	1[b]	100	M3.5	ISO 5
B	3 500	0	350 000	2,000	100	M3.5	ISO 5
C	350 000	2 000	3 500 000	20 000	10 000	M5.5	ISO 7
D	3 500 000	20 000	Not defined	Not defined	100 000	M6.5	ISO 8

[a] 'At rest' should be achieved after a short 'clean-up' period of 15–20 minutes in an unmanned state after completion of operations.

[b] These areas are expected to be completely free from particles greater than or equal to 5 μm. Since it is statistically impossible to demonstrate this, the limit is set to 1 particle/m^3.

chapter when describing cleanrooms in the context of the radiopharmacy or PET facility.

Design properties

A cleanroom (Figure 26.2) may be considered as having the following properties:

- *Air change rate:* Air is usually supplied by an air conditioning plant through diffusers in the ceiling giving an air supply of between 20 and 60 air changes per hour (cf. 2–10 air changes for an ordinary ventilated room) to dilute to an acceptable concentration the contaminants produced in the room.
- *Terminal high-efficiency particulate air (HEPA) filters:* the cleanroom air enters the room via HEPA filters capable of filtering 99.97% of all particles greater than 0.3 μm. These filters are placed at the point of discharge of air into the room.
- *Room pressurisation:* Cleanrooms are positively pressurised to ensure air does not pass from adjacent dirty areas. This is achieved by extracting slightly less air than is supplied. To achieve this, and to ensure air moves from areas of highest cleanliness to less clean in the cleanroom suite, it passes through grilles or extract ducts that are set at low levels in walls and doors.

Table 26.2 EU GMP Guide 2007, recommended limits for microbial contamination

Grade	Recommended limits for microbial contamination[a]			
	Air sample (cfu/m^3)	Settle plates (90 mm) (cfu/4 h)[b]	Contact plates (55 mm) (cfu/plate)	Finger dab 5 fingers (cfu/glove)
A	<1	<1	<1	<1
B	10	5	5	5
C	100	50	25	N/A
D	200	100	50	N/A

cfu, colony-forming unit; N/A, not applicable.

[a] These are average values.

[b] Individual settle plates may be exposed for less than 4 hours, with the colony forming units (cfu) adjusted accordingly.

The type of clean area used in pharmaceutical production usually consists of a conventionally ventilated cleanroom, but in addition to this the product is manipulated within a workstation having a higher quality of air provided by a unidirectional airflow within which the critical or aseptic processing takes place. The workstation options for the aseptic production are usually:

1. A laminar flow workstation housed within a conventional cleanroom
2. An isolator with HEPA filtered air within a dedicated room (minimum GMP Grade D).

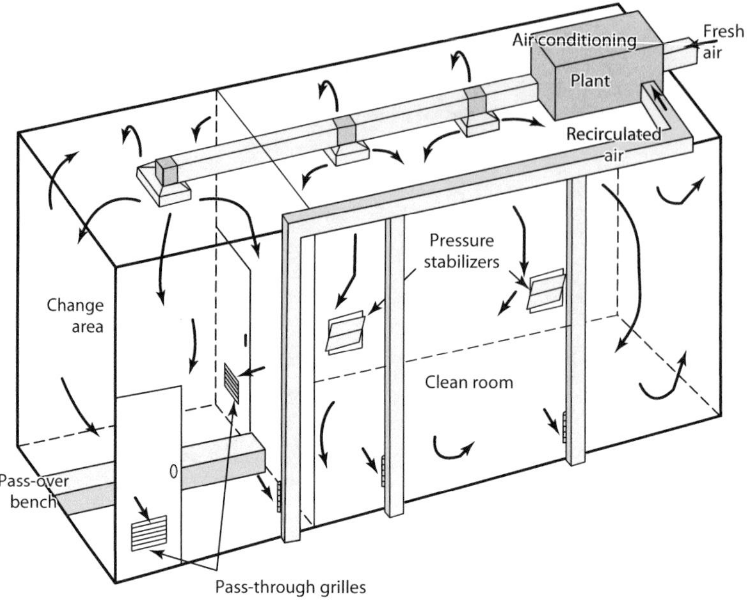

Figure 26.2 A conventionally ventilated cleanroom. Reproduced with kind permission of W. Whyte, © John Wiley & Sons Ltd.

Regardless of which option is chosen, the facilities should produce an environment that satisfies both radiation safety and pharmaceutical quality.

Radiopharmacy design

Conventional cleanroom with laminar-flow workstation

The laminar-flow workstation must provide a controlled internal environment conforming to GMP Grade A and be situated in a cleanroom that is dedicated to aseptic preparation. The latter environment must comply with GMP Grade B. Entry into the cleanroom should use the two-stage method described earlier. The final stages of changing must also operate at GMP Grade B with operators wearing sterile cleanroom clothing (see later).

The laminar flow workstation must be of the type that offers both operator (BS/EN 12469: 2000) and product (BS/EN/ISO 14644: 1999) protection. These were originally designed for the safe handing of microorganisms and can be obtained specifically adapted for radiopharmaceutical production as shown in Figure 26.3 and may incorporate shielding to give additional protection to the operator.

Isolators with a HEPA-filtered air supply

Isolators are contained workstations providing the conditions necessary for aseptically producing sterile injections within which there is an environment complying with GMP Grade A. For radiopharmaceutical preparation it is recommended that isolators operating with negative pressure with respect to the background environment be used. The design of any such facility should comply with the principles laid out in *Pharmaceutical Isolators, a Guide to their Application, Design and Control* (Midcalf 2004). The background environment is generally lower than that required for housing laminar-flow safety cabinets described earlier and should be a minimum of GMP Grade D.

The isolator must be sited in a dedicated room used only for this purpose with surfaces that are smooth, impervious, and non-shedding, allowing easy cleaning and disinfection. Changing facilities along with dedicated clothing must be provided for staff working with the isolator. There are isolators on the market aimed at radiopharmaceutical manufacturing (Figure 26.4) that include designs for technetium dispensing, blood cell labelling, volatile product handling and heavily shielded PET

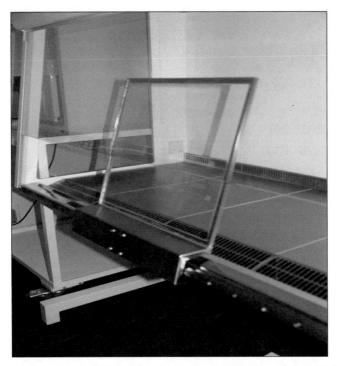

Figure 26.3 Example of a radiopharmaceutical laminar-flow safety cabinet: Mars Class 2, Biohazard Safety Cabinet manufactured by Scanlaf.

isolators. These isolators can have, as an integral part of the enclosure, a lead-shielded area for storage and elution of ^{99m}Tc-generators, centrifuges for performing blood cell separations, and radionuclide calibrators.

Laminar-flow cabinets versus isolators

In the two systems described, cost, convenience and containment properties are the major considerations when weighing up the option of laminar-flow cabinets

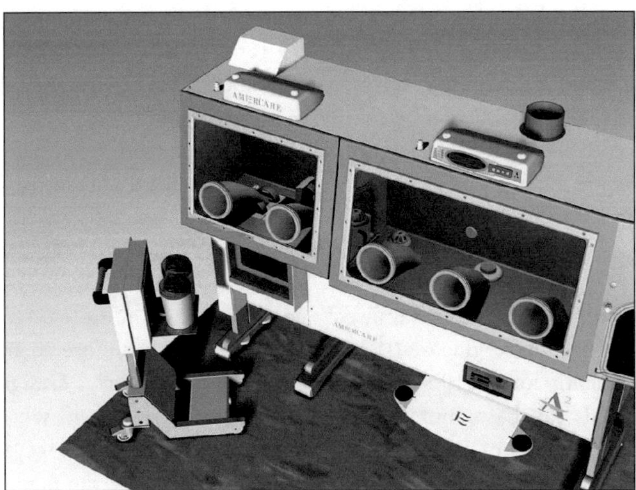

Figure 26.4 Radiopharmaceutical isolator designed specifically for the preparation of ^{99m}Tc-radiopharmaceuticals. The chamber on the left allows safe storage and elution of ^{99m}Tc-generators, whilst the one on the right is designed for aseptic processing. Reproduced with kind permission of Amercare Ltd.

versus isolators. If the scale of the local requirements for radiopharmaceutical production is such that a specialised filter environment is necessary for the siting of an isolator, its major cost advantages may be lost and conventional cleanroom technology may be better.

Special requirements for PET/cyclotron production

The increasing use of positron emission tomography (PET) has led to the development of PET radiopharmacies where short-lived positron-emitting radionuclides are produced in a cyclotron or from a generator and incorporated into carrier molecules. The issue of protection of the operators and product is even more important in the design of these units owing to a combination of working with 511 keV annihilation photons and a higher degree of 'openness' associated with the aseptic preparation procedures adopted. For the purposes of this chapter, we will deal with the cyclotron production method only.

PET radionuclides are produced in a cyclotron by bombarding appropriate target materials with a proton (or deuteron) beam. Utilising automated computer-controlled systems, the radionuclide liquid is 'pushed' along fine-bore tubing by an inert carrier gas to an appropriate automated chemistry synthesis module (housed within hot cells) where the radiochemical is prepared. From there, tubing transfers the product to a steriliser or a dispensing hot cell where it will be manipulated to produce the final radiopharmaceutical suitable for parenteral use. Alternatively, if in close proximity, gaseous radionuclide can be sent directly from the cyclotron to the PET camera room through dedicated high-grade stainless steel piping. In other situations, radioactive gases can be sent via a shielded process cabinet where the gases can be chemically altered.

Currently, the great majority of PET studies utilise fluorine-18 mainly as [^{18}F]fluorodeoxyglucose ([^{18}F] FDG). The half-life is sufficiently long (110 minutes) that the radiopharmaceuticals can be manufactured centrally for distribution to a number of camera sites. However, manufacture of PET radiopharmaceuticals that incorporate the very short-lived radionuclides of carbon-11 (20.4 minutes), nitrogen-13 (9.96 minutes) and oxygen-15 (2.07 minutes) requires the cyclotron and camera to be close to each other.

A number of gases are required in the automation and manufacturing stages of PET radiopharmaceuticals and therefore design should include shielded pipework and a system for the processing of waste gas. Quality control analysis of PET products can be more onerous than for conventional radiopharmaceuticals because of the range and complexity of the tests and the requirement for more testing prior to release. Consideration must therefore be given to the facilities and equipment required to carry out these tests.

Design of the PET facility

Vault, cyclotron and control room

The cyclotron is located inside a vault designed to shield against neutron and gamma radiations to afford adequate radiation protection. Walls are usually made of concrete whose density and thickness will depend on whether the cyclotron has local shielding or not. Most modern medical cyclotrons are negative-ion cyclotrons. One of the advantages of the negative-ion design is that it results in low levels of induced radioactivity within the cyclotron. Surrounding materials are also carefully selected to minimise radiation build-up. Therefore, with the proper safety procedures the exposure to the operating staff should be minimal. The cyclotron room will be part of the radiation controlled area with an interlock to prevent access to the room during periods of high radiation emission. Opening the door to the vault should disable operation of the cyclotron.

The cyclotron itself should provide sufficient energy and beam current to efficiently irradiate the targets and produce a range of radionuclides. Another advantage of the negative-ion design is the simplicity of the extraction process of the beam. It is possible to have multiple extraction systems within the cyclotron and therefore to irradiate more than one target simultaneously. Design of the unit will also include a control room, which should be sited next to the vault where control systems are housed. These include systems for the magnet, radiofrequency, ion source, beam extraction, beam diagnostics, vacuum, cooling water system and power supply.

Gas supplies

Medical and special gases are required for generation of radioisotopes, target cooling and product transfer in the cyclotron area. Gas bottles should be sited external to the vault within a secure ventilated area and pipes can then be led to a gas manifold within the vault. Flammable gases such as hydrogen and deuterium and ammonia should be stored separately from other gases and isolated from sources of ignition. Additionally, the mini-cells housing the chemistry platforms will require a supply of process gases such as compressed air, nitrogen, etc., and these should be regulated and provided from gas manifolds close to the point of use.

Radiation safety

Design of the PET facility must include a system that will minimise radiation hazards to staff and members of the public. This will include effective monitoring and prevention of release of radioactive gases to atmosphere and within the production facility itself. A stack emission monitoring system should be provided from the cyclotron and from the hot cell assembly. Gamma monitoring and warning system for radiation levels within the cyclotron room, including visual display, must be provided as well as radiation monitors within the mini-cells and the dispensing hot cells. Appropriate exit radiation monitoring devices should be provided from the control areas.

Cleanrooms

The majority of PET radiopharmaceuticals are intended for parenteral administration and all processes must be undertaken in accordance with GMP. This requires the construction of a suitably designed cleanroom suite with appropriate support and changing rooms as described earlier, for the housing of the hot cells. Since the hot cell assembly utilises ‘isolator technology’, current MHRA guidance would be to construct a GMP Class D room or better. Guidance provided in Annex 1 of the EU *Guidelines on Current Good Radiopharmacy Practice* (EANM 2007) should be adopted. Most practically, the cleanroom should be constructed adjacent to or close to the cyclotron vault. This will allow target radionuclide liquid to be delivered through short lines of tubing (e.g. fluoroplastic polymer tubing such as ETFE), via shielded conduit, to an entry point in the cleanroom and then on into the production hot cells. Non-radioactive materials and components required for production are disinfected into the cleanroom through an interlocking hatch system.

Hot cells

The hot cell process

Typically, radioactive liquid or gas from the cyclotron is delivered via a shielded conduit to a multipurpose switching valve within the hot cell assembly. Radioactive material can then be passed to one of a number of mini-cells. These cells house the PC-driven proprietary chemistry modules where the target radionuclide is transformed into the desired radiochemical.

From each of the mini-cells, shielded sterilised tubing transports material to a dispensing isolator for further processing. Some systems may incorporate delivery to a steriliser in the first instance, whereas others will rely on an aseptic process that includes a terminal filtration step. Meanwhile, non-radioactive materials and components required for the process are disinfected into a transfer chamber and transferred into an unshielded preparation isolator where all non-radioactive aseptic manipulations are performed. Assembled non-radioactive components can then be transferred via an internal transfer cell into the dispensing isolator.

To minimise operator radiation exposure, an automated dose dispenser (ADD), located in the dispensing isolator, should be used to transfer finished product from the stock vial into individual patient dose vials or syringes. A small sample for quality control testing can also be taken at this point. Together with a radioactivity calibrator sited within the dispensing isolator, the ADD can be programmed to draw the desired volume from the stock vial to the patient dose container. Filled patient containers can be transferred via a transfer device and air lock to shielded transfer containers located outside of the dispensing isolator for shipment.

Hot cell design

Conventional hot cells are heavily shielded enclosures in which radioactive materials can be handled remotely and viewed through shielded windows. This allows extremely radioactive items to be manipulated and worked upon without exposing operators to dangerous amounts of radiation. Hot cells used for manufacturing PET radiopharmaceuticals have the additional element of aseptic processing designed into them. Therefore, a series of sealed and ventilated containments provided with HEPA filters on the supply and extract ducts are required. A variety of configurations of mini-cells and shielded and unshielded isolators are in use. Those used for operations with radioactive materials must be shielded with 75 mm lead (either fixed or moveable shielding) to protect the operator. The design should also include the necessary automation and ergonomic considerations to minimise radiation exposure. Internal materials should be inert and selected to be easily cleaned and withstand regular and frequent application of sanitising agents. Some units have been designed that incorporate a vaporised hydrogen peroxide supply for automated sterilisation. The dispensing isolator will require a dose ionisation chamber, which is best fitted as an integral part of the enclosure to allow measurements of dispensed items prior to removal from the isolator. The preparation and dispensing isolators will require glove ports accessed when the shielding is open, for setting up the production equipment. All internal equipment and doors should be positioned so that they can be reached using remote handling tongs. Access through these ports must be restricted when high levels of activity are present in the isolator. The dispensing isolator, in addition, requires remote handling manipulators and shielded viewing windows. An ADD unit for filling of vials or syringes should also be installed in the dispensing isolator to provide the required operator safety.

Mini-cells will require a supply of process gases such as compressed air, nitrogen, etc., to be piped from the gas manifold. All parts of the hot cell assembly require to be fitted with easily accessed test points for connection of test instruments (particle counter, manometer, filter efficiency test, leak tests, etc.) in order to allow validation and monitoring of the internal environment. Replacement of light tubes or bulbs should be achievable from outside the isolators. Electrical supply will be required for chemistry units, associated PCs and the radioactive calibrator.

There will be a requirement for shielded safe storage beneath the cells for radioactive waste and other radioactive items while they decay. Storage will also be required for accessories such as HPLC components required for the chemistry modules. Consideration must be given to the sterilisation and replacement of product delivery tubing lines, e.g. from the switching valve to each of the mini-cells (tubing to be replaced every few months or so) and from each of the mini-cells to the dispensing isolator (on a regular basis).

Hot cell: air classification and pressure differentials

Advice will differ depending on the regulatory agency of an individual country. The best advice currently is that a pressure drop of 15–20 Pa should be designed between the adjacent elements of the hot cell, with the lowest pressure being in the cell with air at the lowest environmental classification. When a door is opened between adjacent elements, the airflow will be from the higher to the lower air class. Transfer chamber doors should be interlocked to allow a minimum of 2 minutes for clean-down of particles before transfer can occur.

Owing to their potential radiological hazard, mini-cells should operate at negative pressure with air constantly extracted to atmosphere to provide protection. Although served with HEPA-filtered air to the same quality as the rest of the hot cell assembly, air quality can be specified at GMP Grade C to make allowances for the turbulent flow and *in-situ* equipment. The preparation and dispensing isolators should be designed to operate at GMP Class A conditions under positive pressure with partial recirculation. Air pressures in each part of the hot cell assembly should be continuously monitored, along with fan speed and filter pressure drop, and with audible and visual alarms (override for testing). With regard to leak testing, the shielded dispensing isolator and mini-cells must conform to Class 1 as defined in ISO 10648-2 while the unshielded preparation isolator and transfer cell to conform to a minimum of Class 2. Gloves, gaiters and door seals should be monitored by an automated test cycle. Internal pressures of the hot cell assembly components should be continuously displayed, while airflow within the preparation and dispensing isolators should also be displayed and recorded.

Radiochemistry and quality control

A number of commercially available automated (electromechanical) chemistry systems, have been developed for the manufacture of PET radiopharmaceuticals. Many of these systems are dedicated to producing only one radioactive product and require cleaning and refilling with fresh starting materials after each run. Starting materials, complexity of the chemistry, and re-use processes will all have a bearing on the quality control tests required. Basic requirements include radionuclidic identity, radiochemical purity, chemical purity, pH, residual solvent, sterility and bacterial endotoxin level. Therefore, design of a PET production facility must include a quality control laboratory and analytical facilities.

Conventional chemistry modules offer a number of challenges to GMP and the product produced from them requires that a wide range of quality control tests be performed. However, future developments, where the same platform can perform different chemistries using pre-loaded GMP-produced sealed cassettes, may lead to lower risk and greater simplicity of operation.

Commissioning a new facility

At the planning stage of designing any new facility, consideration must be given to how the unit will be commissioned to show that it complies with GMP as well as performing to the design specification. This process is known as validation and it is a documented process wherein a facility, a process or a piece of equipment is tested to demonstrate that it actually performs to give the expected result in a consistent manner. Validation should be carried out against a set of criteria that are defined in advance in a protocol document known as the validation plan. As part of this, re-validation after any change is also required along with periodic re-validation to ensure the systems are operating as originally validated. Qualification is part of validation and may be considered as four separate but related processes that are intended to answer particular questions.

- Design Qualification (DQ) – has it been designed correctly?
- Installation Qualification (IQ) – has it been built or installed correctly?
- Operational Qualification (OQ) – does it work correctly?
- Performance Qualification (PQ) – does it produce the product correctly and reproducibly?

For a fuller description of what might be expected during the commissioning of a facility the reader is directed to Annex 15 of GMP (MHRA 2007) and PIC/S documents PI 006-3, PI 007-3 (PIC/S 2007a,b).

To illustrate the process of commissioning an operation with the validation matrix see Table 26.3.

Table 26.3 Example of validation process: Staff entry from pre-change room to GMP Grade B cleanroom

Element of validation process	Tests to be applied
Design Qualification (DQ)	· Room to comply with GMP Grade B
	· HEPA filtered air supply
	· Interlocking doors to adjacent rooms
	· Room fabric to cleanroom standard
	· Pressure cascade with adjacent rooms (<10 Pa)

(continued overleaf)

Table 26.3 *(continued)*

Element of validation process	Tests to be applied
	• Equipment including, mirror, clothes hooks, step-over bench
Installation Qualification (IQ)	• HEPA installed and is correct grade (H14)
	• Materials used for surfaces are of cleanroom standard
	• Construction gives impervious and smooth surface
	• Equipment is present and is installed correctly
	• Step-over bench made from stainless steel 316L
	• Door interlocks are present and work correctly
Operational Qualification (OQ)	• Filter complies with integrity and leak tests
	• Room particle counts show GMP Grade B unmanned
	• Room pressure differentials comply with design specification
	• Filter pressure differentials comply with design specification
	• Air changes comply with design specification
	• Airflow patterns record no static areas of air
	• After cleaning of the facility, microbiological testing of the room to show compliance with the design specification
	• Airborne microbial contamination using settle plates shows compliance with GMP Grade B unmanned
	• Surface microbial contamination using contact plates shows compliance with GMP Grade B unmanned
	• Active air sampling show compliance with GMP Grade B unmanned
Performance Qualification (PQ)	• Physical and microbiological testing of the room to show compliance with the design specification
	• Room particle counts show GMP Grade B manned
	• Airborne microbial contamination using settle plates shows compliance with GMP grade B manned
	• Surface microbial contamination using contact plates shows compliance with GMP grade B manned
	• Active air sampling shows compliance with GMP grade B manned
	• Operators are able to use the change room to enter the clean room and the changing process can be validated to GMP
	• Process to be performed in the cleanroom is not compromised by the changing process
Performance Re-qualification	• Routine environmental monitoring shows continued compliance with the PQ. Changes in the facility or the changing process may require re-qualification of the facility or process

Good Manufacturing Practice (GMP)

The subject of GMP is dealt with extensively elsewhere. The reader is directed to EU Guidance on GMP (Section II, MHRA (2007), the 'Orange Guide' and PIC/S guidance notes. More specifically the EANM Radiopharmacy Committee have published *Current Good Radiopharmacy Practice* (cGRPP) guidelines (EANM 2007).

In practical terms, the premises and equipment used to manufacture radiopharmaceuticals will have an important bearing on the quality of the products made. However, other essentials including materials used, procedures/documentation, quality control, monitoring and maintenance must be in place. The single most important element in all of this is the personnel themselves. It is vital that sufficient numbers of competent, appropriately qualified and trained staff are available. Only through the effective management of all these elements will we achieve good manufacturing practice. Although GMP is covered comprehensively elsewhere (Chapters 22 and 28), it may be worth while to mention some practical aspects of the aseptic process in more detail.

Cleaning and disinfection

The highest level of cleanliness is required for the manufacture of sterile products intended for injection. It stands to reason therefore that as part of the commissioning of a new unit extensive cleaning and validation is required (in particular the cleanroom suite) prior to hand-over. On an on-going basis, there should be continuity of staff performing cleaning duties and they must be trained and assessed appropriately. Floors, walls, ceilings and work surfaces will require to be cleaned and disinfected regularly. Dedicated cleaning equipment should be used to minimise microbiological contamination and it has become recognised good practice to use sterile disposable mop heads and cleaning solutions. The effectiveness of cleaning should be assessed using contact plates, and the use of alternative disinfectant agents may be required if adverse trends develop.

Cleanroom clothing and changing procedure

The greatest likely source of microbiological contamination introduced into a functioning cleanroom environment will be carried on human skin. Therefore, particularly when dealing with conventional Class B cleanrooms, it is necessary for operators to wear appropriate sterile clothing to cover as much skin as possible. Many contract companies offer services where sterile suits are provided. In addition, the use of pre-sterilised face (and beard) masks and sterile gloves and an effective hand wash/disinfection will be required. Suits are worn for a session, monitored, and sent back for reprocessing (allowing adequate time for decay of any radioactive contamination). As part of operator training, the hand washing procedure should be validated to determine the microbiological status at each stage of the change procedure.

Transfer of materials and microbiological monitoring/validation

Materials such as needles, syringes, lead shields, saline bags, etc., that are used in the dispensing procedure should be sprayed and wiped with a suitable disinfectant, e.g. 70% sterile Industrial Methylated Spirit prior to transfer into the cleanroom. This process should be validated by the use of contact plates.

Settle plates (TSA) should be exposed within the workstation during each dispensing session to determine that microbiological status is within GMP specification (Orange Guide 2007, Annex 1). Sessional plates should also include finger dabs. Regular active air sampling should be used to supplement settle-plate information.

Sterility testing/operator/process validation

Since radioactive samples have to be left to decay for an adequate time the main purpose of testing is to ensure that the procedures used in the radiopharmacy result in sterile products. This test is best supplemented by simulating the aseptic processes using sterile broth. Any contamination will require to be fully investigated and the root cause determined.

Operator safety

The radiopharmacy must be a safe place for staff to work. From a practical point of view, radiation protection can be provided by the appropriate use of shielding and workstation containment. Dispensing techniques must be adopted that prevent the pressurising of closed vials and avoid creation of aerosols during transfer. Extra care will require to be taken with boiled kits, which must be adequately cooled prior to further manipulation. A programme for contamination monitoring and decontamination of work surfaces should be in place. Personnel must monitor their exposure on a continuous basis using appropriate dosimetry devices. Staff must also monitor any direct contamination (clothing or skin) and decontaminate as necessary. On some occasions staff protection through the appropriate use of thyroid blocking may be considered necessary.

Apart from radiation, staff will be subject to other hazards such as chemicals and biohazards. It may be prudent for staff involved in blood labelling, for example, to be immunised against hepatitis virus, while staff will also need to be familiar with the appropriate COSHH (Control of Substances Hazardous to Health) assessments and wear protective clothing when handling hazardous chemicals.

References

BS EN 12469 (2000). *Biotechnology – Performance Criteria for Microbiological Safety Cabinets.* Milton Keynes: British Standards Institution.

BS EN ISO 14644 (1999). *Clean Rooms and Associated Controlled Environments. Part 1: Classification of Air Cleanliness.* (1999). London: British Standards Institution.

EANM (2007) *Guidelines on Current Good Radiopharmacy Practice (cGRPP) in the Preparation of Radiopharmaceuticals.* Vienna: European Association for Nuclear Medicine (EANM). https://www.eanm.org/scientific_info/guidelines/gl_radioph_cgrpp.php?navId=54 (accessed 1 February 2009).

IPEM (2002). *Medical and Dental Guidance Notes. A Good Practice Guide on all Aspects of Ionising Radiation Protection in the Clinical Environment.* York: Institute of Physics and Engineering in Medicine.

MHRA (2007) *Rules and Guidance for Pharmaceutical Manufacturers and Distributors(GMP).* London: Pharmaceutical Press.

Midcalf B *et al.* (2004). *Pharmaceutical Isolators.* London: Pharmaceutical Press.

PIC/S (Pharmaceutical Inspection Convention and Pharmaceutical Inspection Co-operation Scheme) (2007a). PIC/S PI006-3. *Validation Master Plan, Installation and Operational Qualification, Non-Sterile Process Validation, Cleaning Validation.* Geneva: PIC/S. http://www.picscheme.org/publis/recommandations/PI%20006-3%20Recommendation%20on%20Validation%20Master%20Plan.pdf (accessed 1 February 2009).

PIC/S (Pharmaceutical Inspection Convention and Pharmaceutical Inspection Co-operation Scheme) (2007b). PIC/S PI007-3 Recommendation on the validation of aseptic processes. September 2007. http://www.picscheme.org/publis/recommandations/PI%20007-3%20Recommendation%20on%20Aseptic%20Processes.pdf (accessed 1 February 2009).

Stationery Office (1999). *The Ionising Radiations Regulations 1999.* SI 1999, No. 3232. London: The Stationery Office.

Further Reading and Sources

Alexoff D (2001). *Automation for the Synthesis and Application of PET Radiopharmaceuticals.* Upton, NY: Brookhaven National Laboratory.

Beaney AM (2006). *Quality Assurance of Aseptic Preparation Services*, 4th edn. London: Pharmaceutical Press.

Department of Health (2007). *Health Building Note 14-01: Pharmacy and Radiopharmacy facilities.* London: Department of Health. http://195.92.246.148/knowledge_network/documents/HBN_14_01_Exec_summ_20070823130817.pdf (accessed 1 February 2009).

Pharmaceutical Inspection Convention and Pharmaceutical Inspection Co-operation Scheme (PIC/S). (2008). *Guide to Good Practices for the Preparation of Medicinal Products in Healthcare Establishments.* Geneva: PIC/S. http://www.picscheme.org/publication.php?p=guides (accessed 1 February 2009).

Stationery Office (2004). *The Ionising Radiation (Medical Exposure) Regulations 2004.* SI 2000, No. 1059. London: The Stationery Office.

Yu S (2006). Review of ^{18}F-FDG synthesis and quality control. *Biomed Imaging Interv J* 2: e57.

27

Regulation of radiopharmacy practice in Europe

Clemens Decristoforo

Overview

The European Union (EU) provides a system for a common framework harmonising the legal basis for pharmaceutical, radiation protection, transport and other radiopharmacy-related issues. However, many details remain nationally regulated, resulting in great differences in radiopharmacy practice between countries.

This chapter tries to describe all players in the legislation relevant to radiopharmacy practice in Europe and how they interact, and it reviews the main legal issues and documents. This is summarised in Figure 27.1.

Regulatory framework in Europe

Introduction

Historically, legislation in Europe has been the prerogative of national states, enacting legislation being applied only within that state reflecting its tradition and culture. Since World War II and the advent of the European Union, with globalisation of trade but also competition, some harmonisation has taken place. However, the current practice of radiopharmacy in Europe still varies from country to country, to a great extent owing to varying national and sometimes even local interpretation of existing rules. This is possible as not all regulatory documents are mandatory ('hard law') but, strictly seen, are only recommendations for authorities or professionals ('soft law'); however, they are often strictly implemented in some states.

Legislation in the field of medicine has the common goal of protecting the patient, the environment and involved professionals, but, in some cases, also to protect or promote the European market. In the field of radiopharmaceuticals and radiopharmacy practice this is mainly covered by radiation safety and pharmaceutical regulations.

This chapter tries to give an overview of the current European situation, but it should be kept in mind that regulations undergo constant changes. It should

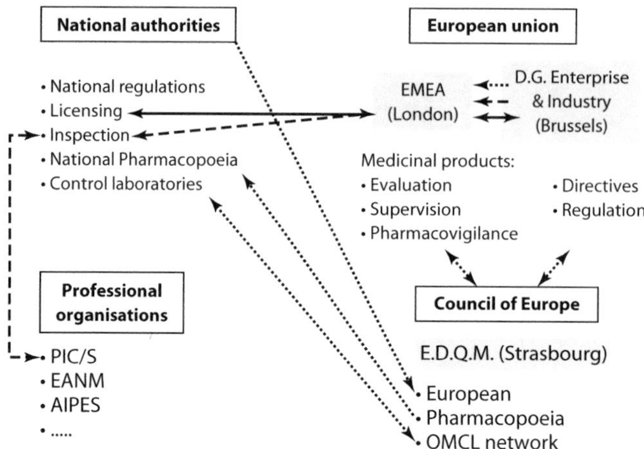

Figure 27.1 Players in pharmaceutical legislation in Europe and examples of interrelation (solid line, marketing authorisation; dashed line, GMP; dotted line, quality requirements).

therefore be read taking into account most recent changes in legislation.

The European Union

The European Union originates from the idea of a common market enabling free trade and exchange within Europe. Currently the EU is composed of 27 member states and a number of European countries have signified their intention to join, with the consequence that they are harmonising their national legislation with that of the EU. Even countries that have declined to join the EU (e.g. Switzerland or Norway) today have, in many aspects, comparable regulations in pharmaceutical issues that enable them to participate in the common market. Thus, EU legislation is important for all European countries, members or not.

The legislative body of the EU is the European Parliament in Brussels and Strasbourg. Its members approve Regulations and Directives that are issued by the EU Commission after consultation with member states. The competences of the European Parliament and the Commission are usually clearly defined and separated from National competences. This means that some topics are still regulated nationally and European legislation plays a minor role. This is the case for regulations regarding magistral and officinal preparations of pharmaceuticals (see below).

European legislative documents are drafted by working parties in the related Directorates General (DGs); for pharmaceutical legislation this is the DG Enterprise and industry, also situated in Brussels. Different legal documents are issued by the Parliament and the EU Commission.

Directives, Regulations and Guidelines

Directives are rules addressed by the EU Commission to the Member States to be translated into the respective national legislation and effectively implemented. Directives are mandatory but leave some room for interpretation at the national level. Deadlines are defined for implementation; however, they are not always met by the national parliaments. European *Regulations* are mandatory in all countries, being directly applied without translation into the national legislation. Besides these 'hard law documents' *Guidelines* may be released by the Commission that are not mandatory but represent recommendations for the effective implementation of Directives and Regulations by the individual Member States. They are intended as advice to interested parties (e.g. applicants for marketing authorisation). Scientific guidelines are often issued to reflect the current scientific knowledge on a certain topic.

The Council of Europe

Besides the European Union, the Council of Europe (CE) has to be mentioned when addressing regulatory aspects of radiopharmacy practice. The CE is situated in Strasbourg and most European Countries including non-EU member states such as Russia or Switzerland are members (currently 46). In contrast to the EU, which has a focus on economy, the CE's mission is to promote and secure human rights. In a convention of the CE of 1964 to promote the free movement of medicines throughout Europe the idea of a common European Pharmacopoeia was born; it is now released by a body of the CE, the European Directorate of Quality of Medicines (EDQM).

National regulations

Although the EU provides a common legal framework, specific issues are still left to be regulated by its member states, unless there is a conflict with EU common interests (free movement of goods, equivalent rights independent from EU nationality, etc.). A typical example is drug preparation. Whereas the industrial preparation is regulated by the EU, pharmacy preparation standards remain the responsibility of the individual member states. However, the interpretation of what is covered by industrial manufacture and pharmacy practice does vary from country to country.

Radiation protection regulations: Euratom

Radiation safety regulation has been standardised in Europe with the implementation of the so called Euratom directives. European Atomic Energy Community (Euratom) is based on a treaty of the members of the European Community mainly to ensure the establishment of the basic installations necessary for the development of nuclear energy in the Community. It is under the responsibility of the Commissioner of Energy with the mandate to draft regulations and directives. The Euratom directives refer to the protection of professionals, patients and the general public from ionising radiation and have changed the perception of radiation protection practices over the last ten years. Directive 96/29/EURATOM (Euratom 1996) sets basic safety standards in the use of radiation in general, whereas Directive 97/43/EURATOM (Euratom 1997) specifically deals with the medical use of radiation ('Medical Exposure Directive'). The directives were released in the late 1990s and came into effect in May 2000, although some countries changed their national legislation to comply with the directives as late as 2002.

The impact on radiopharmacy practice of these directives is manifold. Regarding the facilities of a radiopharmacy, Directive 96/29/EURATOM clearly requires any deliberate addition of radioactive substances in the production of medicinal products as well as their administration to humans to have prior authorisation. This means that any radiopharmacy practice must have an authorisation in accordance with national radiation safety regulations. In some countries this is the main basis for authorisation and inspection of nuclear medicine departments and radiopharmacies, as there are exemptions from the authorisation as drug manufacturer or pharmacy (e.g. Germany). Directive 96/29/EURATOM also defines controlled and supervised areas specifying details on working practices. A major impact of this directive is related to the radiopharmacy personal. This includes classification of workers according to their potential exposure (radiopharmacists have to be classified as Category A workers) and dose constraints. Annual dose limits and age limits are defined but may be stricter in some countries. The need for information and training in radiation protection and medical surveillance is defined as well as procedures/protocols for special cases such as pregnant workers and students.

Directive 97/43/EURATOM is the basis of national legislation to protect the patient and the general public from medical radiation exposure. This includes exposure in occupational health surveillance or health screening or individuals/patients in research programmes. A major impact of this directive was the implementation of strict quality control regimes for devices such as X-ray machines, CT machines or gamma cameras. For radiopharmacy practice, many European countries legally enforce quality control measures of equipment such as dose calibrators and radiation monitors and in some countries even the quality control of radiopharmaceuticals is a legal requirement. Another issue for radiopharmaceuticals in this directive is the requirement to establish national reference levels for administered activities of radiopharmaceuticals. This means that on a national level recommended radioactivities for standard nuclear medicine investigations must be available. For the therapeutic application of radiopharmaceuticals, some EU member states have introduced the requirement of individual dosimetry based on this directive. All these measures can be summarised under Optimisation of Radiation Exposure. In terms of responsibilities this directive defines the need for a medical physics expert recognised by the national authorities. The need for a radiopharmacist or related expert is not defined, however. It also defines the need for additional and continuing education and training programmes of personnel involved in the medical use of radiation, mentioning specifically the need to address quality assurance in the assessment of administered radioactivity.

Marketing Authorisation and EMEA

All documents regarding pharmaceutical legislation in the EU can be found in the so-called EudraLex on-line compendium of the directives and regulations (EudraLex 2010). The major legal document regulating the use of drugs within the European Union is the directive 2001/83/EC (EC 2001a). It clearly states that radiopharmaceuticals, generators, kits and radionuclide precursors (but not sealed sources) are medicinal products (see Table 27.1) therefore falling under this pharmaceutical regulation including a requirement for Marketing Authorisation. Marketing Authorisation is not required when medicines including

Table 27.1 Selection of European legal documents relevant to radiopharmaceuticals

Name of document	Commonly used name	Relevant topic addressed
Regulation		
EC 1394/2007	Advanced Therapy Regulation	Issues related to novel drugs (e.g. cell-based)
Directives		
91/356/EEC	Human GMP	Basics for GMP for medicinal products for human use
96/29/EURATOM	Basic Safety Standards	General radiation safety
97/43/EURATOM	Medical Exposure Directive	Radiation safety in respect to medical application
2001/20/EC	Clinical Trial Directive	General requirements for clinical trials
2001/83/EG		General requirements for pharmaceutical preparation and marketing authorisation, Qualified Person definition
2003/94/EG		GMP requirement for IMP (Annex 13)
2004/27/EC		GMP requirement for API
2005/28/EC		Authorization for IMP preparation
Guidelines		
EMEA/CHMP/SWP/28367/2007	First in Human Clinical Trial Guideline	Recommendation for trials using a new drug for the first time
EMEA/CPMP/ICH/286/95		Requirements on non-clinical safety studies for the conduct of clinical trials.
EMEA/CHMP/QWP/306970/2007	Guideline on Radiopharmaceuticals	Specific requirements for application of marketing authorisation of radiopharmaceuticals
CHMP/QWP/185401/2004	IMPD file	Structure and contents of IMPD

radiopharmaceuticals are prepared in a pharmacy according to a medical prescription by a medical doctor or based on a pharmacopoeial monograph, nor for blood products. Investigational Medicinal Products (IMPs) are exempted as they are regulated specifically (see below). A marketing authorisation can be gained via different routes.

The *centralised procedure* is compulsory for products developed by means of certain biotechnological processes, orphan drugs and new active substances for the treatment of AIDS, cancer, neurodegenerative disorders, diabetes, autoimmune diseases and other immune dysfunctions and viral diseases. However, this applies only for therapeutic products, and only a few radiopharmaceuticals have been authorised via this centralised procedure (e.g. Zevalin) owing to the more complex application process and higher fees payable. Applications for a centralised marketing authorisation are evaluated by the EMA (formerly EMEA) situated in London.

Most radiopharmaceuticals have been granted a national marketing authorisation. Within the so called *mutual recognition procedure* additional member states can approve the authorisation leading to a wider acceptance within the EU without full separate evaluation procedures by each national authority. In the *decentralised procedure* the applicant (the radiopharmaceutical manufacturer) can engage several member states where they would like to apply for a marketing authorisation and chooses one of these as the reference member state for evaluation of their product. This procedure potentially allows simultaneous approval in several member states, but so far has not been used for radiopharmaceuticals.

The European Medicines Agency (EMA) based in London is the EU body dealing with the evaluation, supervision and pharmacovigilance of medicinal products. The Committee for Medicinal Products for Human Use (CHMP) is the responsible body within EMA for preparing documents concerning medicinal products for human use from preclinical requirements to clinical data. For radiopharmaceuticals the CHMP Guideline on Radiopharmaceuticals (EMEA 2007a) gives information on specific documents to be submitted when applying for marketing authorisation of radiopharmaceuticals. Whereas EMA evaluates the documentation and gives guidance, the legal body issuing the marketing authorisation is the European Commission.

Besides Marketing Authorisation, directive 2001/83/EC regulates the manufacture and import of medicinal products. It defines the need for authorisation of manufacturing sites and the requirement of a *Qualified Person*. A qualified person must hold an appropriate university degree and have at least 2 years of practical experience in an authorised institution. However, as radiopharmaceutical preparation is often carried out outside the strict definition of industrial manufacture, these requirements are currently not enforced in many European countries, be it in conventional radiopharmacy or in PET centres.

Additionally directive 2001/83/EC contains detailed requirements for labelling, Summary of product characteristics (SPC), package leaflet and other issues relevant to pharmaceuticals with some specific requirements for radiopharmaceuticals. Specific requirements for the SPC cover the inclusion of additional detailed instructions for extemporaneous preparation and quality control of such preparation. Exact definitions of the content of the label of the container are given and the directive requires the inclusion of an instruction leaflet with safety instructions for patients and users.

Clinical trial regulations

The conduct of clinical trials performed in Europe has changed dramatically with the implementation of the 'Clinical Trials Directive', Directive 2001/20/EC (EC 2001b).

The major change was the introduction of a common procedure of application for clinical trials both to the ethical committee and the competent authority. Application for a clinical trial has to be made supplying a set of documents that is standardised all over the EU. Approval of one national ethical committee can, in the case of multicentre trials, be applied to other centres without the requirement of full re-evaluation nationally. This has simplified the conduct of large multicentre clinical trials for the pharmaceutical industry. On the other hand, it has increased the demands of documentation to be submitted for clinical trials in an academic environment, usually performed in a single centre, as there are no significant simplifications for small studies. When submitting a clinical trial application this has to be entered into a centralised database called EudraCT, where every clinical trial in Europe can be identified by an individual EudraCT number.

A major document for studies with pharmaceuticals is the so called Investigational Medicinal Product Dossier (IMPD). It contains information on the Investigational Medicinal Product (IMP) including chemical and pharmaceutical particulars. A specific guideline on the structure and content of IMPDs has been released by EMA (EMEA 2004). Simplifications to the IMPD may be granted if the pharmaceutical to be used in a clinical trial has a marketing authorisation. In this case a simplified IMPD (mainly the SmPC of the product) can be submitted in the application process. As most radiopharmaceuticals to be used in clinical trials do not have a marketing authorisation this is of no help in the application process unless the radiopharmaceutical is not a central part of the study and is considered as a Non Investigational Medicinal Product (NIMP).

The Clinical Trial Directive also introduced the requirement that IMPs have to be prepared according to GMP. A specific annex to the GMP guidelines was introduced (Directive 2003/94 EC (EC 2003a)). Directive 2005/28/EC (EC 2005) additionally defined the requirement that institutions preparing IMPs have to be specifically authorised to do so.

Specific regulations and guidelines are available for clinical trials with new active substances that have not been tested in patients before. A specific EMA guideline (CHMP/SWP/28367/2007) (EMEA 2007b) describes requirements of the conduct of such 'First in human clinical trials'.

Toxicity requirements for pharmaceuticals to be used in clinical trials can be found in the 'Note for Guidance on Non-clinical Safety Studies for the Conduct of Human Clinical Trials for Pharmaceuticals needed to support human clinical trials of a given scope and duration' (EMEA/CPMP/ICH/286/95) (EMEA 2008). Very important for radiopharmaceuticals, especially when they are used for the first time in clinical studies, is the so called *microdosing* concept. A position paper from EMEA (CPMP/ICH/286/95) (CPMP 2008) defines two microdosing approaches (single or repeated injection) using less than 100 μg and $\leq$1/100th of the pharmacologically active dose per injection.

This can apply to many radiopharmaceuticals, especially if they are prepared at sufficiently high specific activity. Usually these are products that undergo final isolation and purification (e.g. PET products or ^{123}I-labelled radiopharmaceuticals), whereas kit-prepared radiopharmaceuticals and kit components often exceed this limit. Under microdosing conditions, the preclinical information regarding toxicity, genotoxicity and local tolerance required to support the conduct of clinical studies is simplified.

The dosimetry aspects of radiopharmaceuticals to be used in clinical trials are not specifically regulated in European legislation but can be found in corresponding international documents such as publications by the International Commission on Radiological Protection (ICRP).

Regulatory framework concerning GMP

Pharmaceutical production standards in Europe are regulated by 'Guidelines on Good Manufacturing Practice of Pharmaceuticals'. Although called guidelines, their basis is laid down in Directives (91/356/EEC, as amended by Directive 2003/94/EC and 91/412/EEC) (EC 2003b), and therefore changes are not very frequent. This is in contrast to the USA, where the term current Good Manufacturing Practice (cGMP) is used as the guidelines are reviewed annually.

European GMP is published in EudraLex Volume 4 and is composed of two basic parts, one for medicinal products and one for starting materials. Additionally there are a number of annexes covering specific pharmaceuticals. The main annex in the case of radiopharmaceutical preparations is Annex 3 on Manufacture of Radiopharmaceuticals. This annex describes specific issues of GMP related to radiopharmaceuticals and has been revised recently. Other annexes of importance in the field of radiopharmacy are Annex 1 on the 'Manufacture of Sterile Medicinal Products' and Annex 13 on the 'Manufacture of Investigational Medicinal Products'.

However, there is an ongoing discussion as to whether these 'industrial' GMP guidelines are applicable to preparation of radiopharmaceuticals in hospitals. The Radiopharmacy Committee of the EANM has published specific guidelines on the 'Current Good Radiopharmaceutical Practice' (cGRPP) to fill this gap (EANM 2007). To cover the specific needs in current practice, two distinct parts were included, Part A dealing with radiopharmaceuticals prepared from generators and kits, Part B with other radiopharmaceuticals, mainly but not exclusively for PET applications. Several issues have been addressed, allowing a more suitable interpretation of cGMP for small-scale radiopharmaceutical preparation.

Besides such efforts from a professional organisation, another major player in drafting GMP documents is the Pharmaceutical Inspection Convention and Pharmaceutical Inspection Co-operation Scheme (jointly referred to as PIC/S). This international convention of pharmaceutical inspectors has no legal force but in many cases the documents issued by PIC/S have been the basis of GMP guidelines in Europe. An important document in this respect is the PIC/S Guide to Good Practices for the preparation of Medicinal Products in Healthcare Establishments (PIC/S 2008) that describes a specific GMP mainly intended for hospital preparation of pharmaceuticals.

The current interpretation of GMP for radiopharmaceutical practice is very variable throughout Europe. Whereas, for example, the preparation of radiopharmaceuticals from kits and generators is not seen as a pharmaceutical preparation in many countries and therefore GMP is not enforced (e.g. Germany), other countries implement full GMP requirements for radiopharmacy practice (e.g. the UK). The situation is similar for preparation of PET radiopharmaceuticals in hospitals, although some GMP requirements are enforced in most countries.

The European Pharmacopoeia and EDQM

As mentioned above, the European Pharmacopoeia is based on a convention of the European Council to promote free movement of medicines in Europe. It is published by the European Directorate of Quality of Medicines (EDQM) in Strasbourg, which additionally produces and distributes pharmaceutical and biological reference standards, participating in the European Regulatory System by a centralised evaluation of the quality of drug substances and excipients. It runs a European Biological Standardisation programme as well as the European Network of the Official Medicines Control Laboratories (OMCL).

The European Pharmacopoeia convention has been signed by 37 European states, where the pharmacopoeia has a legally binding character, even in non-EU member states such as Switzerland or Norway. This is in contrast to the United States Pharmacopeia (USP) which is an independent, science-based public health organisation and has no direct legal force. The official languages of the European Pharmacopoeia are English and French; however, in many countries it is translated and partly implemented into the national pharmacopoeia. There are 15 additional countries (observer states) who recognise the European Pharmacopoeia outside Europe, such as Canada, the USA and even China.

The European Pharmacopoeia is directed by the European Pharmacopoeia Commission, to which every member state sends delegates who decide on its content, which is reviewed by national pharmacopoeia authorities. The intention of the European Pharmacopoeia is that it be used by manufacturers of medicinal products, suppliers to the pharmaceutical industry, regulatory authorities for medicines, and official medicines control laboratories, and also in the small-scale preparation of pharmaceuticals such as in radiopharmacies. It lays down compulsory standards for medicinal products that have to be met in any form of practice.

The European Pharmacopoeia contains specific monographs on medicinal substances and medicinal products, general methods of analysis to be applied in monographs, and general monographs and chapters on classes of substances and products. The latter are applicable to all medicinal products even if there is no specific monograph.

Monographs are drafted by experts groups dedicated to specific fields. For radiopharmaceuticals this is the so-called Group 14 with radiopharmaceutical experts from several European countries. Currently the European Pharmacopoeia contains a table of physical characteristics of radionuclides and one general monograph on radiopharmaceutical preparations. In this monograph important definitions such as radionuclidic and radiochemical purity or specific radioactivity and their interpretation can be found. Additionally, general information on the identification of a radiopharmaceutical (by half-life, energy) and specific issues of testing such as on endotoxins or sterility as well labelling can be found. Specific monographs on radiopharmaceuticals can be found on conventional radiopharmaceuticals including ^{99m}Tc, radioiodinated materials, other diagnostic radionuclides (^{3}H, ^{51}Cr, ^{57}Co, ^{58}Co, ^{61}Ga, ^{111}In, ^{81m}Kr, ^{201}Tl, ^{133}Xe) and therapeutic radionuclides (^{32}P, ^{89}Sr). An increasing number of monographs deal with PET radiopharmaceuticals (^{18}F, ^{11}C, ^{15}O) and recently monographs on radionuclide precursors (radionuclide formulations that are used for radiolabelling or preparation of generators such as ^{131}I, ^{123}I, ^{99}Mo) and also non-radioactive precursors have been added (mannose triflate, DTPA, MDP). Recent revision of older monographs led to a replacement of some animal testing (identity testing by a biodistribution test) and replacement of pyrogen tests by endotoxin tests in most monographs.

A list of current monographs in the European Pharmacopoeia is given in Table 27.2.

General chapters of importance for radiopharmacy practice are those on biological tests (sterility, pyrogens, bacterial endotoxins) and limit tests (heavy metals, identification and control of residual solvents) as well as on specific dosage forms (parenteral preparations).

The European Pharmacopoeia is important in those cases where radiopharmaceuticals are not prepared from licensed kits and generators. This is especially true for industrial manufacturers who have to show that their products comply with the standards set in the European Pharmacopoeia before marketing authorisation is granted as well as for the release of their products. Here, authorities often demand additional data and testing, and the European Pharmacopoeia is seen as setting the minimum standard. For radiopharmacy practice the European Pharmacopoeia has become of great importance, especially for PET preparations but also for all other preparations made outside normal routine, e.g. in-house kit preparation, radiolabelling for therapeutic applications, deviations from authorised use. The question often arises whether preparations have to undergo all tests described in the European Pharmacopoeia in every case. This is sometimes interpreted differently by authorities, but it is clear that a radiopharmaceutical preparation has to comply if tested.

For daily radiopharmacy practice, the European Pharmacopoeia is a reliable source of validated methods to be used in the analysis of radiopharmaceuticals, e.g. for radiochemical purity determinations.

Table 27.2 Current monographs of the European Pharmacopeia on Radiopharmaceuticals

Title	Monograph no.
General monographs	
Radiopharmaceutical preparations	0125
Table of physical characteristics of radionuclides mentioned in the European Pharmacopoeia	
Parenteral preparations	0520
Bacterial endotoxins	20614
Radiopharmaceutical monographs	
Chromium [^{51}Cr] Edetate Injection	0266
Cyanocobalamin (^{57}Co) Capsules	710
Cyanocobalamin (^{57}Co) Solution	269
Cyanocobalamin (^{58}Co) Capsules	1505
Cyanocobalamin (^{58}Co) Solution	270
Gallium [^{67}Ga] Citrate Injection	0555
Human Albumin Injection, Iodinated [^{125}I]	1922
Indium [^{111}In] Chloride Solution	1227
Indium [^{111}In] Oxine Solution	1109
Indium [^{111}In] Pentetate Injection	0670
Iobenguane [^{123}I] Injection	1113
Iobenguane [^{131}I] Injection for Diagnostic Use	1111
Iobenguane [^{131}I] Injection for Therapeutic Use	1112
Krypton (^{81m}Kr) Inhalation Gas	1533
Norcholesterol Injection Iodinated [^{131}I]	0939
Sodium Chromate [^{51}Cr] Sterile Solution	0279
Sodium Iodide [^{123}I] Injection	0563
Sodium Iodide [^{131}I] Capsules for Diagnostic Use	938
Sodium Iodide [^{131}I] Capsules for Therapeutic Use	2116
Sodium Iodide [^{131}I] Solution	0281

(continued)

Table 27.2 *(continued)*

Title	Monograph no.
Sodium Iodohippurate [^{123}I] Injection	0564
Sodium Iodohippurate [^{131}I] Injection	0282
Sodium Pertechnetate [^{99m}Tc] Injection Fission	0124
Sodium Pertechnetate [^{99m}Tc] Injection Non Fission	0283
Sodium Phosphate [^{32}P] Injection	0284
Strontium [^{89}Sr] Chloride Injection	1475
Technetium [^{99m}Tc] Bicisate Injection	2123
Technetium [^{99m}Tc] Colloidal Rhenium Sulphide Injection	0126
Technetium [^{99m}Tc] Colloidal Sulphur Injection	0131
Technetium [^{99m}Tc] Colloidal Tin Injection	0689
Technetium [^{99m}Tc] Etifenin Injection	0585
Technetium [^{99m}Tc] Exametazime Injection	1925
Technetium [^{99m}Tc] Gluconate Injection	1047
Technetium [^{99m}Tc] Human Albumin Injection	0640
Technetium [^{99m}Tc] Macrosalb Injection	0296
Technetium [^{99m}Tc] Medronate Injection	0641
Technetium [^{99m}Tc] Mertiatide Injection	1372
Technetium [^{99m}Tc] Microspheres Injection	0570
Technetium [^{99m}Tc] Pentetate Injection	0642
Technetium [^{99m}Tc] Sestamibi Injection	1926
Technetium [^{99m}Tc] Succimer Injection	0643
Technetium [^{99m}Tc] Tin Pyrophosphate Injection	0129
Thallous [^{201}Tl] Chloride Injection	0571
Tritiated [^{3}H] Water Injection	0112
Xenon [^{133}Xe] Injection	0133
PET radiopharmaceutical monographs	
Ammonia [^{13}N] Injection	1492
Carbon Monoxide (^{15}O)	1607

Table 27.2 *(continued)*

Title	Monograph no.
Fludeoxyglucose [^{18}F] Injection	1325
Flumazenil (N-[^{11}C]methyl) Injection	1917
Fluorodopa [^{18}F] (Prepared by Electrophilic Substitution) Injection	1918
L-Methionine ([^{11}C]methyl) Injection	1617
Oxygen (^{15}O)	1620
Raclopride ([^{11}C]methoxy) Injection	1924
Sodium Acetate [^{11}C] Injection	1920
Sodium Fluoride [^{18}F] Injection	2100
Water [^{15}O] Injection	1582
Radionuclide precursor monographs	
Sodium Iodide [^{123}I] Solution for Radiolabelling	2314
Sodium Iodide [^{131}I] Solution for Radiolabelling	2121
Sodium Molybdate [^{99}Mo] Solution (Fission)	1923
Precursor monographs	
Iobenguane Sulphate for Radiopharmaceutical Preparations	2351
Medronic Acid for Radiopharmaceutical Preparations	2350
Pentetate Sodium Calcium for Radiopharmaceutical Preparations	2353
Sodium Iodohippurate for Radiopharmaceutical Preparations	2352
Tetra-*O*-Acetyl-Mannose Triflate for Radiopharmaceutical Preparations	2294

Specific national regulations

Despite the common legal framework in Europe a number of member states have released specific documents relating to the small-scale extemporaneous preparation of radiopharmaceuticals. They deal with exemptions of radiopharmaceutical preparations from the requirement for a marketing authorisation, qualification of personnel in radiopharmacy, and in some cases exemptions from GMP. Some examples reflecting the complex situation in Europe are outlined below; the specific regulations in the UK regarding use of radiopharmaceuticals and the rather strict implementation of GMP are covered in Chapter 28.

The preparation of radiopharmaceuticals from generators and kits is, in many European countries such as Germany, specifically exempted from pharmaceutical legislation and performed under the responsibility of the nuclear medicine physician, often without any further requirements except regarding radiation safety. In some countries there is the requirement for a pharmacist to be responsible for this practice. In Spain, France and Belgium radiopharmacy is even recognised as a specific speciality. Other countries have released specific requirements for radiopharmacy premises; in Italy by releasing a monograph within the National Pharmacopoeia, and in Switzerland by indirectly implementing GRPP guidelines as issued by the EANM.

In the field of PET (and other locally produced) radiopharmaceuticals, most European countries enforce pharmaceutical legislation more strictly. This includes at least some GMP requirements, the requirement of pharmaceutical authorisation and inspection and definition of qualified or responsible persons. Specific legislation allowing exemptions for marketing authorisation of (mainly) PET radiopharmaceuticals can be found, for example, in Germany. The recent change in the *Verordnung über radioaktive oder mit ionisierenden strahlen behandelte Arzneimittel* (AmRadV 1987) includes the possibility of using radiopharmaceuticals outside their marketing authorisation or clinical trials, if they are prepared in an authorised institution for not more than 20 applications per week. In Italy a recent change in pharmaceutical legislation (Italian Parliament 2007) includes the possibility to prepare and use 'experimental radiopharmaceuticals' without marketing authorisation but applying specific GMP guidance as outlined in the National Pharmacopoeia. Other comparative pharmaceutical legislation defining specific exemptions for radiopharmaceuticals can be found in Spain, Austria and other European countries. This also reflects an increasing awareness of the characteristics of radiopharmaceuticals regarding their increasingly short lived nature, their preparation on a small scale and the large variety of radiolabelled compounds available for the benefit of the patient.

Definitions and abbreviations in pharmaceutical legislation relevant to radiopharmaceuticals

- *AIPES:* Association of Imaging Producers and Equipment Suppliers (for nuclear medicine in Europe including industrial radiopharmaceutical producers)
- *API:* Active Pharmaceutical Ingredient, e.g. the radionuclide used, the ligand in Tc-kits, but also other materials that are involved in the preparation of the radiopharmaceutical but are not removed during the preparation process (reducing agent, precursor, ligand); has to be prepared under GMP.
- *API-starting material:* Starting material for preparation of an Active Pharmaceutical Ingredient, e.g. precursor for PET preparation if it is separated within the preparation process (e.g. by HPLC)
- *cGMP:* current Good Manufacturing Practice
- *CHMP:* Committee for Medicinal Products for Human Use (EMEA)
- *CPMP:* Committee for Proprietary Medicinal Products for Human Use (EMEA)
- *EANM:* European Association of Nuclear Medicine
- *EDQM:* European Directorate of Quality of Medicines
- *EMA:* European Medicines Agency (formerly European Medicines Evaluation Agency (EMEA)) in London
- *EudraCT:* European database on clinical trials
- *Euratom:* European Atomic Energy Community
- *GRPP:* Good Radiopharmaceutical Practice
- *ICRP:* International Committee on Radiation Protection
- *IMP:* Investigational Medicinal Product
- *IMPD* Investigational Medicinal Product dossier
- *Kit:* Any preparation to be reconstituted or combined with radionuclides in the final radiopharmaceutical, usually prior to its administration.

- *NIMP:* Non Investigational Medicinal Product
- *OMCL*: Official Medicines Control Laboratory (EDQM)
- *PIC/S:* Pharmaceutical Inspection Convention and Pharmaceutical Inspection Co-operation Scheme
- *QP*: Qualified Person
- *Radionuclide generator:* Any system incorporating a fixed parent radionuclide from which is produced a daughter radionuclide which is to be obtained by elution or by any other method and used in a radiopharmaceutical.
- *Radionuclide precursor:* Any other radionuclide produced for the radiolabelling of another substance prior to administration.
- *Radiopharmaceutical:* Any medicinal product which, when ready for use, contains one or more radionuclides (radioactive isotopes) included for a medicinal purpose.
- *SPC* or *SmPC:* Summary of Product Characteristics

References

AmRadV (1987). *Verordnung über radioaktive oder mit ionisierenden Strahlen behandelte Arzneimittel.* Berlin: Das Bundesministerium der Justiz. http://bundesrecht.juris.de/amradv/index.html (accessed 30 January 2009).

CPMP (2009). *Note for Guidance on Non-clinical Safety Studies for the Conduct of Human Clinical Trials and Marketing Authorization for pharmaceuticals.* http://www.emea.europa.eu/docs/en_GB/document_library/Scientific_guideline/2009/09/WC500002720.pdf (accessed 24 August 2010).

EANM (2007). EANM Radiopharmacy Committee. *Guidelines on Current Good Radiopharmacy Practice (cGRPP) in the Preparation of Radiopharmaceuticals* http://www.eanm.org/scientific_info/guidelines/gl_radioph_cgrpp.pdf (accessed 30 January 2009).

EC (2001a) Directive 2001/83/EC. http://ec.europa.eu/enterprise/pharmaceuticals/eudralex/vol-1/dir_2001_83_cons/dir2001_83_cons_en.pdf (accessed 5 February 2009).

EC (2001b) Directive 2001/20/EC. http://ec.europa.eu/enterprise/pharmaceuticals/eudralex/vol-1/dir_2001_20/dir_2001_20_en.pdf (accessed 5 February 2009).

EC (2003a). Directive 2003/94 EG. http://ec.europa.eu/enterprise/pharmaceuticals/eudralex/vol-1/dir_2003_94/dir_2003_94_en.pdf (accessed 5 February 2009).

EC (2003b). 91/356/EEC, as amended by Directive 2003/94/EC and 91/412/EEC. http://ec.europa.eu/enterprise/pharmaceuticals/eudralex/vol4_en.htm (accessed 5 February 2009).

EC (2005). Directive 2005/28/EC. http://ec.europa.eu/enterprise/pharmaceuticals/eudralex/vol-1/dir_2005_28/dir_2005_28_en.pdf (accessed 5 February 2009).

EMEA (2004) CHMP/QWP/185401/2004. http://www.emea.europa.eu/pdfs/human/qwp/18540104en.pdf (accessed 30 January 2009).

EMEA (2007a) EMEA/CHMP/QWP/306970/2007. http://www.emea.europa.eu/pdfs/human/qwp/30697007en.pdf (accessed 30 January 2009).

EMEA (2007b). CHMP/SWP/28367/2007. http://www.emea.europa.eu/pdfs/human/swp/2836707en.pdf (accessed 30 January 2009).

EMEA (2008). *Note for Guidance on Non-clinical Safety Studies for the Conduct of Human Clinical Trials for Pharmaceuticals needed to support human clinical trials of a given scope and duration.* EMEA/CPMP/ICH/286/95. http://www.emea.europa.eu/pdfs/human/ich/028695endraft.pdf (accessed 30 January 2009).

EudraLex (2010). *The Rules Governing Medicinal Products in the European Union.* http://ec.europa.eu/enterprise/sectors/pharmaceuticals/documents/eudralex/index_en.htm (accessed 30 January 2009).

Euratom (1996). Directive 96/29/EURATOM. http://ec.europa.eu/energy/nuclear/radioprotection/doc/legislation/9629_en.pdf (accessed 30 January 2009).

Euratom (1997). Directive 97/43/EURATOM. http://ec.europa.eu/energy/nuclear/radioprotection/doc/legislation/9743_en.pdf (accessed 30 January 2009).

Italian Parliament (2007). Decreto legislativo 6 novembre 2007 N.200. http://www.parlamento.it/leggi/deleghe/07200dl.htm (accessed 5 February 2009).

PIC/S (2008). *Guide to Good Practices for Preparation of Medicinal Products in Healthcare Establishments.* Pharmaceutical Inspection Convention Pharmaceutical Inspection Co-operation Scheme, PE 010-3 October 2008. http://www.picscheme.org/publication.php?id=8 (accessed 30 June 2010).

28

Regulation of radiopharmacy practice in the United Kingdom

Neil G Hartman

Introduction

Radiopharmaceuticals are among the most highly regulated of materials administered to patients because they are controlled both as medicinal products and as radioactive substances.

Some form of medicine regulation has existed in the United Kingdom (UK) since the time of Henry VIII (BP 2009a), and the *Pharmacopoeia Londinensis* of 1618 (possibly Europe's first national pharmacopoeia) listed over 900 compound remedies and 1190 crude drugs (Pharmaceutical Journal 2004). It was, however, important events in the 20th century that brought a plethora of regulatory control not only to medicine, but also to the young discipline of nuclear medicine.

During the 1950s and early 1960s, thalidomide was prescribed first as a sedative, then as an antiemetic to relieve morning sickness during the first few months of pregnancy, but caused serious unpredicted effects (including phocomelia) in children (Encyclopedia 2001). The clangour following the disaster of the thalidomide side-effects resulted in a growing understanding of risk versus benefit, and resulted in the genesis of strict medicines regulation in the UK (MHRA 2008). The overall control of medicines and most previous legislation in this regard were brought together in the Medicines Act 1968. Systems affecting the manufacture, sale, supply and importation of medicinal products into the UK are enabled in the act. At the same time, the then European Economic Community (EEC) sought to control medicines, and this resulted in 1965 in the Directive 65/65/EEC.

In the ensuing years, each member state in Europe contributed to the development and updating of all EEC Directives pertaining to medicines. Each EU member has representation and is involved in consultation before the appearance of new EU directives. The framework and effects of European Union (EU) directives, regulations and guidelines are explained in Chapter 27. EC legislation now takes precedence over the Medicines Act 1968 and its Instruments and Orders. The latter is amended from time to time (to align it with new EC requirements, i.e. Directives).

In the UK, the Medicines Act 1968 (and its regulations) is currently undergoing a review that should take approximately 3 years, and in addition, there is also a review of unlicensed medicines (RUM) assessing the regulatory framework in the light of current EU and UK legislation, in relation to unlicensed products. Amendments to all UK laws pertaining to medicines also reflect three main events:

1. New EU legislation
2. Court cases in the UK and EU
3. A continuous updating of 'good practice'.

The Medicines Act 1968, subordinate legislation arising from the Act, and the Medicines for Human Use (Marketing Authorisations) Regulations are administered and enforced in the UK by the Health Ministers.

Health and safety

The regulations made under the Health and Safety at Work, etc., Act 1974 (HASWA 1974) lay down requirements for the radiation protection of workers and persons affected by ionising radiations at work. These requirements include provisions for the control of radioactive substances used at work. The Health and Safety at Work, etc., Act applies only in Great Britain, but similar requirements exist in Northern Ireland. The Health and Safety at Work Act and the regulations made under that Act are enforced either by the Health and Safety Executive (HSE) or by local authorities. The latter are concerned with premises such as shops, offices, hotels, restaurants and the like. Other premises are the concern of HSE. In particular, it may be assumed that all work involving radiopharmaceuticals will be covered by HSE.

Radioactive Substances Act 1993

The Radioactive Substances Act 1993 requires that premises where radioactive materials are held be registered with the Environment Agency, or Scottish Environment Protection Agency (the equivalent in Northern Ireland is the Department of the Environment for Northern Ireland). The Act also requires authorisation to be obtained for the accumulation, storage and disposal of radioactive waste. For further information, reference should be made to the relevant agency or department. In addition, Euratom Directives oblige member states to take certain measures to protect the health of workers and general public against the dangers of ionising radiation. These EU obligations may be met in each member state by different combinations of primary legislation, statutory regulation and administrative arrangements (or guidance by professional bodies), but the end result should be a harmonised and effective system of safety controls throughout the EU.

The Ionising Radiations Regulations 1999 in the United Kingdom

The Ionising Radiations Regulations 1999 (IRR99) (Ionactive 2009; Radman 2009) were introduced mainly to implement in Great Britain the requirements of Euratom Directive 96/29/EURATOM as from 1 January 2000 (Regulation 5 [Authorisation of specified practices] was only implemented from May 2000). At the same time, they brought British radiation protection legislation up to date by introducing requirements based on the 1977 Recommendations of the International Commission on Radiological Protection (ICRP Publication 26) as well as the more recent ICRP Publication 60, officially adopted in December 1990 (ICRP 1990). (The ICRP Publication 60 was formally replaced in 2007 by the ICRP Publication 103, in which radiation and tissue weighting factors relating to the effective dose have been, amongst others, updated (ICRP 2007)). IRR99 is discussed in Chapter 3.

UK Licensing and Market Authorisation

In the United Kingdom, the primary legislation pertaining to the manufacture, distribution and importation of medicinal products is the *Medicines Act 1968 as amended* (updated/amended nearly every year at the moment). This act is in effect the UK statutory implementation of EU Directive 2001/83/EC (Feldschreiber 2008). There is furthermore secondary legislation (to the Medicines Act) in the UK in the form of Statutory Instruments (SIs), and the SI most appropriately dealing with the licensing of products is SI 1994 No. 3144: *Medicines for Human Use (Marketing Authorisations Etc) Regulations 1994 as amended*. This SI provides "the functions for the Competent Authority of a Member State under the relevant Community provisions Directive 2001/83/EC as amended by 2004/27/EC, except as otherwise provided, to be performed in the UK by the Licensing Authority (LA). They also provide that no medicinal product for human use which is subject to the relevant Community provisions may be placed on the market or distributed in the UK other than in accordance with a current marketing authorisation granted by the Licensing Authority or the European Commission' (MCA 2007).

A new agency was formed in 2002 when the Medicines Control Agency (MCA) and the Medical Devices Agency (MDA) were brought together to form the Medicines and Healthcare products Regulatory Agency (MHRA) (MCA 2007). The main aim of the MHRA is to protect the public health by ensuring that all medical equipment, medicines and healthcare products are safe. One of the many varied roles of the MHRA is to assess all medicines proposed for sale in the UK. The MHRA will authorise the sale/supply of medicinal products (in the UK) once it determines the necessary evidence for such a product. The MHRA is supported by several expert advisory bodies. One of these is the Commission on Human Medicines (CHM), which came into being on 30 October 2005 (MHRA 2009a). The CHM has several functions (MHRA 2009b):

- To advise the Health Ministers and the Licensing Authority (LA) on matters relating to human medicinal products, including giving advice in relation to the safety, quality and efficacy of human medicinal products, where either the Commission thinks it appropriate or where it is asked to do so.
- To consider whether applications that lead to LA action are appropriate (i.e. where the LA has a statutory duty to refer or chooses to do so).
- To consider representations made (either in writing or at a hearing) by an applicant or by a licence or marketing authorisation holder in certain circumstances.
- To promote the collection and investigation of information relating to adverse reactions to human medicines for the purposes of enabling such advice to be given.

The Commission on Human Medicines (CHM) depends on the expert input from Expert Advisory Groups (EAGs) from the early stages of product development, and the statutory EAGs include Chemistry, Pharmacy and Standards; Pharmacovigilance; and Biologicals/Vaccines. The MHRA may also act as rapporteur or co-rapporteur in terms of the verification of radiopharmaceutical dossiers on behalf of other EU members and/or authorities. (The responsibilities of rapporteurs in centralised applications and reference member states in decentralised applications are substantive responsibilities in the assessment of European applications and do not depend on member states' requests (P. Feldschreiber, personal communication, 2010)).

The application/dossier for a marketing authorisation is submitted to the MHRA in a format known as the Common Technical Document (CTD), which is a format that has been agreed upon by the International Conference on Harmonisation (ICH). This form of application for market authorisation is recognised by the three ICH regions: Europe, Japan, and the USA (Feldschreiber 2008).

Since 2009, the MHRA *Special Mail 5* entitled 'Guidelines on submission of applications to the MHRA' specifies that from 2009 eCTDs are accepted by all European countries, and the MHRA will soon make electronic submissions compulsory. The CTD consist of five modules (FDA 1999) which include descriptions, documentation and expert argumentation (FDA 2001): (1) common technical document summaries (national/regional administrative information); (2) common technical document summaries (including the CTD introduction, the quality summary, the non-clinical overview and the clinical overview, all of which include pharmacology, pharmacokinetic and toxicological data summaries); (3) quality; (4) non-clinical study reports; and (5) clinical study reports.

Once the MHRA has granted a marketing authorisation for a product, it regulates a medicinal product and the company that will manufacture it through its Inspection and Standards Division. The Inspectorate

Group of the MHRA consists of five units dedicated to all aspects of Good Laboratory Practice (GLP), Good Clinical Practice (GCP), Good Manufacturing Practice (GMP), Good Distribution Practice (GDP) and Good Pharmacovigilance Practice (GPvP), and furthermore ensures compliance with relevant EU and UK legislation (MCA 2007).

Clinical trial regulations in the UK

In the UK, the licensing provisions of the Medicines Act 1968 required a pharmaceutical supplier to apply for a Clinical Trial Certificate (CTC) before any human administration (SI 2004/1031). This had to include some toxicological evidence to prove to the Licensing Authority that the product would not seriously put patients' lives at risk. Doctors and dentists could initiate trials without a CTC by informing the authorities of their intent, and the LA could object should the proposed trial be deemed unjustified. This proved cumbersome, and in 1981 the Medicines Exemption from Licences (Clinical Trials) Order 1981 (SI 1981/164) came into effect, and a new arrangement for industry-proposed clinical trials came into operation: the Clinical Trials Exemption (CTX) scheme. This scheme exempted the pharmaceutical supplier from the need to hold a CTC for three years, if both the LA had no objection to the trial and certain promises (submission of summaries of pre-clinical drug data, etc.) were kept by the supplier. The LA typically issued the CTX within a 35-day period as specified by the law. The CTX could be renewed after three years, and was widely thought to greatly facilitate industry-sponsored trials again (as compared with doctor/dentist-sponsored initiatives) (Griffin, Stewart 1989).

As already indicated, the publication of EU Directive 2001/20/EC (European Clinical Trials Directive) changed and harmonised the way trials are conducted in Europe. In addition to this EU directive were Commission Directive 2003/94/EC on GMP and the Commission Directive 2005/28/EC of 8 April 2005, which laid down the principles of GCP (EC 2009a). This translated into the Medicines for Human Use (Clinical Trials) Regulations 2004 (SI 2004/1031) in the UK, which was subsequently superseded by the Medicines for Human Use (Clinical Trials) Amendment Regulations 2006 (MHRA 2009c).

These regulations can be summarised as follows (Feldschreiber 2008):

- No clinical trial in the UK can begin or be advertised in any way unless with permission to start from the regulator (MHRA).
- All investigational medicinal products (IMPs) have to be manufactured under good manufacturing practice (GMP; EC 2009b). In the UK this means the correct authorisation is a manufacturer's authorisation for investigational medicinal products, MA(IMP). The MA(IMP) relates to any manufacturing, importation, assembly, etc.
- Each trial has to have a sponsor who takes responsibility for the trial management from start to finish. Sponsors have to give trial medicines (IMPs) free of charge if a subject is not covered by a prescription charge.
- A UK Ethics Committee Authority has been created to form and monitor ethics committees. In practice, these duties are carried out by COREC (Central Office for Research Ethics Committees), which is part of the National Patient Safety Agency (NPSA), and now organised by the National Research Ethics Service (see http://www.nres.npsa.nhs.uk).
- All trials have to be conducted in accordance with the principles of GCP, and the MHRA is to inspect trials on the grounds of GCP and GMP, with the right of enforcement.
- There is a requirement that all serious adverse events are reported, and the MHRA has the right to change or abolish a trial as they see fit upon receipt of such information.
- The Clinical Trials Directive provides protection, in addition to that already granted, for minors and incapacitated adults.

GMP and the 'specials' products in the UK

The UK government's implementation of EU Council Directive 2001/83/EC and EU Commission Directive 2003/94/EC vis-à-vis radiopharmaceuticals differs decidedly from its implementation/scrutiny on the continent. Not only have the UK regulations been adapted to implement the major EU directives, the UK also implements Annex 3 pertaining to the manufacturing of radiopharmaceuticals in both the industrial and hospital environments. The argument often used on the continent that radiopharmaceuticals are sufficiently 'different' (short shelf-life, mostly used diagnostically, very small batch production, etc.) is not accepted within the UK, especially after the publication of the Farwell Report of 1995 (Farwell 1995). All licensed radiopharmacies in the UK, whether industrial or hospital-based, are therefore inspected by the MHRA and held accountable to the same letter of the EU GMP regulations alike, similarly to all other pharmaceutical manufacturers. In practical terms, this ensures full GMP compliance with matters such as quality management, personnel, premises and equipment, documentation, production and quality control (MCA 2007).

In addition to the standard GMP requirements for sterile manufacturing (and in addition to IRR99 regulations), the current Annex 3 of the GMP regulations requires that dedicated/self-contained facilities be used for radiopharmaceuticals preparation, packaging and storage, that negative pressure (in comparison to the surrounding area) be used for radioactive particle containment, that in-process controls and monitoring of process parameters are evident, and that recorded release is necessary even though the quality control of the product might only be completed after its dispatch (EC 2009a). Most radiopharmacies in the UK are thus licensed facilities, and all operations comply with the GMP guidelines (including the manufacturing in Grade A air and the strict specifications for housing isolators/laminar flow cabinets, which is not always the case in continental Europe).

Article 5 of EU Directive 2001/83/EC permits a member state (in line with its own existing legislation) to allow licensed manufacturers to provide medical products that fulfil 'special' needs 'in response to a bona fide unsolicited order, formulated in accordance with the specification of an authorized healthcare professional and for use by an individual patient under her or his direct personal responsibility' (Feldschreiber 2008), and this is implemented in the Medicines for Human Use (Marketing Authorisations Etc) Regulations 1994 in the UK. The provision of 'unlicensed' medicines (when two licensed medicines – for example a licensed Mo-99/Tc-99m generator's eluate and a licensed diphosphonate kit – are aseptically combined, an 'unlicensed' product is formed) is therefore allowed in the UK (when in response to an unsolicited order), and limited distribution is possible if no similar licensed product is available. Most hospital radiopharmacies in the UK thus hold a manufacturer's 'specials licence' under which they manufacture and, to a limited degree, distribute to other hospitals/clinics. The procurement of a 'specials' product is only permitted if a fully licensed product is not available (within the jurisdiction or immediate area). The time/distance from other manufacturers could also play a role (as in the case of short-lived PET radiopharmaceuticals), where one is allowed to procure a 'specials' PET radiopharmaceutical (e.g. [^{18}F]fluorodeoxyglucose) only if there is not a licensed supplier within the immediate vicinity. In the spring of 2009 the MHRA published a consultation document on a re-structuring of the 'specials' manufacturing exemptions within the UK (MHRA 2009d).

The British Pharmacopoeia 2009

The British Pharmacopoeia (BP) has been published since 1864 as the official and comprehensive standard for medicinal substances in the United Kingdom. The latest edition, BP2009, was published in late 2008, pursuant to the Medicines Act 1968, and includes several texts and monographs published in the 6th edition of the European Pharmacopoeia (2007), as amended by supplements 6.1 and 6.2 by the Council of Europe (BP 2009b).

The BP section (monographs) on radiopharmaceutical preparations includes 60 radiopharmaceuticals, all taken from the European Pharmacopoeia, i.e. Chromium [^{61}Cr] Edetate Injection, Flumazenil (*N*-[^{11}C]methyl) Injection, Iobenguane [^{123}I] injection, L-Methionine ([^{11}C]-Methyl) Injection, Technetium [^{99m}Tc] Albumin Injection and Technetium [^{99m}Tc] Succimer Injection.

References

BP (2009a). *British Pharmacopoeia 2009*. London: The British Pharmacopoeia Commission. http://www.pharmacopoeia.gov.uk/the-british-pharmacopoeia-commission.php (accessed 18 November 2009).

BP (2009b). *British Pharmacopoeia 2009*. London: The Stationary Office.

EC (2009a). *Clinical Trials*. European Commission. http://ec.europa.eu/enterprise/pharmaceuticals/clinicaltrials/clinicaltrials_en.htm (accessed 13 November 2009).

EC (2009b) (2009). *EudraLex, Volume 1, Pharmaceutical Legislation*. European Commission.

Encyclopedia (2001). *Thalidomide: Global Tragedy*. http://www.encyclopedia.com/doc/1G2-3468302428.html (accessed 14 February 2010).

Farwell J (1995). *Aseptic Dispensing for NHS patients (Farwell Report)*. London: Department of Health.

FDA (1999). Draft Consensus Guideline. Washington DC: Food and Drug Administration. http://www.fda.gov/OHRMS/DOCKETS/98fr/000186m4gd.pdf (accessed 13 November 2009).

FDA (2001) *M4: Organization of the CTD*. Washington DC: Food and Drug Administration. http://www.fda.gov/RegulatoryInformation/Guidances/ucm129872.htm (accessed 13 November 2009).

Feldschreiber P (2008). *The Law and Regulation of Medicines*. New York: Oxford University Press.

Griffin JP, Stewart AG (1989). Six months experience of new procedures affecting the conduct of clinical trials in the United Kingdom. *Br J Clin Pharmacol* 13: 253–255.

HASWA (1974). Health and Safety at Work etc Act 1974 (chapter 37). http://www.healthandsafety.co.uk/haswa.htm (accessed 14 February 2010).

ICRP (1990). *1990 Recommendations of the International Commission on Radiological Protection*. ICRP Publication 60. Ann. ICRP 21(1–3), 1991. Ottawa, ON: ICRP. http://www.elsevier.com/wps/find/bookdescription.cws_home/29083/description#description (accessed 13 November 2009).

ICRP (2007). *The 2007 Recommendations of the International Commission on Radiological Protection*. ICRP Publication 103 Ann. ICRP 37(2–4), 2007. Elsevier Publishers Ltd.

Ionactive (2009). *IRR99 Guidance*. Ascot: Ionactive Consulting. http://www.ionactive.co.uk/regguidance-parts.html?type=10 (accessed 13 November 2009).

MCA (Medicines Control Agency) (2007). *Rules and Guidance for Pharmaceutical Manufacturers and Distributors 2007*. London: Pharmaceutical Press.

MHRA (Medicines and Healthcare products Regulatory Agency) (2008). *Medicines and Medical Devices Regulation: What you need to know*. London: MHRA. http://www.mhra.gov.uk/Howweregulate/Medicines/index.htm (accessed 14 February 2010).

MHRA (Medicines and Healthcare products Regulatory Agency) (2009a). *Commission on Human Medicines*. London: MHRA. http://www.mhra.gov.uk/Committees/Medicinesadvisorybodies/CommissiononHumanMedicines/index.htm (accessed 13 November 2009).

MHRA (Medicines and Healthcare products Regulatory Agency) (2009b). *Medicines Act 1968 Advisory Bodies Annual Reports 2007*. London: MHRA. http://www.mhra.gov.uk/home/groups/l-cs-el/documents/websiteresources/con2032766.pdf (accessed 13 November 2009).

MHRA (Medicines and Healthcare products Regulatory Agency) (2009c). *Implementation of the Clinical Trials Directive in the UK*. London: MHRA. http://www.mhra.gov.uk/Howweregulate/Medicines/Licensingofmedicines/Clinicaltrials/ImplementationoftheClinicalTrialsDirectiveintheUK/index.htm (accessed 13 November 2009).

MHRA (Medicines and Healthcare products Regulatory Agency) (2009d). *Review of Unlicensed Medications*. London: MHRA. http://www.mhra.gov.uk/Howweregulate/Medicines/Reviewofunlicensedmedicines/index.htm (accessed 13 November 2009).

Pharmaceutical Journal (2004). Treasures of the Royal Pharmaceutical Society's Collections. *Pharm J* 273: 299.

Radman (2009). *Ionising Radiations Regulations 1999. A Guide for Radiation Protection Supervisors*. Macclesfield: Radman Associates. http://www.radman.co.uk/resources/IRR99-ionising-radiation-regulations.aspx#part_ii (accessed 13 November 2009).

29

Regulation of nuclear pharmacy practice in the United States

Joseph C Hung

Introduction

The organisation of this chapter is based on key aspects of nuclear pharmacy practice (e.g. facility design and environmental controls, personnel qualification, preparation, etc.) rather than regulatory and authoritative bodies, for example, States Boards of Pharmacy, Nuclear Regulatory Commission (NRC)/Agreement States, Food and Drug Administration (FDA), and United States Pharmacopeia (USP). Agreement States are those where the NRC provides assistance to States expressing interest in establishing programmes to assume NRC regulatory authority under the Atomic Energy Act of 1954, as amended. On 26 March 1962, the Commonwealth of Kentucky became the first Agreement State. At present, there are 37 states which have entered into an agreement with the NRC, and one is being evaluated. The rules and regulations of the Agreement States must be at least as strict as, if not more rigorous than, those of the NRC.

Related regulations or standards implemented by the regulatory or authoritative agencies for each above-mentioned practice or activity are cited and discussed in this chapter (Figure 29.1).

To avoid unnecessary repetition of listing the same or similar regulations/standards, only unique regulations or standards (not commonly implemented in the European Community) issued by various US agencies that pertain to the listed nuclear pharmacy practice are described in each section.

Personal comments with regard to certain unique and/or 'controversial' regulations and/or standards are included (either described in

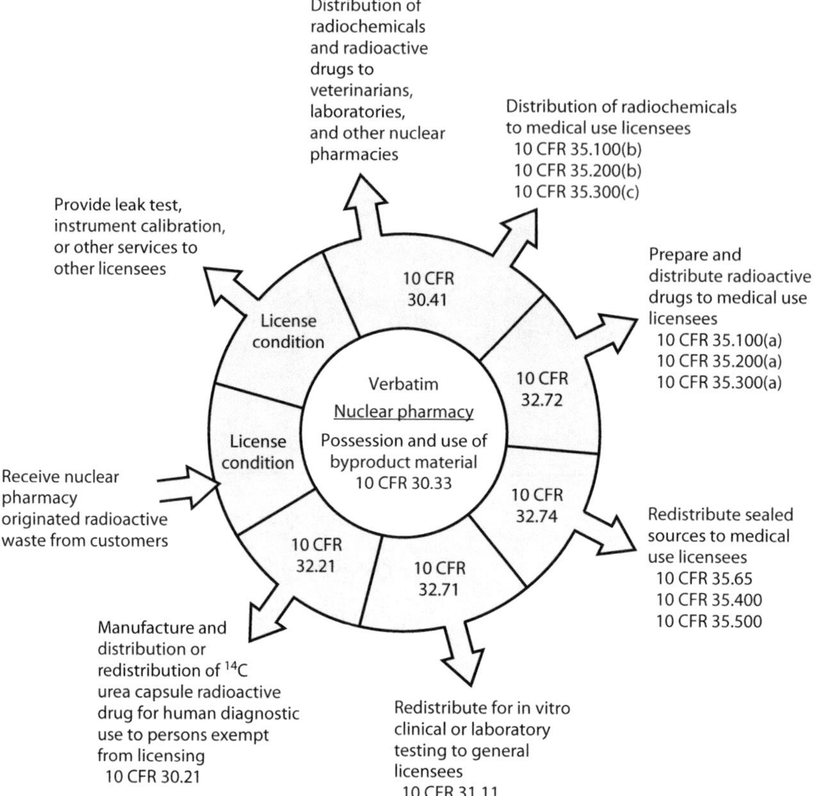

Figure 29.1 'Purpose wheel' – various aspects of nuclear pharmacy operation involving radioactive materials are authorised by several distinct NRC regulations. The appropriate regulation to refer to depends on the nature of the radioactive material, the purpose(s) for which it will be used, and to whom it is sent. CFR = Code of Federal Regulations.

paragraph text or embedded in the regulation/standard as bracketed text) in each practice section. These comments reflect the author's views only, and they have not been endorsed by nor do they necessarily reflect the views of the author's institution or any other entities. This chapter is provided for informational purposes only and is not intended as legal advice.

The regulatory information presented in this chapter is not intended to be all encompassing. Only the essence of the regulatory scene is addressed in order to offer the readers a quick understanding of some fundamental regulatory requirements for nuclear pharmacy practice in the United States. Since the regulatory scenery may be changed owing to professional, social, or political situations, it is prudent for readers to check the latest regulations from their professional and/or regulatory authorities.

Facility design and environmental controls

Requirements from state boards of pharmacy

Typical requirements from various state boards of pharmacy are: (1) adequate space and equipment for storage, manipulation, manufacture, compounding, dispensing, safe handling, and disposal of radioactive material; (2) compliance with all laws and regulations of NRC/

Agreement States and other applicable federal and state agencies; and (3) requirement for proof of the above compliance to be submitted to and approved by the board before a pharmacy licence is issued by the board.

Requirements from NRC or Agreement States

Non-PET nuclear pharmacies

Regulations related to the facility design and environmental control for a nuclear pharmacy that handles only non-positron emission tomography (PET) materials can be found in Title 10, Code of Federal Regulations (10 CFR), Part 32.72(a)(2), 10 CFR 30.33(a)(2), 10 CFR 20.1406, 10 CFR 20.1101(b), 10 CFR 30.35 (g) (NRC Regulations 10 CFR Part 32.72, 10 CFR Part 30.33, 10 CFR Part 20.1406, 10 CFR Part 20.1101, 10 CFR Part 30.35). Similar regulations can be found in each Agreement State.

Facilities and equipment must be adequate to protect health and minimise danger to life or property, minimise the likelihood of contamination, and keep exposures to workers and the public as low as reasonably achievable (ALARA). Items listed below are some of the vital aspects to be considered when designing a nuclear pharmacy.

Sufficient engineering controls and barriers should be provided to protect the health and safety of the public and their employees. Ventilation systems should be verified that effluents are ALARA, are within the dose limits of 10 CFR 20.1301 (NRC Regulations 10 CFR Part 20.1301), and are within the ALARA constraints for air emissions established under 10 CFR 20.1101(d) (NRC Regulations 10 CFR Part 20.1101). Minimum acceptable limits for pertinent airflow rates, differential pressures, filtration equipment, and monitoring systems should be defined and maintained properly.

Exposures to radiation and radioactive materials should be kept ALARA, especially the use or storage of radioactive materials likely to become airborne, such as compounding radioiodine capsules and dispensing radioiodine solutions. Risk from the uses of various types and quantities of radioactive materials should be minimised. Delineation between restricted and unrestricted areas should be marked clearly through the use of barriers, postings, and worker instructions.

The events in the USA of 11 September 2001 have put new emphasis on security to prevent the malicious use of radioactive material, such as in 'dirty bombs'. The NRC and Agreement States have been increasing their enforcement actions to ensure that the radioactive material licensees have proper security and accountability systems in placed for storage, usage, and disposal of the radioactive material in their possession. The drawings and diagrams should provide exact location of materials or depict specific locations of safety or security equipment as, 'Security-Related Information – Withhold Under 10 CFR 2.390' (NRC Regulations 10 CFR Part 2.390).

A diagram and description such as the one shown in Figure 29.2 should be submitted to the NRC or related Agreement State. Until the above review is completed and the application is approved, the construction of the new nuclear pharmacy facility should not be initiated in case change(s) is/are required as a result of the application review.

PET nuclear pharmacies

The establishment of a PET nuclear pharmacy, the facility design, and environmental controls must meet the same regulations and application requirements (including a diagram and descriptions as shown in Figure 29.3) as those for setting up a non-PET nuclear pharmacy. Owing to a much higher energy (e.g. 511 keV) associated with PET radioisotopes, PET nuclear pharmacy applicants should describe the facility, equipment, methodology, and shielding used to physically transfer (e.g. transfer lines) PET radioisotopes to the chemical synthesis equipment for radiopharmaceutical manufacturing and then to the dispensing area. The application should also include a description of shielding used for chemical synthesis and/or dispensing of radiopharmaceuticals. In addition, the type of remote handling equipment used for handling the PET radionuclides and PET radiopharmaceuticals should be described in the application materials.

Owing to the short half-lives of positron-emitting radionuclides, commercial PET radiopharmacies generally produce high amounts of radioactivity, which could lead to the potential for fairly high activities of effluents released into the air if the proper engineering controls are not used. Examples of some engineering

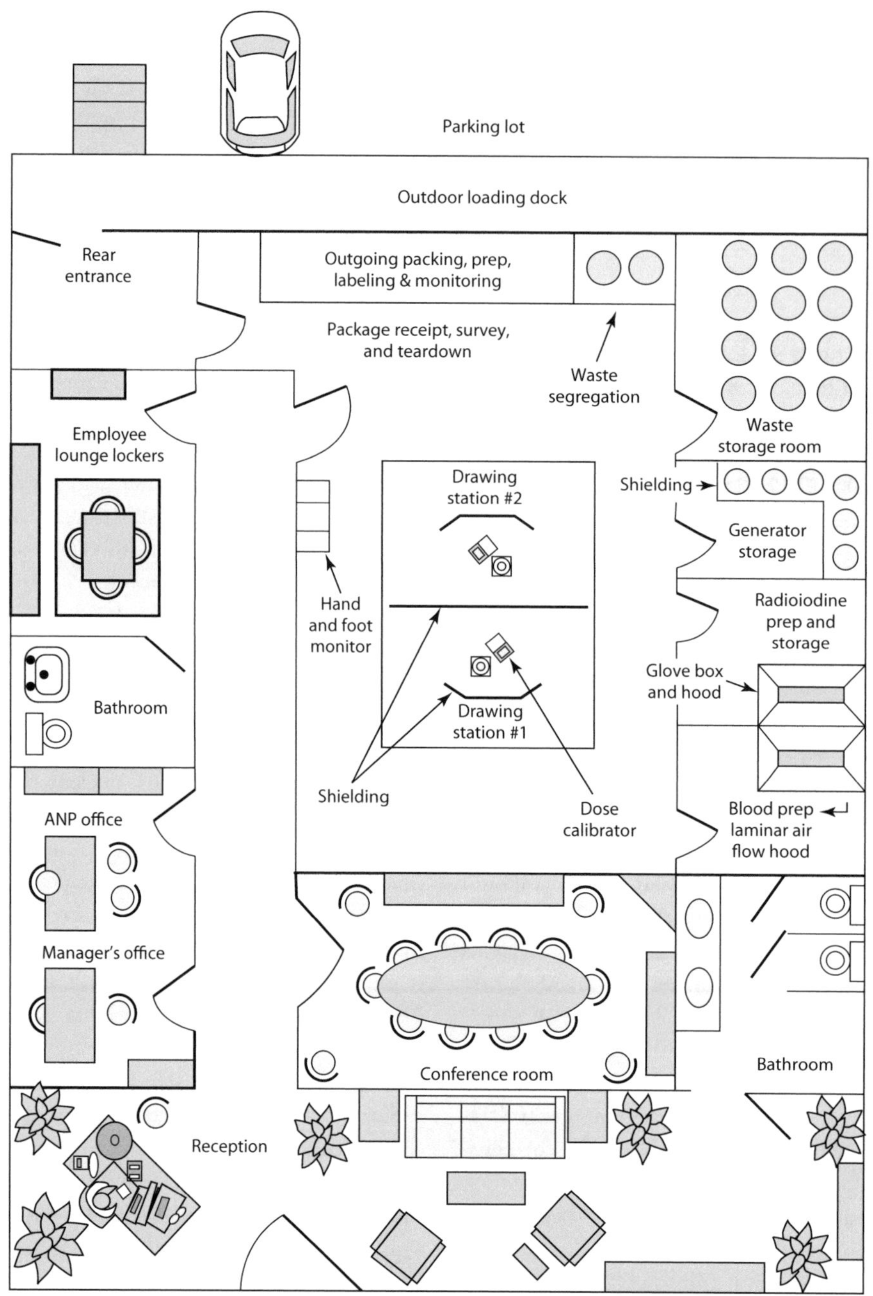

Figure 29.2 A typical non-PET nuclear pharmacy diagram. (Note: this particular diagram does not contain real security-related information.) ANP = authorised nuclear pharmacist.

controls that should be used would include exhaust filtration and/or containment systems for decay of effluents. It is also recommended that a continuous 'real-time' effluent (stack) monitor be installed at the facility.

Requirements from FDA

According to Section 121 of the 1997 FDA Modernization Act (FDAMA) (US FDA Public Law No. 105-115), FDA was directed to establish

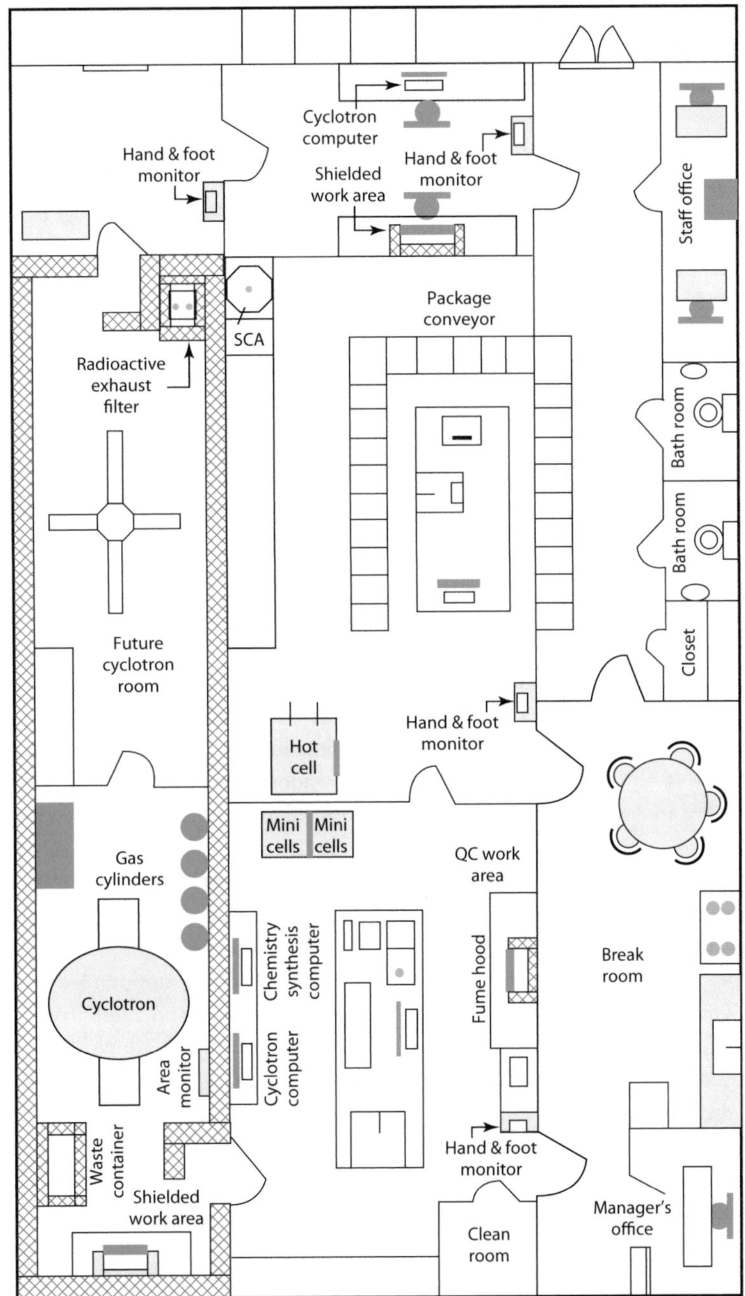

Figure 29.3 A typical PET nuclear pharmacy diagram. (Note: this particular diagram does not contain real security-related information.) SCA = single channel analyser; QC = quality control.

appropriate approval procedures for PET drugs pursuant to section 505 of the Federal Food, Drug, and Cosmetic Act (US FDA Section 505), as well as appropriate current good manufacturing practice (CGMP) requirements. FDA has determined that they will regulate the production and usage of PET drug products as per CGMP requirements and drug approval procedures, respectively, and defer the subsequent dispensing of individual patient doses and use of the PET drug product to be regulated by State and local authorities as FDA generally regards subsequent distribution of the drug product as part of the practice of pharmacy and medicine.

CGMP Rule and Guidance for PET Drugs

Rule

21 CFR 212.30(a) (USFDA Regulations 21 CFR Part 212.30) requires that a PET drug production facility have adequate facilities to ensure the orderly handling of materials and equipment, the prevention of mix-ups, and the prevention of contamination of equipment or product by substances, personnel, or environmental conditions.

Guidance

The recently released guidance for PET CGMP indicates that, in most PET drug production facilities, the same area or room can be used for multiple purposes (e.g. radiochemical synthesis, quality control (QC) testing, and storage of approved components) (US FDA guidance). However, as the complexity in a PET drug production facility increases (e.g. production of multiple PET drug products) or a PET drug production facility is co-located in a research institution, it is important to develop the appropriate level of control required to prevent mix-ups and contamination. It is also important to consider what impact a greater number of personnel and activities could have on the aseptic processing portion of the process.

As per the new guidance, an aseptic processing area is used to assemble sterile components (e.g. syringe, needle, filter and vial) required for sterile filtration of the PET drug product and sterility testing of the finished PET drug product. The guidance also describes the usual precautions to be taken in the design (e.g. no carpet, overhanging pipes or hanging light fixtures) and cleaning (e.g. frequently clean the surfaces of the walls, floors, and ceiling) of an aseptic processing area, as well as to maintain the appropriate air quality of the aseptic workstation (e.g. proper garbing, frequently sanitise the gloved hands, and keep minimum number of items within a laminar airflow workstation).

As an example, a paper written by the Mayo Clinic PET radiochemistry team should be consulted for more information concerning the planning and design of a PET radiochemistry facility, including a cyclotron (Jacobson *et al.* 2002). The suggestions made in this paper for the design of a PET drug production facility were not strictly based on PET regulatory requirements; we also took into consideration production flow, operation objectives, and future growth so that a new PET drug production facility is not only in compliance with the regulations but also provides a safe, efficient, and productive working environment.

Requirements from USP

USP General Chapter <797> 'Pharmaceutical Compounding – Sterile Preparations'

USP General Chapter <797> 'Pharmaceutical Compounding – Sterile Preparations' was published in the 2004 edition of the USP and became official as of 1 June 2008 (US Pharmacopeia 2009). USP General Chapter <797> provides a minimum standard for sterile compounding practices, and is mainly designed to prevent any harm to patients caused by non-sterility, endotoxins, variability of drug quality, chemical/physical contaminants, and sub-optimal quality of ingredients. The impact of USP General Chapter <797> towards the healthcare field is far-reaching – it applies to all persons who prepare compounded sterile preparations (CSPs), all places where CSPs are prepared, and all compounded biologics, diagnostics, drugs, nutrients, and radiopharmaceuticals with the exception of PET radiopharmaceuticals, which are subject to the standards and requirement described in USP General Chapter <823> 'Radiopharmaceuticals for Positron Emission Tomography – Compounding' (US Pharmacopeia 2009).

USP general chapters numbered below 1000, also termed general tests and assays chapters, are considered enforceable (i.e. compliance is required). The USP Convention that develops and publishes USP is a non-governmental, scientific body responsible for setting standards for drug quality and related practices but is not an enforcement agency. Enforcement of compliance with USP General Chapter <797>, therefore, falls upon other agencies such as various state boards of pharmacy, Joint Commission, FDA, and other state agencies (e.g. Department of Health).

Table 29.1 ISO classification of particulate matter in room air (limits are in particles of 0.5 μm and larger per cubic metre)

ISO class	Particle count per m^3
3	35.2
4	352
5	3 520
6	35 200
7	352 000
8	3 520 000

According to USP General Chapter <797>, the compounding facility must be physically designed and environmentally controlled to minimise airborne contamination from contacting critical sites (e.g. vial septa, syringe needles). The risk of, or potential for, critical sites to be contaminated with microorganisms and foreign matter increases with increasing exposed area of the critical sites, the density of contaminants, and exposure time in a non-critical area. A critical area is defined as one complying with ISO (International Organization of Standardization) Class 5 air environment quality (Table 29.1).

The most common sources of ISO Class 5 air quality for exposure of critical sites in nuclear pharmacy practice are biological safety cabinets (BSCs) or isolators that offer unidirectional (laminar) airflow, and these devices are referred to as primary engineering control (PEC) in USP General Chapter <797>. The PEC is typically situated in a buffer area or a clean room that provides at least ISO Class 7 air quality. An ante-area is usually a place where the compounding personnel conduct hand hygiene and garbing procedures; the air quality of an ante-area should be at least ISO Class 8 (US Pharmacopeia 2009).

Figure 29.4 shows a conceptual representation of the arrangement of a facility for preparation of CSPs categorised as low-, medium-, and high-risk level. A simplified listing of USP General Chapter <797> classification conditions for three contamination categories is given below:

- *Low-risk level*: Simple transfers (≤3 sterile products and ≤2 needle entries)
- *Medium-risk level*: Multiple and complex manipulations; long compounding process
- *High-risk level*: Non-sterile ingredients; compounding conditions in a worse than ISO Class 5 environment.

As per the definition of USP General Chapter <797>, radiopharmaceuticals compounded from sterile components, in closed sterile containers, with volume of 100 mL or less for a single-dose injection or not more than 30 mL taken from a multiple-dose container, shall be designated as, and conform to the standards for, low-risk level CSPs. For a PEC used in compounding low-risk level radiopharmaceuticals, USP General Chapter <797> allows the PEC to be located in an air environment with at least ISO Class 8, rather than ISO Class 7 quality.

For sterile radiopharmaceuticals prepared as low-risk level CSPs with 12-hour or less beyond-use date (BUD), USP General Chapter <797> allows these products to be prepared in a segregated compounding area (SCA). The SCA is a demarcated area that is not environmentally controlled; however, compounding practice in

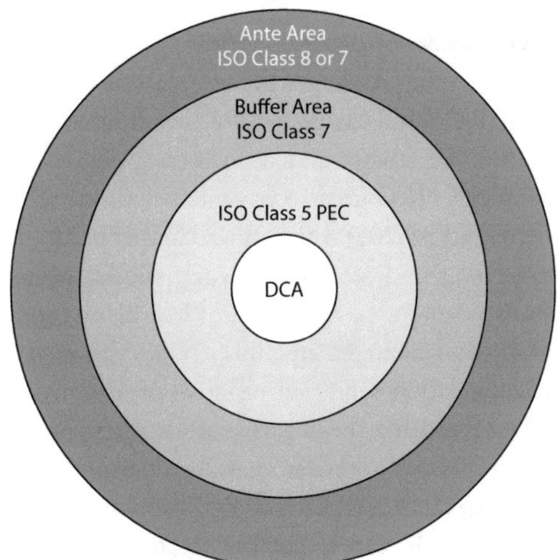

Figure 29.4 Conceptual representation of a typical compounding facility as per USP General Chapter <797>. PEC = primary engineering control; DCA = direct compounding area. DCA is defined as a critical area within PEC where critical sites are exposed to ISO Class 5 air. Reprinted with permission. Copyright 2008 United States Pharmacopeial Convention. All rights reserved.

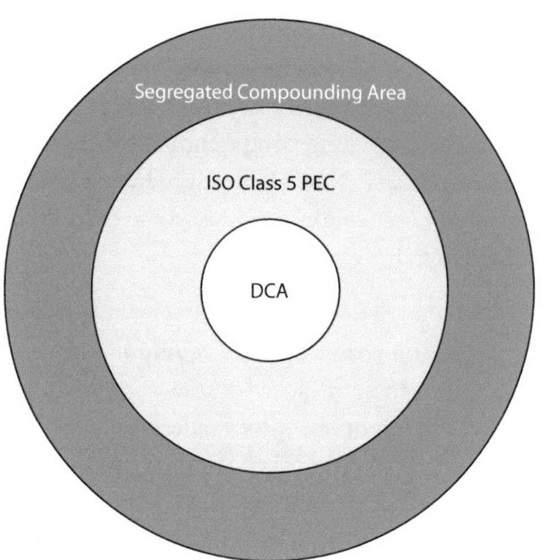

Figure 29.5 Conceptual representation of the placement of an ISO Class 5 PEC in an SCA. Reprinted with permission.

the SCA shall still be carried out in an ISO Class 5 BSC or isolator (Figure 29.5) and personnel cleansing and garbing as stipulated in USP General Chapter <797> shall be observed (US Pharmacopeia 2009).

Negative airflow or positive airflow

According to the 'Radiopharmaceuticals as CSPs' section of USP General Chapter <797>, radiopharmaceuticals shall be compounded in a negative airflow environment. NRC used to have a specific regulation (i.e. CFR, Part 35.205) which indicated that noble gases must be used and stored in a room under negative pressure. When Part 35 – 'Medical Use of By-product Material' was changed in 2002, NRC dropped the specific regulation requiring negative-pressure rooms. However, removing the negative pressure requirement from Part 35 does not mean that one does not have to comply with the ALARA principle as stipulated in Part 20 – 'Standards for Protection against Radiation.' When revised Part 35 was enacted in 2002, NRC stated in its 'Summary of Public Comments and Responses to Comments' that 'Part 35 licensees must comply with the occupational and public dose limits of Part 20' (NRC 2002).

The issue becomes important if there is a spill of a radioactive gas, aerosol, or even fine radioactive powders. A positive-airflow room would spread the radioactive material outside of the room and could potentially contaminate outside areas and/or people. By having this room at negative pressure (or at least negative to the rooms around it), it reduces the potential for the spread of radioactive materials. It is simply good radiation safety practice for areas using such readily dispersible radioactive materials.

Demarcation line or physical barrier

Although USP General Chapter <797> allows a line of demarcation to define the SCA (Figure 29.5) for preparing low-risk level radiopharmaceuticals with 12-hour or less BUD, a demarcated SCA defined by a line of demarcation rather than a physical barrier (e.g. walls, doors and/or a pass-through with interlocking door system) may not be a suitable approach in designing a nuclear pharmacy for the following reasons:

1. For an SCA that is not physically separated from the surrounding area and is simply defined by a line of demarcation, it is a common practice to use the principle of displacement airflow (US Pharmacopeia 2009). The concept (emphasis added) 'utilizes a low pressure differential, high airflow [i.e. an air velocity of 40 ft per minute or more] principle' to move 'dirty' air from the SCA across the line of demarcation into the non-SCA. However, the above 'displacement airflow' concept is only workable if the demarcated SCA has a positive airflow pressure relative to the adjacent non-SCA. Apparently, this is contrary to the negative airflow requirements for a nuclear pharmacy facility.
2. The SCA cannot be used to compound medium-risk level sterile radiopharmaceuticals (e.g. radiolabelled blood cells) or high-risk level sterile radiopharmaceuticals (e.g. Iobenguane I 131 Injection).
3. The SCA can only be used to prepare sterile and non-hazardous radiopharmaceuticals that are classified as low-risk level CSPs with 12-hour or less BUD (US Pharmacopeia 2009): this may not work with certain radiopharmaceuticals that have longer than 12-hour BUD, such as Technetium Tc 99m Mebrofenin Injection (18-hour BUD) (NRC Regulations 10 CFR Part 20.1101), Gallium Citrate Ga 67 Injection (7-day BUD), and Thallous Chloride Tl 201 Injection (4-day BUD).

4 In 2006, the National Institute for Occupational Safety and Health (NIOSH) identified Strontium Chloride Sr 89 Injection and Samarium Sm 153 Lexidronam Injection to be potentially hazardous to healthcare workers who handle them and suggested these two radiopharmaceuticals to be classified as hazardous drugs (NIOSH 2006). According to the requirements stipulated in USP General Chapter <797> for hazardous drugs as CSPs, the ISO Class 5 BSC or isolator for handling the above drugs must be placed in a negative-pressure (≥0.01-inch water column), ISO Class 7 area (e.g., a buffer area/clean room) that is physically separated from the anteroom (Figure 29.3). Optimally, the BSC or CACI for handling hazardous CSPs should be 100% vented to the outside air via high-efficiency particulate air (HEPA) filtration (US Pharmacopeia 2009).

ISO Class 8 versus ISO Class 7

PECs that are used to prepare low-risk level sterile non-PET radiopharmaceuticals, pursuant to a physician order for a specific patient, do not need to be situated in an ISO Class 8 air environment (US Pharmacopeia 2009). However, if the buffer area/clean room is used to prepare medium- and/or high-risk level sterile radiopharmaceuticals or hazardous CSPs, the air environment of the clean room must be ISO Class 7 and physically separated from an ante-area with the same ISO class air quality. This is to preserve the air quality of the buffer area/clean room since it has to meet the negative airflow requirements.

Vented out or recirculating

A Class I BSC provides personnel and environmental protection, but no product protection because unfiltered room air is drawn across the work surface. A BSC with classification of Class II indicates that the hood provides personnel, environmental, and product protection from a biological point of view. Class II BSC Type A2 and Type B1 recirculate 70% and 30%, respectively, of air back through the HEPA filter, whereas Class II BSC Type B2 refers to the hood recirculating no air (i.e. total exhaust).

For compounding hazardous drugs as CSPs, USP General Chapter <797> recommends the BSC and isolator be 100% exhausted to the outside air through HEPA filtration. Although the NRC does not require the air in a BSC or isolator to be 100% exhausted to atmosphere, it is prudent to select a BSC or isolator that does not recirculate air, in order to provide a complete protection to the workers, environment, and product.

Appropriate number of air changes per hour (ACPH)

An adequate HEPA-filtered airflow supply to the anteroom and clean room is required so that the cleanliness classification of these rooms is maintained. The sufficiency of intake air is controlled by the appropriate number of air changes per hour (ACPH). For an ISO Class 7 room supplied with HEPA-filtered air, USP General Chapter <797> stipulates that this room shall receive an ACPH of not less than 30. USP General Chapter <797> allows a minimum ACPH of 15 in the clean room if the area has a PEC that is an ISO Class 5 recirculating device which offers an additional at least 15 ACPH so that the combined ACPH is not less than 30.

Placement of PECs

The locations of PECs should be carefully selected to prevent any cross-contamination and to avoid airflow disruption. The PECs used for a radiolabelling process of a patient's or donor's blood-derived component (e.g. white blood cells) or other biological material shall be clearly separated from routine material-handling procedures and PEC equipment used in other CSP preparations in order to avoid any cross-contamination.

Placement of ^{99}Mo/^{99m}Tc generator systems

USP General Chapter <797> stipulates that ^{99}Mo/^{99m}Tc generator systems shall be stored and eluted in an ISO Class 8 or cleaner air environment.

Environmental and personnel monitoring: radiation safety and aseptic condition

The NRC or Agreement States have the most comprehensive regulations with regard to the environmental and personnel monitoring requirements concerning radiation safety; whereas the monitoring criteria for the aseptic condition of the compounding area and aseptic technique of the compounders are primarily addressed in the USP.

Requirements from state boards of pharmacy

Typical requirements from various state boards of pharmacy are in line with or simply refer to all laws and regulations of NRC/Agreement States (for radiation safety monitoring) and other applicable federal and state agencies, and the USP (for aseptic condition monitoring).

Requirements from NRC or Agreement States

NRC regulations related to the environmental and personnel monitoring for radiation safety are described in 10 CFR 30.53, 10 CFR 20.1501, 10 CFR 20.2103 (NRC Regulations 10 CFR Part 30.53, 10 CFR Part 20.15.01, 10 CFR Part 20.2103). Similar regulations can be found in each Agreement State.

Radiation monitoring (referred to as 'survey' by the NRC) is an evaluation of potential radioactive hazards in the workplace (e.g. restricted or unrestricted areas, equipment, incoming and outgoing radioactive packages and personnel, etc.). These evaluations may be measurements (via various survey instruments), calculations, or a combination of measurements and calculations. Records of survey results must be maintained.

Many different types of monitoring must be performed, and the most important ones are as follows:

- Room survey for possible radioactive contamination on surfaces of floors, walls, furniture, and equipment
- Air sampling measurements for radiopharmaceuticals, especially the volatile ones (e.g. radioiodine), that are handled or processed in unsealed form
- Bioassay measurements – potential radioiodine uptake in a radiation worker's thyroid gland is commonly measured by external counting via a specialised thyroid detection probe
- Surveys of radiopharmaceutical packages entering and departing
- Personnel contamination measurements before radiation workers leave the restricted area.

There have been several instances involving radioactive contamination not being detected (usually owing to radiation workers failing to perform a survey, or not conducting an adequate survey) and radioactive contamination consequently entering public locations and causing public health, regulatory, and public relations problems for the licensees.

Not all survey instruments can measure any given type of radiation (e.g. alpha, beta, and gamma). The presence of other radiation may interfere with a detector's ability to measure the radiation of interest. The energy of the radiation may not be high enough to penetrate some detector windows and be counted. The correct selection, calibration, and use of radiation detection instruments is one of the most important factors in ensuring that radiation monitoring accurately assesses the radiological conditions of the facility and workers. Appendix J, 'General Radiation Monitoring Instrument Specifications and Model Survey Instrument Calibration Program', of the NRC guideline titled 'Program-Specific Guidance About Commercial Radiopharmacy Licenses (NUREG-1556, Vol. 13, Rev. 1)' (US NRC SR1556 #J) is an excellent source to refer to.

The frequency of routine surveys depends on the nature, quantity, and use of radioactive materials, as well as the specific protective facilities, equipment, and procedures that are designed to protect workers from external and internal exposure. Also, the frequency of the survey depends on the type of survey, such as those listed above. Appendix R, 'Radiation Surveys', of NUREG-1556 (US NRC SR1556 #R) contains a model procedure for radiation survey frequencies.

Requirements from FDA

PET CGMP guidance

The PET CGMP rule does not seem to address this particular issue. However, the guidance for PET CGMP has the following general statement in regard to the environmental and personnel monitoring:

> Environmental monitoring is crucial to maintaining aseptic conditions.
> We recommend that microbiological testing of aseptic workstations be performed during sterility testing and critical aseptic manipulation. Methods can include using swabs or contact plates for surfaces and settling plates or dynamic air samplers for air quality.

Requirements from USP

USP General Chapter <797> 'Pharmaceutical Compounding – Sterile Preparations'

Even with the extensive attention to the facility design and environmental controls, the direct or physical contact of critical sites of CSPs with contaminants, especially microbial sources from the improperly cleaned/disinfected gloved hands and/or work surfaces, is paramount. As such, the USP General Chapter <797> institutes several comprehensive monitoring programmes to ensure that the compounding personnel and support personnel (e.g. institutional environmental services) are meticulously conscientious in maintaining a clean compounding environment, as well as in minimising any possible contact contamination of CSPs during their compounding practice.

Viable and non-viable environmental air sampling (ES) testing

The ES testing programme shall be conducted every 6 months in each ISO Class 5 PEC, buffer area/clean room, ante-area, and SCA.

A programme to sample non-viable airborne particles (i.e. total particle counts) differs from that for viable particles in that it is intended to directly measure the performance of the engineering controls used to create the various levels of air cleanliness, for example ISO Class 5, 7, or 8. Evaluation of airborne microorganisms (i.e. viable air sampling) is achieved by employing electronic air sampling equipment to collect a defined volume of air. Impaction is the preferred volumetric air sampling method to collect potential microorganisms with the use of settling plates containing suitable growth media. The recommended action levels for microbial contamination for ISO Class 5, 7, and 8 or worse areas are >1, >10, and >100 colony-forming units (cfu) per cubic metre of air per plate, respectively.

Highly pathogenic microorganisms (e.g. Gram-negative rods, coagulase-positive staphylococci, moulds and yeasts) can be potentially fatal to patients receiving CSPs. Thus, regardless of the number of colony-forming units identified, microorganisms should be identified (to at least the genus level) so that corrective actions can be appropriately taken to address the contamination problem.

Air monitoring

A pressure gauge or velocity meter (preferably with a continuous recording capability) shall be installed to monitor the pressure differential or airflow between the ante area and buffer area/clean room, as well as the ante area and the general environment outside the ante area. ACPHs shall also be properly monitored and documented.

Media-fill test

The skill of personnel to aseptically prepare CSPs shall be evaluated using sterile fluid bacterial culture media-fill verification. An adequate media-fill test shall consist of manipulation steps that represent the most challenging or stressful conditions actually encountered by the personnel being evaluated. Failure to pass the test is indicated by visible turbidity in the media-fill unit on or before 14-day incubation. Media-fill challenge tests can also be used to verify the capability of the compounding environment and processes to produce sterile preparations. All compounding personnel shall have their aseptic technique and related practice competency evaluated initially during the media-fill test procedure and at subsequent annual (for low- and medium-risk level CSPs) or semi-annual (for high-risk level CSPs) media-fill test procedures.

Surface sampling

Surface sampling is an essential monitoring programme to verify whether the compounding area is properly maintained as a suitable microbially controlled environment. It shall be performed in all ISO classified areas on a periodic basis and can be accomplished using contact plates (for regular or flat surfaces) and/or swabs (for irregular surfaces, especially for equipment) and shall be done at the conclusion of compounding. The recommended action levels for microbial contamination detected by surface sampling for ISO Class 5, 7, and 8 or worse areas are >3, >5, and >100 cfu per contact plate, respectively. Regardless of the cfu count, further corrective actions shall be carried out immediately.

Gloved fingertip/thumb sampling

Immediately after the compounder completes the hand hygiene and garbing procedure, the evaluator shall collect a gloved fingertip and thumb sample from both hands of the compounder onto appropriate agar plates by lightly pressing each finger tip into the agar.

Trypticase soy agar with neutralising agents such as lecithin and polysorbate 80 shall be incubated at 35°C± 2°C for 2–3 days. The cfu action level for gloved hands shall be based on the total number of cfu on both gloves and not per hand.

After completing the initial garbing and gloving competency evaluation (to be discussed later), re-evaluation of all compounding personnel shall occur at least annually for low- and medium-risk level CSPs and semi-annually for high-risk level CSPs before they are allowed to continue compounding CSPs. The measuring unit of the environmental microbial bioburden is cfu, and action levels for microbial contamination are determined on the basis of the gathered cfu data. The recommended action levels for viable microbial monitoring, via gloved fingertip sampling, are >3 cfu for sampling location in an ISO Class 5 area as per <797> (US Pharmacopeia 2009). Any cfu count that exceeds action level should prompt a review of hand hygiene and garbing procedures, as well as glove and surface disinfection procedures and aseptic work practices. Employee training may be required to correct the source of the problem.

Personnel qualification

Requirements from state boards of pharmacy

A qualified nuclear pharmacist shall be a currently state-licensed pharmacist with adequate training and experience. Each state may have different requirements for the required nuclear pharmacy training and experience. In Minnesota State, for example, a qualified nuclear pharmacist shall be a currently licensed pharmacist in Minnesota *and* fulfil either one of the following two requirements (Minnesota Office of the Revisor of Statutes 2008):

a be certified as a nuclear pharmacist by the Board of Pharmaceutical Specialties (BPS) – to be discussed later;

or

b have received a minimum of 200 contact hours of instruction in nuclear pharmacy and the safe handling and use of radioactive materials from an accredited college of pharmacy, with emphasis in the areas of radiation physics and instrumentation, radiation protection, mathematics of radioactivity, radiation biology, and radiopharmaceutical chemistry; attain a minimum of 500 hours of clinical nuclear pharmacy training under the supervision of a qualified nuclear pharmacist, and obtain an affidavit of the above training and experience.

Unlike the specific courses to be taken for the required 200 contact hours, there is no mention of the specific areas in which the individual must be trained during the clinical nuclear pharmacy training process (a minimum of 500 hours).

Requirements from the BPS

Nuclear pharmacy was recognised by the BPS as a specialty practice area in 1978. It is the first specialty among a total of five specialties – also including nutrition support pharmacy (1988), pharmacotherapy (1988), psychiatric pharmacy (1992), and oncology pharmacy (1996) – to receive such recognition by the BPS.

Those who are granted certification in nuclear pharmacy specialty may use the designation 'Board Certified Nuclear Pharmacist' and the initials 'BCNP,' as long as certification is valid.

Minimum requirements

The minimum requirements for being certified in nuclear pharmacy are (1) holding a current and active licence to practise pharmacy, (2) obtaining 4000 hours of training/experience in nuclear pharmacy practice, and (3) achieving a passing score on the Nuclear Pharmacy Specialty Certification Examination.

Up to 2000 hours of the required 4000 hours of training/experience may be earned from various academic settings (i.e. undergraduate or postgraduate courses in nuclear pharmacy, MS or PhD degree in nuclear pharmacy, and Nuclear Pharmacy Certificate Program offered by Purdue University, Ohio State University, or the Nuclear Education online programme offered by the University of New Mexico and Arkansas).

The other required 2000 hours can be earned from residency or internship in nuclear pharmacy or nuclear pharmacy practice (hour-for-hour credit in a licensed nuclear pharmacy or healthcare facility approved by state or federal agencies to handle radioactive materials up to a maximum of 4000 hours). If the required

4000 hours have to be earned from didactic training and work experience in the nuclear pharmacy field, the allowable 4000 hours to be obtained in its entirety from 'residency or internship' seems contradictory to the intention of the combined training/experience requirement.

Re-certification for BCNP is required every 7 years, and is a three-step process: (1) self-evaluation, (2) peer review, and (3) formal assessment. The formal assessment is to evaluate the knowledge and skills of the practitioner through (1) achieving a passing score of the re-certification examination, *or* (2) earning 70 hours of continuing education provided by a professional development programme approved by the BPS. The continuing education option for re-certification was implemented in 1996 with BPS, and the University of New Mexico College of Pharmacy's Correspondence Continuing Education Courses for Nuclear Pharmacists, beginning with Volume V, has been designated by the BPS as an acceptable professional development programme.

Requirements from NRC or Agreement States

Authorised nuclear pharmacist

The NRC regulations for a licensed pharmacist to be recognised as an authorised nuclear pharmacist (ANP) can be found in 10 CFR 32.72 (b)(2), (4), and (5); 10 CFR 35.2; 10 CFR 35.55 (a) and (b); and 10 CFR 35.59 (NRC Regulations 10 CFR Parts 35.2, 35.55, and 35.59). Similar regulations can be found in each Agreement State.

Currently, the BPS Nuclear Pharmacist credential is the single board certification recognised by the NRC under Regulation 10 CFR 35.55 (NRC Regulations 10 CFR Part 35.55) for a licensed pharmacist to be classified as an ANP under NRC/Agreement State rules.

The alternative approach for a pharmacist to be recognised as an ANP by NRC/Agreement States is to complete 700 hours in a structured educational programme (i.e. 200 hours of classroom and laboratory training and 500 hours consisting of supervised practical experience in nuclear pharmacy field, similar to the same criteria as stated in the 'Requirements from State Boards of Pharmacy').

In addition, to pass the BPS Nuclear Pharmacy Specialty Certification Examination or to obtain the required 700-hour 'structured education programme', NRC requires that pharmacist who seeks to become an ANP has to obtain a 'written attestation, signed by a preceptor who is an ANP, which indicates that the individual has satisfactorily completed the requirements' as stated above (NRC Regulations 10 CFR Part 35.55) 'and has achieved a level of competency sufficient to function independently as an ANP' (NRC Regulations 10 CFR Part 35.55). NRC also has a 7-year 'recentness of training' requirement (NRC Regulations 10 CFR Part 35.59) to each ANP.

The NRC 'grandfathered' nuclear pharmacists by permitting the licensee to designate a pharmacist as an ANP if the pharmacist used only accelerator-produced radioactive materials, discrete sources of ^{226}Ra, or both, in the practice of nuclear pharmacy for the uses performed before 30 November 2007, or under the NRC waiver of 31 August 2005. These individuals do not have to meet the requirements of 10 CFR 32.72(b)(2)(i) or (ii) (NRC Regulations 10 CFR Part 32.72). However, the applicant must document that the individual meets the criteria in 10 CFR 32.72(b)(4) (NRC Regulations 10 CFR Part 32.72).

Occupationally exposed workers and ancillary personnel

Specific NRC regulations related to occupationally exposed workers and ancillary personnel can be found in 10 CFR 19.12, 10 CFR 20.1101(a), and 10 CFR 30.33(a)(3) (NRC Regulations 10 CFR Parts 19.12, 20.1101, and 30.33). Individuals working with licensed material must receive radiation safety training commensurate with their assigned duties and specific to the licensee's radiation safety programme. In addition, those individuals who, in the course of employment, are likely to receive in a year a dose in excess of 100 mrem (1 mSv) must be instructed according to 10 CFR 19.12 (NRC Regulations 10 CFR Part 19.12).

Personnel involved in hazardous materials package preparation and transport

Applicants must train personnel involved in the preparation and transport of hazardous materials packages in the applicable DOT regulations – 49 CFR 172.700; 49 CFR 172.702; 49 CFR 172.704 (NRC Regulations 10 CFR Parts 172.700, 172.702, 172.704).

Instruction for supervised individuals preparing radiopharmaceuticals

An individual may prepare radiopharmaceuticals for medical use under the supervision of an ANP (NRC Regulations 10 CFR Part 32.72) or a physician who is an authorised user (NRC Regulations 10 CFR Part 35.27). The supervised individual must follow the written preparation instructions and radiation protection procedures established by the supervising ANP or authorised user, as well as the licence conditions and NRC/Agreement State regulations (NRC Regulations 10 CFR Part 35.27).

Requirements from FDA

PET CGMP rule and guidance

Rule

Proposed 21 CFR 212.10 requires a PET drug production facility to have a sufficient number of personnel with the necessary education, background, training, and experience to enable them to perform their assigned functions correctly (US FDA 21 CFR Part 212.10).

Guidance

PET drug production facilities should maintain an updated file (e.g. curriculum vitae, copies of degree certificates, certificate of training) for each employee (US FDA guidance). Each PET drug production facility should have adequate ongoing programmes or plans in place for training employees in new procedures and operations and in the areas where deficiencies have occurred (US FDA guidance).

Requirements from USP

USP General Chapter <797> 'Pharmaceutical Compounding – Sterile Preparations'

This contains a section titled ‘Personnel Training and Competency Evaluation of Garbing and Aseptic Work Practices’.

Personnel training and competency evaluation of garbing, aseptic work practices, and cleansing/disinfection procedures

Personnel training

Compounding personnel shall complete didactic training, pass written competence assessments, and undergo skill assessment using observational audit tools, gloved fingertip/thumb sampling, and media-fill testing (to be discussed later) (US Pharmacopeia 2009) – the skill assessment shall be performed initially before beginning to prepare CSPs and at least annually thereafter for low- and medium-risk level compounding; and semi-annually for high-risk level compounding (US Pharmacopeia 2009).

Cleaning and disinfecting procedures performed by other support personnel shall be thoroughly trained in proper hand hygiene, and garbing, cleaning, and disinfection procedures by a qualified aseptic compounding expert.

An individual who fails the written test or skill assessment shall be re-trained and re-evaluated until he/she passes the above-mentioned evaluation.

Competency evaluation of garbing and aseptic work practices

All personnel shall demonstrate competency in proper garbing procedures (including hand hygiene), as well as in aseptic work practices (e.g. disinfection of component surfaces, routine disinfection of gloved hands). An observational audit form (see Appendix III of USP General Chapter <797>) (US Pharmacopeia 2009) and gloved fingertip/thumb sampling procedures (refer to the section ‘Gloved Fingertip/Thumb Sampling’ above for a full explanation of the sampling procedures) can be utilised to evaluate the compounding personnel’s competency in garbing and aseptic work practices.

Competency evaluation of aseptic manipulation

The skill of all compounding personnel in aseptically preparing CSPs shall be evaluated via an observational audit form (see Appendix IV of USP General Chapter <797> (US Pharmacopeia 2009), as well as using sterile fluid bacterial culture media-fill verification (refer to the section ‘Media-Fill Test’ section for more information about this test).

Competency evaluation of cleansing and disinfecting the compounding area

Surface sampling is a useful evaluation tool to assess whether the area is properly maintained to be a suitable microbially controlled environment for compounding CSPs (refer to the section ‘Surface Sampling’ for a detailed description of this sampling evaluation).

USP General Chapter <823> 'Radiopharmaceuticals for Positron Emission Tomography – Compounding'

According to USP General Chapter <823>, the individuals who are allowed to compound PET radiopharmaceuticals are pharmacists or 'other qualified individuals working under the authority and supervision of a physician' (US Pharmacopeia 2009) – USP General Chapter <823> does not offer any further information about the qualification for the 'qualified individual'. Nevertheless, the compounding and dispensing of a PET drug product can only be carried out by pharmacists or other qualified individuals working under the authority and supervision of a physician 'upon receipt of a prescription for such a preparation' (US Pharmacopeia 2009).

Preparation of radiopharmaceuticals

Requirements from state boards of pharmacy

The majority of state boards of pharmacy do not have specific regulation(s) established for the preparation of radiopharmaceuticals.

Requirements from NRC or Agreement States

The majority of nuclear pharmacy activities involve the preparation of radiopharmaceuticals for commercial distribution to medical users. The title of 10 CFR 32.72 (i.e. 'Manufacture, preparation, or transfer for commercial distribution of radioactive drugs containing by-product material for medical use under Part 35') (NRC Regulations 10 CFR Part 32.72) seems to suggest that it deals with the preparation of radiopharmaceuticals. However, the above regulation only addresses what specific authorisation (e.g. specific licence) is required to manufacture, prepare, or transfer the preparation of radiopharmaceuticals for commercial distribution to medical users. Prior to 1990, the NRC required that radiopharmaceuticals be prepared in strict accordance with package insert instructions.

Pursuant to a petition for rulemaking filed by the American College of Nuclear Physicians and the Society of Nuclear Medicine, NRC revised its regulations to permit licensees to depart from the manufacturer's instructions when preparing reagent kits.

The lack of specific NRC regulations related to the preparation 'process' of radiopharmaceuticals may be due to the following draft policy issued by the NRC on 23 May 2000 (NRC 2000-0113):

> DRAFT FINAL POLICY STATEMENT ON THE MEDICAL USE OF BYPRODUCT MATERIAL (May 23, 2000)
>
> The NRC will continue to regulate the uses of radionuclides in medicine as necessary to provide for the radiation safety of workers and the general public.
>
> The NRC will not intrude into medical judgments affecting patients except as necessary to provide for the radiation safety of workers and the general public.
>
> The NRC will, when justified by the risk to patients, regulate the radiation safety of patients primarily to assure the use of radionuclides is in accordance with the physician's directions.
>
> The NRC, in developing a specific regulatory approach, will consider industry and professional standards that define acceptable approaches of achieving radiation safety.

This draft policy statement appears to be in response to the National Academy of Science/Institute of Medicine's recommendations to the NRC not to interfere with the practice of medicine and pharmacy. The above draft policy ended up becoming the final policy statement (US FDA 21 CFR Part 212.10).

The policy statements issued by the NRC are not regulations, but they are supposed to be the guiding principles that the NRC follows in writing their regulations and implementing their rules through inspection and enforcement.

When submitting an application for a commercial nuclear pharmacy licence, the applicant should indicate the types of radiopharmaceutical preparation activities it intends to perform (e.g. compounding of ^{131}I capsules, radioiodination, chemical synthesis of PET radiopharmaceuticals, and ^{99m}Tc kit preparation).

Requirements from FDA

Package inserts

The package insert (or drug labelling) for each drug approved after 1998 may often be found at Drugs@FDA (US FDA DrugsatFDA). The package insert that accompanies each approved drug products should be the most complete source of information on that drug.

However, there are various deficiencies in package inserts, especially the directions for preparing radiopharmaceuticals and performing QC testing for the reconstituted radiopharmaceuticals. A recent article (Hung et al. 2004) indicates that identified deficiencies in package insert instructions for the preparation of radiopharmaceuticals fall into five categories: (1) absent or incomplete directions (especially with regard to QC procedures); (2) restrictive directions (e.g. specific requirement to use designated needles, chromatography solvents, counting devices), (3) inconsistent directions (e.g. different reconstituted volumes for the same final drug product, unworkable expiration times); (4) impractical directions (e.g. unrealistically low reconstituted activity limits, dangerously high number of radiolabelled particles); and (5) vague directions (e.g. use of the words 'should,' 'may,' 'recommend'). Specific examples for each identified deficiency can be found in the above-cited reference (Hung et al. 2004).

The preparation instructions (i.e. reconstitution, QC testing, and expiration dating) as stated in the package insert for a radiopharmaceutical are intended to ensure, provided these instructions are followed, that the final radiopharmaceutical preparation will be of sufficient quality and purity to meet the label claims regarding safety and efficacy. However, the poor quality or restrictive nature of some manufacturers' directions, as evidenced above, often makes adherence to the preparation instructions not in the best interest of the patient or the nuclear pharmacist and may, in some instances, even compromise therapy or patient safety.

Typically, a drug sponsor conducts clinical trials using radiopharmaceuticals prepared in accordance with specific, usually narrow-range, reconstitution instructions in order to minimise the expense, duration, and complexity of the trials. There is no incentive, economic or otherwise, for the sponsor to conduct trials with radiopharmaceuticals prepared using a broad range of different parameters (e.g. reconstitution activities, volumes, expiration times). The preparation instructions used during clinical trials are incorporated into the package insert, which is submitted to FDA as part of a product's New Drug Application (NDA). Hence, the preparation instructions, being subject to FDA approval, tend to become quite restrictive.

In real life, however, the restrictive nature of package insert instructions, when coupled with a competitive, yet limited, radiopharmaceutical market and geographic constraints on distribution, may well serve to force nuclear pharmacists to deviate from a manufacturer's directions (e.g. to exceed recommended activity, or extend the expiry time). In the event that several patients were to receive doses from a single radiopharmaceutical vial prepared with 'excessive' radioactivity and each patient (or his or her insurance provider) were billed using a standard drug fee based on usage from a vial prepared with a 'standard' amount of radioactivity, the nuclear pharmacist involved would potentially be liable for fraudulent billing under the Federal False Claims Act (US Pharmacopeia 2009) as well as for possible violation of other civil and criminal laws. In addition, such a deviation from FDA-approved preparation instructions may be judged to be misbranding or adulteration.

Clearly, it is necessary to pursue a sensible 'win–win' solution in order to allow nuclear pharmacists to meet the real-world demands of practice and prepare safe and effective radiopharmaceuticals for our patients (maintaining a competitive edge not only in the radiopharmaceutical marketplace but with other imaging modalities as well), while also upholding the interests of the drug manufacturers (in recuperating their operational and research and development costs), and the general public (in curtailing ever-increasing drug costs).

For new drugs, sponsors should be encouraged to determine upper limits for reconstituted radioactivity and expiration times and to include these parameters in the preparation instructions used during clinical trials and, subsequently, in the proposed product labelling for their NDA submissions. Manufacturers should also be encouraged to establish reasonable and fair pricing schedules for multidose vials, offering, if appropriate, prorated refunds for vials that contain a submaximal number of doses.

This solution is a long-shot approach, and it may not materialise in the foreseeable future. The manufacturers' directions for the preparation of radiopharmaceuticals should be viewed as guidance rather than as a mandatory procedure. The examples cited above under the category of vague directions support this view. Deviations from package insert instructions, however, should not be made without careful consideration and professional judgment. FDA, in its *Nuclear Pharmacy Guideline – Criteria for Determining When to Register as a Drug Establishment* (US FDA Nuclear Pharmacy Guideline) allows the compounding of radiopharmaceuticals by discretionary enforcement. Although deviations from package insert instructions are not substantially addressed in this document, FDA noted in its discussion of comments that deviations from instructions or modifications of reagent kits would not require the pharmacy to register as a drug establishment. However, the possibility of misbranding or adulterating a drug product must be considered. Thus, pharmacists must to a large degree rely on their professional judgment as to when and to what extent deviations from preparation instructions are appropriate.

PET cGMP rule and guidance

Control of components, containers and closures

Each PET drug production facility must have a tight and traceable control of various components, containers and closures (US FDA 21 CFR Part 212.40). Qualified vendors should be used for the above-mentioned items – a vendor is qualified when there is evidence to support its ability to supply a material that consistently meets all quality specifications. It is also prudent to have a back-up qualified vendor for each component.

Certification of compliance with the written specifications for reagents, solvents, gases, purification columns, and other auxiliary materials used in the compounding of PET radiopharmaceuticals may be accomplished by inspection of the certificate of analysis (COA) provided by the manufacturer.

For components that yield an active pharmaceutical ingredient and inactive ingredients, COA confirmation for the components is acceptable if finished-product testing ensures that the correct components have been used. If not, identity testing (e.g. melting point determination) would have to be performed on the components.

Production and process controls

Master production and control records are the principal documents describing how a product is made (US FDA 21 CFR Part 212.50). The master production record serves as a template for all batch records, documenting how each batch will be produced.

For a PET drug production facility that has an established history of PET drug production, the process verification can be accomplished using historical batch records, provided that there is adequate accumulated data to support a conclusion that the current process yields batches meeting predetermined acceptance criteria.

Any new processes or significant changes to existing processes must be shown to reliably produce PET drug products meeting the predetermined acceptance criteria before any batches are distributed. This verification should be conducted according to a written protocol and generally include at least three consecutive acceptable production runs.

Under current CGMP regulations in 21 CFR Part 211 (US FDA 21 CFR Part 211), FDA normally requires second-person checks at various stages of production as well as test verification. In a PET production facility with only one person assigned to perform production and quality control tasks, it is recommended that that person recheck his or her own work. Self-checks involve the confirmation of the operator's own action and would be documented. Examples of self-check activities include reviewing batch records (e.g. review the batch record to ensure that all finished-product test results are within the acceptance criteria) before release of the drug product for distribution and verifying calculations in analytical tests.

Stability testing

Proposed 21 CFR 212.61 (US FDA 21 CFR Part 212.61) would require the establishment of a written stability testing programme for each PET drug product. This programme would have to be used to establish suitable storage conditions as well as expiration dates and times.

Examples of stability parameters include radiochemical identity and purity (including levels of radiochemical impurities), appearance, pH, stabiliser or preservative effectiveness, and chemical purity (US FDA guidance). Stability testing of the PET drug product should be performed at the highest radioactive concentration, and the whole batch volume in the intended container/closure should be stored. At least three production runs of the final product should be studied for a period equal to the labelled shelf-life of the PET drug product.

Requirements from USP

USP General Chapter <823> 'Radiopharmaceuticals for Positron Emission Tomography – Compounding

Control of components, materials and supplies

The identities of each lot of components, containers and closures, and materials used in the compounding of PET radiopharmaceuticals are to be verified by defined procedures, tests, and/or documented COA, as appropriate. This is not as specific as the requirements as described in the draft PET CGMP guidance.

Compounding procedure verification

For routine verified processes that are being used with consistent success, a minimum of one verification study (rather three consecutive verification runs as required by the draft PET CGMP guidance) that shows that the product meets acceptance criteria must be conducted on an annual basis.

Quality control (QC) of equipment and radiopharmaceuticals

The QC of equipment and radiopharmaceuticals is addressed in Chapter 23 by Theobald and Maltby (the section 'Quality control of PET radiopharmaceuticals' was contributed in part by J.C. Hung).

Dispensing of radiopharmaceuticals

Written directives

According to 10 CFR 35.40 (NRC Regulations 10 CFR Part 35.40), a written directive must be dated and signed by an authorised user before the administration of sodium [^{131}I]iodide greater than 1.11 MBq (30 μCi), any therapeutic dosage of unsealed by-product material or any therapeutic dose of radiation from by-product material. In addition to the name of the patient or human research subject, the following information must be documented on the written directive:

- For sodium [^{131}I]iodide: the dosage
- For any other therapeutic radiopharmaceutical: the name of the radiopharmaceutical, dosage, and route of administration.

Because of the emergent nature of the patient's condition, an oral directive is acceptable if a delay in obtaining a written directive would jeopardise the patient's health. However, a written directive must be prepared within 48 hours of the oral directive.

An existing written directive may be revised as long as the revision is dated and signed by an authorised user before the administration of the prescribed radiopharmaceutical. An oral revision is permissible because of the patient's condition. The oral revision must be documented as soon as possible in the patient's record, and a revised written directive must be signed and dated by the authorised user within 48 hours of the oral revision.

The licensee shall retain a copy of the written directive for 3 years (NRC Regulations 10 CFR Part 35.2040).

As per 10 CFR 35.2041 (NRC Regulations 10 CFR Part 35.2041), the licensees shall develop, implement, and maintain written procedure for any administration of radiopharmaceutical requiring a written directive. The written procedure shall, at a minimum, address the following issues:

- Verification of the identity of the patient or human research subject.
- Verification that the administration (e.g. name of radiopharmaceutical, prescribed and dispensed dosage, or route of administration) is in accordance with the written directive.
- The licensee shall retain a copy of the procedures for the duration of the licence (NRC Regulations 10 CFR Part 35.2041).

Dosage determination

10 CFR 35.63 (NRC Regulations 10 CFR Part 35.63) requires that the radioactivity of each dosage be determined and recorded before medical use. For a unit dosage, this determination must be made by either a direct measurement or a decay correction based on the

radioactivity determined by a manufacturer, a licensed preparer, or a PET drug producer. For other than unit dosages, the determination must be made by (1) direct measurement, (2) combination of measurement and mathematical calculations, or (3) combination of volumetric measurements and mathematical calculations, based on the measurement made by a manufacturer, a licensed preparer, or a PET drug producer.

Unless otherwise directed by the authorised user, a licensee may not use a dosage if the dosage does not fall within the prescribed dosage range or if the dosage differs from the prescribed dosage by more than 20%. A licensee shall retain a record of the dosage determination for 3 years (NRC Regulations 10 CFR Part 35.2063).

Medical event

NRC defines a medical event as follows (NRC Regulations 10 CFR Part 35.3045):

- The total administered dosage of a radiopharmaceutical differs from the prescribed dosage by 20% or more difference, *and* the difference would result in more than 0.05 Sv (5 rem) effective dose equivalent, 0.5 Sv (50 rem) to an organ, or 0.5 Sv (50 rem) shallow dose equivalent to the skin.
- A dose that exceeds 0.05 Sv (5 rem) effective dose equivalent, 0.5 Sv (50 rem) to an organ or tissue, or 0.5 Sv (50 rem) shallow dose equivalent to the skin from the following:
  - An administration of a wrong radioactive drug containing by-product material
  - An administration of a radioactive drug containing by-product material by the wrong route of administration
  - An administration of a dosage to the wrong individual or human research subject.

The report and notification requirements stipulated by the NRC can be found in 10 CFR 35.3045 (NRC Regulations 10 CFR Part 35.3045).

Labelling of vials and syringes

Requirements from NRC/Agreement States

10 CFR 35.69 (NRC Regulations 10 CFR Part 35.69) indicates that each vial and syringe that contains radioactive material must be labelled to identify radioactive drug (e.g. name of radiopharmaceutical). Each vial shield and syringe shield must also be labelled unless the label on the syringe or vial is visible when shielded.

Requirement from FDA

For PET radiopharmaceuticals, the guidance for PET drug product CGMP (US FDA guidance) indicates that '[b]ecause of radiation exposure concern, it is a common practice to prepare much of the labelling in advance. For example, an empty product vial can be pre-labeled with partial information (e.g. product name, batch number, date) prior to filtration of the radioactive product, and upon completion of QC test the outer shielded container can be labelled with the required information (e.g. radioactivity). Alternatively, a string label can be used to label the immediate container provided that there is a way to associate the label with the vial if the label were to come off. Different approaches can be used as long as the approach ensures that the required information is available on the label. A label identical to that affixed to the container shield can be incorporated into the batch production record. A final check should be made to verify that the correct and complete label has been affixed to the container and the shield.'

Requirements from USP

The PET radiopharmaceutical [^{18}F]FDG (i.e. Fludeoxyglucose F 18 Injection) is used as an example to illustrate the discrepancies of labelling requirements as stated in USP. Overall, the required labelling information as per USP is excessive, especially for a limited-space label of a syringe or syringe shield.

USP General Chapter <823>

> The following information must appear on the label or labeling attached to the final container or dispensing-administration assembly: the identity of the PET radiopharmaceutical, and added substances (e.g., stabilizers and preservatives), an assigned batch or lot number, and the required warning (e.g., radioactive) statements or symbols. The final PET radiopharmaceutical shall also be labeled to include the total radioactivity and radioactive concentration at the stated time of calibration, the expiration time and date, and any required

> or applicable warning statements (e.g., 'Caution-Radioactive Material', 'Do not use if cloudy or contains particulate matter') and/or the radioactivity symbol. (US Pharmacopeia 2009 : 365)

As stated above, the required labelling information is too much for a limited-space label of syringe or syringe shield.

USP Monograph on [^{18}F]FDG

> Label it to include the following, in addition to the information specified for Labeling under Injection: the time and date of calibration; the amount of ^{18}F as fludeoxyglucose expressed as total MBq (mCi) per mL, at time of calibration; the expiration time and date; the name and quantity of any added preservative or stabilizer; and the statement 'Caution—Radioactive Material.' The labeling indicates that in making dosage calculations, correction is to be made for radioactive decay. The radioactive half-life of ^{18}F is 109.7 minutes [not mentioned in USP General Chapter <823>]. The label indicates 'Do not use if cloudy or if it contains particulate matter.' (US Pharmacopeia 2009 : 31)

USP General Chapter <1> `Injection'

The label states the name of the preparation; in the case of a liquid preparation, the percentage content of drug or amount of drug in a specified volume; in the case of a dry preparation, the amount of *active* ingredient; the route of administration (not mentioned in USP General Chapter <823>); a statement of storage conditions and an expiration date; the name and place of business of the manufacturer, packer, or distributor (not mentioned in USP General Chapter <823>); and an identifying lot number. The lot number is capable of yielding the complete manufacturing history of the specific package, including all manufacturing, filling, sterilising, and labelling operations.

Procurement of radiopharmaceuticals

To acquire radioactive materials and reagent kits for the reconstitution of radiopharmaceuticals, the nuclear pharmacy must possess a radioactive material (RAM) licence issued by the NRC or an Agreement State and/or a pharmacy licence issued by a state board of pharmacy (including fulfilment of the specific nuclear pharmacy practice regulations if they exist). The suppliers of radioactive materials require documentation of licensing of the user (e.g. nuclear pharmacy) as to the types and limits of quantities of radioactive material before shipment.

RAM Licences

There are two categories of RAM licences issued by the NRC or the Agreement State: (1) general domestic licence, and (2) specific licences:

General domestic licence (general licence)

As per 10 CFR 31 (NRC Regulations 10 CFR Part 31), a general domestic licence is mainly given for the use of by-product material (in late 2007 the NRC finalised its expanded definition of 'by-product material' to include natural and accelerator-produced radioactive materials) and a general licence for ownership of by-product material used in various devices and equipment. However, the provisions of 10 CFR 31.11 (NRC Regulations 10 CFR Part 31.11) are also applicable for the use of by-product material in certain *in-vitro* clinical or laboratory testing under the general licence.

Specific domestic licences (specific licences)

The specific domestic licences are given in two categories: (1) to manufacture or to transfer certain items containing by-product material (10 CFR 32) (NRC Regulations 10 CFR Part 32) (this part prescribes requirements typically for commercial manufacturers to transfer by-product material for sale or distribution), and (2) to possess, use, and transfer by-product material in any chemical or physical form with the limitations of the maximum activity specified in 10 CFR 33 (NRC Regulations 10 CFR Part 33). The specific licence of the second category is also called specific licence of broad scope ('broad license'). In accordance with 10 CFR 33.11 (NRC Regulations 10 CFR Part 33.11), the broad licence has three types (i.e. Type A, Type B and Type C) which are based on the maximum activity allowed for the receipt, acquisition, ownership, possession, use and transfer of any chemical or physical form of the by-product material specified in the licence.

The Type A broad licence allows specific quantities of radioactivities as specified in the licence. Type B and Type C broad licences must adhere to the maximum activities of by-product materials as specified in 100 CFR 33.100 (NRC Regulations 10 CFR Part 33.100), Schedule A, Column I and Column II, respectively. The majority of commercial nuclear pharmacies apply for the Type A broad licence as it allows the above entities to have a broader latitude to possess, prepare, and transport higher quantity of by-product materials.

Receiving and monitoring of radioactive packages

According to 10 CFR 20.1906 (NRC Regulations 10 CFR Part 20.1906), each licensee who expects to receive a package containing quantities of radioactive material in excess of a Type A quantity shall make arrangements to receive notification of the arrival of the package at the carrier's terminal and to take possession of the package expeditiously. Each licensee shall establish, maintain, and retain written procedures for safely opening packages in which radioactive material is received; and ensure that the procedures are followed and that due consideration is given to special instructions for the type of package being opened.

Monitoring of radioactive packages for possible radioactive contamination is also required as per 10 CFR 20.1906 'Procedures for receiving and opening packages' (NRC Regulations 10 CFR Part 20.1906); the exceptions of the monitoring requirements are if the package contains only radioactive gas or is in special form as defined in 10 CFR 71.4 (NRC Regulations 10 CFR Part 71.4) (e.g. a single solid piece of radioactive material or the material is contained in a sealed capsule that can be opened only by destroying the capsule).

Each licensee should perform the monitoring of the external surfaces of the package for radiation levels as soon as practical after receipt of the package, but not later than 3 hours after the package is received at the licensee's facility if it is received during the licensee's normal working hours, or not later than 3 hours from the beginning of the next working day if it is received after working hours.

Two types of monitoring are performed: survey for external exposure and wipe test for possible non-fixed (removable) contamination. The external survey is done with the use of a GM (Geiger-Müller) survey meter on the surface of the package and at 2 metres, and the readings should not exceed the limits of 2 mSv/hour (200 mrem/hour) and 0.1 mSv/hour (10 mrem/hour), respectively (NRC Regulations 10 CFR Part 71.47). The wipe test for detecting removable radioactive surface contamination is carried out by swabbing areas of 300 cm^2 on the package surface using absorbent paper and counting the swab in a NaI(Tl) scintillation counter. The NRC limit for the wipe test measurement is 6000 dpm/300 cm^2 (NRC Regulations 49 CFR Part 173.443). If any of the readings exceeds the limit, the NRC Operations Center (301-816-5100) and the final delivery carrier must be notified by telephone.

After the completion of the survey, the date of the receipt, the manufacturer, the lot number, name and quantity of the product, date and time of calibration, the survey readings, and the name of the individual performing the tests should be entered into a record book as per NRC rules.

Distribution of radiopharmaceuticals

The distribution and transport of radiopharmaceuticals is covered by international regulations and the topic is addressed in Chapter 30.

Abbreviations and acronyms

ACPH	air changes per hour
ALARA	as low as reasonably achievable
ANP	Authorised Nuclear Pharmacist (USA)
BCNP	Board Certified Nuclear Pharmacist (USA)
BPS	Board of Pharmaceutical Specialties (USA)
BSC	biological safety cabinet (USP)
BUD	beyond use date (USP)
CACI	compounding aseptic containment isolator (USP)

CFR	Code of Federal Regulations (USA)
CFU	colony-forming units
CGMP	current good manufacturing practice
COA	Certificate of Analysis
CSP	compounded sterile preparation (USP)
DCA	direct compounding area
DOT	Department of Transportation (USA)
ES	environmental air sampling
FDAMA	Federal Drug Administration Modernization Act (USA)
HEPA	high efficiency particle arrest/air
ISO	International Standards Organization
NDA	New Drug Application
NIOSH	National Institute for Occupational Safety and Health (USA)
NRC	Nuclear Regulatory Commission (USA)
PEC	primary engineering control (USP)
PET	positron emission tomography
QC	quality control
RAM	radioactive material
SCA	segregated compounding area (USP)
USP	United States Pharmacopeia

References

Hung JC *et al.* (2004). Deficiencies of product labeling directions for the preparation of radiopharmaceuticals. *J Am Pharm Assoc* 44: 30–35.

Jacobson *et al.* (2002). The planning and design of a new PET radiochemistry facility. *Mol Imag Biol* 4: 119–127.

Minnesota Office of the Revisor of Statutes (2008). Chapter 6800-8500 Pharmacist-in-charge https://www.revisor.leg.state.mn.us/rules/?id=6800.8500 (accessed on 3 March 2010).

NIOSH (2006). New FDA drugs and warnings fitting NIOSH criteria for hazardous drugs. Atlanta, GA: The National Institute for Occupational Safety and Health; 2006. http://www.cdc.gov/niosh/docket/pdfs/NIOSH-105/0105-undated-fda%20drugs%20fitting.pdf (accessed on 3 March 2010).

US Food and Drug Administration. Drugs@FDA http://www.accessdata.fda.gov/Scripts/cder/DrugsatFDA/ (accessed on 3 March 2010).

US Nuclear Regulatory Commission. Appendix J – General radiation monitoring instrument specifications and model survey instrument calibration program. In: Program-Specific Guidance About Commercial Radiopharmacy Licenses (NUREG-1556, Vol. 13, Rev. 1) http://www.nrc.gov/reading-rm/doc-collections/nuregs/staff/sr1556/v13/r1/#j (accessed on 3 March 2010).

US Nuclear Regulatory Commission. Appendix R- Model radiation survey procedures. In: Program-Specific Guidance About Commercial Radiopharmacy Licenses (NUREG-1556, Vol. 13, Rev. 1) http://www.nrc.gov/reading-rm/doc-collections/nuregs/staff/sr1556/v13/r1/#r (accessed on 3 March 2010).

US Pharmacopeia. Injections (general chapter 1). http://www.uspnf.com/uspnf/pub/index?usp=32&nf=27&s=2&officialOn=December%201,%202009 (accessed on 3 March 2010, access available only to subscriber).

US Pharmacopeia. Pharmaceutical compounding – sterile preparations (general chapter 797). http://www.uspnf.com/uspnf/pub/index?usp=32&nf=27&s=2&officialOn=December%201,%202009 (accessed on 3 March 2010, access available only to subscriber).

US Pharmacopeia. Radiopharmaceuticals for positron emission tomography – compounding (general chapter 823). http://www.uspnf.com/uspnf/pub/index?usp=32&nf=27&s=2&officialOn=December%201,%202009 (accessed on 3 March 2010, access available only to subscriber).

Legislation

NRC (Nuclear Regulatory Commission) (2002). Medical use of byproduct material; final rule. Fed Regist. 67 : 20302.

US Department of Transportation. Title 49 Code of Federal Regulations Part § 172.700 Purpose and scope. http://frwebgate.access.gpo.gov/cgi-bin/get-cfr.cgi?YEAR=current&TITLE=49&PART=172&SECTION=700&SUBPART=&TYPE=TEXT (accessed on 3 March 2010).

US Department of Transportation. Title 49 Code of Federal Regulations Part § 172.702 Applicability and responsibility for training and testing. http://ecfr.gpoaccess.gov/cgi/t/text/text-idx?c=ecfr&sid=d172ba0c3faf2311976439daa068db45&rgn=div8&view=text&node=49 : 2.1.1.3.7.8 .25.3&idno=49 (accessed on 3 March 2010).

US Department of Transportation. Title 49 Code of Federal Regulations Part § 172.704 Training requirements. http://ecfr.gpoaccess.gov/cgi/t/text/text-idx?c=ecfr&sid=0786e8fffc16fa7f7abb9c24920b54ba&rgn=div8&view=text&node=49 : 2.1.1.3.7.8.25.4&idno=49 (accessed on 3 March 2010).

US Department of Transportation. Title 49 Code of Federal Regulations Part § 173.443 Contamination control. http://cfr.vlex.com/vid/173-contamination-control-19942569 (accessed on 3 March 2010).

US Federal Food, Drug, and Cosmetic Act. Section 505. http://www.fda.gov/opacom/laws/fdcact/fdcact5a.htm#sec505 (accessed on 3 March 2010).

US Food and Drug Administration Act of 1997. Public Law No. 105-115, § 121. http://frwebgate.access.gpo.gov/cgi-bin/getdoc.cgi?dbname=105_cong_public_laws&docid=f:publ115.105.pdf (accessed on 3 March 2010).

US Food and Drug Administration. Guidance PET drug products – current good manufacturing practice (CGMP) http://www.fda.gov/downloads/Drugs/GuidanceComplianceRegulatoryInformation/Guidances/UCM070306.pdf (accessed on 3 March 2010).

US Food and Drug Administration. Nuclear pharmacy guideline – criteria for determining when to register as a drug establishment. http://www.fda.gov/downloads/Drugs/Guidance

ComplianceRegulatoryInformation/Guidances/ucm070293.pdf (accessed on 3 March 2010).

US Food and Drug Administration. Title 21 Code of Federal Regulations Part § 211 Current good manufacturing practice for finished pharmaceuticals. http://frwebgate.access.gpo.gov/cgi-bin/getdoc.cgi?dbname=2009_register&docid=fr10de09-9.pdf (accessed on 3 March 2010).

US Food and Drug Administration. Title 21 Code of Federal Regulations Part § 212.10 What personnel and resources must I have? http://frwebgate.access.gpo.gov/cgi-bin/getdoc.cgi?dbname=2009_register&docid=fr10de09-9.pdf (accessed on 3 March 2010).

US Food and Drug Administration. Title 21 Code of Federal Regulations Part § 212.30 What requirements must my facilities and equipment meet? http://frwebgate.access.gpo.gov/cgi-bin/getdoc.cgi?dbname=2009_register&docid=fr10de09-9.pdf (accessed on 3 March 2010).

US Food and Drug Administration. Title 21 Code of Federal Regulations Part § 212.40 How must I control the components I used to produce PET drugs and the containers and closures I package them in? http://frwebgate.access.gpo.gov/cgi-bin/getdoc.cgi?dbname=2009_register&docid=fr10de09-9.pdf (accessed on 3 March 2010).

US Food and Drug Administration. Title 21 Code of Federal Regulations Part § 212.5 To what drugs do the regulations in this part apply? http://frwebgate.access.gpo.gov/cgi-bin/getdoc.cgi?dbname=2009_register&docid=fr10de09-9.pdf (accessed on 3 March 2010).

US Food and Drug Administration. Title 21 Code of Federal Regulations Part § 212.61 What must I do to ensure the stability of my PET drug products through expiry? http://frwebgate.access.gpo.gov/cgi-bin/getdoc.cgi?dbname=2009_register&docid=fr10de09-9.pdf (accessed on 3 March 2010).

US Nuclear Regulatory Commission. Draft final policy statement on the medical use of byproduct material. http://www.nrc.gov/reading-rm/doc-collections/commission/secys/2000/secy2000-0113/2000-0113scy.html (accessed on 3 March 2010).

US Nuclear Regulatory Commission. Title 10 Code of Federal Regulations Part § 2.390 Public inspections, exemptions, requests for withholding. http://www.nrc.gov/reading-rm/doc-collections/cfr/part002/part002-0390.html (accessed on 3 March 2010).

US Nuclear Regulatory Commission. Title 10 Code of Federal Regulations Part § 19.12 Instruction to workers. http://www.nrc.gov/reading-rm/doc-collections/cfr/part019/part019-0012.html (accessed on 3 March 2010).

US Nuclear Regulatory Commission. Title 10 Code of Federal Regulations Part § 20.1101 (a) Radiation protection programs. http://www.nrc.gov/reading-rm/doc-collections/cfr/part020/part020-1101.html (accessed on 3 March 2010).

US Nuclear Regulatory Commission. Title 10 Code of Federal Regulations Part § 20.1101 (b) Radiation protection programs. http://www.nrc.gov/reading-rm/doc-collections/cfr/part020/part020-1101.html (accessed on 3 March 2010).

US Nuclear Regulatory Commission. Title 10 Code of Federal Regulations Part § 20.1101 (d) Radiation protection programs. http://www.nrc.gov/reading-rm/doc-collections/cfr/part020/part020-1101.html (accessed on 3 March 2010).

US Nuclear Regulatory Commission. Title 10 Code of Federal Regulations Part § 20.1301 Radiation dose limits for individual members of the public. http://www.nrc.gov/reading-rm/doc-collections/cfr/part020/part020-1301.html (accessed on 3 March 2010).

US Nuclear Regulatory Commission. Title 10 Code of Federal Regulations Part § 20.1406 Minimization of contamination. http://www.nrc.gov/reading-rm/doc-collections/cfr/part020/part020-1406.html (accessed on 3 March 2010).

US Nuclear Regulatory Commission. Title 10 Code of Federal Regulations Part § 20.1501 Surveys and monitoring – general. http://www.nrc.gov/reading-rm/doc-collections/cfr/part020/part020-1501.html (accessed on 3 March 2010).

US Nuclear Regulatory Commission. Title 10 Code of Federal Regulations Part § 20.1906 Procedures for receiving and opening packages http://www.nrc.gov/reading-rm.doc-collections/cfr/part020/part020-1906.html (accessed on 3 March 2010).

US Nuclear Regulatory Commission. Title 10 Code of Federal Regulations Part § 20.2103 Records of surveys. http://www.nrc.gov/reading-rm/doc-collections/cfr/part020/part020-2103.html (accessed on 3 March 2010).

US Nuclear Regulatory Commission. Title 10 Code of Federal Regulations Part § 30.33 General requirements for issuance of specific licenses. http://www.nrc.gov/reading-rm/doc-collections/cfr/part030/part030-0033.html (accessed on 3 March 2010).

US Nuclear Regulatory Commission. Title 10 Code of Federal Regulations Part § 30.33(a) (3) General requirements for issuance of specific licenses. http://www.nrc.gov/reading-rm/doc-collections/cfr/part030/part030-0033.html (accessed on 3 March 2010).

US Nuclear Regulatory Commission. Title 10 Code of Federal Regulations Part § 30.35 (g) Financial assurance and recordkeeping for decommissioning. http://www.nrc.gov/reading-rm/doc-collections/cfr/part030/part030-0035.html (accessed on 3 March 2010).

US Nuclear Regulatory Commission. Title 10 Code of Federal Regulations Part § 30.53 Tests. http://www.nrc.gov/reading-rm/doc-collections/cfr/part030/part030-0053.html (accessed on 3 March 2010).

US Nuclear Regulatory Commission. Title 10 Code of Federal Regulations Part § 31 General domestic licenses for byproduct material http://www.nrc.gov/reading-rm/doc-collections/cfr/part031 (accessed on 3 March 2010).

US Nuclear Regulatory Commission. Title 10 Code of Federal Regulations Part § 31.11 General license for use of byproduct material for certain in vitro clinical or laboratory testing http://www.nrc.gov/reading-rm-doc-collections/cfr/part031/part031-0011.html (accessed on 3 March 2010).

US Nuclear Regulatory Commission. Title 10 Code of Federal Regulations Part § 32 Specific domestic licenses to manufacture or transfer certain items containing byproduct material http://www.nrc.gov.reading-rm/doc-collections/cfr/part032 (accessed on 3 March 2010).

US Nuclear Regulatory Commission. Title 10 Code of Federal Regulations Part § 32.72 Manufacture, preparation, or transfer for commercial distribution of radioactive drugs containing byproduct material for medical use under part 35. http://www.nrc.gov/reading-rm/doc-collections/

cfr/part032/part032-0072.html (accessed on 3 March 2010).

US Nuclear Regulatory Commission. Title 10 Code of Federal Regulations Part § 33 Specific domestic licenses of broad scope for byproduct material http://www.nrc.gov/reading-rm/doc-collections/cfr/part033 (accessed on 3 March 2010).

US Nuclear Regulatory Commission. Title 10 Code of Federal Regulations Part § 33.11 Types of specific licenses of broad scope http://www.nrc.gov/reading-rm/doc-collections/cfr/part033-0011.html (accessed on 3 March 2010).

US Nuclear Regulatory Commission. Title 10 Code of Federal Regulations Part § 33.100 Schedule A http://www.nrc.gov.reading-rm/doc-collections/cfr/part033/part/033-0100.html (accessed on 3 March 2010).

US Nuclear Regulatory Commission. Title 10 Code of Federal Regulations Part § 35 Medical product of byproduct material. http://www.nrc.gov/reading-rm/doc-collections/cfr/part035/ (accessed on 3 March 2010).

US Nuclear Regulatory Commission. Title 10 Code of Federal Regulations Part § 35.2 Definitions. http://www.nrc.gov/reading-rm/doc-collections/cfr/part035/part035-0002.html (accessed on 3 March 2010).

US Nuclear Regulatory Commission. Title 10 Code of Federal Regulations Part § 35.2040 Records of written directives. http://www.nrc.gov/reading-rm/doc-collections/cfr/part035/part035-2040.html (accessed on 3 March 2010).

US Nuclear Regulatory Commission. Title 10 Code of Federal Regulations Part § 35.2041 Records for procedures for administrations requiring a written directive. http://www.nrc.gov/reading-rm/doc-collections/cfr/part035/part035-2041.html (accessed on 3 March 2010).

US Nuclear Regulatory Commission. Title 10 Code of Federal Regulations Part § 35.2063 Records of dosages of unsealed byproduct material for medical use http://www.nrc.gov/reading-rm/doc-collections/cfr/part035/part035-2063.html (accessed on 3 March 2010).

US Nuclear Regulatory Commission. Title 10 Code of Federal Regulations Part § 35.27(b) Supervision http://www.nrc.gov/reading-rm/doc-collections/cfr/part035/part035-0027.html (accessed on 3 March 2010).

US Nuclear Regulatory Commission. Title 10 Code of Federal Regulations Part § 35.3045 Report and notification of a medical event http://www.nrc.gov.reading-rm/doc-collections/cfr/part035/part035-3045.html (accessed on 3 March 2010).

US Nuclear Regulatory Commission. Title 10 Code of Federal Regulations Part § 35.40 Written directives. http://www.nrc.gov/reading-rm/doc-collections/cfr/part035/part035-0040.html (accessed on 3 March 2010).

US Nuclear Regulatory Commission. Title 10 Code of Federal Regulations Part § 35.41 Procedures for administrations requiring a written directive. http://www.nrc.gov/reading-rm/doc-collections/cfr/part035/part035-0041.html (accessed on 3 March 2010).

US Nuclear Regulatory Commission. Title 10 Code of Federal Regulations Part § 35.55 (a) and (b) Training for an authorized nuclear pharmacist. http://www.nrc.gov/reading-rm/doc-collections/cfr/part035/part035-0055.html (accessed on 3 March 2010).

US Nuclear Regulatory Commission. Title 10 Code of Federal Regulations Part § 35.59 Recentness of training. http://www.nrc.gov/reading-rm/doc-collections/cfr/part035/part035-0059.html (accessed on 3 March 2010).

US Nuclear Regulatory Commission. Title 10 Code of Federal Regulations Part § 35.63 Determination of dosages of unsealed byproduct material for medical use http://www.nrc.gov/reading-rm/doc-collections/cfr/part035/part035-0063.html (accessed on 3 March 2010).

US Nuclear Regulatory Commission. Title 10 Code of Federal Regulations Part § 35.69 Labeling of vials and syringes http://www.nrc.gov/reading-rm/doc-collections/cfr/part035/part035-0069.html (accessed on 3 March 2010).

US Nuclear Regulatory Commission. Title 10 Code of Federal Regulations Part § 71.4 Definitions http://www.nrc.gov/reading-rm/doc-collections/cfr/part071/part071-0004.html (accessed on 3 March 2010).

US Nuclear Regulatory Commission. Title 10 Code of Federal Regulations Part § 71.47 External radiation standards for all packages http://www.nrc.gov/reading-rm/doc-collections/cfr/part071/part071-0047.html (accessed on 3 March 2010).

30

Packaging and transport of radiopharmaceuticals

Alistair M Millar

Radiopharmacies, whether they are operated by hospitals or commercial organisations, commonly supply radiopharmaceuticals to several hospitals. Transport of these radioactive materials is normally by road. In Europe, an Agreement Concerning the International Carriage of Dangerous Goods by Road (ECE 2008), known as ADR, specifies the requirements for the transport of radioactive materials. As ADR has no provision for enforcement, individual countries have incorporated its requirements into their own legislation. For example, in the UK, the transport of radioactive materials by road is governed by The Carriage of Dangerous Goods and Use of Transportable Pressure Equipment Regulations 2009 (SI 2009). The regulations cover all radioactive materials with a few exceptions such as nuclear weapons and smoke detectors for domestic use. In addition to the Carriage of Dangerous Goods Regulations (CDG), the Carriage of Dangerous Goods: Approved Derogations and Transitional Provisions 2009 (ADTP) sets out circumstances under which particular types of carriage or carriage in particular circumstances are exempt from the provisions of the CDG (DOT 2009). The aim of this chapter is to describe the parts of the regulations that apply to the transport of radiopharmaceuticals and to summarise how a radiopharmacy might comply with these regulations. As with any activity that is regulated by law, there is no substitute for reference to the original legislation. In summary, the regulations specify:

- The types of packaging used for radioactive materials
- The maximum activity in a package
- The maximum level of radioactive contamination on a package
- The labels to be displayed on packages
- The documentation that must accompany a consignment of radioactive material
- The placards to be displayed on a vehicle
- The duties of the driver in the event of an accident
- That a fire extinguisher is carried unless only up to ten Excepted Packages are being transported

Table 30.1 Conditions for package types used to transport radiopharmaceuticals

Category	Package type	Maximum activity	Maximum radiation level at any point on external surface	Transport Index (TI)
Not applicable	Excepted	Yes – see Table 30.2	Not more than 5 μSv/h	Not applicable
I-White	Type A	None	Not more than 5 μSv/h	Not applicable
II-Yellow	Type A	None	More than 5 μSv/h but not more than 500 μSv/h	More than 0 but not more than 1
III-Yellow	Type A	None	More than 500 μSv/h but not more than 2 mSv/h	More than 1 but not more than 10

- That a quality assurance programme exists to demonstrate compliance with the regulations
- That a safety adviser is appointed.

Packages

Although ADR describes eight types of packages for the transport of radioactive material, only two – the Excepted Package and the Type A Package – are relevant to the transport of radiopharmaceuticals. A summary of the conditions relevant to each is shown in Table 30.1.

An Excepted Package contains a limited activity of a radionuclide. The principal requirements for an Excepted package are that:

- The package is designed to retain its contents under routine transport conditions.
- The package bears the marking 'RADIOACTIVE' on an internal surface in such a manner that a warning of the presence of radioactive material is visible on opening the package.
- The activity of the radionuclide in the package does not exceed a specified value. The activity limits for radionuclides that are used in nuclear medicine and might be transported in Excepted Packages are shown in Table 30.2.
- The dose-rate at any point on the surface does not exceed 5 μSv/h.
- The contamination level at any point of the external surface does not exceed 4 Bq/cm^2 for beta emitters, gamma emitters and low toxicity alpha emitters, and 0.4 Bq/cm^2 for all other alpha emitters.

The advantage of using an Excepted Package is that the requirements for transport are minimal. In practice, an Excepted Package is often inappropriate as the activity required for a patient is greater than the package limit.

If a radiopharmaceutical does not meet the requirements of an Excepted Package, it must be transported

Table 30.2 Maximum activities that can be transported in Excepted Packages

Radionuclide	Activity limit (MBq)
Carbon-14	300
Chromium-51	3000
Gallium-67	300
Gallium-68	50
Indium-111	300
Iodine-123	300
Iodine-131	70
Molybdenum-99	600
Rubidium-81	800
Selenium-75	300
Technetium-99m	400
Thallium-201	400

in a Type A Package. The regulations specify many requirements for a Type Package. These include that:

- The package is designed to withstand normal conditions of transport. To demonstrate this, the package design satisfies a series of specified tests that include tests for ingress of water spray, free drop, stacking and penetration.
- The smallest external dimension is not less than 100 mm.
- Sufficient absorbent material is included to absorb twice the volume of the liquid contents or the package has primary inner and secondary outer containment such that liquid contents are retained if the inner container leaks.
- The package is closed with a tamper-evident seal.
- The contamination level at any point of the external surface does not exceed 4 Bq/cm^2 for beta emitters, gamma emitters and low-toxicity alpha emitters, and 0.4 Bq/cm^2 for all other alpha emitters.

A radiopharmacy can undertake the complex process of testing a package of its own design to demonstrate that it complies with the requirements of Type A. The complexity of the tests that must be performed and the evidence that must be kept make this unattractive. A more efficient option is to use commercially available Type A Packages. These are supplied with a certificate of compliance.

Labelling of packages

Packages must be labelled with the name and address of either the consignor or consignee, or both.

The only other labelling requirement on the outside of an Excepted Package is the UN number, i.e. UN 2910 in this case. A warning of the presence of radioactive material must be visible inside the package when it is opened. This can be achieved by the inclusion of a label on top of the contents (Figure 30.1).

Type A Packages must be marked on the outside of the packaging with 'TYPE A', the UN number 'UN 2915' and the proper shipping name 'Radioactive Material, Type A Package'. Type A Packages

CAUTION
This package contains
an excepted quantity of
RADIOACTIVE
MATERIAL

Figure 30.1 Label to be included in an Excepted Package.

are classified into three categories depending upon the maximum radiation level at the surface and at 1 metre from the external surfaces, the latter being used to calculate the Transport Index (TI). To determine the TI, the radiation level in mSv/h is measured at a distance of 1 metre and multiplied by 100. The three categories, which have different identification labels to simplify recognition and to facilitate control during handling, are described in Table 30.1. An example of each is shown in Figure 30.2. The label displays the name and activity of the radionuclide in the package. Those for Category II-Yellow and III-Yellow also display the TI. A Type A Package must bear the appropriate identification label on two opposite sides.

Transport document

Each consignment of packages containing radioactive material must be accompanied by a transport document that contains the following information for each package:

- The name and address of the consignor.
- The name and address of the consignee.
- The UN number – this is 'UN2910' for an Excepted Package and 'UN2915' for a Category I-White, Category II-Yellow or Category III-Yellow Package.
- The Proper Shipping Name – this is 'Radioactive Material, Excepted Package – limited quantity of material' for an Excepted Package and 'Radioactive Material, Type A Package' for a Category I-White, Category II-Yellow or Category III-Yellow Package.
- The United Nations Class Number '7'.
- The name or symbol of the radionuclide.
- A description of the physical form of the material, i.e. Liquid, Solid, Gas or Powder.

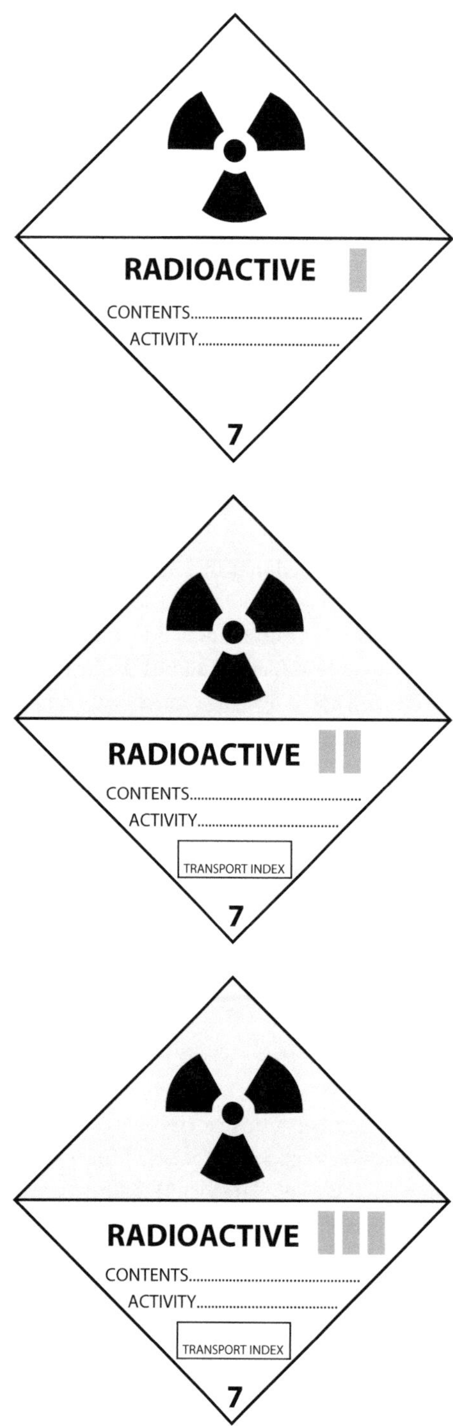

Figure 30.2 (a) Category I – White, (b) Category II – Yellow and (c) Category III – Yellow labels for Type A packages. The shaded areas in the top half of the category II and III labels are yellow. The stripes after 'radioactive' are red.

- A description of the chemical form of the material i.e. Organic Compound or Inorganic Compound.
- The maximum activity of the package contents.
- The category of the package, i.e. I-White, II-Yellow or III-Yellow.
- The Transport Index (for Categories II-Yellow and III-Yellow only).
- A declaration signed and dated by the consignor that the materials are described, packed, marked and labelled in accordance with the relevant regulations. A facsimile signature is acceptable.

The items of information on the Transport Document must be shown in the order in which they are listed above.

For a consignment that consists solely of Excepted Packages, the transport document need show only the UN number. However, to avoid the complication of preparing two types of document depending on the content of the consignment, it may be more practical to issue a full transport document for each consignment. A specimen transport document is shown in Figure 30.3.

Vehicles

Vehicles used for the Carriage of radioactive materials must be equipped with two portable fire extinguishers with a minimum capacity of 2 kg dry powder. If only Excepted Packages are being carried, the vehicle is exempt from the requirement to carry fire extinguishers. The vehicle also is required to be equipped with a wheel chock, two self-standing warning signs and eye rinsing liquid and for each crew member a warning vest, portable lighting equipment, a pair of protective gloves and eye protection.

No placards are required on a vehicle in which only Excepted Packages are being carried. When Category I, II or III Packages are being carried, placards must be displayed on both sides and the rear of the vehicle. The placard design is shown in Figure 30.4. When a small vehicle is used and there is insufficient space to mount 250 mm × 250 mm placards, their dimensions may be reduced to 100 mm × 100 mm.

Vehicles carrying dangerous goods are required to display an orange plate on the front and rear. In

Transport document for Radioactive Materials

in accordance with The Carriage of Dangerous Goods and Use of Transportable Pressure Equipment Regulations 2007

Consignor: Radiopharmacy
Hospital name
Address
City
Telephone number

Despatch date and time: 01-Apr-09 09:00

Package number	Consignee	UN number	Proper shipping name	UN class	Nuclide	Physical form	Chemical form	Activity (MBq)	Package category	TI	Pack type
1005	Dept Nuclear Medicine Hospital name City	UN2915	Radioactive Material, Type A Package	7	Tc-99m	Liquid	Organic compound	5950	I-White	–	A
1006	Dept Medical Physics Hospital name City	UN2915	Radioactive Material, Type A Package	7	I-131	Powder	Inorganic compound	500	III-Yellow	0.6	A
1007	Dept Haematology Hospital name City	UN2910	Radioactive Material, Excepted Package – limited quantity of material	7	Co-57	Powder	Organic compound	0.2	Excepted	–	E

"I hereby declare that the contents of this consignment are fully and accurately described above by the proper shipping name and are classified, packed, marked and labelled and are in all respects in proper condition for the transport by road (ADR) according to the applicable international and national governmental regulations."

Signed *AN Other* (facsimile signature)

Driver's instructions

1. Stow the packages securely in the rear of the vehicle.
2. Carry this certificate in the vehicle while the packages are being transported. It must be shown to the police or transport inspector. Destroy the certificate when you reach your destination.
3. Do not leave the vehicle unattended except when delivering packages. The vehicle must be locked when left unattended.
4. If there is any indication that a package may have been lost or stolen, contact the Radiopharmacy immediately.
5. In the event of an accident, remain with the vehicle until the police arrive then contact the Radiopharmacy.
6. In the event of a breakdown, lock the vehicle and contact the Radiopharmacy.

Figure 30.3 Transport document.

the UK, if a vehicle used to transport radiopharmaceuticals does not exceed 3.5 tonnes, carries no more than 10 packages, and the sum of the transport indexes does not exceed 3, then a fireproof notice, not less than 120 mm × 120 mm, may be displayed in the cab instead of orange plates. A format for the notice is shown in Figure 30.5. The lettering must be embossed or stamped and remain legible after exposure to a fire involving the vehicle. Notices that incorporate the address and telephone number of the radiopharmacy can be ordered from commercial suppliers. Each notice is supplied with a holder for mounting in the cab of the vehicle.

Training of drivers

Drivers of vehicles in which radioactive materials are transported must receive training. If the total number of packages carried does not exceed 10 and the sum of the transport indexes does not exceed 3, attendance at a specialised training course is not required. However,

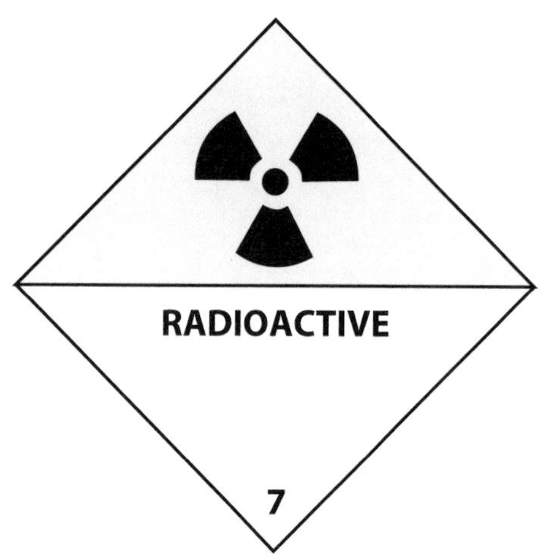

Figure 30.4 Vehicle placard (minimum dimensions 250 mm × 250 mm). The shaded area in the top half is yellow.

This vehicle is carrying

RADIOACTIVE

MATERIAL

In case of accident get in touch at once with

THE POLICE

and

Hospital Name

City, Postcode

Telephone number

Figure 30.5 Fireproof notice.

drivers must receive training relevant to their duties. For drivers involved in the transport of radiopharmaceuticals, this includes knowledge of:

- The need to exercise reasonable care
- How to stow the packages securely in the vehicle
- The restrictions on carrying passengers
- The need to carry the transport document and to produce it for inspection when requested
- The need to remain with the vehicle except when delivering packages
- When to display placards on the vehicle and the fireproof notice in the cab and the need to remove them from display once the radioactive materials have been delivered
- The action to be taken in the event of the loss of a package, an accident or a breakdown.

The provision of this training should be documented. A regular reminder of the main requirements can be provided by including them on the transport document as shown in Figure 30.3.

Quality assurance programme

To demonstrate compliance with the regulations, the radiopharmacy is required to maintain a quality assurance programme. This includes:

- Audit to demonstrate compliance with the regulations
- Maintaining records of all consignments
- Testing of Type A packaging
- Measurements of surface contamination on packages.

Safety adviser

The ADR requires the appointment of a safety adviser who is responsible for helping to prevent the risks inherent in the transport of radioactive materials with regard to persons, property and the environment. The principal duties of the adviser are to:

- Monitor compliance with the regulations
- Advise on the carriage of radioactive materials
- Prepare an annual report on the radiopharmacy's activities in the carriage of radioactive materials.

The adviser may be a member of staff in the radiopharmacy's organisation or may be contracted externally. The adviser is required to undergo training, pass an examination and hold a vocational training certificate.

References

DOT (2009). Carriage of Dangerous Goods: Approved Derogations and Transitional Provisions 2009. Department of Transport.

ECE (2008). UN Economic Commission for Europe –Inland Transport Committee. *The European agreement concerning the international carriage of dangerous goods by road (ADR)*. Geneva: United Nations.

SI (2009). The Carriage of Dangerous Goods and Use of Transportable Pressure Equipment Regulations 2007. Statutory Instrument 2009 No.1348. The Stationery Office.

31

Patient safety and dispensing of radiopharmaceuticals

James Thom

Introduction

Patients in the hospital environment are exposed to a large number of potential hazards, from infection to adverse reactions to name a few. In the Nuclear Medicine Department they may be exposed to additional hazards peculiar to the use of radioactive materials. This chapter will address those aspects under the control and responsibility of the radiopharmacist.

Patient safety begins with the radiopharmaceutical purchased and the facilities and staff preparing the product, i.e. Good Manufacturing Practice (GMP) (MHRA 2007) as well as the training and competence of the staff administering the radiopharmaceutical. In the UK, doses of radiopharmaceuticals are prepared in either a licensed radiopharmacy (licensed and inspected by the Medicines and Healthcare products Regulatory Agency (MHRA), the UK regulatory agency) or a unit preparing them under section 10 exemption of the Medicines Act 1968 (SI 1992a). Both types of unit will be subject to inspection and audit at regular intervals and consequently products will be prepared according to GMP and be fit and suitable for their purpose.

General dispensing of radiopharmaceuticals

Facilities

A radiopharmacy consists of a series of cleanrooms designed to Health Building Note 14-01 (Department of Health 2009), BS/ISO 14644 (BSI 1999, 2004) and incorporating GMP. Air supply to the rooms should be of GMP grade B quality for open-fronted laminar flow cabinets or grade D for isolators. Rooms must be temperature and humidity controlled as well as subject to a minimum of 20 air changes per hour per room. There will also be a cascade of air pressure through the clean rooms to the outside air. Air supply should now be energy efficient and make use of recirculation of air and heat recovery systems. All preparations will be made in either laminar airflow cabinets or isolators with a GMP grade A air quality. The facilities are subject to regular planned preventative maintenance and calibration as well as regular cleaning and environmental monitoring. Operators must wear suitable protective clothing to maintain the environmental conditions and also to prevent contamination of themselves due to spillage. Radiopharmacies are usually sited away from major thoroughfares in the hospital to ensure that radiation exposure to members of the public is reduced.

Radionuclide generators

A full description of generators can be found in Chapter 21. The most common generator system employed is the $^{99}Mo/^{99m}Tc$ generator. These are purchased from commercial suppliers and the quantity of technetium-99m produced by the generator will depend on the original quantity of molybdenum in the generator and its age. The technetium-99m yield of the generators should be suitable and adequate for the dispensing workload of the radiopharmacy.

The generators themselves pose a health and safety risk to staff owing to their weight (up to 18 kg) and they require lifting from the delivery box and manoeuvring to their final position in a clean-air device (isolator or laminar flow cabinet – see Figures 31.1 and 31.2 for examples). Risk assessment should be carried out locally to ensure compliance with manual handling regulations and reducing the radiation risk to staff involved. The generators will also need to be surface cleaned and sanitised before placing in their final position. Additional shielding to reduce the radiation dose from the generators is required and this can lead to further handling issues. Various handling devices are available to aid the lifting of generators, and isolator manufacturers will provide shielding unique to each generator. The generators are usually sited in a module of an isolator or in a separate isolator/clean-air device to reduce their radiation exposure to operators.

The molybdenum/technetium generator is eluted with sodium chloride 0.9% injection on a daily, or twice daily, basis depending on the workload and the eluate is used to prepare the radiopharmaceuticals required, usually from a kit manufactured by a commercial company.

Radiopharmaceutical kits

A radiopharmaceutical kit means any preparation to be reconstituted or combined with radionuclides in a final radiopharmaceutical, usually prior to its administration (SI 1992b). This is generally taken to mean a freeze-dried product containing the product to be labelled as well as other constituents such as pH adjusters, stabilisers, bulking agents and stannous chloride reductant. Commercial products purchased must be licensed within the host country and are subject to

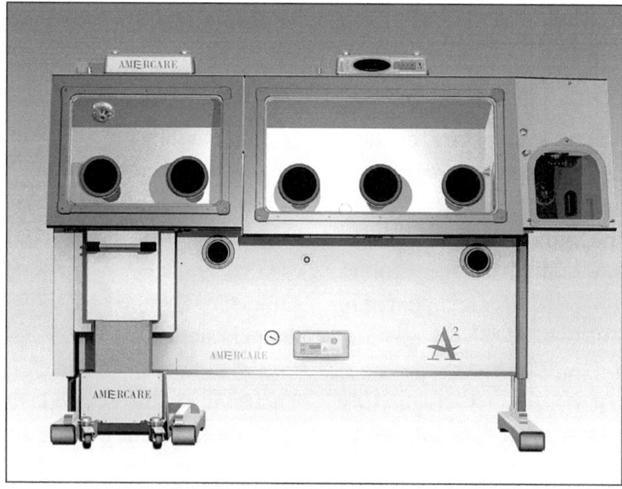

Figure 31.1 Amercare dispensing suite.

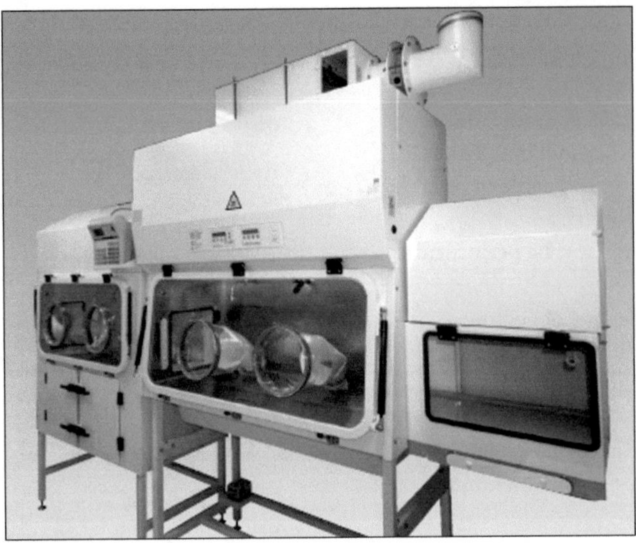

Figure 31.2 Envair dispensing isolator.

the regulations of that country. The rule within the UK is that if a product has a UK product licence it must be used in preference to an unlicensed product.

Where there is no licensed alternative an unlicensed radiopharmaceutical may have to be used, but a clear justification must be provided for its administration by the responsible physician. Clearly, a risk assessment will be required to demonstrate the clinical need versus the risk to the patient for using the product. Again, within the UK the use of unlicensed radiopharmaceuticals should be placed on the institution's risk register and the management board informed. As the product is unlicensed, there may be issues of quality to be resolved before administration to patients. Unlicensed products available in the UK are normally licensed elsewhere in the EU; consequently they will be of a marketable quality according to the standards of that licensing authority and will probably need little testing to validate their quality.

Products without any marketing authorisation within the EU may bring associated problems of quality and efficacy, and a full testing programme will be required to ensure their suitability. The radiopharmacy service will have to satisfy itself of the identity and quality of original material used to produce the patient dose and the quality of the final patient dose itself. The relevant national body will also regulate importation of the product so consequently there may be a delay in obtaining the material. A number of kits licensed in the UK are listed in Chapter 18, to which the reader is referred.

In-house preparations

Preparations that are not commercially available and are made in the host institution are usually intended for research purposes or trials. This type of product often requires multiple manipulations of ingredients and is often an example of an open procedure requiring more stringent manufacturing conditions. In-house preparations are certainly more complex to manufacture than the simple reconstitution of a ready-to-use kit. They require the same, or preferably better, facilities to ensure the quality of the finished product and need a great deal of input from the Quality Assurance and Quality Control staff to ensure their acceptability for use. If they are to be used as part of a clinical trial or research study, they must be produced in an establishment holding an Investigational Medicinal Product licence.

There are a number of disadvantages to in-house preparations:

- The production requires skilled operatives.
- There is the possibility of exposure of the product to the atmosphere and microbiological contamination.
- High radiation dose is received by the operator's fingers.

- They will require additional local shielding, which may be difficult to sterilise and maintain in that condition.
- Unlike licensed radiopharmaceutical kits, in-house preparations are individual and therefore not always reproducible or reliable in quality and or performance.
- Quality control testing must be performed prior to administration.
- The procedures can be extremely time consuming and scheduling them into a busy radiopharmacy timetable may be difficult.
- They require a Qualified Person release if they are classified as an Investigational Medicinal Product.

However, despite many problems these preparations may become the kits of the future if their clinical use becomes popular.

Commercial radiopharmaceuticals

These are products purchased in a ready-to-give formulation, for example Ioflupane [^{123}I] Injection or Iobenguane [^{123}I] Injection. These require no manipulation by the radiopharmacy, but many units will dispense these products as unit-dose preparations. The radiopharmacy will verify that the product and isotope are correct and that the correct dose has been ordered. These products are usually for a single patient dose, so they usually do not contain a preservative.

Open and closed procedures

Aseptic dispensing procedures are often classified as either open or closed procedures.

A *closed* procedure is defined as one whereby a sterile pharmaceutical is prepared by transferring sterile ingredients or solutions into a pre-sterilised sealed container either directly or by using a sterile transfer device, all without exposing the solution(s) or ingredients to the external environment. They form the majority of the procedures for ^{99m}Tc preparations made in most radiopharmacies where kits are reconstituted using the eluate from a sterile ^{99}Mo/^{99m}Tc generator.

Table 31.1 Principal attributes of open and closed of procedures

Closed procedures	Open procedures
Ingredients not exposed to atmosphere or contamination	Ingredients exposed to atmosphere and possible contamination
Less risk of spillage	Increased risk of spillage
Aseptic techniques used	Sterilisation steps may be required
Procedures are rapid and short	Procedures are lengthy
Minimum equipment required	More equipment required
Minimum radiation hazard to operators	Radiation hazard to operators may be high

An *open* procedure is defined as one in which an ingredient or semi-finished product is, at some stage after sterilisation, open to the atmosphere (i.e. not closed in a vial, syringe, generator or other sealed container). Thus, open procedures should be avoided where possible as they carry additional risks of microbial contamination.

Table 31.1 summarises principal attributes of both types of procedures.

Multidose versus unit dose preparations

Presentation

A multidose preparation is, as its name suggests, a vial prepared by the radiopharmacy from which several doses can be withdrawn in the Nuclear Medicine Department. This vial will have been produced in accordance with GMP and be of suitable quality for use.

Multidose preparations are generally cheaper per dose than a unit dose and allow for greater flexibility within the nuclear medicine clinic as additional or larger doses may be withdrawn as required. However, no assurance of the quality of the product can be made after the first dose of the day has been withdrawn because of possible microbiological or chemical contamination in the clinical environment. Training of clinical staff in aseptic technique will reduce the possibility of microbiological contamination of multidose containers. The provision of a suitable clean area within the injection room with reduced access to restrict staff movements into the drawing-up area will also reduce the potential for contamination.

Unit doses are prepared for each individual patient by the radiopharmacy and will be time-specific to compensate for radioactive decay. These are the most expensive dose forms because of the extra time taken to prepare them. However, in a busy department the benefit of having the dose ready to administer may outweigh the possible increased cost.

Table 31.2 summarises the main features of these two types of presentation.

Labelling

All radiopharmaceutical preparations must have an audit trail from manufacture to administration and therefore must be labelled appropriately. Vials and syringes can be labelled prior to preparation with a label detailing, as a minimum, the batch number and name of the product. There is no consensus in the radiopharmacy community as to where the label should be placed once the kit is activated – on the immediate container or the lead pot. The vials and or syringes can be final-labelled after loading, but a risk assessment must be undertaken to assess the finger dose to the operator if this is contemplated.

All outer packages (lead pots) must be labelled with the details as shown in Table 31.3 (see also Chapter 30).

Table 31.2 Main features of unit-dose and multidose preparations

Unit Dose	Multidose
Advantages	
Quick to use	Product presented in nuclear medicine department as per manufacturer's specification
No drawing-up area required, so saves space in department	Cheaper
Maintains sterility	Easy to store
Many syringes in a busy department so there may be a storage problem	One vial for the whole day (providing shelf life allows)
Problems if the patient is late	Easy to adjust the dose
Disadvantages	
Product presented in nuclear medicine department may not comply with manufacturer's specification	Calculation of dose is required by operators
More expensive per dose	Needs to be drawn up
Hard to store	Potential introduction of microbiological contamination
Restricts dose	

Table 31.3 Details for labelling lead pots

POM (prescription only medicine)	Name of preparation
Radioactive trefoil	Route of administration
Radioactive	Activity
Name and address of supplier	Volume
Manufacturer's special licence number	Reference time and date
Storage instructions	Expiry time and date
Batch or reference number	

Doses of radiopharmaceuticals

ARSAC

All doses administered for either a diagnostic or therapeutic application are derived from a set of doses published by the Administration of Radioactive Substances Advisory Committee (ARSAC 2006). The doses listed are for a standard adult and there is a dose adjustment allowance for clinicians to vary the dose depending on weight of the patient and physical size.

Paediatric

Although radiopharmaceuticals are routinely used in paediatrics, few are licensed for this group of patients. Without the appropriate licensing the onus is on the clinician performing the scan to take clinical responsibility for the administration of product outside its licensed application. Children have rapidly growing and dividing tissue which may be more sensitive to ionising radiation and also their organ size to body ratio may be different from the older child or the adult. This, along with the possibility of somatic and hereditary effects from even small amounts of administered radioactivity must be balanced against the possible benefits from the investigation. Before the administration of any radiopharmaceutical to a paediatric patient, due consideration must be given to the following general principles.

- Is this the most appropriate investigation to answer the clinical problem?
- Is the procedure, and the resulting radiation burden, clinically justified?
- Are the facilities within the nuclear medicine department appropriate for children – environment, staffing facilities, etc., – or should child be referred to a specialist centre?

Consequently the activity administered must be reduced by any of the various methods available. The degree of reduction must take into account the smallest activity required to give the desired images and statistics, the test to be performed, the size and weight of the patient, sensitivity to detection equipment, type of examination and acquisition time. The method employed for the activity reduction must be agreed by all clinicians and become a departmental policy or protocol. For most departments a simple chart of the activities to be administered per body weight reduces the chances of misadministration due to calculation errors. Any such chart requires the most up-to-date information and needs to be updated and signed by the responsible clinician.

Activity estimation

Scaling down the adult administration activity in simple proportion to body weight will generally result in the child receiving an effective dose equivalent similar to that an adult would receive.

However, consideration must be given to the procedure in question as infants have a higher uptake in bones, owing to increased growth, and in brain imaging, owing to the organ reaching a high proportion of adult size in young childhood. The method of administering activities to children in individual departments will also vary and so this should also be recognised as a potential complication. Drawing up a small activity for a child involves the use of a needle and syringe and the administration is via a cannula or similar device, and an allowance must be made for the residue left in the devices. Dilution of the radiopharmaceutical may be required for administration to some very small patients; consideration must be given as to where, how, and by whom this is undertaken.

Paediatric activities can be calculated by the following methods.

Fraction of adult administered activity based on child's body weight

This is the method currently approved by ARSAC and has the proviso that no less than 10% of the adult activity is administered. Based upon administering to children by weight, it generally assumes a standard adult weight as 70 kg. The calculation is:

$$\text{Administered activity} = \text{adult amount of activity} \times (\text{child weight in kg}/70)$$

See Table 31.4.

Surface area alone

Surface area can be calculated from the following formulae and the factors taken from Table 31.5.

This method is less favourable owing to the complex calculations involved and the need for the patient to have their correct height and weight measured. Recently the European Association of Nuclear Medicine (EANM) published a new paediatric dosage card (Lassman *et al.* 2007). It is generally recognised that there is a minimum amount of activity that should be administered to a child. This enables the required image to be acquired in a suitable time and, if statistical analysis is being undertaken, sufficient counts to be acquired.

Pregnancy

When it is clinically necessary to administer a radioactive substance to a pregnant patient the dose and therefore the radiation exposure must be kept to a minimum. However it is a delicate balancing act as too little activity administered may lead to an inconclusive

Table 31.4 Fraction of administered adult activity for children

Body weight (kg)	Fraction of administered activity	Body weight (kg)	Fraction of administered activity	Body weight (kg)	Fraction of administered activity
3	0.10	22	0.50	42	0.78
4	0.14	24	0.53	44	0.80
6	0.19	26	0.56	46	0.82
8	0.23	28	0.58	48	0.85
10	0.27	30	0.62	50	0.88
12	0.32	32	0.65	52–54	0.90
14	0.36	34	0.68	56–58	0.92
16	0.40	36	0.71	60–62	0.96
18	0.44	38	0.73	64–66	0.98
20	0.46	40	0.76	68	0.99

diagnostic scan, and therefore potentially require a second administration, or to a misdiagnosis. The request must be justified by the ARSAC licence holder and on this basis a risk assessment must be undertaken as to whether the diagnostic benefit outweighs the risk of exposure to the fetus. When the administration is clinically justified, all possible means should be undertaken to reduce the dose to the fetus; for example, publications have recommended that for a lung perfusion study half a dose of agent be administered.

Table 31.5 Formulae for calculating surface area

Surface area (SA) (m^2)	Divide adult activity by the factor	Approximate age
0.24	7.2	Newborn
0.27	6.4	
0.31	5.6	
0.35	4.9	
0.43	4.0	
0.58	3.0	1 year
0.75	2.3	5 years
1.00	1.7	10 years
1.57	1.1	15 years

$SA = (weight)^{0.425} \times (height)^{0.725} \times 0.007184$.

Therapeutic administration

Notes for Guidance on the Clinical Administration of Radiopharmaceuticals and Use of Sealed Radioactive Sources (ARSAC 2006) gives extensive advice on administration to females of childbearing age concerning how long pregnancy should be avoided after administration of a therapeutic substance.

Breast milk excretion

Administered radiopharmaceuticals have been shown to be excreted into breast milk. It is therefore imperative that before administration a detailed plan is discussed with the mother as to the procedure for breast-feeding. This may include delaying the procedure if that is clinically acceptable until breast-feeding ceases, or choosing the appropriate pharmaceutical to minimise excretion to breast milk, or choosing a different test including a non-nuclear medicine test.

If administration is considered to be acceptable, a number of precautions can be considered.

- A feed should be expressed prior to the test.
- The infant can be fed prior to the test.
- For a suitable period after the test, milk should be expressed and discarded.

Dispensing of therapeutic radiopharmaceuticals

Therapeutic radiopharmaceuticals require specialist expertise for preparation and/or dispensing.

Prior to dispensing a therapeutic radiopharmaceutical, the following must be considered:

- Do staff have any experience of therapeutic radiopharmaceuticals? If not, then training should be sought in an approved centre of excellence prior to undertaking any procedures.
- Once trained, are staff competent to undertake a specific procedure or a range of procedures?
- For each and every procedure dummy runs should be undertaken (without radioactivity) directly mimicking the process.
- Before the dispensing of a therapeutic dose a reduced activity production should be undertaken; this will provide a better indication of the process and help to identify and iron out any problems.
- Finger doses must be monitored while dispensing therapeutic radiopharmaceuticals.

To ensure patient safety the following should be considered:

- Has the prescribed dose been checked? This is important if the dose is dependent on patient weight (dose per kg, etc.)
- Have all calculations used to prepare the dose been checked – and double-checked?
- Has the dose been prepared according to manufacturer's instructions and to national standards and recommendations?
- Has the dose been appropriately labelled and stored in accordance with the manufacturer's instructions?

Patient safety: Other aspects

Have you got the right patient?

The waiting room for a busy nuclear medicine department is a place for possible confusion when patient names are called. It is possible for similar-sounding names to be misheard and the wrong patient to be directed to the injection room before a mistake is discovered. On a similar note, patients should always be asked their full name since, for example, Mrs E. Smith could be Mrs Evelyn Smith, Mrs Edith Smith or Mrs Emily Smith and with more common surnames the mistake is waiting to occur.

Have you got the right isotope/kit?

When products are prepared either in a multidose or unit dose presentation, there is the chance of confusion prior to administration. In a busy injection room with the pressure to inject patients on time, DTPA can easily look like DMSA on a label or a request/referral card.

It is clearly important for patient safety that time is taken for the following:

- Selecting the correct kit/injection
- Taking time to read the referral to establish whether the test is appropriate for the patient.
- Ensuring the correct patient is present
- Ensuring the correct dose is drawn up
- Ensuring that waste is dealt with appropriately.

Side-effects and adverse reactions of radiopharmaceuticals (contributed by N. Hartman)

A record of any adverse events or product defects is only as good as the reports of occurrences. This does not alter the fact that adverse events linked to diagnostic radiopharmaceuticals are rare, and Hesslewood and Keeling, (1997) reported the statistic of 11 events per 10^5 administrations, which is approximately 10^3 times less than the figure anticipated with 'normal' drugs and iodinated contrast media. These infrequent occurrences could be due to the frequently subpharmacological quantities of material administered, but it is also dependent on the stringent management paradigm that encourages reporting. It is also not obvious how to assign an event's cause to the 'target/labelled' molecule or an excipient when a patient receives many other medications concurrently.

The most common adverse events are transient, and include non-specific rashes, urticaria, malaise, tachycardia, hypertension and nausea (Balan *et al.* 2003; Hartman 2005), with very few reports of PET/therapeutic radiopharmaceutical adverse events (Silberstein 1998; UKRG 2009; VirRAD 2009), and no related deaths. Compared to adverse events, product defects are much more infrequent, and mostly relate to generator problems, or issues with therapeutic capsules and their dispensing.

A summary of the adverse events/product defect reported to the UKRG/VirRAD databases for 2007–2008 is given in Table 31.6. The recent increased interest in therapeutic radiopharmaceuticals has not been translated into increased adverse events for these agents.

Adverse events and product defects are typically reported on three levels:

- Within the manufacturer's/user's institution as an event/defect/near-miss.
- Reporting to national/international databases (UKRG, VirRAD, etc.).
- In European (and other) countries there is also a legal requirement to report serious events to the national regulatory authorities responsible for pharmacovigilance or licensing.

In the UK, the national database for reporting is accessed via the United Kingdom Radiopharmacy Group (UKRG) or British Nuclear Medicine Society (BNMS) websites (the latter at http://www.bnms.org.uk/). The EANM (see https://www.eanm.org/) and VirRAD share a European database, which is less comprehensive than the equivalent one in Britain, although events/defects are now commonly stored on both the UKRG and VirRAD databases.

The MHRA supports a national 'yellow card' reporting system where all serious adverse events have to be reported within the UK (see http://yellowcard.mhra.gov.uk). Practitioners do not report directly to the EMEA, although they receive reports from national EU regulatory authorities.

Table 31.6 Summary of adverse events and product defects reported to the UK Radiopharmacy Group and VirRAD databases for 2007–2008

Radiopharmaceutical	Number of reports in UK 2007 and 2008	Summary of concerns
^{99m}Tc-Oxidronate	8	Rash, nausea, metallic taste
Pyrophosphate (as tinning agent)	4	Urticaria/erythema, stomach uptake
^{99}Mo/^{99m}Tc generators	8	Low elution yield
^{99m}Tc-Tetrofosmin	6	No cardiac uptake, itching, blistering
^{99m}Tc- Medronate	11	Dizziness, rash, nausea
^{99m}Tc- Succimer	7	Rash, vomiting, urticaria
^{99m}Tc- Sestamibi	5	Urticaria, metallic taste, vomiting
^{99m}Tc-MAA	2	Blurred vision, uptake in thyroid/stomach
^{99m}Tc-Nanocolloid	1	Itchiness, hypotension
^{99m}Tc-Exametazime	1	Uptake in choroid plexus and thyroid
^{123}I-Iobenguane (mIBG)	3	Painful injection site, lost consciousness
^{123}I NaI solution	1	No activity in vial
^{131}I-Norcholesterol	1	Flushing, chest pain, hypertension
^{131}I NaI therapeutic caps	1	Labelling omission
^{75}Se-SeHCAT	1	Dizziness, nausea

References

ARSAC (2006). *Notes for Guidance on the Clinical Administration of Radiopharmaceuticals and Use of Sealed Radioactive Sources 2006*. London: Administration of Radioactive Substances Advisory Committee.

Balan KK *et al.* (2003). Severe systemic reaction to ^{99m}Tc-methylene diphosphonate: a case report. *J Nucl Med Technol* 31: 76–78.

BSI (1999). BS EN ISO 14644-1 : 1999. *Environmental Cleanliness in Enclosed Spaces. Specification for Clean Rooms and Clean Air Devices*. London: British Standards Institution.

BSI (2004). BS EN ISO 14644-5 : 2004. *Environmental Cleanliness in Enclosed Spaces. Guide to Operational Procedures and Disciplines Applicable to Clean Rooms and Clean Air Devices*. London: British Standards Institution.

Department of Health (2009). *Health Building Note 14-01 Medicines Management – Pharmacy and Radiopharmacy Facilities*. London: Department of Health. ISBN 978-0-11-322795-2.

Hartman NG (2005). Radiopharmacy – problems encountered with the products. *Hosp Pharm* 12: 305–310.

Hesslewood SR, Keeling DH (1997). Frequency of adverse reactions to radiopharmaceuticals in Europe. *Eur J Nucl Med* 24: 1179–1182.

Lassmann M *et al.* (2007). The new EANM paediatric dosage card. *Eur J Nucl Med Mol Imaging* 34: 796–798.

MHRA (2007). *Rules and Guidance for Pharmaceutical Manufacturers and Distributors (2007)*. London: Pharmaceutical Press.

SI (1992a). The Medicines Act 1968 (Application to Radiopharmaceutical-associated Products) Regulations 1992. London: HMSO.

SI (1992b). The Medicines Act 1968 (Amendment) (No. 2) Regulations 1992 Statutory Instrument 1992/3271. London: HMSO. http://vlex.co.uk/vid/medicines-act-amendment-regulations-28347820 (accessed 30 June 2010).

Silberstein EB (1998). Prevalence of adverse reactions to positron emitting radiopharmaceuticals in nuclear medicine. *J Nucl Med* 39: 2190–2192.

UKRG (2009). Database of adverse events and product defects. United Kingdom Radiopharmacy Group. http://www.ukrg.org.uk/ (accessed 30 June 2010).

VirRAD (2009). Database of adverse events and product defects. http://www.virrad.eu.org/ (accessed 30 June 2010).

32

The effect of patient medication and other factors on the biodistribution of radiopharmaceuticals

Sue Ackrill

Introduction

Nuclear medicine scintigraphy has been in practice for around 50 years, and in that time many reports have been made of altered biodistribution of radiopharmaceuticals. It is now known that various factors can alter biodistribution, and several categories of altered biodistribution occur, including altered pharmacokinetics (away from the target organ), or enhanced or reduced uptake in the target organ. An altered biodistribution could make diagnosis difficult, or lead to the wrong diagnosis being made, with serious consequences for the patient.

Many extraneous factors can influence biodistribution, and it is important to identify these and to distinguish the changes they produce from those induced by disease. The factors to be considered are the patient's existing medication, radiation therapy, surgical procedure, and dietary regime. However, most instances of altered biodistribution are due to an interaction between the patient's medication and the radiopharmaceutical. As new radiopharmaceuticals have been introduced that target specific receptors, the effect of patient medication has become even more important.

In this chapter the more important drug–radiopharmaceutical interactions will be described and examples taken from general practice. Also described are other factors that can affect biodistribution, such as radiation therapy and diet.

Classification of drug/radiopharmaceutical interactions

Drug–radiopharmaceutical interactions may be classified by organ of interest, radiopharmaceutical used, the patient's drug, or the type of deviation. In this chapter, abnormal effects will be categorised under the headings of unusual handling of the radiopharmaceutical by an organ as a result of a pharmacological effect, *in vivo* physicochemical interaction, drug-induced disease, and drugs that interfere with cell labelling.

Previously, many reported instances of drug interactions were anecdotal, and it was difficult to establish a direct cause-and-effect relationship. With older classes of drugs and radiopharmaceuticals there was almost complete absence of *in-vitro* testing of the drug with the radiopharmaceutical. It was also difficult to determine modes of action as little work was done on drug interaction at the molecular level. In recent years however, with the introduction of radiopharmaceuticals that target receptors or monoamine transporters such as ioflupane, for example, much work has been done to establish the mechanism of action of significant drug interactions.

Unusual handling of a radiopharmaceutical as a result of a pharmacological effect

A pharmacological interaction occurs when the intended effect of a drug at its usual dose alters the biodistribution of the radiopharmaceutical. These pharmacological interactions are of two types:

- Where the effect is predicted and expected from the mode of action of the drug, i.e. 'class effect' – these have usually been previously reported.
- Where the effect is unexpected, and is not class related, i.e. it is a 'drug-specific effect'.

A large number of reports have been published on the effects of drugs on the adrenal medulla imaging agent iobenguane (*meta*-iodobenzylguanidine, mIBG). There are now European Association of Nuclear Medicine (EANM) guidelines (Bombardieri *et al.* 2003; Giammarile *et al.* 2008) based on the work of Solanki *et al.* (1992), who outlined a pharmacological guide to medicines that interfere with the biodistribution of radiolabelled mIBG. Iobenguane is an aralkylguanidine resulting from the combination of the benzyl group of bretylium with the guanidine group of guanethidine (an adrenergic neuron blocker). It is a noradrenaline (norepinephrine) analogue, and a so-called 'false' neurotransmitter. mIBG images the adrenal medulla (not the adrenal cortex), and sympathetic nervous tissue. mIBG has been shown to have a pronounced uptake in adrenal glands and in neuroectodermal tumours that are derived from the primitive neural crest that develops to form the sympathetic nervous system. Malignant neuroectodermal tumours include phaeochromocytomas, paragangliomas, carcinoid tumours, medullary thyroid cancer and neuroblastomas. mIBG also localises in the heart and salivary glands. Because of the structural similarity with noradrenaline, mIBG is selectively concentrated by tissues with rich adrenergic innervations, essentially neuroectodermal tissue, including tumours of neuroectodermal origin. mIBG may be taken into cells by either the sodium-dependent uptake mechanism (active transport, type I amine uptake mechanism) or by passive diffusion (non-energy-dependent, type II mechanism), and stored in neurosecretory granules. The transfer of mIBG from intracellular cytoplasm into catecholamine storage vesicles (neurosecretory vesicles) is mediated by an ATPase-dependent proton pump. Unlike noradrenaline, mIBG is not metabolised, and is excreted unchanged (Wafelman *et al.* 1994).

Many classes of medicines may theoretically interfere with mIBG uptake and storage (Solanki *et al.* 1992). Ideally, drugs likely to interfere with the uptake and/or retention of mIBG should be withdrawn before treatment and the patient stabilised on alternative medication. However, patients with metabolically active, catecholamine-secreting tumours, e.g. phaeochromocytomas, are likely to require a range of antihypertensive medicines to manage the resulting hypertension, and withdrawal of this medication will not be possible. Patients must be carefully screened for prescription, over-the-counter, herbal and other natural products to prevent a false negative study. Pseudoephedrine or phenylephrine found in over-the-counter cold preparations and decongestants deplete storage vesicle contents.

Drugs that inhibit the sodium-dependent uptake include cocaine, tricyclic antidepressants and antipsychotics and labetolol. A case report from Zaplatnikov *et al.* (2004) discussed drug interference with mIBG uptake in a patient with metastatic paragangliomas. The patient in question had a history of drug consumption, with phases of drug withdrawal. Previous mIBG therapies had shown widespread metastatic uptake on post-therapy whole body scan. In the case of the last therapy dose, the post-therapeutic whole body scan failed to detect the vast majority of metastatic lesions, although these were shown to be still present using FDG-PET. The conclusion drawn was that the patient had taken recreational drugs such as cocaine or an unknown drug mixture immediately prior to the therapy, which caused the long-lasting blockade of the mIBG uptake. This work clearly shows the importance of obtaining an accurate drug history from a patient before therapy, in particular those with a history of drug abuse.

The effect of tricyclic antidepressants on catecholamine uptake into adrenergic storage vesicles is again well known, and in patients taking these drugs uptake of [^{131}I]mIBG may be seriously impaired. Tricyclic antidepressants, such as amitriptyline, have been reported to significantly increase cardiac mIBG washout and inhibit uptake into presynaptic neurons. A study was undertaken by Estorch *et al.* (2004) to determine the effect of a single dose of amitriptyline on regional cardiac mIBG uptake. They demonstrated that a single 25 mg dose of amitriptyline could induce changes in the uptake and retention of cardiac mIBG, with amitriptyline challenge resulting in a significant decrease in regional mIBG uptake in 50% of patients, hence confirming the need to withdraw tricyclic antidepressants prior to a diagnostic scan or administration of therapeutic mIBG. The reduction of mIBG uptake by labetolol in phaeochromocytomas and normal tissues was reported by Khafagi *et al.* (1989). The inhibitory effect of labetolol on mIBG uptake in sympathomedullary tissues is likely to be a result of the drug's additional properties of uptake-1 blockade and depletion of storage vesicle contents, rather than its alpha- or beta-blocking effects.

Reserpine inhibits uptake into neurosecretory vesicles, also depleting the contents of the vesicles, thus reducing uptake and storage of mIBG. Reserpine is no longer used in the UK for treating hypertension, but is a good example of this mechanism for mIBG uptake blockade.

Calcium channel blockers also interfere with mIBG studies, as can some foods. Foods that contain vanillin and catecholamine-like compounds such as chocolate and blue-veined cheese should be avoided in the week prior to an mIBG scan. The paediatric committee of the EANM has also stated in its guidelines for radioiodinated mIBG scintigraphy in children that angiotensin-converting enzyme inhibitors such as captopril may interfere with uptake of mIBG (EANM 2003).

Ioflupane (DaTSCAN) is a dopamine transporter (DAT) imaging agent that was introduced in 2000 as a brain imaging agent to differentiate between Parkinson disease, and essential tremor. It will detect or exclude dopaminergic degeneration in the striatum. Much work has been done to identify those drugs that block the uptake of ioflupane by the dopamine transporter. The effect of paroxetine on quantification of striatal dopamine transporters with [^{123}I]FP-CIT SPECT (DaTSCAN) was reported by Booij *et al.* (2007). However, it has been concluded that the effects of selective serotonin reuptake inhibitors (SSRIs) on an ioflupane SPECT scan are too small to hinder the interpretation of visual assessments. A review by Booij and Kemp (2008) looked at the potential effects of drugs on dopamine transporter imaging with [^{123}I]FP-CIT SPECT (DaTSCAN). Compounds likely to interact with striatal uptake through the dopamine transporter should not be used. The drugs that may influence significantly the visual and quantitative analysis of ioflupane SPECT studies are cocaine, amfetamines, CNS stimulants such as methylphenidate and modafinil, bupropion for smoking cessation, sympathomimetics at high doses, the antimuscarinic drug benzatropine, the opioid fentanyl, and the anaesthetic ketamine, which may be used illicitly. Some drugs mentioned in the literature such as phentermine, mazindol and radafaxine have been withdrawn from use in the UK. The authors conclude that ideally medication that is likely to interfere with the visual interpretation of a scan should be stopped before the administration of the radiotracer, the decision to withdraw any medication being made by the specialist in charge of the patient's care. Drugs such as levodopa, selegiline, haloperidol, risperidone and fluvoxamine are unlikely to affect the uptake of ioflupane by the dopamine transporter. The effect of levodopa therapy on dopamine transporter SPECT imaging with [^{123}I]FP-CIT in patients with Parkinson disease was reported by Schillaci *et al.* (2005). They concluded that levodopa does not affect ioflupane brain imaging, and confirm that it is not necessary to withdraw this medication to measure DAT levels with SPECT. As dopamine agonists (bromocriptine, pergolide and ropinirole) target the post-synaptic dopamine receptor, they are not expected to interfere with dopamine transporter imaging.

It is common practice in many centres to discontinue octreotide therapy prior to a scan with ^{111}In-pentetreotide. However, work by Gunn *et al.* 2006 indicates that this cessation of aqueous octreotide before a diagnostic scan or therapy with radiolabelled somatostatin analogues is not required.

Drugs that alter acid–base ratios can have important sequelae in nuclear medicine and it has been shown that ammonium chloride and sodium bicarbonate may decrease renal uptake and increase hepatic biodistribution of the renal imaging agent technetium-99m dimercaptosuccinic acid (DMSA) (Yee *et al.* 1981).

One of the best-documented drug–radiopharmaceutical interactions is that concerning the suppression of uptake of gallium-67 citrate in cerebral tumours, in patients taking cortisone preparations (Waxman *et al.* 1977). It is thought that this occurs as a result of a decrease in extracellular sodium and water content, leading to a decrease in oedema. The tracer is often associated with the oedematous fluid, so an apparent decrease in the size of the tumour is observed on the scintigram. The effect may be so pronounced as to completely suppress uptake into the tumour, with possible consequences of complete misdiagnosis. Cortisone may also affect the sensitivity of detection of bone trauma in ^{99m}Tc-MDP bone scintigraphy. Animal studies have shown that sensitivity for detecting fractures in rabbits on high doses of hydrocortisone was 48% compared with 85% for control animals (Alazraki *et al.* 1987).

By far the largest numbers of reports of drug/radiopharmaceutical incompatibilities are those in which the functional status of the organ is altered as a result of pharmacological action by the patient's medication. For example, narcotic analgesics such as morphine may cause spasm of the biliary tract due to contraction of the sphincter of Oddi (Pope, Bratke 1981). As a consequence, prolonged transit times of hepatobiliary imaging agents from the liver to the duodenum may occur. Enzyme inducers such as phenobarbitone may enhance biliary excretion of similar imaging agents, and cholinergic drugs may induce gall bladder emptying. Other drugs that may affect hepatobiliary imaging include a number of anaesthetics. Another report showed that total parenteral nutrition (TPN) can influence uptake of tracer into the gall bladder, since during TPN the gall bladder is relatively inactive, resulting in bile stasis and reduced uptake into the gall bladder.

Cytotoxic drugs such as cyclophosphamide, vincristine, bleomycin and cisplatin are reported to affect the pharmacokinetic response of radiopharmaceuticals, particularly the tumour-seeking radiopharmaceutical gallium-67 citrate. This agent localises in some tumours as well as other sites such as the liver, and regions of infection and inflammation. In patients on cyclophosphamide and vincristine, it has been observed that there is very little or no uptake of tracer in the tumour or liver, and very high uptake in the blood pool (Lentle *et al.* 1979). The exact mechanism of interaction is unclear.

Figure 32.1 demonstrates a decrease in skeletal uptake of MDP in a child on a multi-cytotoxic regime. After cessation of therapy the skeletal uptake increases.

An increasing number of drugs are known to alter hormonal status. The effects associated with these changes may produce marked alterations in the expected biodistribution of radiopharmaceuticals. Stilboestrol, digitalis, gonadotrophins, phenothiazines, cimetidine and oral contraceptives all increase the production of oestrogens (Lentle *et al.* 1979) and may induce gynaecomastia. It has been found that

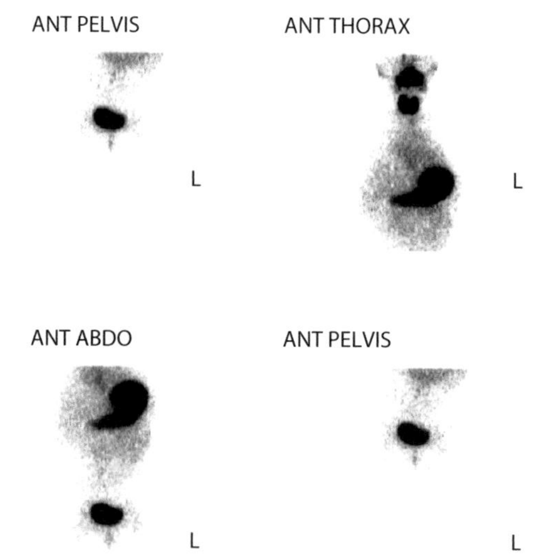

Figure 32.1 Decrease in skeletal uptake of MDP in a child on a multi-cytotoxic regime. After cessation of therapy the skeletal uptake increases. ANT, anterior; ABDO, abdomen.

there is increased localisation of gallium-67 citrate in gynaecomastic breasts.

One of the most important groups of drugs that affect the diagnostic accuracy of nuclear medicine tests is the group that affects the uptake of radiopharmaceuticals into the thyroid. Although diagnostic tests are now much less frequently carried out, the same principle applies to drugs that may interfere with therapeutic radioiodine. Any drug that interferes with the uptake of iodine or blocks its release for the thyroid can interfere with the uptake of therapeutic sodium [^{131}I]iodide. Several drugs in common use have a propensity to affect thyroid uptake of radioiodine. Other drugs include iodine-containing contrast media, antithyroid medications and thyroid supplements.

Table 32.1 summarises many of the drugs and chemicals that interfere with thyroid uptake of iodine-131.

Competing anions such as the perchlorate ions act as competitive inhibitors of the iodine transport mechanism, causing decreased uptake of sodium [^{131}I]iodide. Inorganic iodine-containing medications such as Lugol's Iodine and vitamin and mineral supplements are thought to release iodine, thereby decreasing the specific activity of iodine in the body pool and resulting in decreased uptake of radioiodine into the thyroid gland (Sternthal *et al.* 1980). Similar mechanisms have been proposed for iodine-containing antitussive medicines. Sea foods containing high levels of iodine, e.g. haddock, cod and halibut, may reduce uptake of iodine-131 in the thyroid. Antithyroid drugs such as propylthiouracil and carbimazole inhibit the metabolic synthesis of thyroid hormones, resulting in decreased transport and decreased uptake of iodine-131. (Steinback *et al.* 1979). Phenylbutazone was previously listed with the drugs that interfere with iodine-131 uptake, but is no longer prescribable.

Table 32.1 Drugs and chemicals that interfere with thyroid iodine-131 uptake

Drugs	Contrast media
Lugol's iodine	Hypaque
Iodides	Dionosil
Antitussives	Diodrast
Vitamin preparations	
Anti-thyroid drugs	
Perchlorate	
Sulfonamides	
Steroids	
Antihistamines	

[^{18}F]FDG positron emission tomographic scanning is now a well established imaging technique, which may be affected by a number of factors. Ojha *et al.* (2001) reported on the effect of dietary intake before FDG. The uptake of [^{18}F]FDG by a malignant tumour depends on the blood glucose level. A false-negative scan was reported in a patient who had eaten prior to FDG, whereas a subsequent scan following a fast of 8 hours clearly showed a pulmonary nodule. The authors advocate blood glucose measurement prior to [^{18}F]FDG PET imaging.

The use of diazepam prior to FDG has been questioned. It has been reported that diazepam can inhibit the function of the glucose transporter, and many publications have shown that benzodiazepines can alter the sensitivity of cells to insulin and reduce phosphorylation of glucose by inhibiting hexokinase activity. In a letter to the *European Journal of Nuclear Medicine and Molecular Imaging*, Honming Zhuang (2006) states that oral administration of diazepam before the injection of FDG likely renders dual-phase PET imaging ineffective owing to reduction of the hexokinase/glucose-6-phosphatase ratio. A case was reported by Ashley Groves of gross skeletal muscle uptake of [^{18}F]FDG, it being concluded that the most likely reason for this was the immunosuppressant therapy with tacrolimus and mycophenolate mofetil prescribed following a heart and lung transplant (Groves *et al.* 2004).

A study reported by Israel *et al.*(2007) looked at the effect of patient-related factors on cardiac [^{18}F]FDG uptake. They concluded that cardiac [^{18}F]FDG uptake was lower in patients receiving bezafibrate and levothyroxine, and higher in patients receiving benzodiazepines, and suggested that manipulation of these drugs might represent a tool for optimised PET/CT imaging. An interaction between colony-stimulating factors (CSFs) and [^{18}F]FDG has also been reported (Mayer, Bednarczyk 2002). These authors concluded that administration of CSFs might interfere with accurate [^{18}F]FDG imaging and that a separation of at least 5 days might diminish this interference.

It is well known that caffeine-containing beverages should be avoided prior to an adenosine myocardial perfusion scan. Majd-Ardekani *et al.* (2000) looked into the time required for abstention from caffeine. Results of the study indicate that 12 hours is insufficient and 24 hours is safer to avoid the incidence of a false-negative myocardial perfusion scan.

A report of impaired ^{99m}Tc-MIBI uptake in the thyroid and parathyroid glands in early-phase imaging in haemodialysis patients was made by Özgen Kiratli *et al.* (2004). The study showed that patients with chronic renal failure under haemodialysis are prone to show decreased uptake of radioactivity. An additional finding was that vitamin D supplements could cause diminished uptake of ^{99m}Tc-MIBI, and the authors recommend cessation of vitamin D_3 before parathyroid scintigraphy.

Prior to a captopril renogram study for renal artery stenosis, it is usual to withdraw medication with diuretics, angiotensin-converting enzyme inhibitors, and angiotensin II receptor antagonists. However, a report by Claveau-Tremblay *et al.* (1998) indicates that calcium antagonists can cause false-positive captopril renograms. These drugs should be stopped before captopril renography and physicians should be aware of this possible drug interaction if bilateral symmetrical renal function deterioration is seen on a patient's captopril renogram.

In-vivo physicochemical interaction between the radiopharmaceutical and the patient's medication

Most drug–radiopharmaceutical interactions are associated with a pharmacological change in the organ of interest. However, there are a number of well-defined effects that occur as a result of a genuine physicochemical interaction between the drug circulating in the blood and the administered radiopharmaceutical. It is thought that the formation of local complexes could prevent the normal distribution pattern of the radiopharmaceutical. For example, a number of reports have been published on the effect of intramuscular iron–dextran on the biodistribution of ^{99m}Tc-MDP. Instead of localising throughout the skeleton, a diffuse concentration of activity is usually observed at the injection site, i.e. the gluteal region of the buttock (Mazzole *et al.* 1976). It is thought that local complexing occurs between reduced technetium and ferric hydroxide as this is released from the iron–dextran complex.

Aluminium has also been reported to interact with radiopharmaceuticals. In patients who are taking aluminium-containing preparations such as antacids, the aluminium ion could cause flocculation of colloidal particles of sulfur (used for liver scanning) so that the particles become trapped in the microvasculature of the lungs (Bobbinet *et al.* 1974). There has also been a report of altered biodistribution of gallium-67 citrate in a patient being treated with desferrioxamine for aluminium toxicity. The patient was also undergoing haemodialysis to clear the aluminium. Whole body images obtained 48 hours after injection of the radiopharmaceutical showed poor tissue localisation and complete absence of normal uptake (Brown *et al.* 1990). Desferrioxamine is a chelating agent used primarily to treat iron overload, and is also used to treat aluminium toxicity. Desferrioxamine rapidly forms a complex with aluminium that is readily dialysable (Mulliner *et al.* 1986). However, it also binds gallium, forming a complex much stronger than that of gallium with transferrin (the protein to which gallium usually binds) (Weiner *et al.* 1979). Thus in the patient described, desferrioxamine given prior to gallium would have bound some of the aluminium and would have been removed during dialysis. Excess aluminium desferrioxamine could then have interfered with gallium–transferrin binding and subsequent cellular uptake, thus altering the normal distribution of the gallium. Another aluminium-related case report was that of a patient who was being evaluated for myocardial infarction using ^{99m}Tc-pyrophosphate (Eisenberg *et al.* 1989). The patient was taking 4.8 g daily of Maalox suspension (which contains aluminium hydroxide) for peptic ulcer. Instead of localising in the myocardium, almost all the radioactivity was found to be in the liver and spleen, possibly owing to the formation of colloidal complex of pyrophosphate with aluminium.

There have been many reports in nuclear medicine literature of reduced skeletal uptake of technetium diphosphonates in patients being treated therapeutically with bisphosphonates for Paget disease (DeMeo *et al.* 1991; Chong, Cunningham 1991). It was suggested that technetium-99m could preferentially form complexes with circulating bisphosphonates and thus reduce the amount taken up in the skeleton. Similar effects have been observed in patients treated with calcium, although the cause of the unusual tracer localisation is different (Palmer *et al.* 1992). This topic continues to be debated, and the evidence appears to be equivocal. In theory bisphosphonates could interfere with bone scintigraphy, but the published literature is somewhat anecdotal. There are anecdotal reports of an interaction between bisphosphonates and ^{153}Sm-EDTMP whereby whole body images are of poorer quality when the patient has been prescribed a bisphosphonate. However, Marcus *et al.* (2002) reported that there was no difference in skeletal uptake of ^{153}Sm-EDTMP before or at any time after pamidronate infusion, and they concluded that pamidronate infusion did not interfere with the skeletal uptake of ^{153}Sm-EDTMP.

Drug-induced disease affecting the transport of the radiopharmaceutical: toxicological interaction

It is well known that many drugs in everyday use may cause or aggravate disease, and that iatrogenic (treatment-induced) disease may then produce an unexpected biodistribution of a radiopharmaceutical. If the clinician is unaware of the presence of the iatrogenic disease, it is possible that errors will be made in the assessment of the patient's primary condition.

One group of drugs that can cause iatrogenic disease are those toxic to the liver. These include paracetamol (acetaminophen), aspirin, some cytotoxic agents, and tetracycline. In large doses, these may cause necrosis of liver cells, and a consequent reduction of uptake of a radiopharmaceutical in the liver. TPN therapy has been reported to cause hepatic dysfunction (Hladik *et al.* 1987) including fatty liver disease, and erythromycin hepatotoxicity has been reported to have resulted in a false-positive diagnosis in a patient during scanning with the hepatobiliary imaging agent ^{99m}Tc-DISIDA (Swayne, Kolc 1986). Hepatobiliary tracers accumulate normally and from there pass directly into the duodenum. They depend on the presence of bile and bile flow for their effect. It was thought that erythromycin had interfered with bile production, resulting in altered biliary flow dynamics. Because of the absence of radiopharmaceutical in the gall bladder it was wrongly thought that the patient was suffering from cholecystitis. Another case report (Flynn, Treves 1987) described the diffuse accumulation of ^{99m}Tc-MDP in the liver of a patient with methotrexate-induced hepatotoxicity. The authors postulated that inhibition of protein synthesis by methotrexate caused a disruption of the high cell membrane affinity for calcium of MDP, leading to diffuse uptake of the radiopharmaceutical throughout the liver.

Many drugs are capable of causing acute renal failure, which can cause an abnormal uptake of radiopharmaceutical, or a decrease in glomerular filtration rate. Of particular importance are the aminoglycoside antibiotics, penicillins and sulfonamides (Blathen *et al.* 1978). Other drug-induced renal abnormalities include delayed uptake of gallium-67 citrate in patients taking phenylbutazone or furosemide (frusemide) (Linds *et al.* 1983). It was thought that abnormalities occurred as a result of drug-induced interstitial nephritis. Ciclosporin can cause nephrotoxic effects (Fellstrom 2004)

A few drugs are associated with causing lung disease, the most common of which is bleomycin. Toxicity of this drug is well documented and manifests itself as pulmonary interstitial fibrosis. Abnormally high levels of gallium-67 citrate are observed in the lungs of patients with bleomycin-induced fibrosis; presumably because of leukocyte infiltration (Crystal *et al.* 1976).Other drugs that may produce similar lung uptake abnormalities include amiodarone, busulfan and nitrofurantoin (Hladik *et al.* 1987). Another report suggests that former heroin abusers may have granulomatous lung disease and a resultant abnormal uptake of radiopharmaceutical (Napp 1986).

A number of drugs are cardiotoxic when administered in large doses, e.g. doxorubicin hydrochloride. These agents may impair left ventricular function, resulting in changes in the cardiac biodistribution of heart-seeking radiopharmaceuticals.

A study of the toxicological effect of mitomycin C in mice showed alteration in the biodistribution of radiopharmaceuticals used for renal evaluations (Gomes 2001).

Drugs that interfere with the radiolabelling of blood cells

Radiolabelling of blood cells is a well-established technique, such that it is possible to separate and label erythrocytes, leukocytes, platelets and, in some centres, lymphocytes. Details of the radiolabelling are covered in Chapter 24 and so will not be included here. During cell labelling procedures several factors need to be taken into account to achieve optimal labelling efficiency, including temperature, cell number, and volume of cell suspension. In addition to these criteria it is now established that the drugs circulating in the patient's plasma can also influence the radiolabelling. It has been shown that a number of drugs significantly decrease the labelling efficiency of red blood cells *in vitro*, including hydralazine, methyldopa, prazocin and digoxin. It was shown that the adverse effect with digoxin was associated with the fact that digoxin affects the RBC membrane transport by inhibition of the Na^+/K^+-ATPase-dependent pump (Lee *et al.* 1983).

It is well known that the concentration of stannous ion may have a marked effect on the *in-vitro* labelling efficiency of technetium-99m-labelled red cells and it has been shown that optimum yields are achieved with concentrations in the range 0.03–0.15 μg of stannous ion per mL of blood (Zanelli 1982). Any deviation from that range is likely to cause a decreased labelling efficiency of up to 20%. The same author also showed that propranolol, verapamil, chlorthiazide, and furosemide all had quite significant effects on the labelling efficiency.

An observation was made in 1983 that patients who had previously received iodinated contrast media produced a sub-optimal red cell labelling efficiency (Tatum *et al.* 1983). It was found that the mean labelling efficiency in those patients was 30% as opposed to 90% in patients who had not received the contrast media. It was thought that the poor labelling efficiency could be due to an alteration in the redox potential of the stannous ion and therefore affect its role as a reducer of technetium. Little is known about the effect of different anticoagulants on the labelling efficiency of technetium-labelled red cells, but also in 1983 showed that using acid-citrate–dextrose produced labelling efficiencies of 93.5% ± 3.8 compared with 87.2% ± 4% using heparin. In addition, image quality was improved, with less renal and bladder activity.

In white cell labelling, therapy with antibiotics and corticosteroids may result in a reduction in chemotaxis of leukocytes, which could affect the diagnostic accuracy of the investigation.

Effect of radiation therapy and other extraneous factors

It is well documented that radiation therapy can influence the biodistribution of radiopharmaceuticals, and depending on the dose level the effects may be permanent or transient in nature. In the early phase of treatment soft-tissue uptake of technetium diphosphonate complexes may be observed on skeletal scans within the radiation field. This appears to be associated with an inflammatory response to the radiation and with time this returns to normal. Mineral bone within a radiation field shows a permanently reduced uptake of diphosphonates as a long-term effect. This phenomenon appears to reflect reduced blood flow caused by fibrosis.

Staudenherz *et al.* (2002) reported the effects of irradiation on ^{99m}Tc-sestamibi and thallium-201 uptake in a human papillary thyroid carcinoma cell line. They concluded that sestamibi kinetics in thyroid cancer are not affected by irradiation, and may therefore be superior to thallum-201 in the follow-up of thyroid cancer shortly after radiotherapy.

Renograms reflect altered kidney function in irradiated kidneys with a delayed t_{max} and excretory phase. This effect may be transient or permanent depending upon the radiation dose. In a similar way, sodium pertechnetate uptake in salivary glands and excretion in saliva may be depressed and delayed, reflecting functional damage to these glands. Radiotherapy has also been reported to cause increased bone uptake and enhanced urinary excretion of gallium-67 citrate.

Few tissues are unaffected by radiation. Phagocytosis in the Kupffer cells of the liver, bone marrow and lymph nodes is readily depressed, and is reflected as a reduced uptake of radiocolloid.

The social use of drugs and alcohol should also be taken into account, as these may also affect biodistribution of radiopharmaceuticals. Chronic alcohol abuse is reflected by reduced uptake of radiocolloid. Acute alcoholic poisoning is known to cause rhabdomyolysis in skeletal muscle, which presents as massive uptake of technetium diphosphonate complexes in the affected muscles.

Recent surgery commonly results in the accumulation of radiopharmaceuticals in scars and tissues around the operation site, probably reflecting local oedema.

Effect of nutrition and hydration status

The nutritional status of a patient can exert a considerable influence upon biodistribution characteristics of many radiopharmaceuticals. The degree of hydration influences the rate of renal excretion and should be taken into account when conducting renal studies with agents such as MAG3. The ingestion of beverages containing caffeine, theophylline or theobromine can also influence renal excretion because of their diuretic activity. Similarly, the fasting state influences the rate of absorption and the intestinal transport of orally administered compounds. Hepatobiliary function studies with technetium IDA derivatives are particularly sensitive in this respect. If the subject has not been fasting for at least 4 hours prior to the commencement of the study there is a high probability that the gall bladder will not be visualised. Regional variations in the normal values obtained for bile acid absorption measurements using [^{75}Se]SeHCAT have also been attributed to variations in diet.

Excessive intake of vitamin A has been shown to reduce Kupffer cell uptake of technetium colloids in the liver, as does iron overload. Iron overload also causes enhanced renal uptake of gallium-67 citrate. Nicotinic acid and alcohol both influence the uptake of IDA derivatives in the liver and gall bladder. Iodine-containing foods are well known to affect thyroidal uptake of iodinated compounds as has already been discussed.

Table 32.2 shows a summary of the most frequently reported drug interferences with drugs in common use.

Table 32.2 Summary of the most frequently reported drug interferences with drugs in common use

Drug	Test	Radiopharmaceutical	Deviation
ACE inhibitors	Captopril renogram	Technetium [^{99m}Tc] Mertiatide Injection (^{99m}Tc-MAG3)	Invalidation of study Discontinue before test
Aluminium	Hepatic	Technetium [^{99m}Tc] Sulphur Colloid Injection (Tc-sulfur colloid)	Flocculation of colloid, deposition in lung
Aluminium	RBC labelling	Technetium [^{99m}Tc] Tin Pyrophosphate Injection (^{99m}Tc-PYP)	Poor labelling efficiency, free pertechnetate in thyroid, stomach, salivary gland
Aluminium	Renal	Technetium [^{99m}Tc] Pentetate Injection (^{99m}Tc-DTPA)	Abnormal GFR results
Analgesics (opioid)	Abdominal	Sodium Pertechnetate [^{99m}Tc] Injection ([^{99m}Tc]pertechnetate)	Delay in gastric emptying, unusual pertechnetate transit time
Analgesics (opioid)	Hepatobiliary	Technetium [^{99m}Tc] Etifenin Injection (^{99m}Tc-HIDA)	Constriction of sphincter of Oddi may cause non-visualisation of intestine
Antihistamines	Thyroid	Sodium [^{131}I] Iodide	Abnormal uptake

(continued overleaf)

Table 32.2 *(continued)*

Drug	Test	Radiopharmaceutical	Deviation
Amiodarone	Tumour/abscess	Gallium [^{67}Ga] Citrate Injection (Gallium-67 citrate)	Abnormal uptake in breast
Amiodarone	NE tumour	Iobenguane [^{123}I] Injection ([^{123}I]mIBG)	Abnormal uptake
Ammonium chloride	Renal	Technetium [^{99m}Tc] Succimer Injection Technetium [^{99m}Tc] Pentetate Injection (^{99m}Tc-DMSA)	Reduced uptake
Benzatropine	Brain DAT transporter	[^{123}I]FP-CIT	Reduced uptake in substantia nigra
Beta blockers	MPI	[^{99m}Tc]Tetrofosmin/Technetium [^{99m}Tc] Sestamibi Injection (^{99m}Tc-MIBI)	Prevent treadmill stress patients reaching target heart rate
Bupropion	Brain DAT transporter	[^{123}I]FP-CIT	Reduced uptake in substantia nigra
Busulfan	Tumour/abscess	Gallium [^{67}Ga] Citrate Injection (Gallium-67 citrate)	Abnormal uptake in breast
Bleomycin	Tumour/abscess	Gallium [^{67}Ga] Citrate Injection (Gallium-67 citrate)	Abnormal uptake in lungs
Cisplatin	Renal	Technetium [^{99m}Tc] Succimer Injection ^{99m}Tc-DMSA/DTPA	Abnormal uptake in kidney
Cisplatin	Tumour/abscess	Gallium [^{67}Ga] Citrate Injection (Gallium-67 citrate)	Abnormal uptake in blood pool, kidneys, skeleton
Chlorpromazine	Tumour/abscess	Gallium [^{67}Ga] Citrate Injection (Gallium-67 citrate)	Abnormal uptake in breast
Chlorpromazine and other neuroleptics	NE tumours	Iobenguane [^{123}I] Injection ([^{123}I]mIBG)	Reduced tumour uptake
Cocaine	Brain DAT transporter	[^{123}I]FP-CIT	Reduced uptake in substantia nigra
Cocaine	NE tumours	Iobenguane [^{123}I] Injection ([^{123}I]mIBG)	Reduced tumour uptake
Cortisone	Tumour/abscess	Gallium [^{67}Ga] Citrate Injection (Gallium-67 citrate/^{99m}Tc)	Decrease in apparent tumour size
Corticosteroids	Bone	Technetium [^{99m}Tc] Medronate Injection (^{99m}Tc-MDP)	Decrease in uptake in bone trauma
Corticosteroids	Tumour/abscess	^{111}In-labelled white blood cells	Reduced chemotaxis of labelled leukocytes
Corticosteroids	Tumour imaging	Fludeoxyglucose [^{18}F] Injection ([^{18}F]FDG)	Alters biodistribution of FDG
Cyclophosphamide	Tumour/abscess	Gallium [^{67}Ga] Citrate (Gallium-67 citrate)	Abnormal uptake in blood pool, kidneys, skeleton
Dexamfetamine	Brain DAT transporter	[^{123}I]FP-CIT	Reduced uptake in substantia nigra

(continued)

Table 32.2 *(continued)*

Drug	Test	Radiopharmaceutical	Deviation
Dextrose	Bone	Technetium [^{99m}Tc] Medronate Injection (^{99m}Tc-MDP)	Reduced skeletal uptake
Digoxin	Cardiac	^{99m}Tc-labelled Red Blood Cells	Poor labelling efficiency, presence of free pertechnetate
Doxorubicin	Cardiac	^{99m}Tc-labelled Red Blood Cells	Abnormal cardiac distribution
Erythromycin	Hepatobiliary	Technetium [^{99m}Tc] Etifenin Injection (^{99m}Tc-HIDA)	Increased liver uptake
Fluphenazine	Tumour/abscess	Gallium [^{67}Ga] Citrate (Gallium-67 citrate)	Increased uptake in breast
Frusemide	Tumour/abscess	Gallium [^{67}Ga] Citrate (Gallium-67 citrate)	Reduced uptake
Frusemide	Renal	^{99m}Tc-DMSA/DTPA	Enhanced renal function, misleading diagnosis
Gentamicin	Renal	Chromium [^{51}Cr] Edetate Injection (Chromium-51 EDTA)	Decreased GFR
Haloperidol	Tumour/abscess	Gallium [^{67}Ga] Citrate (Gallium-67 citrate)	Increased uptake in breast
Hydralazine	Cardiac	^{99m}Tc-labelled Red Blood Cells	Poor labelling efficiency, presence of free pertechnetate
Iodides	Thyroid	Sodium [^{131}I]iodide	Abnormal thyroid uptake
Iron salts	Bone	^{99m}Tc-MDP/EHDP	Pronounced abnormal uptake, diffuse accumulation of tracer at site of injection High blood pool, renal activity
Labetolol	NE tumours	Iobenguane [^{123}I] Injection ([^{123}I]mIBG)	Reduced tumour uptake
Lugol's iodine	Thyroid	Sodium [^{131}I] iodide	Abnormal thyroid uptake
Metoclopramide	Tumour/abscess	Gallium [^{67}Ga] Citrate (Gallium-67 citrate)	Increased uptake in breast
Methyldopa	Cardiac/GI bleed	^{99m}Tc-labelled Red Blood Cells	Poor labelling efficiency; free pertechnetate in thyroid, salivary glands, stomach
Morphine (opioids)	Hepatobiliary	Technetium [^{99m}Tc] Etifenin Injection (^{99m}Tc-HIDA)	Abnormal transit time into duodenum
Methotrexate	Hepatic	^{99m}Tc-sulfur colloid	Filling defects in liver due to hepatotoxicity
Methylphenidate	Brain DAT transporter	[^{123}I]FP-CIT	Reduced uptake in substantia nigra
Methylphenidate	NE tumours	Iobenguane [^{123}I] Injection ([^{123}I]mIBG)	Reduced tumour uptake
Modafinil	Brain DAT transporter	[^{123}I]FP-CIT	Reduced uptake in substantia nigra
Modafinil	NE tumours	[^{123}I]FP-CIT	Reduced tumour uptake

(continued overleaf)

Table 32.2 *(continued)*

Drug	Test	Radiopharmaceutical	Deviation
Nifedipine	Cardiac/GI bleed	^{99m}Tc-labelled Red Blood Cells	Poor labelling efficiency, free pertechnetate in thyroid, salivary glands, stomach
Nifedipine	Bone	Technetium [^{99m}Tc] Medronate Injection (^{99m}Tc-MDP)	Reduced skeletal uptake
Nifedipine	NE tumours	Iobenguane [^{123}I] Injection ([^{123}I]mIBG)	Increased uptake in phaeochromocytoma
Nitrofurantoin	Tumour/abscess	Gallium [^{67}Ga] Citrate (Gallium-67 citrate)	Increased uptake in breast
Nicotinic acid	Hepatobiliary	Technetium [^{99m}Tc] Etifenin Injection (99mTc-HIDA)	Abnormal or absence of tracer in gall bladder
Rate-limiting calcium channel blockers (Verapamil, Diltiazem)	MPI	[^{99m}Tc]Tetrofosmin/Technetium [^{99m}Tc] Sestamibi Injection (^{99m}Tc-MIBI)	Interfere with stress testing
Salbutamol	NE tumours	Iobenguane [^{123}I] Injection	Reduced tumour uptake
Sibutramine	Brain DAT transporter	[^{123}I]FP-CIT	Reduced uptake in substantia nigra
Tricyclic antidepressants	NE tumours	Iobenguane [^{123}I] Injection ([^{123}I]mIBG)	Reduced tumour uptake

Registration of instances of abnormal distribution

It is clear that many factors, singly and in combination, can affect the biodistribution of radiopharmaceuticals. There is a clear role for the radiopharmacist to record and document them. The desirability of a centralised registration centre is also evident, with the added advantage of reliably establishing degree of incidence of changes in biodistribution. As national schemes are voluntary, many incidents go unreported. However, the British Nuclear Medicine Society (BNMS) reporting scheme is now integrated with the EANM via VirRAD, the European Radiopharmacy website. This reporting network is multinational and therefore offers the potential for the early detection of adverse reactions, biodistribution problems and quality defects. Currently all instances of adverse biodistribution are collated in the UK by Dr Neil Hartman at St. Bartholomew's Hospital, London.

References

Alazraki N *et al.* (1987). Effect of glucocorticoids on sensitivity of Tc-99m phosphonate bone imaging for detecting bone trauma [abstract]. *J Nucl Med* 28: 606.

Blathen *et al.* (1978). A study of renal biopsies of light electron and imunofluorescence microscopy. *Clin Nephrol* 9: 103–106.

Bobbinet EB *et al.* (1974). Lung uptake of Tc-99m sulphur colloid in patients exhibiting presence of aluminium in plasma. *J Nucl Med* 15: 1220–1222.

Bombardieri E *et al.* (2003). I-131/I-123-metaiodobenzylguanidine (MIBG) scintigraphy: procedure guidelines for tumour imaging. *Eur J Nucl Med* 30(12): BP132–139.

Booij J, Kemp P (2008). Dopamine transporter imaging with [^{123}I] FP-CIT SPECT: potential effects of drugs. *Eur J Nucl Med Mol Imaging* 35: 424–438.

Booij J *et al.* (2007). Quantification of striatal dopamine transporters with ^{123}I-FP-CIT SPECT is influenced by the selective serotonin reuptake inhibitor paroxetine: a double-blind, placebo controlled, crossover study in healthy control subjects. *J Nucl Med* 48(3): 359–366.

Brown SJ *et al.* (1990). Altered biodistribution of gallium-67 in a patient with aluminium toxicity treated with desferrioxamine. *J Nucl Med* 31: 115–117.

Chong WK, Cunningham DA (1991). Case report: intravenous etidronate as a cause of poor uptake on bone scanning, with a review of the literature. *Clin Radiol* 44: 268–207.

Claveau-Tremblay R *et al.* (1998). False positive captopril renography in patients taking calcium antagonists. *J Nucl Med* 39: 1621–1626.

Crystal G *et al.* (1976). Idiopathic pulmonary fibrosis; clinical, histologic, radiographic and biochemical aspects. *Ann Intern Med* 85: 760–788.

DeMeo JH *et al.* (1991). Etidronate sodium therapy – a cause of poor skeletal radiopharmaceutical uptake. *Semin Nucl Med* XXI: 332–334.

EANM (2003). Guidelines for radioiodinated MIBG scintigraphy in children. *Eur J Nucl Med Mol Imaging* 30: 45–50.

Eisenberg B *et al.* (1989). PYP Maalox localisation in liver and spleen. *Clin Nucl Med* 14: 636.

Estorch M *et al.* (2004). Challenging the neuronal MIBG uptake by pharmacological intervention: effect of a single dose of oral amitriptyline on regional cardiac MIBG uptake. *Eur J Nucl Med Mol Imaging* 31: 1575–1580.

Fellstrom B (2004). Cyclosporine nephrotoxicity. *Transplant Proc.* (Suppl 1): S220–S223.

Flynn BMM, Treves ST (1987). Diffuse hepatic uptake of technetium-99m methylene diphosphonate in a patient receiving high dose methotrexate. *J Nucl Med* 28: 532–534.

Giammarile F *et al.* (2008). EANM procedure guidelines for ^{131}I meta-iodobenzylguanidine (^{131}I-mIBG) therapy. *Eur J Nucl Med Mol Imaging* 35: 1039–1047.

Gomes ML (2001). Study of the toxicological effect of mitomycin C in mice: alteration on the biodistribution of radiopharmaceuticals used for renal evaluations. *Hum Exp Toxicol* 20: 193–197.

Gomes ML *et al.* (2002). Drug interaction with radiopharmaceuticals: effect on the labelling of red blood cells with technetium-99m and on the bioavailability of radiopharmaceuticals. *Braz Arch Biol Technol* 45: 143–149.

Groves A *et al.* (2004). Extensive skeletal muscle uptake of ^{18}F-FDG: relation to immunosuppressants? *J Nucl Med Technol* 32: 206–208.

Gunn S *et al.* (2006). in vitro modelling of the clinical interactions between octreotide and ^{111}In-pentetreotide: is there evidence of somatostatin receptor downregulation? *J NuclMed* 47(2): 354–359.

Hladik WB *et al.* (1987). Iatrogenic alterations in the biodistribution of radiotracers as a result of drug therapy. In: Hladik WB, ed. *Essentials of Nuclear Medicine Science.* New York: Williams and Wilkins; 189–219.

Israel O *et al.* (2007). PET/CT quantitation of the effect of patient-related factors on cardiac ^{18}F-FDG uptake. *J Nucl Med* 48: 234–239.

Khafagi FA *et al.* (1989). Labetolol reduces Iodine-131 MIBG uptake by phaeochromocytoma and normal tissues. *J Nucl Med* 30: 481–489.

Lee HB *et al.* (1983). Pharmacologic alterations in Tc-99m binding by blood cells – concise communication. *J Nucl Med* 24: 397–401.

Lentle BC *et al.* (1979). Iatrogenic alterations in radio nuclide biodistributions. *Semin Nucl Med* 9: 131–143.

Linds DS *et al.* (1983). Delayed renal localisation of gallium-67: concise communication. *J Nucl Med* 24: 894–897.

Majd-Ardekani J *et al.* (2000). Time for abstention from caffeine before an adenosine myocardial perfusion scan. *Nucl Med Commun* 21: 361–364.

Marcus C *et al.* (2002). Lack of effect of a bisphosphonate (pamidronate disodium) infusion on subsequent skeletal uptake of SM-153 EDTMP. *Clin Nucl Med* 27(6): 427–430.

Mayer D, Bednarczyk E (2002). Interaction of colony-stimulating factors and fluorodeoxyglucose ^{18}F positron emission tomography. *Ann Pharmacother* 36: 1796–1799.

Mazzole AC *et al.* (1976). Accumulation of Tc-99m diphosphonate at sites of intramuscular iron therapy. *J Nucl Med Technol* 4: 133–135.

Mulliner DS *et al.* (1986). Clerance of aluminium by haemodialysis: effect of desferrioxamine. *Kidney Int Suppl* 29: S100–S103.

Napp I (1986). Inapparent pulmonary vascular disease in ex-heroin users. *Clin Nucl Med* 11: 266–269.

Ojha B *et al.* (2001). Effect of dietary intake before F-18 FDG positron emission tomographic scanning on the evaluation of a solitary pulmonary nodule. *Clin Nucl Med* 26(11): 908–909.

Özgen Kiratli P *et al.* (2004). impaired Tc-99m MIBI uptake in the thyroid and parathyroid glands during early phase imaging in haemodialysis patients. *Rev Esp Med Nucl* 23 (5): 347–351.

Palmer AM *et al.* (1992). Soft tissue localisation of Tc-99m hydroxymethylene diphosphonate due to interaction with calcium. *Clin Radiol* 45: 326–330.

Pope R, Bratke J (1981). Two Tec-99m HIDA cases with delayed emptying into the duodenum. The monthly scan. College of Pharmacy, New Mexico, Monthly Newsletter, May/June.

Porter WC *et al.* (1983). Effect of heparin and acid-citrate-dextrose on labelling efficiency of Tc-99m labelled RBCs. *J Nucl Med* 24: 383–385.

Schillaci O *et al.* (2005). The effect of levodopa therapy on dopamine transporter SPECT imaging with ^{123}I-FP-CIT in patients with Parkinson's disease. *Eur J Nucl Med Mol Imaging* 32: 1452–1456.

Solanki KK *et al.* (1992). A pharmacological guide to medicines which interfere with the biodistribution of radiolabelled metaiodobenzylguanidine (MIBG). *Nucl Med Commun* 13: 513–521.

Staudenherz A *et al.* (2002). Effects of irradiation on ^{99m}Tc Sestamibi and ^{201}Tl uptake in a human papillary thyroid carcinoma cell line. *Nucl Med Commun* 23: 565–568.

Steinbach JJ *et al.* (1979). Simultaneous treatment of toxic diffuse goiter with I-131 and antithyroid drugs: a prospective study. *J Nucl Med* 20: 1263–1267.

Sternthal E *et al.* (1980). Suppression of thyroid radioiodine uptake by various doses of stable iodine. *N Engl J Med* 303: 1083–1088.

Swayne LL, Kolc J (1986). Erythromycin hepatotoxicity: a rare case of a false positive technetium DISIDA study. *Clin Nucl Med* 11: 10–12.

Tatum JL *et al.* (1983). Pitfall to modified in vivo method of technetium-99m red blood cell labelling: iodinated contrast media. *Clin Nucl Med* 8: 585–587.

Wafelman AR *et al.* (1994). Radio-iodinated MIBG: a review of its biodistribution and pharmacokinetics, drug interactions, cytotoxicity and dosimetry. *Eur J Nucl Med* 21: 545–559.

Waxman AS *et al.* (1977). Steroid induced suppression of gallium uptake tumours of the central nervous system [abstract]. *J Nucl Med* 18: 617.

Weiner ME *et al.* (1979). Relative stability of In-111 and Ga-67 desferrioxamine and human transferrin complexes. In: Sodd V, ed. *Radio-pharmaceuticals II. Proceedings of the 2nd International Symposium on Radiopharmaceuticals, Seattle, USA*. New York: Society of Nuclear Medicine. V.Sodd.

Yee CA *et al.* (1981). Tc-99m DMSA renal uptake influence of biochemistry and physiological factors. *J Nucl Med* 22: 1054–1058.

Zanelli GD (1982). Effect of certain drugs used in the treatment of cardiovascular disease on the in-vitro labelling of red blood cells with Tc-99m. *Nucl Med Commun* 3: 155–161.

Zaplatnikov K *et al.* (2004). Drug interference with MIBG uptake in a patient with metastatic paraganglioma (case report). *Br J Radiol* 77: 525–527.

Zhuang H (2006). Effect of diazepam on the efficacy of dual-phase FDG-PET imaging [letter]. *Eur J Nucl Med Mol Imaging* 33: 228–229.

33

Use of drugs to enhance nuclear medicine studies

Helen Whiteside

Introduction

Patients' medication can interfere with nuclear medicine studies but this interference can be used to clinicians' advantage to enhance or extend the diagnostic capability of a nuclear medicine examination (Thrall, Swanson 1989). A specific drug may be administered before, during, or after administration of the radiopharmaceutical(s) as part of the non-invasive nuclear medicine investigation to alter organ function and gain diagnostic information resulting from changes in the biodistribution, uptake or excretion of the radiopharmaceutical. For example, opiate analgesics such as morphine can be used to improve the diagnosis of conditions that delay or prevent gallbladder visualisation, whereas they interfere with hepatobiliary studies by simulating the bile duct obstruction. Over the last 20 years, pharmacological intervention has been increasingly used and dosage regimens have been established to develop reproducible protocols to allow comparison between patients. These regimens allow the desired or critical change in organ function while minimising the exposure of the patient to unwanted pharmacological effects of the drug as well as any potential side-effects. For example, the dose of dipyridamole used in cardiac studies must be large enough to produce a sufficient change in the coronary blood flow but without unacceptable side-effects such as bronchospasm or chest pains. This chapter discusses the rationale behind the interventions for various organ imaging studies and summarises information related to the use of such drugs in a tabular form (Table 33.1) for easy reference.

Cardiac studies

Nuclear medicine of the heart can be divided into two categories: direct imaging of the myocardium to assess regional coronary blood flow and blood

Table 33.1 Drugs used in nuclear medicine interventional studies

Drug and study	Dose and administration	Pharmacokinetics	Comments
Acetazolamide Brain studies	IV: 500 mg–1 g	Rapid onset Peak 25 min Half-life 90 min	No additional increase in rCBF been noted when increasing the dosage from 1 g to 2 g. Caution in patients with acute stroke (may cause deterioration in clinical status of the patients)
Acipimox Cardiac studies	PO: 500 mg 1.5 h before tracer and 250 mg 1.5 mg before FDG	Serum fatty acids fall sharply within 2 h	Aspirin 500 mg may also be given orally with the first dose to limit the vasodilatory effects
Adenosine Cardiac studies	IV: start at 50 µg/kg/min increasing to a maximum of 140 µg/kg/min, maintained for 4 min. Radionuclide injected at 1 min *or* IV: 140 µg/kg/min for 6 min with radionuclide administered at 3 min	Very rapid onset Peak 2 min Half-life <2–10 s	Caffeine containing foods, drinks or medications, dipyridamole and theophylline/aminophylline preparations should be abstained from for a minimum of 24 h before the test. Long-acting methylxanthines require withdrawal for 5 half lives. Contraindicated in patients continuing to take oral dipyridamole because of potential hypotension
Aqueous Iodine Oral Solution BP (Lugol's Iodine)	PO: 0.1–0.2 ml three times a day starting two days before the injection. Duration dependent on type and dose of radionuclide administered		Each 1 mL of the solution contains 50 mg of free iodine and 130 mg of free and combined iodine. Dilute with water or milk before administration to avoid gastrointestinal irritation
Ascorbic acid Salivary gland studies	PO: 500 mg tablet to stimulate the glands to drain into the mouth		
Atropine Cardiac studies	IV: 1 mg maximum dose if required		
Bisacodyl Adrenal studies	PO: Two 5 mg bisacodyl tablets taken the evening before the injection day and two on the evening of the injection day		
Captopril Renal studies	PO: 25–50 mg one hour before radionuclide injection	Onset within 15 min Peak 70 min Half-life 2–3 h	Previous medications of ACE or ACE receptor antagonists should be discontinued before the test; i.e. Captopril for 2 days, Lisinopril for 1 week, Perindopril for 10–14 days, Losartan for 5 days. Diuretics should be withheld for 1 week Caution: First dose hypotension with captopril
Cimetidine Gastrointestinal studies	IV: 300 mg in 100 mL glucose 5% over 20 min with imaging beginning 1 h later PO: 300 mg QDS for 24–48 h before study; children 20 mg/kg QDS	Onset 0.5–1 h Peak 1–2 h Duration 4–6 h	Rapid injections have been associated with cardiac arrhythmias Infusion time and longer patient appointment means IV is used as second line to oral cimetidine or other agents

(continued)

Table 33.1 *(continued)*

Drug and study	Dose and administration	Pharmacokinetics	Comments
Dexamethasone Adrenal studies	PO: 4 mg/kg in divided doses for 7 days prior to administration of radiocholesterol and continue until imaging is complete	Onset immediate Peak 1–2 h Duration 2–3 days following cessation of administration	Take with food to avoid GI side-effects. Patient compliance is required to avoid false-positive results. Before the study, spironolactone should be stopped for 3–4 weeks and diuretics for at least 2 weeks
Dipyridamole Cardiac studies	PO: 300–400 mg crushed and administered in a slurry with 30 mL of water, radionuclide injected after 45 min. Oral suspension also available IV: 0.56 mg/kg diluted in 20 mL of sodium chloride 0.9% administered over 4 min. Radionuclide is injected after completion of the infusion	Onset 1–2 min Peak onset 4 min Half-life 2 min	To reverse chest pain side-effects administer 50–125 mg of aminophylline by slow intravenous injection at a rate not exceeding 25 mg aminophylline per minute, up to a dose of 250–500 mg if symptoms persist. After this, glyceryl trinitrate may be used if aminophylline has not relieved chest pain. Concurrent vasodilation agents may cause severe hypotensive effect. Caffeine-containing foods, drinks or medications, dipyridamole and theophylline/aminophylline preparations should be abstained from for a minimum of 24 h before the test. Long-acting methylxanthines require withdrawal for 5 half lives. Contraindicated in patients continuing to taking oral dipyridamole because of potential hypotension
Dobutamine Cardiac studies	IV: 5–10 µg/kg/min infusion increasing at 3 min intervals to 20, 30 and 40 µg/kg/min. If the patient does not reach 85% of the age-predicted maximal heart rate, atropine will be used	Onset 1–2 min Peak within 10 min Half-life 2 min	Discontinue beta-blockers and other sympatholytic therapy for at least 48 h before the study
Fatty meal	250 mL of proprietary fatty food supplement such as Sandishake® or full-fat milk with a Mars bar or 40 mL of Calogen®		
Furosemide Renal studies	IV: 20–40 mg injected over 3–5 min 15–20 min before (or after) the radionuclide injection Infants and Children: 1 mg/kg up to 20 mg	Onset 5 min Peak 15–30 min Duration up to 2 h	Renal dysfunction can cause absence of responses in cases without significant obstruction Renal maturation is not complete in infants less than 1 year of age and the effect of the diuretic is less predictable
Glyceryl trinitrate	500 µg sublingual tablet or 5 mg buccal tablet		
Lugol's Iodine	See Aqueous Iodine Oral Solution BP		

(continued overleaf)

Table 33.1 *(continued)*

Drug and study	Dose and administration	Pharmacokinetics	Comments
Liothyronine Thyroid studies	PO: 75–100 μg daily in divided doses for 7–10 days	Onset 1–2 days Half-life 1.5 days	
Adrenal studies using radioiodinated compounds	PO: 20 μg every 8 h starting 2 days before the radionuclide injection. Duration of treatment depends on the type and dose of radionuclide administered		
Morphine Hepatobiliary studies	IV: 40 μg/kg diluted in 10 mL of sodium chloride 0.9% administered over 3 min Used if no gallbladder filling has been observed after 40–60 min post radionuclide injection	Onset within 5 min Duration 20–50 min	
Omeprazole Gastrointestinal studies	PO: 40 mg taken the morning before and the morning of the scan in adults	Half-life 3 h	Ranitidine is used for children
Perchlorate Thyroid studies	PO: 1 g for perchlorate discharge test		
Phenobarbital Hepatobiliary studies	PO: 2.5 mg/kg/day twice a day for 5 consecutive days prior to the test	Half-life 1.6–2.9 days in children	
Potassium iodate Adrenal studies and brain studies using radioiodinated compounds	PO: 85–170 mg daily starting 2 h before the radionuclide injection. If first dose is >140 mg the starting time may be reduced to half an hour before the injection. Duration dependent on type and dose of radionuclide administered		Available as 85 mg tablets. 85 mg of potassium iodate is equivalent to 60 mg of potassium iodide. Potassium iodate has a longer shelf-life than potassium iodide
Potassium iodide	PO: See Aqueous Iodine Oral Solution BP and Potassium iodate tablets		
Ranitidine Gastrointestinal studies	PO: Adults 300 mg (children 2–4 mg/kg) taken the morning (or evening) before and the morning of the scan IV: 1 mg/kg. Maximum 50 mg. Infuse over 20 min diluted in 20 mL sodium chloride 0.9%	Half-life 2 h	Rapid injections have been associated with cardiac arrhythmias
Sincalide Hepatobiliary studies	IV: 20 ng/kg given over at least 5 min. To evacuate the gallbladder and optimise subsequent filling with radionuclide: give 30 min before the radionuclide. To study contractile function visualising gallbladder: give 60 min after the radionuclide or when the gallbladder is maximally filled	Onset within 30 s. Peak 5–15 min. Duration 15–20 min. Within an hour, gallbladder returns to resting size	If no gallbladder contraction is observed within 15 min, the dose may be repeated at 40 ng/kg. Avoid rapid injections as this may result in spasm of the gallbladder neck and prevent contracting in a normal gallbladder

pool imaging to determine ventricular function. Cardiac dysfunction and perfusion abnormalities due to coronary artery disease may not occur under resting conditions but can be induced by stress. When stress increases oxygen demand, normal coronary arteries respond; they vasodilate, increasing coronary blood flow and localisation of the radionuclide. Significantly smaller blood flow changes and localisation of the radionuclide are seen in stenosed vessels that cannot dilate. The relative differences in blood flow can be clearly seen. In addition, areas supplied by stenosed arteries develop myocardial wall motion abnormalities provoked by imbalances in the myocardial oxygen supply–demand ratio created by stress (Robinovitch 1985). These can be detected by blood pool imaging, often with dobutamine.

Exercise will induce coronary stress; however, many patients are unable to perform adequate exercise to elicit stress due to anxiety, poor motivation, amputation or medical conditions such as peripheral vascular disease, respiratory, musculoskeletal or neurological disorders and drugs can be used as an alternative. Using standardised drugs provides a reproducible increase in blood flow but does not provide additional clinical information such as exercise capacity and functional status of the patient. Adenosine, dipyridamole and dobutamine are currently used to induce stress (BNMS 2003c).

Dipyridamole is used as an indirect coronary dilator in thallium myocardial perfusion imaging. It inhibits the enzyme adenosine deaminase and blocks cellular uptake of adenosine into the myocardial, endothelial and blood cells, causing increased levels of extracellular interstitial adenosine to react with adenosine receptors that regulate coronary blood flow to meet myocardial metabolic demand. The resulting increase in myocardial cAMP (cyclic adenosine 3′,5′-monophosphate) produces coronary vasodilatation mainly in the small resistance vessels (EMC 2009a). In a healthy person, the coronary blood flow increases by 3–5 times baseline levels. Dipyridamole may be administered orally or intravenously (Taillefer *et al.* 1986). The oral formulation has an erratic absorption profile and gastrointestinal disturbances such as nausea are frequent and can last for several hours (Beller 1991), whereas the intravenous formulation results in a rapid and more predictable response. Up to 47% of patients given intravenous dipyridamole experience adverse events, of which 0.26% would be expected to be severe. Patients receiving oral dipyridamole should withhold their doses for 24 hours before receiving intravenous doses of dipyridamole (EMC 2009a).

Dipyridamole is infused over a 4-minute period at a dose of 0.142–0.56 mg/kg diluted to 20 mL in normal saline. The maximal dilatory effect is achieved about 4 minutes after completion of the infusion and thus the radionuclide is injected between 3 and 5 minutes after completion of the infusion (Hesse *et al.* 2005; EMC 2009a). Dipyridamole is particularly well suited to patients with left bundle branch block. The false-positive rate with this protocol is only 2–5% compared with 30–40% for exercise testing. Adenosine redirects coronary blood flow from the endocardium to the epicardium and may reduce collateral coronary blood flow, inducing ischaemia. If severe ischaemia symptoms and/or orthostatic hypotension occur during infusion of dipyridamole, they may be treated with intravenous theophylline (see Table 33.1) or sublingual glyceryl trinitrate. The antagonistic effect of aminophylline is related to its direct action on the smooth muscle of the coronary vessels (Alfonso 1970; EMC 2009b).

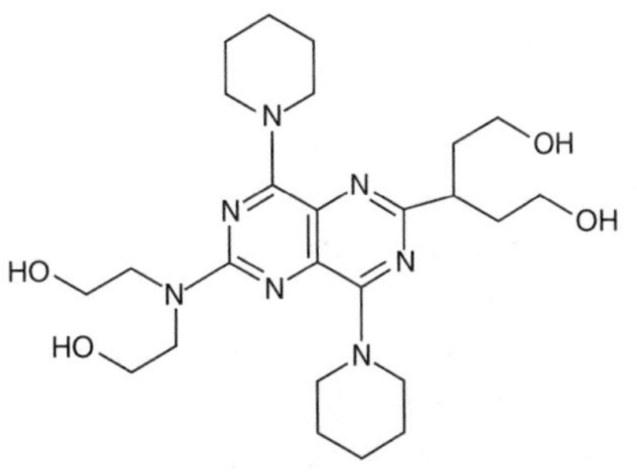

Dipyridamole

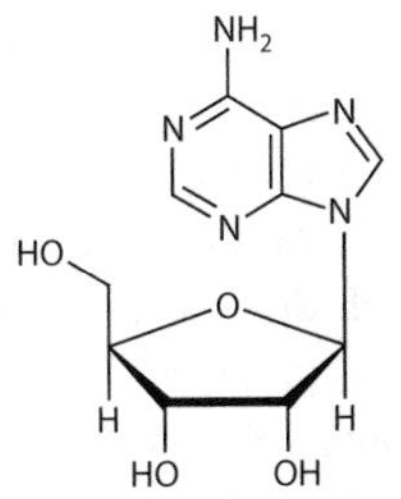

Adenosine

Adenosine is commonly used to induce stress. Along with dipyridamole it is less likely to induce ischaemia than exercise, and both are valuable when investigating patients taking beta-blockers which may blunt the response to exercise-induced stress. Adenosine is an endogenous nucleoside, a natural regulator of coronary blood flow and cardiac demand.

It exerts its pharmacological effects through activation of purine receptors (cell-surface A_1 and A_2 adenosine receptors) (EMC 2009b) and modulation of the sympathetic neurotransmission. There is evidence that adenosine inhibits the slow inward calcium current, reducing calcium uptake, and activation of adenylate cyclase through A_2 receptors in smooth-muscle cells. Adenosine uptake is mediated by an active transmembrane nucleoside transport system. Once inside the cell, adenosine is rapidly phosphorylated to adenosine monophosphate or deaminated to inosine, neither of which is an active metabolite (EMC 2009b).

Adenosine has a half-life *in vitro* of less than 10 seconds and it may be as short as 2 seconds *in vivo* (Verani 1991a,b; EMC 2009b) and is thus administered as a continuous peripheral intravenous infusion using an infusion pump. Doses of adenosine are based on patient weight, with an optimum response of maximum coronary hyperaemia seen in about 90% of cases within 2–3 minutes of the onset of a 140 µg/kg/min intravenous infusion (EMC 2009b). Normally after 3 minutes of infusion the radionuclide is injected at a separate venous site to avoid an adenosine bolus and the adenosine infusion continues for up to a further 3 minutes. For patients at risk the infusion can be started at a lower dose (50 µg/kg/min) and can, if tolerated, be increased to 75, 100 and 140 µg/kg/min at 1-minute intervals and then continued for 4 minutes. The radionuclide should be injected 1 minute after starting the highest dose infusion (Hesse *et al.* 2005). This ability to dose-adjust makes it suitable for stress testing soon after acute myocardial infarction. The short half-life combined with the rapid cessation of side-effects after the infusion is stopped explains the lesser side-effects of adenosine.

Adenosine can decrease the atrioventricular conduction and, as with dipyridamole, patients with sick sinus syndrome, second- or third-degree atrioventricular block or patients with asthma or a tendency to bronchospasm should not receive these products (EMC 2009a,b). In such patients dobutamine could be used as an alternative. Patients must abstain from caffeine and caffeine-containing foods, beverages and medications (e.g. coffee, tea, cola, chocolate, caffeine-containing cold and flu remedies, painkillers and stimulants) for at least 12 hours and preferably 24 hours prior to the study (Majd-Ardekani *et al.* 2000). Treatment with the methylxanthine drugs aminophylline and theophylline must be stopped at least 24 hours before the test as these compounds all have an antagonist effect on adenosine. Treatment with longer-acting formulations should be stopped at least five half-lives of the formulation before the test (Hesse *et al.* 2005). Patients taking oral dipyridamole should discontinue the drug a minimum of 24 hours before the adenosine test (Table 33.2).

Dobutamine is predominantly a beta-1 agonist with very weak alpha and beta-2 properties. In patients with depressed cardiac function dobutamine causes a significant increase in cardiac output and stroke volume with little or no increase in heart rate or peripheral resistance. Coronary blood flow and myocardial oxygen consumption are usually increased owing to increased myocardial contractility (Swanson *et al.* 1985). Dobutamine has been used in association with perfusion imaging (Forster *et al.* 1993; Wallbridge *et al.* 1993). It is also employed in blood pool imaging (Palac *et al.* 1983) as it has been shown to be superior to dipyridamole in inducing myocardial wall motion abnormality; termination of the test owing to ventricular tachycardia or ST segment elevation is more likely with dobutamine than with other stressors (Hesse *et al.* 2005).

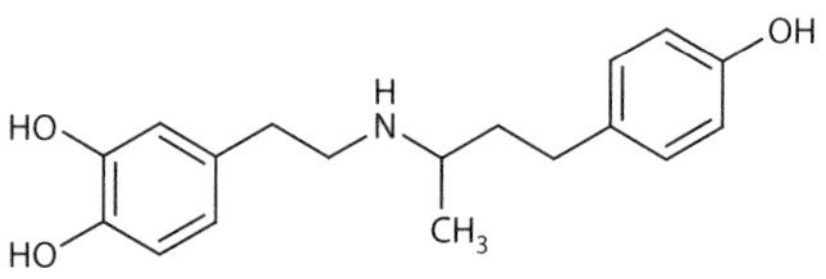

Dobutamine

Dobutamine is infused incrementally starting at a dose of 5-10 µg/kg/min, increasing at 3-minute intervals to 20, 30 and 40 µg/kg/min. If the patient does not reach 85% of the age-predicted maximal heart rate, atropine will be used. A fall in blood pressure occurs in 15–20% of patients receiving the higher doses of dobutamine. This is alleviated by having the patient lie down with their legs elevated, with occasional need for small doses of beta-blockers as an antidote (Hesse *et al.* 2005). The greater risk of cardiac arrhythmias associated with catecholamine stress has limited the use of dobutamine (Robinovitch 1985). Arbutamine hydrochloride is a sympathomimetic with beta-agonist properties and like dobutamine has been used for cardiac stress testing in patients unable to

Table 33.2 Drug, food and drink interruption before stress test perfusion imaging

Drug, food or drink	Exercise	Vasodilator (adenosine, dipyridamole, hybrid tests)	Dobutamine (± atropine)
Nitrates	12–24 hours	12–24 hours	12–24 hours
Beta-blockers Long-acting beta-blockers	48 hours 4–7 days	(+)[a]	48 hours 4–7 days
Calcium antagonists	48 hours	(+) 48 hours	(+) 48 hours
Methylxanthine-containing food, drinks	–	12–24 hours	–
Methylxanthine drugs – theophylline/aminophylline	–	1–5 days dependent on formulation	
Dipyridamole	+	12 or preferably 24 hours	–
Caffeine-containing foods and drinks	–	12–24 hours	–
Fasting insulin	Check blood glucose before exercise to avoid hypoglycaemia	–	–
Digoxin	2 weeks	–	2 weeks
Aspirin/clopidogrel	–	–	–

–, can be continued.
(+), interruption recommended by some but evidence for improved stress test after interruption is limited or not obvious.
[a] Extent and severity of stress defects may be underestimated.

exercise. It is no longer commercially available (MedicinesComplete 2009a).

On some occasions, stomach reflux interferes with the radioisotope pictures of the heart. In these cases, during the examination patients can be asked to take a drink of water to flush the oesophageal radioactivity away from the thorax. In severe cases metoclopramide, a prokinetic agent, has been used to increase gut motility and promote removal of the gastric contents. Cardiac medications that may interfere with the stress test should ideally be withdrawn by at least five half-lives of the drug, although clinically this is not always possible (Hesse *et al.* 2005). In addition to knowledge of the stress-inducing drugs, the clinicians performing these investigations should have a current knowledge of advanced life support and the drug treatments used in national and local current cardiopulmonary resuscitation (CPR) guidelines.

A more recent cardiac scan requiring an adjunctive drug is the MUGA (multigated radionuclide angiography) scan (Figure 33.1). This is a routine test done to assess and monitor the ejection fraction, to estimate the function of the left ventricle pre- and post-heart transplantation and as part of monitoring during breast cancer chemotherapy (NICE 2006a). Around 4% of patients undergoing chemotherapy with trastuzumab can suffer from heart damage. The rare risk is greater if the patient has previously received anthracycline chemotherapy or if they have an underlying heart or lung problem. Red blood cells are labelled *in vivo* with technetium-99m after pre-sensitisation of the cells with an intravenously injected stannous formulation followed 30 minutes later by [^{99m}Tc] pertechnetate intravenously (Nicol *et al.* 2008). Optimum yields are achieved with concentrations in the range of 0.03–0.15 μg stannous ion per mL of blood (Zanelli 1982), with deviations

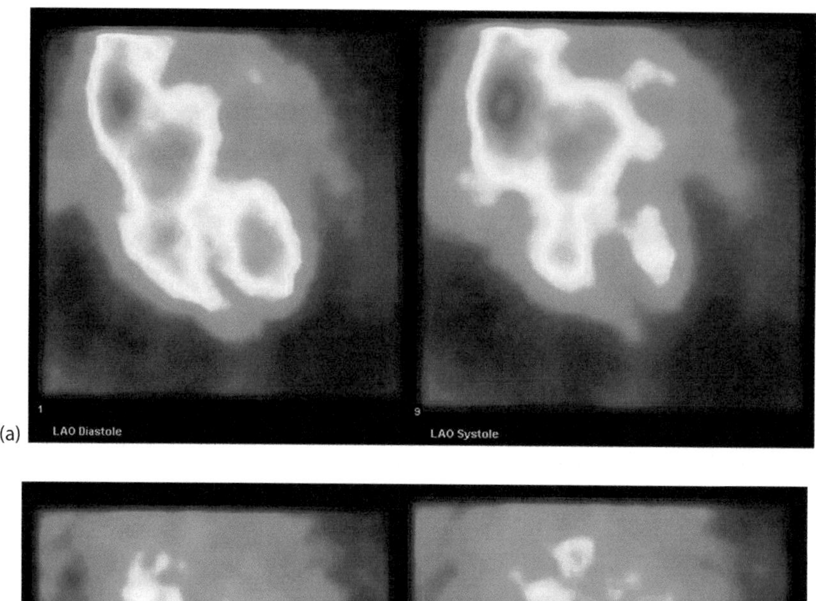

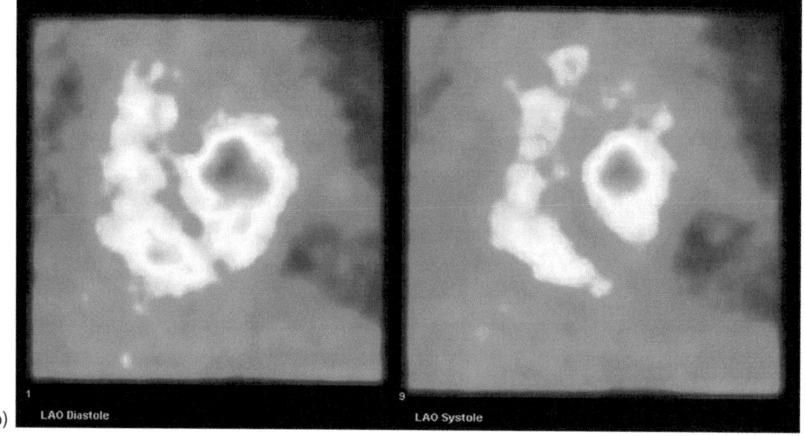

Figure 33.1 MUGA scan: (a) good uptake; (b) poor uptake.

from this range reducing labelling efficiency by as much as 20%.

PET cardiac studies

[^{18}F]Fluorodeoxyglucose (FDG) SPECT imaging has been used to assess myocardial viability in patients with impaired left ventricular function (Bax *et al.* 1997), but more recently has been superseded by developments in FDG PET and PET/CT, where it is used to assess candidates for revascularisation when conventional imaging techniques have not proved helpful. FDG, a glucose analogue, is taken up by cells that use glucose as a primary energy source and is also accumulated in tumours with a high glucose turnover. Cellular uptake is performed by tissue-specific systems such as facilitated diffusion using glucose transporters. [^{18}F]FDG is then phosphorylated by hexokinase into FDG-6-phosphate, which cannot be metabolised and is consequently stored in the cell allowing the tissue to be detected by scintigraphy (MHRA 2006). However, its uptake is affected by a variety of metabolic effects such as diet, lipid and glucose levels and diseases such as diabetes. In the fasting state, uptake is reduced in the septum and anterior wall of the left ventricle relative to the posterior lateral wall since in the fasting state free fatty acids are the preferred substrate for energy production. After glucose loading these differences are less marked, but up to 15% of studies are difficult to interpret because of the regional differences in the uptake in the intraventricular septum. This led to glucose loading being recommended for study of myocardial viability (Walsh, Groppler 1996).

In these investigations of heart function after myocardial infarction, dextrose and insulin are used in a euglycaemic clamp technique to ensure that a specific glucose range is maintained and changes in levels of free fatty acids, insulin and glucose are minimised during the FDG imaging (Knuuti *et al.* 1992) to facilitate uptake of FDG. The technique requires insulin to be infused at a rate of 1 mU/kg/min (mU = milliunits) with the euglycaemic state being maintained by infusion of 20% glucose at a rate determined by serial plasma glucose tests. Niederkohr and Qoun (2007) suggested that insulin glargine, an insulin being used more frequently in the management of diabetes, showed no significant alteration in FDG biodistribution and suggest that these patients may not need to withhold this particular insulin prior to PET scintigraphy. Other drugs suggested to interfere with accurate FDG imaging are colony-stimulating factors (Mayer, Bednarczyk 2002) as well as bezafibrate, benzodiazepines and diazepam (Israel *et al.* 2007). An alternative but simpler technique is to use acipimox, a nicotinic acid derivative that lowers plasma free fatty acid concentrations by inhibiting lipolysis (Bax *et al.* 2002). It also has some vasodilatory effects (Knuuti *et al.* 1994).

Renal studies

One aim of renal studies is to differentiate between dilated, non-obstructed urinary tracts and those with significant mechanical obstruction. The differentiation is important, since renal atrophy can occur if mechanical obstruction is not surgically corrected, whereas muscular atony causing dilatation can be treated with drugs. The prolonged retention of radioactivity seen in non-obstructed dilated systems is due to a 'reservoir effect'. Increasing the urine flow rate with the administration of a diuretic results in a prompt washout of the activity from the dilated structure (Figure 33.2). In contrast, a mechanically obstructed system will demonstrate progressive accumulation of activity that does not respond to diuretic administration. A partial response may indicate partial obstruction or renal dysfunction with an inability to respond to a diuretic. Furosemide is the diuretic of choice because its peak effect is far greater than that observed with other agents (Thrall 1985). Fifty milligrams or less of furosemide can be administered as the undiluted solution, but the rate should not exceed 4 mg/min. This limitation of the rate aims to minimise side-effects such as ototoxicity.

The timing of the furosemide injection may vary. Normally 20–40 mg is given 15 minutes before or after the radionuclide injection (Fine 1991). Since the peak effect of intravenous furosemide occurs at 15–20 minutes after injection, a protocol with furosemide given 15 minutes before the radionuclide reduces imaging time. However, the response to furosemide is determined by measuring the change in activity with time. Measuring the rate of rise of activity before furosemide administration helps to determine whether the rate of fall in activity after administration is appropriate. A moderately poorly functioning kidney would have a moderately impaired rate of rise and a moderately impaired but appropriate rate of fall in response to furosemide in the absence of obstruction. It is necessary to evaluate the furosemide response as good or bad but also as appropriate or not (Britton *et al.* 1991).

Renal studies may also be performed to determine the glomerular filtration rate (GFR) using radiopharmaceuticals excreted by glomerular filtration. Captopril reduces the GFR in patients with renal vascular abnormalities and doses of 25 mg are used to prove the diagnosis of renal vascular hypertension and detect renal vascular disease (Majd *et al.* 1986; Dondi *et al.* 1989, 1991; Fernandez *et al.* 1999). Renal artery stenosis is the most common cause of secondary hypertension and potentially managed by surgery or angioplasty. Captopril, an angiotensin-converting enzyme (ACE) inhibitor inhibits the conversion of angiotensin I to angiotensin II. When renal blood flow falls, angiotensin II constricts efferent arterioles to maintain high filtration pressure in the glomerular vessels, but in the absence of angiotensin II the constriction is lost, the perfusion pressure falls and the GFR drops as in the case of renal artery stenosis. Diagnosis is made by comparing a baseline renal study with a captopril-enhanced study (Figure 33.3). A 50 mg dose may be required if the initial dose has proved unsuccessful. It is important that, prior to the test, other ACE inhibitors, angiotensin II receptor antagonists and diuretics are withdrawn as these may interfere with the results. Claveau-Tremblay *et al.* (1998) also suspect calcium-channel blocking agents are leading to false-positive captopril renography.

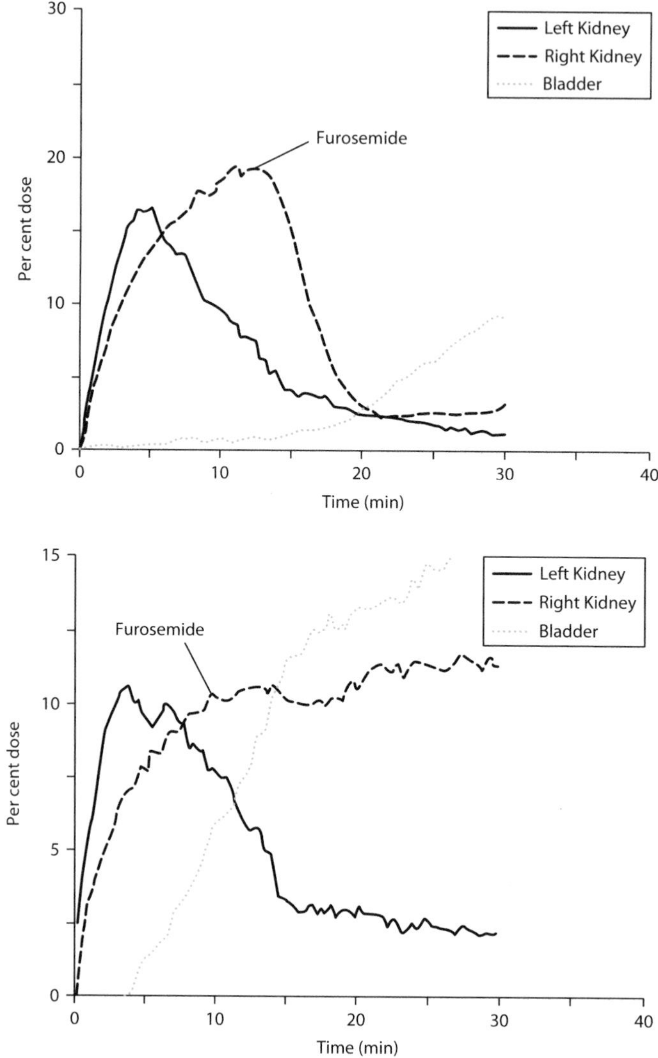

Figure 33.2 Furosemide effect on renal scan: (a) good response; (b) poor response.

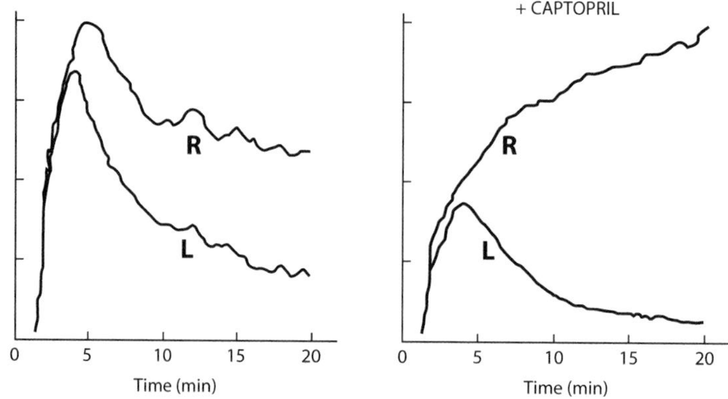

Figure 33.3 Captopril effect on renal study. Excretion curves pre- and post-captopril.

Hepatobiliary studies

Hepatobiliary function is investigated using technetium-99m-labelled compounds of iminodiacetic acid (IDA), which are cleared from the circulation by the hepatic cells and secreted like bilirubin into the bile carrier mechanism. Technetium-99m complexes of IDA derivatives, such as disofenin, etifenin, lidofenin, and mebrofenin are used intravenously in the investigation of hepatic function and in the imaging of the hepatobiliary system. After intravenous injection, radioactivity appears promptly in the liver, followed by movement into the gallbladder and then into the intestine. Various conditions such as the presence of extremely viscous bile in chronic cholecystitis, prolonged fasting or total parenteral nutrition can delay the movement of these radiopharmaceuticals through the hepatobiliary system, resulting in delayed gallbladder visualisation (Thrall, Swanson 1989). To promote earlier visualisation of the gallbladder and reduce the imaging time required for diagnosis, drugs such as morphine are used to optimise filling with radionuclide (Choy *et al.* 1984; Vasquez *et al.* 1988; Fink-Bennett 1991; Fink-Bennett *et al.* 1991a). Morphine causes constriction of the sphincter of Oddi, with a resultant increase in the pressure in the common bile duct, leading to increased flow of bile and radionuclide into the gallbladder if the cystic duct is patent (Murphy *et al.* 1980). This intervention is beneficial in the assessment of acute cholecystitis in the presence of chronic cholecystitis. Conversely, it is well documented that narcotic analgesics such as morphine when taken therapeutically by patients interfere with hepatobiliary studies. They induce contraction of the sphincter of Oddi and prevent release of radiopharmaceutical into the intestine, resulting in prolonged radiopharmaceutical appearance in the gallbladder or common bile duct, which stimulates the appearance of the bile duct obstruction (Chilton, Brown 1990). As such, these analgesics should be withdrawn prior to morphine T-BIDA studies.

In infants with jaundice, hepatobiliary imaging is compromised by poor hepatic uptake and slow biliary excretion. Administration of phenobarbital (phenobarbitone) enhances and accelerates biliary excretion of the radionuclide, increasing the accurate differentiation between extrahepatic biliary atresia and neonatal hepatitis, allowing prompt appropriate treatment to take place. Morbidity and mortality from biliary atresia are decreased when surgically corrected within the first 2 months of life (Majd *et al.* 1981; Fink-Bennett 1991). The choleretic effect of phenobarbital (phenobarbitone) is thought to be due to its effect upon the whole hepatic transport system for organic anions such as radiolabelled IDA compounds and independent of its enzyme-induction effect (Majd *et al.* 1981).

The primary determinant of gallbladder emptying is circulating cholecystokinin (CCK), which is released from the duodenal mucosa in response to the presence of fat and lipolytic products and to a lesser degree to amino acids and small peptides. Originally, CCK prepared from the duodenal mucosa of pigs was available. Two synthetic and more potent preparations containing the active chemical group of CCK, the terminal heptapeptide, were made available in the past. Ceruletide, a synthetic decapeptide amide (Krishnamurthy *et al.* 1983; MedicinesComplete 2009b) originally isolated from the skin of the Australian frog, is still available in Germany but is no longer available or marketed in France. Sincalide, a commercially available synthetic octapeptide of CCK is five times more potent than CCK and is presented as a dry powder for reconstitution and given in doses of 20 ng/kg (BNMS 2003a; MedicinesComplete 2009c). It is used to assess the effectiveness of the gallbladder contraction or ejection fraction (Freeman *et al.* 1981; Fink-Bennett 1991; Fink-Bennett *et al.* 1991b) and is given by intravenous injection over 5 minutes once the gallbladder is visible (Figure 33.4); too rapid an injection may cause spasm of the neck of the gallbladder, preventing contraction of a normal gallbladder (Leung, Hesslewood 1999). Some UK nuclear medicine departments use fatty meal replacements such as full-fat milk, a proprietary fatty meal or a chocolate bar to elicit an effect. They are helpful if a qualitative assessment of gallbladder function is required and an approximate indication of gallbladder emptying is obtained by comparing images obtained before and 20 minutes after the meal (BNMS 2003a). Meals act by nerve stimulation and a direct action on gastrointestinal tract smooth muscle. In inducing gallbladder contractions and emptying of the gallbladder, the response to drugs is quicker and more predictable than that seen following administration of a fatty meal (Freeman *et al.* 1981).

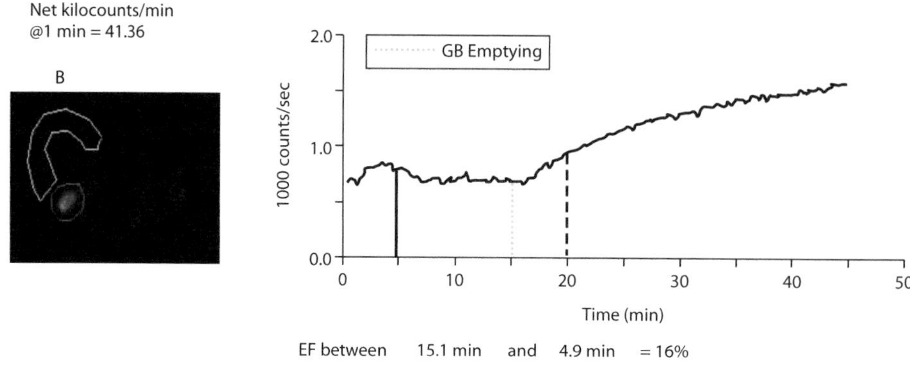

Figure 33.4 Sincalide effect on gallbladder scan: poor response.

Gastrointestinal studies

Meckel's diverticulum is the vestigial remnant of the vitellointestinal duct. It is the most frequent malformation of the gastrointestinal tract, with an incidence of 2–3% in the general population (Stakianakis, Conway 1981). If present, it is located in the distal ileum, usually within 100 cm of the ileocaecal valve. Haemorrhage is a complication in 20–30% of patients and is more common in children under 2 years of age. More than 90% of patients with lower gastrointestinal tract bleeding caused by Meckel's diverticulum have ulcerations secondary to local acid and pepsin secretions by ectopic gastric mucosa within the diverticulum (Froelich 1985). The bleeding site can be imaged by the ability of the ectopic gastric mucosa to trap and secrete [^{99m}Tc]pertechnetate. The detectability of the lesion can be enhanced either by reducing the movement of the radionuclide from the abnormal site or by increasing its uptake at the site.

Researchers proposed that increased intragastric acidity may enhance the transfer of [^{99m}Tc]pertechnetate from mucosal cells in the diverticulum to the gastric lumen by promoting a stable complex formation in the lumen and preventing diffusion back into the mucosa (Froelich, 1985). The use of agents to decrease gastric acidity, such as H_2-antagonists cimetidine (Yeker *et al.* 1984; Datz *et al.* 1991; Diamond *et al.* 1991) or ranitidine (Datz *et al.* 1991; Reeksuppaphol S, *et al.* 2004), resulted in enhanced localisation of the radioisotope at the Meckel's diverticulum because of the accumulation of the tracer by mucosal cells. Proton pump inhibitors such as omeprazole are also used to decrease gastric acidity to improve pertechnetate imaging of Meckel's diverticulum. A dose of 40 mg omeprazole is normally taken by adults in the morning before and the morning of the Meckel scans.

[^{99m}Tc]Pertechnetate is taken up by salivary glands owing to its chemical similarity to other negatively charged ions contained in the saliva, and this can reveal the ability of the glands to take up the activity and the drainage of the saliva. To stimulate the glands to drain into the mouth, patients are asked to suck a slice of lemon or chew an ascorbic acid 500 mg tablet, or to place a drop or two of lemon juice or citric acid solution on the tongue (Schall *et al.* 1981; Croft, Williams 1991). Normal glands accumulate the pertechnetate and then, following stimulation, drain it into the mouth, whereas duct blockage is seen as retention of the pertechnetate proximal to the obstruction. In xerostomia (dry mouth), there is no uptake into the glands and there is no discharge into the mouth.

Adrenal studies

Adrenal studies can be divided into adrenal cortex and adrenal medullary scanning. Radiolabelled cholesterol derivatives are used for scanning the adrenal cortex. It has three histological zones: the outermost zona glomerulosa, primarily responsible for the synthesis and release of aldosterone; the zona fasciculata, which synthesises and releases cortisol; and the innermost zona reticularis, which synthesises and releases androgen and oestrogen hormones. To facilitate scintigraphic evaluation of the zona glomerulosa in hyperaldosteronism or the zona reticularis in hyperandrogenism, dexamethasone is administered to inhibit the release of adrenocorticotrophic hormone (ACTH) from the pituitary and this suppresses the activity of the zona fasciculata (Gross *et al.* 1979). By suppression of the ACTH-dependent component of the radiocholesterol uptake, which normally accounts for 50% of the adrenal uptake, visualisation of the adrenals is delayed (Khafagi *et al.* 1991). Trials of 1,6-β-[^{131}I] iodomethyl-19-norcholesterol (NP-59) in adrenal scans are still ongoing (Pandit-Taskar 2008) in which a dose of 37–74 MBq in 10% ethanol, 0.23% polysorbate-80 and 0.9% sodium chloride is given intravenously slowly over 1–5 minutes. A radiocholesterol product is due to be manufactured in Europe, but currently there is no licensed product available in Europe or the USA (IBA 2010).

The timing of normal adrenal gland visualisation after radiocholesterol administration is dependent on the duration of the dexamethasone suppression (DS) with shorter DS regimens using higher dexamethasone doses resulting in earlier visualisation of normal adrenal activity. The interval between tracer injection and normal adrenal visualisation has been defined for the 4 mg DS regimen (see Table 33.1) as greater than 5 days (Gross *et al.* 1979). Visualisation of adrenal glands earlier than 5 days indicates adenoma or hyperplasia, whereas the pattern of activity defines the abnormality. Bilateral visualisation indicates bilateral hyperactivity or hyperplasia and unilateral visualisation indicates tumour involvement or adenoma (Gross *et al.* 1979). The distinction between adenoma and hyperplasia in the evaluation of primary aldosteronism and adrenal hyperandrogenism is important since the treatment is surgical in the former condition and medical in the latter (Khafagi *et al.* 1991). Hyperplasia can, however, produce marked asymmetry of quantitative uptake so as to suggest unilateral disease (Gross *et al.* 1985). It is therefore useful to quantify the uptake in early unilateral or bilateral visualisation to separate adenoma from hyperplasia. By measuring the level of uptake, adrenal hyperfunction can be separated from normal function as the normal adrenal uptake on DS should not exceed 0.2% of the administered dose (Gross, Shapiro 1985). It is also important to avoid all medications that may affect the adrenal uptake and thus the timing of the normal adrenal gland breakthrough. Spironolactone, diuretics and oral contraceptives have been shown to increase the uptake by the zona glomerulosa by increasing the plasma renin activity (Khafagi *et al.* 1991).

meta-[^{123}I]Iodobenzylguanidine (mIBG) and [^{131}I]mIBG have been used for adrenal medullary scanning in the detection of neuroendocrine tumours such as phaeochromocytoma and neuroblastoma. These neuroendocrine tumours may also be treated with therapeutic doses of [^{131}I]mIBG. The therapeutic dose is determined partly by tumour concentration and retention and partly by elimination. In the past, nifedipine was used by some practitioners to increase retention of mIBG by the tumour, possibly by acting on the tumour kinetics (Blake *et al.* 1988), but its effect was thought to be dependent on the plasma level of nifedipine and it is not routinely used in practice.

Laxatives such as bisacodyl have been used to minimise image interference in adrenal studies by reducing mIBG and radiocholesterol appearance in the colon following excretion from the liver (Gross, Shapiro 1985; Khafagi *et al.* 1991). Two 5 mg bisacodyl tablets are taken the evening before the injection day and the other two on the evening of the injection day. It acts directly on the colon without disturbing the enterohepatic circulation of the radiolabelled cholesterol (Shapiro *et al.* 1983).

In-vivo breakdown of radioiodinated compounds results in the release of free radioiodine, which, along with radioiodine as a radiochemical impurity of the injection, will be taken up by the thyroid unless a blocking agent such as potassium iodate is given (Solanki *et al.* 2004). The administration of the potassium iodate encourages excretion of the unbound radioiodide, reducing the background activity (Petry, Shapiro 1990; Swanson 1990). Aqueous iodine in oral solution BP (Lugol's Iodine) has been used because of the unavailability of iodide tablets. Recently, the more palatable 85 mg potassium iodate tablets have become more widely used. Those patients who are allergic to iodide may be given anions such as perchlorate, which acts as a competitive inhibitor of the thyroid gland anion transport mechanism, or triiodothyronine (Khafagi *et al.* 1991). None of these blocking agents is without side-effects. When administering iodide or triiodothyronine, the risk of inducing hyperthyroidism in elderly patients or those with coronary heart disease must be considered and avoided in these groups where possible. Blood dyscrasias have also been reported following the use of perchlorate (Ellis *et al.* 1977). Although rare, sensitivity to iodine also exists: anaphylactic and allergic reactions in the form of acneiform eruptions, sialadenitis and vasculitis have been reported and it is essential to check patients' allergy status prior to issuing the blocking agents. Despite this, the mortality risk of the blocking procedures is small compared with the estimated risks following these levels of thyroid irradiation. Treatment with the blocking agent should be continued until the estimated level of radioiodine remaining in the body is considered to be at an acceptable level. The duration depends on the radionuclide and the dose of radioactivity administered (Khafagi *et al.* 1991; ARSAC 2006). It can be as short as one day when using the [^{123}I]mIBG for diagnostic purposes or as long as one month when using therapeutic doses in [^{131}I]mIBG (Sisson *et al.* 1994). Children's doses are reduced to percentages of the adult dose. Children at birth to 1 month, 1 month to 3 years, and 3 to 12 years receive 12%, 25% and 50%, respectively, of the adult dose (FDA 2001).

Brain studies

[^{99m}Tc]Pertechnetate does not cross the blood–brain barrier (BBB). It accumulates where the BBB has been damaged, such as brain tumours and intracerebral haemorrhages, but accumulation in the normal choroid plexus causes difficulty in image interpretation and as such is little used now. Radiopharmaceuticals that do cross the BBB can be used to assess regional cerebral blood flow (rCBF) in evaluation of the cerebral vascular disease.

Brain SPECT using hexamethylpropyleneamine oxime (HMPAO; exametazime) provides an image of blood supply to and distribution within the brain that usually reflects brain function. This contributes useful clinical information for evaluation of cerebrovascular disease and stroke. It provides a differential diagnosis of dementia (NICE 2006b), functional localisation of epileptic foci, detection and evaluation of the cause of recurrent headaches and encephalitis (especially herpes encephalitis). It helps to evaluate functional impairment associated with brain trauma and to determine brain death. The acetazolamide test is a test of cerebrovascular reactivity and cerebral perfusion reserve and is indicated in evaluating cerebrovascular reserve in transient ischaemia attacks (TIAs), completed stroke and/or vascular anomalies (e.g. arteriovenous malformation) and to aid in distinguishing vascular from neuronal causes of dementia.(Schwartz, Speed 1993; Dormont *et al.* 2007; Juni *et al.* 2009).

At rest, cerebral blood flow can be normal in many of these patients, although some do also have a lower perfusion on the affected side of the brain. After the administration of acetazolamide, the cerebral blood vessels dilate owing to an increase in local carbon dioxide. In healthy subjects this causes an increase in cerebral blood volume of about 9% while cerebral blood flow increases by up to 50%. Areas of the brain with a good carotid supply respond to this stimulus, while those that are supplied by narrowed (stenosed or occluded) arteries are already dilated and are not able to fully respond. The contrast between the normal, healthy hemisphere and the affected side therefore increases on the SPECT scan. The response in normal brain to an intravenous injection of acetazolamide is not immediate, instead the flow slowly increases over a period of 15–25 minutes and then subsides (Mancini *et al.* 1993). A dose of 1 g of acetazolamide is given by slow intravenous injection. ^{99m}Tc-HMPAO should therefore be administered between 15 and 25 minutes after the acetazolamide, during which time it will reflect the maximum response.

Pharmaceutically, exametazime has limited stability, enhanced by the addition of stannous ions to the formulation. It is available with or without methylene blue stabilisation. Leukocyte labelling must be undertaken using the product without methylene blue stabilisation, resulting in an expiry of only 30 minutes after preparation. Cerebral perfusion imaging can be carried out with either product and ideally should be injected within 15 minutes of preparation.

Movement disorders such as Parkinson disease and other related diseases have common clinical features of tremor, gait disturbance and muscle stiffness, also found in essential tremor. [^{123}I]Ioflupane binds specifically to the nerve cell endings in the striatum, the area of the brain responsible for dopamine transport. If there is a loss of nerve cells containing dopamine as in Parkinson disease, the binding is greatly reduced. This is not the case in essential tremor and thus ioflupane helps to distinguish Parkinson disease and essential tremor (Benamer *et al.* 2000a). Reduced striatal uptake in Parkinson disease correlates with disease duration and severity (Benamer *et al.* 2000b). Ioflupane is also used to differentiate dementia with Lewy bodies from Alzheimer disease (NICE 2006c). To prevent the thyroid gland from taking up the radio-iodine, potassium iodate tablets are administered 1–4 hours before and 12–24 hours after the ioflupane injection (EMEA 2007).

Thyroid studies

Iodine in the form of the [^{123}I]iodide ion is trapped and organified by the thyroid, allowing the anatomy as well as the functioning of the thyroid gland to be measured. Organification is the oxidation of inorganic iodide and attachment to tyrosyl residues, which then couple to form the thyroid hormones levothyroxine and liothyronine. At times, the gland will concentrate iodine normally but will be unable to convert the iodine into thyroid hormone; therefore, interpretation of the iodine uptake is usually done in conjunction with blood tests. Technetium-99m is trapped but not organically bound in the gland and thus is only a useful anatomical test for measuring thyroid physiological functioning. Thyroid nodules that concentrate iodine are rarely cancerous but the same is not true of nodules that take up technetium and all scans are now done with radioactive iodine.

When other laboratory studies show hyper- or hypothyroidism, a radioactive iodine uptake scan is often used to confirm the diagnosis. It is frequently done along with a technetium thyroid scan or other studies to determine the diagnosis. A normal thyroid scan will show a small butterfly-shaped thyroid gland about 5 cm long and 5 cm wide in the appropriate position, with an even spread of radioactive tracer in the gland. An area of increased radionuclide uptake may be called a hot nodule or 'hot spot'. This means that a benign growth is overactive. Despite the name, hot nodules are unlikely to be caused by cancer. An area of decreased radionuclide uptake may be called a cold nodule or 'cold spot'. This indicates that this area of the thyroid gland is underactive. A variety of conditions, including cysts, non-functioning benign growths, localised inflammation, or cancer may produce a cold spot. In addition to diagnosing the cause of hypo- or hyperthyroidism, and measuring the size of the goitre and weight of the gland to provide a more accurate radioactive treatment for Graves disease, scans are used to measure changes in sizes of nodules and to follow up thyroid cancer patients after surgery to check whether cancer has spread outside the thyroid gland. A whole body scan will show whether iodine is in bone or other tissue (iodine uptake) after the cancerous thyroid gland has been removed (Endocrineweb 2009).

Taking thyroid medication reduces iodine uptake by the thyroid gland. Levothyroxine sodium behaves exactly as normal human thyroid hormone. Its half-life of 6.7 days necessitates withdrawal for 4–5 weeks (five half lives) before accurate thyroid testing is possible. Liothyronine sodium has a much shorter half-life of only 48 hours. Often, levothyroxine is changed to liothyronine sodium for one month to allow time for levothyroxine to clear the body while controlling the hypothyroidism features. It is then stopped for 10 days (five half lives) prior to the appropriate test. Even patients with no remaining thyroid function tolerate being off thyroid replacement for 10 days.

When hyperthyroidism is suspected but thyroid hormone blood levels are normal, liothyronine is used to suppress normal thyroid function to evaluate whether functioning nodules are autonomous (Hurley, Becker 1981; Swanson *et al.* 1985). A second interventional study is the thyroid stimulation test (Swanson 1990), which has been used to differentiate between primary and secondary hypothyroidism.

Pendred syndrome is a rare autosomal recessive condition characterised by incomplete oxidation of trapped iodide prior to organification. Clinical features include sensorineural deafness and often a mild primary hypothyroidism with a non-toxic diffuse goitre. It can be confirmed by a positive perchlorate discharge test. Perchlorate displaces non-organified iodide; about 20 MBq of radioactive iodine (RAI) is given to the patient, time is allowed for its accumulation, and its loss from the thyroid gland is observed after the administration of 1 g of oral perchlorate. An abnormally rapid loss of RAI confirms the organification defect in patients with Pendred syndrome (General Practice Notebook 2009).

Patients on levothyroxine sodium should stop treatment 4 weeks prior to the test and patients on liothyronine (T_3) should stop treatment 2 weeks before the test if adequate images are to be obtained.

Relevant clinical history should be obtained including thyroid medication, investigations with contrast media (especially iodine-containing media), previous surgery, other relevant medication including amiodarone and lithium, and diet including kelp intake.

Other tests

The Schillings test is performed with [^{57}Co]cyanocobalamin to investigate vitamin B_{12} malabsorption and pernicious anaemia. As part of the protocol, 1 mg of vitamin B_{12}, hydroxycobalamin is used as a flushing dose several hours after the radionuclide with 100 µg of intrinsic factor. To prevent interference with the test, patients should not have had a vitamin B_{12} injection in the previous 4 days or an oral dose in the previous 7 days.

Conclusions

The diagnostic capability of nuclear medicine testing has expanded through the development of equipment, computers and radiopharmaceuticals and through the development of new physiological and pharmacological interventions. The changes and additional information obtained from these interventional studies allow clinicians to differentiate between various disease conditions and treat them appropriately. This chapter summarises the more widely used pharmacological interventions used in current practice.

Acknowledgment

Images illustrating this chapters were provided courtesy of the Nuclear Medicine Department, Leeds Teaching Hospitals NHS Trust.

References

Alfonso S (1970). Inhibition of coronary vasodilating action of dipyridamole and adenosine by aminophylline in the dog. *Circ Res* 26: 743–752.

ARSAC (2006). *Notes for Guidance on the Clinical Administration of Radiopharmaceuticals and Use of Sealed Radioactive Sources*. Didcot, Oxon: Administration of Radioactive Substances Advisory Committee. http://www.arsac.org.uk/notes_for_guidance/documents/ARSACNFG2006Corrected06-11-07.pdf (accessed 29 January 2009).

Bax JJ *et al.* (1997). FDG SPECT in the assessment of myocardial viability. Comparison with dobutamine echo. *Eur Heart J* (Jun 18; Suppl D): D124–129.

Bax JJ *et al.* (2002). Safety and feasibility of cardiac FDG SPECT following oral administration of Acipimox, a nicotinic acid derivative: comparison of image quality with hyperinsulinemic euglycaemic clamping in nondiabetic patients. *J Nucl Cardiol* 9(6): 587–593.

Beller GA (1991). Pharmacological stress imaging. *JAMA* 265: 633–638.

Benamer TS *et al.* (2000a). Accurate differentiation of Parkinsonism and essential tremor using visual assessment of [^{123}I]-FP-CIT SPECT imaging: the [^{123}I]-FP-CIT study group. *Mov Disord* 15(3): 503–510.

Benamer HT *et al.* (2000b). Correlation of Parkinson's disease severity and duration with ^{123}I-FP-CIT SPECT striatal uptake. *Mov Disord* 15(4): 692–698.

Blake GM *et al.* (1988). Modification by nifedipine of I-131-metaiodobenzylguanidine kinetics in malignant phaeochromocytoma. *Eur J Nucl Med* 14: 345–348.

BNMS (2003a). *Hepatobiliary Scintigraphy*. London: British Nuclear Medicine Society. http://www.bnms.org.uk/images/stories/downloads/documents/microsoft_word_-_hepatobiliary_scintigraphy_.pdf (accessed 28 June 2010).

BNMS (2003b). *Radionuclide Thyroid Scans*. London: British Nuclear Medicine Society. http://www.bnms.org.uk/images/stories/downloads/documents/microsoft_-word_-radionuclide_thyroid_scans_.pdf (accessed 28 June 2010).

BNMS (2003c). *Procedure Guidelines for Radionuclide Myocardial Perfusion Imaging Adopted by the British Cardiac Society, the British Nuclear Cardiology Society, and the British Nuclear Medicine Society*. (2003). http://www.bnms.org.uk/images/stories/downloads/documents/mpi_20guidelines_20jun_2003.pdf (accessed 28 June 2010).

Britton KE *et al.* (1991). Renal radionuclide studies. In: Maisey MN *et al.*, eds. *Clinical Nuclear Medicine*, 2nd edn. London: Chapman and Hall Medical, 91–130.

Chilton HM, Brown ML (1990). Radiopharmaceutical for abdominal and gastrointestinal imaging: reticuloendothelial, hepatobiliary and intestinal. In: Swanson DP *et al.*, eds. *Pharmaceuticals in Medical Imaging*. New York: Macmillan, 462–500.

Choy D *et al.* (1984). Cholescintigraphy in acute cholecystitis: use of intramuscular morphine. *Radiology* 151: 203–207.

Claveau-Tremblay R *et al.* (1998). False-positive captopril renography in patients taking calcium antagonists. *J Nucl Med* 39: 1621–1626.

Croft DN, Williams JG (1991). The gastrointestinal tract. In: Maisey MN *et al.*, eds. *Clinical Nuclear Medicine*, 2nd edn. London: Chapman and Hall Medical, 292–314.

Datz FL *et al.* (1991). Physiological and pharmacological interventions in radionuclide imaging of the tubular gastrointestinal tract. *Semin Nucl Med* 21: 92–101.

Diamond RH *et al.* (1991). The role of cimetidine-enhanced technecium-99m-pertechnetate imaging for visualising Meckel's Diverticulum. *J Nucl Med* 32: 1422–1424.

Dondi M *et al.* (1989). Evaluation of hypertensive patients by means of captopril enhanced renal scintigraphy with technecium-99m DTPA. *J Nucl Med* 30: 615–621.

Dondi M *et al.* (1991). Use of technecium-99m-MAG3 for renal scintigraphy after angiotensin-converting enzyme inhibition. *J Nucl Med* 32: 424–428.

Dormont D *et al.* (2007). ACR Appropriateness Criteria® Dementia and Movement Disorders. Expert panel of neurologic imaging. Dementia and Movement disorders. Reston, VA: American College of Radiology. http://www.acr.org/SecondaryMainMenuCategories/quality_safety/app_criteria/pdf/ExpertPanelonNeurologicImaging/NeurodegenerativeDisordersUpdateinProgressDoc9.aspx (accessed 28 June 2010).

Ellis RE *et al.* (1977). The use of thyroid blocking agents. A report of a working party of the M.R.C. Isotope Advisory Panel. *Br J Radiol* 50: 203–204.

EMC (2009a). *Persantin Ampoules®*. http://emc.medicines.org.uk/emc/assets/c/html/displaydoc.asp?documentid=303 (accessed 23 January 2009).

EMC (2009b). *Adenoscan®*. http://emc.medicines.org.uk/emc/assets/c/html/displaydoc.asp?documentid=6940 (accessed 28 January 2009).

EMEA (2007). Datscan®. European Public Assessment Report. EMEA/H/C/266. London: EMEA. http://www.emea.europa.eu/humandocs/PDFs/EPAR/Datscan/072200en1.pdf (accessed 23 January 2009).

Endocrineweb (2009). *Thyroid Gland Function.* http://www.endocrineweb.com/tests.html (accessed 28 June 2010).

FDA (2001). *Guidance: Potassium iodate as a thyroid blocking agent in radiation emergencies.* Siver Spring, MD: FDA. http://www.birdflumanual.com/resources/Self_Defense/files/Guidance%20for%20use%20of%20KI%20for%20nuclear%20emergency%20USG.pdf (accessed 28 June 2010).

Fernandez P *et al.* (1999). Value of renal scintigraphy in hypertensive patients with renal failure. *J Nucl Med* 40 (3): 412–417. jnm.snmjournals.org/cgi/reprint/40/3/412.pdf (accessed 29 January 2009).

Fine EJ (1991). Interventions in renal scintirenography. *Semin Nucl Med* 21: 116–127.

Fink-Bennett D (1991). Augmented cholescintigraphy: its role in detecting acute and chronic disorders of the hepatobiliary tree. *Semin Nucl Med* 21: 128–139.

Fink-Bennett D *et al.* (1991a). Morphine-augmented cholescintigraphy: its efficacy in detecting acute cholecystitis. *J Nucl Med* 32: 1231–1233.

Fink-Bennett D *et al.* (1991b). Cholecystokinin cholescintigraphy: detection of abnormal gallbladder motor function in patients with chronic acalculous gallbladder disease. *J Nucl Med* 32: 1695–1699.

Forster T *et al.* (1993). Simultaneous dobutamine stress echocardiography and technetium-99m isonitrile single photon emission computed tomography in patients with suspected coronary artery disease. *J Am Coll Cardiol* 21: 1591–1596.

Freeman LM *et al.* (1981). Role of cholecystokinetic agents in Tc-99m-IDA cholescintigraphy. *Semin Nucl Med* 11: 186–193.

Froelich J (1985). Gastrointestinal studies. In: Thrall JH, Swanson DP, eds. *Diagnostic Interventions in Nuclear Medicine.* Chicago: Year Book Medical, 195–225.

General Practice Notebook (2009). *Perchlorate Discharge Test.* Stratford-upon-Avon: Oxbridge Solutions. http://www.gpnotebook.co.uk/simplepage.cfm?ID=-87031762 (accessed 28 January 2010).

Gross MD, Shapiro MB. (1985). Pharmacological manipulation to enhance diagnostic imaging in adrenal gland scintigraphy. In: Thrall JH, Swanson DP, eds. *Diagnostic Interventions in Nuclear Medicines.* Chicago: Year Book Medical, 76–117.

Gross MD *et al.* (1979). The normal dexamethasone suppression and adrenal scintiscan. *J Nucl Med* 20: 1131–1135.

Gross MD *et al.* (1985). Limited significance of asymmetric adrenal visualization on dexamethasone-suppression scintigraphy. *J Nucl Med* 26: 43–48.

Hesse B *et al.* (2005). EANM/ESC procedural guidelines for myocardial perfusion imaging in nuclear cardiology. *Eur J Nucl Med Mol Imaging* 35(4): 851–885.[Available at http://www.ecnc-nuclearcardiology.org/pdf_docs/EANM_ESC_guidelines_radionuclide_imaging.pdf (accessed 9 June 2010)].

Hurley JR, Becker DV (1981). Thyroid suppression and stimulation testing: the place of scanning in the evaluation of nodular thyroid disease. *Semin Nucl Med* 11: 149–160.

IBA (2010). *Norchol-131*. Dulles, VA: IBA Molecular. http://www.iba-molecular.com/products/norchol-131 (accessed 28th June 2010).

Israel O *et al.* (2007). PET/CT quantification of the effect of patient-related factors on cardiac F-18 FDG uptake. *J Nucl Med* 48: 234–239.

Juni J *et al.* (2009). Procedure Guideline for brain perfusion SPECT using Tc-99M Radiopharmaceuticals 3.0. *Society of Nuclear Medicine Practice Management Procedure Guidelines Manual.* Reston. VA: Society of Nuclear Medicine. http://interactive.snm.org/docs/Brain_SPECT_Guideline_2003.pdf (accessed 28th June 2010).

Khafagi FA *et al.* (1991). The adrenal gland. In: Maisey MN *et al.*, eds. *Clinical Nuclear Medicine*, 2nd edn. London: Chapman and Hall Medical, 271–291.

Knuuti MJ *et al.* (1992). Euglycaemic hyperinsulinaemic clamp and oral glucose load in stimulating myocardial glucose utilization during positron emission tomography. *J Nucl Med* 33: 1255–262.

Knuuti MJ *et al.* (1994). Enhancement of myocardial (fluorine-18) flurodeoxyglucose uptake by a nicotinic acid derivative. *J Nucl Med* 35: 989–998.

Krishnamurthy GT *et al.* (1983). Optimization of ceruletide intravenous dose for gallbladder emptying. *J Nucl Med* 24: 38–39.

Leung SCE, Hesslewood SR (1999). Use of drugs to enhance nuclear medicine studies. In: Sampson CB, ed. *Textbook of*

Radiopharmacy: Theory and Practice, 3rd ed. Amsterdam: Gordon and Breach, 321–335.

Majd M *et al.* (1981). Effect of phenobarbital on Tc-99m IDA scintigraphy in the evaluation of neonatal jaundice. *Semin Nucl Med* 11: 194–204.

Majd M *et al.* (1986). Captopril enhanced renal scintigraphy for detection of renal artery stenosis and uptake [abstract]. *J Nucl Med* 27: 962.

Majd-Ardekani J *et al.* (2000). Time for abstention from caffeine before an adenosine myocardial perfusion scan. *Nucl Med Commun* 21: 361–364.

Mancini M *et al.* (1993). Transcranial Doppler evaluation of cerebrovascular reactivity to acetazolamide in normal subjects. *Artery* 20: 231–241.

Mayer D, Bednarczyk E (2002). Interaction of colony stimulating factors and fluorodeoxyglucose 18F positron emission tomography. *Ann Pharmacother* 36: 1796–1799.

MedicinesComplete (2009a). *Arbutamine.* http://www.medicinescomplete.com/mc/martindale/2007/14332-y.htm?q=%22arbutamine%22#_hit (accessed 23 January 2009).

MedicinesComplete (2009b). *Ceruletide.* http://www.medicinescomplete.com/mc/martindale/2007/2124-t.htm?q=%22ceruletide%22#_hit (accessed 23 January 2009).

MedicinesComplete (2009c). *Sincalide.* http://www.medicinescomplete.com/mc/martindale/2007/2148-b.htm?q=%22sincalide%22#_hit (accessed 23 January 2009).

MHRA (2006) *Public Assessment Report. Metatrace FDG Solution for Injection 200mBq/ml. Fludeoxyglucose (18-F) PL 21750/0001.* London: Medicines and Healthcare products Regulatory Agency. http://www.mhra.gov.uk/home/groups/l-unit1/documents/websiteresources/con2033925.pdf (accessed 11 February 2009).

Murphy P *et al.* (1980). Narcotic anaesthetic drugs. Their effects on biliary dynamics. *Arch Surg* 115: 710–711.

NICE (2006a). *Trastuzumab for the adjuvant treatment of early-stage HER2-positive breast cancer.* London: National Institute for Clinical Excellence. http://www.nice.org.uk/nicemedia/pdf/TA107guidance.pdf (accessed 30 January 2009).

NICE (2006b). *Dementia: Supporting people with dementia and their carers in health and social care.* London: National Institute for Clinical Excellence. http://www.nice.org.uk/nicemedia/pdf/CG042NICEGuideline.pdf (accessed 30 January 2009).

NICE (2006c). *Parkinson's Disease. Diagnosis and management in primary and secondary care.* London: National Institute for Clinical Excellence. http://www.nice.org.uk/nicemedia/pdf/cg035niceguideline.pdf (accessed 30 January 2009).

Nicol A *et al.* (2008). *Procedure Guidelines for Planar Radionuclide Cardiac Ventriculogram for the Assessment of Left Ventricular Systolic Function* http://www.bnms.org.uk/images/stories/downloads/documents/microsoft_word_-_rnvg_revised_2_acc_changes.pdf (accessed 28 June 2010).

Niederkohr RD, Qoun A (2007). No apparent alteration of F-18 biodistribution when injected shortly after insulin glargine. *Clin Nucl Med* 32(4): 302–303.

Palac R *et al.* (1983). Exercise versus dobutamine infusion during radionuclide ventriculography in patients with coronary disease. *J Am Coll Cardiol* 1: 642. (abstract).

Pandit-Taskar N (2008). Adrenal scans with radioiodine-labeled norcholesterol (I 131 1, 6-beta-iodomethyl-19-norcholesterol) (NP-59). Bethesda, MD: ClinicalTrial.gov/NLM. http://clinicaltrials.gov/ct2/show/NCT00591643 (accessed 30 January 2009).

Petry NA, Shapiro B (1990). Adrenomedullary imaging. In: Swanson DP *et al.*, eds. *Pharmaceuticals in Medical Imaging*. New York: Macmillan, 368–386.

Reeksuppaphol S *et al.* (2004). Ranitidine-enhanced 99m-technetium pertechnetate imaging in children improves the sensitivity of identifying heterotopic gastric mucosa in Meckel's Diverticulum. *Pediatr Surg Int* 20 (4): 323–325.

Robinovitch MA (1985). Pharmacological interventions in nuclear cardiology. In: Thrall JH, Swanson DP, eds. *Diagnostic Interventions in Nuclear Medicine.* Chicago: Year Book Medical, 31–35.

Schall GL *et al.* (1981). Radionuclide salivary imaging usefulness in a private otolarynology practice. *Arch Otolaryngol* 107: 40–44.

Schwartz JA, Speed NM (1993). SPECT imaging in medical psychiatry. In: Stoudmire A, Fogel BS, eds. *Medical Psychiatric Practice*, Volume 2. Washington DC: American Psychiatric Publishing, 141–166.

Shapiro B *et al.* (1983). Value of bowel preparation in adrenocortical scintigraphy with NP-59. *J Nucl Med* 24: 732–734.

Sisson JC *et al.* (1994). Radiopharmaceutical treatment of malignant phaeochromocytoma. *J Nucl Med* 25: 197–206.

Solanki KK *et al.* (2004). Thyroid blocking policy – revisited. *Nucl Med Commun* 25: 1071–1076.

Stakianakis GN, Conway JJ (1981). Detection of ectopic gastric mucosa in Meckel's diverticulum and in other aberrations by scintigraphy: I. Pathophysiology and 10-year clinical experience. *J Nucl Med* 22(7): 647–654.

Swanson DP (1990). Adrenocortical imaging. In: Swanson DP *et al.*, eds. *Pharmaceuticals in Medical Imaging.* New York: Macmillan, 360–368.

Swanson DP *et al.* (1985). Formulary: Pharmacological interventions in nuclear medicine. In: Thrall JH, Swanson DP, eds. *Diagnostic Interventions in Nuclear Medicines.* Chicago: Year Book Medical, 247–267.

Taillefer R *et al.* (1986). Thallium-201 myocardial imaging during pharmacologic coronary vasodilatation: comparison of oral and intravenous administration of dipyridamole. *J Am Coll Cardiol* 8: 76–83.

Thrall JH (1985). Diuresis renography in hydroureteronephrosis. In: Thrall JH, Swanson DP, eds. *Diagnostic Interventions in Nuclear Medicine.* Chicago: Year Book Medical, 124–150.

Thrall JH, Swanson DP (1989). Diagnostic interventions in nuclear medicine. *Curr Probl Diag Radiol* 18: 1–37.

Vasquez TE *et al.* (1988). Intravenous administration of morphine sulphate in hepatobiliary imaging for acute cholecystitis: a review of clinical efficacy. *Nucl Med Commun* 9: 217–222.

Verani MS (1991a). Adenosine thallium-201 myocardial perfusion scintigraphy. *Am Heart J* 122: 269–278.

Verani MS (1991b). Pharmacological stress with adenosine for myocardial perfusion imaging. *Semin Nucl Med* 21: 266–272.

Wallbridge DR *et al.* (1993). A comparison of dobutamine and maximal exercise as stress for thallium scintigraphy. *Eur J Nucl Med* 20: 319–323.

Walsh JF, Groppler RJ (1996). Positron emission tomography of the cardiovascular system. In: Henkin RE *et al.*, eds. *Nuclear Medicine*, Volume 1. St. Louis, MO: Mosby Year Book, 772–797.

Yeker D *et al.* (1984). Radionuclide imaging of Meckel's Diverticulum: cimetidine versus pentagastrin plus glucagon. *Eur J Nucl Med* 9: 316–319.

Zanelli GD (1982). Effect of certain drugs used in the treatment of cardiovascular disease on the in-vitro labelling of red blood cells with Tc-99m. *Nucl Med Commun* 3: 155–161.

SECTION F

Techniques in research and development

34

Molecular biology techniques in radiopharmaceutical development

Jane Sosabowski

Introduction

The field of radiopharmaceutical development encompasses a wide range of disciplines, from molecular and cell biology to chemistry, physics, bioinformatics and medicine. The technologies that currently drive the field forward in terms of new targets and targeting molecules come largely from the areas of genomics and proteomics. It is therefore highly advantageous for those scientists who work in the forefront of radiopharmaceutical development to have an understanding of these techniques when selecting the targets and targeting molecules that will be most useful for molecular imaging. Since the pace of innovation within these fields and the seemingly vast amounts of information generated can seem daunting to non-experts, this chapter aims to give a simplified overview of genomic and proteomic technologies to assist the non-biologist.

Molecular imaging represents a shift from largely non-specific diagnostic imaging techniques to targeting genes or proteins that are known to be linked to human disease. Molecular biology and molecular imaging have become intertwined. Nuclear medicine molecular imaging can be used to monitor *in-vivo* delivery of targeted molecules such as siRNA (short interfering RNA, which binds to complementary messenger RNA (mRNA) causing a targeted translational block) (Merkel *et al.* 2009) or to visualise reporter gene expression (see below). Equally, molecular biology techniques such as phage display have been used to discover ligands that, when radiolabelled, can be used to image receptors *in vivo* (see below). The decoding of the human genome has led to a huge acceleration in identification of molecular targets for diagnosis and treatment of disease. These targets may be at the genomic or at the proteomic level and in both cases, high-throughput screening techniques are commonly utilised to discover molecules that bind to or are substrates for these targets.

Genomics

While genetics looks at single genes one at a time, genomics has been defined as the large scale analysis of gene expression. This analysis may be on the scale of a whole organism, a whole tissue or a whole cell and is a snapshot of the gene expression under the prevailing conditions. Since gene expression changes constantly according to the requirements of the cell, experiments are usually conducted as a comparison of cells under two different conditions (i.e. analysis of differential gene expression). A major driving factor behind the enormous growth of genomics has been the emergence of DNA microarray and chip technologies, which have provided a means of measuring gene expression on a massive scale.

DNA microarrays and chips

DNA microarrays and chips are either low- or high-density arrays of DNA molecules used for parallel hybridisation analyses. Hybridisation is the binding together of two complementary polynucleotides by base pairing (for example, a DNA molecule with the sequence –A-A-C-G-T-C- will bind to another with the sequence –T-T-G-C-A-G- to form double-stranded DNA). This technique can be used to identify which DNAs or RNAs are present in different cells and ideally their relative abundances.

Strictly speaking, microarrays and chips are two distinct types of matrix that differ in the way they are created and hence in the density (i.e. the number of DNA sequences per cm^2) of the array. Both are based on older molecular biology techniques that use DNA hybridisation to detect specific molecules (e.g. northern blotting, which uses DNA–RNA hybridisation), but are transformed into a genomic technology by the ability to screen very many DNA sequences in parallel. The DNA sequences can be PCR products (the polymerase chain reaction is a method for exponentially amplifying sections of DNA) or cDNA sequences (DNA copies of mRNA sequences) or synthetic oligonucleotides. To create a gene array, for example, a large number of DNA sequences for known genes are applied to a surface (such as a glass slide), thus creating an array of spots. Each DNA sequence has a defined location in the array. This gene array is then treated with a test sample (e.g. fluorescently labelled total RNA extracted from cells). The RNA molecules bind to complementary DNA sequences in the array by DNA–RNA hybridisation. The amount of RNA bound to each DNA spot is measured (by densitometry or fluorescence techniques) and reflects the relative expression levels of different genes within the RNA test sample.

A microarray is simply a miniaturised gene array with the DNA sequences applied robotically in very tiny spots. Despite this, the typical 18 × 18 mm, 6400-spot array (i.e. 80 × 80) that can be achieved using this method is still regarded as a low-density array (see Figure 34.1).

DNA chips on the other hand provide a really high-density array as the oligonucleotides are synthesised *in situ* on the surface of a glass or silicon wafer. The technique used to create these chips was first developed for synthetic combinatorial peptide libraries (see below) but the applications for DNA synthesis were recognised immediately (Fodor *et al.* 1991). Usually, oligonucleotide synthesis involves attachment of nucleotides one at a time to the growing end of an oligonucleotide. The sequence is determined by the order of addition of the nucleotides to the reaction

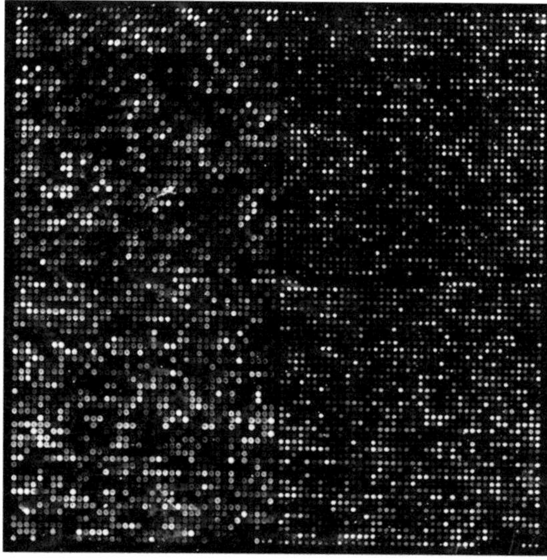

Figure 34.1 A DNA microarray.

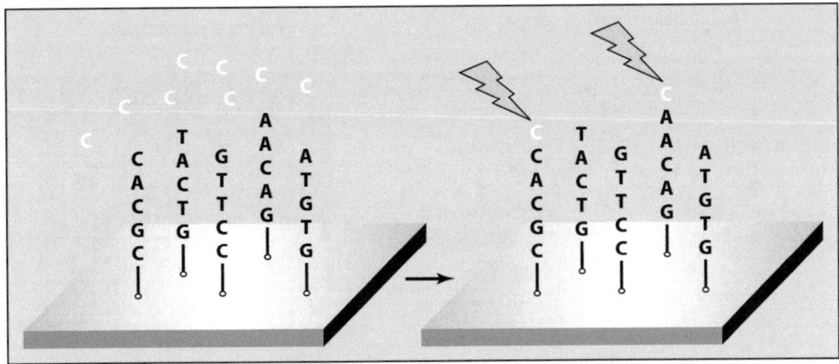

Figure 34.2 Creation of a DNA chip using photolithography. Light-activated nucleotide reagents are added to the growing DNA sequences only at the illuminated positions.

mixture. If this method were to be used for synthesising DNA chips, all the DNA spots would display the same oligonucleotide as each would have been exposed to the nucleotides in the same order. To overcome this, modified nucleotide substrates are used that require light activation to attach to the end of the growing oligonucleotide. Individual positions on the chip are illuminated with pulses of light to activate attachment of the nucleotide added to the reaction mixture at each step (a technique known as photolithography) (see Figure 34.2). This results in attachment of the nucleotide substrate to only certain of the growing oligonucleotides at each step. When the next nucleotide is added to the reaction mixture, different positions will be illuminated, with the result that each of the final DNA sequences attached to the chip is unique. The density of oligonucleotides attached in this way can be up to 300 000 per cm^2.

Gene expression arrays: mRNA expression profiling

The transcriptome is the initial product of genome expression and is made up of RNA copies of genes whose secondary products (proteins) are required by the cell at a particular time (see Figure 34.3).

Thus the transcriptome is made up entirely of messenger RNA (mRNA) (protein-coding RNA) which comprises less than 4% of the total cell RNA. To analyse the transcriptome using chip or microarray technology, the total mRNA of a cell is reverse-transcribed into cDNA (complementary DNA), which is then fluorescently labelled and hybridised to a DNA chip or microarray containing thousands of different probes (corresponding to different genes). The labelled cDNAs that bind are detected by laser scanning (the laser excites the dye at a certain wavelength and the dye in turn emits a fluorescent signal). Signal intensity is depicted by a pseudocolour scale with red indicating the greatest level of hybridisation. Since this method provides only relative intensities, it is usual to compare two different transcriptomes (for example, two different disease states). Using two arrays, however, can increase the level of complexity of the experiment in that it is difficult to ensure that the different levels of fluorescent intensities reflect differences in the two transcriptomes rather than any experimental factor. This problem can be overcome by labelling the two transcriptomes with different fluorescent dyes and binding them to the same array. This can then be scanned using two appropriate wavelengths to obtain the relative intensity of the fluorescence signal at each position on the array (see Figure 34.4).

Gene expression can also be quantified relative to a housekeeping (reference) gene (which must be

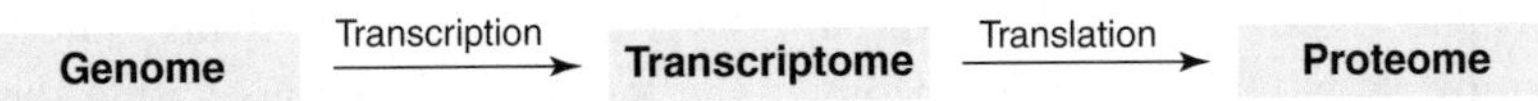

Figure 34.3 The products of genome expression.

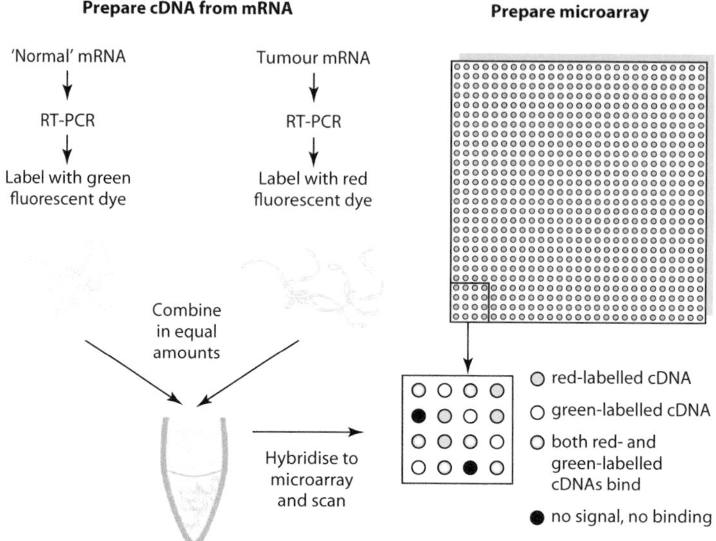

Figure 34.4 Schematic showing the procedure for differential gene expression analysis in two different cell states, e.g. diseased versus normal or dividing versus rested. Calculation of the red-to-green fluorescence ratio in each spot reveals the relative expression of the gene in the two samples.

carefully picked as its expression should be constant across the samples to be compared). This can be done using quantitative real-time PCR (qPCR) which allows the researcher to simultaneously amplify and quantify the DNA through the use of fluorescent dyes and fluorescent oligonucleotide probes. Using the reverse transcriptase polymerase chain reaction (RT-PCR), minute amounts of mRNA can be reverse-transcribed into cDNA and then amplified using qPCR to give a quantitative measurement of gene transcription.

Laser capture microdissection

Laser capture microdissection (LCM) is essentially a cell purification technique allowing single cells to be harvested from tissue sections. This addresses the problem of tissue heterogeneity in disease and provides a means of isolating cells that display characteristic disease morphology.

The method was developed in 1996 (Emmert-Buck *et al.* 1996) as an extension of manual microdissection methods and greatly improved the speed and accuracy of removing cells from a heterogeneous sample. A thin tissue slice is mounted on a glass slide and a thermoplastic transfer film is applied to the surface of the tissue section. The tissue section is viewed under a microscope and cells are selected for capture. A near-IR laser (which is integrated with the optics of the microscope) is activated and, with great precision, fuses the transfer film to the selected cells. The transfer film is then removed from the tissue section along with the bound cells, leaving the unwanted cells on the slide. The cells are not damaged or altered by this process and can be used for DNA, RNA or protein analysis.

Proteomics

Genomic technologies look at differential gene expression arising from changes in cellular states on the mRNA level. However, there is a poor correlation between the message and the final product (the protein) as mRNA levels are not the only determinant of protein levels (factors such as translational controls and regulated degradation may have equally important effects) (Cox, Mann 2007; Gygi *et al.* 1999). Proteins almost always control the biological functions within the cell and therefore it can be argued that protein expression levels (rather than mRNA levels) are the most relevant factor when characterising a biological system, be it healthy or diseased. This leads us into the field of proteomics.

The proteome is the complete set of proteins encoded by the genome. For example, the proteome of a cell is made up all the proteins present in a cell at a particular time. Therefore, the field of proteomics incorporates any technology that characterises large sets of proteins. This is a much more complicated task than analysis of the genome for a number of reasons. Firstly, proteins have a much greater variability than DNA or RNA. They are subject to post-translational modifications such as glycosylation and phosphorylation, as well as proteolytic cleavage. Secondly, proteins cannot be amplified in the same way as oligonucleotides, and therefore the problem of small sample size and sensitivity becomes an issue. The technologies that have emerged to deal with separation and characterisation of large sets of proteins are two-dimensional gel electrophoresis and mass spectrometry.

Two-dimensional gel electrophoresis

Although advances in mass spectrometry have been most instrumental in moving towards the goal of proteomics, i.e. characterising all the proteins that make up a particular proteome, even the most advanced mass spectrometry techniques cannot analyse entire complex proteomes. Therefore, the sample is usually divided up into smaller, more manageable subsets of proteins that can then be more effectively analysed by mass spectrometry. Two-dimensional gel electrophoresis (involving two separations at right angles to each other) allows far greater resolution of mixture components than separations in one dimension. The technique of 2D-PAGE (two-dimensional polyacrylamide gel electrophoresis) under denaturing conditions, capable of separating hundreds of proteins, was introduced by O'Farrell in 1975 (O'Farrell 1975). This demonstrated that proteins could be separated in the first dimension by isoelectric focusing (IEF) and then in the second dimension (at right angles to the first) on the basis of molecular weight using sodium dodecyl sulfate (SDS). Further developments over the years have made it possible for a variation of O'Farrell's technique to be used to separate large numbers of proteins. Protein charge depends on amino acid composition, covalent modifications and the pH of its environment. The isoelectric point (pI) of a protein is the pH at which it carries no charge (i.e. it is neutral). If proteins are electrophoresed in a gel containing a pH gradient between two oppositely charged electrodes, each protein will travel towards its oppositely charged electrode until it reaches the point within the pH gradient where its charge becomes zero (i.e. the pI of the protein). When each protein reaches the point of neutrality, it will cease to move in the gel (i.e. it becomes 'focused') as it is not attracted towards either electrode. In 1982, immobilised pH gradients (IPGs) were introduced (Bjellqvist *et al.* 1982). Here ampholytes were attached to acrylamide molecules and cast into the gel and this greatly improved drift and reproducibility. This in turn led to the development of narrow pH band IEF strips, which allowed the resolution of larger numbers of proteins in a sample. For instance, the use of several narrow band strips (4–5, 5–6 and 5.5–6.7) outperformed single strips of either pH 3–10 or pH 4–7 (Wildgruber *et al.* 2000). However, the use of several strips requires more sample.

Once the proteins have been separated by IEF, they are electrophoretically transferred from the pH focusing strip gel onto a resolving polyacrylamide gel where they are further separated (at right angles to the first separation) according to molecular weight using SDS. All of the proteins assume an equal negative charge-to-mass ratio in the presence of SDS and are electrophoretically separated, with the higher-mass proteins migrating more slowly through the gel. Therefore the final result of a 2D-PAGE separation is a stained gel (via silver or Coomassie blue staining) that has pH on the first axis and molecular weight on the second (see Figure 34.5).

The sensitivity of 2D-PAGE can be enhanced by fluorescently labelling the proteins prior to separation. It also allows the comparison of up to three different protein samples on the same gel, an advantage as spot-to-spot comparisons between different gels is not easy. This technique is known as two-dimensional difference gel electrophoresis (2D-DIGE) (Minden 2007). The fluorescent cyanine dyes

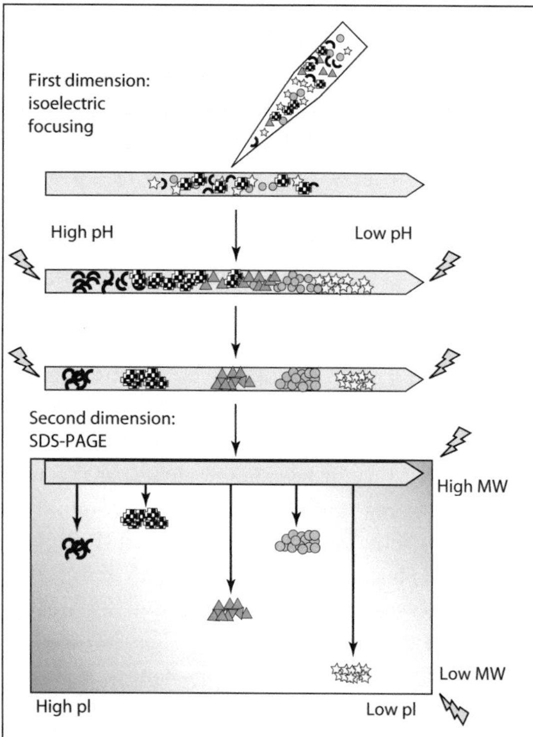

Figure 34.5 Schematic showing the separation of proteins using two-dimensional gel electrophoresis. Separation in the first dimension is according to isoelectric point (pI) and in the second dimension according to molecular weight.

(Cy3, Cy5 and Cy2) are commercially available and have different excitation and emission wavelengths. They are usually used to label protein extracts from healthy and diseased samples as well as a control consisting of a mixture of equal amounts of protein from each of the two samples. The sample, consisting of equal concentrations of the differently labelled proteomes and the control, is added to a gel plate and separated using 2D-PAGE. The resulting gel can be scanned with a fluorescence imager using three different wavelengths to give the relative abundances of the proteins in different disease states compared with the control. The control also allows normalisation of protein abundance with other gels. 2D-DIGE therefore halves the number of gels used and also eliminates the experimental error incurred by running two samples for comparison on different gels. Interesting proteins can be excised from the gel and analysed by mass spectrometry (see below).

Mass spectrometry

The use of mass spectrometry (MS) for analysis of biological macromolecules became possible with the development of soft ionisation techniques such as electrospray ionisation (ESI) and matrix assisted laser desorption ionisation (MALDI) that do not cause fragmentation of the fragile protein molecules. This was the vital step forward in the characterisation of biomolecules that has become the basis of proteomics. In recognition of this, the inventors, John Fenn (ESI) and Koichi Tanaka (laser desorption) were awarded the Nobel Prize for Chemistry in 2002.

ESI relies on evaporation of aqueous droplets of protein, which are usually positively charged. As the droplets reduce in size, the electrostatic charges begin to repel each other, causing each droplet to explode. This produces a spray of tiny droplets each with their own electrostatic charges. The protein molecules in various states of protonation are desorbed (freed) from the droplets and pass into the mass analyser where their mass-to-charge ratio (m/z) is determined in a vacuum. ESI-MS is commonly coupled with high performance liquid chromatography (HPLC) (LC-MS), whereby a mixture of peptides or proteins is separated by HPLC and the components pass directly into the MS instrument, often in tandem, i.e. MS/MS for mass analysis. In tandem MS, the first MS analysis scans all the ions in the sample to find the most intense peaks. In the second analysis, selected m/z species are further fragmented and analysed according to their m/z ratio. The use of LC-MS/MS in proteomics research has been reviewed by Listgarten and Emili (2005).

MALDI uses a low-energy laser at a wavelength that is not absorbed by the protein (direct absorption of the laser energy would destroy the protein molecule). The laser energy is instead absorbed by a matrix comprising small, UV-absorbing, acidic molecules such as 2,5-dihydroxybenzoic acid (gentisic acid) or cinnamic acid. The matrix solution is mixed with the protein and spotted onto a metal plate where the matrix and protein co-crystallise when the solvent evaporates. After the laser is fired, the energy is absorbed and transferred from the matrix to the protein, causing ionisation. The vaporised mixture enters the mass analyser, usually a time-of-flight (TOF) analyser, where the m/z ratio is determined by accelerating the ionised proteins in an electric field and measuring the time it takes for each particle to cover a known distance to a detector (heavier molecules travel more slowly).

MALDI-TOF is the most frequently used mass spectrometry technique in the field of proteomics. A typical proteomics experiment might involve separation of one or more proteomes by 2D-PAGE or 2D-DIGE (see above) and excision of individual proteins from the gel. These are usually then subjected to a protein digestion (using trypsin), which cuts the protein up into small pieces. These peptides are identified by MALDI-MS and the parent proteins from which they originated are identified by searching for the peptide sequences in protein databases.

Protein–protein interactions

As well as studying protein expression levels, proteomics techniques can be used to examine protein–protein interactions using protein microarrays and global yeast two-hybrid methods.

Protein microarrays are an adaptation of DNA microarrays in which the substances immobilised onto the slide can be proteins, peptides, antibodies, antigens or small molecules. This spotting can be done manually or robotically, or the compounds can be synthesised onto the slide (see combinatorial libraries below). The slide is then exposed to the test mixture and the compounds that bind to the targets on the slide are identified.

In simple form, the yeast two-hybrid system uses a yeast protein that regulates the expression of an enzyme and consists of two independent domains. One domain is a DNA activator (which binds to a DNA sequence near to the promoter that causes the enzyme to be expressed) and the other activates transcription. In the yeast two-hybrid system, one protein (the bait) is fused to the DNA-binding domain while the proteins that are to be used as the 'prey' are fused to the activation domain. If the prey and the bait interact, the functional yeast protein can then activate expression of the reporter gene, which provides the detection method. For example, the expression of the *lacZ* reporter gene by this method can be detected by growing yeast in the presence of the chromogenic substrate X-gal – if β-galactosidase (the protein product of the *lacZ* gene) is present, it will hydrolyse the X-gal and cause the yeast cells to turn blue. There are many forms of the yeast two-hybrid system presently in use and the method can be scaled up to screen libraries of proteins. This is a method that has some similarity to the phage display library system (see below).

Biological combinatorial libraries: phage display

Phage display is a technique that allows proteins, peptides or DNA that bind specifically to predefined molecular targets to be isolated from a mixture (or library) of billions of such molecules. It has been used in the field of nuclear medicine by workers seeking to develop novel receptor- or antibody-targeting radiopharmaceuticals (Ladner 1999; Engfeldt *et al.* 2007; Zitzmann *et al.* 2007). Phage display allows not only selection of binding molecules from a library but also is a means of amplifying and identifying the selected few so they may be synthesised and undergo further testing. This is down to the nature of the phage itself.

A bacteriophage (or phage) is a virus that infects bacteria. Phages have a long history of use in medicine, especially in the former Soviet Union (mainly as an alternative to antibiotics) (McGrath, van Sinderen 2007). Filamentous bacteriophages are phages that have a rod filament shape and infect Gram-negative bacteria. M13 and fd are filamentous phages and are most commonly used for phage display systems, although other types of phages are also used (e.g. T4, T7 and lambda). M13 phage consists of circular single-stranded (ss) DNA, enclosed in a protein coat (see Figure 34.6) and is 1 μm long and 5–7 nm wide. The protein coat consists of about 2700 copies of a 50-amino-acid protein called p8 and 3–5 copies of

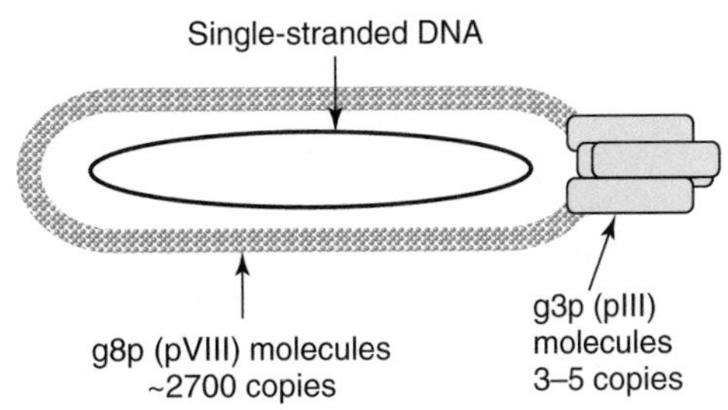

Figure 34.6 Schematic of M13 phage.

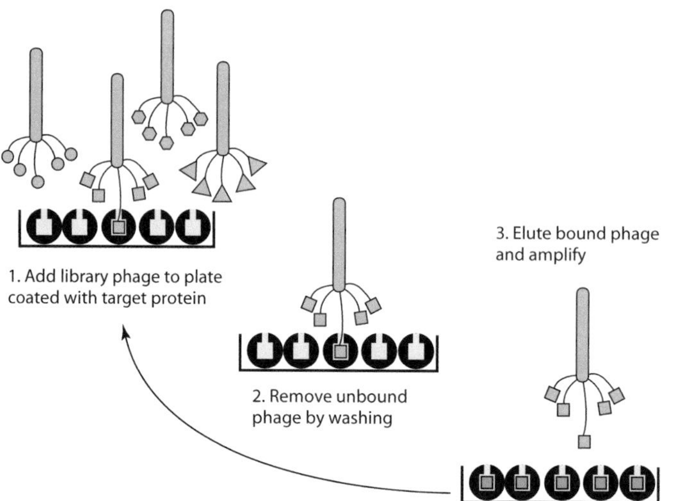
1. Add library phage to plate
coated with target protein
2. Remove unbound
phage by washing
3. Elute bound phage
and amplify

Figure 34.7 Schematic of the phage screening process.

a minor coat protein (p3) at its end. These proteins are encoded in its genome as geneVIII and geneIII. It is a non-lytic phage that infects *Escherichia coli* and induces the bacteria to reproduce and secrete phages.

The technique of phage display was conceived with the discovery that foreign DNA inserted into filamentous phage geneIII is expressed as a fusion protein and displayed on the surface of the phage (Smith 1985), hence the term 'phage display'. By inserting DNA sequences of interest into the phage DNA, the gene product is displayed as a fusion protein with the minor coat protein of the phage. Libraries of phages can be constructed, each particle displaying a different protein/peptide on its outer coat. The gene encoding each protein or peptide is physically attached to its product; if particular ligands are selected out of this library, DNA sequencing can be carried out to identify them. In the case of cDNA libraries the concept is the same except that, since the cDNA has been reverse-transcribed from mRNA and inserted into the phage gene (usually T7 phage), the libraries are limited to naturally occurring proteins.

The molecular target may be a receptor, antibody or enzyme and is immobilised in some way (e.g. purified receptors/antibodies, immobilised on a plate). Cell membranes or intact cells may also be used, although this is much more complicated as they express hundreds of different receptors. The immobilised target is exposed to the phage library. The phages that carry molecules that bind to the target are retained when the rest of the non-binding library phages are washed away (see Figure 34.7). These phages with binding proteins or peptides are then removed (or eluted) from the target with an acid wash or by competitive displacement with an excess of a ligand known to bind specifically to the receptor/antibody. The eluted phages are amplified (in *E. coli*) and the screening process is repeated. Therefore, in each round of screening, phages that do not bind to the target are discarded while those that do bind are kept. This leads to a pool of phages that is enriched with displayed proteins that bind to the target.

After three rounds of screening have been carried out, the phage pool is plated out. A number (typically 12–24) of individual phage colonies are picked and each one is amplified in *E. coli*. This amplification provides enough material for extraction of the DNA of the individual phage clones. The DNA of each of these clones is sequenced and, because the protein/peptide displayed on the outer surface of the phage is encoded in its genome, the displayed molecules are identified. The amino acid sequences of these 12–24 molecules are compared to see whether there are any similarities between them (see Table 34.1 for an example). For instance, if a particular amino acid sequence is necessary for binding to the target, this sequence would be expected to be present in a number of otherwise different sequences. Sequences that show a degree of similarity within the group of selected phages are known as consensus sequences. If no

Table 34.1 Biopanning of a commercially available 7-mer peptide library against streptavidin results in consensus sequences after three rounds (New England Biolabs (Ltd), Technical bulletin #8100)

First round sequences	Second round sequences	Third round sequences
Q L D R L P V	S L L A H P Q	T L L A H P Q
Y C Q A L R C	T L L A H P Q	N L L N H P Q
S L W L H T P	L P L Y V P Q	S L I A H P Q
M S G P L S V	T L L A H P Q	T L I N H P Q
A A L S K A S	S L L A H P Q	S L L A H P Q
S D H R W A S	N L L N H P Q	T L L A H P Q
Q P M L V A S		S L I A H P Q
Consensus: no consensus	**Consensus:** S/T L L A H P Q	**Consensus:** S/T L L/I A H P Q

consensus sequences exist, further rounds of screening, amplification and sequencing are carried out. The peptides or proteins encoded by the consensus DNA sequences are then synthesised and tested for target affinity.

It is possible to construct one's own phage display libraries, but they are also commercially available at a fraction of the price of synthetic chemical libraries, and with greater diversity.

Up until the year 2000, the vast majority of published studies detailing the successful use of phage display libraries were those that used antibody phage libraries (Szardenings 2003). However, more recently increasing numbers of high-affinity peptide ligands have been identified through phage display (Aina *et al.* 2007). The targets for peptide phage display can be purified cell surface molecules, whole cells in culture, or the intact vasculature through *in-vivo* screening (where phage libraries are injected into live animals or humans). *In-vitro* screening against purified cell surface molecules is the simplest and generally the most successful approach. Screening against whole cells in cell culture has been carried out in cases where a functionally folded soluble extracellular domain of the target protein cannot be obtained, for example G protein-coupled receptors (GPCRs) which have seven transmembrane domains. This is much more complex than using purified immobilised protein as a target as there are hundreds of different cell membrane receptors to which the phage peptides can bind. However, the results can be improved by eluting the phage with a known competitive ligand for the receptor of interest and the use of subtractive panning (exposing the phage display library to cells that are exactly the same as the target cells, except that they do not contain the receptor of interest). In this way, peptides that bind to other cell targets can be eliminated. To increase the success rate of biopanning on whole cells, it is recommended that initial screening be done on at least 15 randomised amino acid positions and that the target should be in the correct conformation (Szardenings 2003). Alternating between different cell lines containing the same target molecules can also increase the chances of success. Consensus peptides obtained via this method should be regarded as lead compounds and a further library may be constructed based on the lead compound (via mutagenesis) and further screening carried out.

When applying peptide phage display techniques to the field of radiopharmaceutical development, it is useful to bear in mind that small peptides are most likely to make good radiopharmaceuticals and it is a good idea to start with a large linear library (e.g. 10^{10}) of 12–15-mer peptides. Although a good lead is unlikely to come out of the first screening of the library, it may be that a binding motif can be identified that can be used to construct a new library. Small peptides are generally unstable *in vivo*, so progression to the use of cysteine-constrained peptides (i.e. cyclic peptides) can be advantageous. This is because they are less susceptible to exopeptidases (enzymes that degrade peptides from their ends). Another strategy that can be used for increasing the *in-vivo* stability of lead compounds is to substitute natural L-amino acids with D-amino acids, which are again less susceptible to peptidases. Homo- or hetero-dimerisation of the peptide leads can be investigated as a means of increasing affinity.

In-vivo screening by intravenous injection of phage-displayed peptide libraries in mice is a technique pioneered by Pasqualini and Ruoslahti (1996), who identified peptide ligands for targets found on endothelial cells of blood vessels supplying various organs (as well as tumour). The advantages of using this technique include depletion of phages displaying peptides that bind to plasma and cell surface proteins as well as preferential selection of peptides that are stable *in vivo*. These workers and colleagues have also used this technique in humans, showing that the tissue distribution of circulating peptides was not random (Arap *et al.* 2002) and went on to isolate a mimic of IL-11 from prostate biopsies after IV administration of a peptide library (Zurita *et al.* 2004). Thus, *in-vivo* phage display selection is a powerful technique for identifying peptides that bind to the vasculature of specific tumours. It also opens up the possibility of patient-specific therapeutics. For example, a study by Krag *et al.* (2006) on eight patients with late-stage tumours of different kinds identified a peptide that was specific to an individual patient's melanoma. This peptide did not bind to human melanocytes and bound to only one of a cohort of other melanoma cell lines. In addition to peptides that bind to the vasculature of tumours, it has also been possible to identify peptides that bind to the tumour lymphatic vessels (Laakkonen *et al.* 2008).

Synthetic combinatorial libraries

Combinatorial chemistry is a technique whereby a set of starting materials is reacted in all possible combinations to obtain a collection of between 10^4 and 10^8 molecules that can be screened. While synthetic combinatorial libraries do not fall within the category of molecular biology techniques, their use allows the high-throughput screening of molecules with non-biological moieties such as D-amino acids and other unnatural amino acids or structural features. In this respect, their use in lead optimisation is extremely valuable. Unlike the traditional chemistry methods of synthesising and purifying one molecule at a time, combinatorial chemistry uses the same reaction conditions to make large numbers of structurally distinct molecules at the same time, either in parallel or in mixtures and using either solid- or solution-phase techniques.

There are many different ways of generating synthetic combinatorial libraries, but the field as a whole originated with Merrifield's development of solid-phase peptide synthesis in the 1960s (Merrifield 1963). Up until that time, peptide synthesis had been extremely laborious as, after the addition of each amino acid, rigorous purification of the growing peptide was required prior to reaction with the next amino acid, and final yields (especially of longer peptides) were low. Merrifield's innovation was to attach the C-terminus of an amino acid to a solid material. Excess amounts of the next amino acid could then be added to react with the N-terminus of the attached amino acid, ensuring a rapid completed reaction. Purification involved simply washing the solid material (and the attached peptide chain) to remove the excess reactants. Then the next amino acid was added and the peptide chain was built up. Merrifield received the Nobel Prize for Chemistry in 1984 for this work. In the 1980s Mario Geysen used this technique to create the first combinatorial library where hundreds of different peptides were synthesised in parallel, each on the head of a 'pin' (a polyethylene rod) (Geysen *et al.* 1984). The pins were arranged in an array in the format and on the scale of a microtitre plate. The pin array was aligned with a tray containing hundreds of wells arranged in the same matrix format, each containing different reactants. The pins were dipped into the wells and once the reactions were complete, the array was washed and dried before dipping it once more into the wells, which now contained different reactants. The final synthesised peptides were then reacted with antibody targets without removal from the array. This early limited combinatorial library is an example of a spatially addressable parallel library in which compounds that are positive in the screening step can be positionally located and identified. Other such examples are chemical microarrays (Fodor *et al.* 1991), which use photolithography and paved the way for the development of DNA chips (Pease *et al.* 1994) (see above) and SPOT synthesis (Frank 2002).

A further step in the development of combinatorial libraries came with the mix-and-split approach, which allows the synthesis of much larger libraries. This method was pioneered by Furka and colleagues (Furka *et al.* 1991) and involves splitting a sample of resin solid-phase support material into a number of equal portions. A single different reagent is added to each of these portions and, when the individual reactions are complete and washing of excess reagent has been carried out, the portions are combined and mixed. The mixture is again divided into equal portions and the process is repeated with a further set of activated reagents to give the complete set of dimeric units and so on. Although the reagents could be any kind of chemical precursor or monomeric unit, in the case of a peptide library the reagents would be amino acids. Taking the simple case of using three amino acids to create a library of all possible combinations, the result would be three mixtures of nine peptides each, i.e. 27 different tripeptides. It is clear that, using this method, each individual piece of resin would only display one chemical entity. Lam *et al.* used this method to create a one-bead one-compound (OBOC) peptide library containing close to 2.5×10^6 pentapeptides from 19 amino acids (Lam *et al.* 1991). The peptides were then successfully screened for binding to streptavadin or a monoclonal antibody against β-endorphin using a colorimetric assay whereby binding beads were identified visually and picked out using micromanipulation. The compounds can also be cleaved from the beads for solution-phase testing as a mixture. Activity in any one mixture reveals the residue coupled last (usually the N-terminal residue) of the active compound as the last added is unique to each mixture. Having retained samples of beads from the previous reaction step, these mixtures are screened to reveal the mixture containing the most active amino acid at the second-to-last position in the chain and so on. Deconvolution (the process of identifying an active compound by tracing it back through the synthetic mixtures used to make it) of the active mixtures through further synthesis and screening eventually identifies the most active compound. Since deconvolution can be more time consuming than synthesising the library itself, encoding is also used. Encoding is a strategy for marking compounds with physical or chemical tags so that the compounds can easily be identified and includes techniques such as peptide nucleic acid (PNA)-encoded chemical microarrays (Winssinger *et al.* 2004) and radiofrequency tagging (Xiao *et al.* 2000).

Combinatorial chemistry is a field in which developments are rapid, including dynamic combinatorial chemistry, polymer-supported reagents and improved deconvolution methods.

References

Aina OH *et al.* (2007). From combinatorial chemistry to cancer-targeting peptides. *Mol Pharm* 4: 631–651.

Arap W *et al.* (2002). Steps toward mapping the human vasculature by phage display. *Nat Med* 8: 121–127.

Bjellqvist B *et al.* (1982). Isoelectric focusing in immobilized pH gradients: principle, methodology and some applications. *J Biochem Biophys Methods* 6: 317–339.

Cox J, Mann M (2007). Is proteomics the new genomics? *Cell* 130: 395–398.

Emmert-Buck MR *et al.* (1996). Laser capture microdissection. *Science* 274: 998–1001.

Engfeldt T *et al.* (2007). Imaging of HER2-expressing tumours using a synthetic Affibody molecule containing the ^{99m}Tc-chelating mercaptoacetyl-glycyl-glycyl-glycyl (MAG3) sequence. *Eur J Nucl Med Mol Imaging* 34: 722–733.

Fodor SP *et al.* (1991). Light-directed, spatially addressable parallel chemical synthesis. *Science* 251: 767–773.

Frank R (2002). The SPOT-synthesis technique. Synthetic peptide arrays on membrane supports – principles and applications. *J Immunol Methods* 267: 13–26.

Furka A *et al.* (1991). General method for rapid synthesis of multicomponent peptide mixtures. *Int J Pept Protein Res* 37: 487–493.

Geysen HM *et al.* (1984). Use of peptide synthesis to probe viral antigens for epitopes to a resolution of a single amino acid. *Proc Natl Acad Sci U S A* 81: 3998–4002.

Gygi SP *et al.* (1999). Correlation between protein and mRNA abundance in yeast. *Mol Cell Biol* 19: 1720–1730.

Krag DN *et al.* (2006). Selection of tumor-binding ligands in cancer patients with phage display libraries. *Cancer Res* 66: 7724–7733.

Laakkonen P *et al.* (2008). Peptide targeting of tumor lymph vessels. *Ann N Y Acad Sci* 1131: 37–43.

Ladner RC (1999). Polypeptides from phage display. A superior source of in vivo imaging agents. *Q J Nucl Med* 43: 119–124.

Lam KS *et al.* (1991). A new type of synthetic peptide library for identifying ligand-binding activity. *Nature* 354: 82–84.

Listgarten J, Emili A (2005). Statistical and computational methods for comparative proteomic profiling using liquid chromatography-tandem mass spectrometry. *Mol Cell Proteomics* 4: 419–434.

McGrath S, van Sinderen D, eds. (2007). *Bacteriophage: Genetics and Molecular Biology*. Norwich: Caister Academic Press.

Merkel OM *et al.* (2009). In vivo SPECT and real-time gamma camera imaging of biodistribution and pharmacokinetics of siRNA delivery using an optimized radiolabeling and purification procedure. *Bioconjug Chem* 20(1): 174–182.

Merrifield RB (1963). Solid phase peptide synthesis. I. The synthesis of a tetrapeptide. *J Am Chem Soc* 85: 2149–2154.

Minden J (2007). Comparative proteomics and difference gel electrophoresis. *Biotechniques* 43: 739–745.

O'Farrell PH (1975). High resolution two-dimensional electrophoresis of proteins. *J Biol Chem* 250: 4007–4021.

Pasqualini R, Ruoslahti E (1996). Organ targeting in vivo using phage display peptide libraries. *Nature* 380: 364–366.

Pease AC *et al.* (1994). Light-generated oligonucleotide arrays for rapid DNA sequence analysis. *Proc Natl Acad Sci U S A* 91: 5022–5026.

Smith GP (1985). Filamentous fusion phage: novel expression vectors that display cloned antigens on the virion surface. *Science* 228: 1315–1317.

Szardenings M (2003). Phage display of random peptide libraries: applications, limits, and potential. *J Recept Signal Transduct Res* 23: 307–349.

Wildgruber R *et al.* (2000). Towards higher resolution: two-dimensional electrophoresis of *Saccharomyces cerevisiae* proteins using overlapping narrow immobilized pH gradients. *Electrophoresis* 21: 2610–2616.

Winssinger N *et al.* (2004). PNA-encoded protease substrate microarrays. *Chem Biol* 11: 1351–1360.

Xiao XY *et al.* (2000). Solid-phase combinatorial synthesis using MicroKan reactors, RF tagging, and directed sorting. *Biotechnol Bioeng* 71: 44–50.

Zitzmann S *et al.* (2007). Identification and evaluation of a new tumor cell-binding peptide, FROP-1. *J Nucl Med* 48: 965–972.

Zurita AJ *et al.* (2004). Combinatorial screenings in patients: the interleukin-11 receptor alpha as a candidate target in the progression of human prostate cancer. *Cancer Res* 64: 435–439.

35

Chemical characterisation of radiopharmaceuticals

Philip J Blower

The importance of structural characterisation of radiopharmaceuticals

This chapter provides background and examples to show why careful and critical characterisation of structure and properties of radiopharmaceuticals of all kinds is extremely important if reliable image interpretation is to be achieved, whether the radiopharmaceutical is a small organic molecule, a small metal complex, a labelled peptide or protein, or a particulate tracer. Experimental methods are discussed in subsequent sections.

Small molecules and complexes

Although several highly effective and valuable technetium-99m radiopharmaceuticals that are still regarded as the day-to-day stock-in-trade of nuclear medicine were developed more than three decades ago, and although the contents (chelators, reducing agents, buffers, etc.) of the cold kits used to prepare them are well-defined, in many cases the chemical structures of these technetium-99m complexes remain unknown. Regulatory approval and marketing authorisation requirements are now more demanding than at the time these tracers were developed, and it is unlikely that active constituents of radiopharmaceuticals (i.e. the technetium-99m or other radionuclide-containing molecules) being developed now and in the future would gain clinical acceptance as readily with such meagre knowledge of structure. In addition, the refinement of new molecular imaging approaches to optimise imaging quality, specificity, sensitivity, etc., in modern pharmaceutical chemistry depends on the ability to identify and exploit structure–activity relationships so that rational structural modifications can be suggested and evaluated. Structure–activity relationships self-evidently require knowledge of structure. In the modern era of tracer and contrast agent development, it is therefore necessary to have a much greater understanding of the structure of radiopharmaceuticals than in the past.

Radiopharmaceuticals based on metal coordination complexes (e.g. ^{99m}Tc complexes of DMSA, MDP, DTPA, etc.), especially, are subject to criticism from this perspective, because their structures are less predictable and less bound by well-understood 'rules' than those of small organic molecules (e.g. [^{123}I]mIBG, 2-[^{18}F]fluoro-2-deoxyglucose). Reasons for the lack of structural knowledge are manifold. In the past it may not have been regarded as a regulatory requirement because the complexes are administered in trace amounts; by the same token, the small amount/concentration has also made it difficult to determine molecular structures because conventional analytical and spectroscopic techniques do not have the necessary sensitivity. Scaling up the quantity/concentration to levels amenable to these methods often changes the chemical nature of the complexes, due to polymerisation or oligomerisation. For example, rhenium-188 complexes of bisphosphonates prepared at the no-carrier-added level do not show any bone affinity *in vivo*, whereas if carrier rhenium is added to increase the concentration, bone affinity is observed (Verdera *et al.* 1997).

A pertinent example highlighting the need for structural characterisation of the labelled complexes as well as cold-kit constituents is that of the ^{99m}Tc-DMSA complexes. Mixing the dimercaptosuccinic acid chelator with stannous chloride and pertechnetate at the acidic pH (3–4) induced by the dimercaptosuccinic acid gives rise to the well-known renal perfusion imaging agent, whose structure, and metal oxidation state, are uncertain. It is commonly known as 'trivalent' ^{99m}Tc-DMSA, although there is no definitive evidence that the metal is in fact trivalent. The mechanism by which the complex is trapped in the kidney is also uncertain (Vanlicrazumenic, Petrovic 1981, 1982a,b; Vanlic-Razumenic 1999). Attempts to characterise the active species by increasing the concentration and applying spectroscopic techniques have not proved conclusive (Ikeda *et al.* 1976). On the other hand, mixing the same ligand and reducing agent with pertechnetate at mildly basic pH (8–9) yields new complexes with completely different *in-vivo* biodistribution, showing reduced uptake in kidney and high affinity for bone metastatic sites and certain soft-tissue tumours, notably medullary thyroid carcinoma (Ohta *et al.* 1984) (Figure 35.1). The structure of this

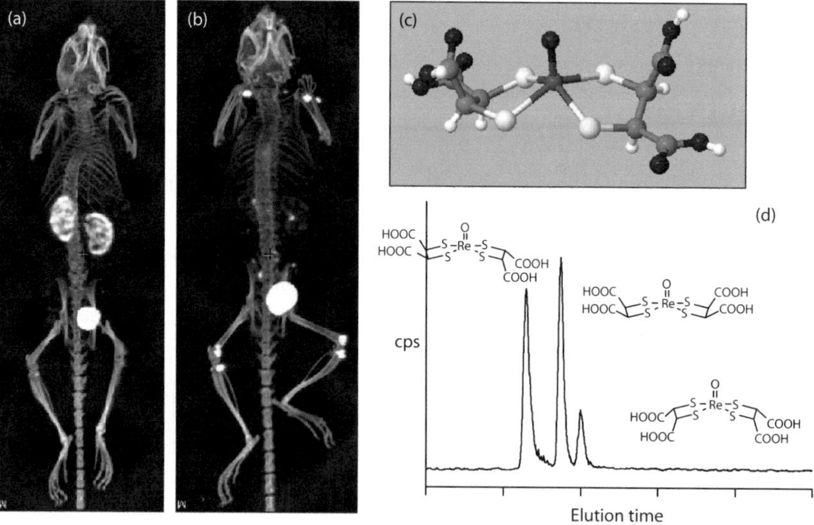

Figure 35.1 Characterisation of ^{99m}Tc-dimercaptosuccinic acid complexes. (a) SPECT/CT scan of a mouse injected with 'trivalent' ^{99m}Tc-DMSA complex showing renal perfusion. (b) SPECT/CT scan of a mouse injected with pentavalent ^{99m}Tc-DMSA complex showing uptake in regions of bone metabolism. (Images courtesy of Dr Fijs van Leewen, Netherlands Cancer Institute.) (c) Structure of pentavalent rhenium–DMSA complex determined by X-ray crystallography. (d) HPLC radiochromatogram of pentavalent ^{188}Re-DMSA complexes, showing isomerism; the UV-visible chromatogram and the ^{99m}Tc analogue show an identical pattern of peaks, confirming the structural identity of the radioactive complexes (Blower *et al.* 1991).

complex was subsequently determined by comparing its chromatographic behaviour (see methods later in this section) with spectroscopically characterised samples of the 'cold' technetium and rhenium analogues (Blower *et al.* 1991, 1992, 1998; Singh *et al.* 1993). (In fact, technetium has no stable isotopes – the isotope ^{99}Tc, which is the gamma-decay product of ^{99m}Tc, is available in relatively bulky quantities as a fission waste product from nuclear reactors. It has proved extremely useful for studying the structural coordination chemistry of technetium using conventional chemical spectroscopic and analytical methods (Tisato *et al.* 2006). This was feasible because, unlike the case with the 'trivalent' form, the chromatographic behaviour of the complex was easily studied and was not affected by scaling up.

Similar issues remain with other 'first-generation' technetium radiopharmaceuticals: the bisphosphonate complexes (e.g. MDP, HDP) used for bone scans, and the DTPA complex (see Figure 35.2 for chelator structures) used for dynamic renal scanning and lung ventilation studies are not structurally defined and not homogeneous (that is, the solutions contain a mixture of complexes of variable structure), because the ligands were not purpose-designed to match the coordination requirements particular to technetium.

Other complexes in current use that were developed more recently (1980s onwards), such as the mercaptoacetyl triglycine (MAG3) complex (Figure 35.2) are generally better-defined and exploit chelators that are more specifically designed to form stable complexes. However, even the case of ^{99m}Tc-MAG3 raises another structural issue, that of stereoisomerism and chirality, which is a frequent complication (albeit one that is too often ignored). Although the MAG3 ligand has no stereoisomers, once it is complexed to

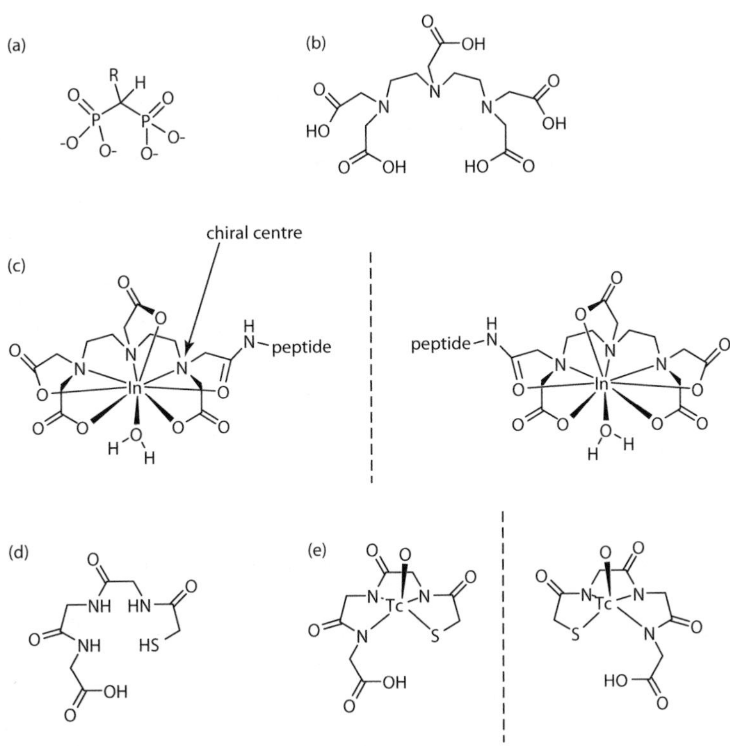

Figure 35.2 Structures and isomerism of ligands and complexes. (a) 1,1-Bisphosphonate ligands used in ^{99m}Tc bone imaging agents; when R = H, the ligand is methylene diphosphonate (MDP). (b) Diethylenetriamine pentaacetic acid (DTPA). (c) ^{111}In complex of DTPA-peptide conjugate showing chirality induced by complexation of the metal. The two mirror image forms are non-superimposable, chemically separable and may behave differently *in vivo*. (d) Mercaptoacetyltriglycine (MAG3) used as a ligand for ^{99m}Tc in dynamic renal scanning and as a bifunctional chelator for ^{99m}Tc and ^{188}Re. (e) Chirality induced by complexation with technetium; the mirror image forms are not superimposable.

technetium two enantiomers (non-identical mirror images of one another, see Figure 35.2) form that could, in principle, have different biological behaviour in the chiral *in-vivo* environment (although, in this particular case, the manufacturers state that the two enantiomers behave the same, at least insofar as dynamic renal scanning is concerned).

Proteins and peptides

Proteins (e.g. antibodies) and peptides are becoming increasingly important as a basis for molecular imaging. Modification of these molecules for attachment of a radiolabel must as far as possible preserve the binding affinity for the target, and ensure homogeneous structure. This in turn requires site-specific labelling methods. Many proteins and peptides have been investigated, sometimes without due regard for these principles, leading to the risk that molecular targeting strategies that are sound in principle may fail (and be abandoned) when the products tested give sub-optimal performance because of lack of attention to molecular design and characterisation. The importance of these considerations, and the approaches to dealing with them, depend on the size of the biomolecule. Very small peptides with just a few amino acid residues (molecular weight <2000) may be very strongly affected in both binding affinity and pharmacokinetics by the modifications required for labelling. However, control over the bioconjugation chemistry to achieve the desired properties, including homogeneity, is relatively easy to achieve in these cases because the synthesis is straightforward. There is likely to be only one reactive site in the smallest peptides; and if this is not the case, solid phase peptide synthesis with chelator-derivatised amino acids can be used to incorporate the prosthetic group specifically at the chosen location (Greenland *et al.* 2003; Surfraz *et al.* 2007; Armstrong *et al.* 2008). At the other end of the scale, very large proteins such as monoclonal antibodies (molecular weight >150 000) have so many potential sites for conjugation of chelators or prosthetic groups that modification of a small number of them (e.g. one or two) is very unlikely significantly to alter target binding affinity or pharmacokinetics; site-specificity is difficult to achieve but is often unnecessary. The most challenging molecules lie in between these extremes. Two examples of labelled proteins in this range are provided here to illustrate the challenges: tissue inhibitor of metalloproteinase (Giersing *et al.* 2001) and annexin-V (Tait *et al.* 2006).

N-TIMP-2 is the N-terminal domain of tissue inhibitor of metalloproteinase-2, a small protein (molecular weight ~14 000) that binds with high affinity to the active site of some classes of matrix metalloproteinases (MMPs). MMPs become highly expressed and active in various tissue pathologies involving breakdown of the extracellular matrix, such as cancer metastasis and atherosclerosis. N-TIMP-2 was selected for labelling as the basis of a radiopharmaceutical for imaging MMP activity. Its labelling with indium-111 using DTPA as a bifunctional chelator presents a good example to illustrate the importance of site-specific labelling. Incubation of the protein with DTPA cyclic anhydride gave rise to a mixture of conjugates (Figure 35.3) with different numbers of lysine-DTPA modifications in the molecule. Using methods described later in this section, it was shown that molecules carrying only one DTPA are modified at a region of the protein not involved in MMP binding, whereas those that carry two are modified in addition at a lysine within the MMP-binding region of the protein and thus have lost all activity (Figure 35.3). Thus, radiolabelling of the mixed conjugates would give a product in which a significant fraction of the radioactivity will not bind to the target. Moreover, the problem is amplified because each molecule of the doubly-modified fraction of the protein would carry twice as many indium-111 labels as the singly-modified form, so a disproportionately high fraction of the imaging signal would derive from inactive protein. The problem was solved in this case because it was possible to separate the different labelled forms by ion-exchange chromatography and discard the unmodified and doubly-modified protein (Giersing *et al.* 2001).

Often it is difficult or impossible to separate the differently modified forms of the protein, and in such cases it is necessary to devise bioconjugation methods that are site-specific. The design of a site-specifically modified annexin-V illustrates both the problem and a possible solution. Annexin-V is a protein that binds to phosphatidylserine (PS) residues exposed by cell membrane fragmentation during apoptosis, and labelled forms have been of interest for imaging cell

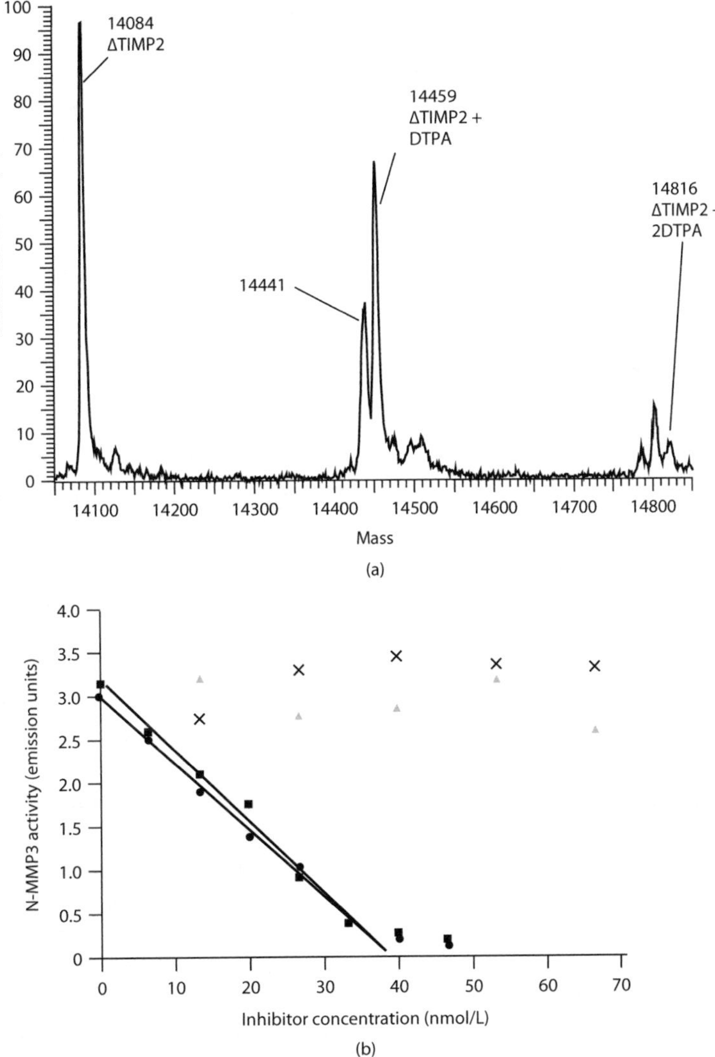

Figure 35.3 (a) Deconvoluted electrospray mass spectrum of N-TIMP-2 protein after incubation with the cyclic anhydride of DTPA. Unmodified protein gives a peak at $m = 14\,084$; a group of peaks around 14 459 appears due to conjugates with one DTPA; the additional peaks are due to DTPA cross-linking between two lysines (14 441) and to trace metal ion complexation by the DTPA (peaks around 14 500) (b) Stromelysin inhibition assay of the separated protein conjugates: unmodified N-TIMP-2 (♦); singly modified protein DTPA-N-TIMP-2 (■); doubly modified protein $(DTPA)_2$-N-TIMP-2 (×); myoglobin negative control (▲). This assay shows that the second modification abolishes the stromelysin-inhibiting activity and hence that site specificity of protein modification can be critical. Reprinted (in part) with permission from Giersing B K *et al.* (2001). Synthesis and characterization of In-111-DTPA-N-TIMP-2: A radiopharmaceutical for imaging matrix metalloproteinase expression. *Bioconjugate Chemistry* 12: 964-971. Copyright 2001 American Chemical Society.

death, for example during cancer treatment. It has four distinct target binding domains, each requiring calcium binding to facilitate interaction with PS. To preserve maximum target affinity, all four domains must remain active after labelling. Modification with bifunctional chelators at lysine residues in the conventional way leads to mixtures of products including unmodified protein, and singly-, doubly-, triply- etc., modified proteins. The presence of unmodified protein reduces the achievable specific activity, while multiple modification causes some inactivation of protein because the calcium-binding domains have several lysine residues that can be modified. This reduces target affinity and leads to poor biodistribution. Once again, the more heavily modified protein molecules, and hence those with the least binding affinity, are disproportionately represented in the radioactive imaging signal because they carry more radiolabel per molecule. The distribution of the various species in the mixture of products (whose frequencies in the mixture depend statistically on the average stoichiometry), and the consequent distribution of radioactivity among these species, is shown in Figure 35.4 (Tait *et al.* 2006). These figures illustrate quantitatively the potentially large deleterious effect on imaging quality caused by statistical mixtures of differently labelled species. The approach taken by the authors was to engineer an amino acid sequence into the protein at a location remote from the four PS-binding sites to allow site-specific labelling (Tait *et al.* 2006). The affinity data shown in Figure 35.4 demonstrate the value of this approach, compared with the non-site-specifically labelled mixtures, in ensuring the highest possible affinity. The importance of a well-characterised, homogeneous molecular tracer is clear, as in turn is the need for methods of determining the structure and homogeneity.

Small peptides and stereoisomerism

Even a homogeneous biomolecule that can be site-specifically labelled can become inhomogeneous as a result of the labelling process. The bioconjugate reaction between cysteinyl thiol and maleimide, for example, generates a chiral centre which, since the protein or peptide is itself chiral, will give rise to two diastereomers with potentially different biological behaviour. Even when the attachment of a prosthetic group does not induce such isomerism, the labelling might. For example, the MAG3 ligand shown in Figure 35.2 is often used as a bifunctional chelator for ^{99m}Tc and $^{186/188}$Re. It has no isomerism and does not induce any on conjugation to proteins by amide bond formation at a lysine or N-terminal amino group. However, on formation of the technetium complex, a chiral centre is formed (Figure 35.2), which gives rise to two diastereomers by virtue of the chiral protein or peptide to which it is attached. These are in principle chromatographically separable and may have different biological behaviour. Another example is ^{111}In-labelling of DTPA derivatives. Reaction of DTPA cyclic anhydride with peptide amino groups generates a DTPA conjugate without chirality because the nitrogen atoms invert rapidly at room temperature. However, complexation with the In^{3+} locks the nitrogen configuration without any control over which of the two enantiomers is formed (Figure 35.2). Thus, once again two separable and chemically distinct diastereomers are formed. Clearly, then, it is potentially important to be able to separate and identify these isomers to confirm that one does not degrade the performance of the other.

Particulates and nanoparticles

Particulate radiopharmaceuticals utilise particle size as part of the mechanism of biological targeting. Control and uniformity of particle size is therefore critical to function, and methods for measuring the distribution of particle sizes are accordingly needed. Particle size distribution is difficult to control, but the advent of the specialist science of nanotechnology has generated improvements in this field. An example of its importance is the rather variable cell-labelling behaviour of the particulate tracer ^{99m}Tc-SnF_2 colloid, developed for the phagocytic labelling of white blood cells for imaging of infection and inflammation (McClelland *et al.* 2003) (Figure 35.5). Labelling of isolated leukocytes with this agent gave highly irreproducible labelling efficiency, and studies of particle size and aggregation behaviour were performed to seek a cause of this irreproducibility. The fraction of radioactivity trapped on selected filter membranes with selected pore sizes, and light scattering measurements, gave a high degree of variation in effective particle size among different samples and within individual samples. Electron microscopy showed a wide variety of effective particle sizes caused by aggregation. These results highlighted that even small changes in the particle size distribution between samples can be greatly amplified when this is analysed in terms of the fraction of radioactivity, rather than the number of particles, associated with particular size ranges. It is quite possible that a cubic relationship may exist between particle diameter and radioactivity per particle, so that a small number of large particles could harbour a very large fraction of the radioactivity.

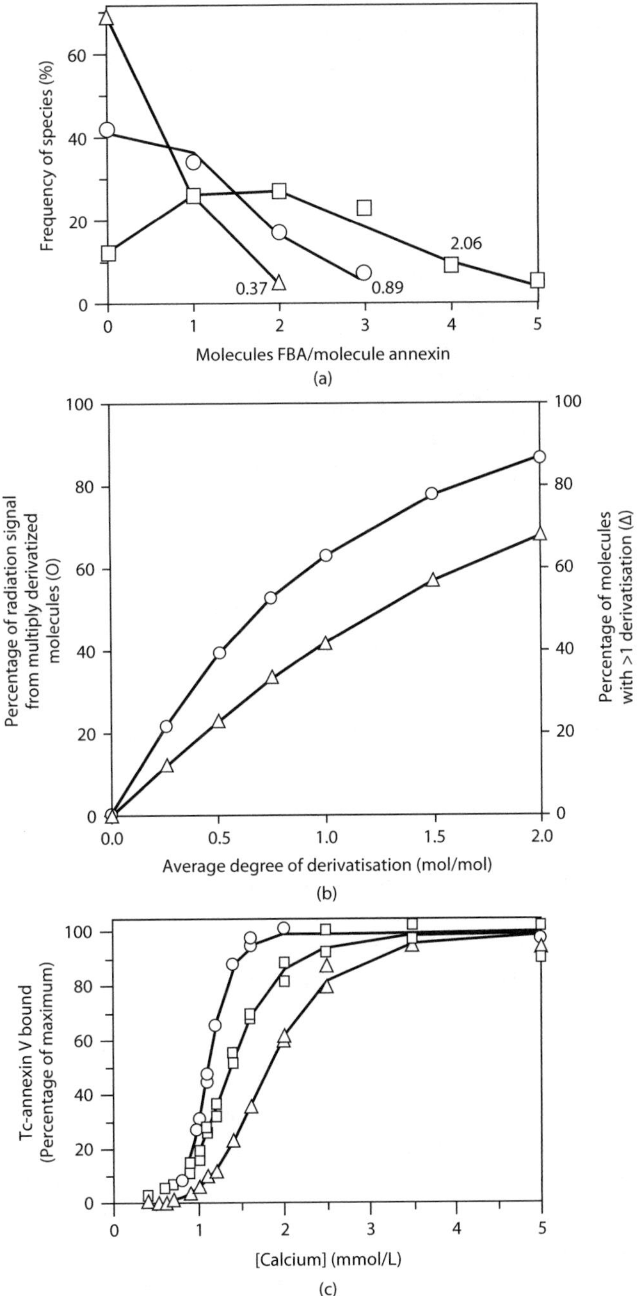

Figure 35.4 Site-specific and non-site-specific labelling of annexin V. (a) Frequency of protein molecules containing different numbers of prosthetic groups in mixtures with various average stoichiometric ratios of prosthetic group to protein, indicated by numerical labels 0.37 (Δ), 0.89 (○) and 2.06 (□). The lines represent the statistical model, while the data points represent the experimental values. Even with an optimal prosthetic group:protein ratio, there is a large contribution from unconjugated and/or multiply conjugated species, both of which are undesirable. (b) Chart showing the relative amplification of signal from multiply conjugated species in the mixture; these species are the least functional but contribute a disproportionately high radioactive signal. (c) Target binding affinity curves for singly, site-specifically ^{99m}Tc-labelled annexin V, labelled via designed N-terminal sequence (○); non-site-specifically ^{99m}Tc-labelled annexin V, labelled using HYNIC (□); and the HYNIC derivative with additional non-site-specific biotinylation (Δ). This comparison shows the benefits of minimal, site-specific modification of proteins. Reproduced with permission from Tait *et al.* (2006).

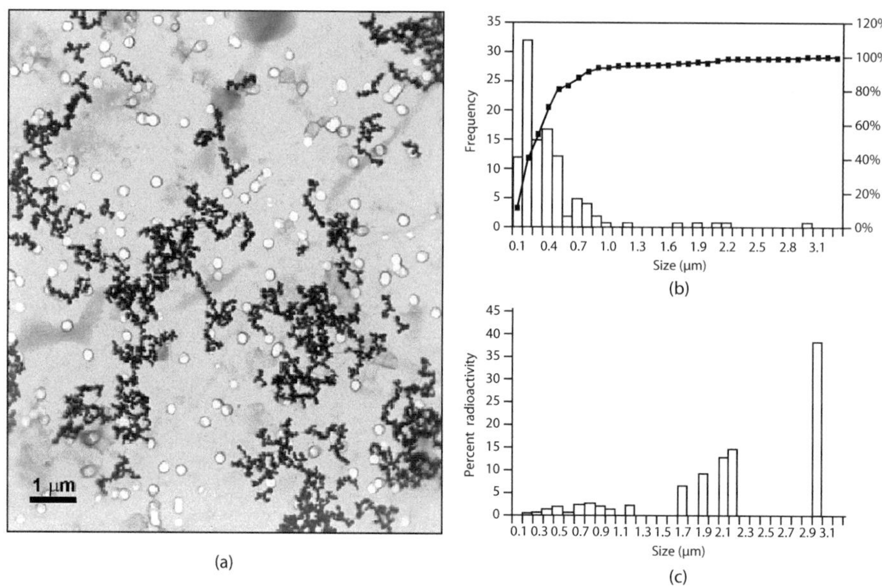

Figure 35.5 Importance of uniform particle size in particulate radiopharmaceuticals. (a) Electron micrograph of ^{99m}Tc-SnF_2 particles captured on a 0.22 μm filter, showing variation in aggregate sizes. (b) Aggregate size distribution measured from electron micrographs such as those on the left (bars) and cumulative distribution (percentage of particles below particle size limit). (c) Particle size distribution in the same sample, expressed as radioactivity bound to specific aggregate sizes rather than numbers of aggregates, showing the disproportionate amplification of signal from the larger particle sizes and that a small irreproducibility in particle size distribution could have very critical effects on biodistribution of radioactivity. From McClelland *et al.* (2003). Reproduced with permission from Wolters Kluwer Health.

If particles of different sizes give different labelling efficiency, this small irreproducibility in particle size distribution could lead to a very wide variation in labelling efficiency from sample to sample. Therefore, application of these methods (filtration, light scattering, electron microscopy) for careful characterisation of particle size distribution is required not just to measure frequency of particle size but more importantly, percentage radioactivity associated with each particle size (Figure 35.5).

Experimental methods for studying molecular structure and function of radiopharmaceuticals

The challenge in molecular characterisation throughout all areas of radiopharmaceutical chemistry arises mainly from the very small (tracer) quantities of material – the very same attribute that gives radionuclide imaging its extraordinary sensitivity for imaging molecular processes without perturbing them. For example, a typical technetium-99m generator eluate contains about 10^{-8} mol/L technetium with a radioactive concentration of several GBq per mL. A typical patient dose may contain of the order of a picomole of technetium. These quantities are well below those required for conventional analytical techniques such as nuclear magnetic resonance (NMR), UV-visible spectroscopy, IR spectroscopy, X-ray crystallography, extended X-ray absorption fine structure (EXAFS), etc. It has already been pointed out above that at the low concentrations involved, the molecular structure may differ from that which prevails at higher concentration. Nevertheless, structural characterisation must involve studying the structure of 'cold' analogues, with due regard for checking that the chemistry is the same at the tracer level (carrier-free or no-carrier-added) as it is at the macroscopic level at which spectroscopic methods are applicable, by comparing them side-by-side. At these concentrations, the only way to reliably detect radiopharmaceuticals in order to perform these comparisons is by means of their radioactivity. To take advantage of this, methods of characterising

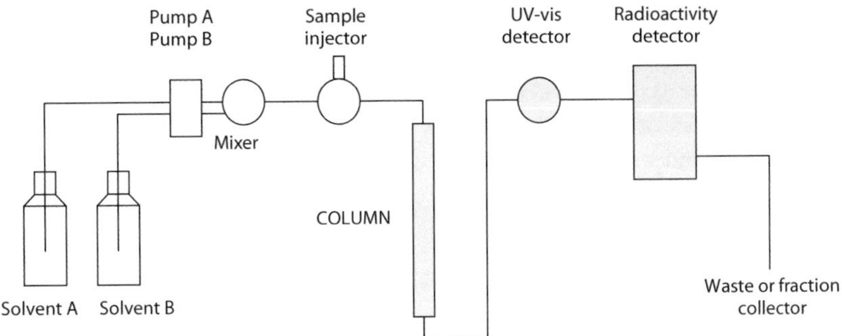

Figure 35.6 Typical HPLC configuration for use with radioactive samples.

radiopharmaceuticals rely on studies of their chromatographic, solubility and electrophoretic properties. The most discriminating methods are various forms of high performance liquid chromatography (HPLC), with a gamma-ray detector to monitor the radioactive tracer component (which usually cannot be detected by other methods) and a UV detector to monitor the cold or carrier-added analogue (see Figure 35.6).

An example of the application of this analytical approach is that shown in Figure 35.1. The technetium oxobis(dimercaptosuccinate) complex was synthesised and purified using technetium-99 along with its rhenium analogue. The identity of the complex was confirmed by NMR, elemental analysis, IR and UV-visible spectroscopy, and the rhenium complex was crystallised and its structure confirmed by X-ray crystallography. The three isomers were distinguished by a combination of NMR and crystallography. The technetium-99 and rhenium complexes were compared with the technetium-99m (no-carrier-added) complex by several chromatographic techniques including reversed-phase HPLC. Since the latter has the necessary discriminating power to separate all three isomers, the similarity of the visible-wavelength chromatogram with the radiochromatogram provided a high level of confidence that the complexes formed at the tracer and bulk levels were identical. To strengthen the conclusion, other chromatographic methods including size-exclusion chromatography and electrophoresis were applied (Blower *et al.* 1991, 1992).

An important deficiency of HPLC is that radioactive compounds that have very long elution times, or that fail to elute at all, are not detected, because it is not easy to measure column-bound radioactivity. Therefore, additional techniques that guarantee to capture all of the radioactivity in the sample should be applied. These include thin-layer chromatography (TLC) and instant thin-layer chromatography (ITLC), in which all activity on the chromatogram is accounted for by scanning or counting, and column chromatography using small disposable columns that can be counted in the gamma counter or dose calibrator. This advantage comes at the cost of relatively poor resolution, so it is always advisable, or essential, to combine these methods with HPLC.

The methods used in this example are among those discussed in more detail in the following sections. The equipment used to detect the radioactivity for these techniques (e.g. flow-through gamma detectors, TLC plate scanners, phosphor imaging devices, etc.) is described in Chapters 4 and 5.

High performance liquid chromatography

High performance liquid chromatography (HPLC) is a form of column chromatography (Baldas *et al.* 1989; Franssen *et al.* 1994; Hyllbrant *et al.* 1999) that gains its extremely powerful separating capability from use of solid phases consisting of very small, uniform, tightly packed particles, which consequently offer a very high surface area for analyte binding and exchange, but which also imposes a high resistance to flow. The resulting high backpressure requires high-pressure pumps capable of delivering a very uniform and reproducible flow rate, as well as fittings and tubing capable of withstanding the high pressures. A typical set-up is illustrated schematically in Figure 35.6. The main components are the column itself, one or more solvent (mobile phase) reservoirs, one or more pumps, a mixing device, flow-through detectors for both bulk (usually UV-visible absorbance) and radioactive (usually gamma) components of the effluent from the column, and a waste receptacle or fraction collector. The detectors are typically in tandem with one another so that data are collected in two channels a few seconds apart (the time-lag depending on the flow rate and the volume of tubing between the two detectors).

The data streams from these detectors are captured simultaneously by a two-channel chart recorder, or more often nowadays an analogue–digital converter interfaced with a computer. Two or more solvents are usually used together, with the relative proportions controlled by the programmable, microprocessor-controlled pumps. This arrangement permits solvent gradients to be used, so that the sample can be loaded into the column and eluted with solvents of gradually changing composition to ensure, where possible, full elution of all analytes. For optimal reproducibility, isocratic elution (i.e. with a mobile phase of constant composition) is generally preferred, but for many practical purposes it is faster and more convenient to use a gradient.

If relatively high levels of radioactivity are used, and sensitivity is not a limiting factor, in-line flow detection of radioactivity is preferred for reasons of convenience, time economy and good resolution. This requires a simple set-up in which the tubing carrying the eluate from the column is passed in front of a gamma detector (e.g. sodium iodide crystal), usually after passing through the UV-visible absorbance detector. This generates a data stream of counts/second versus time that can be plotted together with or superimposed on the UV-visible chromatogram in real time. Where this method offers insufficient sensitivity (because the radioactivity is in front of the detector for only a fraction of a second, limiting counting statistics), it may be necessary to collect fractions using a fraction collector, and count them later in a gamma counter. This method provides high sensitivity but is time consuming and resolution is severely limited by the fraction size. In general, radiochromatography is a perpetual compromise between resolution and sensitivity.

The separation of analytes on the column relies on the relative affinity of the analyte molecules for the stationary phase and the mobile phase. The most common mode is reverse phase, in which the stationary phase particles are coated with a hydrophobic material e.g. 'C_{18}' (a $C_{18}H_{37}$ or C_8H_{17} alkyl derivative) while a more polar solvent is used as the mobile phase (often mixtures of methanol or acetonitrile with water). The analytes are separated according to their lipophilicity – in the dynamic equilibrium, the most lipophilic compounds spend the most time associated with the hydrophobic stationary phase and elute relatively late, requiring a higher proportion of non-polar solvent in the mobile phase. Less often used is 'normal phase' in which, conversely, the stationary phase is polar (usually silica or alumina) and the mobile phase is less so.

In recent decades a much wider range of stationary phase functionality has become available, such as ion exchange (cation or anion) for separation according to charge and ion-pairing properties, size exclusion for protein and polymer separation according to molecular size, and mixed modes. The best source of information about these is the manufacturers' catalogues and web sites. In size-exclusion chromatography, the stationary phase consists of a porous material in which the pores are too small to accommodate molecules above a certain chosen diameter (typically with a molecular weight of a few thousand) but can accommodate mobile phase molecules and small molecules and ions. This makes part of the volume of the mobile phase inaccessible to the larger molecules, which therefore have a smaller volume of distribution throughout the column and elute faster, while the smaller analytes are delayed because they can enter the pores. A typical reversed-phase HPLC method involves loading the sample in an aqueous or partly aqueous solution, and eluting with a gradient starting with a high proportion of water with gradual increase in the percentage of a less polar solvent such as acetonitrile or methanol. 'Modifiers' such as organic-soluble salts and acids (e.g. tetrabutylammonium salts, trifluoroacetic acid) are often used to allow the more hydrophilic ions to form ion pairs, allowing them to associate more strongly with the non-polar stationary phase and thus giving better separation. In ion-exchange chromatography, the gradient often involves a gradual change of pH and/or ionic strength.

The advantages of HPLC are its high discriminating power and resolution, giving confidence in assignment of chemical identity with non-radioactive standards, and versatility by virtue of the range of packing materials. Very closely similar molecules can be separated, such as the isomers of the pentavalent technetium-DMSA complex described above (Figure 35.1), and diastereomers of indium-111-DTPA peptide conjugates (Figure 35.2). The disadvantages are that it is expensive and demanding on bench space and operator time, as well as the aforementioned difficulty in accounting for radioactivity that may not have eluted from the column.

These attributes make radioHPLC an essential item in the radiochemistry development laboratory, but it is of no major value in the day-to-day quality control of radiopharmaceuticals. This purpose is better served by cheaper and quicker methods that may not have the resolving power of HPLC but are much more practical for day-to-day use when the purpose is to determine the presence of likely impurities of known identity, with confidence that all radioactivity is accounted for. These methods (e.g. TLC, ITLC, paper or membrane electrophoresis, solvent extraction, filtration, disposable mini-chromatography columns), which have important uses in the research laboratory too, are described fully in Chapter 23.

Mass spectrometry

It has been said already that conventional methods of spectroscopic characterisation of molecules are difficult to apply to radiopharmaceuticals at the tracer level because they lack the necessary sensitivity. However, one analytical method has developed in recent years to the point where tracer-level labelled molecules are within its analytical powers – mass spectrometry. Particularly since the advent of electrospray ionisation (ESI) and atmospheric pressure chemical ionisation (APCI), mass spectrometry has become an extremely useful analytical tool in radiopharmaceutics, and a few laboratories now perform mass spectrometry on radiolabelled compounds (Franssen *et al.* 1994; Hyllbrant *et al.* 1999; Liu 2005). Since these ionisation modes ionise the analytes directly from solution (rather than requiring deposition onto a solid probe or matrix), they can be used in conjunction with liquid chromatography (LC) to give the 'hyphenated' technique LC-MS, offering the possibility to combine UV-visible and gamma detection (as described above) with mass spectrometry. The eluate from the HPLC column passes through each sequentially (and through the mass spectrometer last), offering an unprecedented quantity of information from a single sample.

The process of ESI (El-Aneed *et al.* 2009) involves first the mobile phase and analyte being nebulised (broken into small droplets) as it emerges from the tip of a charged capillary. The mobile-phase solvent evaporates from the droplets (desolvation), and the charge density in the droplets increases until the Rayleigh limit (10^8 V/cm^3) is reached, whereupon the droplet undergoes coulomb explosions and breaks into smaller droplets. Under the influence of the electrostatic potentials in the spray chamber, the analyte ion is desorbed from the droplet as ions. This process is rapid and the ionisation efficiency depends largely on the extent to which the analyte molecules were ionised in solution. Although no ionisation technique analyses ions truly in their native solution state, ESI is the nearest approximation to this ideal. The ions formed are then analysed and separated according to their mass-to-charge ratio (m/z) by the spectrometer (e.g. quadrupole, time of flight (TOF), ion trap, ion cyclotron resonance, magnetic sectors), and then detected (by a photomultiplier, electron multiplier, microchannel plate, or image current plate). Ionisation can be in positive or negative mode to optimise detectability of species that ionise most readily as cations or anions, respectively. Ionisation can also be tuned to be more or less energetic, leading to more or less fragmentation, by altering the energy of collisions with the collision gas or by controlling the accelerating voltage or the temperature or pressure of the collision gas.

Data from the detectors are output to a computer to produce a mass spectrum. If the mass spectrometer is in tandem with liquid chromatography, an additional chromatogram can be produced corresponding to the total ion current (TIC) detected as a function of elution time, giving an indication of the relative sensitivity of the mass spectrometer to the different analytes present in the sample, by comparison with the UV-visible and radioactivity detector chromatograms. The mass spectrum of all or part of the TIC chromatogram, including a single selected chromatographic peak, can be analysed separately.

Small molecules/ions usually give singly charged anions or cations, with m/z numerically equal to m, unless multiply-ionisable groups are present (e.g. multivalent metal ions, polyanions such as phosphonates, etc.) with m/z numerically equal to $m/2$, $m/3$, etc. Large molecules such as proteins may ionise by multiple protonation, in which case ions with m/z

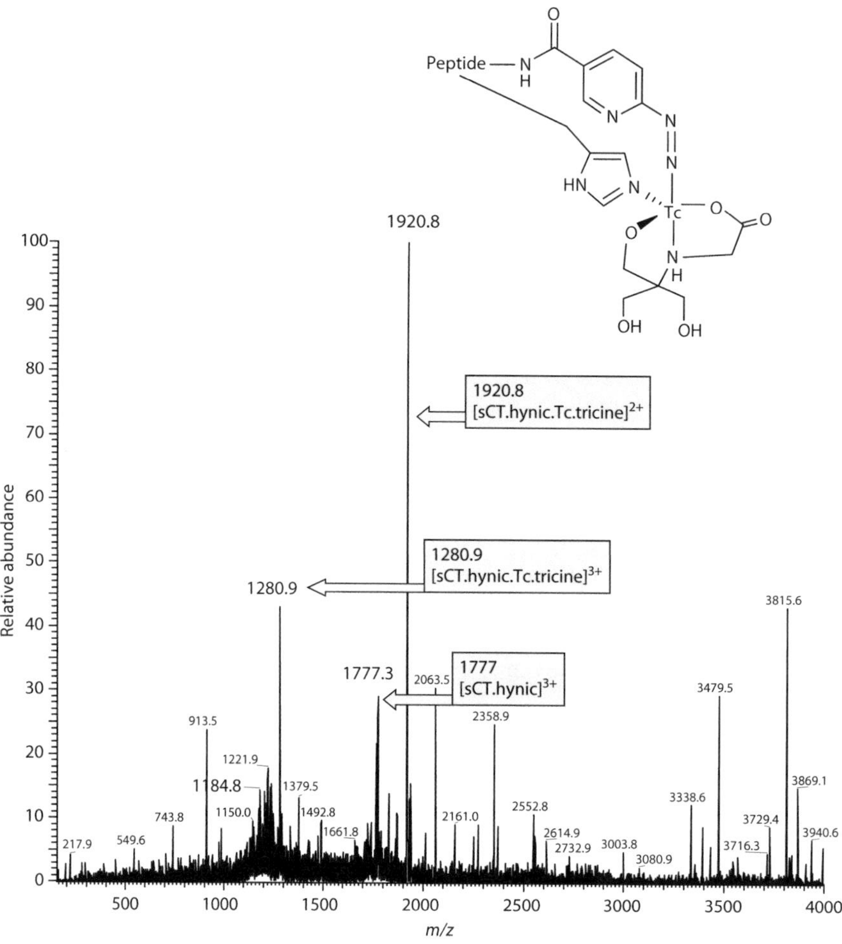

Figure 35.7 Electrospray ionisation mass spectrometry (ES-MS) of salmon calcitonin-HYNIC conjugate labelled with ^{99m}Tc in the presence of tricine co-ligand. The ES-MS spectrum showed that the mass added to the peptide upon labelling corresponded to one technetium, and one tricine ligand with the loss of five protons, suggesting a coordination sphere similar to that shown on the right.

corresponding to $(m+H)^+$, $(m+2H)^{2+}$, $(m+3H)^{3+}$, etc., are detected. Spectra with these multiple *m/z* peaks originating from the same molecular species can be 'deconvoluted' mathematically to give a spectrum of parent molecule masses (El-Aneed *et al.* 2009).

The value of LCMS is illustrated in the following examples of different types of radiopharmaceutical molecules. The examples of ^{111}In-DTPA-N-TIMP-2 given above (Figure 35.3) show how mass spectrometry can be used with proteins to identify structural features of the modification, such as the number of bifunctional molecules attached (Giersing *et al.* 2001) It can also detect occupancy of the bifunctional chelator by trace metal ions (Figure 35.3) and, by fragmenting the protein using, for example, trypsin digestion, it can be used to identify the location of modifications within the molecule. Where there is uncertainty about the nature of the metal-binding site (e.g. in the case of protein labelling with ^{99m}Tc-HYNIC, the number of ancillary ligands such as oxo, chloro, or ancillary chelators such as tricine), the mass spectrum can provide the missing information. If resolution is good enough to count accurately the number of protons displaced by the radioactive metal, it can even determine the oxidation state of the metal. For example, ES-MS showed that technetium labelling of HYNIC-derivatised proteins was accompanied by loss of five protons, leading to a

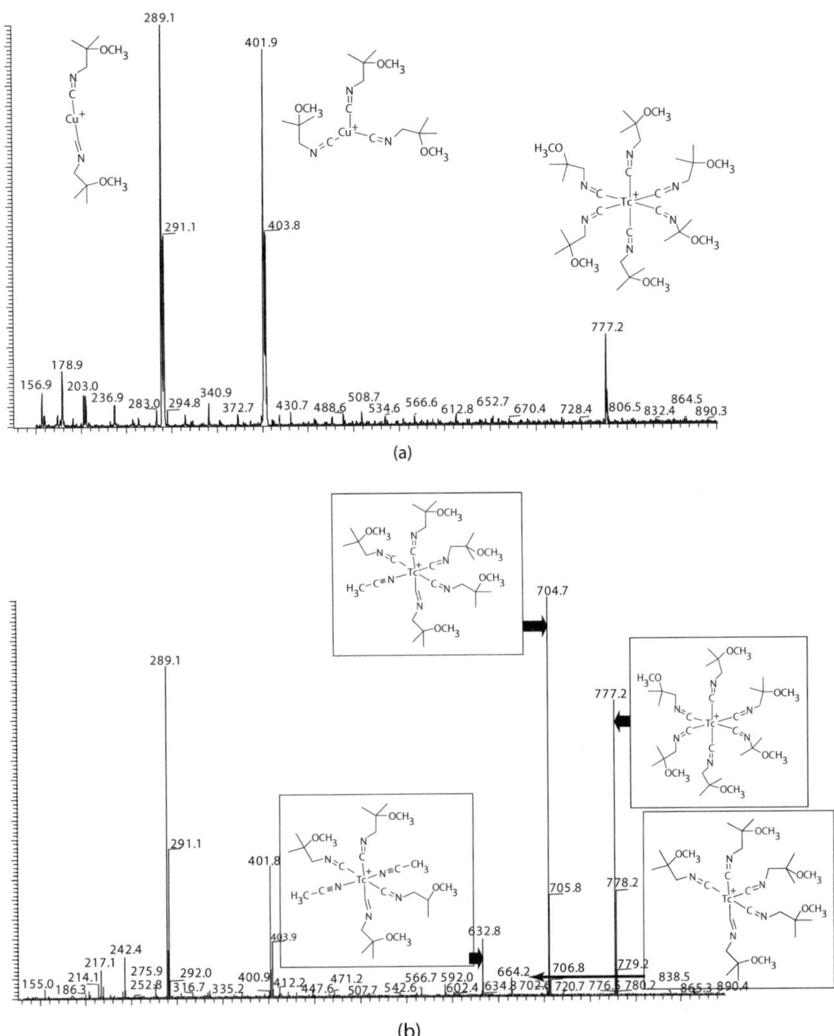

Figure 35.8 Electrospray ionisation mass spectrum of ^{99m}Tc-sestamibi. (a) Kit prepared in the normal way with boiling, showing only one Tc-containing species $[Tc(MIBI)_6]^+$, along with the copper-MIBI complex precursor that is a constituent of the cold kit. (b) Highest-lipophilicity eluate from HPLC of a kit prepared at room temperature, showing additional Tc(I) complexes with five and four MIBI ligands, which cannot be separately detected by the TLC/ITLC quality control procedure.

formal oxidation state assignment of +5 for the technetium. It also showed that the coordination sphere of the technetium did not include chloro or oxo ligands (Figure 35.7) (Greenland *et al.* 2003; King *et al.* 2007). Mass spectrometry of proteins with reduced disulfide groups directly labelled with Tc or Re, by reduction in the presence of water soluble phosphines (as reducing agent), showed that the two metals did not form structurally analogous complexes: the bound technetium was in oxidation state +3 and retained a phosphine in its coordination sphere, whereas the bound rhenium was in oxidation state +5 and it retained an oxo ligand but no phosphine. Dimers of protein bridged by the metal were observed in both cases along with labelled monomers (Greenland, Blower 2005).

An example of application of ES-MS to small molecules is the insight gained into possible impurities present in the ^{99m}Tc-sestamibi complex. Positive mode ES-MS of a properly prepared kit showed that the cationic Tc(I) complex with six MIBI ligands is readily detected and is the only significant technetium-containing species (Figure 35.8). However, if the kit is not subjected to its normal boiling procedure but is instead prepared at room temperature, a number of intermediates are detected in which the Tc is reduced to Tc(I) but fewer than six MIBI ligands are present; species such as $[Tc(MIBI)_5]^+$, $[Tc(MIBI)_5(MeCN)]^+$, $[Tc(MIBI)_4(MeCN)_2]^+$ are detected along with the required complex $[Tc(MIBI)_6]^+$. The acetonitrile was not present in the kit and was probably recruited from the LC solvent, suggesting that a labile ligand (e.g. water) may have been present in the coordination sphere of the Tc(I) complex en route to the final product. The presence of these multiple species, which are separable by HPLC but not by the TLC/ITLC methods used for quality control, shows that in this case the quality control methods are not adequate to detect likely radioactive impurities in the product.

Summary

Conventional analytical techniques, on the whole, are not directly applicable to tracer-level radiopharmaceutical molecules because they lack the required sensitivity. Instead they have to be applied to cold analogues prepared in relative bulk in order to characterise the products and use them as bona fide chromatographic standards. These are compared by various separation methods with the radioactive tracer-level compounds. The central, most important and most widely used method for this is HPLC, which has become an indispensable tool in radiopharmaceutical research. An exceptional technique is electrospray ionisation mass spectrometry which is often capable of detecting molecular ions in solution at the tracer level (10^{-6}–10^{-12} mol/L). This promises to be a valuable tool leading to the improved molecular characterisation of radiopharmaceuticals in the coming years. The ability to determine the molecular structure of radiopharmaceuticals is improving and it is important for radiopharmaceutical chemists to exploit this by adopting a critical approach to, and asking the questions about, molecular structure and how it can be controlled to improve the quality of radionuclide imaging.

References

Armstrong AF *et al.* (2008). A robust strategy for the preparation of libraries of metallopeptides. A new paradigm for the discovery of targeted molecular imaging and therapy agents. *Chem Commun*, 5532–5534.

Baldas J *et al.* (1989). Use of high performance liquid chromatography for the structural identification of technetium-99m radiopharmaceuticals at the NCA level. *J Nucl Med* 30: 1240–1248.

Blower PJ *et al.* (1991). The chemical identity of pentavalent technetium-99m-dimercaptosuccinic acid. *J Nucl Med* 32: 845–849.

Blower PJ *et al.* (1992). The chemical identity of pentavalent technetium-DMSA and editorial – small coordination-complexes in tumor imaging. [Comment on: *J Nucl Med* 1991 May;32(5):849–850]. *J Nucl Med* 33: 469–469.

Blower PJ *et al.* (1998). Pentavalent rhenium-188 dimercaptosuccinic acid for targeted radiotherapy: synthesis and preliminary animal and human studies. *Eur J Nucl Med* 25: 613–621.

El-Aneed A *et al.* (2009). Mass spectrometry, review of the basics: electrospray, MALDI, and commonly used mass analyzers. *Appl Spectrosc Rev* 44: 210–230.

Franssen EJF *et al.* (1994). Application of liquid-chromatography combined with mass-spectrometry (LC-MS) to establish identity and purity of PET-radiopharmaceuticals. *Appl Radiat Isot* 45: 937–940.

Giersing BK *et al.* (2001). Synthesis and characterization of ^{111}In-DTPA-N-TIMP-2: A radiopharmaceutical for imaging matrix metalloproteinase expression. *Bioconjug Chem* 12: 964–971.

Greenland WEP, Blower PJ (2005). Water-soluble phosphines for direct labeling of peptides with technetium and rhenium: Insights from electrospray mass spectrometry. *Bioconjug Chem* 16: 939–948.

Greenland WEP *et al.* (2003). Solid-phase synthesis of peptide radiopharmaceuticals using Fmoc-N-e-(Hynic-Boc)-Lysine, a technetium-binding amino acid: application to Tc-99m-labeled salmon calcitonin. *J Med Chem* 46: 1751–1757.

Hyllbrant B *et al.* (1999). On the use of liquid chromatography with radio- and ultraviolet absorbance detection coupled to mass spectrometry for improved sensitivity and selectivity in determination of specific radioactivity of radiopharmaceuticals. *J Pharm Biomed Anal* 20: 493–501.

Ikeda I *et al.* (1976). Chemical and biological studies on Tc-99m-DMS—II. Effect of Sn(II) on formation of various Tc-DMS complexes. *Int J Appl Radiat Isot* 27: 681–688.

King RC *et al.* (2007). How do HYNIC-conjugated peptides bind technetium? Insights from LC-MS and stability studies *Dalton Trans* 4998–5007.

Liu S (2005). 6-Hydrazinonicotinamide derivatives as bifunctional coupling agents for Tc-99m-labeling of small biomolecules. In: *Contrast Agents III: Radiopharmaceuticals – from Diagnostics to Therapeutics.* [Topics in Current Chemistry 252: 117–153]. Berlin: Springer-Verlag.

McClelland CM *et al.* (2003). Tc-99m-SnF_2 colloid 'LLK': particle size, morphology and leucocyte labelling behaviour. *Nucl Med Commun* 24: 191–202.

Ohta H *et al.* (1984). A new imaging agent for medullary carcinoma of the thyroid. *J Nucl Med* 25: 323–325.

Singh J *et al.* (1993). Studies on the preparation and isomeric composition of Re-186-pentavalent and Re-188-pentavalent rhenium dimercaptosuccinic acid complex. *Nucl Med Commun* 14: 197–203.

Surfraz MBU *et al.* (2007). Trifluoroacetyl-HYNIC peptides: Synthesis and Tc-99m radiolabeling. *J Med Chem* 50: 1418–1422.

Tait JF *et al.* (2006). Improved detection of cell death in vivo with annexin V radiolabeled by site-specific methods. *J Nucl Med* 47: 1546–1553.

Tisato F *et al.* (2006). The preparation of substitution-inert Tc-99 metal-fragments: Promising candidates for the design of new Tc-99m radiopharmaceuticals. *Coord Chem Rev* 250: 2034–2045.

Vanlic-Razumenic N (1999). Radiopharmaceutical complexes of technetium and tin: physicochemical and biochemical research. *J Radioanal Nucl Chem* 242: 235–240.

Vanlicrazumenic N, Petrovic J (1981). Biochemical-studies of the renal radiopharmaceutical compound dimercaptosuccinate.1. Subcellular-localization of DMS-Tc-99m complex in the rat-kidney in vivo. *Eur J Nucl Med* 6: 169–172.

Vanlicrazumenic N, Petrovic J (1982a). Biochemical studies of the renal radiopharmaceutical compound dimercaptosuccinate. II. Subcellular localization of 99Tc-DMS complex in the rat kidney in vivo. *Eur J Nucl Med* 7: 304–307.

Vanlicrazumenic N, Petrovic J (1982b). Preparation of technetium-99-DMS renal complex in solution and its chemical and biological characterization. *Int J Appl Radiat Isot* 33: 277–284.

Verdera ES *et al.* (1997). Rhenium-188-HEDP-kit formulation and quality control. *Radiochim Acta* 79: 113–117.

36

Evaluation of radiopharmaceuticals using cell culture models

Daniel Lloyd

Overview

Preclinical development of radiopharmaceuticals requires a thorough understanding of how the agent under investigation works at the cellular level. This is increasingly important in the field of targeted radionuclide therapy, in which agents are being developed to interact with and kill target cells. In order to fully understand, refine and improve such therapies, their interaction with, and effects upon, normal cellular process must be fully understood so that the full potential of targeted radiation can be harnessed for maximum therapeutic benefit.

A number of experimental technologies have emerged in recent years that facilitate the use of cell culture models. While many of these have been developed for the needs of other areas of scientific research, such as detecting occupational exposure to DNA-damaging agents or monitoring DNA damage response mechanisms, they are highly applicable to the evaluation of the cellular response to radiopharmaceuticals. This chapter introduces some of these useful technologies, and demonstrates how they can be applied in radiopharmaceutical research to help build a picture of how target cells respond to radiopharmaceuticals and to understand the mechanisms by which radiopharmaceuticals work. The chapter focuses largely on the development of therapeutic radiopharmaceuticals, but the technologies described can equally be applied to reagents for imaging.

Cell culture

The use of cell culture is a cornerstone of modern biology. It allows scientists to address fundamental research questions in a focused manner and in the absence of other complicating factors associated with whole animal physiology. There are fundamental aspects of radiopharmaceutical evaluation, such as biodistribution and therapeutic efficacy, that cannot be addressed in cell culture. However, there are important elements of preclinical development that benefit from experiments in isolated cells; for example, affinity, specificity for particular molecular targets, understanding of biological and cellular effects, and cytotoxicity can all be assessed in cell culture. Also, the effects of minor changes in radiopharmaceutical chemistry can often be evaluated most appropriately in cell culture prior to animal studies.

Cell culture can be roughly divided into two types. *Monolayer culture* is based on the ability of cells to grow on an adherent surface. Typically, modern adherent cell culture involves the use of disposable plasticware coated with a positively-charged growing surface; this allows adhesion molecules on certain cells to attach to the growing surface and grow and divide normally. *Suspension culture* involves the growth of cells in solution without surface attachment; this is more typically used for blood-derived cell lines such as lymphocytes. Both types of cell culture require appropriate growth media containing essential salts and minerals, amino acids, vitamins, and serum derived from animal sources; precise recipes vary according to the cell type. In some instances antibiotics, antimycotics and fungicides are used to prevent contamination, however, this is regarded by some as poor practice since long-term culture in the presence of antibiotics can promote the growth of resistant infection.

While cell culture is a valuable tool for preclinical evaluation, it is important to recognise the differences between cells growing in cultured conditions and those growing in their natural physiological environment. The loss of interactions between cells in the same tissue, and the matrix in which the cells are held, affects cell–cell communication processes. Bioavailability of nutrients to cells within tissues will be different from that for cells grown in media, and the ability to spread, migrate and proliferate in culture is much greater owing to the absence of constraining factors. None of these characteristics of the tissue environment can be reproduced in the laboratory, and this must be borne in mind when interpreting the results of cell-based studies and applying them to the whole organism.

Selection of appropriate cell culture models

Primary cell lines offer the closest match to cells found in the tissue environment. They have been subjected to no genetic modification or mutagenising treatments to alter cell growth characteristics. They have a limited growth span of between 30 and 50 doublings, which can limit their usefulness in laboratory studies; furthermore, at later stages of growth normal cellular processes can alter, which may affect study results. When primary cells are received from commercial sources they arrive with a 'passage number' that indicates the stage of growth as indicated by the number of doublings the cells have been through since being harvested from the tissue. When using primary cell lines (such as WI38 fetal lung fibroblasts) it is important that experiments within a study are undertaken on cells with the same or similar passage numbers; this ensures that results are not compromised by altered cellular characteristics at later stages of growth. This can be challenging when replicate experiments take place over a long period of time and are subject to the availability of radiopharmaceuticals. For this reason, few studies have used primary cells to evaluate radiopharmaceuticals, apart from blood cells, which arguably lose slightly less of their tissue environment in the transfer to cell culture.

A more convenient type of cell line to work with in the laboratory is one that has been 'transformed', i.e. one that will grow indefinitely in culture conditions. Transformation can be inherent within the cell line if it has been derived from a tumour. Many cells commonly used in biology have been derived from human tumours, partly because of their convenient growth characteristics that make them more suitable for experiments than primary cell lines. This circumvents the problem of undertaking experiments at similar stages of growth. However, it presents other problems in that cancer and cancer-like cells are often genetically unstable, and high spontaneous mutation rates can lead to significant changes in cellular characteristics. Since these cells grow in a continuous and unregulated manner it is tempting for individual laboratories to grow and maintain their own collections of cells. Over time, this may lead to cell collections in different laboratories having different phenotypes, or indeed contamination with other cell lines, affecting reproducibility of work between those laboratories. Regular sourcing of cell lines from reliable collections promotes good practice and increases the likelihood of robust and reproducible data.

Another option is to use primary cell lines that have been transformed in the laboratory; for example, primary WI38 fibroblasts can be transformed using simian virus-40 (SV40) so that the characteristics of the primary cell line are retained but desirable growth characteristics are introduced. However, such transformation usually has other cellular effects and, depending on the nature of the study, may be unsuitable. For instance, SV40 transformation is known to abrogate p53, an important regulator of growth and DNA damage response (Bargonetti *et al.* 1992; Sheppard *et al.* 1999). Much care therefore needs to be exercised in selecting appropriate cell models, balancing the scientific underpinning of the research question and the rigorous sourcing and maintenance of the cells, alongside the ease with which experiments can take place.

Advances in molecular biology have facilitated some of these issues and provided scientists with appropriate alternatives to existing cell lines by engineering in or out certain characteristics that help to address the research question. For instance, it is possible to genetically engineer cells to express proteins that are not usually present or which are present at very low levels. This is achieved by incorporating a cloned gene, encoding the protein of interest, into an appropriate DNA vector and then introducing the vector into the cells so that it can express the gene. This is accompanied by preparation of the control cell line in which the vector is introduced to the cells without the gene of interest. The advantage of using this recombinant technology is that it permits a direct comparison between cell lines that are identical apart from production of the single protein of interest. For instance, in a study by Parry *et al.* (2007), the lung cancer cell line A427 was transfected with the cloned DNA of the somatostatin receptor subtype 2 (sst2) to generate individual cell line clones that had differing levels of sst2 expression on the cell surface. These were then used to correlate binding, internalisation and other characteristics of a copper-64–octreotide complex *in vitro* and in an *in-vivo* mouse model.

Using the opposite approach of reducing the amount of a specific protein within a cell, a technique called RNA interference, or RNAi, has been developed in the last few years (reviewed by Martin and Caplen (2007)). Short fragments of RNA, complementary to the RNA produced during the transcription of specific genes, bind to the messenger RNA transcripts and target them for degradation. Thus it is also possible to target specific genes at the mRNA level and reduce their expression. So far this approach has not been widely applied to the study of radiopharmaceutical targeting although its widespread use in cell biology has opened up a very adaptable and powerful new avenue of radiopharmaceutical research and evaluation.

Cell binding, uptake and distribution analysis of radiopharmaceuticals

A fundamental principle in the successful development of radiopharmaceuticals is the matching of the physical emission properties of the radioactive isotope with the targeting mechanism. This is particularly crucial for therapeutic radiopharmaceuticals. There is increasing interest in radioactive isotopes emitting high-LET, short-path-length radiations such as Auger electrons and alpha emitters, which deposit energy over a very short range, and their potential application in targeted radionuclide therapy. The short path lengths of these radiations may ensure greater specificity to target tissue as their path length does not allow them to penetrate surrounding healthy tissue. However, it also means that appropriate mechanisms must be used to maximise proximity to target cells. Furthermore, the distribution of the radiopharmaceutical/radionuclide *within* cells can have significant effects on efficacy. For instance, adding a nuclear localisation peptide sequence to an anti-CD33 antibody conjugated to the Auger emitter indium-111 directs more isotope to the nucleus and increases cytotoxicity (Chen *et al.* 2006).

Since many radiopharmaceuticals target proteins expressed on the cell surface (for example, receptors), many radiopharmaceuticals comprise ligands for these cell surface proteins that are conjugated to an appropriate radionuclide. The binding of the radiopharmaceutical to cells that express this molecular target can be measured in relatively simple experiments. Cultured cells can be treated with the

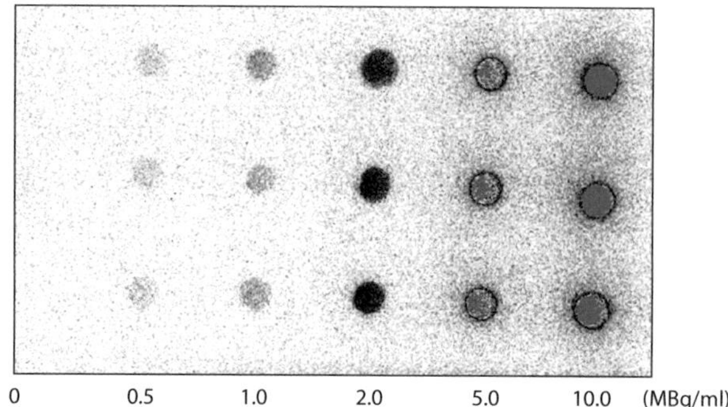

Figure 36.1 Measuring cell binding or uptake of radiopharmaceuticals using a phosphorimager. In this experiment, the uptake of the lymphocyte labelling agent ^{111}In-oxinate into HT1080 fibrosarcoma cells was measured. Cells were cultured as monolayers in 24-well plates before incubation with between 0 and 10 MBq/mL ^{111}In-oxinate for 1 hour at 37°C. Media containing the ^{111}In-oxinate was then removed and the cells were rinsed twice with phosphate-buffered saline. The multiwell plate was then placed on a Multisensitive Phosphor Screen (Perkin Elmer), separated by 3 × 1 mm lead collimators. The exposed phosphor screen was then placed in a Cyclone Phosphorimager (Perkin Elmer) and subjected to analysis by Cyclone software. A standard curve of known ^{111}In-oxinate activities, combined with separate cell counting, allows a calculation of cellular uptake in becquerels per cell (Bq/cell). (Image produced by Dr. Amanda Weeks, University of Kent.)

radiopharmaceutical and washed with phosphate-buffered saline solution, and subjected to appropriate radioactivity measurement using a dose calibrator, gamma counter or scintillation counter. It is also possible to use phosphorimager technology (i.e. exposure to a phosphor screen) to monitor binding of radiopharmaceuticals to adherent cell cultures in a multiwell plate format (Figure 36.1); this expedites the process in large experiments but owing to crossover activity between wells it requires the use of collimators between the multiwell plate and the screen. A calibration curve is required for the particular radionuclide, which is used to establish the response of the machine and convert raw data into activity in becquerels, while counting the number of cells also allows a calculation of cell binding in becquerels/cell. Specificity of the radiopharmaceutical for a given molecular target can be measured by conducting identical experiments with cells that do not produce that particular protein, or by blocking the protein with an excess of unlabelled ligand. These are essential control experiments that need to be considered in evaluating specific binding of radiopharmaceuticals to target cell surface proteins.

In some instances, it may be desirable to supplement cell binding data with an investigation of whether radiopharmaceuticals are taken into the cell. This is particularly of interest for evaluating therapeutic radioconjugates emitting short-path-length radiations such as Auger and alpha emitters. In these instances it may be desirable for the radiopharmaceutical to internalise, thereby concentrating the isotope within the target cell and ensuring its proximity to the most radiosensitive parts of the cell. Since the key target of internalised radiation for cancer treatment is the DNA, it is particularly important to maximise the radiation dose to the nucleus. Nuclei can be isolated from cells using buffers containing specific detergents, such as Igepal, that disrupt the plasma membrane but leave the nuclear membrane intact (Greenberg, Ziff 1984); several commercially available kits perform the same function. Thus it is possible to isolate the nuclear fraction and determine how much radionuclide is contained in this fraction using the procedures outlined above. It is also possible to verify the quality of the nuclear preparation and exclude cytoplasmic contamination by probing for abundant cytoplasmic proteins such as calpain (Hu *et al.* 2006).

Subcellular fractionation, as described by Cox and Emili (2006) can also be used to determine the proportion of radionuclide associated with particular subcellular organelles (plasma membrane, mitochondria, etc.); since many radiopharmaceuticals remain bound to cell surface receptors it is particularly useful to determine the radionuclide fraction bound to the cell membrane. Microautoradiography techniques have also been applied to study the detailed subcellular distribution of radioisotopes (Puncher, Blower 1995), although the resolution of this technique, while impressive at around 2 μm, may ultimately be more valuable in determining distribution within tissues rather than cells. Nevertheless, the ability to determine the subcellular distribution of radioactivity permits microdosimetry modelling to estimate the absorbed dose to the cell; published models for particular radionuclides, for example by Goddu *et al.* (1994), allow an estimation of absorbed dose based on levels of nuclide found in the cytoplasm, on the cell surface or in the nucleus.

Measuring cellular responses to radiopharmaceuticals

Internalised radiation targets the cellular DNA to cause a number of chemical changes. The extent of the resulting 'DNA damage' and the way in which human cells respond to it is an important factor when considering the effectiveness of radiopharmaceuticals for imaging or therapeutic purposes.

Ionising radiation results in a range of DNA lesions (Figure 36.2). Among the most common are DNA strand breaks, in which the sugar phosphate backbone of DNA is cleaved by ionising radiation or oxygen free radicals derived from radiolysis of water. Usually these are single-strand breaks, in which only one strand of DNA is compromised and the complementary strand remains intact; these are relatively easily processed and repaired by the cell provided they are present in low numbers. Double-strand breaks are more serious and more difficult to repair as the two 'ends' of DNA, flanking the break, lose contact with each other. In addition to strand breaks, a number of structural modifications can occur in the DNA bases that encode the genetic sequences. These can range from simple hydroxylations to more complicated ring-opened base products. Collectively, these ionising radiation-induced DNA lesions cause significant problems for the cell, causing errors in replication, blocking transcription, and interfering with other essential cellular processes. These cellular responses either will represent safety concerns for imaging radiopharmaceuticals or will be an encouraging indication of cell killing potential for those developed for therapeutic purposes.

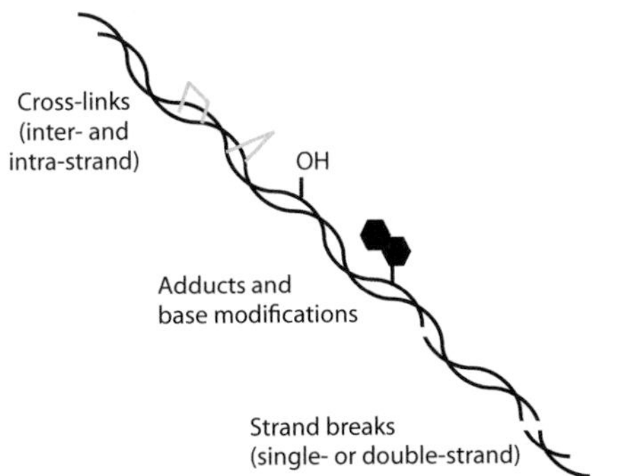

Figure 36.2 Chemical changes induced in DNA by exogenous agents. DNA is subjected to DNA damage induced by a range of chemical and physical agents, leading to a number of discrete structural modifications. Breaks in the sugar-phosphate backbone in one or both DNA strands lead to the formation of single- or double-strand breaks. Cross-links can be formed between adjacent DNA bases on the same or opposing DNA strands, while 'adducts' can be formed by the addition of chemical groups to DNA bases. These groups can range from large organic molecules to simple oxidation and methylation products. Ionising radiation induces a mixture of oxidised DNA bases and single- and double-strand breaks.

The cellular response to DNA damage

The way in which cells respond to radiation-induced DNA damage is crucial to the therapeutic effects of radiopharmaceuticals. There are three major responses to DNA damage, as outlined in Figure 36.3. A number of excellent reviews have given a comprehensive account of these processes; for example, Su (2006) provides a comprehensive overview of the response to double-strand breaks. Given the broad scope of this subject area, the complex range of DNA damage responses will be covered only briefly here. They are pivotal mechanisms that ensure genomic integrity and prevent the replication of a damaged DNA template, which can lead to mutation and the onset of tumorigenesis if mutations are located in key genes that regulate growth. They have an important protective effect in human cells and have evolved to prevent the deleterious effects of genetic damage.

Cells that are subjected to radiation-induced DNA damage can initially undergo cell cycle arrest. In this tightly regulated process, a number of proteins

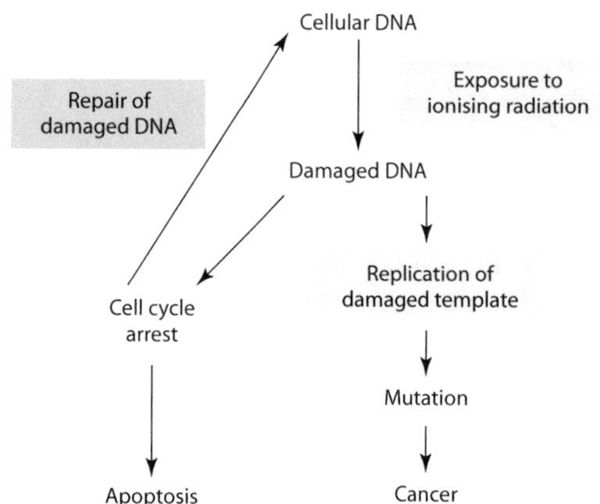

Figure 36.3 Biological responses to DNA damage. DNA damage promotes errors in replication of the genetic code. In response to DNA damage, cells inhibit proliferation by inducing cell cycle arrest, thereby preventing entry into the replication phase of the cell cycle. Cells will then either undergo DNA repair or activate the cell suicide mechanism apoptosis. These mechanisms coordinate to maintain the integrity of the genome.

coordinate together to act at the transitions between key stages of the cell cycle known as cell cycle checkpoints (Figure 36.4). A particularly important checkpoint is at the junction between the initial growth stage of the cell cycle (G_1) and the stage in which DNA is replicated (S-phase), known as the G_1S checkpoint. Activation of this checkpoint prevents cells from entering the S-phase of the cell cycle and replicating a damaged genome, and gives the cell time to activate other DNA damage responses.

Depending upon how extensively the genome has been damaged, the cell may activate mechanisms that repair DNA damage and restore an intact genome. Radiation-induced oxidative base modifications and single-strand breaks can be processed by base excision repair (BER). In this highly efficient repair process, any oxidised bases are removed from the sugar phosphate backbone to leave an abasic site, a process catalysed by glycosylase enzymes. The abasic site is subjected to hydrolytic cleavage to leave a single nucleotide gap, which is filled with the appropriate nucleotide and covalently linked into the double helix. Single-strand breaks are repaired in a similar way; while they usually do not require glycosylase activity, the strand break does require processing in the same way as abasic sites, sometimes with the assistance of additional proteins, to allow the gap-filling stage to take place. Double-strand breaks present more of a problem for the cell. The ends of the breaks are often unable to be joined together without further modification, and the two ends of the break need to be in sufficient proximity and alignment to allow them to be ligated together. A number of proteins act in concert to rejoin the two ends of a double-strand break in a mechanism known as non-homologous end joining (NHEJ). An altogether more accurate mechanism of double-strand break repair is homologous recombination (HR), in which an area of sequence homology in another region of the genome is used as a template to resynthesise DNA more accurately.

DNA repair processes are costly to the cell in that they require energy in the form of cellular energy 'currency', adenosine triphosphate (ATP). If cellular damage is extensive enough that the energy cost to the cell is prohibitive, the cell is able to undergo a 'cell suicide' mechanism known as apoptosis. Radiation-induced DNA damage is an important signal for apoptosis and, through activation of proteins called caspases, stimulates a characteristic series of events: shrinkage of the cell, ruffling or 'blebbing' of the

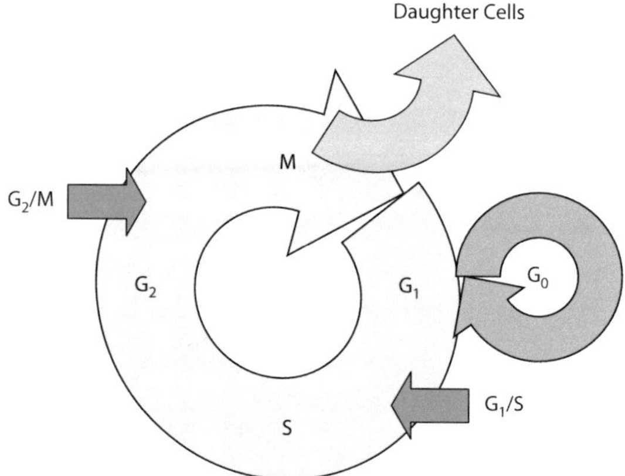

Figure 36.4 The cell cycle. In order for cell division to take place, cells must proceed once through the cell cycle. The cell cycle contains two growth phases (G_1 and G_2), separated by the synthetic (S) phase in which the genome of the cell is copied during a process of semiconservative replication. The second growth phase is followed by the mitotic (M) phase in which chromosomes are separated into each daughter cell. The G_1S and G_2M cell cycle checkpoints, involving the coordinated action of several proteins, are activated by DNA damage and prevent entry into the critical S-phase and M-phase of the cell cycle.

plasma membrane, fragmentation of the nucleus and of chromosomes, and the division of the cell into numerous 'apoptotic bodies' that can be targeted and destroyed by the immune system. This cellular mechanism is an important contributor to radiation-induced cytotoxicity and is to be exploited in the development of therapeutic radiopharmaceuticals.

The aim of therapeutic radiopharmaceuticals is to induce sufficient DNA damage to overwhelm protective cellular mechanisms such as DNA repair, and promote apoptotic mechanisms within target cells to ensure maximum toxicity. These can be carefully evaluated in cell culture using a range of experimental procedures, which collectively represent a robust experimental platform with which to evaluate therapeutic potential.

Measuring radiopharmaceutical-induced damage to DNA

Comet assay

The single-cell gel eletrophoresis assay, or 'comet' assay, is a highly sensitive method for the detection of DNA damage. In simple terms, it takes a 'snapshot' of the total amount of DNA damage present in a single cell, including the oxidative base modifications and single- and double-strand breaks induced by ionising radiation. It uses the same basic principle of agarose gel electrophoresis; shorter fragments of negatively charged DNA, resulting from DNA damage, migrate towards the cathode when an electric field is passed through a solid matrix. The extent of DNA fragmentation can be analysed to determine the amount of DNA damage present. This analysis is typically undertaken for 100 individual cells derived from at least two independent experiments. First described by Ostling and Johanson in 1984, the comet assay has benefited from international workshops that have led to a widely accepted experimental protocol (Hartmann *et al.* 2003). This prevents variation in the technique used and gives added confidence in the interpretation of results from different laboratories.

The most widely used variation is the alkaline comet assay, because it combines high sensitivity with relative simplicity. In this assay, cells treated with radiopharmaceuticals are mixed with a liquid agarose matrix and applied to a microscope slide. This mixture solidifies and forms a mini-agarose gel in which cells are embedded. These cells are lysed *in situ* in a high-salt solution containing detergent, to degrade the plasma membrane of the cell, and are then subjected to an alkaline solution. This alkaline solution unwinds the DNA by breaking the hydrogen bonds between complementary bases in DNA. The separation of the DNA strands is an important factor in the sensitivity of the assay as there are likely to be more single-strand breaks in an irradiated cell than double-strand breaks. The sensitivity can be increased further by ensuring the alkaline solution has a pH above 12.6; this allows the conversion of oxidative base modifications to single-strand breaks and therefore reveals more DNA damage per cell. When the cells are subjected to an electric field under these alkaline conditions, DNA fragments migrate towards the cathode. The DNA in the cells can subsequently be stained with DNA-specific dyes such as propidium iodide, which reveals the characteristic 'comet' shape of a cell that contains DNA damage (Figure 36.5). Using fluorescence microscopy, it is possible to evaluate the proportion of DNA contained in the 'tail' of the comet compared with the 'head'. There is some disagreement in the literature regarding the best way of doing this (Collins *et al.* 2008); some favour giving scores to individual cells based on the extent of tail staining, others measure the length of the comet tail, but the most common is use of the Olive Tail Moment, a calculation that takes into account the proportion of DNA in the tail and the mean distance migrated and which is a standard feature of comet assay software packages (Olive *et al.* 1990).

The comet assay is a very versatile technique, with applications in human and environmental biomonitoring, regulatory genotoxicology, and translational medicine, and is widely accepted as an appropriate indicator in these diverse fields. It can be applied to cultured cells and primary cell sources, and requires only a limited number of cells to give statistically significant results, thereby sparing precious radiopharmaceutical and reducing handling exposure. It is a multistage process and the analysis can be laborious, although a number of commercially available software packages have been developed to facilitate automated analysis. Despite its sensitivity, the comet assay has rarely been used to determine radiopharmaceutical-induced DNA damage; one study used the

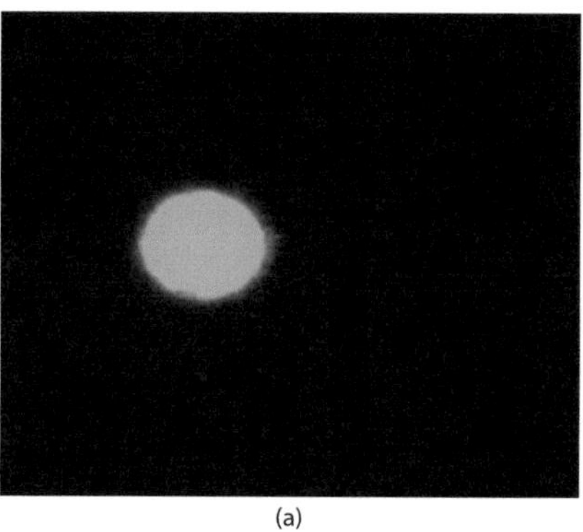
(a)

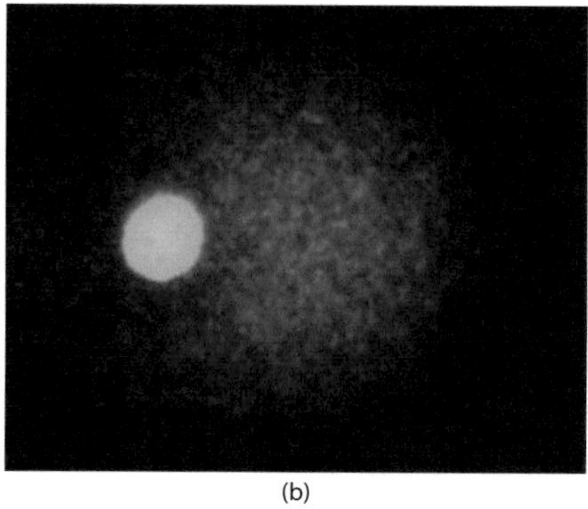
(b)

Figure 36.5 The single-cell gel electrophoresis (comet) assay. Cells are embedded in agarose, lysed and subjected to alkaline electrophoresis before staining with a DNA-specific stain (e.g. propidium iodide) and visualisation under a microscope. (a) Staining of nuclear DNA that has not been subjected to DNA damage; thus the DNA remains in the 'head' of the comet under the conditions of electrophoresis. (b) The nucleus of a cell that had previously been treated with ^{64}Cu-ATSM, a hypoxia-selective radiotracer. This has resulted in significant DNA fragmentation, as shown by DNA staining in the comet 'tail', which represents shorter fragments of single-stranded DNA. Relative staining in the head and tail are used to calculate the degree of DNA damage present in a single cell. Typically, 100 cells are analysed per data point. (Images produced by Dr Amanda Weeks, University of Kent.)

assay to demonstrate DNA damage in hypoxic cells after exposure to hypoxia-selective ^{64}Cu-ATSM (Obata *et al.* 2005; Weeks *et al.* 2010). While the alkaline comet assay gives the total amount of DNA damage present in a cell, it is perhaps limiting for radiopharmaceutical analysis in that it does not specifically detect double-strand breaks, a key factor in radiation-induced toxicity. Use of the neutral comet assay does detect double-strand breaks, although sensitivity is much reduced and it is likely that other types of analysis are more suitable for this application.

H2AX assay

The H2AX immunofluorescence method has been developed for the sensitive detection of double-strand breaks (DSBs). Within the nucleus, DNA is packaged into nucleosomes. These are composed of DNA and histone proteins, which are crucial for packaging of large amounts of genomic DNA in the nucleus and are also involved in gene regulation. The formation of DNA DSBs, following exposure to ionising radiation, induces the rapid phosphorylation of a specific histone called H2AX (or γ-H2AX) in the chromatin, flanking the site of the break (Rogakou *et al.* 1998). This phosphorylation site on γ-H2AX is four amino acid residues from its C-terminus at serine 139; phosphorylation at this site is thought to be involved in the recognition and/or repair of DNA DSBs. An antibody directed against γ-H2AX can be used to detect specific phosphorylation at this site; detection of the bound antibody with fluorescence microscopy shows the formation of a γ-H2AX focus at the site of the DSB that increases in size over 10–30 minutes and remains until after the break is repaired (Nakamura *et al.* 2006). Image analysis of immunofluorescence microscopic detection of γ-H2AX is a sensitive method of measuring DSB formation; furthermore, the disappearance of γ-H2AX foci over time may be used to detect DNA repair events. Formation of γ-H2AX foci is generally regarded as the most sensitive method currently available for detection of DNA DSBs from low doses of ionising radiation. Some studies suggest that this approach can detect individual DSBs with one γ-H2AX focus representing one DSB. DNA damage elicited by radiation doses as low as 1 mGy can be detected using this method (Rothkamm and Lobrich 2003).

Measuring radiopharmaceutical-induced toxicity

When is a cell dead? On the surface, this might appear to be a straightforward question. However, the number of biological endpoints used to determine the survival of cells can lead to a confusing picture regarding the toxicity and biological activity of a radiopharmaceutical. There are a large number of experimental techniques that are used to determine the toxicity of a range of agents including radiopharmaceuticals. Each has its own advantage, but the fact that they measure 'death' in different ways means that there can be large variation in stringency and sensitivity, which should be borne in mind when interpreting experimental data.

Colorimetric assays

Some of the simplest methods of establishing the viability of a cell culture are colorimetric assays that rely upon a change in colour or uptake of a chromophore into cells. The use of trypan blue is commonly used to establish viability of cell cultures. Trypan blue is a negatively charged molecule that will not enter cells unless the cell membrane is compromised. Thus it is possible to visually inspect cell cultures using a haemocytometer and inverted light microscope, and determine a percentage viability by counting the number of cells that have taken up the blue chromophore (non-viable) and those that exclude it (viable). Since membrane damage can result from radioactive emissions and cellular responses to radioactivity, the trypan blue method of cell viability can be used as a rapid indicator of cellular survival. For instance, trypan blue exclusion was used successfully to determine viability of mouse haematopoietic progenitor cells after labelling with ^{111}In-oxinate. The study aimed to evaluate whether this radiopharmaceutical could be used as an imaging agent to track the fate of transplanted cells in mice. The assay was sufficiently sensitive to determine statistically significant differences in viability according to dose and retention (Nowak *et al.* 2007). However, membrane damage can be a relatively late event in cell death processes, and so the trypan blue 'exclusion' test may underestimate toxicity. This method might not, therefore, offer the necessary sensitivity for evaluating the cytotoxicity of all radiopharmaceuticals, although it does give a useful indication of the general 'health' of a cell culture prior to undertaking experiments.

Other colorimetric assays work on the basis that viable cells retain metabolic activity. For instance, 3-(4,5-dimethylthiazoyl-2-yl)-2,5-diphenyltetrazolium bromide (MTT) is reduced to a purple formazan crystalline product by the mitochondrial enzyme succinate dehydrogenase; this can be solubilised and measured by spectrophotometry. The MTT assay (and similar colorimetric assays using related tetrazolium compounds such as XTT (2,3-bis-(2-methoxy-4-nitro-5-sulfophenyl)-2H-tetrazolium-5-carboxanilide) and water-soluble tetrazolium salt (WST)-1) was developed as a cell proliferation assay to monitor cellular growth, although it has been applied successfully to evaluate the cyototoxicity of DNA damaging agents including radiopharmaceuticals. The assay involves growth of a fixed number of cells with a range of radiopharmaceutical doses, followed by a suitable recovery time, incubation with MTT and solubilisation in a suitable solvent such as dimethyl sulfoxide. It is a rapid process for establishing a baseline indication of cytotoxicity, and the process can be further automated by processing of samples in 96-well cell culture plates, which allows spectrophotometry in automated microplate reader devices.

Johnson and Press (2000) used the MTT assay, in combination with trypan blue exclusion, to reveal synergistic cytotoxic effects of an ^{131}I-labelled anti-CD20 antibody, when combined with the pharmaceuticals cytarabine and fludarabine, in human lymphoma cell lines expressing the cell surface protein CD20. Like the trypan blue exclusion method, the MTT assay can underestimate cytotoxicity; cells undergoing cell death mechanisms such as apoptosis may retain metabolic competence for some time after lethal exposure to a radiopharmaceutical. This may be particularly significant in evaluating radiopharmaceuticals for imaging purposes in which low toxicity is desired; the MTT assay may reveal limited toxicity while other assays, such as clonogenic survival, are more stringent in their evaluation of cytotoxicity. The assay is also less able to reveal subtle differences in toxicity between different radiopharmaceuticals.

Colony-forming assays

Perhaps the most stringent way to establish whether a cell is dead or not is to determine whether it is able to grow and divide to form a colony. This is the basis of the clonogenic survival assay, a very stringent measure for establishing the cytotoxicity of radiopharmaceuticals and other DNA-damaging agents. The classical technique is simple in principle; it requires the seeding of single cells at a very low density (for instance, around 500 cells in a 10 cm diameter adherent cell culture dish), treatment of cells with the test reagent in an appropriate culture medium, and leaving them to grow for 7–14 days to allow viable cells to multiply and form discrete colonies. The colonies are then fixed in methanol, stained with an agent such as methylene blue, and counted. Owing to the limited availability of test compound and, in the case of radiopharmaceuticals to reduce radiation exposure to the worker, the treatment with the test reagent can be undertaken in a small volume prior to seeding at low density into larger volumes, which reduces the amount of reagent needed.

The clonogenic assay is a stringent measure of cytotoxicity because the 7–14-day period required for colony growth is sufficient for the completion of cell death mechanisms in cells that have sustained lethal cellular damage. It is technically simple to set up and, while somewhat laborious and slow to generate results, it is a highly reproducible assay and regarded as something of a gold standard for assessing cytotoxicity of DNA damaging agents of all types, not only radiopharmaceuticals. The cell counting can be expedited by a number of commercially available software packages and freeware (Niyazi *et al.* 2007) and further allows the user to set threshold levels for automated counting and preventing user error. While the assay works best for adherent cell lines, it is possible to undertake clonogenic analysis on suspension cell lines too, using semi-solid methylcellulose growth media. For example Methocult was used as the basis for clonogenic evaluation of an internalising, non-labelled peptide that acts as a potent inducer of apoptosis in malignant blood cells (Marks *et al.* 2005). The clonogenic assay usually indicates greater cytotoxicity of a given concentration of toxic chemical than colorimetric assays such as the MTT assay; furthermore it reveals greater differences in cytotoxicity between experimental conditions (Bhana, Lloyd 2008). This assay is considered to reflect more accurately the true cytotoxicity (Brown, Wouters 1999), although it is worth bearing in mind for therapeutic radiopharmaceuticals in particular that the lethal dose to cells in culture may be significantly less, as measured by the clonogenic assay, than in tissues.

Measuring apoptotic markers

There is a range of methods for the detection of apoptotic markers that can be applied to the measurement of the biological effects of radiation. Protein complexes with important functions in apoptosis, such as caspases and conjugates of annexin V, can be detected in relatively straightforward procedures developed commercially. Caspases are a group of cysteine proteases that have initiator and effector roles in apoptosis. Several commercial kits are available for analysis of apoptosis based on caspase function. Caspase assays may utilise the enzyme activity of caspase to cleave a bioluminescent substrate, or an antibody directed against caspase that can be used in flow cytometry or cell based multiwell plate assays. For example, Urashima *et al.* (2006) used a fluorogenic substrate of caspase-3, which is induced under conditions of apoptosis, to compare the apoptotic response of Auger-emitting radioisotopes and gamma radiation in human tumour cell lines. Apoptosis can also be detected by flow cytometry using fluorescent conjugates of annexin V. Phosphatidylserine residues are located on the inner surface of the cell membrane in healthy cells. During apoptosis, phosphatidylserine is translocated to the outer surface of the membrane, where it can be detected by annexin V staining. A late event in apoptosis is degradation of the genome, and a relatively crude way of determining apoptosis is to isolate DNA and perform agarose gel electrophoresis, which reveals a characteristic 'ladder' of DNA fragments of defined size. This is, however, less sensitive than other assays and not quantitative.

Conclusion

This chapter has reviewed some of the key considerations in applying cell culture techniques to the thorough evaluation of radiopharmaceuticals. Clearly, given the relative advantages and disadvantages of each of the technologies described, care must be taken in selecting the most appropriate approach for a particular research question. The continuing advances in cell-based technologies will furnish nuclear medicine with even more powerful tools. It is important that radiopharmaceutical scientists take the opportunity to exploit this emerging knowledge base and apply it to their own investigations in nuclear medicine.

References

Bargonetti J *et al.* (1992). Site-specific binding of wild-type p53 to cellular DNA is inhibited by SV40 T antigen and mutant p53. *Genes Dev* 6: 1886–1898.

Bhana S, Lloyd DR (2008). The role of p53 in DNA damage-mediated cytotoxicity overrides its ability to regulate nucleotide excision repair in human fibroblasts. *Mutagenesis* 23: 43–50.

Brown JM, Wouters BG (1999). Apoptosis, p53, and tumor cell sensitivity to anticancer agents. *Cancer Res* 59: 1391–1399.

Chen P *et al.* (2006). Nuclear localizing sequences promote nuclear translocation and enhance the radiotoxicity of the anti-CD33 monoclonal antibody HuM195 labeled with ^{111}In in human myeloid leukemia cells. *J Nucl Med* 47: 827–836.

Collins AR *et al.* (2008). The comet assay: topical issues. *Mutagenesis* 23: 143–151.

Cox B, Emili A (2006). Tissue subcellular fractionation and protein extraction for use in mass-spectrometry-based proteomics. *Nat Protoc* 1: 1872–1878.

Goddu SM *et al.* (1994). Cellular dosimetry: absorbed fractions for monoenergetic electron and alpha particle sources and S-values for radionuclides uniformly distributed in different cell compartments. *J Nucl Med* 35: 303–316.

Greenberg ME, Ziff EB (1984). Stimulation of 3T3 cells induces transcription of the c-fos proto-oncogene. *Nature* 311: 433–438.

Hartmann A *et al.* (2003). Recommendations for conducting the in vivo alkaline Comet assay. 4th International Comet Assay Workshop. *Mutagenesis* 18: 45–51.

Hu M *et al.* (2006). Site-specific conjugation of HIV-1 tat peptides to IgG: a potential route to construct radioimmunoconjugates for targeting intracellular and nuclear epitopes in cancer. *Eur J Nucl Med Mol Imaging* 33: 301–310.

Johnson TA, Press OW (2000). Synergistic cytotoxicity of iodine-131-anti-CD20 monoclonal antibodies and chemotherapy for treatment of B-cell lymphomas. *Int J Cancer* 85: 104–112.

Marks AJ *et al.* (2005). Selective apoptotic killing of malignant hemopoietic cells by antibody-targeted delivery of an amphipathic peptide. *Cancer Res* 65: 2373–2377.

Martin SE, Caplen NJ (2007). Applications of RNA interference in mammalian systems. *Annu Rev Genomics Hum Genet* 8: 81–108.

Nakamura A *et al.* (2006). Techniques for gamma-H2AX detection. *Methods Enzymol* 409: 236–250.

Niyazi M *et al.* (2007). Counting colonies of clonogenic assays by using densitometric software. *Radiat Oncol* 2: 4.

Nowak B *et al.* (2007). Indium-111 oxine labelling affects the cellular integrity of haematopoietic progenitor cells. *Eur J Nucl Med Mol Imaging* 34: 715–721.

Obata A *et al.* (2005). Basic characterization of 64Cu-ATSM as a radiotherapy agent. *Nucl Med Biol* 32: 21–28.

Olive PL *et al.* (1990). Heterogeneity in radiation-induced DNA damage and repair in tumor and normal cells measured using the "comet" assay. *Radiat Res* 122: 86–94.

Ostling O, Johanson KJ (1984). Microelectrophoretic study of radiation-induced DNA damages in individual mammalian cells. *Biochem Biophys Res Commun* 30: 291–298.

Parry JJ *et al.* (2007). Characterization of somatostatin receptor subtype 2 expression in stably transfected A-427 human cancer cells. *Mol Imaging* 6: 56–67.

Puncher MR, Blower PJ (1995). Frozen section microautoradiography in the study of radionuclide targeting: application to indium-111-oxine-labeled leukocytes. *J Nucl Med* 36: 499–505.

Rogakou EP *et al.* (1998). DNA double-stranded breaks induce histone H2AX phosphorylation on serine 139. *J Biol Chem* 273: 5858–5868.

Rothkamm K, Löbrich M (2003). Evidence for a lack of DNA double-strand break repair in human cells exposed to very low x-ray doses. *Proc Natl Acad Sci U S A* 100: 5057–5062.

Sheppard HM *et al.* (1999). New insights into the mechanism of inhibition of p53 by simian virus 40 large T antigen. *Mol Cell Biol* 19: 2746–2753.

Su TT (2006). Cellular responses to DNA damage: one signal, multiple choices. *Annu Rev Genet* 40: 187–208.

Urashima T *et al.* (2006). Induction of apoptosis in human tumor cells after exposure to Auger electrons: comparison with gamma-ray exposure. *Nucl Med Biol* 33: 1055–1063.

37

Animal models: preclinical molecular imaging, why and how?

Richard Southworth

Introduction

Non-invasive imaging of physiological and molecular processes in patients has the potential to drive many improvements in medical practice, providing better information for clinical decision-making, aiding the execution of interventional procedures, and providing better indices of the effectiveness of therapy (Weissleder, Mahmood 2001; Massoud, Gambhir 2003; Conti *et al.* 2008). Molecular imaging, alongside structural and functional imaging, is also assuming great importance in the development and evaluation of new drugs, through the use of imaging biomarkers to replace patient survival and other non-specific clinical endpoints (Willman *et al.* 2008). This increasing importance is reflected in burgeoning clinical imaging activity and the continuing construction of both new clinical PET centres and comprehensive imaging centres by the pharmaceutical industry and in academia.

In basic science, the ability to image biochemical processes non-invasively in humans and in animal models is also being used increasingly to understand the molecular basis of disease from its earliest onset (Riemann *et al.* 2008) and guide the design and development of new therapies with many advantages over existing methods. These include: (i) real-time monitoring, (ii) accessibility without tissue destruction, (iii) low invasiveness, (iv) multiple time points over wide ranges of time scales, and (v) multiscale information, i.e. from the cellular level to organ systems, to the complete organism. This chapter summarises why and how animals are used in basic scientific research, and how this is currently regulated. It then explains why preclinical imaging is increasingly being used in basic research using animals, what are its advantages over existing methods, and how preclinical imaging has the potential to reduce the number of animals required for medical and scientific research in the future.

Why are animals used in medical research?

The use of animals in scientific research is a controversial subject and a major issue in the public perception of the biomedical sciences. Before focusing on preclinical imaging and its merits, it is important to first appreciate the context in which animals are used in scientific research in general, and the regulations that govern their use in the UK.

In an ideal world, disease would be detected in patients from the moment of its onset and characterised and monitored accurately, safely and non-invasively, most likely using medical imaging techniques. The same techniques employed to diagnose and track the progression of a disease would then be used to guide and evaluate the effectiveness of its treatment. Therapeutic drugs would be designed by computerised molecular modelling to specifically target each disease process; their efficacy, toxicity, potential interactions and adverse effects would be accurately predicted by computer simulation, and treatment and monitoring regimes would be routinely tailored for each individual patient. While advances in medical imaging technology continue to make great strides towards realising many of these ambitions, we are still a long way from being able to employ this kind of medical and scientific approach. We are confounded by a number of problems that cannot currently be answered directly by the study of patients for physical, practical, ethical, and often legal reasons.

Animals are used in medical research for two fundamental purposes: to elucidate the biological mechanisms of health and disease, and to provide proof of principle and safety testing for new methodologies and treatments. While every effort is made to limit the use of animals, or replace them with alternatives where possible, animal experimentation unfortunately remains the most practical and useful means of studying many disease processes, establishing product toxicity, and developing new medical treatments. It must be understood that under no circumstances is animal experimentation perceived as the sole means of understanding a disease process in humans; it is one of a range of approaches that, in combination with clinical observation (*in situ* or by biopsy), *in-vitro* human cell studies, and computer modelling approaches, contribute to the slowly accumulating knowledge base to provide understanding of, and ultimately clinical solutions for, the diseases of our time. An overview of some of the difficulties in obtaining *relevant* data from the clinic, or human-derived tissues, and how and why animals or animal tissues are used as a surrogate in each case is detailed below.

Understanding disease initiation

Most diseases start and progress for a long time before they are detectable by any of our existing technologies (and before patients themselves are aware of them) – how are we to understand, and thereby prevent, the onset of these diseases if they are already well advanced by the time the patient presents in the clinic?

Animal models allow the study of many disease processes from their earliest beginnings; in the study of the progression of many cancers, for example, the implantation of just a few cancer cells into the thigh of a mouse, or the endogenous generation of cancer cells using well-characterised carcinogens or genetically predisposed animals can be used to study the very early stages of tumour development and metastasis far earlier than they could be detected and studied in patients (Frese, Tuveson 2007). Similarly, the development of atherosclerotic plaque in arteries, a major contributor to heart disease and sudden cardiac death, is a long, complex and multifactorial process. By using animal models such as the ApoE knockout mouse, which is predisposed to developing these plaques when fed a high-fat diet, studies of the early stages of plaque development and the evaluation of plaque-limiting/stabilising therapies can be performed (Kolovou *et al.* 2008). Using approaches such as these, where animals are studied before, during, and after the experimental induction of a disease process, the early pathways of a disease process can be characterised, providing us with the best hope of treatment – prevention rather than cure.

Inter-patient variability

The progression of disease varies greatly from patient to patient, and is affected by numerous factors, including age, sex, diet, lifestyle, ethnic origin, and genetic susceptibility. With so many external factors, it becomes extremely difficult to understand the basic mechanisms of a disease process in isolation.

Experimental animals are pure-bred strains; the general scientific approach is to use animals of the same strain, sex and age, which have all been maintained under the same environmental conditions, and on the same diet. By limiting the number of external variables in this manner, the progression of disease in an animal model can be examined in isolation, whereas such study is confounded by external factors too numerous to count in patients. Increasingly, even the time of day that an experiment is performed is taken into account; circadian variation in the expression of different proteins and hormones during the day can have profound effects on experimental outcome, particularly considering the fact that most rodents are nocturnal, while (most) scientists are not! Light cycles are often reversed in animal holding facilities to counter this. While excluding the effects of such confounding factors and narrowing down the experimental question can provide insight into the molecular basis of a disease process, careful experimental design can then be used to broaden the knowledge base, by repeating experiments with different animal models to characterise the effect of age, sex, diet, etc., on the parameters under investigation.

Availability and relevance of biopsy material

To fully understand a disease process, or to validate a therapeutic approach, we need to obtain tissue samples upon which we can perform a multitude of biochemical tests. Not only is the obtaining of such biopsy tissue from humans potentially difficult and dangerous (or just not possible), the relevance of the tissue samples obtained is subject to inter-patient variation (age, sex, diet, stage/type/severity of disease, and so on) and sampling errors (the tissue obtained in the biopsy is not necessarily representative of the diseased organ as a whole). The large amount of tissue required from large numbers of patients to conduct a full disease characterisation in this manner is generally prohibitive, and obtaining multiple biopsies from the same patient to study the progression of a disease process is very difficult to justify ethically. Practically, once biopsy tissue is removed from an organ, it is no longer functioning as part of that organ; even if available, the information that biopsy tissue can provide is therefore limited.

Tissue from healthy animals and disease model animals provides biological material for research purposes in much greater quantity than is possible with the collection of human biopsy tissue. Not only is there physically more tissue available, but we can obtain much more reproducible tissue samples in terms of disease progression, subject age, dietary status, etc. Biopsy tissue is usually taken from patients in a relatively advanced stage of disease, so it provides little insight into disease onset and progression, where therapeutic approaches would be more effective. Using animal models with well-defined disease progression patterns, we can obtain tissue samples from much earlier in the disease process. Biopsy sampling errors and limitations of post-excision viability can be avoided by sampling and investigating changes in intact excised animal organs. As described in the next section, not only can entire organs be studied post mortem, but also these organs can potentially be maintained viable outside of the body for several hours, providing us with a very powerful manipulable model for scientific study and therapy development.

Multifactorial nature of disease

Many diseases are by their very nature multifactorial; understanding their progression requires the ability to simultaneously measure and quantify changes in numerous parameters. We do not currently have anything like the arsenal of non-invasive clinical techniques required to characterise a disease process in this manner in patients.

Ischaemic heart disease is characterised by a disparity between blood supply and blood demand, usually caused by a narrowing of the coronary arteries, leading to myocardial infarction, heart failure, and ultimately, death (Lee 1995). It is a complex, progressive and very dynamic disease process that is very difficult to study in its early stages; a cardiac patient's first presentation to a hospital is commonly their last. The asymptomatic early stages of the disease are therefore still poorly understood. The blood supply to the heart performs numerous functions, not only delivering fuel, nutrients, oxygen, hormones and immune cells, but also removing the waste products of metabolism. The hydrostatic pressure that blood exerts on the coronary arteries also has an important structural and functional role in maintaining heart cells at their optimal level of stretch for efficient cardiac contraction. An insufficient blood supply therefore has numerous inter-related consequences, initiating an 'ischaemic cascade', comprising hypoxia, loss of cellular energy, acidosis, ionic imbalance, electrophysiological changes, oedema, inflammation, and changes in structural integrity at the cellular and gross tissue levels (Schrader 1985). It is impossible to accurately model all of these inter-related parameters simultaneously in cells in culture, and very difficult to study them directly *in vivo* because of the heart's inaccessibility, and the lack of biophysical techniques available to quantify them all. The isolated Langendorff perfused heart model is particularly useful in this respect, and has been the main test-bed for experimental cardiology for over 100 years. By removing the heart (typically rat or mouse hearts are used), and retrogradely perfusing it via the aorta with a warmed oxygenated physiological salt solution, the heart can be maintained viable and contracting outside of the body for several hours (Skrzypiec-Spring *et al.* 2007). The effects of various direct interventions on the function, pharmacology and biochemistry of the heart can be observed directly, without the associated problems of systemic innervation, hormonal influence or drug metabolism. Ischaemia, impossible to study at its onset in humans, and difficult to accurately model in isolated cells, can be induced in a Langendorff perfused heart as simply as turning off a tap (Hearse, Sutherland 2000). The progression of the ensuing ischaemic cascade can then be studied by numerous biochemical and biophysical techniques ranging from the force that the heart can generate by compressing a latex balloon, to a full real-time biochemical profile by NMR spectroscopy, PET imaging (Southworth, Garlick 2003), or genomic profiling (Wiechert *et al.* 2003).

Relevance of cultured human cells

While human cultured cells are used to model and study various disease processes, the relevance of the data obtained has to be carefully considered. These cells are maintained in a completely different environment from that of their disease 'analogues' in patients *in situ*; even the cell lines themselves (such as immortalised cancer cell lines) can be different from those found *in vivo*. Many disease processes are complex and multifactorial; it is very difficult to accurately reproduce these conditions *in vitro*.

Isolated cell culture techniques, using both human and animal cell lines, are used in almost every field of biomedical research, providing much detailed information about cellular biochemistry during health and disease. While useful, these approaches are limited in that they provide very little insight into how cells interact with each other on a whole organ/organism basis. The environment in which cells reside has a very significant effect on their behaviour, and this is often very difficult to reproduce in culture. If one considers the environment within a tumour, for example, cancer cells exist in a state of patchy intermittent hypoxia, subject to a changing extracellular environment with fluctuating concentrations of hormones, extracellular messengers and growth factors, under varying degrees of attack from the immune system (Mbeunkui, Johann 2009). All of these factors will have a dynamic effect on the growth and progression of the tumour, which is something very difficult to characterise and then model *in vitro*.

Even more difficult to study *in vitro* is metastatic migration and its development of a new tumour blood supply through angiogenesis. In terms of therapy, it is very easy to kill cancer cells in a culture dish; killing them when ensconced within a living organism without harming the organism is a significantly more difficult problem. *In-vivo* animal models therefore provide a much more relevant, practical and meaningful means of studying these processes for many approaches aimed at understanding the pathology and treatment of cancer.

Clinical toxicity testing

The testing of new drugs and treatments directly on humans is highly regulated, and dosing of patients with novel agents without any toxicological insight from animal studies is strictly prohibited. The high-profile near-fatal clinical trial of the monoclonal antibody TGN1412 at Northwick Park Hospital in 2006 highlights how potentially dangerous toxicity testing in man can be (Ho, Cummins 2006).

Many animals used for research purposes in the UK are used for toxicity testing. This is a legal requirement for the licensing of any new drug. This, again, is due to the fact that animals can be bred and maintained in such a manner as to provide reproducible data on the mode of action, efficacy, and toxicity of chemical entities in a strictly controlled environment. Using highly sensitive nuclear imaging techniques, 'first in human' studies examining biodistribution and targeting of new drug/imaging agents at sub-pharmacologically relevant 'safe' concentrations are becoming increasingly common; it is hoped that this approach may ultimately lead to a reduction in the number of animals required for toxicity/biodistribution studies. As is the case in first in human studies, imaging of experimental animals is increasingly being used to study drug biodistribution, and obtain structure–activity relationships non-invasively, with the potential to dramatically reduce the number of animals required for toxicity testing worldwide. This is discussed later in this chapter.

Overview of animal usage statistics in scientific research

After peaking at around 5.5 million per year in the mid 1970s, the absolute numbers of animals used in scientific procedures in the UK declined year on year to a value of just above 3 million in 2007 (Home Office 2007; Figure 37.1). This reduction has been attributed to a combination of improvements in scientific technique, technology and experimental design, and higher levels of control and regulation from the Home Office, which oversees the use of animals in research in the UK. In recent years, the numbers of animals being used have started to rise again, due mainly to the increasing use of transgenic mice for the investigation of gene function. However, it could be argued that the power of the experimental data acquired from the use of such models is so great that they are responsible for the reduction of a large number of animal experiments that would be required if this technology were not available.

The vast majority of animals used in scientific procedures (84%) are rodents, primarily mice (82% of total rodents used; Figure 37.2). Most of the remaining scientific procedures are performed on fish and birds. Dogs, cats, horses and non-human primates collectively are used in less than 1% of all procedures. Mice are preferentially used because of their relevance to human biology, their relative cheapness to obtain and house, and their short breeding cycles. The gestation period for a mouse is 20 days, and they reach sexual maturity after approximately 50 days. This makes them very suitable for various breeding procedures, including the production of mutant and genetically modified animals, which accounted for 37% of all scientific procedures performed in 2006. Approximately 38% of all procedures used anaesthesia to alleviate the adverse effects of the procedure; for the majority of the remainder, the act of administering anaesthesia would have been more severe than the procedure itself. Procedures evaluating product toxicity have fallen in recent years from 25% of all procedures in 1995 to 14% in 2006. Of all the toxicological studies conducted on animals in 2006, 86% were performed to satisfy legal or regulatory requirements.

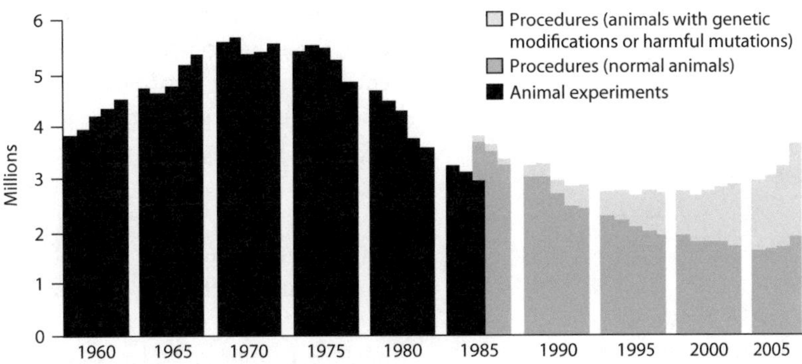

Figure 37.1 Numbers of animals used in scientific procedures in the UK between 1960 and 2008. Data from http://www.understandinganimalresearch.org.uk//

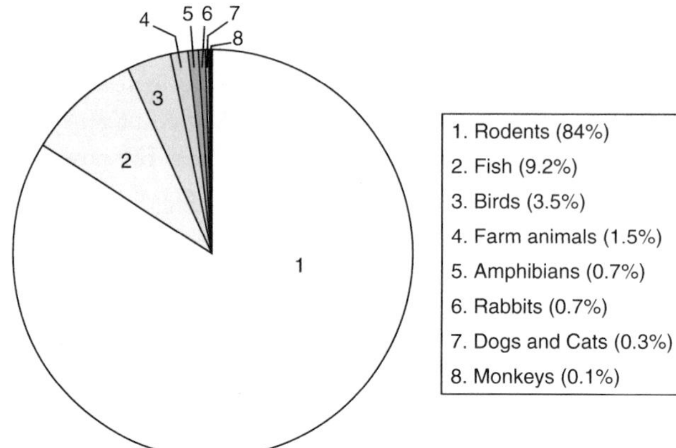

Figure 37.2 Animals used in scientific procedures by species, in the UK in 2006. Source data: *Statistics of Scientific Procedures on Living Animals, Great Britain.* Home Office 2007.

While 3 million animals a year is a considerable number, as a means of providing a little perspective, it is interesting to compare the numbers of animals used in scientific procedures in the UK with those used for food in the same year (Table 37.1). Even excluding animals used in food production whose products were imported into the UK, animal experimentation accounts for a little over 0.1% of the nation's consumption of animals for food.

Table 37.1 Comparison of the use of animals in the UK for scientific procedures and for food in 2007

Use	Number of animals killed in the UK in 2007
Animals in scientific procedures	3 million
Animals for food	
Cattle	5 million
Pigs	10 million
Sheep	15 million
Turkeys	15 million
Chickens	798 million
Total animals used for food (including fish and excluding imported meat)	2500 million

Data sources: Home Office and DEFRA.

Public perception and the anti-vivisection lobby

As scientists, it is important that we are able to defend the value of, and need for, animal experimentation, both to our critics and to the general public, who may be swayed by emotive rhetoric in the absence of a balancing voice. Historically in the UK, this voice has been muted through fear of the intimidatory tactics of the radical wings of the anti-vivisectionist lobbies, and informed televised debates on the subject are rare. The danger of such a climate of fear, ignorance and apathy was recently demonstrated in Rio de Janeiro, Brazil, where a local law was pushed through by a charismatic actor-come-politician in the face of a weak and complacent counter-lobby by the academic and pharmaceutical community, resulting in the prohibition of all animal experimentation by local private companies (Enserink 2008). While not currently being enforced, and likely to be overruled at the federal level, this local law is putting at risk the activities of companies like Fiocruz, a major vaccine producer in the region. However, it seems that in the UK at least, the tide is turning. In 1990, the British Association for the Advancement of Science coordinated a declaration affirming the importance of animal experimentation in the advancement of science and medical treatment, which was signed by more than 1000 scientists and clinicians, including 31 Nobel laureates. In 1996 an online campaign called the

'People's Petition' was launched by the Coalition for Medical Progress, stating that:

> Medical research is essential for developing safe and effective medical and veterinary treatments, requiring some studies using animals. Where there is no alternative available, medical research using animals should continue in the UK.
>
> People involved in medical research using animals have a right to work and live without fear of intimidation or attack

By the end of that year, the petition had amassed upwards of 21 000 signatories, including an unprecedented letter of support by the then Prime Minister Tony Blair. In February 2006, Pro-Test, a student organisation supporting animal testing in research organised the country's first pro-vivisection rally in Oxford, in response to the campaign by the organisation SPEAK against the building of the Biomedical and Animal Research Facility at Oxford University to be held on the same day. The Pro-Test rally outnumbered the SPEAK rally by over 5 to 1 (Demopoulos 2006). While affirmation of the necessity for animal experimentation by the public and scientific community is becoming more vocal in the UK, the anti-vivisectionist lobby seems to be losing much credibility and public support through the actions of their extremist factions, such as the highly publicised grave-robbing of the grandmother of the owners of the Darley Oaks guinea-pig farm by animal liberationists in 1996 (Woolcock 2006). This relative shift in tactics by the two camps already seems to be impacting on the public perception of animal use in scientific research. According to a recent MORI survey, the largest change in the public consciousness with respect to this issue is that of trust. In 1999, 65% of the public agreed that they had 'a lack of trust in the regulatory system about animal experimentation'. In the 2005 survey, this number had fallen to 36%. Similarly, in 1999, 29% of the public trusted scientists not to cause unnecessary harm to animals. By 2005, this had risen to 52% (MORI 1999, 2005). These figures can only be explained by increased openness and transparency by the scientific and legislative communities (in a climate of declining militancy by the anti-vivisectionists), and while these figures are encouraging, public mistrust of scientific procedures being carried out 'in an unregulated manner, behind closed doors' is still disappointingly high. This can only be combated with greater transparency and openness on our part. For further material on the ethical debate over the use of animals in experimentation, the following discussions may be of interest: Baumans (2004), Senior (1995), Langley *et al.* (2007), and Rollin (2007).

Britain was the first nation in the world to introduce legislation to regulate animal experimentation (the Cruelty to Animals Act of 1876). This was replaced in 1986 by the Animals (Scientific Procedures) Act, which is overseen by the Home Office, and is widely accepted to maintain the highest standards of regulation and care for animals used in scientific procedures in the world. While many countries employ an ethical review process, in the UK project licences are subject to two separate review processes: first local ethical review (which is subject to scrutiny by the Home Office), and then review by the Home Office itself. After a licence has been granted, the conditions and working practices are overseen and inspected by a team of Home Office Inspectors with unlimited access to all facilities housing or using protected animals, and the power to make unannounced visits to facilities and suspend or revoke licences or instigate criminal prosecution in the event of a breach of protocol.

Legislation and regulations

The Animals (Scientific Procedures) Act 1986 regulates the use of 'protected animals' in 'regulated procedures'. The protected animals that are covered by the Act are any living vertebrates other than humans and include mammals, birds and reptiles from halfway through their gestation period, and fish, amphibians and octopuses from when they become capable of independent feeding.

Regulated procedures

A regulated procedure is defined as 'any experimental or other scientific procedure applied to a protected animal which may have the effect of causing that animal pain, suffering, distress or lasting harm'. This includes disease, injury, physiological or psychological discomfort, either immediately or in the longer term. The lower threshold for a regulated procedure is the 'skilled insertion of a hypodermic needle', and equivalents for other experimental/procedural approaches such as psychological stress, or withholding food or water have been established by the Home Office. The generation, breeding, and maintenance of genetically manipulated animals are considered regulated procedures, where such modification will result in pain, distress or lasting harm either to that animal or to its offspring. Procedures are also regulated when performed under general anaesthesia if pain, distress, or lasting harm would be caused by that same procedure to an unanaesthestised animal. This includes procedures in which animals are not allowed to recover consciousness. The administration of anaesthetics themselves for experimental purposes, rather than for the alleviation of pain, is also considered a regulated procedure.

Procedures that are not regulated by the Act include the ringing or tagging of protected animals if it causes no more than momentary pain or distress and no lasting harm; procedures applied in the course of recognised veterinary or animal husbandry practice; and the humane killing of an animal by a method appropriate for that animal listed under Schedule 1 of the 1986 Act. While such killing does not require a specific project licence or personal licence, Schedule 1 killing must be carried out by a competent person, appropriately trained, within a designated establishment. A description of these licences and permissions is as follows.

Licences and certification

The regulation of the 1986 Act is governed by the Home Office through three points of control, the personal licence, the project licence and the certificate of designation. All of these licences are held by individuals, rather than organisations, and each individual is personally responsible and liable to either the certificate holder for the institution, or the Home Office directly for compliance and accountability.

Personal licences

A personal licence is the Secretary of State's endorsement that the holder is a suitable and competent person to carry out, under supervision if necessary, specified procedures on specified classes of animal. It does not, in itself, authorise the holder to carry out any regulated procedure on any protected animal; permission to carry out each and every procedure must be specifically sought from and granted by the Home Office in the form of a project licence. Similarly, a personal licence only grants permission for the holder to perform regulated procedures at the designated establishment, known as the 'primary availability'.

Personal licence holders are personally responsible to the Home Office for compliance with the terms and conditions of the licence that they hold; they must also be familiar with, and ensure that they are adequately trained to adhere to, the terms of the project licence under which they will be working, including the objectives, protocols, endpoints, and conditions of use. The primary responsibility of the personal licence holder is for the welfare of the protected animals upon which regulated procedures are being performed. They should have appropriate knowledge of the techniques involved and their consequences, and be able to recognise, minimise and prevent any signs of pain or distress in the animals in their care. They should obtain veterinary advice where appropriate, and advise the project licence holder immediately should the severity limit of a protocol be exceeded, or be close to being exceeded. It is their responsibility to ensure that should an animal in their care be in severe pain or distress that cannot be alleviated, it should be painlessly killed by an appropriate Schedule 1 method. They are also responsible for maintaining adequate records and cage labelling to allow the efficient monitoring of the animals and of their own technical competence.

Applicants for a personal licence must be over 18 years of age, have appropriate education and training, typically at least five GCSEs, and have completed training modules 1, 2 and 3 of a Home Office-accredited Animal Welfare course. Personal licence applicants are usually sponsored by a more senior personal licence holder in a position of authority at the institution where the applicant is to work.

Project licences

Project licences specify a programme of work. They are essentially a contract between the project licence holder and the Home Office, describing the regulated procedures to be used for a specific defined purpose, during a discrete period of time, at a designated location. Project licences are held and overseen by an individual personal licence holder with a position of authority within the host institution. A project licence may cover the focused project of an individual, or the work of an entire academic research division, covering a team of many personal licence holders using many protocols on many species. Project licences have a maximum duration of 5 years, after which time further permission must be sought from the Home Office for work to continue, in the form of a new project licence application. The key features of a project licence application are that it states the specific aims and objectives of the proposed work; defines the likely benefits of the work; describes the regulated procedures to be used, including likely adverse effects and how they shall be minimised and dealt with should they occur; and sets the severity band of the project.

In the first instance, a project licence will not be granted by the Home Office unless it falls within one or more of the following purposes:

- The prevention (whether by the testing of any product or otherwise) or the diagnosis or treatment of disease, ill-health or abnormality, or their effects, in humans, animals, or plants.
- The assessment, detection, regulation or modification of physiological conditions in humans, animals or plants.
- The protection of the natural environment in the interests of the health or welfare of humans or animals.
- The advancement of knowledge in biological or behavioural sciences.
- Education or training other than in primary or secondary schools.
- Forensic enquiries.
- The breeding of animals for experimental or other scientific use.

Upon receipt, and confirmation that the project licence application meets the above criteria, the Home Office will then evaluate it with respect to the following considerations

Cost–benefit analysis: What is the likely benefit of the work with regard to the likely harm to the protected animals being used? This is specific to the project application itself, rather than the importance of the general area of study. Every effort must be made to maximise benefit and minimise cost in each case. Each protocol is assigned a severity limit, which is the upper expected adverse effect that may be encountered by a protected animal – essentially a 'worst-case scenario', even if it is only experienced by a small number of the animals used in the project. The severity limit is the most important part of the project licence application – no matter what the potential benefit; a project licence will not be granted if the severity limit is extreme. Any procedure likely to cause severe pain or distress that cannot be alleviated will not be granted a project licence by the Home Office.

Likelihood of success: Each project application is reviewed for its scientific merit, the suitability of its approach, and how likely it is to achieve the objectives it proposes.

Consideration of alternatives: Replacement, reduction and refinement. Consideration of the 'three Rs' as they are termed is becoming an increasingly important part of the project grant evaluation process. Applicants must demonstrate that they have considered all means of minimising the numbers of animals, and the severity band of the procedures used, that are required to meet the objectives of the project, such as:

- Alternatives to using animals, including cultured cells and computer modelling approaches.
- Minimising the numbers of animals necessary to obtain meaningful data.
- Using animals with the lowest capacity to experience pain, suffering or distress; e.g. the use of rats will not be permitted when an established insect model capable of addressing the same research question is equally applicable.
- Protocols and endpoints that cause the least pain, suffering and distress are used.
- Protocols and endpoints that yield the most appropriate data are used.

Certificate of designation

Establishments where regulated procedures are to be performed must obtain a certificate of designation. Within this certificate are detailed the areas to be used for animal accommodation, care and use, and lists of the persons responsible for the day-to-day care of the animals, including the veterinary surgeons. Again, the licence is held by an individual, the certificate holder, who assumes overall responsibility for the establishment to the Home Office. The certificate holder has a number of duties:

- To provide and oversee the Ethical Review Process.
- To prevent unauthorised procedures being carried out.
- To oversee animal care and accommodation.
- To recruit and train staff and maintain staffing levels to ensure high standards of animal care. This includes the recruitment of Named Animal Care and Welfare Officers (NACWOs), who are intimately involved in, and primarily responsible for, the day-to-day care of the animals, and Named Veterinary Surgeons.
- To ensure that project licence holders adequately identify the animals in their care
- To maintain daily records of animal environment, animal sources, use and disposal of animals used in regulated procedures, including a health record, obtained under the supervision of a Named Veterinary Surgeon. These records must be kept for at least five years after the animal's death, and made available for Home Office inspection upon request.

Why do we need preclinical imaging?

Recent advances in medical/preclinical imaging technology, and in particular molecular imaging, have the potential to revolutionise the way much basic research is done, with many implications for the manner in which animals are used for research purposes. Preclinical imaging is increasingly being used either to supplement or even to replace other basic science techniques, and can provide unique information on numerous biological processes during health and disease.

Proof of principle/quantification of response to therapy: biomarkers

Possibly the largest focus of research in preclinical imaging is in the identification, development and validation of biological markers, or 'biomarkers'. Biomarkers have previously been defined as 'cellular, biochemical or molecular alterations in biological media such as human tissues, cells, or fluids' (Hulka 1990). They are used to screen for the appearance of, or predisposition to, a disease (predictive biomarkers); to classify or stage a disease (diagnostic biomarkers); to predict clinical outcome regardless of therapy (prognostic biomarkers); or to predict the efficacy of a therapy ahead of time (surrogate biomarkers) (Mayeux 2004; Ludwig, Weinstein 2005; Stadler 2007; Gerszten, Wang 2008).

Imaging technology has made available a host of new biomarkers, which have many potential advantages over existing techniques. In cardiology, for example, the appearance of the cardiac-specific protein creatine kinase–MB in serum is a widely used diagnostic biomarker of myocardial infarction, but it provides little information on the size, severity and location of the infarcted tissue. Using imaging biomarkers, however, we can obtain quantitative information on a disease process, as well as identify exactly *where* disease or injury exists. Multiple imaging biomarkers can also be used sequentially (or simultaneously as will be discussed later) to provide a more detailed diagnosis. While a relatively non-specific $^{15}NH_3$ PET scan can delineate a region of low myocardial blood flow (as a diagnostic biomarker), a follow-up ^{64}Cu-ATSM PET scan could then be used to determine the pathophysiological consequence of that low flow, by delineating the regions of the heart that are biochemically hypoxic but still viable, and would therefore benefit from revascularisation (a prognostic biomarker) (Lewis *et al.* 2002). The other advantage of employing imaging to obtain prognostic biomarkers is that imaging techniques have sufficient sensitivity to detect subtle biochemical changes well in advance of gross tissue changes that occur in advanced disease. Numerous molecular imaging approaches are being explored to specifically image angiogenesis, for example, by targeting VCAM-1 or $\alpha_v\beta_3$ integrins, which are expressed on the vascular lumen very early in disease processes like atherosclerosis and metastatic tumour growth (Provenzale 2007; Cai *et al.* 2008).

While our ultimate goal is to develop these tools for clinical exploitation, we must first more fully understand the behaviour and relevance of our new imaging biomarkers (Smith *et al.* 2003). This is where the various advantages of using animal experimental models and molecular imaging techniques form a truly powerful technology, significantly aiding biomarker validation. While patient data are invaluable, they generally represent disease in a progressed form. For the development and validation of diagnostic imaging approaches for *early* disease detection, and to accurately predict therapeutic outcome, we need to develop agents that target molecular or cellular biomarkers *predating* clinically apparent disease. For true validation of imaging biomarkers, their appearance must be correlated with the disease they represent, which must be evaluated by comparison with tissue histology and biodistribution data, blood measurements, changes in physiological function, morbidity, mortality, etc. All of these parameters are most widely available for study in animal models. While imaging provides a unique range of biomarkers for providing new biological insight, the optimal approach is to combine imaging datasets with biomarkers using other techniques such as histology, biochemical assay, or genomic profiling. As previously outlined, patient data are heterogeneous and are influenced by a vast array of extraneous factors such as age, maturity of disease, diet, existing medication, etc. We therefore need to be able to observe biomarker expression in well-characterised, reproducible animal models at the earliest possible time points.

While the use of molecular imaging to investigate disease processes in animal models has great potential to reduce animal use in drug discovery and development, it is unfortunately the case that identifying therapeutic molecular targets for these drugs, and identifying and validating biomarkers for disease processes and their therapies, will continue to require animal models. However, preclinical imaging of animals offers a means of drastically reducing the numbers of animals required for such work. Traditionally, therapeutic efficacy and drug targeting have been evaluated in animal disease models by postmortem analysis and biodistribution studies in excised organs. If appreciation of a time course is required, multiple animal groups will be employed in parallel, and each group sequentially culled and compared for examination of changes in various parameters over time. If 10 time points were required, for example, typically 60 animals would be used (with replicated animal groups of 6 per time point). With longitudinal non-invasive imaging, however, time courses can be non-invasively tracked over the same time period in just one group of animals. Not only does this significantly reduce the number of animals required in a study (from 60 to just 6 in our example), but it also increases the statistical power of the study because each animal can commonly act as its own control. Conventional biodistribution information is only accessible in the specific organs that are collected and counted; thus unexpected but valuable biodistributions in other targets can potentially be missed. Imaging provides whole body data, allowing the detection of such unexpected results and, moreover, providing biodistribution patterns between organs as well as within the target organ itself, and giving indications on drug clearance routes and potential non-target organ toxicity, etc. Preclinical imaging therefore offers better information quality, greater information yield per animal, and the possibility of detecting unexpected and unsought observations, all of which are highly advantageous in most if not all biomedical and clinical fields.

Drug development and toxicity testing

A significant proportion of novel drug candidates are rejected because of poor specificity and selectivity, and inappropriate uptake or metabolism in other critical organs (most commonly the liver or gastrointestinal tract). Evaluation and rejection of candidate compounds in this manner is expensive, both financially and in terms of animal lives. Molecular imaging provides the means to visualise 'first in human' radiolabelled drug biodistributions at concentrations several orders of magnitude lower than those which would cause a pharmacological effect. Confirming appropriate drug targeting and pharmacokinetics at the earliest possible opportunity in human subjects is a very attractive proposal to the pharmaceutical industry (Weber *et al.* 2008). However, this approach is not without its limitations. Nuclear imaging techniques cannot distinguish between tissue accumulation of the tracer itself and the accumulation of its metabolites; the latter may bear no relation at all to the biology under investigation. A potentially useful adjunct to first in human imaging studies in this respect is a technique known as 'microdosing' (Bauer *et al.* 2008). While not widely used currently, microdosing has recently been recommended by EMEA as a potentially attractive means of providing an early evaluation of the pharmacokinetics of lead pharmaceutical candidate compounds (Kimmelman 2007). With appropriate ethical clearance, a ^{14}C-labelled microdose of a lead compound can be injected into a human subject at 1/100 of the concentration expected to induce a pharmacological effect. The detection of the drug and its metabolites in plasma and excreta can then be accurately quantified by the exquisitely sensitive technique of accelerator mass spectrometry (AMS). While microdosing provides no information on biodistribution, in combination with radiolabels appropriate for nuclear imaging, a combined approach using PET or SPECT imaging and AMS microdosing offers significant promise in simultaneously determining biodistribution and pharmacological fate in humans in a 'Phase 0' setting, providing a 'go/no go' decision on a drug candidate before it has been evaluated in a single animal. A further major problem remains, however; the behaviour of a drug may not be the same at therapeutic concentrations as it is at trace concentrations. Many receptors and transporters may become saturated at these therapeutic concentrations, but not at tracer concentrations. Tracer pharmacokinetics may not necessarily accurately represent therapeutic drug pharmacokinetics. It is likely therefore that subsequent efficacy/toxicity testing in animals would still be required at some level, to determine concentration-dependent toxicity effects prior to advancing to Phase I clinical trials. Nevertheless, first in human imaging/microdosing studies have the potential to significantly reduce the number of animals required in this early stage of drug discovery and evaluation.

The future of preclinical imaging

Preclinical imaging has expanded as an experimental tool hand-in-hand with the development of imaging hardware, such that imaging of small animals (and particularly mice) with sufficient sensitivity and resolution to provide reproducible, meaningful data is now routine. As is reviewed in Chapters 4 and 5, most current preclinical PET scanners employ crystals as small as $1 \times 1 \times 12$ mm, and can obtain voxel volumes as low as 1.1 mm^3 (Pichler *et al.* 2008; Tay *et al.* 2005). While clinical SPECT systems suffer from lower sensitivity than PET, due to significant attenuation from the patient and the necessary use of collimators (reviewed by Rahmim and Zaidi (2008)), preclinical SPECT scanners have many advantages over preclinical PET scanners that may make them a more favourable modality for many applications. Current state-of-the-art small-animal SPECT scanners employ four large detector heads with multi-pinhole collimators, which provide a multiplexed image that is then reconstructed into a single image. With use of multiple pinholes, far less of the radiation is collimated, resulting in significant improvements in sensitivity. Preclinical SPECT scanners currently have a resolution of less than 0.5 mm, and because of the small size of the animal are far less hampered by tissue attenuation. Such resolutions are currently not possible with preclinical PET systems because they are below the positronic range of the PET isotopes used. For experimental purposes, SPECT also has a significant advantage in being able to perform spectral analysis to simultaneously image more than one isotope, allowing the tracking of multiple biological processes.

Most preclinical imaging systems are now multimodal, being equipped with high-resolution CT systems ($<100\,\mu$m resolution) as standard, allowing the generation of fused structural/functional images. Multimodality is becoming an increasingly important consideration in the development of these systems, the next generation of which is likely to bring together PET and MR imaging technologies (Pichler *et al.* 2008; Rowland, Cherry 2008). While CT has excellent spatial resolution, it is limited to providing structural information and delivers a significant radiation dose to the animal (in addition to the dose received from the nuclear imaging agent), which limits scan time and frequency for longitudinal studies. MRI, on the other hand, has no restrictions with respect to radiation dose, and is significantly more versatile, providing both structural and biological information. Not only does MRI provide native *in-vivo* biomarkers, such as measurement of blood oxygen saturation (BOLD MRI; Egred *et al.* 2006), or intracellular energetics (by quantifying intracellular ATP or pH by ^{31}P NMR spectroscopy; Jung, Dietze 1999), but there are also numerous injectable MRI contrast agents available and in development, for both traditional and molecular imaging approaches. These range from the essentially simple, such as iron-containing

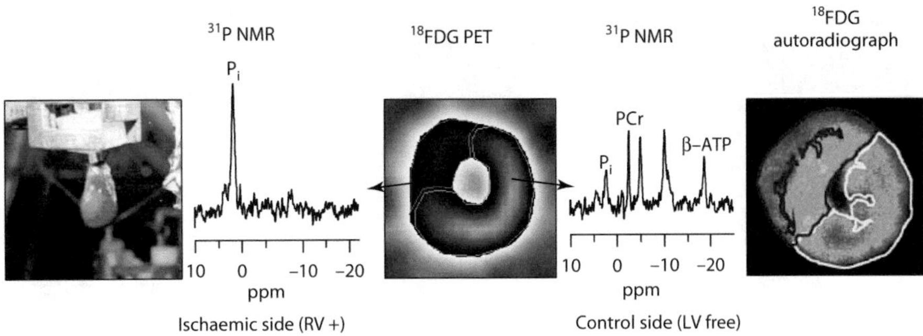

Figure 37.3 A PANDA (dual PET/MR spectroscopy) dataset from an isolated perfused rat heart. The rat heart is maintained viable inside the PANDA system by perfusing it with a physiological salt solution, and [^{18}F]FDG can be either infused constantly or injected as a bolus. The left and right sides of the heart can be independently perfused to induce regional ischaemia (the two vascular beds are delineated by dye in the left panel). Mid-ventricular PET scans are then acquired throughout the experiment to quantify [^{18}F]FDG-6-P accumulation (centre panel), and ^{31}P NMR spectra from the ischaemic and control sides acquired at the same time to quantify intracellular ATP, phosphocreatine and inorganic phosphate levels. At the end of the experiment, hearts are frozen and sectioned, and the [^{18}F]FDG-6-P accumulation is confirmed by high-resolution autoradiography (right) (Southworth, Garlick 2003; Southworth et *al.* 2002).

nanoparticles (superparamagnetic iron oxides, or SPIOs), which are phagocytosed by macrophages and thereby delineate inflammation (Mun *et al.* 2008), to the more complex and experimental, such as lipid-encapsulated perfluorocarbon-cored nanoparticles (quantifiable by ^{19}F magnetic resonance spectroscopy and visualised by either ^{19}F or ^{1}H MRI; Southworth *et al.* 2009; Lanza *et al.* 2005), which are targetable to specific vascular binding sites by peptide binding sequences on their surface, and capable of delivering a payload of a site-targeted drug (Winter *et al.* 2008).

The combination of PET and magnetic resonance technology can give added biological and mechanistic insight through the simultaneous provision of complementary biological data. The first prototype system, PANDA (**P**ET **and** **N**MR **d**ual **a**cquisition), built in the mid-1990s as a collaborative project between King's College London and UCLA, consists of a single-slice PET detector positioned within the bore of a 9.4-tesla NMR spectroscopy magnet (Shao *et al.* 1997). The magnetic field-sensitive photomultiplier tubes of the PET system are housed outside of the magnetic field, and coupled to the detector ring by a series of long fibre-optic cables. Biological samples or isolated organ preparations can then be inserted into the magnet bore and interrogated simultaneously by both techniques. PANDA has been used extensively to correlate changes in myocardial glucose uptake (obtained by PET) with changes in myocardial energetics (by ^{31}P NMR spectroscopy) in Langendorff perfused hearts (Garlick *et al.* 1999; Figure 37.3).

This apparatus shows great potential in the validation and characterisation of novel imaging agents, whereby the tissue accumulation of a candidate tracer can be quantified by one modality and simultaneously correlated with biomarkers quantified by the other modality, giving a biological readout that relates to the uptake of the tracer of interest. For example, the tissue accumulation of a hypoxia-specific tracer like ^{64}Cu-ATSM could be followed by PET, and the hypoxia dependence of its uptake validated by measuring intracellular oxygen levels by ^{19}F NMR oximetry at the same time. The uptake of the PET tracer could also be related to the loss of intracellular ATP (by ^{31}P NMR spectroscopy) to provide insight into the biological relevance of the level of hypoxia at which PET tracer accumulation occurs.

Combining modalities can also serve to overcome their respective weaknesses. PET has extremely high sensitivity (less than nanomolar), but relatively poor resolution ($>1\,mm^3$). MRI has extremely high resolution ($>0.1\,mm^3$), but relatively poor sensitivity (>millimolar). By combining the imaging modalities,

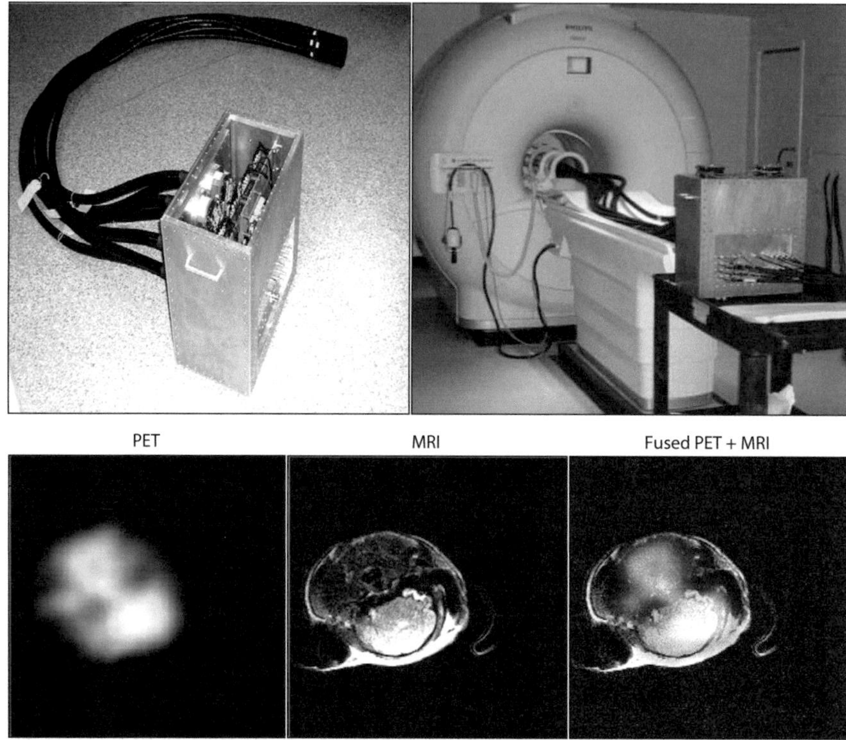

Figure 37.4 Simultaneous PET/MRI of a mouse brain. This prototype system is based on a similar design to the PANDA system, with the PET detector crystals connected to the electronic components of the system by fibre-optic cables, allowing the electronics to operate outside of the magnetic field (top left). This system is compatible with a 3-tesla Philips Achieva clinical MRI system (top right). Bottom panels: preliminary dataset from a mouse brain using this system showing the [^{18}F]FDG PET image, magnetic resonance image, and overlaid images respectively. Photographs and images courtesy of Drs Jane Mackewn and Paul Marsden, King's College London.

and using dual labelling approaches (perhaps simultaneous labelling with ^{18}F/^{19}F, or ^{18}F/gadolinium), it would be possible to co-register these images to provide high-sensitivity PET guidance to a high-resolution magnetic resonance imaging for numerous molecular imaging applications. It is because of its obvious potential and flexibility, that PET/MR has become an increasingly desirable technology. Several preclinical dual imaging prototypes have been successfully developed (Mackewn *et al.* 2005 (Figure 37.4); Werhl *et al.* 2009), and a prototype system for imaging the human brain has recently been demonstrated (Schlemmer *et al.* 2008). The race is now on to complete the world's first commercial full-body clinical system, which is likely to drive the development and validation of a new generation of dual-modality imaging tracers.

Summary

It is apparent that, for the foreseeable future, animal models remain our best hope of developing and advancing our understanding of and treatment for human disease. Until better replacements can be refined, we are duty bound to afford the animals that we use the best standards of care possible, and to ensure that these standards are monitored and enforced to guarantee compliance across the entire scientific community. However, we are currently at the dawn of an exciting new scientific revolution fuelled by advances in medical and molecular imaging, which not only has the potential to reduce the number of animals required to provide the scientific insight we need but in many applications has the potential to replace animal experimentation altogether. It is essential that we continue to engage both the public and our peers in the prospective benefits that both clinical and preclinical imaging can provide.

References

Animals (Scientific Procedures) Act 1986. London: The Home Office. Available at: http://scienceandresearch.homeoffice.gov.uk/animal-research/publications-and-reference/ (accessed 11 June 2010).

Bauer M *et al.* (2008). Microdosing studies in humans: the role of positron emission tomography. *Drugs R D* 9(2): 73–81.

Baumans V (2004). Use of animals in experimental research: an ethical dilemma? *Gene Ther* 11: S64–S66.

Cai W *et al.* (2008). Imaging of integrins as biomarkers for tumor angiogenesis. *Curr Pharm Des* 14(28): 2943–2973.

Conti PS *et al.* (2008). Molecular imaging: the future of modern medicine. *J Nucl Med* 49(6): 16N–20N.

Demopoulos K 2006. Oxford prepares for first pro-vivisection protest. *The Guardian* February 24.

Egred M *et al.* (2006). Blood oxygen level dependent (BOLD) MRI: a novel technique for the detection of myocardial ischemia. *Eur J Intern Med* 17(8): 551–555.

Enserink M (2008). Brazilian scientists battle animal experimentation bans. *Science* 319: 1319.

Frese KK, Tuveson DA (2007). Maximizing mouse cancer models. *Nat Rev Cancer* 7(9): 645–658.

Garlick PB *et al.* (1999). Differential uptake of FDG and DG during post-ischaemic reperfusion in the isolated, perfused rat heart. *Eur J Nucl Med* 26(10): 1353–1358.

Gerszten RE, Wang TJ (2008). The search for new cardiovascular biomarkers. *Nature* 451: 949–953.

Hearse DJ, Sutherland FJ (2000). Experimental models for the study of cardiovascular function and disease. *Pharmacol Res* 41(6): 597–603.

Ho MW, Cummins J (2006). London drug trial catastrophe – collapse of science and ethics. *Science in Society* 30: 44–45.

Home Office (2007). *Statistics of Scientific Procedures on Living Animals Great Britain.* London: Stationery Office.

Hulka BS (1990). Overview of biological markers. In: Hulka BS *et al.*, eds. *Biological Markers in Epidemiology.* New York: Oxford University Press, 3-15.

Jung WI, Dietze GJ (1999). ^{31}P nuclear magnetic resonance spectroscopy: a noninvasive tool to monitor metabolic abnormalities in left ventricular hypertrophy in human. *Am J Cardiol* 83(12A): 19H–24H.

Kimmelman J (2007). Ethics at phase 0: clarifying the issues. *J Law Med Ethics* 35(4): 727–733.

Kolovou G *et al.* (2008). Apolipoprotein E knockout models. *Curr Pharm Des* 14(4): 338–351.

Langley G *et al.* (2007). Replacing animal experiments: choices, chances and challenges. *Bioessays* 29: 918–926.

Lanza GM *et al.* (2005). ^{1}H/^{19}F magnetic resonance molecular imaging with perfluorocarbon nanoparticles. *Curr Top Dev Biol* 70: 57–76.

Lee JA (1995). The pathology of cardiac ischaemia: cellular and molecular aspects. *J Pathol* 175(2): 167–174.

Lewis JS *et al.* (2002). Delineation of hypoxia in canine myocardium using PET and copper(II)-diacetyl-bis (*N*(4)-methylthiosemicarbazone). *J Nucl Med* 43(11): 1557–1569.

Ludwig JA, Weinstein JN (2005). Biomarkers in cancer staging, prognosis and treatment selection. *Nat Rev Cancer* 5: 845–857.

Mackewn JE *et al.* (2005). Design and development of an MR-compatible PET scanner for imaging small animals. *IEEE Trans Nucl Sci* 52(5): 1376–1380.

Massoud TF, Gambhir SS (2003). Molecular imaging in living subjects: seeing fundamental biological processes in a new light. *Genes Dev* 17: 545–580.

Mayeux R (2004). Biomarkers: potential uses and limitations. *J Am Soc Exp Neurother* 1: 182–188.

Mbeunkui F, Johann DJ Jr (2009). Cancer and the tumor microenvironment: a review of an essential relationship. *Cancer Chemother Pharmacol* 63(4): 571–582.

MORI (1999) *Animals in Medicine and Science.* Research study conducted for the Medical Research Council. London: MORI.

MORI (2005) *Use of Animals in Medical Research.* Research study conducted for Coalition for Medical Progress. London: MORI.

Mun HS *et al.* (2008). Graft rejection in the xenogeneic transplantation of mice: diagnosis with in-vivo MR imaging using the homing trait of macrophages. *Xenotransplantation* 15(4): 218–224.

Pichler BJ *et al.* (2008). Latest advances in molecular imaging instrumentation. *J Nucl Med* 49(Suppl 2): 5S–23S.

Provenzale JM (2007). Imaging of angiogenesis: clinical techniques and novel imaging methods. *AJR Am J Roentgenol* 188(1): 11–23.

Rahmim A, Zaidi H (2008). PET versus SPECT: strengths, limitations and challenges. *Nucl Med Commun* 29: 193–207.

Riemann B *et al.* (2008). Small animal PET in preclinical studies: opportunities and challenges. *Q J Nucl Med Mol Imaging* 52(3): 215–221.

Rollin B (2007). Animal research: a moral science. *EMBO Rep* 8(6): 521–525.

Rowland DJ, Cherry SR (2008). Small-animal preclinical nuclear medicine instrumentation and methodology. *Semin Nucl Med* 38(3): 209–222.

Schlemmer HP *et al.* (2008). Simultaneous MR/PET imaging of the human brain: feasibility study. *Radiology* 248(3): 1028–1035.

Schrader J. Mechanisms of ischemic injury in the heart. *Basic Res Cardiol* 80(Suppl 2): 135–139.

Senior K (1995). Defending the use of animals to research human disease. *Mol Med Today* 7: 308–309.

Shao Y *et al.* (1997). Simultaneous PET and MR imaging. *Phys Med Biol* 42(10): 1965–1970.

Skrzypiec-Spring M *et al.* (2007). Isolated heart perfusion according to Langendorff – still viable in the new millennium. *J Pharmacol Toxicol Methods* 55(2): 113–126.

Smith JJ *et al.* (2003). Biomarkers in imaging: realizing radiology's future. *Radiology* 227(3): 633–638.

Somers GF (1962). Thalidomide and congenital abnormalities. *Lancet* 1(7235): 912–913.

Southworth R, Garlick PB (2003). Dobutamine responsiveness, PET mismatch, and lack of necrosis in low-flow ischemia: is this hibernation in the isolated rat heart? *Am J Physiol* 285(1): H316–H324.

Southworth R *et al.* (2002). Dissociation of glucose tracer uptake and glucose transporter distribution in the regionally ischaemic isolated rat heart: application of a new autoradiographic technique. *Eur J Nucl Med Mol Imaging* 29 (10): 1334–1341.

Southworth R *et al.* (2009). Renal vascular inflammation induced by western diet in ApoE-null mice quantified by ^{19}F NMR of VCAM-1 targeted nanobeacons. *Nanomedicine* 5(3): 359–367.

Stadler W (2007). Fuzzy thinking on biomarkers. *Urol Oncol Semin Orig Invest* 25: 97–100.

Tay YC *et al.* (2005). Performance evaluation of the microPET focus: a third-generation microPET scanner dedicated to animal imaging. *J Nucl Med* 46: 455–463.

Weber WA *et al.* (2008). Technology insight: novel imaging of molecular targets is an emerging area crucial to the development of targeted drugs. *Nat Clin Pract Oncol* 5 (1): 44–54.

Wehrl HF *et al.* (2009). Pre-clinical PET/MR: technological advances and new perspectives in biomedical research. *Eur J Nucl Med Mol Imaging* 36: 56–68.

Weissleder R, Mahmood U (2001). Molecular imaging. *Radiology* 219: 316–333.

Wiechert S *et al.* (2003). 24-h Langendorff-perfused neonatal rat heart used to study the impact of adenoviral gene transfer. *Am J Physiol* 285(2): H907–H914.

Willmann JK *et al.* (2008). Molecular imaging in drug development. *Nat Rev Drug Discov* 7(7): 591.

Winter PM *et al.* (2008). Minute dosages of alpha(nu)beta3-targeted fumagillin nanoparticles impair Vx-2 tumor angiogenesis and development in rabbits. *FASEB J* 22(8): 2758–2767.

Woolcock N (2006). Animal rights grave-robbers are jailed for 12 years each. *The Times* May 12.

Zaidi RA, Habib YR (2008). PET versus SPECT: strengths, limitations and challenges. *Nucl Med Commun* 29(3): 193.

Appendix

The radioactive decay law and some practical applications

The basic principles of radioactive decay are discussed in Chapter 2. This appendix deals with some of the practical consequences of the decay law. The rate of disintegration or decay of radionuclei, dN/dt, is determined by the decay constant λ (or probability of decay) and the number N of radionuclei in the sample:

$$\frac{dN}{dt} = -\lambda N = A \quad (A.1)$$

The rate of disintegration is known as the *radioactivity* A and is measured in disintegrations per second (dps) or becquerels (Bq, where 1 Bq represents an average disintegration rate of 1 dps). Integration of the rate equation leads to

$$A_t = A_0 e^{-\lambda t} \quad (A.2)$$

and taking natural logarithms gives

$$\ln(A_t) = \ln(A_0) - \lambda t \quad (A.3)$$

where A_t is the radioactivity at time t and A_0 is the radioactivity at the reference time $t = 0$. This is a simple exponential decay.

The decay can also be characterised by the half-life $t_{1/2}$, defined as the time required for the radioactivity to be halved from its starting value. The relationship between λ and $t_{1/2}$ is

$$\lambda = \frac{\ln(2)}{t_{1/2}} = \frac{0.693}{t_{1/2}} \quad (A.4)$$

The half-lives of some medical and pharmaceutical radionuclides are tabulated in Chapter 2.

The half-life gives an immediate appreciation of the radioactivity remaining in a sample. For example, after two half-lives the radioactivity has fallen to one-quarter of the starting level; after 10 half-lives it has fallen to $(1/2)^{10} = 1/1024$ or approximately 0.1% of the original radioactivity. The '$10 \times t_{1/2}$' rule of thumb is a very useful guide when considering the disposal of radioactive waste.

There are three practically important consequences of the radioactive decay law. The first is to calculate the *number of radionuclei* in a radioactive sample; the second is to calculate the *radioactive dose* of radiopharmaceuticals (which are dispensed beforehand and must contain excess radioactivity at the time of dispensing) and to ensure that material has decayed sufficiently for disposal. The third consequence is the reliability of radioactivity measurements through the *statistics of counting*.

The number of radionuclei or atoms in a sample

Equation (A.1) can be used to calculate the radioactivity, or *specific activity* (S), of a sample of pure radionuclide, given the number of atoms (radionuclei) and the decay constant. For example, the maximum specific activity in Bq/mol is

$$S_{max}(Bq) = \lambda(s^{-1}) \times 6.02 \times 10^{23}\ (mole^{-1})\ Bq/mol$$

Using half-life instead:

$$S_{max}(Bq) = (0.693 \times 6.02 \times 10^{23})/t_{1/2}\ (s) = 4.173/t_{1/2}\ (s)$$

The BP gives the following formula for calculating maximum specific activity (S_{max}):

$$S_{max} = \frac{1.16 \times 10^{20}}{W \times t_{1/2}} Bq/g \qquad (A.5)$$

where W is the atomic weight and $t_{1/2}$ is expressed in hours.

For example, 1 mole of pure ^{99m}Tc contains 6.02×10^{23}atoms and its decay constant, expressed in seconds, is 3.198×10^{-5} per second. Substituting these values into equation (A.1),

$$A = (3.198 \times 10^{-5}) \times (6.02 \times 10^{23}) = 1.93 \times 10^{19} Bq$$

which is a very large quantity, better expressed as 19.3 EBq (exabecquerels).

Performing the same calculation using the BP equation (A.5) gives us

$$S_{max} = \frac{1.16 \times 10^{20}}{99 \times 6.02} = 1.946 \times 10^{17} Bq/g$$

and multiplying this result by the atomic weight (i.e. $99 \times 1.946 \times 10^{17}$) gives the same result.

The calculation can be done in reverse, to determine the mass of ^{99m}Tc corresponding to a known quantity of radioactivity. For example, a patient dose of 400 MBq of a ^{99m}Tc radiopharmaceutical will contain

$$N = \frac{400 \times 10^{6}}{3.21 \times 10^{-5}} = 1.25 \times 10^{14}\ atoms$$

Converting this to mass, we divide by the number of atoms in a mole, then multiply by the atomic weight (99 in this case) to get

$$m = \frac{(1.25 \times 10^{14}) \times 99}{6.02 \times 10^{23}} = 2.05 \times 10^{-8}\ grams$$

This can be expressed as 20 nanograms, showing that the physical mass of the radionuclide is incredibly small in a radiopharmaceutical, and that an injection of Sodium Pertechnetate [^{99m}Tc] Injection is indistinguishable from isotonic saline, except for the radioactivity. This result is typical of all medical radionuclides as shown in Table A.1.

Table A.1 Specific activities and masses of some medical radionuclides

Radionuclide	Half-life	S_{max} (Bq/g)	Mass of 37 MBq (g)
^{81m}Kr	13 seconds	3.21×10^{22}	1.16×10^{-15}
^{11}C	20.3 minutes	2.87×10^{19}	1.29×10^{-12}
^{51}Cr	27.7 days	1.74×10^{17}	2.13×10^{-10}
^{57}Co	271 days	1.78×10^{16}	2.08×10^{-9}
^{58}Co	70.8 days	6.83×10^{16}	5.42×10^{-10}
^{75}Se	118.5 days	4.08×10^{16}	9.07×10^{-10}
^{99m}Tc	6.02 hours	1.93×10^{19}	1.92×10^{-12}
^{111}In	2.8 days	1.73×10^{18}	2.14×10^{-11}
^{123}I	13.2 hours	8.79×10^{18}	4.21×10^{-12}
^{125}I	60.1 days	8.04×10^{16}	4.60×10^{-10}
^{131}I	8.04 days	6.01×10^{17}	6.16×10^{-11}

Corrections for radioactive decay

The second application is to calculate the volume of radiopharmaceutical to be administered when some time has elapsed between preparation (T) and administration (t). For this we use equations (A.2) or (A.3) to determine the fraction of radioactivity remaining at the time t. Using (A.2) we can calculate the fraction F remaining from the expression

$$F = 1 \times e^{-\lambda(T-t)} \qquad (A.6)$$

where $T-t$ is the elapsed time between preparation and administration. In practice this expression is not used; a table of pre-calculated fractions is employed instead.

Taking the technetium-99m example again, suppose a radiopharmaceutical containing 400 MBq per 1 mL dose is prepared at 08:00 but is not administered until 10:30. The elapsed time ($T - t$) is 2.5 hours and the decay constant is 0.1151 per hour. Substituting these values into the equation, we obtain $F = 0.75$, so that the preparation now contains $400 \times 0.75 = 300$ MBq per 1 mL dose. A larger volume of $(1/0.75) = 1.33$ mL must be administered to give the required dose of 400 MBq. A typical worksheet for this calculation is shown at the end of this appendix.

The linear form of the integrated equation (A.3) can also be used to calculate the amount of radionuclide remaining after a specified time as the following examples show.

Example 1

Calculate the fraction (or percentage) of radioactive atoms remaining after 3 weeks for a sample of ^{32}*P* ($t_{1/2} = 14.3$ *days) and* ^{24}*Na* ($t_{1/2} = 15$ *hours).*

The procedure here is to express the decay time in *exactly* the same units as half-life, then apply the equation to convert from half-life to decay constant (i.e. $\lambda = 0.693/t_{1/2}$), and finally substitute into the logarithmic form of the equation (i.e. $\ln(N_t) = \ln(100) - \lambda t$).

For ^{32}***P we have:***

- Elapsed time: 3 weeks = 21 days.
- Decay constant: $\lambda = \ln(2)/t_{1/2} = 0.693/14.3 = 0.04847$ day^{-1}.
- Per cent remaining: $\ln(N_t) = 4.605 - (0.04847 \times 21) = 3.1365$. Therefore, $N_t = 36.14\%$.

The calculation shows that an appreciable quantity of ^{32}P remains after 3 weeks; it could be used for clinical purposes in the radiopharmacy and is far too radioactive for disposal.

For ^{24}***Na we have:***

- Elapsed time: 3 weeks = 504 hours.
- Decay constant: $\lambda = \ln(2)/t_{1/2} = 0.693/15 = 0.0462$.
- Per cent remaining: $\ln(N_t) = 4.605 - (0.0462 \times 504) = -18.675$. Therefore, $N_t = 7.7 \times 10^{-9}\%$.

This calculation shows that there is practically no ^{24}Na left, and the decayed material can be safely disposed of. Such calculations are necessary in the radiopharmacy to ensure that the material disposed of contains less than the permitted disposal activity.

The statistics of counting

The third application is to the precision of radioactivity measurements. Most measurements of radioactivity depend on counting the number of events from a sample of the material with an appropriate detector. Radioactive decay is a random process and this is reflected in the variation in the counts observed when a sample is repeatedly counted. Consequently there is no absolute count rate and we can only measure the average count rate. The distribution of counts within a specified time interval is described by the Poisson distribution. This statistical distribution deals with rare events (such as disintegration of a nucleus, which can only happen once in the lifetime of the nucleus, so is very rare). All we know is that the event did occur, but have no information about the number of times it did not occur.

The important fact derived from the Poisson distribution is that the reliability of the counting measurement depends on the number of counts actually recorded. The variance of the count is the count itself, and consequently the standard deviation is the square root of the count. In other words, for a count of N events, the standard deviation will be $\sqrt{N}$. This leads us to defining the relative standard deviation (RSD) as $(\sqrt{N})/N$ and the coefficient of variation (CV) as $100 \times$ RSD. It can be seen from Table A.2 how the relative standard deviation decreases as the total number of counts increases. Thus, to determine the radioactivity with a relative standard deviation of 1% it is necessary to accumulate at least 10 000 counts.

For counts above 100 the distribution of repeated counts approaches a normal distribution and so we can apply normal statistical tests such as a chi-square test to our observed counts to see whether the data are

Table A.2 Relative standard deviation ($\sqrt{N}$)/N in relation to total number of counts N

N	$\sqrt{N}$	$\sqrt{N}/N$	% RSD
10	3.16	0.316	31.6
100	10	0.1	10
1000	31.6	0.0316	3.16
10 000	100	0.01	1

really normally distributed. Sometimes, because of instrument breakdown, or excessive activity in the sample, the distribution is not normal and we have to investigate the cause.

In any set of replicated counts the observed values will be scattered about a mean count and the scatter can be expressed as variance V or standard deviation s:

$$V = \frac{\sum (x-\overline{x})^2}{n-1} \quad s = \sqrt{\frac{\sum (x-\overline{x})^2}{n-1}}$$

As stated above, for a Poisson distribution the standard deviation is the square root of the true mean, or our estimate $\overline{x}$, of this quantity. Thus the standard deviation of individual counts can be calculated by taking the square root of that count, and it follows that the standard deviation varies with the size of the mean. This could cause difficulties when comparing different-sized counts and so the relative standard deviation RSD or coefficient of variation CV are used:

$$\text{RSD} = s_{\overline{x}} = s/\overline{x} \quad \text{CV} = 100(s/\overline{x})$$

In a set of replicated counts, each greater than about 100, we expect the scatter to follow a normal distribution. Any faults in the detector or electronics may be detected by comparing the observed scatter with that expected from a normal distribution through the *chi-square test* (χ^2), which may be calculated in this case from the expression:

$$\chi^2 = \frac{\sum (x-\overline{x})^2}{\overline{x}} = \frac{\sum x^2 - (\sum x)^2/n}{\sum x/n}$$

For a total of $n = 50$ replicates the value of chi-square should lie between 34.75 and 67.49. For $n = 10$ the corresponding values are 3.35 and 16.92. If the calculated value of χ^2 lies above the upper limit, excessive variation is occurring; and if it is below the lower limit then there is not enough variation. In both cases the detector and electronics are suspect and the causes of abnormal performance must be investigated.

Counting statistics must be considered whenever two counts are to be compared, as in radiochemical purity testing where the impurity has a low count rate compared with the major component, and in biodistribution studies where the accumulation may be small in some critical organs. Here, the strategy is to keep counting the sample until sufficient counts are accumulated to achieve statistical accuracy.

Since all counting measurements are corrected for the background count it is important to know something about the statistics of the sample and background counts and how they affect the final corrected result. The corrected count (C_R) is obtained by subtracting the background count (C_B) from the observed sample count (C_{S+B}), using the counting times t_B and t_S, respectively:

$$C_R = C_{S+B} - C_B$$

The propagation of error theory states that the standard deviation (σ) of the corrected count is the geometric mean of the standard deviations of the background and sample count rates:

$$\sigma_R = \sqrt{(\sigma_{S+B}^2 + \sigma_B^2)}$$

If the standard deviation of the background count rate C_B is

$$\sigma_B = \sqrt{\frac{C_B}{t_B}}$$

and the standard deviation of the observed count rate C_{S+B} is

$$\sigma_S = \sqrt{\frac{C_{S+B}}{t_S}}$$

then the standard deviation of the corrected count rate is

$$\sigma_R = \sqrt{\left(\frac{C_{S+B}}{t_S} + \frac{C_B}{t_B}\right)}$$

This shows that the standard deviation of the corrected sample count rate depends on the precision of both sample and background measurements. When the observed sample count rate is large compared with background then the background contribution to the error is negligible. On the other hand, when the sample and background count rates are both low then a long counting time is needed for both and the background count makes an appreciable contribution to the error. In radiopharmacy practice, count rates are often embarrassingly high and so the question of erroneous background counts is not a problem. But in quality control laboratories and radiopharmacology studies the question of background correction must be addressed.

Technetium Dispensing Calculation Worksheet

Radiopharmaceutical

Dose required = D ______________ MBq

Time required = T ______________ (hh:mm)

Volume required = R ______________ mL

Stock Pertechnetate Details

Pertechnetate total radioactivity = P ______________ MBq

Pertechnetate volume = v ______________ mL

Time of measurement = t ______________ (hh:mm)

Radioactive concentration = $C = P/v$ ______________ MBq/mL

Pertechnetate Dose Volume Calculation

Elapsed time = $T - t$ ______________ (hh:mm)

Decay factor F (from lab chart – reprinted below)

Pertechnetate volume required

$$V = \frac{D}{C \times F}$$ ______________ mL

Final Dispensing Volumes

Pertechnetate ______________ mL

Diluent saline ______________ mL

Total volume ______________ mL

Batch number

Dispensed by

Checked by

Date

STICK LABEL HERE

Technetium-99m decay factor table

Calculated from the expression $F(Tc) = e^{-0.1151t}$

	Hours						
Minutes	**0**	**1**	**2**	**3**	**4**	**5**	**6**
0	1.0000	0.8909	0.7937	0.7072	0.6300	0.5613	0.5000
2	0.9962	0.8875	0.7907	0.7044	0.6276	0.5591	0.4982
4	0.9923	0.8841	0.7877	0.7017	0.6252	0.5570	0.4962
6	0.9885	0.8807	0.7846	0.6990	0.6228	0.5549	0.4943
8	0.9847	0.8773	0.7816	0.6964	0.6204	0.5527	0.4924
10	0.9809	0.8739	0.7786	0.6937	0.6180	0.5506	0.4905
12	0.9772	0.8706	0.7756	0.6910	0.6156	0.5485	0.4887
14	0.9734	0.8672	0.7726	0.6884	0.6133	0.5464	0.4868
16	0.9697	0.8639	0.7697	0.6857	0.6109	0.5443	0.4849
18	0.9659	0.8606	0.7667	0.6831	0.6086	0.5422	0.4830
20	0.9622	0.8573	0.7638	0.6805	0.6062	0.5401	0.4812
22	0.9585	0.8540	0.7608	0.6778	0.6039	0.5380	0.4793
24	0.9546	0.8507	0.7579	0.6752	0.6016	0.5360	0.4775
26	0.9512	0.8474	0.7550	0.6726	0.5993	0.5339	0.4757
28	0.9475	0.8442	0.7521	0.6701	0.5970	0.5318	0.4738
30	0.9439	0.8409	0.7492	0.6675	0.5947	0.5298	0.4720
32	0.9403	0.8377	0.7463	0.6649	0.5924	0.5278	0.4702
34	0.9366	0.8345	0.7434	0.6624	0.5901	0.5257	0.4684
36	0.9330	0.8313	0.7406	0.6598	0.5878	0.5237	0.4666
38	0.9295	0.8281	0.7378	0.6573	0.5856	0.5217	0.4648
40	0.9259	0.8249	0.7349	0.6548	0.5833	0.5197	0.4630
42	0.9223	0.8217	0.7321	0.6522	0.5811	0.5177	0.4612
44	0.9188	0.8186	0.7293	0.6497	0.5789	0.5157	0.4595
46	0.9153	0.8154	0.7265	0.6472	0.5766	0.5137	0.4577
48	0.9117	0.8123	0.7237	0.6447	0.5744	0.5118	0.4559
50	0.9083	0.8092	0.7209	0.6423	0.5722	0.5098	0.4542
52	0.9047	0.8061	0.7181	0.6398	0.5700	0.5078	0.4524
54	0.9013	0.8030	0.7154	0.6373	0.5678	0.5059	0.4507
56	0.8978	0.7999	0.7126	0.6349	0.5656	0.5039	0.4490
58	0.8944	0.7968	0.7099	0.6325	0.5635	0.5020	0.4472

Glossary

The material in this glossary has been compiled, with permission, from a number of sources including the VirRad website, the UK Radiopharmacy Group website, and private individuals.

^{125}I-Albumin	Albumin radiolabelled with iodine-125 in order to make it traceable *in vivo*. Used clinically for plasma volume studies.
Absorbed radiation dose	The energy deposited in a body by the absorption of ionising radiation, which is measured in units of energy absorbed per unit mass. The SI unit is the *gray* (q.v.) which replaces the older *rad* (q.v.)
Absorber	Any material used to absorb radiation for a specific purpose; absorbers are used in the determination of radiation characteristics and as shields for reducing the intensity of radiation for safe handling and storage.
Absorption	A process in which all or some of the energy of a radiation beam is transferred to the material through which it passes by interactions with electrons or atomic nuclei.
Absorption coefficient	The rate of change in the intensity of a radiation beam as it passes through matter. The *linear absorption coefficient* is the fractional decrease in beam intensity per unit distance and the *mass absorption coefficient* is the fractional decrease in beam intensity per unit of surface density (cm^2/g).
Accelerator	A device used to accelerate charged particles for bombardment of targets and production of radionuclides. Cyclotron, synchrotron, betatron and LINAC are examples of particle accelerators.
Accelerator-produced radionuclides	Radionuclides artificially produced by exposing stable nuclei to a beam of accelerated protons (p or $^1H^+$), deuterons (d or $^2H^+$), helium-3 ions ($^3He^{2+}$), particles (alpha (α), or $^4He^{2+}$) or electrons. Most accelerator-produced radionuclides decay by electron capture or positron emission, mostly followed by photon (γ-ray) emission.
Activity	The strength of a radioactive source and a term often used loosely for radioactivity; it refers to the number of nuclear transformations occurring in unit time.
Adverse reaction	Any noxious and unintended drug reaction that occurs after administration of therapeutic or diagnostic drugs. The term usually excludes accidental exposure or attempted suicide. Because the majority of radiopharmaceuticals do not have therapeutic or pharmacological effects, there are some difficulties in adapting

the term from currently used medicines to radiopharmaceuticals. It is usually accepted that radiopharmaceuticals adverse reactions are associated with the vehicle carrying the radiation and not with the radiation itself, overdose or any administration injury.

Agreement State — A state that has signed an agreement with the Nuclear Regulatory Commission under which the state regulates the use of by-product, source, and small quantities of special nuclear material in that state. (USA)

ALARA — As Low As Reasonably Achievable – a concept widely used in radiation protection and health and safety; each exposure situation is evaluated in terms of achievement of lowest exposure commensurate with reasonable cost and effort, rather than avoidance of maximum permissible exposure values.

ALARA principle — The general principle that exposure to radiation emitted by radionuclides must be kept As Low As Reasonably Achievable

Albumin [^{99m}Tc] colloid injection — Sterile suspension for injection, containing a colloidal dispersion of heat-denatured human serum albumin (particle dimensions $<1\,\mu m$) labelled with technetium-99m. The use of such preparations depends on the size of the colloidal particles. Preparations with very small particles < 50 nm, also called nanocolloids, are used for lymphoscintigraphy, bone marrow scintigraphy and detection of infection. When the particles are larger, the colloid preparation can be used for liver scintigraphy (although this is largely obsolete), labelling of solid meals and sentinel node scintigraphy.

Albumin [^{99m}Tc] microspheres — Heat-denatured human serum albumin in the form of small, uniform spheres with dimensions of between 10 and 100 μm and labelled with technetium-99m. Such particles have the same use as ^{99m}Tc-labelled aggregated particles, i.e. lung perfusion studies with gamma camera imaging.

Albumin [^{99m}Tc] nanocolloid injection — See Albumin [^{99m}Tc] colloid injection.

Albumin [^{99m}Tc], aggregated — Aggregated heat-denatured human serum albumin (HSA) labelled with technetium-99m. The dimensions of the aggregates are of the order of 10–100 μm and the particles have an irregular shape. Used for evaluation of lung perfusion using gamma camera imaging.

ALI — Annual Limit on Intake – defined as the annual intake of a radionuclide that would result in an absorbed radiation dose equivalent to the dose limit. Data on ALIs are given in the Ionising Radiation Regulations.

Alpha decay — A radioactive decay, transformation, or disintegration process in which the unstable nuclide emits an alpha (α) particle, consisting of two neutrons and two protons (a $^{4}He^{2+}$ ion). The resulting daughter nucleus has two protons and two neutrons fewer than the mother nucleus. All alpha particles from a given transformation will have the same energy; this can be used to identify alpha emitters. Alpha decay occurs in the natural radioactive elements heavier than lead ($Z = 82$), which is often the final product from a natural radioactive decay series.

Alpha emitters
: Alpha emitters are unstable nuclei or radionuclides that decay to more stable daughter nuclides through the emission of an alpha particle ($^{4}He^{2+}$ ion). They are mostly found in the elements with atomic number >82. Typical alpha emitters are radium-226 and radon-222.

Alpha particle
: A helium nucleus ($^{4}He^{2+}$ ion), having 2 protons and 2 neutrons, hence a mass of 4 AMU and a charge of +2. These particles are emitted during *alpha decay* (q.v.)

Alpha radiation
: Ionising radiation consisting of emitted alpha particles. Alpha particles have the least penetrating power, move at a slower velocity than other types of radiation, and are deflected slightly by a magnetic field in a direction that indicates a positive charge. Alpha rays are nuclei of ordinary helium atoms (see alpha particles). Alpha decay reduces the atomic weight, or mass number, of a nucleus, while beta and gamma decay leave the mass number unchanged. Thus, the net effect of alpha radioactivity is to produce nuclei lighter than those of the original radioactive substance. Alpha radiation produces significant ionisation (formation of free electrons and positive nuclei) in the absorbing material.

Aluminium breakthrough
: Aluminium contamination in the eluate of a technetium-99m generator, derived from the alumina bed of the generator. The presence of aluminium in the ^{99m}Tc-eluate interferes with, for example, the preparation of ^{99m}Tc-sulfur colloid, which tends to precipitate with excessive aluminium. It also interferes with the labelling of red blood cells with ^{99m}Tc, causing their agglutination.

amu
: Atomic mass unit, equal to 1/12 the mass of an atom of ^{12}C, approximately 1.66×10^{-27} kg.

Anger camera
: Named for its inventor, Hal Anger, also called a gamma camera, the Anger camera is an apparatus to detect and localise electromagnetic radiation (X-rays and gamma rays) emitted from the body after administration of a radiopharmaceutical. The detector material is a rather large thallium-activated sodium iodide (NaI(Tl)) scintillation crystal (thickness about 1 cm) that emits light internally when ionising radiation is deposited. This light is converted into electronic signals by multiple photomultiplier tubes situated behind the NaI(Tl) crystal. There is a lead collimator in front of the sodium iodide crystal that permits passage of only those gamma rays and X-rays emitted perpendicularly from the patient in relation to the crystal. The generated electronic signals are converted into an image that shows the distribution of the radioactive compound in the viewed area of the body.

Annihilation radiation
: The radiation produced by the reaction between a particle and an anti-particle resulting in the annihilation of both. The radiation normally consists of photons having a total energy equivalent to the masses of the particles annihilated. For the negatron–positron annihilation the photons have energies of 0.511 MeV.

Anthropogenic radionuclides
: Those radionuclides introduced into nature by human activity.

Antimatter
: Fundamental and nuclear particles that are unstable in our universe; they combine with ‘normal’ particles by annihilation and the mass of the two particles is converted to energy.

Antimony sulfide [^{99m}Tc] colloid injection	Colloidal suspension of antimony sulfide and technetium-99m sulfide, prepared by heating a mixture of [^{99m}Tc]pertechnetate solution and antimony sulfide. It is mainly used for lymphoscintigraphy.
Antineutrino	A very small nuclear particle, almost impossible to detect, which is presumed to be emitted during negatron decay and which carries off the decay energy not given to the negatron.
ARSAC	Administration of Radioactive Substances Advisory Committee, the UK organisation responsible for advising ministers on applications from physicians to administer radioactive substances.
Atomic number	The number of protons in a nucleus. Symbol Z.
Attenuation	The decrease in the intensity of radiation caused by absorption and scattering of the radiation as it passes through matter.
Auger effect	A process involving the transition of an orbital electron from an excited state to a lower energy level, resulting in the production of an X-ray. The X-ray does not escape from the sphere of influence of the atom before colliding with a second orbital electron to which it imparts all of its energy.
Auger electron	Electron ejected from an atom following an internal photoelectric effect. It absorbs the characteristic X-rays that are emitted as outer orbital electrons fill the vacancies left in deeper energy levels after internal conversion.
Autoradiograph	A photographic record showing the location of radioactivity in an object prepared by placing the object in contact with unexposed photographic film followed by the usual developing processes.
Background	Intrusive radiation that interferes with recorded electronic signals; a more or less steady level of noise above which the effect (e.g. radioactivity) being measured by an apparatus (e.g. a Geiger counter) is detected; a somewhat steady level of radiation in the natural environment (such as from cosmic rays). In measurements of radioactivity, it is the observed count in the absence of the sample. It is caused by cosmic radiation, instrument noise, and naturally occurring radionuclides. In general, background includes electronic noise from instruments, power supplies, etc.
Background count	Number of counts per unit time originating from background radiation under the conditions of measurement of radioactivity.
Background subtraction	Correction of the measured radioactivity (counts per unit time) for the counts due to background radiation to obtain the net radioactivity of a sample or object.
Barn	A unit for expressing the area of nuclear cross-sections. 1 barn = 10^{-24} cm^2, or 10^{-28} m^2; 1 millibarn = 10^{-31} m^2.
BAT	1,2-Dithia-5,8-diazacyclodecane, a ligand that forms stable lipophilic complexes with ^{99m}Tc, used for brain imaging.
Becquerel	The SI unit of radioactivity, abbreviated Bq. An activity of 1 Bq implies an average disintegration rate of 1 disintegration per second. This unit replaces the

curie (q.v.). For radiopharmaceuticals, radioactivity is mostly expressed in kilobecquerels (1 kBq = 1000 Bq), megabecquerels (1 MBq = 1 million Bq) and gigabecquerels (1 GBq = 10^9 Bq).
An older unit of radioactivity is the curie (Ci), 1 Ci being equal to 3.7×10^{10} Bq.

Beta decay — A radioactive decay process in which a beta (β) particle is emitted from the nucleus of an atom, raising the atomic number of the atom by 1 if the particle is negatively charged, lowering it by 1 if the particle is positively charged. The negatively charged particle is also called an electron (or negatron); the positively charged particle is called a positron. In beta decay, an additional particle with no electric charge and a vanishingly small mass is emitted, called the antineutrino in the case of electron emission and a neutrino in the case of positron emission. Detection of the (anti)neutrino is extremely difficult. The energy of the (anti)neutrino is equal to the difference between the energy of the accompanying beta particle and the maximum energy dissipated during the beta decay of a radionuclide.
A general term for three transformation processes in which the nuclide gains stability by emission of a negatron or positron, or by electron capture.

Beta emitter — A radioisotope that decays with emission of beta particles

Beta particle — Electron (β^-) or positron (β^+) emitted from an atomic nucleus during radioactive decay. Beta radiation was first identified and named by Ernest Rutherford, who found that it consists of high-speed electrons (negatrons). Positrons were discovered later by Carl Anderson in 1932.

Bifunctional chelate — A metallic chelating agent that will also react with active groups on proteins and other macromolecules. In the field of radiopharmaceuticals, this term is used to indicate a compound that on the one hand can form a stable complex with a (radioactive) metal ion and on the other hand contains a functional group via which it can be coupled to biologically interesting compounds (such as a peptide that binds to receptors on tumour cells).The bifunctional chelate is usually reacted with the macromolecule and the compound is purified and then labelled with the radionuclide by chelation. Bifunctional chelates are used widely with monoclonal antibodies and the commonest radionuclides are ^{99m}Tc and ^{111}In.

Binding energy — The energy that binds a particle to an atom or nucleus. Electron binding energy is a synonym for ionisation potential; nuclear binding energy is equal to the difference in mass of the nucleus and the sum of masses of its constituent particles.

Biodistribution — Distribution of a chemical (radioactive or stable) in the body of a living being.

Biological half-life — The time required for one-half of an administered substance to be eliminated from the body, or from an organ or section of living tissue.

Body burden — The amount of radioactive or toxic material present in a human or animal body.

Bone scan — A bone scan is performed by intravenously injecting a small amount of radioactive marker (usually a ^{99m}Tc-labelled bisphosphonate). Some hours later the patient is scanned (usually with a gamma camera) and the radioactive marker will be concentrated in any region where there is high bone turnover. A bone scan is sometimes performed to rule out an inflammatory process (such as a tumour or infection) or an occult fracture (small fracture not seen on an X-ray). A bone scan is a highly sensitive test to pick up tumours, infections, or very small fractures because these conditions all result in high bone turnover. It can also be used to determine whether a compression fracture of the vertebral body is old or new, as an old fracture will not light up but a new one will.

Bone-seeking tracers	Radioactive compounds that concentrate in bone in proportion to the bone turnover rate.
Bq	Abbreviation for the unit *becquerel* (q.v.)
Branched decays	Decay schemes in which the radionuclide may undergo one of several possible decay modes. Each nucleus can undergo only one decay, but the percentages of a population decaying through each mode are usually marked on a decay scheme.
Branching ratio	The proportion of radionuclide that decays by a given mode.
Bremsstrahlung	Literally 'braking radiation'; X-rays emitted when an electron slows down in passing through a substance. The kinetic energy is transformed to the photon energy. The fraction of the electron energy transformed to bremsstrahlung will depend on the density and atomic number of the absorber and the energy of the electron beam
BSC	Biological safety cabinet.
BUD	Beyond use date.
Build-up	The increase in radiation flux through a shield arising from scattering, thus making the shield less effective than predicted from its attenuation properties.
CACI	Compounding aseptic containment isolator.
Calibration	The act of standardising a measuring instrument by determining the measurement deviation from a standard so as to ascertain the proper correction factors. In the radiopharmacy, instruments for measuring the radioactivity (e.g. an ionisation chamber used as a dose calibrator) and balances (used to weigh an accurate amount of a compound for pharmaceutical or chemical use) have to be calibrated frequently. The daily calibration of dose calibrators is recommended to ensure accurate and reproducible instrument response. Calibration is easily achieved and maintained by the use of long-lived radioactive reference sources.
Cardiolite	Trade name for the labelling kit used to prepare ^{99m}Tc-sestamibi. ^{99m}Tc-Sestamibi is a radiopharmaceutical for diagnosing coronary artery disease and identifying patients at risk for heart attacks and heart disease. The Cardiolite kit contains a complex of copper(I) with 4 molecules of methoxyisobutylisonitrile (MIBI). When this Cu-(MIBI)$_4$ complex is heated with ^{99m}Tc in the form of pertechnetate in the presence of a reducing agent such

as stannous ion, the copper ion is replaced by a Tc^+ ion and a complex is formed in which one Tc^+ ion is bound to six molecules of MIBI (called technetium-sestamibi). It is injected into a patient intravenously and travels through the bloodstream to the heart. A patient undergoing a rest-and-stress examination receives two injections of ^{99m}Tc-sestamibi, one while at rest and one while vigorously exercising on a stationary bike or treadmill. Images obtained from each of the two sessions can be compared to determine whether the blood supply to the heart is being blocked.

Cardiotec — Brand name of a labelling kit to prepare ^{99m}Tc-teboroxime, a myocardial perfusion tracer agent. The kit has been withdrawn from the market.

Carrier — A substance added to a radionuclide preparation to ensure that the radioactivity is 'carried' through a process and does not become fixed to containers, etc. The carrier must have very similar chemical properties to the radioelement being investigated, and is frequently the non-radioactive material itself.

Carrier-free — Applied to a radioactive isotope the term denotes a preparation of a radioisotope that does not contain any other isotopes (stable or radioactive) of that element as carrier. For instance, a carrier-free preparation of fluorine-18 does not contain any stable fluorine-19. A carrier-free preparation is thus one in which only the stated radionuclide is present without its corresponding stable isotope. However a truly carrier-free state is seldom attained. A *no-carrier-added* preparation is one in which unlabelled tracer or precursor is not added intentionally during radionuclide production, radiosynthesis and final product formulation.
A ^{99m}Tc preparation always contains a small amount of the same compound(s) labelled with long-lived ^{99}Tc and thus is not carrier-free. However, if no ^{99m}Tc was added intentionally to this preparation, it would be 'no-carrier-added'.

CASI — Compounding aseptic isolator.

Cell labelling — Radioisotope labelling of blood cells, normally taken from a patient. The radiolabelled cells are then re-administered to the same patient for a radioisotopic measurement.

Ceretec — Trade name for the labelling kit used for the preparation of ^{99m}Tc-exametazime (HMPAO) – see also *exametazime*. Used for visualisation of cerebral blood flow in stroke patients and also for labelling of white blood cells to localise intra-abdominal infection and inflammatory bowel disease.

CFR — Code of Federal Regulations (USA)

cGMP — Current Good Manufacturing Practice

Chain reaction — A situation in which a radionuclide undergoes fission, releasing neutrons that cause fission of another radionuclide and so on in a chain. A controlled chain reaction is realised in an atomic reactor, and an uncontrolled one in a nuclear weapon.

Chelation — The formation of a closed ring of atoms by attachment of a chelator or ligand to a central metal atom.

Cherenkov radiation	Visible light emitted by charged particles as they pass from a transparent medium of low refractive index to a transparent medium of high refractive index, when their velocity in the first medium exceeds the velocity of light in the second medium.
[^{57}Co, ^{58}Co, ^{60}Co]Cyanocobalamin solution	A solution containing cyanocobalamin (vitamin B_{12}) in which the central non-radioactive cobalt atom is replaced by a radioisotope of cobalt. Vitamin B_{12} radiolabelled in such a way is used in the so-called Schilling test. This test is performed to determine the origin of pernicious anaemia.
Coincidence counting	A method of counting that employs coincidence circuits so that the event is recorded only if both detectors simultaneously detect it. The method is used to reduce background counts or scattered counts.
Colloidal albumin	Albumin that has been denatured by the action of heat into water-insoluble aggregates. In nuclear medicine, ^{99m}Tc-labelled macroaggregated albumin (particle size 10–100 μm) is used to measure lung perfusion.
Colloidal rhenium sulfide	A colloidal solution of technetium-99m heptasulfide Tc_2S_7, in which Re_2S_7 acts as carrier molecule for colloidal sulfur and Tc_2S_7 particles
Colloidal sulfur	In ^{99m}Tc-labelled sulfur colloid, technetium is present as (almost insoluble) Tc_2S_7 (Tc has a valency of +7 as in TcO_4^-) in the presence of colloidal particles of sulfur. This can be preparing by heating an acidic solution of sodium thiosulfate in the presence of [^{99m}Tc]pertechnetate solution.
Colloidal tin	Technetium–tin colloid is a co-precipitate of $^{99m}TcO_2$ with different tin species ($SnOF_2$, $Sn(OH)_2$), as carrier. This colloid is made by reduction of pertechnetate with Sn(II)F_2, or Sn(II)Cl_2, in an alkaline environment.
COMARE	Committee on Medical Aspects of Radiation in the Environment.
Complexing agents	Organic compounds that are able to form complexes with metal ions. Examples of such complexing agents used in radiopharmacy to complex metallic radionuclides include *DTPA*, *EDTA*, *MDP*, *MAG*$_3$ and *exametazime*.
Compton effect	Inelastic collision of a photon and an electron in which the direction of the photon is changed and its energy reduced. The electron is set in motion by the collision and is called the Compton recoil electron.
Controlled area	A defined area where workers must follow written procedures in order to control their radiation exposures.
Cosmic rays	Radiation originating outside the earth's atmosphere, consisting of particles capable of producing ionising events, mainly protons and nuclei.
Cosmogenic nuclide	A nuclide formed by bombardment by cosmic rays.
CPB	Competitive protein binding; a saturation radioassay in which labelled drug or hormone competes with endogenous material for sites on a binder protein added to the system. The radioactivity of the protein is then inversely proportional to the amount of endogenous material in the system.

Cross-section, nuclear	The target area presented by a nucleus to an approaching particle. It varies with the type of nucleus, type and energy of the projectile particle and the specified interaction, and is measured in *barns* (q.v.).
CSP	Compounded Sterile Preparation (USP).
CT	Computed axial tomography; an imaging technique in which a collimated beam of X-rays is directed through an axial slice of the subject and the attenuation measured each time as the beam is rotated slightly. The data from each complete circle are computer-processed to reconstruct an image of that slice of the subject.
Curie	The older unit of radioactivity, originally intended to represent the disintegration rate of 1 g of radium, but agreed internationally to be equivalent to 3.7×10^{10} disintegrations per second. The curie (symbol Ci) is too large a unit for many purposes and the sub-multiples nCi, μCi, mCi are used in practice; these are equivalent to 37 Bq, 37 kBq, 37 MBq, respectively.
Cyclotron	A machine that accelerates charged particles in a spiral or circular path and deflects them onto a target.
DADS	Diamide disulfur ligand; *N*,*N*′-bis(mercaptoacetamido)ethylenediamine. A diamine dithiol-containing chelating system for labelling with technetium. The ^{99m}Tc-complex is used in renal imaging.
Daughter activity	Radioactivity emitted by daughter radionuclide.
Daughter radionuclide	The nuclide immediately resulting from the radioactive decay of a parent or precursor nuclide.
DDTC	Diethyldithiocarbamate; complexes with ^{201}Tl and ^{99m}Tc are used as brain imaging agents.
Dead time	The length of time immediately following an electrical impulse for which a detector remains insensitive and unable to record another ionising event.
Decay (disintegration, radioactive decay)	Spontaneous transformation of the nucleus of a radioactive atom into a new nuclear form, accompanied by the emission of radiation.
Decay chain	The sequence of radioactive atoms produced by successive transformations from an original or primordial radionuclide, ending when a stable form of atom is finally achieved.
Decay constant	Synonym for *disintegration constant* (q.v.).
Decay scheme	A diagram showing the energy levels, decay modes and branch percentages for a radionuclide, often including daughter radionuclides and their decay.
Decay tables	Systematic presentation of amount of radionuclide remaining at tabulated points during the decay processes.
Decay-corrected radiochemical yield	The radiochemical yield corrected for decay after synthesis and processing to the time of measurement.
Decontamination (radioactive)	Making an object or area safe for personnel by removing radioactive material by means of cleaning.

Delta rays	Secondary electrons with sufficient energy to create an ionisation track of their own.
Deterministic effects	Effect on the body caused by exposure to radiation. The severity increases with dose above a threshold level. Called *non-stochastic effects* in ICRP.
Deuteron	Nucleus of deuterium containing one proton and one neutron.
DFP	Diisopropylfluorophosphate; the ^{18}F compound has been used for PET imaging and tomographic studies.
Diagnostic radiopharmaceutical	A radioactive drug that is administered to the subject by injection, ingestion, instillation or inhalation, with its radioactive emissions being used for the analysis or detection of diseases or other medical conditions.
DIDA	Diethyliminodiacetic acid; a small analogue of the HIDA series of hepatobiliary imaging agents. It forms a stable complex with ^{99m}Tc.
Diethylenetriaminepentaacetic acid (DTPA)	A chelating agent with many industrial and analytical applications, e.g. water treatment, pulp and paper manufacture, synthesis of polymers, etc. Formula: $C_{14}H_{23}N_3O_{10}$; MW 393.35. In radiopharmacy, DTPA is used as a chelating agent for several radiometals. When radiolabelled with ^{99m}Tc, it is used clinically as a renal imaging agent.
Dimercaptosuccinic acid (DMSA)	*meso*-2,3-Dimercaptosuccinic acid. Formula: $HO_2CCH(SH)CH(SH)CO_2H$; $C_4H_6O_4S_2$; MW 182.21. In radiopharmacy it is labelled with ^{99m}Tc to be used as renal imaging agent.
DISIDA	Diisopropylphenyliminodiacetic acid; the ^{99m}Tc complex is used as a hepatobiliary imaging agent.
Disintegration	Transformation of a nucleus, either spontaneous or by bombardment with particles or photons.
Disintegration constant	The decay or disintegration constant (λ) is a measure of the rate of radioactive decay. It is equal to the reciprocal value of the average lifetime (τ).
DMSA	Dimercaptosuccinic acid; the $^{99m}Tc(III)$ complex is used in renal imaging while the so-called $^{99m}Tc(V)$ complex will image a number of tumours.
Dose commitment	The future radiation dose inevitably received by a person or group.
Dose equivalent	The absorbed dose multiplied by a quality factor (ICRP 26) or a radiation weighting factor (ICRP 60) to take account of the differing effectiveness of radiations to cause biological damage.
Dose limits	Limits placed on the equivalent dose received by workers or members of the public. The limits are 20 mSv per year averaged over defined periods of 5 years to workers and 1 mSv per year to members of the public.
Dose rate	The absorbed dose received in unit time, typically mGy per year.
Dose, radiation	The quantity of radiation energy absorbed.
Dosemeter, dosimeter, dose rate meter	Instruments that measure radiation doses or dose rates. These must be calibrated annually against certified standards.

DTPA	Diethylenetetraminepentaacetic acid (q.v.), pentetic acid
Edetate	The acid radical corresponding to EDTA.
EDTA	Ethylenediaminetetraacetic acid (q.v.), edetic acid.
Effective dose	The sum of the equivalent doses in all tissues and organs in the body multiplied by the tissue weighting factors that allow for the differing relative sensitivities of the various tissues and organs.
Effective half-life	The half-life of a radionuclide in a biological system as a result of the combined effects of the biological and physical half-lives.
EHDP	Ethane-1-hydroxy-1,1-diphosphonate, editronate; a complex with ^{99m}Tc is used for bone and skeletal imaging.
EHIDA	Abbreviation of 2,6-diethylphenyl carbamoylmethyl iminodiacetic acid, or etifenin, used as the ^{99m}Tc complex for hepatobiliary imaging.
EIDA	The diethyl analogue of HIDA; used as the ^{99m}Tc complex for hepatobiliary imaging.
Electron	A negatively charged particle (charge $= 1.602 \times 10^{-19}$ coulomb, mass $= 9.11 \times 10^{-31}$ kg) present in all atoms.
Electron capture	A beta decay process in which radionuclides having excess protons gain stability by capturing an orbital electron (usually from a K shell and hence the alternative name K-capture) and converting a proton to a neutron. The general equation is identical to that for *positron decay* (q.v.) but the main difference is that no particles are emitted, only X-radiation characteristic of the daughter nuclide: $^{51}_{24}\text{Cr} \rightarrow ^{51}_{23}\text{V} + 0.005$ MeV X-ray Electron capture (abbreviated EC) is an alternative to positron decay and some radionuclides will undergo both processes as a *branched decay* (q.v.), e.g. ^{68}Ga β^+ 86%; EC 13%.
Electronvolt	A unit of energy used in radiation science that corresponds to the energy acquired by an electron accelerated through a potential difference of 1 volt. One electronvolt is equivalent to 1.6×10^{-19} joules. The multiples keV and MeV are widely used in describing the energies of ionising radiations.
ELISA	Enzyme-linked immunosorbent assay. An assay that measures the binding of an antibody to *epitope*-carrying preparations in multiwell plates.
Emission probability	The probability that a specified particle or photon is emitted during the decay of a nucleus. Often expressed as a fraction or percentage.
EOB	End of bombardment: within a cyclotron or other accelerator machine.
EOS	End of synthesis of a radiochemical.
EPD	Electronic personal dosemeter. A device that gives an instant readout of dose rate or accumulated dose.

Epitope	That part of an antigenic molecule to which an antibody binds.
Equivalent dose	The absorbed dose averaged over an organ or tissue multiplied by the radiation weighting factor. The SI unit of equivalent dose is the sievert (Sv).
ERPF	Effective renal plasma flow
Ethylene hydroxydiphosphonate (EHDP)	A complexing agent that after labelling with ^{99m}Tc is used for visualisation of pathologies of the skeleton. Formula: $(HO)_2P(=O)-C(OH)(CH_3)-P(=O)(OH)_2$.
Ethylenediaminetetraacetic acid (EDTA)	A colourless compound, with the molecular formula $C_{10}H_{16}N_2O_8$, structural formula $(HOOC-CH_2)_2N-CH_2-CH_2-N(CH_2-COOH)_2$, capable of chelating a variety of polyvalent (2+, 3+, 4+) metal cations; as a salt used as an anticoagulant, antioxidant, blood cholesterol reducer, food preservative; as a calcium-disodium salt used in the treatment of lead and other heavy-metal poisonings. The radiopharmaceutical ^{51}Cr-EDTA is used to measure glomerular filtration rate.
Etifenin	See EHIDA.
Exametazime	The rINN for *d,l*-hexamethylpropyleneamine oxime or *d,l*-HM-PAO. It is a racemic mixture of (3*RS*,9*RS*)-4,8-diaza-3,6,6,9-tetramethylundecane-2, 10-dione bisoxime. This ligand is a constituent of the Ceretec labelling kit which, upon addition of a saline solution containing sodium [^{99m}Tc]pertechnetate, yields the technetium-99m–exametazime complex (^{99m}Tc-*d,l*-HMPAO).
Exametazime [^{99m}Tc] injection	Technetium [^{99m}Tc] Exametazime Injection is indicated for brain scintigraphy. The product is used for the diagnosis of abnormalities of regional cerebral blood flow, such as those occurring following stroke and other cerebrovascular disease, epilepsy, Alzheimer disease and other forms of dementia, transient ischaemic attack, migraine and tumours of the brain and also used for *cell labelling* (q.v.).
Exchange ligand	In the preparation of technetium-99m radiopharmaceuticals, an exchange ligand is used to form a temporary and relatively weak complex with the reduced technetium. This occurs almost instantaneously after reduction of pertechnetate (Tc(VII)) to a lower oxidation state (usually +5). As the labelling reaction proceeds, a stronger complexing agent becomes available in the solution and an exchange takes place in which the ^{99m}Tc leaves its complex with the weak chelating agent (the exchange ligand) to bind with the stronger complexing agent. Examples of such exchange labelling reactions are the preparation of ^{99m}Tc-mertiatide, ^{99m}Tc-MAG$_3$, in which tartrate is used as the exchange ligand, and the preparation of ^{99m}Tc-sestamibi in which cysteine acts as the exchange ligand.
Excited state	A system having excess energy compared with its normal or ground state; the energy being emitted commonly as radiation, when it returns to the ground state.
Exponential decay	A decrease in the amount of radioactivity through a first-order rate reaction: $A_t = A_0\, e^{-\lambda t}$

where A_t is the radioactivity at time t, A_0 is the radioactivity at $t = 0$ and λ is the decay constant.

Exposure	The process of being irradiated with or exposed to radiation and potentially receiving an absorbed dose.
External dose rate	Absorbed dose or dose equivalent per unit time, on the outside of the body.
Fall out	Deposition of radioactive material from the atmosphere as a result of accidental release of radioactive material to the atmosphere, or from a nuclear explosion.
Fast neutrons	Neutrons travelling close to the speed at which they were ejected from a nucleus, typically around 2×10^7 m/s, with energy greater than 100 keV, and distinguished from slow or *thermal neutrons*.
Fatty acid	Any of a class of aliphatic carboxylic acids, such as palmitic acid, stearic acid, and oleic acid. Compounds of fatty acid structure are quite simple. There are two essential features: (1) A long hydrocarbon chain. The chain length ranges from 4 to 30 carbons; 12–24 is most common length. The chain is typically linear, and usually contains an even number of carbons. (2) A carboxylic acid group. The many fatty acids that occur naturally differ primarily through variation of chain length and degree of saturation.
FDA	Abbreviation for the US 'Food and Drug Administration' (see http://www.fda.gov). The FDA is the US federal agency responsible for ensuring that foods are safe, wholesome and sanitary; that human and veterinary drugs, biological products, and medical devices are safe and effective; that cosmetics are safe; and that electronic products that emit radiation are safe. The FDA also ensures that these products are honestly, accurately and informatively represented to the public.
FDG	2-Fluoro-2-deoxy-D-glucose, often labelled with the positron emitter fluorine-18 and used in PET scintigraphy of the brain and heart. FDG is taken into cells by normal routes for hexoses but the metabolite remains trapped within the cell, thus allowing imaging of metabolically active cells.
Ferrous [^{59}Fe] citrate injection	Ferrous [^{59}Fe] citrate injection is a sterile solution with a pH ranging between 3.5 and 5.5, a specific activity ranging between 370 and 2220 MBq (10–60 mCi) per mg of iron and a radioactive concentration of 7.4 MBq/mL (0.2 mCi/mL) at the reference date stated on the label (calibration date). When administered intravenously, [^{59}Fe]ferrous citrate is used to determine various parameters of the kinetics of iron metabolism, including plasma iron clearance, plasma iron turnover rate, and the utilisation of iron in new red blood cells. The values of serum iron obtained from these studies provide diagnostic information in patients with anaemias. [^{59}Fe]Ferrous citrate is also useful to assess the role of the spleen in red blood cell production and destruction, and thus to help determine the advisability of splenectomy. Also, organ uptake measurements are used to measure the sites of red cell production (or lack thereof) in extramedullary erythropoiesis in myeloproliferative disorders. When administered orally, [^{59}Fe]ferrous citrate is used to measure the absorption of iron from the intestine.

Fibroma	A benign, usually enclosed neoplasm composed primarily of fibrous tissue.
Film badges	A film badge is used for measuring exposure of individuals to radiation. It is usually made of metal, plastic, or paper and loaded with one or more pieces of X-ray film. Through the use of such dosimeter badges, employees working in areas where radiation or radioactive materials are present can be monitored to ensure that exposure does not exceed safety standards.
First-pass cardiac imaging	Radionuclide ventriculography in which a bolus of radionuclide is injected and data are recorded from one pass through the heart ventricle. Left and right ventricular function can be analysed independently during this technique. First-pass ventriculography is preferred over gated blood pool imaging for assessing right ventricular function.
Fission	Nuclear fission is the splitting of a nucleus of a heavy atom such as uranium or plutonium into two or more parts after absorption of a neutron. When such an occurrence takes place, a very large amount of energy is released.
Fission yield	The percentage of fissions that produce a particular nuclide.
Fluence	The total number of photons or particles crossing a sphere of unit cross-section surrounding a point source of radioactivity.
Food and Drug Administration	See FDA.
Free radical	In chemistry, a molecule or atom that contains an unpaired electron but is neither positively nor negatively charged. Because they have a free electron, such molecules are highly reactive. Radicals seek to receive or release electrons in order to achieve a more stable configuration, a process that can damage the large molecules within cells.
Functional group	A group of atoms that represents a potential reaction site in an organic compound. It is the portion of a molecule responsible for its specific chemical properties.
Functional imaging	Functional imaging represents a range of measurement techniques in which the aim is to extract quantitative information about physiological function from image-based data.
Furosemide	A powerful diuretic used especially to treat oedema. Furosemide is a potent diuretic that, if given in excessive amounts, can lead to a profound diuresis with water and electrolyte depletion. Therefore, careful medical supervision is required and dose and dose schedule must be adjusted to the individual patient's needs. In nuclear medicine, furosemide (trade name Lasix) is used in dynamic renal radionuclide studies to obtain a maximum diuretic response.
FWHM	Full width at half maximum; a term used to characterise peaks in gamma spectrometry and other techniques. It refers to the width of a peak at half the maximum height.
Gallium	Metallic chemical element; symbol Ga; atomic number 31; atomic weight 69.72; melting point. 29.78°C; boiling point 2403°C; valence +2 or +3. It is the only metal, except for mercury, caesium, and rubidium, which can be

liquid near room temperatures; this makes possible its use in high-temperature thermometers. It has one of the longest liquid ranges of any metal and has a low vapour pressure even at high temperatures. Ultra-pure gallium has a beautiful, silvery appearance, and the solid metal exhibits a conchoidal fracture similar to glass. The metal expands on solidifying; therefore, it should not be stored in glass or metal containers, as they may break as the metal solidifies. High-purity gallium is attacked only slowly by mineral acids. Gallium arsenide is capable of converting electricity directly into coherent light and gallium arsenide is a key component of LEDs (light-emitting diodes).

Gallium-67 Gallium-67 is a radioisotope of gallium with a half-life of 78.27 hours. It decays by electron capture to zinc-68 with the emission of gamma rays of 91 keV, 93 keV, 185 keV, 300 keV, 394 keV. It can be produced by the irradiation (with protons of suitable energy) of a zinc target, preferably enriched with zinc-68. Gallium-67 can be separated from zinc by solvent extraction or column chromatography.

Gallium-67 citrate injection Gallium [^{67}Ga] Citrate Injection is a sterile solution of gallium-67 in the form of gallium citrate. It may be made isotonic by the addition of sodium chloride and sodium citrate and may contain a suitable antimicrobial preservative such as benzyl alcohol. [^{67}Ga]Gallium citrate is used to demonstrate the presence and extent of lymphoma, bronchogenic carcinoma, acute myelocytic leukaemia, chronic myelocytic leukaemia, hepatoma and bone sarcoma. It may also be useful in the detection of epithelial, head and neck carcinoma; malignant melanoma; malignant fibrous histiocytoma and testicular tumours. [^{67}Ga] Gallium citrate is also used for the localisation of focal inflammatory lesions, such as abscess, osteomyelitis, pneumonia, pyelonephritis, and granulomatous diseases (sarcoidosis). It may also be useful in the detection of active tuberculosis; and for assessing the activity of the inflammatory process in certain interstitial pulmonary diseases, including sarcoidosis and fibrosing alveolitis. Gallium [^{67}Ga] citrate is useful in the diagnosis and monitoring of *Pneumocystis carinii* pneumonia, tuberculosis, and other infections in acquired immunodeficiency syndrome (AIDS) patients. [^{67}Ga]Gallium citrate is useful as a diagnostic screening test in cases of prolonged fever, when physical examination, laboratory tests, and other imaging studies have failed to disclose the source of the fever.

Gallium-68 Gallium-68 is a positron emitter with a half-life of 67.63 minutes that can be used in PET imaging.

Gallium-68 radiopharmaceuticals Tracer agents labelled with gallium-68 via a metal chelating moiety in the molecule of biological interest or via a metal chelating bifunctional agent coupled to the molecule of biological interest. No gallium-68 radiopharmaceuticals have been officially approved up to 2010, but several such agents have been developed and are being evaluated, e.g. ^{68}Ga-labelled peptides for tumour detection.

Gallium–germanium generator A generator that produces gallium-68 from the parent radionuclide germanium-68. Germanium-68 has a half-life of 280 days, and ^{68}Ga, with a half-life of 68 minutes, decays by positron emission and hence 511-keV annihilation radiation. This generator can be eluted quite frequently because the maximum yield is obtained in a few hours.

Gamma camera	A medical apparatus that detects the radiation (gamma rays) from a radioactive tracer injected into a person's body after the administration of a radioactive drug and produces images of the organ being investigated. It is used especially in medical diagnostic scanning. Also called an *Anger camera* (q.v.) or a scintillation camera.
Gamma emitters	A radioactive isotope that emits gamma radiation during radioactive decay.
Gamma radiation	High-energy photons emitted as one of the types of radiation resulting from natural radioactivity. It is the most energetic form of electromagnetic radiation, with a very short wavelength (high frequency), and originates from the nucleus during radioactive decay, electron–positron annihilation and nuclear fission. The energies of gamma photon range from thousands of electronvolts (keV) to millions of electronvolts (MeV), and their wavelengths are correspondingly very short (10^{-11} m to 10^{-13} m).
Gamma ray dose constant	A specific gamma ray dose constant (SGRDC) is a value for correlating the dose-equivalent rate (per unit of activity) for a radionuclide at a specified distance. For example, the SGRDC (in tissue) for a point source containing ^{137}Cs at a radial distance of 1 metre of air is 1×10^{-4} mSv/h/MBq. Using this value, a 1 MBq point source of ^{137}Cs will generate a dose rate of 1×10^{-4} mSv/h at 1 metre. These constants are calculated by estimating the energy deposition rate for all significant modes of interaction for gamma and X-ray emissions from a radionuclide. For the most part, the constant for an otherwise fixed geometry will increase with photon energy and gamma-emission probability.
Gamma ray spectroscopy	Gamma ray spectroscopy measures, identifies and quantifies the gamma rays emitted from natural or synthetic radioactive elements that are present in solid and liquid samples. Gamma ray spectra are (mostly) recorded using a scintillation detector (e.g. NaI(Tl) crystal) or a semiconducting detector (e.g. intrinsic germanium detector) coupled to a multichannel analyser. Gamma ray spectroscopy is used by scientists in many disciplines to determine what radionuclides are present in a sample.
Gamma spectrum	Graphic representation of the number of gamma (and X-) rays of different energies detected and recorded when the electromagnetic radiation of a sample is absorbed by a suitable detector (scintillation or semiconducting detector). As gamma rays can be absorbed by the detector in different ways (photoelectric effect, Compton scattering, pair formation) and special effects can occur during conversion of the absorbed electromagnetic energy into an anode pulse (such as escape of part of the energy, summation of two gamma rays, summation of a gamma and an X-ray), more than one peak may be observed in the spectrum even if the source emits only one type of gamma rays.
Ge(Li)	Germanium (lithium-drifted) detector; a high-resolution semiconductor ionisation detector used for gamma spectroscopy.

Geiger counter or Geiger–Müller (GM) counter	An instrument for the detection and quantitative determination of ionising radiation such as alpha particles, beta particles, X-rays and gamma rays. It was first developed by Hans Geiger and later improved by Geiger and A. Müller. Variously designed for different uses, it consists commonly of a gas-filled metal cylinder that acts as one electrode (cathode), and a needle or thin wire along the axis of the cylinder that acts as the other electrode (anode). Glass caps used to seal the ends of the tube serve as insulators. A voltage applied to the device is so adjusted that it is almost strong enough to cause a current to pass through the gas from one electrode to the other. The gas becomes ionised whenever the counter is brought near radioactive substances, however small the quantity and however faint the emanations. The resulting ionised particles of gas are able to carry the current from one electrode to the other, thus completing a circuit. Once established, the current is amplified by an electronic device so that it can indicate by an audible click the presence of ionised particles. The gas quickly returns to its normal non-ionised state, permitting each new particle or ray to register, making counting possible. The instrument can also register ionisation by a pointer and scale called a rate meter. The Geiger counter is used in the detection of cosmic rays and for locating radioactive minerals. Counters enable radioactive tracers to be followed as they make their way through complex organisms such as the human body; in medicine Geiger counters have found several successful uses in the location of malignancies. They are used also to follow radioactive isotopes in chemical reactions. For a number of research applications the Geiger counter has been largely replaced by scintillation detectors and solid-state detectors.
Generator	A device in which a short-lived daughter radionuclide is separated physically and periodically from a long(er)-lived parent radionuclide adsorbed onto a column. For example in a ^{99}Mo/^{99m}Tc-generator ^{99}Mo ($t_{/12} = 66$ hours) is adsorbed in the form of molybdate onto an alumina column. The technetium-99m ($t_{1/2} = 6$ hours) formed by the decay of molybdenum-99 in the form of pertechnetate (TcO_4^-) can be separated from the ^{99}Mo by elution of the column with a 0.9% saline solution.
Genetic effects	Effects produced in the descendants of persons or organisms exposed to radiation.
GFR	Glomerular filtration rate; the volume of plasma undergoing ultrafiltration in the glomerulus of kidney tubules per unit time.
GHA	Glucoheptonate; the ^{99m}Tc complex is used for brain imaging and also as an *exchange ligand* (q.v.).
GM detector	Geiger–Muller detector; a gas filled ionisation detector used for beta and gamma radiations; see *Geiger counter*.
Gray	The SI unit of absorbed radiation dose, equivalent to an energy deposition of 1 joule per kilogram.
Ground state	The lowest energy state of a system.

GSD — Genetically significant dose; an index of presumed genetic impact of radiation on the whole population from radiation received by individuals; it is determined by the gonadal dose to the exposed populations, population size, and the number of children to be expected from this population.
For 1964 in the USA the GSD for radiological procedures was estimated as 0.16 mSv; in 1970 the GSD was estimated at 0.2 mSv despite the increase in the number of radiological procedures performed. Natural background radiation contributes about 0.9 mSv to the overall GSD.

Haematocrit — The ratio of the volume of red blood cells to a given volume of blood, expressed as a percentage.

Haemoglobin — A red, iron-containing protein present in red blood cells largely responsible for the blood's oxygen-carrying capacity. Haemoglobin is composed of four polypeptide chains, two alpha (α) and two beta (β) chains.

Haemolysis — Disruption of the membranes of red blood cells leading to loss of haemoglobin.

Half-life — The time required for the amount of substance to be reduced to one-half. Several half-life concepts are used in radiopharmacy: physical, biological, and effective half-life. Half-lives are also used in kinetic studies and have a similar meaning, but when the substance in question is also a radionuclide then both the physical and kinetic half-lives must be considered.

Half-life, biological — Biological half-life (t_B): the time in which the amount of a radioactive nuclide clears from the body to half its initial value (also used to describe the clearance of non-radioactive materials and drugs).

Half-life, effective — Effective half-life (t_E): The half-life resulting from the combination of t_P and t_B, where $1/t_E = 1/t_P + 1/t_B$.

Half-life, physical — Physical half-life (t_P): time in which the amount of a radioactive nuclide decays to half of its initial value.
Values range from milliseconds to tens of millions of years. This half-life, often written simply as $t_{1/2}$, is related to the decay constant λ by the expression $t_{1/2} = 2.303/\lambda$, both expressed in the same time units.

HAM — Human albumin microspheres; when labelled with ^{99m}Tc they are used for lung imaging.

HAMA — Human anti-mouse antibodies (q.v.).

HAS — Human serum albumin; can be labelled with ^{99m}Tc or preferably with an iodine radioisotope for measurement of plasma volume by isotope dilution analysis.

HCAT — Homotaurocholate; the selenium-75 compound, SeHCAT or selenohomotaurocholate, is a radiopharmaceutical used for measurement of bile acid pool loss in, for example, Crohn disease.

Health physics — The study and administration of radiation protection.

Heavy metal — Any metal with a specific gravity of 5.0 or greater, especially one that is toxic to organisms. Examples include lead, mercury, copper, and cadmium.

HEDP	Hydroxyethylidenediphosphonate; the ^{99m}Tc complex is used for skeletal imaging.
HEDSPA	1-hydroxyethylidene-1,1-disodium phosphonate; see HEDP.
HEDTA	*N*-Hydroxyethylethylenediaminetetraacetic acid; a chelating agent. The ^{99m}Tc chelate has a stability constant of $10^{20.8}$.
Hepatitis	Inflammation of the liver.
Hepatobiliary imaging	This is one of the common emergency procedures performed in nuclear medicine and is carried out for the evaluation of biliary function of the liver. The procedure might also be called a HIDA (hepatic iminodiacetic acid) or a DISIDA (dimethyl iminodiacetic acid, labelled with ^{99m}Tc) scan, or cholescintigraphy (examination of the gallbladder and bile ducts).
Hereditary effects	Stochastic effects expressed in the offspring of an exposed person.
HIDA	*N*-(2,6-dimethylphenyl)carbamoyliminodiacetic acid; the ^{99m}Tc complex is used as a hepatobiliary imaging agent and is the parent complex of a series of hepatobiliary agents such as EHIDA and PiPIDA.
High performance liquid chromatography (HPLC)	A variation of liquid chromatography that utilises fine particle stationary phases and high-pressure pumps to increase the efficiency of the separation. Liquid chromatography is used to separate analytes in solution including metal ions and organic compounds. The mobile phase is a solvent and the stationary phase is a liquid on a solid support, a solid, or an ion-exchange resin.
HIPDM	2-Hydroxy-3-methyl-5-iodobenzyl-1,3-propanediamine. The iodine-^{123} compound is used in brain imaging.
Hippuran	2-Iodohippuric acid labelled with iodine-123 or iodine-131; used for radioisotopic measurement of renal function and determination of effective renal plasma flow.
HMDP	Hydroxymethylene diphosphonate; the ^{99m}Tc complex is used for bone and skeletal imaging.
HMPAO	Hexamethylpropylene amine oxime (exametazime (q.v.)).
Hormones	Naturally-occurring substances produced by specialised cells, which act on receptors present in other cells to influence their metabolism or behaviour. If the hormones are hydrophilic (such as insulin) the receptors are on the cell surface. If the hormones are lipophilic, the receptors may be intracellular.
HPLC	High performance liquid chromatography (q.v.), a technique now being used in radiochemical purity testing.
Human anti-mouse antibodies (HAMA)	Antibodies produced in humans during an immune response against administered mouse proteins. HAMA responses are often seen when mouse monoclonals are used as therapeutics, and can lead to the immune rejection of the mouse monoclonal.

HVL	Half-value layer; the shield thickness required to absorb 50% of a gamma or X-radiation beam. It is related to the linear absorption coefficient, x, by $HVL = (\ln 2)/x$.
Hypertension	A condition in which the patient has consistently high arterial blood pressure. The primary factor is an increase in peripheral resistance resulting from vasoconstriction or narrowing of peripheral blood vessels.
Hyperthyroidism	A condition characterised by accelerated metabolism caused by excessive functional activity of the thyroid gland (overproduction of thyroid hormones).
Hypothalamus	A region in the brain which lies beneath the thalamus; it consists of many aggregations of nerve cells and controls a variety of autonomic functions aimed at maintaining homeostasis.
Hypoxia	A condition in which there is a decrease in the oxygen supply to the tissue despite adequate blood perfusion of the tissue.
IAEA	International Atomic Energy Agency (q.v.).
IC_{50}	Concentration resulting in a 50% reduction in response to agonist, or binding of ligand to receptor.
ICRP	International Commission on Radiation Protection.
ICRU	International Commission on Radiation Units and Measurement.
IDA	Iminodiacetic acid, a chelating agent.
Immunoglobulins	Immunoglobulins, also known as antibodies, are glycoproteins found in blood and in tissue fluids. Immunoglobulins are produced by cells of the immune system called B-lymphocytes. Their function is to bind to substances in the body that are recognised as foreign antigens (often proteins on the surface of bacteria and viruses). This binding is a crucial event in the destruction of the microorganisms that bear the antigens. Immunoglobulins also play a central role in allergies when they bind to antigens that are not necessarily a threat to health and provoke an inflammatory reaction.
Immunoreaction	An immunological reaction between an antigen and an antibody (especially *in vitro*).
IMP	*N*-Isopropyl-*p*-iodoamfetamine; a radioiodinated analogue of amfetamine which localises in brain tissue and has been used for brain imaging.
In vitro	Outside the living body and observable in a test tube or an artificial environment.
IND	Investigational New Drug (USA).
Indium-111	Radioisotope of indium, decaying by electron capture to cadmium-111with a half-life of 2.804 days. It emits gamma radiation of 171 keV and 245 keV. Its uses in nuclear medicine include ^{111}In-labelled octreotide (for detection of tumours), ^{111}In-labelled leukocytes (obtained by incubation of isolated leukocytes with ^{111}In-oxine and used for detection of infection and imaging) and ^{111}In-DTPA (for cisternography).

Infarct	An area of tissue death (such as in the heart or kidney) due to local lack of oxygen.
Infection	Invasion and multiplication of body tissues by microorganisms, e.g. bacteria and viruses.
Inflammation	A local protective response to cellular injury that is marked by capillary dilatation, leukocytic infiltration, redness, heat, and pain and that serves as a mechanism initiating the elimination of noxious agents as well as damaged tissue.
Inorganic	Pertaining to compounds that are not hydrocarbons or their derivatives (i.e. are not of organic origin).
Internal conversion	The transition between two energy states of a nucleus where, instead of the energy difference being emitted as a photon (gamma ray), it is transferred to an orbital electron, which is then ejected from the atom.
Internal conversion coefficient	The ratio of conversion electrons to the number of gamma photons emitted.
International Atomic Energy Agency (IAEA)	Intergovernmental organisation established in 1957 under the aegis of the United Nations to promote the peaceful uses of atomic energy. Its headquarters are in Vienna. It may purchase and sell fissionable materials, offer technical assistance for peaceful nuclear energy uses, and establish safeguards preventing diversion of nuclear materials to military use. It inspects for compliance with the Non-Proliferation Treaty. The organisation is made up of a general conference, consisting of representatives of all member states, a board of governors of 35 members, and a secretariat headed by a director-general. In September 2003 there were 137 members. (See http://www.iaea.org.)
International Union of Pure and Applied Chemistry (IUPAC)	The International Union of Pure and Applied Chemistry serves to advance the worldwide aspects of the chemical sciences and contribute to the application of chemistry in the service of humankind. (See http://www.iupac.org/dhtml_home.html.)
Intra-arterial injection	Injection of a substance into the bloodstream through an artery (less common than intravenous delivery).
Intrathecal injection	The injection of a substance into the spinal fluid.
Intravenous injection	Injection of a substance into the bloodstream through a vein.
Iodine-123	A radioisotope of iodine having 53 protons and 70 neutrons. Decays by electron capture to stable tellurium-123. Half-life: 13.27 hours; energy of principal gamma ray: 159 keV. Used as radiolabel in different radiopharmaceuticals for diagnostic imaging.
Ion	An electrically charged atom or group of atoms formed by the loss or gain of one or more electrons, such as a cation (a positive ion which is created by electron loss and is attracted to the cathode in electrolysis), or an anion (negative ion which is created by an electron gain and is attracted to the anode). The valence of an ion is equal to the number of electrons lost or

	gained and is indicated by a plus sign for cations and a minus sign for anions, thus: Na^+, Cl^-, Ca^{2+}.
Ion pair	A positively charged ion and the electron removed by ionising radiation.
Ionisation	The process of removing electrons from atoms and molecules to create ions. High temperatures, electrical discharges and radiation can cause ionisation.
Ionisation chamber	An instrument for measuring radiation, operating by measurement of ions produced by the radiation in a given volume between charged electrodes.
Ionising radiation	Any radiation, particulate or non-particulate, that causes ionisation in materials through which it passes. Alpha and beta particles cause more ionisation than gamma rays or X-rays of equivalent energy. Neutrons do not cause direct ionisation.
IRMA	Immunoradiometric analysis; an immunological assay method based on the same principles as *RIA* (q.v.).
Irradiate	To expose to radiation, particularly penetrating X- and gamma radiations.
IRRS	UK legislation on Radiation Protection based on the *ICRP* (q.v.) recommendations.
Isobar	Nuclides sharing the same number atomic number, e.g. ^{40}K, ^{40}Ca and ^{40}Sc.
Isoelectric point	The isoelectric point is the pH of a solution or dispersion at which the net charge on the macromolecules or colloidal particles is zero. In electrophoresis there is no motion of the particles in an electric field at the isoelectric point.
Isomeric transition (IT)	A transition between two isomeric states of a nucleus. Examples are ^{99m}Tc to ^{99}Tc, and ^{137m}Ba to ^{137}Ba.
Isomers	Nuclides having the same mass and atomic numbers, but differing nuclear binding energies. A good example is the ^{99m}Tc–^{99}Tc pair.
Isotopes	Nuclides having the same atomic number but differing in atomic weight and mass number. The nuclei of isotopes contain identical numbers of protons, equal to the atomic number of the atom, and thus represent the same chemical element, but do not have the same number of neutrons. Examples are ^1H, ^2H and ^3H, known as hydrogen, deuterium and tritium.
Isotopic abundance	The fraction or percentage of a specified isotope in a mixture of isotopes of an element.
Isotopic dilution	An analytical technique in which a radiochemical is added to an unknown quantity of the normal chemical, mixed, and the radioactivity of the mixture is determined. From the result the amount or concentration of the chemical can be determined.
Joule	Abbreviation: J; a unit of work or energy. It is the work done or energy expended by a force of 1 newton acting through a distance of 1 metre. The joule is named after James P. Joule.

Joule per kilogram	The SI unit of absorbed dose is the joule per kilogram (J/kg), termed the gray (Gy). (1 J/kg = 1 Gy = 100 rad.)
K capture	See *electron capture*.
Karyocyte	Any cell that possesses a nucleus. A neuron (nerve cell) is a karyocyte; it has a nucleus. A mature erythrocyte (red blood cell) is not a karyocyte; it lacks a nucleus.
KERMA	Kinetic energy released per unit mass.
keV	kilo-electronvolt; 1000 electron volts, 10^3 eV.
Kidney imaging	See Renal scan.
Kinetics	Kinetics (with an ‘s’ at the end) refers to the rate of change in a biochemical (or other) reaction, the study of reaction rates. *Kinetics* is a noun. It is distinct from ‘kinetic’ (an adjective) meaning with movement. The opposite of kinetic is *akinetic* meaning without movement. In neurology, kinetic and akinetic serve to denote the presence or absence of movement.
Kits	Especially in radiopharmacy, kit is the short name for ‘labelling kit’. A labelling kit is composed of one or two vials containing the reagents in appropriate quantity for the preparation of a radiopharmaceutical. To enhance stability, the reagents are often in lyophilised form. Example: a labelling kit for the preparation of ^{99m}Tc-medronate (^{99m}Tc-MDP) is a vial that contains under an atmosphere of nitrogen a mixture of 5–15 mg medronic acid (MDP), 0.5–1.0 mg stannous chloride and possibly an antioxidant such as ascorbic acid, in the form of the lyophilised residue of a solution. Upon addition of a solution of sodium [^{99m}Tc]pertechnetate to such vial, Tc^{99m}-medronate is formed almost instantaneously.
Knockout mouse	A mouse missing a single gene (the gene that has been ‘knocked out’). Knockout mice are used in biomedical research.
Krypton-81m	A radioisotope of krypton, a noble gas. It contains 36 protons and 45 neutrons and is in metastable form. It decays with a half-life of 13 seconds to krypton-81. Krypton-81m is used as a ventilation agent in nuclear imaging and is generated by radioactive decay of rubidium-81. Rubidium-81/krypton-81m generators are commercially available and have a useful life of one day.
KTS	Kethoxal-bis(thiosemicarbazone); it forms a neutral lipophilic chelate with ^{99m}Tc useful for labelling substances that must cross cell membranes.
Label	A term used to indicate isotopic replacement of one or more atoms by a stable isotope (e.g. ^{2}H, ^{13}C) or radioisotope (e.g. ^{3}H, ^{14}C).
Labelled compound	A molecule in which one or more of the atoms are replaced by radionuclides, either isotopes or foreign elements. By observations of radioactivity or isotopic composition this compound or its fragments may be followed through physical, chemical or biological processes.
LAFW	Laminar air flow workstation

LAL	The *Limulus* amoebocyte lysate, used as one of the main components in a test for bacterial endotoxins.
Laminar-air flow work spaces	An air filtering system in which the entire mass of air within a designated space moves with uniform velocity in a single direction along parallel flow lines with a minimum of mixing.
Lasix	A proprietary preparation of *furosemide* (q.v.). A sulfonamide-type loop diuretic, with a pK_a of 3.9, it is soluble in alkali hydroxides. It is used in radioisotopic kidney studies.
LD_{50}	A standardised measure for expressing and comparing the toxicity of chemicals. The LD_{50} is the dose that kills half (50%) of the animals tested (LD = lethal dose).
Lead shielding	A material interposed between a source of radiation and people for their protection.
LET	Linear energy transfer; the energy (in keV/mm) transferred from a radiation beam to a body during passage of the beam. The LET value depends on the energy and type of radiation, being largest for low-velocity large charged particles and least for high-velocity light particles and photons.
Leukocytes	The leukocytes, or white blood cells, help the body defend itself from infecting organisms and other diseases, both in the tissues and in the bloodstream itself. Human blood contains about 5000 to 10 000 leukocytes per cubic millimetre and this number increases in the presence of infection.
Leukopenia	A condition in which the number of white blood cells circulating in the blood is abnormally low.
LFOV	Large field of view, a term applied to a gamma camera.
Ligand	Any molecule that binds to another; for example, in the case of a hormone binding to its receptor, the hormone would be classed as the ligand. In complexation chemistry, the ligand is usually a molecule or ion that (along with other molecules) is bound to a central metal ion. All ligands are lone pair donors (and thus function as Lewis bases). Simple ligands include water, ammonia and chloride ions (these are all monodentate ligands, i.e. they have only one bond to the central metal ion). More complicated ligands can be bidentate (e.g. ethylenediamine) or polydentate (e.g. EDTA).
Ligand exchange	A reaction in which one ligand in a complex ion is replaced by a different one.
LINAC	Linear accelerator: a device that accelerates particles in a straight path.
Lipophilic compounds	Molecules that are preferentially soluble in lipids or non-polar solvents.
Liposomes	Liposomes (lipid vesicles). Synthetic closed structures of curved lipid bilayers (vesicles) that entrap in their interior a part of the solvent in which they freely float. Developed for the delivery of relatively toxic drugs – the drug is trapped inside the liposome, which may be tagged with an organ-specific antibody.

Liposomes range in size from 20 nm to several tens of micrometres, while the thickness of their membranes is about 4 nm.

Liquid scintillation counting/detection — A technique for measuring samples of radioisotopes that are low-energy beta or auger electron emitters. In biology, liquid scintillation counting is mainly used for emitters such as carbon-14, sulfur-35, tritium (hydrogen-3) and phosphorus-32. The samples are dissolved in a liquid scintillant that converts the energy of the nuclear emission into UV light, the intensity of which is proportional to the initial energy of the beta particle. The counting instrument converts this UV light into an electrical pulse and then into a measurement of the radioactivity of the sample.

Liquid scintillator — A liquid formulation in which the absorption of radiation causes emission of visible photons.

Lithium fluoride — The crystal used in a thermoluminescent dosimeter. After being exposed to radiation, the material in the dosimeter (lithium fluoride) luminesces on being heated. The amount of light that the material emits is proportional to the amount of radiation (dose) to which it was exposed.

LSF — Line spread function; a measure of the resolution of a gamma camera.

Lugol's solution — Solution of potassium iodide and iodine used to block uptake of radioactive iodide into the thyroid in examinations in which radioiodine labelled compounds are used. It is also used as a disinfectant.

Luminescence — The production of light without emission of accompanying heat.

MAA — Macroaggregated albumin (q.v).

Macroaggregated albumin — Macroaggregated albumin (MAA) is prepared by heating a mixture of human serum albumin, which denatures the protein. In nuclear medicine, these water-insoluble aggregates (particle size 10–100 μm and irregular shape) labelled with technetium-99m are used for lung perfusion imaging.

Macrosalb [^{99m}Tc] injection — Sterile white suspension of albumin in the form of irregular aggregates of human albumin produced by heat denaturation. Macrosalb is supplied as a lyophilised kit formulation to be labelled with ^{99m}Tc. It may contain reducing agents, antimicrobial agents, buffers and macroaggregates of human albumin. ^{99m}Tc-MAA is used clinically for lung perfusion studies.

MAG_3 — Mercaptoacetyltriglycine (q.v.).

Magic numbers — The charge and neutron numbers 2, 8, 20, 28, 50, 82, that are characteristic of many stable nuclei.

Mass defect — The difference between the mass of a nucleus and the sum of the masses of its constituent nucleons. It is related to the binding energy by $E = mc^2$ where E is the energy corresponding to mass m and c is the velocity of light.

Mass number — The number of neutrons and protons within the nucleus of an atom. Symbol A.

MCA — Multichannel analyser; a device for measuring the energy spectrum of a radiation source. Electric pulses from a detector are sorted into channels according to the pulse height and the number of counts in a channel is related to the energy of the radiation giving rise to the pulse.

MDA — Minimum detectable activity: the lowest radioactivity of a sample that can be distinguished from background by a specified counter.

MDP — Methylene diphosphonate; the ^{99m}Tc complex is used for bone and skeletal imaging.

MDP labelled with ^{99m}Tc — A solution of methylene diphosphonate (MDP) and stannous salt labelled with ^{99m}Tc. MDP is supplied as a lyophilised kit formulation to be labelled with ^{99m}Tc. It may contain antimicrobial agents, antioxidants and buffers. ^{99m}Tc-MDP is used clinically for bone imaging.

Mebrofenin [^{99m}Tc] injection — A solution of mebrofenin (bromotrimethyl derivative of iminodiacetic acid) labelled with ^{99m}Tc. It contains a stannous salt as the reducing agent. Mebrofenin is supplied as a lyophilised kit formulation to be labelled with ^{99m}Tc. It may contain antimicrobial preservatives. This ^{99m}Tc-radiopharmaceutical is used clinically for hepatobiliary imaging. The BP preparation is Technetium [^{99m}Tc] Mebrofenin Injection.

Medronate [^{99m}Tc] injection — Solution of sodium medronate (methylene diphosphonate (MDP)) and stannous salt labelled with ^{99m}Tc. MDP is supplied as a lyophilised kit formulation to be labelled with ^{99m}Tc. It may contain antimicrobial agents, antioxidants and buffers. This ^{99m}Tc-radiopharmaceutical is used clinically for bone imaging. The BP preparation is Technetium [^{99m}Tc] Medronate Injection.

Mercaptoacetyltriglycine (MAG_3) — Mercaptoacetyltriglycine, a commonly-used ligand for ^{99m}Tc. The resulting ^{99m}Tc-complex is used for clinical monitoring of renal function. Kits normally contain the more stable precursor betiatide (*S*-benzoylmercaptoacetyltriglycine) which is debenzoylated under the conditions of labelling to form the complex with ^{99m}Tc. The BP preparation is Technetium [^{99m}Tc] Mertiatide Injection.

Metabolism — The biological process whereby ingested foreign materials are broken down or converted to less toxic and easily excreted products called metabolites.

Metabolite analysis — The process of determining the identities, quantities and rates of production of metabolites.

Metastable state — Isomeric nuclear states with energies above the ground state. ^{99m}Tc is the familiar example.

Methylene diphosphonate (MDP) — A diphosphonate compound that localises in bone. When labelled with ^{99m}Tc, the complex is used in nuclear medicine for bone imaging.

MeV — Mega-electronvolt, 10^6 eV; used to describe energies of ionising radiations.

mIBG — Abbreviation for *meta*-iodobenzylguanidine, a noradrenaline (norepinephrine) analogue now known as Iobenguane in official preparations. Among the three isomers of iodobenzylguanidine, the *meta* isomer (mIBG) is the most stable to *in-vivo* deiodination. Thus, it has been radioiodinated with $^{123/131}$I by isotope exchange and it is clinically used for imaging of the adrenal medulla and in radionuclide treatment of neuroblastoma (^{131}I).

Millicurie (mCi)	One thousandth of a curie (Ci), a unit of radioactivity still widely used although formally replaced by the SI unit becquerel (Bq). 1 mCi = 3.7×10^7 disintegrations per second = 37 MBq
MIRD	Medical Internal Radiation Dose (committee); a scheme for calculating the absorbed radiation doses due to radiotracers and radiopharmaceuticals.
Molecular imaging	The use of gamma-emitting radiolabelled biochemicals or drugs that bind to specific receptors in the body and can be imaged by SPECT or PET cameras.
Molybdenium-99 breakthrough	Contamination of a ^{99m}Tc generator eluate with the ^{99}Mo parent radionuclide.
Molybdenium-99/technetium-99m breakthrough test	Test (usually required by regulation) to evaluate any contamination of the ^{99m}Tc eluate with ^{99}Mo before use in making up kits for clinical use. A technique used to determine the radionuclide purity of the eluate can easily be performed in a dose calibrator. The eluate vial is shielded in a lead pot (about 6 mm thick) to stop all ^{99m}Tc 140 keV photons and to count only ^{99}Mo 740 keV and 780 keV photons. The shielded vial is then assayed in the dose calibrator. The acceptable limit of contamination with ^{99}Mo is $\leq 0.1\%$.
Molybdenum-99	A radioactive nuclide of molybdenum. It is a β^- emitter with $t_{1/2} = 66$ hours; 87% of its decay goes ultimately to the metastable state ^{99m}Tc and the remaining 13% to the ground state ^{99}Tc. It has photon transitions of 740 keV and 780 keV. Owing to its decay properties, it is the parent nuclide in the widely used $^{99}Mo/^{99m}Tc$ generator. The molybdenum for early generators was produced by thermal neutron activation reaction in a reactor, but almost all current generators make use of fission-produced molybdenum-99. The resulting molybdenum-99 is carrier free and of very high specific activity, allowing the production of high-activity, small-volume columns for the generator and permitting elution in a small volume.
Molybdenum-99/technetium-99m generator ($^{99}Mo/^{99m}Tc$)	The most commonly used generator system, in which ^{99}Mo ($t_{1/2} = 66$ hours, usually produced by fission of ^{235}U) decays to ^{99m}Tc ($t_{1/2} = 6$ hours) by β^- emission. The generator consists of an alumina column onto which the ^{99}Mo is adsorbed in the chemical form of molybdate. The ^{99m}Tc is eluted as sodium pertechnetate ($Na^{99m}TcO_4$) with 0.9% NaCl solution. These generators are available from several commercial suppliers. There are two types of generators: wet column and dry column. In the dry column generators, all the saline is drawn through the column during routine elution, leaving the column dry. This prevents any radiolysis of water, which may be possible in a wet generator.
Mössbauer effect	Emission of gamma photons without loss of energy to recoil of the emitting nuclide, leading to very narrow energy bands.
MPBB	Maximum permissible body burden; the amount of a radionuclide that can be present in the body throughout a working lifetime without exceeding the maximum permissible dose to specified organs or tissues.
MWPC	Multiwire proportional counter; a device for imaging positrons.

Myoview	Brand name of tetrafosmin (6,9-bis(2-ethoxyethyl)-3,12-dioxa-6, 9-diphosphatetradecane). This compound is supplied as a kit to be labelled with ^{99m}Tc. The resulting ^{99m}Tc-tetrafosmin complex is used clinically mainly for myocardial imaging. Myoview is useful in the diagnosis and localisation of regions of reversible myocardial ischaemia in the presence or absence of infarction under exercise and rest conditions.
NaI(Tl) crystal	Sodium iodide crystal doped with a very small amount of thallium. This crystal is the detector most commonly used for gamma ray detection.
Natural decay series	Three series of naturally occurring radionuclides starting with uranium-238, thorium-232 and uranium-235, with a fourth artificial series starting with neptunium-237.
n.c.a.	Abbreviation of the term 'no carrier added'.
NCR	Nuclear Regulatory Commission (USA).
NDA	New Drug Application (USA).
Negative pressure system	A system used in one of the two types of chromatographic radionuclide generator. It is operated using an evacuated elution vial. The vacuum in the elution vial draws the eluent (solvent) from the reservoir through the generator column.
Negatron	An electron, having a mass of about 0.00055 amu, emitted during *negatron decay* (q.v.).
Negatron decay	A beta decay process in which radionuclides having excess neutrons gain stability by conversion of a neutron to a proton and negatron.
Neospect	A trade name for depreotide, a somatostatin analogue. This compound is supplied as a kit to be labelled with ^{99m}Tc. The resulting ^{99m}Tc-depreotide is used clinically for somatostatin receptor imaging, in particular, those receptors that are over-expressed in lung cancer (small cell and non-small cell lung cancer).
Neurolite	Brand name of the ethyl cysteinate dimer (ECD), also known as bicisate. This compound is supplied as a kit to be labelled with ^{99m}Tc. The resulting ^{99m}Tc-ECD is used mainly for brain perfusion imaging.
Neurotensin	Neuropeptide involved in intracellular communication, both in the central nervous system and in the intestine. This linear tridecapeptide has been defined as a potential growth factor in different human cancer cell lines and tumours. Consequently, radiolabelled neurotensin synthetic analogues may be used to target neurotensin receptor-positive tumours, with potential applications as tumour imaging agents or therapeutic radiopharmaceuticals.
Neutrino	A neutral particle of very small (possibly zero) mass. P.A.M. Dirac proposed the neutrino to account for that part of the beta decay energy not associated with the beta particle.
Neutron	A nuclear particle having a mass of about 1.00898 amu. The number of neutrons in a nucleus is determined partly by the number of protons and by the

stability of the nuclide. Neutrons are emitted from unstable nuclei during the process of spontaneous fission; when not bound in the nucleus, they are unstable particles with a half-life of about 12 minutes.

Neutron activation analysis	A technique for determining the composition of samples by measuring the radionuclide activities produced on neutron irradiation of the sample.
Neutron capture reaction or (n,γ) reaction	A reaction to produce radionuclides, carried out in a nuclear reactor. In this nuclear reaction the target nucleus captures one thermal neutron and emits gamma (γ) rays to produce an isotope of the same element.
Neutron number	The number of neutrons in a nucleus, equal to the mass number minus the atomic number ($A - Z$). Symbol N.
NIOSH	National Institute for Occupational Health and Safety (USA).
No carrier added (n.c.a.)	Term used to characterise the state of a radioactive compound to which no stable isotope of the compound has been added purposely.
Non-imaging studies	Nuclear medicine studies using radiopharmaceuticals that provide information about physiology and pathophysiology of an organ system by external detection of the radioactivity without any imaging detection. Information about the uptake or clearance of the radiopharmaceutical is obtained by external counting of samples taken from the patient. General examples of these studies are the measurement of red cell or plasma volumes or measurement of glomerular filtration rate.
Non-specific binding	Binding of a drug or hormone to non-specific tissues, membranes or receptors.
Non-stochastic effects	Radiation effects with severity increasing with dose above a threshold level. No effects are seen at doses below the threshold.
NP-59	6β-Iodomethyl-19-norcholesterol. This compound has been used in adrenal gland scanning after radioiodination with ^{131}I.
NTA	Nitriloacetic acid; a chelating agent.
Nuclear medicine radionuclides	Radioactive nuclides with suitable physical and chemical characteristics to be used in the preparation of radiopharmaceuticals for diagnostic or therapeutic purposes. Most are artificially produced in cyclotrons or reactors and their usefulness is limited by several factors: radiation dose, detectability, reactivity with carrier molecules, availability and cost. In the preparation of diagnostic radiopharmaceuticals there are two main groups of radionuclides: short lived positron emitters (e.g. ^{18}F, ^{11}C) and single gamma photon emitters (mainly ^{99m}Tc). Ideal radionuclides for therapy are those with abundance of non-penetrating radiation (charged particles) and lack of penetrating radiations (gamma rays and X-rays), and that can be bound to carrier molecules to be taken up selectively by diseased tissue.
Nuclear pharmacist	A pharmacist specially trained to prepare radiopharmaceuticals according to the rules of Radiation Protection and Good Manufacturing Practice for Medicinal Products.

Nuclear pharmacy A laboratory suite in which radiopharmaceuticals are prepared, analysed, stored and dispensed in a suitable form for human administration. It has facilities for the preparation of radiopharmaceuticals that satisfy both radiation safety and pharmaceutical quality requirements. Staff in a nuclear pharmacy have special training to handle radioactivity in unsealed sources and to prepare sterile and pyrogen-free pharmaceuticals according to those requirements.

Nucleon Either of the constituent particles (protons and neutrons) of the atomic nucleus.

Nuclide An atomic species characterised by its atomic number Z and mass number A. Nuclides are distinguished in print by the use of subscripts and superscripts, ${}^{A}_{Z}N$: for example ${}^{14}_{6}C$ and ${}^{2}_{1}H$. In practice the atomic number Z is omitted since the same information is contained implicitly in the chemical symbol.

Occupational dose The dose received by an individual during the course of employment in which the individual's assigned duties involve exposure to radiation or to radioactive material from licensed and unlicensed sources of radiation, whether in the possession of the licensee or other person. Occupational dose does not include doses received from background radiation, from any medical administration the individual has received, from exposure to individuals administered radioactive material and released, from voluntary participation in medical research programmes, or those incurred as a member of the public.

Octreoscan Trade name of pentetreotide (octreotide conjugated to DTPA). This compound is supplied as a lyophilised kit to be labelled with ^{111}In. The resulting ^{111}In-pentetreotide binds to somatostatin receptors. It is particularly useful in the detection of primary and metastatic neuroendocrine tumours such as carcinoids, islet cell tumours, vipomas, gastrinoma, neuroblastomas and pituitary adenomas.

Octreotide Synthetic analogue of the human hormone somatostatin that binds to some somatostatin receptors on body tissues that are over-expressed in several pathologies. It is used therapeutically to suppress growth hormone secretion in acromegaly. This octapeptide can also be labelled with gamma-emitting radionuclides such as ^{111}In and ^{99m}Tc, to image primary and metastatic neuroendocrine tumours. It can also be labelled with β^- emitters (e.g. ^{90}Y) to be used as therapeutic radiopharmaceutical.

OIH *ortho*-Iodohippurate, an iodinated analogue of *p*-aminohippuric acid used for ERPF (effective renal plasma flow) studies in nuclear medicine.

Oncology The study of new growths (tumours) in the body.

Opsonin A blood serum protein that combines with foreign cells or particles and makes them more susceptible to the action of phagocytes. For instance, it binds to the surface of colloid particles in order that they may be recognised by phagocytes for ingestion.

Oral radiopharmaceuticals Radiopharmaceuticals that are orally administered for diagnosis or therapy. An example of this type of formulation is given by capsules for the administration of therapeutic doses of ^{131}I. In studies of gastric emptying, hepatobiliary reflux, transit time or oesophageal reflux the radiopharmaceutical can be combined with a solid or a liquid, depending on the requirements of the study.

Oxidation	Chemical process by which an atom or a group of atoms loses electrons to become more positively charged.
Oxidation state	The formal charge on an atom within a molecule if, hypothetically, the entire molecule were composed of ions.
Oxidizing agent or oxidant	A compound that induces an oxidation reaction.
Oxidronate [^{99m}Tc] injection	A solution of sodium oxidronate or hydroxymethylene diphosphonate (HDP or HMDP) labelled with ^{99m}Tc. HDP is supplied as a kit formulation to be labelled with ^{99m}Tc. This ^{99m}Tc-radiopharmaceutical is used clinically for bone imaging.
Oxine	8-Hydroxyquinoline, chelating agent that forms lipophilic complexes with indium. Radiolabelled with ^{111}In, it has been used to radiolabel blood cells (red cells, leukocytes and platelets).
Pair production	Term indicating a process by which an incident photon with energy greater than 1.022 MeV passing through the electrostatic field of a nucleus creates an electron–positron pair whose total energy is just equal to the energy of the photon (which ceases to exist). Thus, this is a process whereby energy is transformed into matter. The electron and positron lose their kinetic energy by ionisation and excitation and the positron combines with an electron to create the annihilation radiation of two 511 keV photons travelling at 180° to each other. This annihilation reaction is the inverse reaction to pair production.
Parent nuclide	A radioactive nuclide that undergoes radioactive decay to form the daughter nuclide. For example, ^{99}Mo is the parent nuclide in the ^{99}Mo/^{99m}Tc generator.
Particle sizing	In radiopharmacy, particle sizing is used for the evaluation of the particle size of colloidal or aggregate preparations, the two major types of particulate suspensions used as diagnostic radiopharmaceuticals. The particles in suspension should have a size range suited to the purpose of the study, but this may vary considerably from batch to batch. For visualisation of the reticuloendothelial system, colloids should have a mean size of 0.1 μm. Size can only be accurately checked with electron microscope, but filtration through polycarbonate membranes gives useful data for quality control. In aggregated preparations, the particle size range should be 20–80 μm with no particles larger than 100 μm or smaller than 20 μm. This can be checked using a haemocytometer under a light microscope. Alternatively, a Zahlstreifen eyepiece that has adjustable parallel counting lines can be used to count particles and to detect oversized particles.
Particulate agents or particulate preparations	Terms referring to the two major types of particulate suspensions used as diagnostic radiopharmaceuticals: colloidal and aggregated suspensions. Colloidal preparations are used for investigation of the reticuloendothelial system. Macroaggregates or microspheres of human serum albumin are used in lung perfusion studies.

PEC — Primary Engineering Control (USA).

Pentetate [^{99m}Tc] injection — A solution of sodium diethylenetriaminepentaacetic acid (DTPA) or calcium trisodium DTPA labelled with ^{99m}Tc. DTPA is supplied as a kit formulation to be labelled with ^{99m}Tc. This ^{99m}Tc-radiopharmaceutical is used clinically, mainly for renal flow study, glomerular filtration rate measurement and aerosol preparation. The BP preparation is Technetium [99mTc] Pentetate Injection.

Pentetreotide — A cyclic octapeptide analogue of somatostatin coupled with a DTPA moiety for radiolabelling. The octapeptide portion of pentetreotide confers the receptor recognition properties of the radiopharmaceutical, while the DTPA portion enables labelling with ^{111}In. The resulting ^{111}In-pentetreotide is used for the scintigraphic localisation of neuroendocrine tumours bearing somatostatin receptors.

Peptide hormones — Hormones with polypeptidic structure that bind to specific receptors on body tissues. Some of these receptors are also expressed in certain tumour types, especially neuroendocrine tumours. Polypeptide hormones consist of a specific group of regulatory molecules whose functions are to convey specific information among cells and organs. Some synthetic analogues of peptide hormones or even the native peptides (e.g. somatostatin, bombesin, neurotensin, vasoactive intestinal polypeptide (VIP)) are used for treatment of neuroendocrine pathologies and some have been radiolabelled to visualise receptors in primary and metastatic neuroendocrine tumours or for use as therapeutic radiopharmaceuticals.

Perfusion agent — Any molecule used to measure the passage of a fluid through the vessels of an organ in conjunction with imaging. Good perfusion agents have one of the following characteristics: they are trapped by the perfused tissue in proportion to the perfusion; they remain strictly intravascular; or they diffuse freely throughout the tissue of interest. Examples of perfusion agents in clinical use are ^{99m}Tc-HMPAO and ^{99m}Tc-ECD (brain scanning by trapping of the radiopharmaceutical); ^{99m}Tc-MIBI and ^{99m}Tc-tetrafosmin (heart scanning by trapping of the radiopharmaceutical); ^{99m}Tc-MAG_3 (kidney scanning with the intravascular radiopharmaceutical); ^{133}Xe (regional blood flow measurements where the radiopharmaceutical freely diffuses).

Perfusion imaging — Any method that provides regionalised maps of tissue perfusion. The usual imaging modality is nuclear medicine imaging including PET imaging. In this instance, perfusion imaging is the visualisation of the process by which a radiopharmaceutical penetrates within or passes through an organ, tissue or tumour, especially by way of the blood vessels. The methods used can be categorised as wash-in, wash-out and bolus tracking methods.

Perfusion scans — Scanning of a perfusion radiopharmaceutical by a tomographic system that provides regionalised maps of tissue perfusion.

PET — Positron emission tomography (q.v.).

PHA — Pulse height analyser; a device for measuring pulse heights and counting the number occurring in each range selected.

Phosphorus-32	A radioactive nuclide of the element phosphorus (P). Phosporus-32 is a pure beta emitter ($t_{1/2} = 14.3$ days) produced by irradiating sulfur with neutrons in a nuclear reactor. It is then separated from the melted sulfur by leaching with a solution of NaOH.
Phosphorus-32 sodium phosphate injection	A solution of sodium and disodium orthophosphates containing phosphorus-32. The clinical uses of ^{32}P include the therapeutic treatment of polycythaemia vera, leukaemia and other haematological disorders. It was the first radioactive material to be widely employed to alleviate the pain of osseous metastatic disease since the phosphate is incorporated into hydroxyapatite. The BP preparation is Sodium Phosphate [^{32}P] Injection.
Photoelectric effect	A process in which the absorption of a photon ejects a bound electron from an atom.
Photon	A quantum of electromagnetic radiation having energy $h\nu$ (where h is Planck's constant and ν is the frequency).
PIPIDA	N-(*p*-Isopropylanilino)iminodiacetic acid; the ^{99m}Tc complex is used for hepatobiliary imaging.
PMT	Photomultiplier tube.
Poisson statistics	A statistical distribution of random events wherein the probability of each event is very small. Radioactive decay is a rare event and counting is governed by Poisson statistics. In brief, the variance of a count is equal to the count, while the standard deviation is the square root of the count.
POP	2,5-Diphenyloxazole; a primary scintillator in liquid scintillation cocktails.
POPOP	1,4-Bis(5-phenoxazole)benzene; a secondary scintillant in liquid scintillation cocktails.
POPUMET	Regulations governing the radiation doses to the population as a whole.
Positive pressure system	A system used in one of the two types of chromatographic radionuclide generators. In this system the elution vial is at atmospheric pressure and, instead of an eluent reservoir, a pressurised vial containing the desired volume of eluent is connected to the inlet of the generator column.
Positron	A nuclear particle having a mass of about 0.00055 amu and bearing a positive charge; it is emitted during *positron decay* (q.v.). It has properties similar to the electron (negatron) except for the sign of the charge and is regarded as an antimatter particle that undergoes annihilation on encounter with an electron, the combined mass being converted to two 0.511 MeV photons that are emitted in opposite directions. The directional distribution of the photons is used in PET and positron cameras.
Positron decay	A beta decay process in which radionuclides having excess protons gain stability by conversion of a proton into a neutron and a positron.
Positron emission tomography (PET)	Positron emission tomography is a tomographic nuclear imaging procedure that uses a radiopharmaceutical labelled with a positron emitter (e.g. ^{11}C, ^{13}N, ^{15}O, ^{18}F) and positron–electron annihilation reactions to locate

them. It is based on coincidence detection of the two 511 keV photons emitted in opposite directions due to the decay of a positron-emitting radionuclide. Clinical applications of PET imaging include assessment of cerebral and cardiac function, metabolism, detection of foci of inflammation and tumour staging. [^{18}F]Fluorodeoxyglucose is the most commonly used PET radiopharmaceutical, others being [^{15}O]water and [^{13}N]ammonia.

Positron emitter	A radionuclide that decays by *positron decay* (q.v.).
Positron-emitting radiopharmaceuticals	Radiopharmaceuticals that incorporate a positron-emitting radionuclide. The biodistribution of these radiopharmaceuticals is detected by PET.
Positron range	The distance that a positron travels in matter before annihilation.
PPi	Pyrophosphate; the ^{99m}Tc complex is used as a bone and skeletal imaging agent.
PPX	Polyphosphate; the ^{99m}Tc complex was the first used for bone imaging.
Proportional counter	A radiation detector producing electrical pulses proportional in height to the energy of the radiation.
Proton	A nuclear particle having a mass of about 1.00759 amu. The number of protons in a nucleus determines the chemical properties of that element.
PYP	Pyrophosphate; see PPi.
QF	Abbreviation of the term *quality factor* (q.v.).
Quadramet	Trade name of ^{153}Sm-ethylenediaminetetramethylene phosphonic acid. Samarium-153 is produced in reactor and reacted with ethylenediaminetetramethylene phosphonic acid (EDTMP) to form the ^{153}Sm-EDTMP complex. This radiopharmaceutical is supplied as solution and it is used mainly for the palliation of pain arising from metastatic bone cancer. The 103 keV photons (28%) allow scintigraphic imaging of the whole body.
Quality assurance	A concept that covers all matters which individually or collectively influence the quality of a product. The aim of quality assurance is to ensure that the result of a working procedure meets predefined quality standards. The quality of radiopharmaceuticals must be assured by a quality assurance system that ensures they are manufactured, prepared and controlled in such a way that they comply with the required specifications throughout their shelf-life.
Quality control	Specific tests and measurements that ensure the purity, potency, product identity, biologic safety and efficacy of a drug. All quality procedures that are applied to non-radioactive pharmaceuticals are also applicable to radiopharmaceuticals but these require in addition tests for radionuclidic and radiochemical purity.
Quality factor (QF)	A factor dependent on linear energy transfer multiplied by absorbed dose (rads or grays) to calculate the dose equivalent in rems. It is used in radiation protection to take into account the relative radiation biological damage caused by different radiations to an exposed individual. The QF is 1 for X, gamma, and beta radiation, 10 for neutrons and protons; and 20 for alpha, multiply charged

and heavy particles and fission fragments. Quality factors are now replaced by Radiation Weighting Factors under ICRP60.

Quantum

An irreducible unit most often of energy or another physical quantity describing an object obeying quantum physics. Photons are quanta of electromagnetic energy.

Quenching

A mechanism required in Geiger counters to prevent a single ionisation event causing the counter to go into a pulsation series of discharges. It is achieved by addition of a suitable quenching gas. Multiple pulsing in Geiger counters is caused by a secondary discharge that arises when the positive ions created by the passage of radiation drift away from the anode wire and arrive at the cathode. Most of the ions will be neutralised by combination with an electron from the cathode surface. However, it is possible that a free electron will be liberated from the cathode by the arrival of the ions and then will drift towards the anode wire. Once there, a single electron can trigger another avalanche, leading eventually to a continuous output of pulses. With the addition of a quenching gas, the positive ions from the initial ionisation will collide with the gas molecules and, as consequence of the difference in ionisation energies, there will be a tendency to transfer the positive charge to the gas molecules. If the gas concentration is sufficiently high, all positive ions arriving at the cathode will be those of the quenching gas and, when they are neutralised, the excess energy is channelled into disassociation of the more complex quenching gas molecules and not in liberation of electrons. Organic liquid scintillation counters also suffer from quenching, although here it refers to the mechanism that reduces the amount of light output from the sample. Liquid scintillation quenching consists of three types: chemical quenching, colour quenching and dilution quenching.

Rad

Radiation Absorbed Dose: a measure of the energy deposited per unit mass of any material by any type of radiation. One rad is equal to 100 ergs of radiation deposited per gram of matter, or equal to an absorbed dose of 10^{-2} J/kg of any medium (10^{-2} gray).

Radiation dose (D)

The amount of radiation energy absorbed per gram of material. As well as the quantity of ionising radiation received, the term dose is often used in the sense of exposure dose, expressed in roentgens or grays.

Radiation exposure

Exposure to any source of radiation. Exposure in radiopharmacy may be internal or external radiation exposure. With unsealed radiation sources, the major concern is internal exposure since the resulting radiation doses are difficult to predict because of varying biochemical and physiological factors. External exposure can usually be more readily measured and controlled. The greatest risks occur from spillage and contamination during the preparation of the radiopharmaceuticals. The hazards depend on the total activity, radiotoxicity, nature and physical and chemical form of the radioactive material.

Radiation monitor

A survey meter used to check radioactivity levels, an essential part of a radiation safety programme. In radiopharmacy and nuclear medicine departments, two types of survey instruments are used: (1) an ionisation chamber to measure high fluxes of radiation; (2) a Geiger counter for low-level surveys because of its long dead time.

Radiation monitoring — Specific tests and measurements of radiation performed to estimate or control the level of radiation exposure. It is an essential part of a radiation safety programme.

Radiation protection — The safe handling of radioactive materials and exposure to radiation according to established legislation. The implementation of such regulations is important since radiation can cause damage to living systems. In view of the potentially adverse health effects of radiation a number of national and international organisations have set guidelines for the safe handling of radioactive materials. Any level of radiation, even small, can theoretically cause damage to living tissue at the cellular level and therefore there is no threshold below which exposure to radiation can be considered safe. Alpha particles are among the most damaging because of their great mass and charge, followed by beta particles and gamma rays. The main parameters to consider when minimising exposure to external radiation are time, distance, shielding and activity. It is recommended that you minimise the duration of your exposure to the radiation source; that you maximise the distance between yourself and the source; that you use shielding whenever possible; and that you avoid working with high levels of activity where possible.

Radiation shielding — Barriers or containers used to provide protection from radiation. Radionuclides and radiopharmaceuticals should be stored and handled in shielded areas. The material for such barriers or containers depends on the radionuclide. While alpha- and beta-emitting radionuclides produce radiation with short ranges, gamma rays are highly penetrating. Therefore, gamma-emitting radionuclides require the use of highly absorbing materials for shielding, such as lead. However for alpha- and beta-emitting radionuclides the containers themselves could act as shield.

Radiation sources — Artificial sources that contribute to the population's exposure to radiation. They include a wide variety of radioactive and X-ray sources mainly used in medicine and industry. This description is generally used for human-made sealed sources of radiation in radiation therapy or radiography, but natural radionuclides, radionuclide generators or particle accelerators are also considered to be radiation sources.

Radiation weighting factor — In ICRP60 these are used to correct for the dependence of stochastic effects on radiation quality. The absorbed dose is multiplied by the radiation weighting factor to give the equivalent dose.

Radiation–matter interactions — Processes by which radiation interacts with matter. These processes depend on the properties of the radiation, mainly its charge and mass. The major processes involved in the interaction of charged particles (alpha particles, negatrons and positrons) with an absorbing material are ionisation and excitation of atomic electrons. X-ray and gamma ray photons incident upon matter do not cause ionisation directly but can transfer all or part of their energy to atomic electrons by scattering or absorption and it is these electrons that produce ionisation.

There are several interactions with atomic electrons or nuclei that can cause scattering or absorption of an X-ray and gamma ray. The main ones are elastic (Raleigh) scattering; inelastic (Compton) scattering; the photoelectric effect; and pair production.

Radioactive concentration	The radioactivity per unit quantity (mass or volume) of any radioactive material; examples of units in common use are MBq/mg and kBq/mL.
Radioactive contamination	Defined as an undesirable radioactivity level in the working environment (usually above 5–50 Bq/cm^2). The handling of radiopharmaceuticals or radionuclides incurs the possibility of radioactive contamination since, with the use of unsealed sources, spillage can never be discounted. Such spillage could result in direct contamination of personnel or surfaces. In the event of a contamination incident (measured or suspected), immediate decontamination procedures must be undertaken according to a contingency plan. Routine contamination surveys are required to be carried out in radiopharmacies.
Radioactive decay	A first-order process in which radionuclides are transformed from a parent to a daughter species. The decay rate depends on the probability of decay, the decay constant (k). Decay processes are characterised by the radiations (and their energies emitted) and the decay constant or half-life. The daughter nuclide may be unstable and undergo further decay processes until the final nuclide is a stable one.
Radioactive equilibrium	A steady-state condition in which the rate of decay of daughter is equal to its rate of production from parent.
Radioactivity	The spontaneous transformation of an unstable *radionuclide* (q.v.) to a more stable nuclide, which may also be radioactive. Energy released in this process may appear as particles (alpha and beta particles, neutrinos, neutrons) or as electromagnetic radiation (X-rays and gamma rays).
Radiobiology	The study of interactions of radiation or radioactive substances with biological systems.
Radiocarbon dating	A technique for determining the age of a material from its residual ^{14}C content.
Radiochemical purity	The proportion of the total radioactivity present in the stated chemical form.
Radiochemical yield	The fraction or percentage of the original radionuclide incorporated into the radiochemical at the end of the synthesis.
Radiochemistry	The chemistry of radioactive materials including the production and purification of radionuclides, synthesis of labelled compounds and the use of these materials in chemical studies.
Radiography	A method of non-destructive testing in which a beam of penetrating radiation is passed through an object. The dense parts absorb the radiation and the spatial variations in radiation intensity can be recorded on film. Examples include medical X-ray diagnosis and industrial gamma radiography.

Radioimmunotherapy	The delivery of a therapeutic radiation dose to a cancer by labelling a site-specific monoclonal antibody with an alpha- or beta-emitting radionuclide.
Radioisotope	An isotope containing an unstable arrangement of protons and neutrons that will, at some stage, be transformed to either a completely stable or a more stable combination of nucleons.
Radiolabelling	The labelling of compounds with radionuclides. Radiolabelled compounds are used in medical, biochemical and other fields. In the radiolabelled compound, atoms or a group of atoms of a molecule are substituted by or coupled to similar or completely different radioactive atoms. In any radiolabelling process a variety of selected physicochemical conditions must be employed. There are different methods employed in the preparation of radiolabelled compounds for clinical use depending on the radionuclide and the molecule to be labelled, but the most commonly used are direct incorporation into a molecule of a radionuclide by the formation of covalent bonds or coordinate (dative covalent) bonds, often by chelation (e.g. ^{99m}Tc-radiopharmaceuticals, iodinated proteins), and labelling with bifunctional chelating agents (e.g. ^{111}In- or ^{99m}Tc- labelled proteins or peptides).
Radiology	Medical use of radiation for diagnosis.
Radiolysis	The decomposition of material by radiation.
Radionuclide	An unstable or radioactive nuclide that decays by spontaneous fission, or emission of alpha particles, beta particles or electromagnetic radiation.
Radionuclide generator	A system used to generate a radionuclide for routine clinical practice. The most widely used generator system is the ^{99m}Tc generator. See *generator*.
Radionuclidic purity	The proportion of the total radioactivity present in the stated radionuclide.
Radiopharmaceutical	Any pharmaceutical preparation that includes a radionuclide in its composition. Radiopharmaceuticals can be used for the diagnosis or therapeutic treatment of human diseases and have two basic components: a chemical moiety and a suitable radionuclide to provide the signal for detection outside the body after administration. This enables assessment of the morphological structure or the physiological function of a target organ or system or radiation of tissues for treatment purposes. A radiotracer or radiochemical, specially formulated and tested for suitability in human studies that (in the UK) complies with the provisions of the Medicines Act. Radiopharmaceuticals are used both for diagnosis and therapy.
Radiopharmacist	A pharmacist with specific training in the preparation of radiopharmaceuticals according to Radiation Protection Requirements and Good Manufacturing Practice for Medicinal Products.
Radiopharmacy	A laboratory suite in which radiopharmaceuticals are prepared, analysed, stored and dispensed in a suitable form for human administration. It has facilities for the preparation of radiopharmaceuticals that satisfy both radiation safety and pharmaceutical quality requirements. Staff in a radiopharmacy are trained in the handling of unsealed radioactive sources and in the preparation of sterile and pyrogen-free pharmaceuticals.

Radiotherapy	Treatment of disease by the use of ionising radiation.
Radiotracer	A tracer labelled with radioactive material.
Ratemeter	A rate-counting meter used to determine the average count rate of ionising events.
RBE	Relative biological effectiveness; different radiations have quantitatively different biological effects and the RBE must be incorporated as a quality factor when assessing radiation doses.
RDRC	Radioactive Drug Research Committee (USA).
Rem	The older unit of biologically effective radiation dose; essentially the absorbed radiation dose (rad) multiplied by a *quality factor* (q.v.) to account for the different biological effects of various radiations.
Renal perfusion studies	Kidney scanning that provides a map of how the radiopharmaceutical passes through the kidney. An example of a commonly used renal perfusion radiopharmaceutical is ^{99m}Tc-MAG_3.
Renal scan	A scan of the kidney. There are two main types of kidney scans, those which provide information about relative function of the kidneys and urine outflow (renogram) and those which demonstrate functioning renal parenchyma. Some commonly used radiopharmaceuticals for dynamic renal imaging are ^{99m}Tc-DTPA for the measurement of glomerular filtration rate and renographic studies; ^{99m}Tc-MAG_3 and ^{123}I- or ^{131} I-hippuran used for both flow and function studies of the kidneys. ^{99m}Tc-DMSA is the commonest radiopharmaceutical used as a renal imaging agent, allowing the diagnosis of renal scarring, space-occupying lesions and renal trauma.
Renogram	Renal function imaging study in which an activity-versus-time curve is produced demonstrating the passage of radiopharmaceutical through the kidney. This provides information about the relative function of the kidneys and urine outflow.
RIA	Radioimmunoassay; an immunological assay technique in which a radiolabelled substrate competes with the unlabelled analogue for binding sites on an antibody. The radioactivity of the antibody–substrate complex is inversely proportional to the concentration of substrate in the sample.
Roentgen	An obsolete unit of exposure of X- and gamma radiation.
ROI	Region of interest (on a scintigram).
Samarium-153	A radioactive nuclide of the element samarium (Sm). It is a beta emitter produced in the reactor by neutron irradiation of ^{152}Sm. It has a half-life of 1.9 days. Samarium-153 is used to radiolabel ethylenediaminetetramethylene phosphonate (EDTMP) and used mainly in the palliation of pain arising from metastatic bone cancer (see also Quadramet).
SCA	Segregated compounding area.
Scaler	A device for indicating the number of counts registered by a detector.

Scan	An image of the distribution of radioactivity in part or the whole of the body or organ produced (e.g. by computer) by combining data obtained from several angles or sections.
Scintigram	An image or other record of the whole or part of the body obtained by measuring radiation from an administered radioactive tracer.
Scintigraphic agent	A radioactive tracer used to image the whole body or an organ by detection and recording of the radioactivity distribution. A radiopharmaceutical used for diagnostic imaging.
Scintigraphy	Production of a scintigram by administration of a radioactive tracer.
Scintillation	A flash of light produced within a phosphor or scintillator upon absorption of radiation. The intensity of the light is proportional to the energy of the radiation.
Scintillation counter	A detector in which the scintillations are amplified and recorded.
SDS-PAGE	Sodium dodecyl sulfate–polyacrylamide gel electrophoresis. A method of analysis for proteins based on unfolding and negatively charging, then sieving of different-sized molecules through a cross-linked gel under the influence of an electric field gradient. The smaller molecules migrate faster.
Sealed source	A totally enclosed radiation source constructed to prevent leakage of radioactive material.
Secular equilibrium	A condition in which the radioactivity of a daughter is equal to the parent. This can only occur when the daughter half-life is much shorter than the parent.
Semiconductor detector	A radiation detector that uses the effects of radiation on the properties of a semiconductor material.
Sestamibi [^{99m}Tc] injection	A sterile solution of hexakismethoxyisobutyl isonitrile [^{99m}Tc]technetium(I) chloride (Sestamibi or ^{99m}Tc-MIBI). The lyophilised kit is supplied as a copper(I) complex under the brand names Cardiolite (for myocardial imaging) or Miraluma (for breast imaging). The BP preparation is Technetium [^{99m}Tc] Sestamibi Injection.
Side-effects	A term indicating an unexpected or unusual and undesirable clinical manifestation resulting from administration of a radiopharmaceutical. There are some difficulties in adapting the term currently used for medicines in general to radiopharmaceuticals, mainly because the majority of radiopharmaceuticals do not have therapeutic or pharmacological effects. It is usually accepted that radiopharmaceuticals' adverse reactions are associated with the vehicle carrying the radiation and not with the radiation itself, overdose or any administration injury.
Sievert	The SI unit of biologically effective radiation dose; the absorbed radiation dose (in grays) multiplied by a *quality factor* (q.v.) to account for the different biological effects of various radiations.

Single-photon emission computed tomography (SPECT)
A tomographic radionuclide imaging technique that uses gamma-emitting radiopharmaceuticals. SPECT systems usually consist of a gamma camera with one or two NaI(Tl) detector heads mounted on a gantry, which rotate around the patient to acquire data that can be processed into three-dimensional images. Acquisition and processing of data is done by an on-line computer.

Skeletal imaging
Bone scan. ^{99m}Tc-Diphosphonates (MDP, HDP) are the current agents of choice for bone imaging. They exhibit similar behaviour *in vivo* with rapid bone uptake, low background uptake in non-skeletal areas and urinary clearance of non-bound activity. Various diseases are diagnosed by increased uptake of ^{99m}Tc-diphosphonates including bone tumours, metastatic lesions and rheumatoid arthritis.

Sodium [^{99m}Tc]pertechnetate ($Na^{99m}TcO_4^-$)
A chemical form of ^{99m}Tc available from a ^{99}Mo/^{99m}Tc generator. Chemically the ion $^{99m}TcO_4^-$ is rather unreactive and has to be reduced to a lower oxidation state in order to use it for radiolabelling.

Soft radiation
Radiation having little penetrating power. Examples are the beta radiation from ^{14}C and the alpha radiation from ^{238}U.

Specific activity
The radioactivity per unit mass of a radioactive substance, usually expressed as MBq/mg or GBq/mmol.

Specific binding
Binding of a drug or hormone to a receptor specific for that molecule. The binding may be reversible and be subject to competition for similar molecules. In most cases there is an upper limit to the amount bound owing to saturation of available receptors.

Specific gamma ray constant
The exposure rate produced by the gamma rays from a unit point source of a radionuclide at unit distance.

Specific ionisation
The number of ion pairs produced per unit distance along the track of an ionising particle, usually expressed as keV/mm.

SPECT
Single-photon emission computed tomography (q.v.).

SPPS
Solid-phase peptide synthesis. The fundamental premise of this technique involves the incorporation of *N*-α-amino acids into a peptide of any desired sequence, with one end of the sequence remaining attached to a solid support matrix. While the peptide is being synthesised, usually by stepwise methods, all soluble reagents can be removed from the peptide–solid support matrix by filtration and washed away at the end of each coupling step. After the desired sequence of amino acids has been obtained, the peptide can be removed from the polymeric support.

SSTR
Serotonin subtype receptor.

Stochastic effects
Used in relation to radiation exposure, for effects where the probability of occurrence is proportional to dose without any threshold. Such effects include genetic effects and the induction of cancer.

Strontium-89
A radioactive nuclide of strontium (Sr). It is a pure beta emitter produced in a nuclear reactor ($t_{1/2} = 50.6$ days). It is supplied in the

form of $^{89}SrCl_2$ solution for the relief of bone pain in skeletal metastases. It is incorporated into hydroxyapatite like calcium. Its trade name is Metastron.

Succimer [^{99m}Tc]injection — A solution of dimercaptosuccinic acid (succimer; DMSA) labelled with ^{99m}Tc. Succimer is supplied as a lyophilised kit formulation to be labelled with ^{99m}Tc. The ^{99m}Tc-DMSA complex is used mainly for renal imaging. The BP preparation is Technetium [^{99m}Tc] Succimer Injection.

Sulfur colloid — ^{99m}Tc-labelled sulfur colloid was used for liver and spleen imaging but is now replaced by tin and albumin colloids, which are easier to label.

Sulfur colloid [^{99m}Tc]injection — A suspension of sulfur micelles labelled with ^{99m}Tc. The colloid may be stabilised with a protecting substance. The particle size range of the colloid is 100 nm–3 μm. ^{99m}Tc-Sulfur colloid is used for liver and spleen imaging. The BP preparation is Technetium [^{99m}Tc] Colloidal Sulphur Injection.

Supervised areas — Areas for radioactive work where conditions are monitored but where special procedures are not necessary.

Target, target material — The material that is bombarded by an accelerated beam of charged particles to produce a radionuclide.

Target organ — An organ intended to be imaged and expected to receive a high concentration of administered radioactivity.

Target-to-background ratio or target-to-non-target ratio — The ratio between the radioactivity uptake in target tissue and that distributed in blood and soft tissue (background), measured at a certain time post administration. To obtain adequate visualisation of the tissue, target tissue uptake should be high while blood and soft-tissue levels are low.

Tc-BIN — A complex of ^{99m}Tc with *t*-butylisonitrile, used for cardiac imaging.

Teboroxime — Lipophilic mixture of cyclohexanedione dioxime, methylboronic acid, cyclodextrin, stannous chloride, citric acid, pentetic acid and sodium chloride to be radiolabelled with ^{99m}Tc.

Technetium — A group 7 transition metal with atomic number 43. No stable isotope of technetium exists in nature. All the isotopes of this metallic element are radioactive and artificially produced. Technetium-99m (^{99m}Tc), a gamma emitter, is used in diagnostic nuclear medicine. The ground-state isotope (^{99}Tc) has a half-life of 2.1×10^5 years and is the only isotope available in macroscopic concentrations. Thus, most of what we know about the chemistry of technetium has been discovered using ^{99m}Tc.

Technetium-99m — The most commonly used radionuclide in diagnostic nuclear medicine. Nearly 80% of all radiopharmaceuticals are ^{99m}Tc-labelled owing to its favourable physical characteristics ($t_{1/2} = 6$ hours, gamma emitter; monochromatic 140 keV photons; no emission of alpha or beta particles). Furthermore, ^{99m}Tc is readily available in a sterile, pyrogen-free state from a ^{99}Mo/^{99m}Tc generator. ^{99m}Tc, a metastable state of technetium, is the daughter radionuclide of the parent ^{99}Mo and decays by isomeric transition to ^{99}Tc.

Tetrafosmin [^{99m}Tc] injection	A solution of tetrafosmin (6,9-bis(2-ethoxyethyl)-3,12-dioxa-6,9-diphosphatetradecane) labelled with ^{99m}Tc. Tetrafosmin is supplied as a lyophilised kit formulation to be labelled with ^{99m}Tc under the brand name of Myoview and the ^{99m}Tc-tetrafosmin complex is used for myocardial imaging. It is indicated for the detection of reversible myocardial ischaemia and myocardial infarction.
Thallium-201	A radioactive nuclide of the element thallium (Tl). It is produced in a cyclotron ($t_{1/2} = 73$ hours) and is supplied in isotonic saline solution for intravenous administration. It decays by electron capture and emits X-rays and gamma rays with a maximum energy of 167 keV.
Thallous [^{201}Tl] injection	Thallium chloride solution used clinically for myocardial perfusion imaging. The BP preparation is Thallous [^{201}Tl] Chloride Injection.
Thermal fission	Nuclear fission induced by thermal neutrons.
Thermal neutrons	Neutrons in thermodynamic equilibrium with (i.e. having the same mean kinetic energy as) their surroundings at room temperature, when their mean energy is around 0.025 eV and their speed around 2.2×10^3 m/s.
Thyroid scan	Thyroid imaging, useful in detecting any palpable mass (nodule). Some radiopharmaceuticals commonly used for thyroid scanning are [^{99m}Tc] pertechnetate and sodium [$^{123/131}$I]iodide. In addition to imaging the thyroid, radioactive iodine can be used to quantify thyroid activity.
Tiatide [^{99m}Tc] injection	A solution of mercaptoacetyltriglycine (MAG_3 (q.v.)) labelled with ^{99m}Tc.
Tin colloid [^{99m}Tc] injection	Suspension of colloidal tin labelled with ^{99m}Tc. The colloid may be stabilised with a protecting substance and contains fluoride ions. The particle size range of the colloid is 50–600 nm. Tin colloid suspension is supplied as a lyophilised kit formulation to be labelled with ^{99m}Tc. The resulting ^{99m}Tc-tin colloid is used for liver imaging. The BP preparation is Technetium [^{99m}Tc] Colloidal Tin Injection.
Tin pyrophosphate [^{99m}Tc] injection	A solution of stannous pyrophosphate labelled with ^{99m}Tc. It is supplied as lyophilised kit formulation to be labelled with ^{99m}Tc. The ^{99m}Tc-pyrophosphate is used for myocardial infarct and bone imaging, as well as in red blood cell labelling. The BP preparation is Technetium [^{99m}Tc] Tin Pyrophosphate Injection.
Tin-117m-diethylenetriamine pentaacetic acid	Tin-117m decays by isomeric transition. Labelled to diethylenetriamine pentaacetic acid (DTPA), it can be used for metastatic bone pain palliation. It is one of the newer bone-seeking radiopharmaceuticals that have been evaluated, but some authors claim it has the advantage of being less myelotoxic than other radiopharmaceuticals used for the same application.
TLD	Thermoluminescent dosimeter. A type of personal dosimeter in which the radiation energy is absorbed and is released as visible photons when heated. The amount of light emitted gives a measure of the radiation absorbed.
Tracer	A labelled molecule used to trace a chemical reaction or to follow the passage of a substance through a biological or physical system.

Transient equilibrium	A condition in which the ratio of daughter to parent radioactivity is constant. The daughter half-life must be less than the parent for this to occur.
TSK	A trade mark that refers to a type of silica-based HPLC column originating from Tosoh Bioscience.
Tungsten-188/rhenium-188 ($^{188}W/^{188}Re$) generator	Generator system in which ^{188}W ($t_{1/2} = 65$ days) produced by double irradiation (n,α) of ^{186}W decays to ^{118}W ($t_{1/2} = 17$ hours). This generator is made of an alumina column containing ^{188}W in the form of acidified tungsten oxide.
Unrestricted area	An area where the access is neither limited nor controlled for the purpose of protection of individuals from exposure to radiation and radioactive materials.
Unsealed source	Radioactive material that is not encapsulated or sealed and is used as a tracer or source of radiation.
USP	United States Pharmacopoeia.
Vapreotide	Also called RC160. Vapreotide is a synthetic analogue of the human hormone somatostatin, and binds to a somatostatin receptor subtype in some tumours that do not bind the commonly used somatostatin analogue, octreotide. It is a potential alternative to octreotide as a radionuclide carrier, although clinical studies performed with this radiolabelled analogue do not appear to show any advantage over radiolabelled octreotide.
Vasoactive intestinal peptide (VIP)	A linear 28-residue peptide with a broad spectrum of functions in a variety of tissues, present in human lung in high concentration. Originally VIP was characterised as a vasodilatory substance with effects on pulmonary blood pressure, but the secretion of a variety of hormones is also stimulated by VIP. VIP receptors are expressed in a variety of human tumours. Radiolabelled ^{123}I VIP has been used for tumour imaging. However, these studies were hampered by the potent pharmacological effects of VIP and its short *in-vivo* half-life.
Ventilation	Exchange of air between the lung and the ambient air.
Ventilation imaging of lungs	Study of lung ventilation function using a radiopharmaceutical such as ^{133}Xe gas, ^{81m}Kr and ^{99m}Tc-aerosols (commonly produced by nebulising ^{99m}Tc-DTPA) to detect any obstructions.
Ventilation scans	Study of lung ventilation function using a radiopharmaceutical.
Ventilation/inhalation studies	Study of lung ventilation function by inhalation of a radioactive gas or aerosol of radiolabelled preparation.
Ventilation-perfusion ratio (v/q or v_a/q_c)	A ratio that correlates the patterns of lung ventilation (using a radioactive gas or aerosol) and lung perfusion (using an intravenously administered radiopharmaceutical) in the same patient. Most often used to diagnose pulmonary embolism.
VIP	Vasoactive intestinal peptide (q.v.).
Washout of tracer	Removal of radioactive tracer from a certain organ or tissue.

WBC	White blood cells.
Weighting factor (W_T)	W_T for an organ or tissue is the proportion of the risk of stochastic effects resulting from irradiation of the organ or tissue to the total risk of stochastic effects when the whole body is irradiated uniformly.
Whatman paper chromatography	A chromatography technique in which a small aliquot of the sample is applied to a strip of Whatman paper (stationary medium) and developed with an appropriate solvent (mobile phase). During chromatography, different components of the sample distribute themselves between the adsorbent paper and the solvent depending on their distribution coefficients.
White blood cells (WBC) or leukocytes	White or colourless circulating blood cell that have nuclei, do not contain haemoglobin and are mainly concerned with body defence mechanisms and repair. These cells can be radiolabelled with gamma-emitting compounds (e.g. ^{111}In-oxine or ^{99m}Tc-HMPAO) to detect their accumulation in the reticuloendothelial system (RES) or inflammatory sites.
Whole body	A term that for purposes of external exposure refers to the head, trunk (including male gonads), arms above the elbow and legs above the knee. For the purpose of weighting the external whole body dose, $W_T = 1$.
Whole body monitors	An assembly of large scintillation detectors used to identify and measure the total gamma radiation emitted by the human body.
Workstation	A work bench or small working enclosure/cabinet that has its own filtered air supply (usually a unidirectional air flow) and complies with standard protection requirements. The cabinet is contained so that radiopharmaceuticals can be prepared in a safe way to prevent contamination of the operator, the product or the environment.
X-ray	High-energy electromagnetic radiation with shorter wavelength than ultraviolet radiation or visible light. X-rays are generated by the interaction of highly energetic electrons with matter where the electrons eject inner shell electrons of the target nuclei.
Xenon [^{133}Xe] gas	Radioactive gas supplied for inhalation. It may be diluted with air or oxygen. This radiopharmaceutical is used for lung ventilation studies.
Xenon [^{133}Xe] Injection	A solution of ^{133}Xe in sodium chloride. This radiopharmaceutical is used for regional blood flow measurements.
X-ray film badges	Common device used for monitoring radiation doses received by personnel exposed to radiation. It consists of a piece of X-ray film inside a paper envelope. The badge is contained within a plastic holder. The monitoring period depends on the level of exposure. At the end of that period the film badge is processed by a dosimetry service.
X-ray fluorescence	An analytical technique for identifying and quantitating elements from the characteristic X-rays they emit when irradiated by radiation of a higher energy.
Yield	The fraction or amount of final product produced from raw materials at the end of a chemical synthesis.

Yttrium [^{90}Y] silicate injection	A solution of yttrium silicate containing ^{90}Y. It is clinically used as a radiation synovectomy agent.
Yttrium-90	A radioactive nuclide of the Group 3 element, yttrium (Y). Yttrium is a pure β^- emitter and is reactor or generator produced ($t_{1/2} = 2.7$ days). ^{90}Y has been used in therapeutic studies in oncology. ^{90}Y-acetate is the preferred radiochemical form used for labelling peptides and antibodies conjugated with bifunctional chelating agents (usually DTPA or DOTA analogues).

Index

Note: Page numbers with suffix 'f', 'sc', 'st', 't' and 'ws' refer to figures, schemes, structures, tables and worksheets, respectively.